HANDBOOK
of Health Care
Human Resources
Management

HANDBOOK
of Health Care
Human Resources
Management

Edited by

NORMAN METZGER

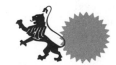

AN ASPEN PUBLICATION
Aspen Systems Corporation
Rockville, Maryland
London
1981

Library of Congress Cataloging in Publication Data

Handbook of health care human resources
management.

   Includes bibliographies and index.
   1. Health facilities—Personnel
management—Addresses, essays, lectures.
2. Hospitals—Personnel management—Addresses,
essays, lectures. I. Metzger, Norman, 1924-
[DNLM: 1. Personnel management. 2. Health
manpower—Organ. W88 H236]
RA971.35.H36   362.1'1'0683   81-3473
ISBN 0-89443-363-6   AACR2

Library of Congress Catalog Card Number: 81-3473
ISBN: 0-89443-363-6

Printed in the United States of America

1   2   3   4   5

To my wife, *Marcia,*
a professional in the personnel field and an unwavering supporter

The society is constantly changing; the economy is being transformed; workers enter employment with a higher level of education and with aspirations and goals quite different from those of their parents and grandparents. In the face of these radical changes, management cannot possibly discharge its functions effectively by a rigid adherence to a body of rights that reflect an earlier period and different conditions. Management can meet the new challenges which it confronts and those which it will encounter in its functions that will enable it to keep the company vital and profitable as the boundaries over rights—its rights, the rights of workers, and the rights of the government—continue to shift. Static rights are incompatible with an expanding economy and a dynamic society.

ELI GINZBERG AND IVAR E. BERG
Democratic Values and the Rights of Management

CONTENTS

PREFACE

This *Handbook* is a comprehensive compilation of articles in the field of human resources management, benefits administration, and labor relations. It is one of the most complete books of its kind in the areas of health care personnel and labor relations. The first article is titled "There's More To It Than People Shuffling." That is the theme of this collection. Readers will find a potpourri of articles by experts covering such diverse subjects as theories of motivation, antecedents of employee satisfaction, organization development, fundamentals of employee benefits administration, ERISA benefit funds, maintenance of nonunion status, negotiation with the collective bargaining unit, house staff unionization, arbitration from the arbitrator's view, multiemployer bargaining, and how to discipline.

The distinguished Editorial Advisory Board was instrumental in bringing together experts in the field, both scholars and practitioners. It was this board that nominated contributors, recommended and selected subject matter for coverage, and reviewed and evaluated the entries. Bill Abelow worked tirelessly to obtain high-quality articles. Mike Macdonald, who has always been a source of knowledge and inspiration for me as a peer and adviser, made invaluable contributions. Sam Levey brought together some outstanding scholars and practitioners to put into words their invaluable knowledge and experience. Sam Oberman and Larry Bassett, both outstanding consultants in the health care field, attracted the highest quality contributors. Addison Bennett, the most prolific writer in our field, was an invaluable contributor to this collection. Jack McGervey brought us the flavor and expertise that so typify his career. Joel Douglas rounded out what I must refer to as a brilliant Editorial Advisory Board.

When my publisher solicited my interest in developing such a handbook, I viewed it as an excellent opportunity for contributors to include key articles in what I anticipated would be one of the worthiest books of its kind in the field. In addition to the many articles being printed for the first time here, I would like especially to acknowledge the cooperation of Aspen Systems Corporation for permitting me to reprint outstanding articles from earlier manuals and books it has published. I also would like to acknowledge similar cooperation by S. P. Medical and Scientific Books, Division of Spectrum Publications, Inc., New York; *Hospitals, JAHA*, American Hospital Association, Chicago; International Foundation of Employee Benefits, Inc.; and the American Arbitration Association, New York.

The enormity of this project did not escape a key individual in assembling, organizing, and following through on the material. To Irene Wehr goes my everlasting gratitude. She labored diligently in typing and editing what seemed to be a continuous stream of "first drafts," "second drafts," and "final drafts." She sent out "dunning" letters and obtained all of the necessary legal forms and releases. Her energy was boundless and her understanding limitless.

To the many experienced teachers in the field of health care personnel and labor relations, I recommend this collection as an invaluable source for student research. I, personally, shall make good use of it with my graduate students in the Health Care Administration Program at Bernard M. Baruch College of the City University of New York, and at the New School for Social Research. To my many close associates and admired peers in the field of hospital personnel and labor relations, I recommend this *Handbook* as a simple and available storehouse of up-to-date ideas and usable wisdom, providing both theoretical and practical understanding and application. I am proud that what finally has been assembled is a convenient and comprehensive compendium of knowledge and experience in personnel administration and labor relations of use to students, scholars and researchers, practitioners, and all others who have the awesome responsibility of maintaining a high level of employee-employer relationships.

Norman Metzger
June 1981

PART I
HUMAN RESOURCES MANAGEMENT

The primary aim of hospitals and homes is providing the highest quality of patient care. Often overlooked, yet nevertheless true, efficient patient care develops not from the quality of medical knowledge alone nor from modern medical equipment nor drugs alone, but from a combination of all of these things *and* a well-motivated, well-administered, and well-rewarded work force. It has been noted that the personnel practices of not-for-profit health care institutions are characterized by a high degree of informality and paternalism. The personnel function continues to expand. It includes wage and salary administration, grievance handling, recruiting and interviewing, benefits administration, training, staffing planning, organizational development, and the broad area of human relations.

Modern human resources managers must ensure that personnel programs are integrated into the larger system. They play a key role in developing programs that will utilize human resources better. In the final analysis, these administrators must be concerned with making the health care institution more effective. This includes reviewing the use of the institution's existing personnel at the present level of development and creating programs that will enhance the skills of these individuals and will contribute to a more productive and rewarding environment. Dale Yoder, the dean of the field of personnel administration, challenged human resources executives by stating that personnel management must give more attention to the satisfaction of fundamental psychological and social needs of employees if it is to perform its function with greatest effectiveness.

One of the authors points out that if personnel administrators are to gain their rightful place on the hospital management team, they must be prepared to offer services well beyond the traditional technical aspects of their function. To begin to provide these services, they must be willing to make difficult choices. Still another author points out that he has found the personnel department viewed by hospital management as nothing more than an employment or recordkeeping function. The personnel function often was disjointed, with nursing maintaining its own records and departments doing their own hiring and even setting their own wage rates.

Employee satisfaction may be important both because of its possible relationship to turnover and absence rates and because of its potential impact upon employee productivity. Addressing the needs of the work force is an integral part of human resources management. The personnel director in a health care institution is an important member of the administrative team that must direct its attention to arranging organizational conditions and methods of operation, so that individuals can achieve their goals by directing their efforts toward organizational objectives. This is the process primarily of creating opportunities, releasing potentials, removing obstacles, encouraging growth, and providing guidelines. It is finally accepted now that one of the more important responsibilities of the health care institution is that of personnel administration.

People provide care to the sick and the needy. Health care institutions are in the business not of manufacturing things but of offering service. Service industries are far more dependent than others upon employee morale and commitment. Institutions that provide medical care are criticized more for the *attitudes* of their personnel than for the *quality* of care. It may be difficult to accept, but nevertheless, it is a valid observation that patients and visitors are more impressed, and concerned with the attentiveness, empathy, and responsiveness of the health care worker than with the financial aspects of their exposure to an institution. The highly sophisticated and complex environments now operative in health care institutions mandate that the individuals responsible for the human resources function no longer communicate and implement by the seat of their pants. They must focus the attention of administrators and medical staff upon the social and psychological side of the enterprise.

1. There's More To It Than People Shuffling

ADDISON C. BENNETT

Reprinted with permission from *Hospitals*, J.A.H.A., Vol. 52, No. 23, © December 1, 1978, published by the American Hospital Association.

Whether most administrations fully accept or understand the notion that "the real difference is people" (often heard expressed in the familiar claim that "people are our most valuable asset"), they continue to expend considerable time and dollars to support it: orienting new employees, conducting job training, maintaining competitive wage and salary policies and programs, and providing acceptable levels of employee benefits. Much of this "investment in people," however, tends to be a consequence of economic and legislative happenings. In more instances than not, they are uncontrollable sources of action impinging on the managerial prerogatives of administration and summoning additional displays of technical expertise on the part of the personnel executive.

If there is a revolution taking place, it is in the realm of attitudes and values of people—a transition of thinking on the part of the average worker, who has left behind old notions and assumptions and moved toward the adoption of new beliefs and expectations. This transition, contends Louis Banks, adjunct professor at MIT's Sloan School of Management and former managing editor of *Fortune*, is not antibusiness or antiorganization per se. While employees are becoming increasingly "skeptical about 'the company'—any company—they are still motivated by opportunity, excited by prospects of development and growth, and concerned about the corporation's well-being as long as it deserves their concern."[1] Unfortunately, this "transition of thinking" has not been paralleled by any observable tendencies on the part of all too many administrations to keep their thinking and action process in touch and in tune with the times—processes of a quality that is in keeping with the advice of Lodge, who offers the thought that, "It behooves managers to clear their heads, to inspect all old assumptions, to identify as precisely as possible what is happening and what new ideas and definitions of values are germinating, and then to look objectively at the choices that remain."[2]

Six decades have passed since the formal inauguration of personnel recruitment and management in the U.S. Army—a step that paved the way for modern personnel systems and development in all fields of endeavor. Over the years, the development of the personnel administration function in both service and nonservice industries has been characterized by evolutionary change, with the health care sector falling sharply and consistently behind personnel progress being made on many fronts.

Looking back to the 1950s, for example, what was found in our nation's hospitals, with but few exceptions, was the bare maintenance of an employment office. The changes that were introduced subsequently, during the '60s and '70s, in the personnel function were still not sufficiently progressive to take us any further than a contemporary profile of the personnel director's position that continues to reveal the inadequacy of the function in terms of meeting new demands and problems in the health care workplace.

Without question, a historical account of the development of the personnel administration activity in health care shows a degree of stagnancy that has caused this key function to be ill-equipped to deal with many of the current problems of a human service industry.

Symptoms of the functional malady that have persisted over the past several years remain with us today. Most often when we look at top management behavior, we see:

- The absence of respect for the personnel function.
- The tendency to be penurious in providing resources for the function, the result being foolish economy in an area requiring expert knowledge and professionalism.
- The holding of the personnel executive at arm's length from corporate policy and strategic decisions.

At the same time, a high sense of frustration continues to be expressed by personnel directors, who claim that their feelings of discouragement and disillusionment stem from such obstacles as:

- The lack of support of top administration.
- The problem of the organizational position, status, and influence of the personnel function.
- The attitudes of "line" management, at all levels, toward the personnel function.
- The fragmentation of personnel activities (nursing department doing its own thing, professional service units hiring and firing, and the like).
- The economic problems of the hospital.

Personnel department deficiencies, in the past, have given the appearance of defying satisfactory solutions because administrations and their personnel executives have not reconciled their perspectives consistent with the larger and more meaningful role of personnel administration. There are reasons enough for the members of top management to consider the development of human resources one of their chief concerns, but it is chiefly the personnel directors themselves who give all indications of being the perpetuators of traditional approaches to conducting personnel affairs. Their preoccupation with regulatory compliance as an end purpose of their existence, their identification with employee welfare rather than with the balancing of institutional and employee needs to the beneficial outcome of both, their concern with single employee relations activities (such as picnics) rather than with total employee relations programs typify this. It is, without question, this persistent narrowness in their view that sustains their problems, as well as the continuance of

the behavior and attitudes of administration toward the personnel function.

NEW PERSPECTIVES

To go beyond the traditional bent of contemporary personnel work found prevalent within the health care industry, a wider range of vision on the part of both administrations and their personnel executives will need to be brought to bear on the personnel function. These visionary extensions must see the function from new and different perspectives. They must reflect a consciousness of its potential contributions and influence not as yet realized in terms of institutional outcomes, organization and management development, and economic performance.

Institutional outcomes and the personnel executive's role need to find greater linkage. If this relationship is not achieved, business will be the preoccupation of the personnel function, rather than performance that is contributory to the desired outcomes of the institution. The personnel executive can take on a more active role in this direction by:

- Providing needed input to top management during the hospital's goal-setting process so as to bring a humanistic dimension to organizational goals.
- Exercising imagination in establishing human resources objectives that affect the organization as a whole, rather than on a single aspect of the personnel function, and that integrate existing personnel programs into a long-term plan for institutional growth.
- Going directly to employees via attitude surveys, group discussions, and individual interviews aimed at discerning employee attitudes, beliefs, and values which, in light of the complexities of today's world, may lack clear delineation without the presence of an organized effort on the part of the personnel executive.
- Providing leadership in the development of an appraisal process that ties rewards to attainment of organizational objectives and to levels of individual performance.

Organization development implies management development as a main mission of personnel administration. The point to be made here is that the personnel executive's involvement in and contribution to the effort of developing managers at all levels in the hospital will return the greatest payoffs in terms of optimizing the effectiveness of the personnel department's performance. To be successful in adding strength to the management effectiveness of the organization, the personnel executive himself must be an effective manager.

Because "people" problems cut across all functional lines, the hospital must remain steady on one basic course: extending managerial competence throughout the organization. Here again, the personnel executive must create opportunities for action aimed at contributing to the development of the organization and its management. For example, the personnel executive may:

- Assist in the design and implementation of mechanisms to enhance internal communications, such as administration/department head forums, small group sessions for employees, departmental meetings, training in counseling, and evaluative feedback to top management regarding its communicative effectiveness.
- Work with the hospital's training staff to develop and sponsor educational programs targeted toward strengthening the managerial skills of individuals and the working relationships of people from different functional areas of the organization.
- Exercise leadership in problem-solving activities directed toward improving the human affairs of the hospital. These activities can take the form of task forces, committees, training groups, or individual assignments aimed at broadening manager sensitivities and skills.
- Be the architect of a process that provides the hospital with a continuing capability for management manpower planning and development that embraces (1) an analysis and evaluation of the organization as it now exists, (2) a projection of the organization three to five years into the future, (3) a forecast of organizational changes such as new positions, elimination or combination of functions and tasks, and anticipated turnover, (4) an inventory of existing talent at high as well as low levels, and (5) specific action plans to develop talent to meet the future needs for replacement and expansion.

Economic performance of the personnel function in today's hospital is given surprisingly little attention, in spite of the fact that people resources compose the largest cost element of operating the enterprise. It is believed that a part of this problem is a disparity that exists between the priorities of the personnel officer and the priorities of administration. What needs to be seen is that personnel administration, by its very purpose and function, is centrally placed in the "mainstream of profitability" where cost containment op-

portunities can be uncovered and, at the same time, the needs of people can be fulfilled. With the realization of these two compatible goals, the dilemma of ordered priorities dissolves.

Opportunities for improving the economic performance of the personnel unit can be found in such actions as:

- Setting personnel unit objectives that express measurable expectations in terms of savings.
- Entering into a "partnership" with key department managers with the purpose of assisting them in achieving cost containment objectives for their units.
- Working closely with department managers and supervisors, as well as with the hospital's management engineer, on problems of staffing and productivity.
- Exercising continuing efforts to question the ways in which the personnel unit currently performs its work and to search for more effective methods for getting the job done. A wide spectrum of improvement opportunities are available to the personnel executive, ranging from implementation of the self-funding concept for various benefit programs to simplification of routine record-keeping activities.
- Engaging in shared programs, such as courses of training and education, data management systems, and multifacility recruitment activities.
- Controlling the total personnel system through periodic audits. There are cases to prove that the employment of part-time college students to do a thorough annual auditing job on such cost-contributing factors as absenteeism, turnover, overtime, timecard entries, unemployment insurance, sick leave, and differential pay practices can be a significant cost-effective undertaking, one that can cause both administration and the "staff" executive to get a new perspective on how the personnel function relates to the bottom line.

The February 1976 issue of *Fortune* contained an article titled: "Personnel Directors Are the New Corporate Heroes." Observably, hero-worshipping of the personnel officer is far from being a popular pastime in most health care institutions. Yet, the needs and conditions do exist to set the stage for making personnel people in hospitals "the new corporate heroes." At a time when the attainment of cost-effective outcomes is imperative and more workers are dissatisfied with their jobs than at any other time in the past 25 years, surely the need for personnel heroes is at hand. Achieving such heroism requires hard work and the making of some difficult choices. Most of all, it requires fresh thinking and new perspectives about managing human resources in a people-serving-people environment.

NOTES

1. Louis Banks, "Here Come the Individualists," *Harvard Magazine*, 80 (September-October 1977): 24.

2. G.C. Lodge, "Business and the Changing Society," *Harvard Business Review*, 52 (March-April 1974): 59.

2. Personnel Administration in the Health Care Field

RALPH F. ABBOTT, JR., BRIAN E. HAYES, JAY M. PRESSER,
MARTIN E. SKOLER, AND JAMES N. TRONO

Reprinted with permission from *Health Care Labor Manual*, Vol. II, Chapter 11, by Skoler & Abbott, P.C.,
attorneys at law, Springfield, Mass. (Martin E. Skoler, Ralph F. Abbott, Jr., Brian E. Hayes, editor-in-chief;
Jay M. Presser, and James M. Trono, published by Aspen Systems Corporation, Germantown, Md. © 1981.

1 INTRODUCTION

Personnel administration is the function of management concerned with the intelligent acquisition, development, and use of human resources. Unfortunately, the function of today's personnel administrator is neither as easy nor as concise as this bare-bones definition would imply. Within the past five years alone, changes in the economy and in the law have transformed the personnel department into a melting pot where the objectives of the employer, worker, and society must somehow blend into a dish palatable to all. The health care field, with its unique characteristics and demands, presents special challenges to today's personnel administrator.

The health care field is unique in at least the following aspects:

- It is enormous and constantly growing. In 1980, health-related expenditures in this country totaled almost $200 billion, close to $1,000 per capita. Between 1965 and 1980, the percentage of the U.S. Gross National Product (GNP) consumed by health expenditures increased by more than half. Office of Management and Budget statistics project that in 1985, the health care field will consume

10.5 percent of the GNP, rising to 11.5 percent in 1990. It is the largest service industry in dollars spent and is exceeded in numbers of people employed only by the field of education.

- It is a fragmented industry, ranging from physicians in independent practice to hospitals employing many thousands. Yet the average size of the nation's approximately 5,800 short-term hospitals is relatively small. More than half have less than 100 beds.

- It is labor intensive—as distinguished from oil refining, for example, which is capital intensive. Community hospitals spend 60 percent or more of their income on wages and benefits. In major medical centers and teaching hospitals this figure may escalate to 70-75 percent of each income dollar. Pay and benefit levels, once marginal, have become highly competitive during the past decade.

- Depending upon who is counting, some 200-300 distinct jobs or major job classifications can be identified.[1] The array of specialized skills required to operate even an institution of modest size is overwhelming. The number and kinds of occupations are increasing, with the traditional doctor, nurse, and technician augmented with draftsmen, biomedical engineers, anthropologists, systems and computer engineers, etc.

- Despite recent changes in attitude towards sexual stereotyping in employment, the health field is still predominantly female (65-75 percent of the work-

---

Note: All references to other chapters or sections in this article are references to chapters or sections in the *Health Care Labor Manual*, Vol. II, published by Aspen Systems Corporation.

force). The 1.4 million registered nurses who hold active licenses to practice in this country make up, by far, the largest group of professional health care providers. Men represent less than 30,000 of this total. However, women, who represent over 50 percent of the population, still represent less than 12 percent of all physicians, dentists, and optometrists. Thousands of minorities are also entering health professions where they have been traditionally underrepresented. It is estimated, however, that less than 7 percent of the registered nurse population have racial and/or ethnic minority backgrounds. The Department of Labor statistics for 1979 reveal that less than 3 percent of the nation's physicians are black, while Hispanics and American Indians represent just over 1 percent of all dentists and optometrists. As the racial-ethnic complexion of the health care industry changes, so do the requirements of professional and preprofessional training, registration, and licensing—areas of special concern to the personnel administrator.

- The health care industry workforce is young (with the majority under 35) and highly mobile, contributing to rapid turnover rates. A large New England hospital was alarmed to discover its own nursing graduates remained only 23 months after completion of their studies. A check of neighboring hospitals showed that most employed newly graduated nurses remained for only 19 months. This may help to explain the predominance of career-oriented men in senior management posts. Yet, women are widely represented in the ranks of top administrators, and they clearly predominate as directors of nursing, dietetics, medical records, social services, and some other key areas.

- The health care field is highly fragmented and compartmentalized by function and occupation. Between 50 and 70 departments and identifiable work groups can be counted in most major short-term hospitals. Further fragmentation occurs by occupation. Guildlike societies and associations, often national in scope, have increased in influence in recent years. Most have as their avowed purpose the maintenance of high professional standards through education, certification, and licensure. Frequently such groups have been subjected to criticism for establishing artificially inflated standards so as to keep new aspirants from being able to join their ranks and thereby improve their bargaining position in the job market.

- In recent years, substantial inroads in the health care field have enabled certain labor unions to preserve their viability as bargaining agents. While the past several years have witnessed a steady decline in general unionization, unionization in the health care field has increased. In 1979, the percentage of union victories among white collar workers alone was the highest in well over a decade. Thirty-four percent of these newly organized white collar workers were in the health care industry. The prudent personnel administrator must be keenly sensitive to organizing trends—trends that, one way or another, can shape and influence the entire workplace.

- Serious, and indeed successful, inquiry into the nature, cause, and cure of disease is often carried out under physical, financial, and managerial constraints that other industries could not tolerate. Researchers themselves contribute to these inefficiencies by lack of preparation for or interest in their administrative responsibilities. Yet the entire system progresses, and the three-legged stool of patient care, research, and teaching continues to provide the basis, albeit fragile, for an enterprise now far removed from its ecclesiastical beginning.

- A new kind of national expectation is the final unique characteristic of the health care industry. Specifically, how may all Americans, regardless of where they live, be assured of access to uniformly high quality health care at a price they can afford to pay? The dilemma is largely a systemic one. Numerous experiments and working models, here and abroad, suggest alternatives to our present modes of patient care. Even the terminology used to describe or identify these changes is in flux. Health Maintenance Organizations (HMO), Prepaid Group Plans (PGP), and Professional Standards Review Organization (PSRO) have become part of the new vocabulary. "Peer review" as a method of assuring quality health care has gradually emerged from an experimental status to a widely used method of performance analysis. Hospitals and clinics are called health care providers or deliverers. Insurance companies are called third party payors. Patients are called health consumers. One must develop and maintain an acute ear for the subtleties of change, because the personnel administrator will be called upon to play an increasingly important role in making the health enterprise more responsive to the public demand for better care.

Historically, the personnel practices of nonprofit health care institutions were characterized by a high degree of informality and paternalism, particularly in smaller institutions. Many important personnel questions were never dealt with in terms of the institution's best policy interests; instead, administrators made *ad hoc* decisions in individual cases, which may have been inconsistent with those made in prior cases. Problems relating to compensation, for example, were often resolved on a personal basis. Moreover, management of personnel matters was frequently entrusted to persons whose major assignments were in financial management and recordkeeping and who lacked training, temperament, and commitment to act effectively in the personnel field. There was a prevailing sense that nonprofit health care organizations were so different from profit-making organizations that the procedures and experiences of the latter not only could not, but *should* not be applied to the former.

These attitudes have changed markedly in the last decade or two. Health care institutions, on the whole, have become committed to professional personnel management by persons whose training and skills qualify them to act effectively in this field.

The personnel function is an expanding one. No longer is it concerned solely with such traditional matters as wage and salary administration, grievance handling, recruiting and interviewing, benefit administration, and training. In some institutions it has come to include manpower planning, organizational development and community relations. And, where some of the institution's employees have been organized for purposes of collective bargaining, the personnel function may include responsibility for labor relations as well.

One indication that personnel administration has achieved a new level of importance in the health care field is that an increasing number of institutions have elevated the principal personnel officer to the level of a vice-president or an associate administrator. As the movement toward collective bargaining gains momentum, the personnel function will be heightened further. In short, the personnel office, which at one time did not have very much importance, has become one of the most significant departments in a health care institution serving varied and notable functions.

This chapter addresses the major issues confronting the modern health care personnel administrator. Where prevailing industrial models may be applied usefully, they have been noted. Likewise, distinctions have been pointed out where necessary. This chapter is not intended to be an exhaustive treatment of the subject. Sources of more complete information are appropriately listed in the discussion and in the bibliography.

The health care employer must be aware that the application of labor laws to the industry's employees is in a state of flux. It is imperative that the personnel director read Chapter 9 of the Manual, which deals with the Equal Employment Opportunity Law and the necessity for the institution's compliance with an affirmative action program. The employer must be mindful that such employment criteria as educational requirements, testing policies, pregnancy leave, inquiries as to arrest records, or height and weight of applicants, for instance, have been held to perpetuate policies of past discrimination, even though they may appear to be neutral as to sex and race. In 1980, the Equal Employment Opportunity Commission (EEOC) also finalized firm guidelines that would hold the employer liable for sexual harassment in the workplace. Other 1980 EEOC guidelines call for the employer to make accommodation where reasonable for the religious preference of the employee or job applicant. In short, the responsibilities of the personnel administrator today far exceed the rudiments of hiring and firing. The employer and personnel administrator should assess personnel policies carefully, since results and consequences of subtle employment practices matter, rather than the employer's intent.

In order to maintain a flowing discussion, the following terms are defined. The personal pronoun "he" is meant to include "she" as well. "Personnel director" also means personnel administrator or officer. Hospital, unless specifically identified as such, is intended to mean clinic, group practice, or any similar institution offering health care.

2 THE PERSONNEL DEPARTMENT AND ITS ROLE

In the past the personnel director was often thought of as the kindly soul who said he liked people, could do a reasonable job of screening out applicants deemed unsuitable, and keep minimal records. Little else was expected or even desired.

More frequently the top administrator or individual department heads performed personnel functions themselves as part of their duties. In larger hospitals these uncoordinated efforts occasionally led to the discharge of an employee from one department and his subsequent hire by another without challenge or question. More serious than the absence of even elemental procedures or concern for legal niceties was that there were striking variations in personnel practices among the different departments. Personnel directors, when they existed, reflected the senior administrator's perplexity over how to best utilize the diverse skills needed in the cure of the ill.

The introduction to this chapter suggests some of the factors which have propelled personnel administration within the health establishment into significant influence and visibility during the past twenty-five years. As subsequent topics are discussed in the following pages, the reasons for so dramatic a shift in emphasis should become even more apparent. To see the personnel function in contemporary perspective, we will digress briefly and examine the organization in which it must operate.

2-1 The Health Care Organization

Hospitals and related facilities like to view themselves as patient-oriented. To portray this graphically they often show a series of concentric circles with the patient surrounded by skilled men and women representing many disciplines. Following is a simplified version of one such chart.

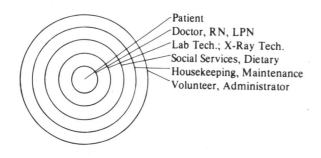

- Patient
- Doctor, RN, LPN
- Lab Tech.; X-Ray Tech.
- Social Services, Dietary
- Housekeeping, Maintenance
- Volunteer, Administrator

A more conventional approach tacitly assumes the patient's best interest is foremost in everyone's mind. But, in reality, two separate and sometimes competing organizations report to the Board of Trustees. Such a structure is illustrated below.

In recent years, the complexity of health organizations and the need for more centralized control of day-to-day operations have forced larger hospitals to adopt an approach modeled along corporate lines. Part of one such chart is on page 11.

Large hospitals, especially those with medical school affiliations, seem to have ambivalent feelings regarding the value of the physician as chief operating officer versus the "lay" administrator who is not an M.D., but who has completed a master's program and internship in hospital administration. It is argued on one hand that the physician can cope with and gain the respect of his sometimes unruly colleagues, while counting on his priestly qualities to awe the heads of housekeeping, pharmacy, purchasing, accounting, etc. Adherents of the trained nonphysician school point with equal vigor to the need for a person especially prepared to deal with the economics of health care and the mechanics of weaving the bits and pieces of a delivery system into one effective whole. Those entering health care administration for the first time should expect to see either model and perhaps some hybrid between the two. The personnel director may, in fact, be asked to examine and recommend changes in the organization. If he is new, he should proceed with particular caution. All alternatives, including political factors within the institution, must be analyzed with considerable care before fundamental changes are suggested.

2-2 Organization of the Personnel Department

In organizing his own department or making major changes in it, the personnel director would do well to

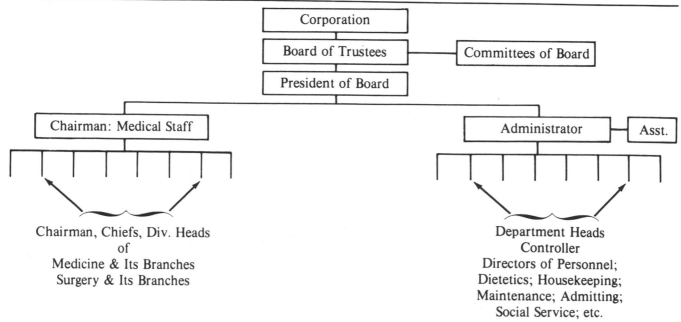

Corporation

Board of Trustees — Committees of Board

President of Board

Chairman: Medical Staff

Administrator — Asst.

Chairman, Chiefs, Div. Heads
of
Medicine & Its Branches
Surgery & Its Branches

Department Heads
Controller
Directors of Personnel;
Dietetics; Housekeeping;
Maintenance; Admitting;
Social Service; etc.

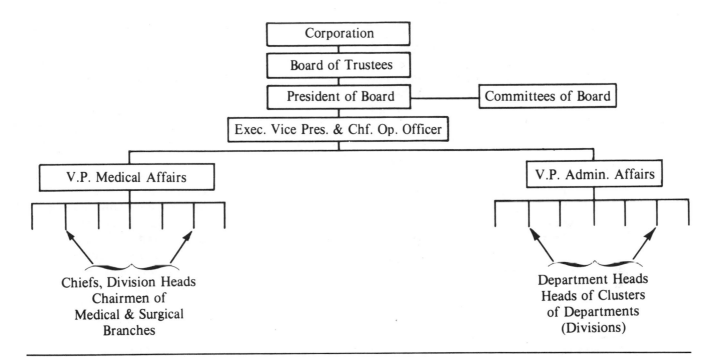

forget, at least briefly, everything ever learned about chart making, and concentrate on the final result he hopes to achieve for the institution. More than a few personnel directors have met sorry ends because they wasted precious time chasing the wrong problem while basic and often serious internal difficulties went unattended. Let us be specific and examine a list of broad areas in which personnel expertise might be profitably directed. No significance should be attached to the order in which the following are listed.

Employee Relations: What do employees and prospective employees think of your institution? (Facts are less important than feelings.) What is your turnover rate compared with neighboring hospitals? Does the average employee feel that his needs, opinions, and complaints are given a fair hearing?

Labor Relations: Does the hospital now have union contracts? If not, is unionization or an organizational drive near at hand? (Either of the foregoing can demand enormous amounts of time from the personnel director and his staff.)

Recruitment: Is the recruiting staff sufficiently large and professionally competent to do the job expected of it? Do department heads recruit through personnel or through sources developed on their own? After spending money to bring in candidates, are the good ones lost in a storage and retrieval system which is inadequate by present day-standards?

Personnel Policies: Does a policy manual exist? Is it written clearly and concisely? Are the policies it enunciates fair and defendable by modern standards? Are employees aware of its existence?

Salary Administration: Does a formal plan of any kind exist? Does it reasonably reflect the different requirements of different jobs? Does a sampling of job descriptions show careful analysis of present demands for each position? Are salary levels consistent with those prevailing in the local area for the same work?

Benefits: How do they compare with the community and within the occupational family in which recruitment will take place? Are benefits used as recruiting tools, productivity incentives, employee relations, or have they just accumulated over the years without conscious effort or planning? How much do benefits cost? Are they fairly and effectively administered by the personnel department? Has a profile of workforce by age, sex, or length of employment been undertaken?

Personnel Records: Are they complete, correct, and confidential? Are changes of employee status (insurance beneficiary changes, for example) handled promptly and accurately? Do employees trust the personnel department's recordkeeping abilities? Can data processing be more profitably employed in maintaining records and providing a comprehensive data base for future needs?

Training: Are employees adequately trained for their jobs? Where is training done—outside or internally? Are there provisions for continuing programs to keep employee skills up-to-date? How much does training cost? Can economy be realized through cooperative programs among groups of neighboring hospitals?

Organization should follow need. And the employee, institutional, and community perception of need can provide only bemusement and frustration for a personnel administrator who has not built flexibility and sensitivity into his own department.

Because of their tendency to be rigid, organization charts do not easily adapt to the rapid shifts in emphasis now required in health care institutions. Should charts be drawn at all? By all means. But they can do little to educate or motivate a personnel staff who are already well trained, bright, adaptable, and able to perform many different jobs within the department.

Basic as it may seem, everyone should know how to answer a telephone and record a message correctly. Not all personnel people do. Everyone should know how to greet an applicant, visitor, or employee with warmth and grace. Every personnel employee should consider himself at center stage while performing his job and reflect the institution through his manner, dress, and competence.

The organization needed to carry out these multifaceted roles might be portrayed in the following example from a medium-size hospital's personnel department. (See following diagram.)

the next. Yet now that health employers are competing more actively in the same commercial, trade, and service pool as other industries, the terminology gap is actually narrowing. Although the reverse is true in a few highly specialized areas of medicine where new jobs are constantly being created, whatever gap does exist can be surmounted. Even experienced health care recruiters must unceasingly refresh their knowledge of this growing field.

More serious—even dangerous—is the belief that recruitment can somehow be carried out in splendid isolation from the image and reputation among patients, community, and employees with which the institution has already cloaked itself.

Hospitals, nursing homes, clinics, and similar enterprises often discover too late that they live in a goldfish bowl of public scrutiny and that shoddy treatment of one part of their constituency may seriously impair their acceptance by the other parts. Psychiatrist Karl Menninger once observed that attitudes are more important than facts. This is especially so at the front door of any hospital, where the reputation it has developed in the past is clearly reflected in the numbers

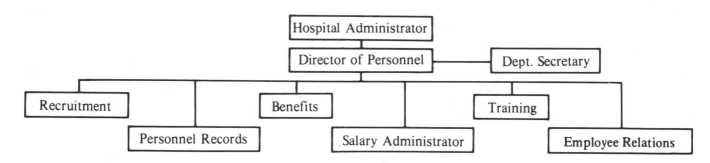

The alert personnel director will explore a number of alternative structures, relate them to his institution's unique requirements, and make appropriate changes well in advance of crisis.[2]

2-3 Recruitment

Certain unwarranted anxieties face anyone entering health care recruitment for the first time. Among these is the notion that the hundreds of interrelated jobs and exotic terminology can never be sufficiently understood without a prolonged training period. Fears of this sort often come from those who already feel comfortable in complex fields such as electronics, insurance, or manufacturing. But these same people are later surprised to learn that good recruiting techniques are transferable to medicine. Job titles, specification, vocabulary, and the like will vary from one industry to

and quality of job applicants appearing at the personnel department.

One seasoned personnel director may have oversimplified by suggesting that if you watch the back door, the front door will take care of itself. The recruitment process, while vital to the creation of jobs and replenishment of staff, can never be safely viewed except as a fractional part of the total institutional image. As recruiting techniques are discussed, therefore, it should be remembered that most will represent time and money wasted unless a thoughtful plan of modern employee relations is concurrently developed and carried out. Finally, the institution's posture in this vital area must be clearly articulated from the most senior administrator to every manager and employee. The message will be repeated through all communications media, but especially in the day-to-day actions of those who are entrusted with supervisory responsibilities.

2-4 *The Setting*

The emergency room, admitting office, main lobby, reception desk, and employment office are windows through which an entire institution receives instant, yet lasting appraisal. Because it is not unusual for a busy hospital personnel department to be visited by many outsiders each year, facilities for reception, waiting, testing, and interviewing should be easily accessible from the street or parking area. This usually means a good ground floor location, preferably with its own entrance and exit. The flow of applicant traffic should follow a logical pattern which makes verbal directions and signs unnecessary under most circumstances. Carpeting, curtains, acoustical ceilings, and other sound-reducing furnishings and equipment should be used to create a businesslike, dignified atmosphere. Finally, an element of welcome and warmth in furniture arrangement, use of color, wall hangings, and lighting can turn the customary drabness of an employment office into an unspoken statement of friendly efficiency. Reception areas become untidy very quickly. The receptionist should be sensitive to the message your facility is intended to convey and should keep reception and testing areas neat during the day. In larger inner city hospitals, receptionists, interviewers, and others who have continuous off-the-street public contact often have silent "panic buttons" under their desks. In the event of trouble an alarm can be rung which sounds in the security department or in the personnel director's office.

Privacy is essential to a successful interview. Rooms and offices used for this purpose should have doors, just enough modern furniture to avoid a cluttered look, and a telephone that does not ring unless intended for the interviewer. Bulletin boards, cute desk signs, and personal memorabilia of the interviewer can be distracting, especially in a small office, and ought to be avoided. An ideal traffic pattern is one which permits the applicant to be ushered into other parts of the hospital or directly to the street without passing back through the reception area. Interviews, even for those already employed, are stressful experiences. The physical setting you provide for this purpose can do much to remove needless anxieties, and thereby make the visit more productive.

2-5 *Sources of Applicants and Their Relative Value*

Those in personnel frequently use the word "traffic" to express applicant flow. To the less experienced, high traffic is good, low traffic is bad. The reverse may in fact be true. Much wasted time and disappointment to job seekers can be avoided if recruiters first identify with some precision the kinds of skills they are seeking and then learn where to look.

Application forms should contain a question asking the candidate how he learned of the position he seeks. A daily log of applicants seen and résumés received by mail permit a separation by source and should indicate whether a hire will ultimately take place. For Affirmative Action purposes, the log should also incorporate information on race, sex, and type of position sought.[3] Logs, if kept in a three-ring binder chronologically by date, may be easily reviewed and summarized.

A personnel director and his recruiting staff are limited only by their own imagination and energy in selecting and utilizing sources likely to produce the kind of job candidates they wish to attract. Among the sources commonly used to recruit job applicants are: newspaper, professional journal, radio, and television advertising; search firms; employment agencies (public and private); public transportation ads on bus routes passing the hospital; contacts in other personnel departments; walk-ins from the street; recommendations by employees; department head contacts among their peers in other institutions; social agencies; trips to high schools and colleges; and payment to employees who refer successful applicants. Each has its advantages and each extracts a price from the limited personnel reservoir of money and time. For reasons of space, only limited comments will be made on the major sources and it is suggested that results be constantly monitored. Experimenting with the wrong medium is not so disastrous as failing to recognize when a change in either the source or its use is called for.

2-6 Advertising. When he was with the large New York advertising agency, Batten, Barton, Dursten, and Osborne (B.B.D.&O.), Bruce Barton used to say that he wasted half of each advertising dollar. Pausing to let this sink in, Barton would add that unfortunately he didn't know which half it was. Since advertising in newspapers and journals is often the largest item in a hospital's recruitment budget, it should be undertaken with special concern for results. There is no believable body of canon law, nor are there dogmas that will last for all time. Tuesday, Wednesday, and Thursday aren't always the best days to advertise, but no one can say that Saturday and Sunday are always the best days. Below the newspaper fold rather than above it isn't fatal. Black borders, two or three column widths, large rather than small ads—may pull on Monday and bomb on Thursday just as easily as a tiny ad placed on a supposedly wrong day may draw the one candidate who is hired.

Applicants often make the problem of effective advertising more murky by insisting that they saw your notice in a publication you have not used in months. Successful recruiters already know this. Yet they often fall into the rut of complacency and expect the momentum of past advertising successes to continue producing walk-in traffic sufficient for their needs. Lazy recruiters do not last long in a heads-up organization.

Local newspapers will ordinarily provide the best advertising exposure when recruiting in neighboring communities. For certain positions, however, perhaps only a limited number of people in the United States may qualify. Hospitals, medical schools, and similar institutions frequently by-pass the local market and resort to advertisements in professional journals. Research investigators and department heads can save the recruiter time and possibly money by helping to zero in on the appropriate publication. Most journals are published biweekly or monthly, are not unusually expensive but have copy deadlines of two to eight weeks before an advertisement will appear. Therefore, the vacant position will often be filled before publication of the advertisement. Moreover, publications often expect payment in advance. When considering the use of a national publication, personnel administrators should note that studies have shown that workers such as nurses or lab technicians are not likely to relocate great distances just to accept a similar position at a comparable salary.

To be counted among the personnel director's best friends is a good advertising agency. The account executive of an agency should be given a complete tour of the facilities and be encouraged to stop and talk with people. This will help him capture the atmosphere of the health care center to be used in advertising copy. For example, pediatric hospitals might consider a theme involving children's art work; institutions being enlarged could make use of cranes and point to growing job opportunities in the future. Advertising agencies can easily lose the creative spark that is essential to effective, compelling ads. Therefore, the personnel director should periodically monitor his advertising as it finally appears in print, even if day-by-day ad decisions are delegated to someone else. Each ad makes a statement about the entire institution. The personnel director must be sure the ad is saying what he wants it to say. Moreover, he should be certain that he is receiving the full range of services the agency can offer.

Regardless of who prepares final copy for publication, certain points should not be overlooked. The ideal ad is one which produces a number of well qualified candidates for the jobs to be filled. Vaguely worded advertisements waste time. A thorough representation of the job to be filled, its prospective minimal as well as ideal requirements, and the salary range give an applicant a clearer understanding of the position available. Salary levels and significant benefits belong in most ads. Be wary of precise salaries of, for instance, $21,615.83. They bespeak rigid pay structures with little room for the creative applicant to feel he can negotiate.

Verbiage suggestive of bureaucracy is to be avoided. "Salary commensurate with education and experience" really means the employer does not yet know current pay rates for the job, or does know the rates and hopes to buy cheaper. "Closing date for applications is . . ." is another unfortunate phrase common in agencies of government. Some employers still use "challenge" to describe jobs with no other visible merit. Make a list of worn out words and phrases, and avoid them when possible. "Equal Opportunity Employer M/F" and/or "Affirmative Action Employer" are tag lines which may be required of your institution under federal and certain state civil rights laws. Certain phrases no longer impress civil rights investigators who, nevertheless, still insist upon their use in one form or another. Those who have felt the sting of discrimination are deceived even less. A more imaginative approach is to work an equal opportunity posture into the body of the ad through fresh words and illustrations.[4]

Advertising copy should quickly address the institution's real needs, as simply as possible. But effective simplicity takes time to create, so allow adequate time to prepare and review the ad. Twenty minutes before deadline is too late to start writing a good advertisement for anything.

Agencies will ordinarily write or assist with the task of ad preparation. They will also provide copies of ads as published. These should be posted on plain white pages and inserted in a three-ring binder so that notes can be made on what results were achieved. Changes in format or wording must not be delayed for several reasons: if the ad did not reach the person you seek, it represented valuable time wasted in filling the position. Secondly, the cost of advertising has been rising much faster than most other expenses in personnel department budgets. Finally, constant advertising, especially of one or two positions, tends to create the impression of high turnover. Readers do not know that the position was never filled when it ran weeks ago. Repetitive ads suggest that someone was hired, was fired shortly thereafter, and now there is a search for another victim.

Blind ads, in which the name of the hospital has been omitted, should almost always be avoided. A blind ad might be considered in a situation where morale of current employees would be affected were it known the hospital was trying to fill a position from outside.

Hospitals in large cities and those in the midst of building programs sometimes use display cards in buses and transit terminals. Because the cards normally entail the expense of art work, color plates, and silk screening, they are changed only after three months or so. For this reason it is generally wiser to omit reference to specific jobs unless it is clear that technicians, nurse's aides, secretaries, registered nurses, etc. represent *types* of positions that may be available rather than current vacancies. Many hospitals have found display cards a useful backup to more specific ads. The theme often used is simply that the institution is growing, or it is a good place to work, or possibly that it is close to home. Results of this kind of advertising are hard to measure and the cost can be high. However, the idea should not be discarded without some thought and possibly a three-to-six-month trial period using selected routes and stations.

Radio or television advertising has the obvious advantage of allowing one to describe specific openings and sometimes reach a different market. Cost is a factor which has limited wider use of these media.

Additional sources to be considered are regional, minority, and foreign language newspapers and radio stations. Results are unpredictable, but the relatively low cost makes experimentation worthwhile, and further helps the institution reach groups of people untouched by the more conventional methods.[5]

2-7 Search Firms; Employment Agencies. Although they operate differently, search organizations and employment agencies offer several common advantages. They provide a measure of confidentiality and enable the employer to limit his advertising expense and exposure. With good fortune and competence, the number of applicants ultimately interviewed by the employer is limited to those likely to be offered work. In the identification and selection process, good search firms and agencies will check references and otherwise do a skillful job of "prepackaging" each candidate, thereby making selection easier.

Search organizations normally operate on either a fixed fee to the employer or offer an estimate of cost based upon a daily charge plus out-of-pocket expenses. Often, an hourly charge is made in addition to expenses and a placement fee. They will also provide some idea of how long the search should last. In most cases you can terminate the arrangement if you either decide not to fill the position or locate a suitable candidate from some other source. As is true with search firms, private employment agencies normally charge only the employer. The shift from employee-paid to employer-paid fees began in the early 1960s and was virtually complete by 1970. However, some agencies still charge only the employee or will arrange to have the charge shared between both parties. Agencies customarily operate on a contingency basis—no placement, no fee. As a rule, they screen a larger volume of candidates and tend to refer greater numbers of applicants for employer consideration.

Search firms bear the undignified sobriquet of "head hunters" because they do only minimal advertising and use their considerable contacts to reach into competing organizations—including yours—for likely candidates. The ritual requires, among other things, that the candidate react first with surprise and then reluctance to change jobs. This is calculated to sweeten the compensation package, and if played with adroitness, does. Search firms have reached a level in recent years which has made them increasingly useful adjuncts to the difficult task of locating and recruiting scarce professional talent. Their charges have more than kept pace, however, and tend to run upwards of 25 percent of the successful candidate's first year gross salary. Employment agency fees have also increased rapidly. They usually run 10 to 25 percent of the initial annual rate of pay, and are contingent upon a successful placement. Some guarantee of satisfaction on the employer's part is customary.

If not carefully monitored, search fees and agency charges can quickly get out of hand. Overall, they should represent a small portion of the recruitment budget and should be confined to hard-to-fill positions. Otherwise, the employment manager and his staff simply are not doing the job for which they were hired.

Both the competence and integrity of search firms and private agencies have often been called into question, and not without reason. Unfortunately the business is easy to get into and out of. The initial investment is not high, and although state licensure is becoming widespread, the industry still suffers fools and scoundrels. On balance, a high order of professionalism together with trade association sanctions have wrought beneficial changes to a business long plagued with a fringe of quick-buck operators whose theory was that heavy applicant flow through their offices, quick interviews, and referrals to employers meant that someone was bound to get hired and a fee thus earned. In dealing with search firms and employment agencies, it is well to use the same set of precautions one might employ in picking an advertising agency, a stockbroker, or an attorney. What are the obligations of each party? How long has the firm been in business? Can the owners give you the names of client firms they now serve? Are the people you will be dealing with sensitive to the needs of the health field as well as the specialized jobs for which they will be asked to recruit? Do you and your people understand that by using an outside source for recruiting purposes you cannot abdicate your responsibility to critically examine the credentials and representations of all job candidates however referred?

Health care institutions have available the facilities of the state employment service in their area as well as the services of social, religious, and welfare agencies—all eager to place their clients. Minority-sponsored employment offices have sprung up in recent years. They offer an entry into a potentially valuable market. Some hospitals have offered the services of their own interviewing staffs to help such agencies become established and stay afloat.

State employment services make no charge to employer or applicant. They have testing facilities, are connected by computer with other state job banks throughout the country, and until very recently were sufficiently financed through taxes to do a most satisfactory job. As is true with other agencies, however, results are highly variable. Because of their size, it is frequently difficult to establish a one-to-one relationship with a state employment service interviewer and thus have someone who fully understands your needs.

Hospitals have occasionally found it quite valuable to hold an open house complete with tours, speeches, and refreshments for outside placement agencies of all kinds. Guests have an opportunity to develop a better notion of the hospital's present and future needs. They can also suggest measures you might take to help them serve you better. Their candid criticism can prove highly valuable. Listen to them because they are constantly comparing you with other employers.

2-8 The Front Door. Walk-ins provide a most important pool of applicants, and many hospitals rely heavily upon this source despite the fact that the majority of inquirers cannot be employed on the day they appear. However, these men and women deserve the same courtesies accorded those who called for appointments. They should be preinterviewed by a receptionist and unless clearly unsuitable for any position, be asked to complete an application. If an interviewer is not available, a subsequent appointment should be arranged. Meanwhile, the visit should be logged in and some inquiry made as to how they heard of you. This latter information can provide a useful clue regarding your institution's image in the community. A good storage and retrieval system is essential in making certain that this valuable human resource is not overlooked when positions become available. Be aware, however, that placing reliance on walk-ins may have a discriminatory effect if it has the tendency to perpetuate an existing segregated make-up within the hospital.

2-9 Employee Referrals. When your employees go to some effort to recommend their relatives and friends, they are paying your institution a compliment it cannot ignore. While it is a good practice to acknowledge all new applications by letter, one of the most appreciated added touches is a personal note of thanks to any employee who refers a friend or relative. A telephone call is even better, for it permits the interviewer to ask questions about the candidate. Institutions need not feel compelled to hire those recommended by employees. In fact, if a supervisory relationship between friends is likely to occur, this is a situation more easily avoided prior to employment than after.

Sensing the value of employee referrals, some hospitals have offered cash bonuses (*e.g.*, $25, $50, or $100) when the person hired as a result of this type of recommendation stays on the job a specified number of months. Before adopting such a system, consider the possible negative effect on employee relations of appearing to offer bounties as inducement to work within your walls. If you believe that employment should remain a privilege not lightly conferred, avoid payments for this purpose. Moreover, be aware that a health care employer who relies on word of mouth or nepotistic hiring may well be violating antidiscrimination laws if the effect of this practice limits the number of minority applicants or employees.

2-10 Promotions and Transfers. People are often the most visible yet overlooked resource within any health care organization. The heavy initial costs of recruiting, orienting, and training have already been borne, some degree of loyalty and stability has been demonstrated, and work appraisal, however informal, has at least begun. In short, you know much more about the present employee and his potential than you will ever learn from a telephone call to his last employer. Furthermore, bringing in an outsider at the same or higher pay level than that paid to an existing employee who is performing what he believes to be work of equal value, can do violence to all of your progressive employee relations. The overlooked worker would do you a favor if he complained. More often he remains silent and vents his frustrations upon patients, supervisors, new employees, and the institution itself.

Opportunity for internal promotion and transfer should be an established and functioning privilege. It is normally the personnel department's responsibility to exercise leadership in articulating the policy and making it work. Managers will not ordinarily oppose interdepartmental transfers and promotions—so long as they themselves do not feel injured in the process. But there is a pervasive natural instinct to use such a policy to "unload bad apples" (without the pain of discharge) while keeping good ones. Earnest support must begin at the top and filter down through the organization. It never works from the bottom up.

Specific ideas will be discussed later in this manual. But, in general, the ingredients of a sound transfer/promotion program include the following:

1. An up-to-date skills inventory of your present workforce.
2. A fair, easily understood policy along with forms and procedures to make it work.
3. A tuition assistance program together with on-site opportunities for skill improvement.
4. A personnel staff who can counsel employees who were considered for better things but found unqualified.
5. Good statistics on the number and kinds of people who were transferred or promoted during each quarter of the year.

2-11 Other Sources. The recruiting of new employees ought to be a cooperative effort on many levels. Supervisors and department heads are among those who are best informed and have the broadest outside contacts. Solicit their advice and support in your recruiting efforts. Instead of viewing them as rivals in a race to fill technical positions in their own departments, actively seek their help in establishing new sources of already trained people. In the long run you will be well down the road toward another goal—that of firmly establishing the personnel department as the one gate of entry for new employees.

Many recruiting officers have found their contacts with peers in other hospitals a useful way of making and obtaining cross-referrals. Profitable though this may be, it can also backfire if you allow the referral of unsuitable applicants to a neighboring institution just to get rid of them. In short, do not recommend anyone to another institution whom you deem unemployable in your own.

College recruiting trips, attendance at job fairs, symposiums, and open house functions are windows into markets of professionals, young people, and minority groups. They are often overlooked by traditional recruiting techniques. Be prepared to discuss your institution and its goals intelligently; know your future manpower needs in some detail; bring application forms and any available literature promoting your employment opportunities; and finally, do not overlook the potential of gentle gimmicks such as "smile" buttons, Chinese fortune cookies containing short messages about your hospital, and the like.

News releases and feature stories about your institution, its plans, and people are a way of establishing a public understanding of who you are, where you are headed, and the kinds of numbers of people you will need in the future. Personnel and public relations directors have found repeatedly that, while their functions may overlap, each has much to gain from a close working relationship.

As pointed out earlier, the only real limit on recruiting ideas is the imagination of the personnel director and his staff. And the only major sin, aside from incompetence and bad taste, is unwillingness to try a new approach when old ones no longer produce the desired results. Remember also that successful recruitment and retention can only take place where there are well-cultivated employee and community relations.

2-12 Tools of Recruitment

Personnel management has over the years developed a number of useful devices to aid in the hiring process. These include a broad assortment of forms, brochures, tests, and reference checking techniques. All offer some degree of utility; none can replace the perceptiveness of a skilled interviewer.

2-13 Forms

As a means of saving time in the reception and interviewing rooms, some hospitals use a "preemployment" form. It may be half of an 8½" x 11" sheet in size and may contain the most basic information, such as type of position(s) desired, years of experience in the field, highest school grade level attained or degree received, name of most recent employer, source of referral (ad, friend, walk-in, etc.), earliest date of availability for work, and finally, name, address, and telephone number. This form can be completed by either the applicant or the receptionist. The preemployment form is designed to elicit the most useful information in the shortest time. Care must be taken to avoid appearing perfunctory, even on a busy day with a full reception room and all of the telephones ringing. However, if one vacancy exists and twenty people have already applied who seem qualified, new candidates might find it to their advantage to look elsewhere. Any who wish to stay and complete formal applications, or perhaps take them for completion and return them later, should be permitted to do so. If this prescreening process is handled with grace and sincerity, applicants will be grateful to you for not wasting their job-hunting time with one more application and interview proffered in the name of courtesy.

Formal applications are as numerous and diverse in content as each personnel director's notions and legal strictures can make them. All are intended to elicit objective information in a manner which can be quickly read and evaluated. The application form is designed for the employer's convenience. The resumé is the job candidate's mechanism to expand on accomplishments, shift the reader's attention from one set of facts to another, and otherwise solicit more job offers. Both forms are useful preliminaries to the offer and acceptance of employment. Returning to the application, we will make a few sparing recommendations, issue several caveats, and suggest that you examine the selection of samples found in Chapter 16 of this Manual.

Often personnel directors will continually change their employment applications in order to produce the perfect form. But, most expect the applications to carry a greater burden than two sides of an 8½" x 11" sheet of paper can adequately bear. More useful are two or even three separate forms: one aimed at service, trade, non-professional nursing and clerical applicants; another for technical and professional nursing candidates wherein registration numbers may be needed; and finally, one for professional applicants from whom titles of publications, teaching activities, and examples of managerial accomplishment may be important. No single piece of paper will address itself adequately to all three categories, so compromises are inevitable.

However you choose to design your forms, what is not asked can be almost as important as what is asked. For example, the names and addresses of elementary schools can safely be omitted, as can "separated" and "engaged" under marital status. Names and ages of children take space better used elsewhere. But be aware of the federal and state laws and regulations regarding questions dealing with the candidate's age, race, national origin, sex, maiden name, criminal record and the like. The EEOC has taken the position that preemployment inquiries regarding race, color, religion or national origin are not per se violations of the law, but are generally irrelevant in determining a job applicant's ability or qualifications. Indeed, such inquiries—unless related to a bona fide occupational qualification (see Chapter 9)—and other inquiries which tend to disclose such information, including the requirement of having a photograph accompany applications, may constitute evidence of discrimination. However, preemployment inquiries made pursuant to the requirements of local, state or federal law or regulations will not be considered evidence of discrimination. Employment inquiries necessary for reporting purposes or equal opportunity evaluations are not il-legal if the material thus gathered is maintained separately from an employee's personnel file.

Employment applications should request only the information you really must have to make an intelligent employment judgment. Questions should be specific, and adequate space should be allowed for answers to each one. The experience and opinions of those who interview regularly can prove highly valuable in sifting through the maze of possible inquiries. Your interviewing staff should therefore play an important hand in question selection and location of the form. The same people will have definite views on the amount of open space to provide for their comments and record of referrals to department heads. Finally, competent legal counsel should be consulted to assure conformity with current legislation protecting applicants' rights against unlawful inquiry.

Other useful forms for which samples have been provided in Chapter 16, Volume II include those dealing with job requisitions, reference checks, terminations, terminal interviews, and applicant logs. Useful as the job requisition is, interviewers should be trained to critically scrutinize each one as it comes to their attention. Is the position a new one? Who authorized its creation? If it is a replacement, who is leaving and when? Has an appointment been made by personnel for a terminal interview and return of hospital property? Has the job changed sufficiently to require a new job description? Would a phone call or visit to the department give better information on the type of person needed?

The other forms, revised for your own needs, can aid the recruitment process and make the hire-no hire judgment easier.

2-14 Literature

Not to be forgotten is that the decision to hire also involves a decision to be hired. The health field is especially vulnerable to seasonal changes in the supply of trained people. The need for manpower is relatively constant throughout the year. However, secretarial and technical schools as well as universities and schools of nursing tend to graduate their students at certain times of the year. Large numbers of medical secretaries, for example, graduate in June. Many are discouraged by the few jobs available and by their numerous competitors, yet these same secretaries may have been eager for employment had they finished their training in January when jobs may have been open. Variations of this tale are repeated to different degrees by nurses, laboratory and radiologic technologists, respiratory therapists, clinical chemists, social workers, and others.

Added to the above situation, a job market peopled by many different but related skills and salary and benefit levels that change rapidly can cause you to be competitive one week and behind in your personnel needs the next. Therefore, you must do some merchandising to be assured of a steady flow of suitable applicants to meet present and future needs. Colorful brochures describing your institution, the services it offers and the kinds of people it seeks as employees as well as employee handbooks and summaries of major benefits can enhance the prospective employee's understanding of your institution and what it might offer him. Even well-written tastefully designed pieces may evoke questions which ought to be answered before rather than after hiring (*e.g.,* pay ranges, merit increases, vacation and sick leave allotments, smoking rules). Literature of this nature involves a considerable initial investment for art work, layout, writing of copy, and printing. Be sure it meets at least the following tests before going to the printer:

—Will the information, style of presentation, illustrations, and phrases look as fresh and timely two years from now as they do today?

—Can the piece function equally as a personnel department handout, envelope stuffer when answering employment inquiries, and attention grabber at professional meetings, job fairs, recruiting trips to schools, and even on the coffee table in your own main lobby? Also, be sure that, if you include photographs of employees, minority employees are pictured as well.

2-15 Tests

To the extent that they can predict job success with reasonable accuracy and fairness, tests are a useful recruitment tool. They were hailed in personnel circles not many years ago as the wave of the future. More recently, tests have elicited much concern. Tests used as allies and not in substitution of good judgment, can sometimes offer a rational basis for evaluation when selecting new employees and promoting existing ones. They have not always succeeded in this measure. But this is less a condemnation of tests than of our failure to recognize their limitations. They may not be used to discriminate against some classes and races of people even though they were intended only to remove human error from the selection process.

On the other hand, while it is true that the courts and regulatory agencies have approved of an employer affirmatively working to increase the number of minority employees by hiring minorities with lower test scores than non-minorities, this approval has always been conditioned on the employer tying its testing practices to a *bona fide* affirmative action plan. Thus, by not giving these tests to minority applicants, the employer remains vulnerable to a successful charge of racial discrimination inasmuch as its reluctance to administer a "biased" test has not been directly coupled with an affirmative attempt to recruit and hire more minorities. The watchword in testing is "caution."[6]

The design and use of tests involves a number of distinct steps. These can be summarized as follows:

1. *Purpose to be served.* For which jobs or skills can tests prove most valuable? Should they be used where national or state board examinations are required or where professional societies conduct their own accrediting exams? The answer is probably no. This does not mean that retesting should never take place. But personnel departments are not likely to have the capability for periodic retesting however much it may be needed. Testing should largely be confined to clerical aptitude, mechanical skills, and the abilities to weigh, measure and count if these are clearly related to the job which must be done. There should be a compelling reason for testing and the hoped for benefit ought to be well defined in advance.

2. *Identification of skills and job elements to be tested.* Here the questions that should be asked are: what constitutes an appropriate skill level in each job or job element to be tested? (*e.g.,* typing at 60 w.p.m. in the psychiatry department, where good spelling is also necessary, versus 40 w.p.m. but numerical accuracy in the accounting department). In short, which skills, knowledge, and aptitudes are critical to the successful performance of the job? Further, is it possible to examine and test for potential as well as existing skills?

3. *Selection of norms against which test results may be measured.* Here it is important that criteria be reviewed and changed just as the job to be done is changed by external forces. A prosaic example: tests may still be given on a manual typewriter long after the institution has converted to electric. Another example: are the skills for which the applicant is being tested (*e.g.,* arithmetic, filing, sorting, measuring) still a bona fide occupational qualification (BFOQ) for the job?

4. *Validation.* The issue of validation is a complex one. Some of the problems involved have already been discussed in Chapter 9, the relevant portion of which should be reread in conjunction with this section.

Some final suggestions regarding tests follow:

- Because the design, installation, and validation of tests are complex, federally regulated and time consuming, outside help should be sought in starting such a program.
- Final employee selection should not hinge upon the results of any series of tests, much less upon any single test within a series. Tests, when used at all, should be viewed as only part of the total selection process. They can be highly valuable tools but are far from infallible predictors of work performance. It is important that no test can purport to be a valid measure of human motivation or enthusiasm for training.
- The work environment cannot be ignored in validating test results. Ineffective supervision, poor physical conditions, low wages, and benefits—all are reflected in absenteeism, illness, and poor productivity, and are totally unrelated to how well an individual might have scored on a carefully controlled test. The classic example is the typist who tested at 80 words per minute but comes to work late and takes long lunch hours. The test may have been valid, but it failed to measure the employee against the work environment.
- The risks of injury to patients, damage to equipment, cost of training and lost time should be considered before deciding whether tests become part of the selection process. It may be that the number of people hired in any one year is so small and the consequences of failure on the job so insignificant as to make testing uneconomical.
- Be certain that tests are not used to exclude those who are untrained but who may, once trained, be capable of high productivity. Rigid cut-off points should be avoided.
- Racial, sexual, and cultural bias can easily destroy or seriously damage an otherwise sound testing program. Discriminatory hiring practices are against federal law and the advancing tide of state legislation.
- Do not overlook the valuable source of manpower in your own institution. As part of an ongoing internal promotion and transfer policy, existing employees should be made fully aware of job vacancies (bulletin boards, newsletters, etc.) and given an opportunity to take the same tests as offered to new candidates for employment.

2-16 References

When factual and reasonably free from personal whim, references can prove highly useful in predicting success on the job. But when they mislead, no matter how honestly given, they can prove costly to the employer who places undue faith in them in arriving at a hire-no hire decision.

References are normally received two ways: by telephone and by letter. Each has value and limitations which will be discussed. In descending order of reliability, customary reference sources are as follows:

1. Former employers
2. Professional or business associates
3. Personal friends and acquaintances
4. Clergymen and public officials

The two major kinds of information to be expected from former employers are those relating to facts (e.g., typing speed, length of employment, number of days absent) and those dealing with the employee's personality (loyality, competency, lazy, friendly, unkempt, and the like).

A key fact—almost an article of faith—is that a reference is a statement by a fallible person about another fallible person to a third fallible person. It is subject to all the incalculable emotions and prejudices lying within the human breast. Worse, it can vary with the passage of time, the intended recipient, and whether conveyed by the spoken or written word.

People cannot work together for one, five, ten years without developing highly subjective opinions about each other. It would be folly to dismiss the importance of such views when checking references. The risk, of course, is that the inquirer may rely unduly on feelings when he should also be sorting out and weighing questions of fact. Some additional cautions: most employers want their remarks held in strict confidence—especially even if mildly uncomplimentary statements are to be expressed. Since the receiver of such information is inclined to accept confidentiality as a price for getting the reference at all, the job candidate is never given a chance to find out what is being said about him, much less dispute it or offer comment. Reference checking thus becomes cocooned in enforced secrecy. This can hurt the job applicant and deceive the employer who depends upon information not easily verified by open inquiry.

Unless time is a compelling factor, written references tend to be preferred. Derogatory statements will ordinarily not be consigned to paper unless valid, and employers tend to weigh feelings more equitably and with less emotion in a letter. Naturally your chance to ask additional questions is limited, but this may be a reasonable price. Moreover, a subsequent telephone call seeking clarification is still possible. Beware of "To Whom It May Concern" letters. They are always complimentary if carried by job applicants.

Form letters are widely used in soliciting references. They are commonly ignored or elicit a noncommital response. If they must be used at all, have them at least personally signed by the personnel director or employment manager to indicate their importance. The form or checklist type of request has some value. It makes response easier by asking directed questions. It also can be answered by a clerk from a termination notice that may have been completed months before when the supervisor's memory was fresher. Courtesy as well as speed dictate enclosing a stamped, self-addressed reply envelope marked for the attention of a specific individual in the personnel department.

Whether received by letter, phone or other contact, the reference source is just as important as the judgment given. A department head who has just fired the fourth person in a year from the same job and who gives a poor recommendation should not be completely believed. It may be difficult for one to work for him. Perhaps his selection or training methods are inadequate. Or perhaps he has just had a run of bad luck. Whatever the reason, high turnover and poor references often go hand-in-hand. Unusually good references may have a deadening effect on the hearer's senses. They too bear further inquiry. The most reliable reference is usually one received from an employer whom you have known and dealt with on other matters for some time. He knows whether you can be trusted with sensitive information, and he is able to balance off the good and bad comments somewhat more fairly. He may also give you useful clues regarding working conditions and supervisory competence in his own institution.

Length of service and how recently employed are important factors in evaluating references. The applicant who just left a position after five years should have that reference judged more heavily than from a job lasting for three months.

The candidate himself may have given you insights as to the relative value of his references. If he asks you to check some employers but not others, if he tells you a certain supervisor (or all supervisors) did not like him, or if his visible work history shows a succession of short term positions, caution is in order. Similarly, a series of steadily more responsible positions rising to a crest and then diminishing could suggest caution in hiring him for particularly demanding work. A few well-directed questions of the applicant during his interview will help in assessing which reference sources deserve primary attention.

Professional or business associates may be valuable sources of additional help. Their opinions ought to be solicited and weighed against those of former employers. The same is true of personal friends and acquaintances. Because the element of subjective feeling—usually favorable but not always—enters the picture, opinions of friends and acquaintances are not ordinarily given the importance of work references. Probably least valuable are clergymen and public officials whose names constantly appear on application forms. They frequently know little about the candidate and are inclined to given statements of support to a parishioner or constituent seeking work.

References, standing alone, should never be taken as *prima facie* evidence of virtue, fault, skill, or ineptness. Yet they have a way of fleshing out and coinciding with information and impressions given during an interview. It is important to use them with great care and, wherever possible, rely primarily on factual information which can be verified from other sources. If references are to be relayed to someone else within your institution, it ought to be on a need-to-know basis only. Under no circumstances should references or their source be a topic of idle conversation.

2-17 Terminal Interviews

To find out whether your employee relations goals are being achieved ask those who are leaving. At few other times can you expect more candor in such matters as training, supervision, working conditions, pay, cafeteria meals, and the like. Aside from the opportunity it offers to take the institution's "temperature," a terminal interview can reveal information about the employee-work environment which may help in selecting his replacement. Perhaps he should never have been hired in the first place; possibly he was right, but the job was wrong. Even though the match may have been nearly perfect, he can still provide you with insights that should help you select the next incumbent with greater precision.

The terminal interview should take place on neutral territory—preferably in the personnel department and with the officer who originally placed the employee in his job. It should be emphasized that after months or years of evaluation by his superiors, you are now asking the employee for his frank, confidential appraisal of your institution. He should do most of the talking, you the listening. Start off with a clean desk free from questionnaires or forms. Initial questions ought to steer away from his known reasons for leaving. Personalities should be avoided until the employee feels he can confide in you. But also remember when it is time to discuss individuals and possible conflicts, your role is that of fact finder and not inquisitor or sympathizer. Among the insights to be gained from a careful terminal interview are: over-or-under education for the job, vocational expectations that may not have been realized, subtle personality clashes, pay or benefit levels below those prevailing in the marketplace, or possibly a dozen other aspects of the employee's relationship with your institution that might have been detected during the initial interview had you been more alert. The terminal interview should conclude with a further assurance that the employee's remarks will be held in confidence and indeed they must be. However, some record should be kept of this discussion. A sample form may be found in Volume II, Chapter 16.

Used discreetly, interviews with departing employees will enable you to capture your institution's strengths and weaknesses. While still protecting the confidence individual employees have placed in the personnel department, remedial action should be taken promptly to correct clear patterns of poor supervision, noncompetitive pay or benefits, or evidence of unacceptable working conditions. The terminating employee can, if listened to carefully, provide numerous early warning signals to those areas where your employee relations stance needs shoring up. But more immediately, he should be able to help you zero in on the kind of person who should replace him.

2-18 The Recruitment Interview

We have now set a stage for the most difficult aspect of recruitment—the job interview. Difficult because it attempts to divine and measure a future none of us can foretell, leaning upon evaluation techniques still not fully understood. Crucial because the level and quality of patient care, research and teaching may well hinge upon judgments growing out of the recruitment interview.

Why interview at all? Convincing studies have shown that decisions based on interviews alone are no better than would be expected by chance. Equally believable statistics draw a positive correlation between interview data and subsequent job success. It can at least be said that the personnel director is in good company. For all its advance billing, computer diagnosis of disease is incomplete without sound clinical judgment.

The selection task is complicated by a number of factors the personnel administrator may not care to acknowledge to his laboratory, engineering, or accounting-based associates: people behave unpredictably; department heads seem to hire the "wrong" people and reject the "right" ones; there is never a time or place to interview free from distractions; agencies of government hamper the selection process with an increasingly heavy hand; the most critical jobs must be filled immediately; job specifications never seem to

be up-to-date; the one best candidate has two other offers at more money; and finally, the employment interviewer, having allowed himself to be set up as the resident expert on people, is given precious little margin for error.

But there are some steps the personnel director can take to define his risks—or at least cut his losses. Briefly stated, he must select his employment staff with great care, train them thoroughly and continuously, monitor their results, and support them fully.

2-19 Selection of Interviewers

There is no set of skills fitting all circumstances or tastes. Those qualities of their recruiters most often mentioned by senior personnel administrators in a number of major medical centers include the following.

1. Degree: at least a bachelor's degree; probably, but not necessarily, in liberal arts or the behavioral sciences. Scientific, health-related fields (*e.g.*, nursing), or economics are also considered acceptable.
2. Age: at least 25 and preferably older.
3. Experience: two or more years working closely with people, although not necessarily in personnel. Sales, social work, nursing, training, publishing, advertising are just a few fields to consider.
4. Intelligence: demonstrated ability to think quickly, verbalize with fluency, write clearly, sort priorities and know which problem to tackle first, retain and evaluate facts with relative ease, and follow through with sometimes endless details.
5. Emotional qualities: high degree of personal warmth, sincere desire to serve both institutional objectives and needs of job applicants, keen interest in each candidate without emotional involvement, understanding and awareness that gossip and idle chatter concerning candidates, employees or supervisors have no place in personnel, and ability to accept disappointment graciously.
6. Stamina: good health and energy to work longer than usual hours, a high level of motivation, and the wish to succeed.
7. Special qualities: Some of the best interviewers lack degrees or the kind of prior experience detailed above. Certain attributes college degrees and experience are supposed to confer do not always. Look for intellectual curiosity, a broad range of interests, sufficient self-confidence to converse and work with the physician and dish-

washer equally well, personal integrity with a sense of right and wrong (even though it may differ from yours), a working vocabulary in which the words "please" and "thank you" come easily, and a gentle sense of humor that does not harm others.

2-20 Training Interviewers

Just as throwing a person into the water to teach him how to swim is not a good method, neither is "throwing" a new interviewer into his work a good idea. The consequences of error in judgment can have lasting effects on the interviewer himself, the applicant, the personnel department, and the institution. A good individualized training program should be developed for each new employment officer before the day he begins interviewing. The key word is "individualized." Rather than detail a training program, we will list some of its key elements and suggest that it be adapted, twisted, speeded, or prolonged as required.

First Week

1. The new employee should attend an institution-wide orientation.
2. There should be a one-half to full day personal tour of major departments with introductions to department heads, but no long visits.
3. Arrange for private conversations of 15-60 minutes with key personnel department members—including heads of salary administration, benefits, records, etc.
4. Orient the new employee to personnel department procedures (recruiting, hiring, signing onto payroll, testing, etc.) including required backup forms. Allow ample time for questions. Encourage your new employee to challenge procedures. He will never be more objective than during these early weeks of employment, and may innocently force you to improve.
5. The personnel director should set aside one or two 30-60 minute uninterrupted periods for further questions and to critique the progress of his new employee.
6. Outside reading:
   a. Selected chapters of *The Lives of a Cell—Notes of a Biology Watcher,* by Lewis Thomas (1974). This book is a series of essays originally published in the *New England Journal of Medicine.*
   b. Your institution's personnel manual, description of benefits, work rules, recruitment flyers, brochures given to patients, recent is-

sues of the house newsletter, public relations department releases, etc. should be read.
   c. Select readings from Chapters 16, 17, and 19 of the *Health Care Labor Manual,* with current supplements.
   d. Select articles from *Hospitals (JAHA).*

Second Week

1. Early in the second week, for not more than 2 hours, the new employee should review his first week with his employment supervisor or personnel director. Also discuss the description of the program for the second week, including information on the major departments and how they function (*e.g.,* nursing, housekeeping, clinical laboratories—all sections including special procedures), radiology (diagnostic and radio therapy), dietetics, medical records, emergency services, and clinics. Introduce special terms used by the above departments. Avoid ponderous details to conserve time and reduce confusion. Make ample use of literature or booklets generated by these departments (*e.g.,* lab handbooks, instructions to new house officers, "special diet" manual).
2. The new employee should now extend his visits to key members of the departments. Encourage department heads to discuss the kind of people they hire as well as the skills needed. Have the new employee prepare for these visits by reading pertinent job descriptions.
3. Encourage or arrange luncheon dates with staff members of departments to develop more personal working relationships.
4. He should observe selected interviews with applicants' permission. If possible, interviews should be for positions in those departments where visits have taken place. The interviewer should review each discussion immediately afterward and invite questions.
5. There should be further discussion with the personnel director allowing ample time for questions. The new employee should also be given an introduction to labor relations.
6. Outside reading:
   a. Continue with same list as outlined in first week.
   b. Select readings from *The Personnel Journal* and reprints from *The Harvard Business Review.*
   c. Introduce the Prentice Hall Series, Bureau of National Affairs publications, etc.

d. Select chapters of the *Health Care Labor Manual*—especially the section on "Interviewing Techniques" in Chapter 16, followed by Chapters 1, 2, and 3 on Labor Relations.

Third Week

1. Review first and second weeks.
2. Your employee should attend as a guest at selected management meetings, job evaluation meetings, etc.
3. Have the employee visit additional departments and meet with key managers and supervisors and visit research laboratories, the morgue (why not?), and the power plant. His escort should be encouraged to stop, make introductions, and chat briefly with employees at all levels.
4. Introduce senior administrators and medical staff members on a time available basis.
5. He should observe additional interviews followed by critiques. Let him conduct selected interviews for departments already visited. The experienced interviewer should observe, answer questions, if asked, and review techniques after the applicant has left. The section entitled "Interviewing Techniques"[7] in this manual should be reviewed in light of actual problems arising during discussion with applicant. The new interviewer should evaluate the applicant and be asked to explain his evaluation in detail.
6. Outside reading:
   a. All foregoing materials cited for weeks one and two.
   b. Review and select the remaining texts and periodicals in the personnel department and, if it exists, present the administration section of the hospital library.
   c. Review key reference sources (*e.g.*, physicians' desk book, directory of medical specialists—with particular reference to the role of each specialty). (Guide issue of *Hospitals*, directory of hospital administrators.)
   d. *Health Care Labor Manual*, Chapters 4, 5, 6, 12, and 13.
   e. *Wage and Salary Administration In A Dynamic Economy*, by Leonard R. Burgess, *Health Care Labor Manual*, Chapters 16 and 17.

Fourth Week

1. Hold a review and discussion with the employment supervisor and personnel director and an informal but detailed oral examination of reading materials, experiences during preceding three weeks, terminology, personnel policies, labor relations, functions of major departments and their relationship to patient care and each other.
2. Observe additional interviews (administrative, professional, technical) is suggested.
3. He should conduct selected interviews under guidance. The interviews should be without observation, but critiqued immediately after.
4. When ready, possibly late in the week, begin full interviewing and placement schedule.
5. Visits to smaller departments by appointment.
6. Outside reading:
   a. *Health Care Labor Manual*, Chapters 7, 8, 9, 10, 14, and 15.
   b. Other texts, articles and periodicals as assigned by the personnel director.

Training is a process, not an event. The personnel director has a clear and ongoing responsibility to encourage his entire staff to keep abreast of developments in health care. This includes patterns of delivery of health services; new positions, their titles and requirements; changes in terminology; new equipment and services the institution is or will be using; changed financial circumstances; new personnel policies; labor relations developments; etc. In addition to departmental meetings and the routing of appropriate publications to various personnel employees, a formal and continuous reading program should be expected, attendance at outside conferences and symposiums encouraged and special meetings arranged to discuss interviewing techniques, salary administration problems, new ideas, and so on. Were it possible to hold such meetings off premises and over dinner, so much the better.

2-21 Monitoring Results

To varying degrees, most busy executives are inclined to plan with some care and then select trusted subordinates to carry out the plan, safe in the knowledge that all is well. Often all is not. And nowhere is this more true than in the development of a competent recruiting staff. The cardinal question is, "Did I actually achieve the goal I envisioned?" In collaboration with his employment manager or senior interviewer, the personnel director should regularly review all recruitment activities. Key elements must include:

1. Advertising: does it say what you want it to? Is it timely? Does it produce the response you need in

relation to cost? Are the media used still drawing the applicants you need?

2. Are recruiting handouts and other materials current? Do they still sound bright and fresh?

3. Is your receptionist sensitive to the institution's recruiting objectives? Do all recruitment staff members know your posture regarding equal opportunity and affirmative action?

4. Are interviewers projecting the kind of image you want—neat appearance, clean offices, avoidance of personal telephone calls, friendly helpful manner to all, positive approach to problem solving?

5. Do interviewers use good judgment? Do they exercise care and not recommend applicants who are not qualified? Do they call just to make appointments for candidates to see department heads or do they follow up and facilitate decision making? Do they check references carefully?

6. Do department heads trust your interviewers and have an understanding of their problems?

7. Is your employment staff considered both competent and discreet?

None of the above questions should have an easy answer. The skilled personnel administrator should have a regular program of reviewing his plans and sampling the opinions of employees and medical staff members. He should make it clear to the entire institution that he expects the members of his own department to set an example of personal behavior, competence and motivation all others could well emulate.

2-22 *Supporting the Recruitment Effort*

Because their work involves difficult judgments, the results important and the pressures intense, interviewers are sometimes subjected to more personal criticism than other employees. Of course, if you have established an ongoing system of monitoring their efforts and are convinced that you have not chosen wisely or trained well, nothing is gained by permitting unsuitable interviewers to impair the entire recruitment program. A transfer or separation should be decided upon and carried out quickly. In most cases such drastic measures are not necessary. What *is* necessary is a conscious strategy of support. Test the following questions against your present efforts to provide the back-up your interviewers need.

1. Are interviewing rooms or offices neat, pleasant, reasonably modern, and well furnished?

2. Do you demand high professional standards of all personnel employees? Are they proud to work for you? Do they regard you as competent and

fair in your dealings with them and others throughout the institution?

3. Have you provided the forms, procedures, policies, brochures, etc. that they need to do a thorough job?

4. Do you come to their defense when they are unfairly criticized outside of the department?

5. Do you avoid taking sides in petty intraoffice squabbles? Do you praise in public and criticize in private?

6. Do you let it be known throughout the institution that you are proud of your people and the way they function?

7. Do you ask for their counsel and give them credit when their ideas are adopted?

The recruitment interview is ultimately the responsibility of the senior personnel administrator, who must:

1. Carefully select the interviewing staff.

2. Effect a program of thorough and continuous training.[8]

3. Monitor results.

4. Consciously and firmly support the entire recruitment effort.

3 ORIENTING THE NEW EMPLOYEE

A new employee will always become oriented to his job, but the quality and timeliness of this orientation is the real challenge. The new employee should be accurately informed about the hospital's policies and the programs that affect him and his individual status there. He should be properly introduced to his duties and to the assignments of others. Finally, the hospital should insure a good first impression. It must show its concern with the quality of services provided and indicate that the hospital will be demanding of him, yet at the same time be demanding *for* him in such matters as salaries, benefits, and fair treatment and will encourage him to grow in his work.

These first impressions will very likely persist. They may affect an employee's success or support of the hospital. A sound orientation is the institution's best opportunity to insure a positive employee relations climate while developing productive and knowledgeable workers.

Although this section is directed toward the ideal program for new employees in a large hospital setting, certainly the smaller health care institution should find material which can be adapted successfully to its own needs and abilities to provide a positive orientation experience for its newly hired employees.

3-1 The First Orientation

Orientation is of great importance once a person has been hired, yet it begins while he is still a candidate for employment. As a candidate, he should receive the courtesies of a visitor. A member of the personnel department should coordinate appointments and make certain that the applicant is escorted and properly introduced to his interviewers. The personnel officer should insure that the candidate has a clear understanding of what the job is and is not, together with information on supervisory relationships, promotional opportunities, and salary potential. This is important so as to avoid an employee being surprised at the conditions of the job. Such misunderstandings can seriously impair a working relationship and injure an otherwise well-conceived employee relations program.

When a job offer has been made and accepted, the new employee should be referred back to the personnel department to review and confirm conditions of employment. These include the agreed starting salary and salary review dates, major benefits for which the employee is eligible, his starting date and time, the location and the person to whom he should report, working hours, and workdays. To avoid broken promises, whether real or imagined, that can impair future relationships, all such information should be in writing with copies to the department head and for the employee's file. Finally, employee handbooks and written information on benefits should be given to the new employee at this time. This will allow the new employee to learn about the hospital even before he begins working.

3-2 Orientation to the Department

The second stage of orientation begins on the employee's first day at work and may take one of two directions. The emphasis may be on introducing the new employee to the total hospital or just the department in which he will work and his own job in it.

Introduction to the total hospital on the first day usually takes the form of a hospital-wide orientation meeting for all employees who begin work on that day. This has the practical advantage of allowing complete concentration in his own department afterwards, thus minimizing disruption of work schedules later.

There are, however, significant drawbacks to this approach. Psychologically, people are more successful getting used to smaller groups before being exposed to larger groups. Moreover, it is difficult to convey all of the information necessary to acquaint an employee with the total hospital on that first, often confusing day at work. There is indeed an early saturation point for the employee, brought on, in part, by apprehension and preoccupation with the normal traumas of a new position. Smaller institutions have often found weekly orientation programs impractical, and therefore wait until five or ten new employees begin work.

Because of these problems, the material which follows is organized on a departmental basis first, to be followed by a hospital-wide orientation within two weeks of the employee's starting date.

The orientation to the department varies with the specific nature of the work environment but usually includes an introduction to five general areas:

1. the *role and function* of the department;
2. its *organization*, including various supervisors; fellow employees and a brief look at their functions;
3. *departmental policies*, rules and procedures;
4. the *various facilities* in and around the department;
5. and to the *general job functions* the new employee will be performing.

Much of this information is important detail. It is, however, sometimes neglected since it is well understood and taken for granted by other employees. To properly introduce the new employee to this often bewildering information, the department head should meet with him immediately upon arrival. A supervisor or senior employee should be responsible for completing the orientation and should be available to answer questions.

The new employee should be introduced to fellow employees and their functions and should be informed of such things as hours of work, workdays, meal and rest breaks, time-clock and payroll procedures, calling-in requirements when absent, accident reporting procedures, and other department rules. It is imperative that each new piece of information support rather than contradict what the employee may have already been told during the hiring process.

He should also be made familiar with the location of various facilities. The employee will be more effective when he has learned where he must go for personal or job needs.

Once the employee has an overview of the department and his role in it as well as some initial impression of the various personalities, policies, and facilities, he will be better able to focus on his job and become a more productive and efficient member of the department.

3-3 Orientation to the Hospital

Institution-wide orientation takes on increasing importance with the recognition that hospitals appear to be such complicated organizations. Their size and complexity tend to generate insecurity on the part of some employees, along with misunderstanding about policies, and frustrations in meeting personal goals and needs.

The situation is further complicated by the relatively high turnover in hospitals, and the comparative inexperience of new employees. Specifically, hospital turnover is often thirty to sixty percent annually. Moreover, since approximately fifty percent of the employees are under thirty, it is probable that many will be starting their first full-time job with no real experience in the world of organization. Of the other new workers, a surprising number will be starting a hospital job for the first time. In light of these factors, a thoughtful and well managed hospital-wide orientation is essential for a productive and knowledgeable work force.

The hospital-wide orientation is designed to familiarize a new employee with hospital goals, history and development, organization and facilities, and with the policies, programs and benefits that affect the employee. It should also introduce him to the administrator, to the personnel department staff and to others in leadership positions. Orientation is also designed to reflect the employee relations posture of the hospital. It should set the tone for future relationships with employees as useful and respected members of the health care team.

The design and management of this program will usually be the responsibility of the personnel director, in cooperation with the administrator and senior operating management. They will, in fact, be integrating the hospital-wide program with their own department orientation activities.

A model for this orientation program provides for a 75 to 90 minute meeting followed by a 30 to 40 minute tour of major areas of the hospital, with emphasis on areas an employee may not see in the course of his work.

This orientation should be scheduled on the least busy day of the week. Groups of new employees should be invited within two weeks of their first day of work. Departments should be advised that the release of employees for the full two hours is required. Success of the program will depend on its regularity, on the priority it is given by departments, and, of course, on the quality of the presentation.

The program itself should include the following subjects:

Introduction of the program and participants;

A welcome by the administrator;

A review of hospital roles, objectives, history, and development;

A pictorial tour of the hospital (slide or movie presentation);

A discussion in summary form of:

Hospital-wide policies and procedures (flip chart presentation);

Fire prevention and safety rules (fire extinguisher and alarm procedure demonstration);

Employee relations policies and programs (flip chart presentation);

Employee benefits, services, and activities (slide presentation);

A general question and answer period and review of previous handouts (employee handbook, benefit booklets, etc.)

A tour of major hospital areas.

The tenor of this meeting should be relaxed with an informal seating arrangement and refreshments (at least coffee). It should radiate a concern for each employee and suggest that there are many who wish to help him succeed.

Participants in the meeting should include the administrator (or his assistant if his schedule will allow more regular attendance), the director of personnel, and his specialists who are responsible for salary and benefits administration. The group should be welcomed by the administrator who then discusses the hospital generally, its activities, the services it provides, its place in the community, its growth and development, trends that will have an impact on it, and the employees' roles in achieving the hospital's goals.

The staff of the personnel department should be responsible for the other topics with each member discussing his specialty (*e.g.,* salary administrator on salary administration, payroll, premiums). The personnel director will host the program and be responsible for presentations on policies, rules, and procedures.

The use of several participants is an important factor in the program's success. A variety of voices keeps the group alert and this method also introduces employees to those people they may approach for assistance.

Visual aids and handouts are other ways of stimulating interest in the program. Films, film strips, tapes, and slide presentations have been used effectively to insure consistency in the presentation and to provide a professional program. A less professional but more personal approach can be achieved with artistically designed color slides, overhead transparencies, or flip charts narrated by a person using outline notes. In any event, it is important to keep up with changes in policies and benefits.

The tour of the hospital will be a particularly memorable part of the program for many, particularly for those in nonclinical jobs, who will rarely have another opportunity to see areas such as the radiology department, laboratories, operating rooms and other patient-related facilities. This will be especially effective if a representative from each major area can be introduced and discuss the operation of his department.

Hospital-wide orientation completes an employee's introduction to his new employer. However, if the program has succeeded it will not end at this point. There should be a follow-up contact by the employing personnel officer in the first few weeks of work to reinforce the relationship developed during the hiring process. The new employee's supervisor will also be involved in follow-up in the course of job instruction training.

The new employee, then, has been exposed to a variety of information important to him and has a clearer indication of what will be expected of him. Just as important, he now is familiar with a variety of people who are there to help him succeed. For its part, the hospital has underlined the fact that every employee and every department is vitally important to effective patient care.

4 SALARY ADMINISTRATION IN HEALTH CARE INSTITUTIONS[9]

4-1 Goals and Perspectives

One of the most critical and far-reaching roles for the personnel director is that of salary administrator, manager of the institution's greatest single expenditure, which could comprise sixty to seventy-five percent of its total cost of operation. For the employee, his salary is the heart of his economic well-being, and it has also a major noneconomic impact on his life and status in the community.

To satisfy the needs of both the hospital and the employee, today's personnel director must provide expertise to achieve three objectives of salary administration:

1. a *salary system* that insures equity to all employees through the institution.
2. a *salary policy* that provides a basis for determining individual salary levels, irrespective of where the person is employed in the hospital, and
3. *salary ranges and levels* that are affordable yet competitive with those of other employers.

In its present complex form, salary administration is a relatively new function for the hospital and its personnel professionals. To understand why, a perspective on the immediate past is important. In the 1960s there was an entirely different outlook toward salaries in the health field than at present. Hospital employees had been traditionally rather poorly paid, a fact not overlooked by union organizers. Medicare, Medicaid and other dependable third party payors had not made their full impact, and hospital charges historically had been unrealistically low relative to costs.

Pressures to raise salaries had also been minimal. Inflation had a nominal impact upon most families in the 1960s. Federal laws regarding minimum wage and overtime compensation did not apply to hospitals. Collective bargaining as a force was not available to most hospital employees, who were also excluded from the protection of many state and federal laws.

As a result, professional salary administration was minimal or nonexistent, even in the most forward-looking hospitals. Salaries often were not competitive with community norms, nor did they have to be. Internally, there were often extreme inequities between comparable jobs and employees in different departments. Frequently an "un-system" existed for determining the financial worth of an employee, based strictly on a department manager's judgment and unfettered by institution-wide guidelines.

This situation began to change quite rapidly during the 1960s, with many forces emerging to stimulate both salaries and salary demands. Between the early 1960s and the early 1970s, the technological demands upon both hospitals and their employees became increasingly complex. Hospitals began competing with each other and with higher paying industries for scarce nonclinical professionals, and on occasion, those skilled in the life sciences. Shortages of professional nurses and other skilled specialists became acute as demands for increased health care grew. These pressures forced hospitals and similar institutions into an uncomfortable catch-up position regarding both salaries and benefits.

In 1967 minimum wage and overtime payments became necessary when the federal wage-hour law was extended to include hospitals. Finally, new pressures developed with increased inflation, and particularly with the inclusion of employees under the various state and federal collective bargaining laws. On the income side, third party payment of hospital charges increased substantially, providing new sources of funds for competitive salaries.

In a single decade, hospitals confronted changes that were introduced in other industries over a period of thirty-five years. The need for rational salary management programs has become increasingly apparent. Today's salary administrator must deal with an inherited array of *ad hoc* salary systems.

4-2 The Components of Salary Administration

The four major components of salary administration reflect the importance of this subject to the hospital and the magnitude of it as a personnel management responsibility. Basic to these components is a comprehensive salary philosophy which will be the basis for the program as well as for decisions relating to individual salaries.

A draft recommendation of this statement is often developed by the personnel director. Since the success of hospital-wide salary administration depends largely on the department heads, they, too, are asked to contribute comments and suggestions to this draft. It is then reviewed by the administrator and his associates, submitted for approval at the highest organizational level of the hospital, and the final statement is communicated to managers and employees, as well as to the affiliating medical staffs and other interested parties. Though there are many possible variations to such a salary philosophy, "Suggested Statement of Philosophy Regarding Salaries" (see Chapter 17) is an example of current thinking on the subject.

Two major methods of salary administration are of particular interest to health care administrators: the job evaluation approach and the salary approach.

Both include technical aspects and special areas for management's attention. Although the techniques will be introduced below, the emphasis of this section will be on the management problems.

4-3 The Job Evaluation Program

In an effort to create an even-handed, cost effective, yet equitable approach to measuring the financial worth of jobs, an increasing number of hospitals are turning to the mechanism of job evaluation. There are several approaches: ranking, grading, the point system, and factor comparison.

The point system is by far the most common and is used both in hospitals and industry. This is a quantitative approach by which job factors (*e.g.*, education, experience, responsibility, working conditions) are established, numerical point values are assigned to each factor, and all jobs are evaluated based upon the sum of the points. A detailed description and set of specifications is developed for each job. The description is then evaluated in relation to the predetermined job factors, which are assigned the point values. The salary grade is based upon the total point value;[10] thus, salary ranges are systematically determined for each salary grade.

4-4 Developing the Hospital's Job Evaluation Program

Developing a hospital-wide system of pay grades involves some sensitive issues. Past practice often represented the uncoordinated wisdom of many managers, all making decisions on grades and salaries with little or no centralized control. Formal salary administration plans thus represent the first major limitation on management's authority, since the grade will circumscribe the range of salaries that may be paid for a position. Similarly, apprehension may occur among employees who, for the several months of the project development, will be uncertain about their salary levels.

Despite obvious drawbacks, the point evaluation method will introduce an element of participation and credibility to a previously mystical process. Apprehension by employees over "what are they trying to pull on me now?" is to be expected and must be dealt with early, clearly, and openly.

Managers will ordinarily see the advantages of a formal program providing some guidance for difficult salary decisions where inequities within their own and other departments may be resolved by some central authority.

Employees also can be reassured successfully and will be inclined to support the program since they recognize the same inequities, once they are convinced that no employee's salary will be reduced after the program has begun.

Coincident with the decision to undertake hospital-wide job evaluation is the decision of who will be responsible for the program's development. Some hospitals engage a consulting firm to establish such a program. There are many such firms. Many possess excellent technical competence and knowledge of hospital positions and functions. There should, however, be involvement from within the hospital as well. Ideally, the personnel director should provide in-house direction dor the program. Under the guidance of the consultant he should develop and oversee evaluation of job descriptions and establishment of grades and ranges. Initial introduction of the system is the personnel director's responsibility.

The writing of job descriptions is a time-consuming yet important task. A standard format is normally used and information input by managers and employees is required.[11] Since job descriptions are the foundation for a sound program, it may be worthwhile to temporarily assign a junior manager as a full-time job analyst or possibly hire a person on a project basis who is skilled in interviewing and writing, and who may have knowledge of hospital personnel. The consultant should provide technical training and guidance but would ordinarily not be responsible for the detailed preparation of individual job descriptions.

The next major task is to select the person who will evaluate the job descriptions and determine the salary grade. Various approaches may be suggested. Some consultants, in their proposal, suggest that for the sake of consistency they be permitted to evaluate all jobs. This provides a significant advantage if salary surveys are later conducted with other hospitals who use the same consultant. Although the consulting fee may be higher, the validity of position comparisons is improved substantially by this approach.

An alternative is to establish a broadly-based committee within the institution. Such a group is usually chaired initially by the consultant and later by the personnel director or his representative. The committee usually includes 8 to 10 managers and senior supervisors from various hospital departments. Its function is to decide on point values for each factor in each position being evaluated. This precedes the determination of what point totals will relate to which salary grades. The committee should retain the same members throughout the initial evaluation of hospital positions (4 to 8 months). Committee members will gradually develop expertise with the point system and provide a consistency of judgment that is important. Given the proper leadership the committee will also be able to expand on and improve upon the description content by the members' knowledge of hospital functions and interrelationships.

Once the descriptions and evaluation are complete it is possible by using the point totals, the existing average salaries for each job, and salary survey information to develop appropriate point and salary ranges for each grade.

It may be necessary to review a few positions that are graded either too high or too low, based upon evaluations and the proposed salary range structure. It is quite important that these changes be made in conjunction with the committee and to the satisfaction of the hospital, avoiding at the same time arbitrary action. Credibility of the committee as job evaluators must be established to balance against the impact of possible grading errors.

The final stage in job evaluation is fixing of grades, inaugurating salary change policies, and assigning individual employees to a schedule for merit review. This often results in a substantial one-time expenditure if the hospital accepts as it should some basic premises:

- Employees should be paid no less than the minimum of their salary range. Adjustments up to the new minimum may be necessary.
- There should be a merit and service related spread of individual employee pay rates throughout the salary range. Adjustments may result when a position is graded higher than reflected by many of the salaries previously paid or when there is a crowding around the minimum at the time when many jobs are brought up to the minimum.
- Merit review schedules should be initiated coincident with the job evaluation program, irrespective of adjustments as noted above.

Acceptance of all these premises can result in substantial increases for some employees and none for others. The principles are sound. But budget constraints together with employee perception of who should earn what may dictate phasing in the program over a period of months. A consultant can advise, but the hospital administration must face the timing judgment alone and stand by its decision.

A useful approach may include the following sequence:

1. A general pay increase coincident with initiation of the salary system, replacing any increase previously planned for the near future;
2. Raising the salary of any employees below the new minimum to that minimum;
3. Allowing spread adjustments on an exceptional basis only;
4. Initiating merit review increases effective within 6 months or longer from the date of the adjustments.

Job evaluation is a major step forward; needless to say it is a subject of particular interest to employees. Communication to supervisors and employees must be extensive prior to the date the program is initiated. The following sequence is suggested.

1. Department heads receive lists of their employees indicating the new grades, salary ranges, and the new salaries before the effective date of the program. There should then be discussion between the personnel department and department heads to create a mechanism for appeals and to reinforce the department heads' understanding of the program.
2. A comprehensive briefing for all managers and supervisors should be held a week before the effective date of the program. Policies and other general information should be distributed.

3. A brochure should be distributed to employees describing in full the program, its immediate impact on salaries, and provisions for future salary reviews. Each employee should also be advised of his salary grade and salary range.

An additional note on establishing the salary system concerns those to be included and excluded. What has been discussed deals principally with nonexempt hospital positions, although some job evaluation programs include exempt positions at the B.A./M.A. professional level and at the first level of supervision. There is an increasing tendency to establish separate compensation programs for managerial employees, at least from department heads and above. (There is further discussion of compensation for managers in a separate section below.)

A final note is in order also about the salary grades and ranges. The ideal salary system gathers all jobs of equal point value within the same grade. Situations do occur, however, when even temporary shortages of employees with a certain skill so escalate a salary requirement that, if retained in the overall salary system, the job would substantially raise the grade of all positions at that level. Traditionally, these positions have been established in a separate grade with a unique salary range. Staff RNs and LPNs have been treated in this fashion, particularly during times of acute and continuous shortages.

4-5 Maintaining the Job Evaluation Program

The stability and acceptance of any salary system involves continuing job evaluation to maintain up-to-date salary grades. The job content of health-related positions changes substantially over time, especially if the hospital is involved in new programs or in research. Large institutions have found it desirable to employ a job analyst who is charged with constantly reviewing job descriptions. Smaller organizations include the job analysis function with those of other personnel professionals. One useful approach is to provide for it as an annual project. Planned conferences with department heads and employees can add substantial benefits by exposing other problems.

Job grade changes may take effect either when they are resolved or at the beginning of the next budget year. This latter approach, while convenient financially, may have some negative effects upon employee relations that should be avoided unless the savings are substantial.

Another significant decision involves the method of continuing evaluation. There is a tendency to centralize this procedure between the concerned department head and either the personnel director or the job analyst. Unquestionably the job analyst will soon be able to predict accurately an appropriate salary grade. In the short run there should be no great difficulty. However, a problem of credibility may arise. Pressure will come from department heads to upgrade jobs in order to obtain raises for individuals who are at their maximum salaries or perhaps to attract a certain candidate, or for status reasons. Eventually such pressures can lead to expedient decisions and increasingly hard feelings toward the personnel department. An alternative is to appoint a standing job evaluation committee, meeting at regular intervals. This group should be smaller than the original committee so that it may meet without delays and should have representation at the second level of supervision from the nursing, technical, clerical, and service areas. It should be chaired by a personnel officer. Although the committee's decisions would normally stand unchallenged, review and final determination ought to remain a prerogative of the personnel director.

4-6 Some Approaches to Salary Policies

Now that the various jobs have been established in an array of salary grades and the initial competitive salary levels established, attention is turned to another long-term question important to both the employee and to the hospital. What will be the basis for individual salary determination and salary increment? There are two major alternatives for consideration: the merit system and the longevity system.

4-7 The Merit Approach

This system is characterized by the ranges of salary increase that an employee may receive, based on relative achievement reflected by his supervisor's recommendation at predetermined review times.

Also common to this approach are the concepts of salary minimum, midpoint, and maximum. The salary minimum is the starting rate for employees not having exceptional experience. The employee then moves to the midpoint by 2 to 3 increases, often occurring at, let us say, six month intervals. The midpoint of the range is also the competitive rate for similar work being done in the community. The spread between minimum and midpoint reflects the learning period necessary to become job competent. Once an employee arrives at the midpoint of the range, salary review periods are longer (at least 12 months), and the basis for any change is exceptional, rather than competent performance. The maximum salary is the highest that can be received by a person in a particular salary grade.

To many, the merit system has a very logical theoretical base. Should not the hard-working employee be rewarded for his superior effort and ability? Should not the resources of the organization be directed primarily to substantial contributors, rather than to the indolent and mediocre?

Some administrators have taken exception to the merit system and its salary range concept based on problems they have experienced in its operation. For instance:

- If the midpoint is the competitive salary in the community, and particularly if many employees in the area are on a single rate (union) system, how can employees be recruited at less than that midpoint rate?
- If the range between minimum and midpoint is the learning period, does not the learning period differ from job to job and person to person? Can there be an arbitrary time between minimum and midpoint?
- Can the hospital remain competitive and deny employees some annual increase after they arrive at midpoint? If not, the notion of exceptional performance is in jeopardy.
- Finally, the most common criticism of the merit system is management's imprecise ability to determine degrees of merit, and the resulting small differences in salary between employees. In practice, can management effectively measure the differences in contribution? Is it possible that the employee who is less of a rival to the supervisor and is more deferential, receives the larger increase?

This latter criticism is particularly common at entry level positions where degrees of merit are more difficult to determine.

In reinforcement of these fears, there has been a growth in the number of people who challenge the effectiveness of small differences in pay. Do these differences evoke a positive effort to excel or do they evoke resentment by employees against both the supervisor and the higher paid employee, thus resulting in a negative effect on performance? Equally important, some employers question the very ability of money to motivate in our current work environment.

These challenges to the basic merit system have resulted in conversion by some hospitals to other systems such as longevity.

However, many who retain a belief in the efficacy of rewarding merit have developed modifications to meet the weaknesses in the merit program. These include:

- Establishment of step increments rather than a range of possible increase and a "go-no-go" decision by the supervisor as to whether a raise is merited or is to be delayed to another specified review date. This decision often must be approved at the next level of supervision.
- Establishment of quantitative bases for evaluation wherever possible (*e.g.,* attendance, typing production speed, etc.).
- Development of participating approaches to performance evaluation, including self-appraisal, objectives-related appraisal, or appraisal by several supervisors.
- Moving to a longevity approach for entry level positions, where differences in performance are difficult to assess.

Under this program, employees would receive modest longevity increases to midpoint, then be reviewed on the merit system. Other employees, in positions whose achievements are more measurable, would be eligible for merit increases from the minimum.

Before leaving the merit idea, another management concern is worth mentioning. In recent years inflation and competitive pressures have frequently resulted in hospitals increasing their hiring salaries at the beginning of each budget year. The effect is to increase the entire salary range to maintain the relationships within each grade and to provide across-the-board increases to employees which are equal to changes in the range. To the extent that these increases exceed the value of the merit raise, the emphasis on merit is undermined. In addition, some hospitals have had difficulty funding both across-the-board and merit increases. Compromises have been made in which merits are maintained on a more exceptional basis, retaining the philosophical base to the program as well as significant merit rewards.

4-8 The Longevity Approach

Much of the structure described under the merit system also applies to any pay increase program based upon longevity. There is still the minimum, midpoint, maximum concept, with a person eligible for salary reviews at stated intervals. The principal difference is that increases are based upon length of service only, irrespective of achievement. The employee's supervisor has no significant say in determining the amount or appropriateness of the increase.

An interesting factor about longevity is its recent growth and application with various groups. Historically, there has been an emphasis on longevity for nonprofessional groups. Presently, there is a tendency toward a longevity base also among many professional groups, including public school teachers, university professors, medical house staff physicians, and many hospital professionals.

The growth of the longevity system suggests some important advantages that should be noted here.

- It eliminates a source of real stress between employer and employee, to the extent that employees have been dissatisfied with the supervisor's salary recommendations.
- It effectively counteracts union organizing claims of arbitrary management, by adopting the salary increase approach espoused by unions.
- Finally, it demands that supervisors concentrate on other ways of motivating employees.

There are also disadvantages attributed to any longevity program including the following.

- There is no tangible way to reward excellence within a particular job.
- There is no way to encourage the resignation of marginal employees by withholding increases.
- Longevity foregoes any leverage provided by the merit program for a continuous, formalized performance appraisal program. This could also lead to a breakdown in the informal day-to-day performance appraisal process. Without this, employees who have taken their jobs for granted may be terminated, without what they feel is adequate warning.
- A supervisor has little opportunity to assume responsibility and authority in a highly judgmental area.
- Finally, longevity creates the tendency to have narrow salary ranges (minimum to maximum) to avoid overpaying the modest performer. The regrettable effect of this decision is that exceptional performers are also limited. The exceptional people may leave for a better paying opportunity, whereas the less capable will tend to remain.

4-9 Managing the Salary System

The job evaluation/salary system provides a structure and a rational, equitable approach to salary administration. Once it is established, however, there is still the need to: (1) establish policies and procedures for its use; (2) update the salary levels on a continuing basis; and (3) integrate the program with the salary budgeting and control process.

4-10 Salary Policies

The principal problems in the administration of a salary program deal with the timing and authority to increase wages and the assigning of power to make exceptions to the salary administration policy.

Candidates present themselves with varying levels of experience and to some extent deserve salary variations reflecting their experience in their *starting salaries*. Evaluating the significance of work experience for starting salary purposes entails a delicate interface between the department head, the expert on technical ability, and the personnel director, who is often responsible for the salary system and its objective of hospital-wide equity. With this in mind, the question of who decides starting salaries is usually compromised.

A common approach is that the department head, with prior notice to the personnel department, may authorize salaries up to one-half of the midpoint of the salary range. Salaries beyond that point are authorized individually by the personnel director. Coordination of starting rates under these circumstances is frequently a source of confusion, and it is important that there be an employment representative to announce the starting salary. This flexibility in starting salary also has an impact on the date for the first merit increase review date; the higher the starting salary, the longer the period before first salary review.

The second major policy area in salary administration is that of *merit increases*. Basic to many programs is an initial salary review after 6 months followed by either 12-month work spans between reviews or successive 6-month work period to midpoint. The initial 6-month salary review includes a careful appraisal of the employee to make an early determination whether there is a suitable match between the employee and his position. This is usually considered to be the employment probation period.

Salary reviews beyond the midpoint for exceptional performance are usually on an annual basis with longer periods as a person approaches the maximum of the salary range (up to 18 months). This concept of "stretchout" recognizes both the need for a salary maximum and the negative implications of a long-service superior employee being passed over for merit increases.

An additional problem concerns the date of such salary reviews, particularly beyond midpoint. The common alternatives to the anniversary date include a specified date monthly, quarterly, semi-annually, or annually. The further away a review date is from the anniversary date, the more unfair and unwieldy the system becomes. Annual review dates do therefore offer some advantages. Logistically, it greatly simplifies the processing of salary reviews to have employees uniformly considered and makes sure no one is overlooked due to an awkward control system.

It further provides an opportunity for department heads to review all employees at the same time and so balance a merit and service-related salary spread throughout their departments.

Finally, a single date provides management flexibility. At a time when general increases are necessary, it is important to determine total funds available for merit increases after general increase decisions are made and to insure hospital-wide fairness in use of those funds. Some programs provide for an annual merit review date in the middle of the fiscal year, so as to maximize the impact of two salary increases in a given year.

4-11 Job Changes

Changes in position also require salary administration policies. These can include promotions, lateral transfers, demotions, and re-evaluation of positions.

Promotions, by implication, usually involve a higher salary. Frequently, however, due to salary range overlap, an employee already is within the salary range for the new position. Nevertheless, most programs will provide an increase unless the employee is higher than the midpoint of the new salary range, which is a rare situation.

Lateral transfers demand salary review and thorough communications. Usually the employee will transfer to the new position at the same salary, assuming that the same skills are used in the new position. If, however, he is using a new set of skills, the salary should be negotiable. It may even be less than before, in fairness to the co-workers in the new department.

An employee may be demoted for cause or because of personal preference; the difference is important. Commonly, health care institutions may employ a senior employee who is no longer able to perform his old job, whether due to personal disability or a change in the demands of the position. Under these circumstances, many programs allow the employee to transfer, retaining his previous salary level, but exclude him from merit review raises until the new salary range catches up to his salary level.

When an employee requests a change to a lower graded position (*e.g.*, the RN who wishes to treat patients rather than supervise), the salary should be adjusted to a level no higher than the maximum of the grade for the new position. This is a negotiated process and may result in a salary level lower than the maximum.

Finally, when a job is re-evaluated, employees should be treated as though promoted. They should be brought at least to the new minimum. To provide a proper spread, increases should also be allowed within the new range up to midpoint.

4-12 Maintaining Salary Ranges and Levels

The salary ranges and levels are key ingredients to a successful salary program. They must be substantial enough to attract and retain the most able employee yet modest enough not to waste the hospital's resources. The ranges and levels are primarily the responsibility of the personnel director and justifiably, are scrutinized carefully by the hospital since they represent such a substantial impact on its funds.

The salary ranges provide for a minimum, a midpoint and maximum. The minimum must be high enough for 80 to 90 percent of the candidates to accept it as a starting salary. It must be competitive. The midpoint must be enough to retain the employee once he has become thoroughly skilled and contributing to the job. The maximum must be sufficient to retain the best employees, avoiding their loss by piracy or disenchantment.

To achieve these objectives the salary range will usually be narrower at entry-level positions, broadening out either on a dollar or percentage basis at higher grades. A common variance in salary ranges is from 20 percent (minimum to maximum) at entry-level positions to 35 to 40 percent at the senior positions (department head). This reflects a greater need at senior levels for salary flexibility to reward a greater variety of skills and to minimize turnover, the impact of which increases dramatically at high levels. Such differences in the breadth of ranges and salary levels introduce a great emphasis on market requirements as opposed to equity requirements.

The salary levels within a system are the "moment of truth" to that program and are the most important factor to both employer and employee. Determining optimum salary levels depends most on management judgments rather than on a system. In arriving at these judgments many questions must be resolved by the hospital, only some of which can be answered in objective terms.

What is the hospital's philosophy toward salaries? Should it be the highest paying employer? Should it be competitive or slightly over or under the competition? Also, do cost of living changes play a role in salary level determination?

What are the present market forces? Are neighboring hospitals and other employers raising salaries, or do they expect to? Is there a labor shortage or a surplus?

What are the prevailing union salaries? If you are a nonunion hospital, what levels will be necessary to discourage collective bargaining?

What have been the cost of living changes? Are they fully represented by the market forces? Do they suggest even higher salaries than the market might dictate?

Finally, what about the hospital's ability to pay? If it is limited does this ability result in adjustments only in areas of most critical need within budget limitations?

The answers to many of these questions will modify the answer to the basic question: what salary levels will be demanded of us by the marketplace if we are to attract and retain competent staff?

Salary surveys can be particularly valuable in answering this question, although they are only part of the answer. Most hospital associations have reliable salary information, particularly about jobs involving large numbers of employees or for which there is a labor shortage. Additionally, survey information from nonclinical sources should be reviewed for managerial, business, craft and service positions. A common mistake made by hospitals is to ignore the fact that many employees can sell their abilities to nonhospital employers.

Surveys, unfortunately, cannot be taken simply on face value. Comparability of positions is approximate at best. Inaccuracies can occur in data, particularly if minimums are not utilized consistently. Frequently, small survey information from those with whom you have particularly good rapport is often more valuable than larger broadly based formal surveys. Note that survey results, no matter how accurate when compiled, become quickly out of date.

There are factors that modify these basics which should be included in the total evaluation. If the physical plant is in a prime location and is new and attractive, it provides an edge that can offset some salary limitations. Conversely, if your facility is in an undesirable area and out of date, there is need for at least competitive salaries to offset your disadvantage.

Additional evaluation points are at your "front door" and your "back door." An alert employment officer will be aware of the extent that his hospital is less competitive than others. Employment officers should ask themselves the following. What vacancies are open for lengthy periods? What candidates for what jobs turn down the position because of salary? For what jobs must the salary range minimum be raised to attract the candidate?

The "back door" relates to turnover. Although someone may accept a job with a comparatively low salary, the more able employee will not be satisfied with it for long. Turnover will provide information not only about salary levels, but also about adequacy of salary ranges, or the placement of a position on a particular grade.

Lastly, it is important in determining salary levels to forecast the future, recognizing that salary rates normally must be adequate for the fiscal year. This means a forecast of 16 or more months, lead time included.

4-13 Salary Planning, Budgets, and Controls

The personnel organization should work closely with the controller in salary planning, budgets and controls. All are integral parts of the budgeting process, in which managers must project the timing of salary changes for each individual in each position based on the salary administration policy. An accurate projection must incorporate a review by the personnel department to insure effective administration of that policy.

Throughout the year, the salary administration section of the personnel department is responsible for insuring that employees are considered for salary increases at the proper time, that such increases are in accord with the salary administration policy, and that variances from the salary plan are brought to the attention of the department head, personnel director, and controller. Though this is in part a controller's responsibility, salary administration employees are in the best possible position to exercise before-the-fact control.

The hospital-wide program as described provides guarantees that an employee will receive salary review consideration on a programmed basis. It also provides certain discretionary authority by the various managers (*e.g.*, starting levels, increases under merit programs). The control of the program must insure the integrity and fulfillment of both objectives, usually by way of a review conducted by the salary administration section.

This division of the personnel department is charged with:

- Reviewing all information on new hires for compliance with the established salary policy and for establishing the proper job code and salary grade (and step, if appropriate);
- Reminding each department periodically of salary reviews that are imminent;
- Insuring that salary changes, in compliance with policy and the salary plan, and/or performance appraisal forms are received on each employee involved; and

● Insuring that employees are aware of the salary increase possibilities.

The salary administration section and the procedures under which it operates are essential elements in the salary program. The staff of this section must be totally familiar with policy and the salary program and the forms and methods designed to implement the policy. The senior employee here will occasionally be required to deal with all levels of management under stressful situations, and he must be able to effectively communicate the salary policy of the institution.

4-14 Unions and Salary Administration

Few would contest the notion that a hospital which has established and maintained a salary program is less likely to be a target for union organizers than one without. While achieving operating efficiency and effectiveness, with a salary system the hospital also provides much of what unions offer to employees: relative freedom from arbitrary management; equal pay for equal work; consistency in the approach to salaries; and to some extent, a commitment to provide the highest possible salary levels.

But the record shows that there are other reasons why employees choose collective bargaining, and so hospitals with good salary programs may still be organized despite their attention to salary administration. For example, recent studies have shown that one way in which labor unions are stimulating interest is to key on issues such as greater worker participation in corporate decision making and input into methods of patient care.

Whatever the reasons for organizing, unions are viewed as agents for economic security, and usually they promise to increase salaries and benefits for their members. The organized hospital should therefore plan on a union having a significant impact on its salary administration program. The union will affect not only the members of the collective bargaining unit, but also the nonunion employees and supervisors of the hospital. Management will have to determine its new role in salary administration, what aspects of the existing salary program must be salvaged, and the impact of the union's presence on nonunion wages.

Collective bargaining is much more than negotiations and newsworthy strikes. The term encompasses a whole complex of human interaction that cuts to the very core of the hospital's internal function. What is truly vital is what occurs *after* the contract is signed.

4-15 Union vs. Management Philosophies about Salary Administration

In a flamboyant moment a union official defined collective bargaining with the comment, "You bargain; we collect." Though something of a simplification, he made the important point that union officials are under substantial pressure to get *more;* the salary administration component is a very secondary consideration.

Many unions share basic philosophies about salaries. Some are in accord with current management thinking, while others conflict. Unions generally believe that a worker should be compensated for his job's complexity, that employees should receive equal pay for equal work, that length of service is a significant factor in deciding pay levels, and that there should be a consistent approach to salary decisions. Beyond these areas of agreement with management, however, are areas of conflict. The most significant difference concerns salary determinations based on management's evaluation of the complexity of a position and the merit of an employee's performance. The unrestricted use of management judgments is in basic conflict with the collective bargaining process. A corollary to this is that unions believe they need at least equal power over salary decisions and that employees must look to the union, instead of a salary system, for economic gains.

Often these areas of conflict lead to management's "throwing the baby out with the wash water," scrapping its salary objectives and system and simply playing adversary, a role that often is counter-productive.

There is in fact a larger part that management should take to best achieve its objectives of salary efficiency and equity. Elements of the salary system can support this new role, be compatible with collective bargaining, and help achieve objectives that the union may also wish to see. For instance, the system should:

1. Insure that salary levels are based on position complexity rather than manager biases or political pressures within the union;
2. Insure that salary increase criteria do not encourage lethargy and behavior that increases the workload of others (*e.g.,* excess absenteeism); and
3. Insure that excessive salary levels do not result in restriction of staffing levels or laying off employees to meet budget requirements.

The introduction of a union into salary administration thus complicates the achievement of salary objectives and requires additional effort on management's part.

4-16 *Salvaging Elements of the Salary System under a Union Contract*

Each of the various elements of a salary system—job evaluation, salary grading, approaches to salary review and general salary policies—require review to once again determine: (1) if they still support salary administration objectives, and (2) if they are compatible with the collective bargaining process.

Job evaluation for salary grading is the basis for most salary systems in nonunion organizations. This is compatible with a unionized operation to the extent that it is systematic and minimizes qualitative judgments by managers. Hence, a point system should have a greater possibility of surviving in some form than would a ranking system.

Often, a preunion job evaluation and grading system and the existing grades will be acceptable unless there is major pressure to correct alleged inequities. New positions will be graded based on one of three approaches:

1. A union-management agreement on where a job ranks (without specific criteria) in an existing array of grades;
2. A joint job evaluation via the point system or ranking, but with specific criteria; or
3. A determination of the salary grade by management, presumably based on the preexisting job evaluation program.

The third approach has the advantage of maintaining management initiative. Too, the union will often wish to avoid participating in a decision that will always be unpopular with some segment of its membership.

A major concern when incorporating job evaluation into the collective bargaining process involves the job description. When used for job evaluation and for recruiting, it was probably designed to show *examples of functions* indicating the level of complexity of a position but did not include all job functions.

Such a job description should *not* be the basis for limiting the functions performed by an employee, except for major variations involving significant time, effort, and contribution. If jurisdictional agreements are made, job descriptions should be written carefully to avoid unreasonable disputes and unjustified reluctance by employees to perform certain functions.

4-17 *Salary Ranges, Job Rates, and Merit Raises*

Since merit programs involving management's unrestricted judgments conflict with collective bargaining, the two bases for salary determination most common under a union contract are the salary range involving longevity-related incremental steps and the single job rate. Additionally, there is the use of *quantitative* criteria to determine merit salary increases. This usually occurs beyond the traditional midpoint of the salary range and considers such factors as attendance, punctuality, or measured productivity.

The use of the salary range has significant advantages over the job rate for the employee and for the hospital but is of less advantage to the union. Not only does it allow management to hire at a rate reflecting the new employee's modest knowledge of the hospital and its practices and then advancing him as his value to the hospital is increased; the range concept also tends to reduce turnover by providing something to look forward to that is guaranteed rather than simply a possibility. It allows an employee to rely on a system rather than on managers or union officials.

A salary range allows management flexibility in the starting salary to cope with market pressures and to attract more experienced job candidates. Usually the established practices involving specific credit for durations of related experience will be acceptable to a union.

A complicating factor with the salary range approach relates both to the longevity base and to the bargaining process. Since merit is usually not a factor, salary ranges under union contracts tend to be narrow to avoid excess payments to the modest performer (15 to 20%). At the same time, however, the high achiever can become dissatisfied by a "low ceiling" and leave. Hopefully, this can be avoided by quantity-based merit reviews as described earlier.

There is also a tendency for negotiations to focus on the minimum salary in the range and pressure to raise that minimum. Because salary scale increases are frequently on a percentage basis, the cascading effect on the range will make it an increasingly expensive system. Such pressures commonly result in negotiating increases in dollars, rather than in percentage terms. The expenses of the salary range basis should be balanced with the economies and advantages suggested above weighed against the potential that the alternative of a higher job rate for union employees will become the minimum rate in a range for nonunion employees.

The job rate approach forces high starting salaries to be paid before a person is actually making a contribution. It eliminates the incentive for longevity-based growth, and the employee must rely on the union and on the sometimes traumatic negotiation process for any salary improvement. Such disadvantages would be less significant for a bargaining group with long service, with most employees moving to the top of the range in a short period. However, in groups where turnover is substantial the economic effect of job turnover rate versus salary range should be considered carefully.

4-18 Impact of the Union Presence on Nonunion Salary Administration

One of the problems resolved by a hospital-wide salary program is the elimination of separate plans for separate work groups. The different sets of rules may be costly and can also create serious morale problems with employees always viewing the more generous aspects of the *other* plan, the "greener pastures." Such a situation also makes the development of a hospital-wide positive employee relations climate nearly impossible.

The coming of collective bargaining to a group of any size in a hospital can have the same effect on employee relations. Suddenly there is a separate group where the rules are different; the rules for behavior, the rules for performance, and the rules for salary. In salary administration this creates several major hazards. Some possible hazards are as follows:

- That union settlements will be the sole determinant for salary scale changes for nonunion employees;
- That a change from a merit base to a longevity base or job rate for union employees will encourage dissatisfaction with the merit program among nonunion employees;
- That salary increases for mediocre work will encourage similarly mediocre work by others;
- That the benefits in salary under collective bargaining will encourage further collective bargaining.

Such pressures have an impact on nonunion employees, particularly those who are at salary levels similar to the union employees, and also on supervisors, particularly those supervising union employees.

4-19 The Impact on Nonunion Employees

In some large urban hospitals a problem appears when a segment of the employee group is organized, and there is a change from a salary range to a job rate for the unit employees who are covered by the collective bargaining agreement of the union. If the starting salary is escalated to what had previously been the midpoint of the range for that group, the hospital then must make some difficult choices concerning nonunion starting salaries. It still must attract candidates to nonunion positions, maintain equity with union payscales, and avoid encouraging others to bargain collectively.

In those circumstances, the hospital may choose to eliminate the salary range for nonunion employees and substitute a similar job rate. It can establish the job rate as a minimum of the range for comparable nonunion positions, but by escalating salaries for other positions accordingly, starting salaries eventually will be distorted community-wide. The hospital can retain the original (or other) lower entry rate, but increase the opportunity for rapid merit-based salary improvement to the existing midpoint of the range.

Local conditions must dictate the decision. The hospital must carefully assess the degree of hazard of increased collective bargaining if nonunion starting rates are too low and the economic impact of the various alternatives.

A more common problem arises where salary ranges are retained which are longevity-based for union employees and merit-based for nonunion employees. Nonunion employees then ask the question, "Is the merit-based program so attractive that it is more palatable than the guarantees of the longevity system?"

Hospitals which want to retain the merit-based approach and minimize interest of nonunion employees in collective bargaining often attempt to sell merit raises based on: (1) greater opportunity for more liberal reward, teamed with (2) a more personalized approach to the employee, plus (3) the intangible status-related qualities of the approach.

In specific terms, one or more of the following modifications can be made to a merit-based program which features a range of increase provision.

- Change to an increment increase provision with a "go-no-go" decision. This would eliminate the former system's characteristic small salary differences, often challenged as indefensible because of the supervisor's limited ability to assess levels of merit.
- As suggested earlier, insure that ranges for merit-based programs are broader than for longevity plans. Increments also could be larger.
- Combine the longevity and merit approaches, with nonunion employees being eligible for longevity increases to the ceiling of the union scale and being eligible for merit increases to a more liberal maximum; and/or
- Insure that salaries of nonunion employees increase at least to the extent of the union em-

ployees when negotiations resulted in salary scale changes.

Because employees presently not organized may later choose to do so, using these more generous salary programs as an economic base for upward negotiations makes the prudent hospital avoid depending entirely on these economic means to avoid further collective bargaining.

Changes can be made recognizing the intangible reasons for which employees join unions. These include:

- Improving the quality of performance evaluations and the judiciousness with which they are carried out. This should involve clearly established review procedures which separate the timing of performance evaluations from the timing of salary increases and allow an opportunity for performance improvement;
- Communicating energetically the opportunities implicit in the merit program;
- Insuring that there is attention given to management of the nonunion salary program, at least in the same proportion as the notoriety involved in union negotiations. The hospital might convene *ad hoc* nonunion employee committees to develop employee suggestions and to insure continuous dialogue with nonunion employees to cope with their grievances;
- Consider the use of time sheets rather than time clocks for nonunion personnel, raising them to a quasi-salaried status; and
- Finally and possibly most importantly, protect nonunion employees from overzealous or arbitrary supervision which is often the principal cause of the dissatisfaction which ultimately leads to collective bargaining.

4-20 *The Impact on Supervisory Employees*

The supervisor of newly organized employees experiences the impact of collective bargaining most directly. The demands of his job and his relationship with his employees change radically, and some will conclude that the job is far less satisfying. Complicating the situation further is the modest attention given in many hospitals in the past to supervisors' salaries. In many cases the salary system was the same as for nonsupervisory employees, including such provisions as overtime pay and premiums for such things as working on other shifts, on weekends and through lunch. But this system provided no significant recognition for the responsibilities of being in charge.

First level supervisors must be paid adequately for their more demanding positions by a method which encourages their association with the management rather than with the union. Paying supervisors on a salary basis, rather than on an hourly basis, is the usual solution. On the other hand, the hospital must be careful that increasing salaries of supervisors will not necessitate salary increases in other high-level positions, such as its professionals.

If supervisors are to be continued on the same merit-based system of the nonunion, nonmanagement employees, the same systemic changes should be applicable for them as were mentioned above for other nonunion employees. Also, there should be a grade adjustment for supervisors coincident with placing them on a salaried basis, basically exempt from premium overtime and premium benefits. The grade adjustment could be kept minimal if supervisors were authorized straight-time for overtime for lengthy periods. This would retain peer relationships under the grading program but compensate supervisors sufficiently and by an appropriate method.

Other forms of "compensation" can also be effective in recognizing the supervisor's contribution and maintaining his essential support. Some hospitals do this with a liberalized benefit program for supervisors (and other managers), focusing on the needs of this group. Insurance benefits (health, disability, and life) and/or vacations can be provided in more generous measure at minimum cost but with significant impact.

Once again, economic improvement will not completely insure the support of supervisors in a unionized organization, yet it is an essential underpinning which will insure the credibility of noneconomic measures.

4-21 Salaries for Hospital Managers

4-22 *Salary Objectives*

Salary programs designed for managers, principally from the level of department head up, are replacing the casual approaches of the past or reliance on the salary systems designed for nonexempt employees. It used to be possible to administer the salaries of a small group of management decision makers on an informal basis. Now, the demands for improved hospital administration have increased the number of management professionals and have involved department heads in more management decision making than before. The increased numbers and more demanding roles suggest the need for a systematic approach to determine appropriate salary levels when recruiting individuals and for providing optimum rewards and incentives.

Any approach should support the same philosophies and objectives as the nonexempt program, of internal equity plus the efficient use of salary dollars. Further, in the face of a trend away from merit-based programs caused by inflation and collective bargaining, there is an overriding need for hospital management to be both merit and change oriented.

Creating the necessary vigor and change-oriented climate in an organization involves many details. They should include the communication of the institution's directions and goals by the trustees and administrator, the effective selection and development of managers, and the formal recognition of managers as agents of change for the organization. These efforts must necessarily be augmented by a salary program that attracts and rewards excellence, reinforcing the hospital's objectives of excellence and innovation in all management functions. Using objectives and systematic methods, the program should be designed to relate the salary range of a position to its level of management and professional responsibility and relate an individual's salary to his achievement of objectives within his level of responsibility. In doing so it will focus the total hospital's attention on quality and improvement.

4-23 The Salary Program Structure

Basic to a management salary program is a structure that will answer several primary questions:

1. What are the levels and areas of responsibility for each management position?
2. What is the relative value of each management position compared to that of other such positions, hospital-wide?
3. What is a reasonable grouping based on position value, generally at the same salary level?
4. Finally, what is the least and most that the hospital should pay for various management services?

These questions are not unlike those answered by other salary programs. The structure, too, will be similar and will include position descriptions, position evaluation, salary grading, and salary ranges.

Yet the similarity ends with this basic structure. The content and administration of the program differ by their dominant concentration on the hospital's goals and objectives.

4-24 The Position Description

The management position description is the foundation which provides the basis for salary grading and ultimately the salary for the individual. It is also a management tool with several other objectives.

It may include quantitative standards of performance. When teamed with an effective appraisal program and a periodic review of management goals, the standards will provide a tool for performance evaluation. These several programs also provide a basis for determining management development needs and evaluation. Finally, the position description is a tool used to improve the effectiveness of manager selection.

For evaluation purposes, the management position description emphasizes the professional and managerial responsibilities of the position as well as the background normally demanded by the position. There is a noticeably greater emphasis on the processes and functions in the manager's area of responsibility than in the nonexempt job descriptions.

Though the evaluation criteria stressed in a description vary with the system adopted (normally established by a management consultant) some common evaluation criteria include:

- The level of managerial and professional expertise required;
- The level of impact that the incumbent has on the quality goals of the hospital;
- The potential that the incumbent has for influencing hospital-wide policies and practices;
- The level of budget (or facilities) responsibility; and,
- The level of responsibility for personnel (in numbers, in a variety of positions, and in skills).

Additionally, standards of performance are built into the position descriptions for purposes of manager evaluation and development. They should include such quantitative measures as: (1) budget efficiency; (2) staffing level efficiency; (3) controllable turnover; and (4) quality control measures. Of the four, quality control measures are least used, yet often available, and may include such measures as the following:

For the Nursing Service: The extent and effectiveness of patient care planning, the continuity of patient care, the reported level of patient or physician satisfaction (or dissatisfaction) with nursing services, the extent of staff technical improvement (via in-service training, etc.), the efficiency of staff schedule, and the level of staff absenteeism.

For the Medical Records Department: The transcription lead time and record availability lead time.

For the Housekeeping Department: The bacteria count in critical areas of the hospital, the housekeeping manhours per square foot of space, and the level of employee grievances.

For the Business Department: Billing lead time and level of accounts receivable.

The process of developing the management position description is the keystone to the management salary program. The description can and should clarify interdepartmental relationships and responsibility roles and will often lead to a clearer definition of who is and who is not a "department head" based on newly defined levels of expectations. It should give both superior and subordinate personnel an opportunity to clearly understand the roles and expectations of the parties.

4-25 Position Evaluation

The evaluation and grading of management positions may be accomplished in a variety of ways, dependent on the size and inclinations of the institution. For a small management group of 15 to 20 (beginning with the senior supervisor or department head) the grading objective may be achieved by an informal ranking, using the position description as a general guide. The ranked positions are grouped (graded) based on a system provided by the consultant, and salary ranges are then established.

However, when large numbers are involved, or where sensitivities dictate a more objective approach, then a more systematic ranking or modified point system will be appropriate. Such systems are available from professional consultants who evaluate criteria from the position description similar to those described above. An example from one such system that evaluates job factors by their level of complexity is given in Chapter 17.

The process of evaluation and grading of department heads is usually conducted by a senior management committee, including or reporting to the administrator. By so doing, many of the status relationships can be worked out and functions clarified by consensus of senior management rather than by the action of a remote consultant or by a single administrator. This should lead to a greater acceptance of the grading system by those affected. Grading recommendations for immediate associates of the administrator are usually worked out by him with his consultant and submitted with all salary ranges to the trustees for approval.

The salary ranges for management positions deserve particular comment. They are particularly broad, with department heads commonly at the 35-40% level from minimum to maximum, extending to 55-60% for the administrator. This reflects the need for flexibility when determining salaries for managers using a merit-based approach and the varied levels of contribution that can be made even by managers in a single salary grade. It also acknowledges the need for flexibility to attract the most talented candidates to a position.

4-26 Administration of the Management Salary Program

The most notable variations from the nonexempt program occur in the administration of the management salary program. With regard to beginning salaries, it is customary for the administrator and his associates, when filling a position, to exercise salary discretion up to midpoint of the salary range, or 20% of minimum for a department head (*e.g.*, from $15,000 to $18,000 for a range of $15,000 to $21,000). Discretion beyond the midpoint is discouraged to avoid damaging the basic program.

Merit salary reviews for managers usually occur annually on a date distinct from that for other employees. Managers at higher salary levels (*e.g.*, $20,000 and above) are often reviewed less frequently, possibly at 18-month intervals as specified by policy. It is also common for policy to provide for a "stretch out" process, whereby salary review intervals will also be longer (perhaps 15 to 18 months) beginning when a manager reaches a certain level of his salary range (*e.g.*, 75% to maximum). This recognizes the need for continued salary growth to encourage performance for a salary maximum, but it may have a negative impact on a person who has reached his maximum.

Budgetary provisions for salary increases usually include either (1) a salary increase budget based on a percent of the total management payroll or (2) a wage increase budget based on a previously accepted salary increase plan. In either case, the total budget should reflect a merit component and a component for across-the-board changes provided other employees, which is not directly shared by the management group. This latter component is the amount by which all salary ranges would be increased as required by market or cost-of-living factors.

When a range of increase is established, the average, if given hospital-wide to managers, should amount to the salary increase budget.

Higher than average increases to high achievers will necessarily have to be offset by lower than average increases to lesser achievers in order to function within budget limitations. This encourages implementation of the merit approach. Variations to this limiting feature are subject to the administrator's approval.

The above salary determinations are *merit-based* and often use some, or all, of the following evaluation tools.

- The appraisal of overall manager performance (see sample appraisal forms, Chapter 16);
- The review of the manager's achievement of *performance standards* indicated in the position description;
- The review of *goals and objectives* previously established for the year as part of the "management by objectives" program.

One recent approach to the performance appraisal process begins with the manager reporting his accomplishments for the previous year to his supervisor. This is followed by a discussion between the two and a final recommendation by the supervisor for a merit salary change. This recommendation is subject to approval at a second level of authority. This dialogue provides a unique two-way communication in the appraisal process and also sets the stage for development of management objectives for the forthcoming year, both for the manager and hospital-wide.

Separate management salary programs are still uncommon in hospitals. As a result, their introduction may be particularly disturbing to those used to a more tenure-based program. The individual institution will determine if it is necessary to implement the program in stages, to insure its success. Over time, however, its initiation will provide an achievement-oriented climate within the management group to complement growing demands for improved administrative management in health care facilities.

5 BENEFITS[12]

Benefits, when viewed as a significant part of total compensation, are relatively new to the health care delivery system. Yet during the past decade alone they have achieved so high a level of importance—and cost—that health administrators and third party payors have been forced to take a fresh look at what the dollar is actually buying. It is anachronistic that the adjective "fringe" is still used to describe a substantial and increasing portion of total manpower costs.

During the wage control years of 1942-1947, benefits, because they were not regulated, received special impetus. In the intervening 30 years, they have escalated to 32-33% of payroll costs according to a 1973 U.S. Chamber of Commerce study of American industry. Social Security, Unemployment and Workmen's Compensation account for some 10% of the payroll,

with much of the remaining 22-23% coming under increased governmental scrutiny and regulation. High income taxes, spiraling inflation, union demands, and competition for skilled employees have enriched benefit programs and, it is agreed, hastened the decline of cash compensation as the sole motivator of work performance.

5-1 Benefits Versus Cash

Employees—administrators too—occasionally dream of how simple life could be were all benefits converted to cash and stuffed into the pay envelope. That this glistening fantasy rests atop an iceberg is soon apparent.

In brief:

Certain benefits are legislatively ordained and have become a fixed part of labor costs (*e.g.*, Social Security, Unemployment Compensation and Workmen's Compensation).

Tax laws favor the deferring of some income until retirement, when reduced tax rates will apply to lower gross income. Many not-for-profit institutions have taken advantage of this portion of the Internal Revenue Code to set up tax deferred annuity plans for their employees. More recent legislation permits employees to establish individual plans for sheltering income from immediate taxation if they choose.

Group purchases of life, health and accident, retirement, disability and similar insurable benefits can be made with before-tax dollars. Individuals buying the same protection would be denied the cost advantage of group rates and would further be required to pay premiums using after-tax dollars.

Over the years management has evolved the notion of benefits as a kind of social contract, lending stability to the employment relationship and offering the employee some base line of protection against economic catastrophe. Despite occasional charges of paternalism, benefits have become inextricably woven into the total payment for services, creating a blur between cash and noncash compensation. Rising employee expectations have further aimed benefits in one clear direction—more and better.

At issue then is not benefits *versus* cash, but rather establishing a mix of both that is affordable, competitive, and responsive to employees' changing perceptions of need.

5-2 Planning a Benefit Program

Benefits have mushroomed as a response to legal requirements, competition from neighbors, and employee demands. Further, they are easy to create, difficult to pay for, and are virtually impossible to revoke. It thus behooves the health care employer to sit down and carefully assess what it is buying, what it is costing, and in which direction future benefit programs ought to be aimed.

At the beginning of this chapter we saw that the health care industry and its workforce had certain unique characteristics. These cannot be safely overlooked in benefit planning. Specifically, hospitals and similar institutions:

- have matched industry in salary and benefit levels only in recent years,
- have financial constraints imposed upon them by third party payors, including government agencies,
- are labor intensive, with wages and benefits representing two-thirds or more of operating budgets and creating substantial cost impacts as new benefits are introduced,
- have more women than men in their workforces,
- have more young people than old,
- have a high labor turnover, and
- employ increasing numbers of skilled people who compare their wage-benefit packages with national

or regional norms rather than local norms.

Benefit planning entails a series of questions that must be answered in relation to the objectives and special needs of each institution and work group. Some of the more important questions are listed below.

5-3 Benefit Planning Questions

1. What is the workforce profile?

Experience has shown that young, single women, who numerically dominate the average hospital payroll, seek compensation packages emphasizing cash and time off (*i.e.*, vacations, holidays, sick leave.) Older women supporting households and married men with families appear more interested in health and accident, life, and disability insurance, as well as retirement plans. It should not be surprising that the typical employee, as he grows older and his personal circumstances change, will alter his benefit expectations a number of times. However, with the passing of the Civil Rights Act of 1964, it is mandatory that insurance benefits be the same for men and women.

In a talk before the New England Hospital Assembly, Anne V. Cronin, Director of the Personnel Division at Boston's Beth Israel Hospital, cited some results of the attached hospital study she has completed. It showed the following:

Full-time Workforce Distribution by Sex and Age

Sex	% Of Total	% Under 30	% 30-39	% 40-49	% 50-59	% 60-69
Female	70.8	46.9	17.9	13.0	13.8	8.4
Male	29.2	45.7	19.4	13.1	13.1	8.7

Full-time Workforce Distribution by Sex and Age Employment

Sex	% Of Total	% Under 2	% 2-4	% 5-9	% 10-14	% 15-19	% 20-24	% 25 & over
Female	70.8	51	19	14.8	4	2	2	
Male	29.2	53	17	18	8	2	1	1

Miss Cronin cited a 2,025 full-time employee community hospital in another city with a female to male ratio of 76:24 and found the following age distribution:

	% Under 30	% 30-39	% 40-49	% 50-59	% 60 & over
Male & Female Combined	51.1	17.6	12.8	14.3	5.1

The same institution had the following distribution by years of employment:

	% Under 2	% 2-4	% 5-9	% 10-14	% 15-19	% 20-24	% 25 & over
Male & Female Combined	42.7	24.8	19.5	6.8	3.9	1.3	.7

The two sets of figures are surprisingly close yet different enough to suggest that each hospital develop its own workforce profile and update it at least annually.

2. Should emphasis be placed upon recruitment or retention?

Both are important. The prospective employee will compare your entire compensation package with those he may now be receiving, and as questions arise, the alert interviewer must be prepared to discuss the merits of each. In addition, many candidates are aware of benefit programs in other companies and institutions. Again, personnel officers must know the marketplace. A word of caution: an influx of applicants expressing interest in a single benefit may indicate that you are attracting the people for the wrong reasons. A sound, comprehensive benefit program can greatly augment other recruiting efforts, although it should not be the major means for attracting applicants.

Without question, benefits serve not just to attract new employees but to stabilize a workforce by articulating the institution's genuine concern for its staff. Unfortunately, some otherwise sophisticated employers expect benefits to carry a far greater employee relations burden than they can ever bear. Louis XIV, who did much for the cathedral building industry in France, was heard to cry after a disastrous battlefield defeat, "How can God do this to me after all I've done for Him!" Employers still express stunned disbelief that their employees could consider starting unions "after all I've done for them."

3. Which benefits must be offered to all as a reward for service and a protection from hazards?

In general, vacations, holidays, and sick leave fall into this category. Although waiting periods for vacations and sick leave are both customary and defensible, institutions more and more view these as benefits to be earned and accrued from date of hire—not to be taken away even in the event of discharge. Health and accident insurance goes far toward protecting employees from the consequences of serious illness. Such coverage has become increasingly costly, and although it would be an enormous help were the entire cost borne by the employer, there is an important symbolic value in having the employee realize even in some small way the price of this protection by contributing to its cost. Group life insurance on the other hand, is relatively inexpensive if bought under a "no name" blanket term policy with a refund provision for favorable experience. The minimum coverage should be $2,000 with the institution paying the entire cost. More and more hospitals are increasing term life insurance protection to one or more times the employee's annual rate of pay.

The above benefits should be considered basic and minimal. In general, they represent an underpinning to any more comprehensive package. For further information and sample policy statements on these and other benefits, see the sample personnel policies found in Chapter 16.

4. Which benefits are legally required?

Social Security, Unemployment and Workmen's Compensation must, for legal reasons, be added to the cost of those benefits suggested above. In addition, retirement plans under the Employee Retirement Income Security Act of 1974 (ERISA)[13] and antidiscrimination laws at both the federal and state level (e.g., maternity leave) entail further direct and overhead costs properly chargeable to benefits.

5. Which benefits did you inherit?

There was a time when it was felt that x-ray technicians should receive four weeks' vacation instead of two or three; this was because of presumed radiation hazards. Both equipment and people are now adequately protected, yet the policy remains. Most personnel administrators find that they have acquired a number of benefit programs ranging from the frivolous to the unaffordable. Often the benefits appear inspired by caprice or social pressures no longer identifiable. Many seem unevenly applied to various groups of employees. All bear the sanctity of time.

The astute personnel director must first identify these aberrations, eliminate some, select what is useful and can be made to fit into a more practical package and make certain that benefits are fairly applied throughout the institution.

The personnel director should list benefits now prevailing in his own recruiting market (nationally as well as locally). He might take the initiative by organizing or joining with other hospitals, manufacturers, stores, banks, and the like in surveying existing benefit programs, seek the opinions of department heads, employees, and especially his own interviewers. He should categorize each benefit in order of probable importance and further break each down by degree and potential cost (*e.g.,* 100% versus 75% tuition assistance; $2,000 life insurance versus coverage of one year's gross salary). What should emerge is an imperfect but valuable starting point. Again, it is important to remember that employees attracted or kept largely because of benefits represent a poor investment.

6. *Which benefits are motivators?*

It is not within the purview of this manual to cover the broad field of motivational theory. Instead we would call your attention to the Bibliography in Chapter 19 and particularly to the basic writings of A. H. Maslow (*A Theory of Human Motivation*), Douglas M. McGregor (*The Human Side of Enterprise*), and Rensis Likert (*Motivation and Increased Productivity*). In listing his now-famous "hierarchy of needs," Maslow draws a number of conclusions all personnel directors dealing with benefits will understand: man is a perpetually wanting animal; the appearance of one need usually rests on the prior satisfaction of another, more pressing need.

Human needs have been labeled as "maintenance" (*e.g.,* food, clothing, shelter) and "motivational" (these range from a new insurance plan or pay increase to the threat of discharge if performance does not improve). With respect to benefit planning, it is well to remember that what motivated yesterday is expected today and may evoke boredom tomorrow.

Should the possible motivational effects of benefits be ignored in the face of our imprecise understanding of shifting human needs and expectations? Not at all. Instead, the present and potential effect of each benefit ought to be identified and, wherever possible, used to the advantage of both employer and employee. Unless some attempt is made to isolate the factors making people *want* to do superior work, benefits will continue to spiral in response to pressures management will pay for but not control.

7. *Need all benefits be costly?*

Very young employees tend to be indifferent to pension, hospitalization, and other insurance plans. But group travel at discount rates to Europe, sporting events, and ski weekends often run a close second to vacations and holidays as benefits of major interest to this age group. Aside from the administrative expense of arranging such activities, they are virtually cost

free. In addition, it is possible to spread the dollar impact of temporary vacation relief among workers by featuring winter group travel and long holiday weekends. Benefits such as the above can never take the place of a sound program of paid leave and insurance. But they do provide an interesting and imaginative icing to an otherwise comprehensive benefit package.[14]

5-4 *Analyzing Your Present Benefit Program*

Once you have identified the various benefits, their cost and probable value to employees, it is possible to arrange them in some logical sequence. By so doing, the more glaring gaps and instances of overemphasis become apparent. Unless you have selected more appropriate general categories, try the following:

1. Old Age
   a. Social Security
   b. Medex
   c. Pension
   d. Life Insurance (reduced coverage)
   e. Deferred Compensation
2. Loss of Income
   a. Health Insurance (include maternity and outpatient coverage)
   b. Life Insurance (full coverage)
   c. Long- and Short-Term Disability
   d. Sick Leave
   e. Workmen's Compensation
   f. Unemployment Compensation
   g. Paid Leave (*e.g.,* jury and national guard)
3. Pursuit of Happiness
   a. Vacations
   b. Holidays
   c. Free Days
   d. Time Off in Lieu of Sick Leave
   e. Subsidized Assistance
   f. Educational Assistance
   g. Picnics, Christmas Parties, Sports Events, Bowling Teams
   h. Awards for Long Service
   i. Four Day (or "Rearranged") Workweek

5-5 *Trends in Benefit Programs*

It is not possible to detail the exact direction individual benefits will take in the years ahead. But it is safe to echo the late Walter Reuther of the United Auto Workers who, when asked at a bargaining session with General Motors' negotiators what the U.A.W. really wanted, is reputed to have said simply, "More!"

We have listed below some of the benefits that will appear on the scene, be expanded, or receive increased attention by labor unions and other employee groups in the near future. It is suggested that you add others for future reference.

1. Old Age
   a. Social Security—increased benefits; equalized male survivor benefits
   b. Medex—increased benefits
   c. National Health Insurance
   d. Retirement Programs—trend toward non-contributing plans; increased regulations under ERISA; broader coverage, earlier vesting, trend toward full portability, early retirement, cost of living escalators, tie-in with life insurance and deferred annuity programs
   e. Life Insurance—full coverage
   f. Sick Leave—use of unused accrued sick leave
   g. Vacation—increased allotment in years before retirement
2. Loss of Income
   a. Health Insurance—trend toward full payment by employer; psychiatric, maternity, diagnostic, "health maintenance," dental, optical coverage, increased dollar maximums, catastrophic illness coverage
   b. Employee Clinics—expanded on-premises health facilities, captive HMOs, routine health care including immunizations for family members, discounts for prescription drugs and professional services
   c. Long- and Short-Term Disability—employer paid, shorter waiting periods (180 to 90 to 30 days for LTD), increased benefits including inflation hedge and some payment to surviving spouse
   d. Life Insurance—increased coverage from flat $2,000 to $5,000 toward multiples of annual salary, privilege of conversion from term to straight life, shorter, waiting period for coverage
   e. Unemployment Compensation—continuation of group health insurance, life insurance, sick pay, strike benefits
   f. Workmen's Compensation—increased individual and family allowances
   g. Business Travel Accident—24-hour coverage during a business trip
   h. Sick Leave—unlimited accrual or tie-in with long or short term disability and Social Security disability, payment for unused sick leave
   i. Miscellaneous Leave—marriage, birthday, maternity, paternity, divorce, educational, relocation, sabbatical, etc., all with full or partial employer payment
   j. Severance Pay—informal program based upon salary level and length of employment
3. Miscellaneous Benefits
   a. Expansion of "Pursuit of Happiness" Benefits previously listed [15]
   b. Group Purchasing—personal and household articles
   c. Free or Low Cost Legal Services
   d. Group Auto & Homeowner's Insurance
   e. Day Care Centers
   f. Automatic Bank Deposit of Pay Checks
   g. Traveler's Checks
   h. Foreign Travel Immunizations
   i. Vocational Counseling
   j. Subsidized Parking and Public Transportation
   k. Suggestion Programs with suitably attractive awards
   l. Pre-Retirement Counseling
   m. Flexible Work Schedules—outgrowth of the 3 day/40 hour work week
   n. Social/Recreational Activities—expanded programs with increased financial support by employer
   o. Relocation Expense Reimbursement
   p. Sabbatical Leave—partly or fully paid
   q. Educational and Management Training Leave on work time
   r. Business Travel Expenses—increased mileage, meal, hotel, public transportation reimbursement
   s. Cafeteria or Supermarket Benefit Plans [16]
   t. Employee Store—partially subsidized
   u. Tax Deferred Annuities—increased flexibility and broader investment vehicles
   v. Blood—available as needed by employee and family
   w. On-premises banking

5-6 Self Insurance Benefits [17]

To varying degrees, every health care employer operates his own informal insurance company. This is most evident in the contingency liability he bears for sick leave that may never be taken, vacation leave for which he may have to hire temporary help, experience-rated unemployment compensation, workmen's compensation, and health insurance programs. If he is thinking any distance into the future, the hospital personnel director is attempting simultaneously to serve employee needs and reduce costs by establishing ongoing programs for training of new skills and rehabilitation of partially disabled individuals. He is further promoting safety activities and carefully documenting both unemployment compensation and workmen's compensation cases to avoid needless liability.

He should examine premium costs carefully and solicit proposals from outside consultants specializing in self-insurance plans. The question of self-insurance does not lend itself to one easy answer for all employers. A good rule-of-thumb, whether you choose to self-insure, coinsure, reinsure, or simply pay standard or "book" rates, is to regularly reexamine the chosen vehicle in light of changing costs, losses, and encumbered capital to support losses. The advantages of dealing at arm's length and changing or eliminating carriers are obvious.

5-7 Communicating Benefits

With the advent of the Employment Retirement Income Security Act of 1974 (ERISA)[18] every employee in a covered institution must receive regular notification of the status of his pension, annuity, stock bonus, profit sharing, or other qualified plan benefits "written in a manner calculated to be understood by the average plan participant." If you have already established a continuous system for both communicating and explaining such benefits, this portion of the law may require only a supplemental statement or two. You have company if you have agonized over and tinkered with benefits to assure both adequacy and fairness—and then neglected to tell your employees clearly and regularly what you have done. A number of consulting firms have rushed to fill this gap and provide counsel on the complexities ERISA has created. If you have not already been approached, an initial no-obligation consultation with one of these firms in your community is recommended.

Beyond what is now required by law in the pension area, the problem of communicating benefits generally should be addressed on a number of successively detailed levels and specific questions should be encouraged from those employees who wish more information. You may wish to consider the following:

Level 1:

a. Required ERISA summary to each employee's home with cover letter from the personnel department or hospital administrator inviting questions.
b. Bulletin boards calling attention to specific benefits and costs but avoiding detailed explanations. Feature name and telephone extension of the benefits manager. Invite questions.

c. A brief list and description of benefits in institution's newsletter.
d. Letters home (no more than one per month), devoting several each year to brief explanation of benefits. Invite questions.
e. Employee handbook. Keep it up-to-date and restrict benefit explanations to a few lines for each.
f. Personal visits (by department head invitation) to meetings of employees. Personnel director accompanied by administrator or benefit-manager should briefly describe major benefits, answer questions, seek directions for the future.

Level 2:

a. Personnel Policy Manual summary of each benefit. The manual normally goes only to department heads because of frequent changes. Each benefit should be sufficiently explained to enable department heads to discuss it intelligently. Employees should know of manual's existence and their privilege to examine it at reasonable times.
b. Meetings with department heads to brief them on benefits, inform them that original insurance policies may be studied by them, and the personnel benefits manager will be available to answer more questions. Inform them that following your explanation and answers to questions, future communications to employees will suggest that they consult their department heads first on all personnel policies including benefits.
c. By letters and meetings (if necessary), inform department heads first of any new benefits or major changes in existing benefits. They will never forgive you for being told of changes or additions after everyone in the cafeteria already knows.

Level 3:

a. The administrator is preoccupied with many concerns other than benefits. Yet the cost may be high and the return difficult to measure as each new benefit is suggested or an existing one improved. Be prepared to offer considerable detail if requested—including which employees could be affected, probable cost over a 2-5 year period, expected improvements in productivity (or morale or competitive stance), major provision of the benefit, proposed beginning date, etc. Be prepared to discuss with board of trustees if requested.
b. Establish working file of all blanket insurance policies, riders, changes, correspondence, notes of telephone calls, etc. that occurred during

negotiations with outside vendors. Key policies and documents should be kept in institution safes. Maintain files of claims forms, procedural instructions and signed beneficiary cards for all insurance benefits.

5-8 Summary

Benefits have become an integral part of the employer-employee relationship. They serve an important office in cementing the fortunes of both parties more amicably and securely. But they can never replace competitive salary levels, equitable relationships between pay grades, fair incentive systems, adequate working conditions, responsive yet firm managers, an operating grievance or complaint mechanism, clearly stated evenly applied rules of conduct, and finally a system of internal communications that effectively works in both directions.[19]

6 PERSONNEL RECORDS ADMINISTRATION[20]

Frequently there are danger signals that personnel management is not what it should be. These warnings include the department that somehow becomes overstaffed; the employee who is hired at an excessive (or inadequate) salary, or who is not paid on time; the salary increase that is lost or bears little resemblance to what is expected; or complaints about inequities or lack of responsiveness.

Such problems may be the result of faulty policies or programs, but often they are caused by fragmented administration. They can be the outcome of decentralized interpretation and administration of policy together with inadequate procedures and personnel records which do not insure consistent and efficient policy implementation.

In years past formal personnel policies and programs were few, and government agencies and regulations made even fewer demands on the employer-employee relationship. But with the mushrooming of demands on health care institutions, the days of the informal handwritten personnel record and the autonomy of each department are rapidly coming to an end.

The concept of centralized personnel administration and records management has three primary hospital objectives. They are:

1. to insure the expeditious and consistent application of hospital personnel policies,

2. to develop and provide data for purposes of reference, information and analysis, and
3. to insure compliance with legal recordkeeping and reporting requirements.

6-1 Centralized Personnel Administration

Personnel policies must be carried out efficiently and uniformly; at the same time necessary information must be stored and retrieved and legal requirements must be met. All personnel actions should be administered by the personnel department to implement hospital-wide policies. This would be an efficient and economical way to improve administrative quality by establishing full-time specialists in complex clerical and professional tasks. It would also limit access to confidential information to the few who need to know.

As soon as personnel departments were established in hospitals some centralization of clerical functions occurred. More recent is the transfer of authority for interpreting personnel policy from the department head to the personnel director, with right of appeal to the hospital administrator.

6-2 Major Personnel Administrative Functions

The administrative section of the personnel department makes no policy decisions. Instead, it processes routine requests according to policy. Unresolved questions are forwarded to the right person. It is the repository for personnel records, and it develops and maintains periodic reports, usually from the computer, for use on a need to know basis. One particularly valuable characteristic of the administrative section is its homogeneous nature. It is concerned with the relationship of all personnel actions to existing hospital policy. Amidst the continuous demand for change and the need to cope with individual problems, the administrative section should be primarily concerned with procedures which efficiently and dependably handle routine matters.

The position control program, employment processing and termination, salary and benefit administration are duties of the administrative section. A number of common but not all-inclusive methods which hospitals have found useful in this area follows.

6-3 Position Control Administration

Large hospitals with substantial turnover (50 to 60 percent) which have internal mobility and fast changing staffing needs require a position code number assigned for each authorized full or part-time position or an authorization in full-time equivalency for each type of position (*e.g.,* 13.5 RNs in I.C.U.) in an expense center. The staffing is agreed upon at the beginning of the fiscal year and usually retained throughout the year. When the administrative section receives a request to fill a vacancy it verifies the opening, possibly on a computer-produced position control report that compares authorized versus actual current staffing. If there is a vacancy, the request will be forwarded to the employment section for action.

One effective *form for requesting a new employee* (see Chapter 16, pages 16:15 and 16:103 which were originally on one sheet of paper) is a full size page perforated in the center with two forms. One form is the request for a new employee and the other is the notification of the vacancy. This supports the position control process and also often alerts the administrative section to a pending termination.

An additional important form *authorizes a new position* in an expense center. Midyear authorization changes upset budget planning but often are necessary to meet unpredicted needs. Position control also requires an orderly process to communicate the updated authorization to both the fiscal and personnel departments. This form doubles as a justification for increased (or decreased) staffing and is retained in the personnel records section.

6-4 Employment Processing

Time is quite critical in processing the newly employed person. Furthermore, if using a computerized payroll system more time is needed to ensure the timely payment of salaries. In many states there is a requirement that a person be paid during the week following the end of the first payweek occurring after he began working.

The employment officer should be made aware promptly of employment decisions and should be a part of those decisions. By the first day of work there should be a folder of information about the new employee sufficient to establish him on both the personnel-payroll computer file and the master employment file. This should be forwarded to the administrative section and should include the employment application and resumé, federal, state, and hospital benefit withholding authorization forms (health insurance), benefit declination forms, any reference checks, and a copy of the employment information form. The request form for a new employee should also be returned to the administrative section for its permanent records.

After once again verifying the availability of the opening, the administrative section should prepare and forward the computer payroll input, simultaneously verifying job code, salary grade, and starting salary as being in accord with hospital policy.

The forms referred to earlier are similar to those used by and familiar to most hospitals. Several forms, however, deserve comment. The *benefit declination form* is one that is more frequently used as benefit programs increase. Where there is a contributory program available all employees should be aware of it and offered the opportunity to participate or to decline in writing. Beyond being good administrative practice, federal agencies want assurances; it also protects the hospital against claims by an employee alleging that the programs were not made available to him.

The *employment information form* is designed to avoid misunderstandings at a time confusing to an employee. It is given to the employee with information about his pay and benefit provisions, the names of his department head and supervisor, work location and starting time on the first day of work.

Finally, it is best to obtain *beneficiary cards* for life insurance along with enrollment forms during the employment procedure, explaining that the benefit is deferred pending a waiting period.

A final comment concerns the impact of temporary employees on position control. Such employees should always be employed for a specific period of time, despite the uncertainty of the situation. The administration section as part of its position control function should periodically review the status of temporary employees to avoid them somehow becoming permanent, obtaining any necessary approvals for continuation. Temporary workers should be made aware that this is established procedure.

6-5 Termination Processing

The process of terminating employment has become an imperfect and sometimes costly operation requiring centralized administration. Hospital workers often leave their jobs without giving notice. In addition to the inconvenience to the work schedule, new cost elements are introduced. Where insurance benefits (health, life and disability) are administered on a self-billing basis, the hospital is responsible for reporting additions to and terminations from the plan. Commonly a hospital inadvertently pays for an employee's coverage after he is no longer employed.

A lack of knowledge can also be unnecessarily costly in unemployment compensation. Since states often require an employer to inform them promptly of the reason for termination or lose appeal rights for liability, it is necessary for the hospital to have the information completed quickly—ideally before the last date of work.

Additionally, other operational factors make it important to improve processing of terminations. Not the least of these factors is the accuracy of the payroll file. There is always the possibility of paying a salary to one who is no longer actually working.

Finally, long-range improvement in employee relations and in hospital operations can be suggested by listening carefully to employees during exit interviews. The person who is leaving has a particularly interesting perspective of alterations which might be valuable to hospital policies.

The formal approach to termination begins with the employee's department head. The combined form for termination/recruitment of replacement is forwarded to the administration section. This form is reviewed for completeness, including a coded reason for the termination. The administration section is responsible for a clear and complete reason and may request greater detail.

Copies of the form are then forwarded both to payroll and to the employment officer; the former as authorization to remove the person from the payroll and the latter for the purpose of a terminal interview. If the employee has left, a questionnaire can be forwarded to his last address.

The master copy of the termination notification is retained for coding computer cards for turnover analysis. It is also used by the insurance billing clerk to adjust the enrollment in the insurance programs.

6-6 Salary Administration and Salary Planning

The administration section's most important activity is salary administration. No personnel function is more crucial to the hospital or the employee than accurate and prompt management of the salary program.

Most salary programs call for pay increases, either in increments or within a range of increase at appointed review dates. Important to this process is the reminder notice sent to department heads alerting them to salary reviews coming due during the following month. This notice, though laborious if done manually, can be justified as a computer operation because it eliminates discontent caused by omission. The master file should include the date of last salary increase and the schedule for salary reviews will have to be established by the computer programmer.

The same computer list can be returned with a change form indicating the recommended new salary for the employee. This becomes the change request and computer input.

Whether the response from the department is by computer list or by individual request for salary increase, the administrative section must determine if it is within salary administration policy and approve it. Coincident with this review, the section compels the completion of any performance appraisals expected at the time of increase. A common problem in relating performance and salary review is the surprising number of situations in which they are seemingly unrelated. The correlation should be reviewed by the administrative section and if at all questionable should be brought to the attention of the personnel director.

Increases should also be correlated with salary plans that were submitted at the beginning of the fiscal year. Variances are brought to the attention of the controller and personnel director if the department budget is likely to be exceeded.

Hospitals employing a single annual salary review date will find an additional advantage in using a computer-generated reminder and request list. This will allow a review of the relative salaries of all employees in a department at the same time; it will also facilitate the review of raises for a large number of employees.

After checking thoroughly for compliance with policy, correlation to performance appraisal, and for relationship to the department's salary plan, salary change requests are transferred to computer input format and forwarded to the payroll section or directly to the computer. A copy of the request form will be returned to the personnel department for the permanent records affirming the change.

Following salary reviews there should be a formal notice to the employee concerning the amount of salary increase, the reason, and the effective date. This may be by memorandum either from the personnel director or from the department head. In a large organization, there is probably need for this to be done centrally. There should, however, be a reference to the part played by the department head (by name) in the salary decision.

6-7 Benefits Administration

The area of insurance and retirement benefits is growing so rapidly that its administration is becoming a specialty of its own. As a result, some hospitals have established separate benefit administration offices. Whether or not this is done in your hospital, a specialist probably is required to administer enrollments, claims, billing procedures and other procedural matters dealing with such benefits.

This specialist's most common responsibilities are health, life, and long- and short-term disability insurance, workman's compensation, unemployment compensation, and pension and tax-deferred annuity programs.

To provide timely enrollment and clear understanding of the various provisions, the insurance paper work should be completed on or before the date of employment, even if there is a waiting period for eligibility. It should be part of the employment process for a new employee to come to the administrative section for a personal briefing and form-signing session conducted by the specialists. Each employee will thus be familiar with the person best able to answer his questions in the future. In addition to the mechanics of enrollments, new employees should be thoroughly briefed on workmen's compensation, unemployment compensation and given some introduction to the pension plan. Insurance forms are forwarded to the insuror as necessary, and deduction authorizations are forwarded to the payroll department. Beneficiary cards are best retained in the administrative section as permanent records.

Claims for life and disability insurance and workmen's compensation should be handled by the administrative section within the hospital. Though the procedures and forms of the insurance carrier are used, several internal matters are of particular concern to the hospital. Since long-term disability insurance is so infrequently used and is often fully paid by the hospital, there is a possibility that employees may not recall its availability. Even department heads have ignored or forgotten the program and terminated an employee for excessive absence. This should be considered by the administrator handling the termination and considered a signal of a possible claim. If they qualify, employees should be retained on the payroll at least until initiation of LTD benefits, and possibly thereafter, if pension benefits are a consideration.

There is probably no single fool proof method of recognizing all employees who should file claims for LTD insurance. It is therefore important that several approaches be used, including:

a. cooperation by department heads in contacting the administrative section about employees with lengthy absences;
b. notification by the payroll department of employees on a no-pay status for longer than a month;
c. check up by the administrative section when a replacement is requested for an ill employee;
d. informal conversation about illnesses.

A reminder file should be maintained by the administrative section concerning the timely filing of LTD claims. It is important for the specialist on benefits to follow up LTD claims to expedite receipt of doctor's certificates, etc., and to insure prompt payments to the employee. Because of complicated procedures and the fact that the employee may be bedridden, there is sometimes a need to physically "walk papers" through the various stages of processing.

The same file may be used as a reminder of such matters as protracted workmen's compensation claims, pending investigations of accidents, employees who are eligible for preretirement counseling and retirement. All require particularly conscious concern and a system to be administered efficiently.

A second claims responsibility requiring systematic management is that of workmen's compensation. Again, it is important for administrative matters to be handled thoroughly and swiftly to assure a disabled employee a continuity of income. Laws in many states also require speedy reporting of work-related injuries and speedy payment of legitimate claims.

Policies should require the department heads to report to the administrative section any work-related injury or disease on the day of occurrence. An accident report form should be submitted on that same day. Procedures designated by the insurance carrier should be followed through swiftly. The benefits specialist should assume the role of advocate to insure timely investigation, acceptance or challenge of the claim, and prompt payment whenever appropriate.

A third claims responsibility occurs in the event of the death of an employee. Though it is difficult to establish formal channels for notification, department heads should contact the personnel director if an employee dies. After briefing by the benefits specialist, the personnel director should notify the hospital administrator, arrange for flowers if appropriate, and for representation at the funeral. He should file claims for life insurance after determining the appropriate beneficiary from the hospital files. Proof of death is normally required in the form of certified copies of the death certificate.

Another administrative task in the benefits area involves billing. For the most part this is governed by the procedures of the carriers; however, a conscious effort must be made to enroll participants as soon as eligible and terminate them as soon as they leave.

The process for including new participants is an extension of the employment procedure. The termination of participants is an extension of the termination procedure. Additionally, a periodic list of new hires and terminations should be prepared on the computer as a cross-check on manual records.

6-8 Uses of the Computer

In recent years, computers have become commonplace in health care institutions as in many other business organizations. One of the most common uses has been to provide personnel management with a substantial opportunity to improve its administrative effectiveness as well as to develop programs and decisions based on a quantitative analysis.

As the largest single area of expense in a hospital, the payroll system is frequently the first major computer application. The expansion of the payroll master file to include personnel information that is not payroll-related results in an ability to improve personnel administration in three major areas, including:

1. Administration of the economic provisions of personnel policy (*e.g.,* salary and premium programs) or similar provisions of collective bargaining agreements, by the go-no-go abilities of the computer (excluding value judgments);
2. Maintenance of personnel records, at least in part, by computer-generated information; and
3. Providing statistical information for analysis, program control and individual reference.

6-9 Computerized Administration of Economic Policies

Before computers, department heads often had to specifically request the payment of overtime and shift premiums by requesting the total amount actually due. Accuracy depended upon their recalling that a premium was called for by policy. Frequently the exact hourly rate was also subject to individual recollection.

This was a source of continual error because of both memory lapse and misunderstanding of policy by the department head. It resulted in poor employee relations despite thoughtful policies, in the tarnished image of the department head, and often in the violation of the federal wage and hour law.

A well-programmed computerized payroll should exclude the department head from all interpretation of amounts payable except where value judgments are involved. Shift premiums are based on established quantitative criteria, not personal judgments.

While the computer is able to make such "interpretations," it is necessary to provide the proper programming and payroll input. A test should be made to compare each employee's payroll entries for eligibility for a shift premium based on the hours worked against the hours when the premium is payable. If the hourly premium rate is based on the employee's job or salary grade, reference should be made to this information, available in coded form on the employee's master file.

In summary, given the proper payroll data and programmed to be aware of such policies as overtime, premiums, paid meal breaks, and vacation and sick leave accruals and usage, the computer should be used to determine what amount of payment is due. This should take place without manual intervention. There should be automatic updating of such information as vacation and sick leave accruals. A computer application is a major step toward centralizing the more mechanical yet highly important aspects of personnel administration in a large health care facility.

6-10 The Computerized Personnel Record

The maintenance of personnel records has been greatly modernized by computer technology. Prior to electronic data processing, record maintenance involved substantial manual posting and filing operations. The personnel department kept up the employee's record card, which included all basic information including entries of salary and other status changes. The same records were often duplicated in various departments.

This was not only unwieldy and expensive, it was often inaccurate because of transcribing errors, omissions, and erroneous interpretation.

The expanded personnel/payroll master file of information has a mirror image in the computer of practically all pertinent information maintained manually at the personnel and department levels. This provides the potential for major reduction in clerical work at both of these locations.

Much of the need for reference information concerns an employee's current status (*e.g.,* department, salary, job, grade). This data is readily available on a periodic computer-prepared list, with copies kept in the personnel and department offices. Only historical information is not available directly from the computer.

There is limited use for historical employee information, particularly where high turnover and short service exist. The need does exist, however, to document incidents such as grievances; it is thus important that a complete history be available. The most efficient method of storing this information is again in the computer.

As changes in status occur and the master file is updated, a card output should be produced reflecting the updated file, listing the old and new information. By serially numbering cards for each employee, a complete historical record will be available. In addition, there will be feedback to the personnel department of all status changes.

6-11 The Computerized Report

The personnel/payroll master file can provide a wealth of information, but there can be a significant amount of misjudgment involved in using it. It is tempting to request a large amount of trivial information and provide it to managers without sufficient introduction to its possible use or to refrain from using data that could be of substantial help if provided in a different format.

Three general types of reports are particularly useful in personnel administration, and can be justified economically by reducing the manual process, improving management controls, or (most difficult to quantify) providing analysis that supports the decision-making process, particularly in salary and benefit matters.

The *listing-type* report has already been mentioned as a substitute for traditional recordkeeping. Such reports may be used not only for individual reference but can also identify employees in selected jobs, salary grades, expense centers, minority groups, ages, lengths of service, sex, marital status, or any other characteristic on file.

The *summary-type* report is an outgrowth of the employee list, but it focuses on numbers rather than individuals and involves only the adding of data. The federal EEOC report on minority and female representation can be compiled quickly and automatically. Other examples include:

- Comparison of staffing authorizations with staffing complements;
- Total employees in full-time equivalent (F.T.E.s) classifications.

Such summaries disclose trends, and can be used for analyses on which to base management decisions.

Analytical reports are often underutilized, although they have the potential for substantial contribution. Computers can be programmed to make simple decisions. Substantial computer generated assistance is available to analyze large amounts of data that are unmanageable with manual methods, to compute even a smaller volume of data, or to project and propose a model based on data already built into an existing computer program.

There is often great disparity between the amount of analysis preceding decisions on one-time capital expenditures and the casual review that sometimes precedes personnel decisions involving substantial ongoing expenses. With computer capability there is now little excuse for proposing such economic personnel changes based strictly on subjective analysis without supportive quantitative evaluation.

Of the many such proposals and questions, some that lend themselves particularly to computer analysis include:

a. What would be the impact, direct and indirect, of selected salary scale adjustment to various salary grades?

b. What effect would the submitted salary planning proposals have on the hospital's salary expenses?

c. What would be the financial impact of a market basket approach to benefit options, given various assumptions of employee response?

d. What would be the effect of increased vacation or sick leave programs on absence and staffing needs, or a short-term disability program integrated with limited sick leave?

e. What progress has been made in affirmative action regarding employment, retention, promotions, and levels in the organization?

f. Where is the controllable turnover occurring— and for what reasons?

The variety of questions subject to quantitative analysis is substantial and dependent primarily on the analytical abilities of the personnel and systems staff and the extent of coded information maintained in the master file. Though each hospital has unique information needs, there are some reports that provide particularly basic information. A list of such computer reports can be found in Chapter 17.

There is a tendency in some organizations to develop computer reports in large numbers without full assessment of their value. This is not only uneconomical, it is also unjustified.

There are questions which should be asked before requesting computer support. How frequently will your report be used? How valid is the data? If it is for a one-time need can the request be amended to anticipate future needs? Better yet, can information be used from other completed reports with the final product being done manually? Finally, what is the cost of developing the information to furnish the report?

The computer report should be made as useful as possible. Often such reports supply a large volume of information in coded form, which may be understandable to the computer-oriented specialist in personnel or fiscal services, but is, however, quite mysterious to many department heads and often to administrators as well.

If it is sometimes necessary to distribute coded lists or reports, an explanation of all codes and of the most significant data on the list should be included with the distribution. It is more desirable to distribute computer information in a noncoded report form. This is clearer, more concise, more useful, and minimizes the amount of extraneous and often confidential material that is circulated.

6-12 Staffing the Administration Section

There are three distinct areas needed in the administration section of a personnel department. In a larger hospital, staffing would require a supervisor who may be called Manager of Personnel Administration, who is responsible for the operational functions described in this chapter. In a smaller hospital this person may well be the "number two" person in the department, either the Assistant Personnel Director or the Salary Administrator.

The holder of this position will probably have a four-year college background in personnel management or business administration. By training or aptitude he should be knowledgeable in the analytical and systems areas. He should also have a working knowledge of salary administration and personnel policies and procedures and a sensitivity to their objectives. By instinct he should be able to get results and particularly able to interact with all levels of management in stress situations. He should have full responsibility for administration of personnel changes, should handle as many matters of interpretation as proper coordination and his abilities permit, and be responsible for manual and computer systems development.

The other two important people in the administration section are senior clerical specialists in the areas of salary administration and benefits administration. Both need post high school training, but just as importantly should have extensive experience in their specialties, hopefully in hospitals. They should bring to their positions knowledge of procedures and objectives, an analytical ability, and a sensitivity to deadlines. Most important is their ability to interact with employees as knowledgeable and understanding management representatives, willing and able to be employee advocates achieving results through the administrative system.

With a little creativity, the contribution of this trio to the total personnel program can be magnified substantially. Too often this group finds itself limited to work within the office area. Yet they are the people best able to answer the questions most frequently asked by and most important to individual employees. It is often effective employer relations for these staff members to meet periodically with small groups of employees in informal question and answer sessions at the various departments. Not only are employee questions resolved, but the interest levels of the staff members are raised by their personal contacts, resulting in a more responsive department.

6-13 Personnel Files

As well as being the central administrator of personnel activity, the administrative section is responsible for records relating to hospital-wide personnel management. Though these increasingly involve computerized records, the manual record will remain important.

The master *employee file* is the primary record. It assembles all original documents relating to an employee from his application to his termination. It includes all status changes, salary and otherwise, and is available to back up any question or challenge to the hospital, legal or otherwise. Such documentation is especially important with noneconomic and EEO regulations, where management may be required to justify promotions, layoffs, and disciplinary actions including terminations for cause. Therefore, copies of performance appraisals and reprimands are an important part of the file.

The *employee history record* has traditionally been a hand-posted card-type record of employee status changes. As discussed in the section on "Use of the Computer," there are now alternative approaches to maintaining this manual status record. Current status information is available from computerized reports, which diminishes the importance of a manually maintained card for that purpose. Other alternatives are possible if the history is retained in the computer and produced periodically or when a change occurs. The computer can accumulate a chronology of change.

Some hospitals have elected to eliminate the manual card as a continuing record of employee status. If so, it is doubly important to insure the integrity of the computer master file and to provide a standard format for reconstructing a physical record when individual situations require it.

The administrative section maintains *the computerized report* including both listing format and statistical analysis. By keeping these reports in a central location, authorized persons will have access to them for diverse purposes. Such a library should reduce requests for computer reports for information that is already available. Ideally, the manager of personnel administration should insure the most efficient approach to information gathering. The large and awkward size of the documents tends to promote careless handling, so the administrative section should have facilities to store computer lists as confidential documents, eliminating the hazard of private information becoming common knowledge.

The administrative section has responsibility for other special-purpose files, such as:

Department Salary Plans—indicating when increases of various amounts are planned for individual employees, as estimated in the hospital-wide salary budget policy.

Master Position Control File—indicating the authorized staffing levels for each job and department. Authorized mid-year changes should also be filed here.

Master Personnel Policy Files—including any important backup.

Beneficiary Card Files—for employee life insurance.

A Reminder File—to follow up on such matters as salary reviews, benefit claims outstanding and deadline-related projects.

Claims Files—including separate files for data relating to disability and workmen's compensation claims.

Termination Information—often key-punched onto IBM cards for periodic analysis using the termination reason codes.

Job Evaluation Files—retained in this section unless there is an authorized person with day-to-day need for the information.

6-14 Accessibility of Information

Employees of hospital personnel departments share the same unique responsibility as most other hospital employees; the information they deal with is privileged and confidential. This is as true for the salary clerk with employee information as it is for the physician or RN with patient information. Just as in clinical areas, a breach of confidential information by personnel department employees is a major infraction often resulting in disciplinary action. It is with this thought in mind that the question of accessibility to information takes on major significance.

Three general rules are often adopted by personnel departments to protect confidentiality.

1. Information about individual employees is available to managers only on a strict need-to-know basis, with very few having unlimited access (*e.g.*, the administration and personnel director). Thus, managers ordinarily have access only to information on their own employees. Statistical information is available to managers on a need-to-manage basis, with far fewer limitations than personal information;

2. Government agencies may acquire access to information about individuals based on a court order and have access to statistical information to ascertain compliance with laws and regulations with the full cooperation of the hospital, where requests appear reasonable;

3. Other outside parties have access to factual information on individual employees (*e.g.*, salary, length of service) other than management information, only with the consent of the employee. Statistical information is available if specifically authorized by the personnel director.

Personnel department staff members work within these three constraints to insure that necessary information is available for purposes of implementing personnel management programs and also in accordance with legal requirements. In this era of public concern over unauthorized intrusion, sound employee relations and court decisions suggest that employers refrain from maintaining data not related to employment or legal requirements.

Though much of the information developed is used internally, there are occasions when information is needed by managers outside the personnel department. The question then arises as to how, and to what extent, information should be provided. This is when the "need-to-know" concept should be applied, remembering that original records should not ordinarily be released from the department. Following this policy not only safeguards information but also lessens a manager's responsibility for sensitive information not essential to his needs.

The personnel record file should be retained in the personnel department. Authorized personnel should have access to it and copy pertinent information when necessary, in lieu of allowing the record outside the department. This will sometimes be an unpopular policy, but it is necessary to insure the integrity and confidentiality of the file.

If this limitation causes unhappiness, it may be that departments are not receiving sufficient information on a periodic basis. This can be corrected by developing a computer report for department heads with up-to-date pertinent information on their personnel. Though some hospitals are reluctant to distribute such information for fear of its falling into the wrong hands, others suggest that a department head must be trusted to handle sensitive information which better enables him to do his job.

If additional information is required, the department can provide the specifics needed. This can be done for senior officers in the hospital as well as department heads.

The health care facility must also develop a policy of handling outside requests for employee information, usually reference checks by other employers or credit information for firms and banks.

Employers nation-wide are increasingly reluctant to cooperate with such reference checking, as a result of the public's outcry at the careless provision and misuse of reference information. With this in mind it is important to observe strict procedures for disclosure.

Telephoned reference requests from employers are not ordinarily honored without verifying the caller's identity. This is done by calling the organization allegedly making the request at a number the hospital's representative finds listed. The reference information is limited to the last appraisal that the employee has seen and been allowed to comment on. Particularly damaging evaluations should be handled by the manager of personnel administration or his superior.

Written references from employers are handled in much the same fashion. Addresses of firms are verified and information is based on the last substantive evaluation made available to the employee. Such references deal with the hospital's assessment of the person as a past employee, and do not focus on confidential factual information.

Retailers' requests concern information which should not be volunteered. Rather, the personnel department should only verify information disclosed to the caller by the employee, following authentication of the caller's identity.

6-15 Security of Information

A final consideration in records management concerns the physical security of records. Although not a new problem, it has become more significant due to the increase in volume of information and the way it is packaged.

The security of manual records, particularly personnel files, requires that a check-out procedure be established when records are elsewhere even in the department. Follow-up and retrieval should be diligent. Within the section, where large numbers of records are in constant use, particular attention is needed at the close of each business day to be sure they are returned to a locked file cabinet.

There should be a schedule for disposal of no longer needed records to minimize the volume handled and substantially ease the security problem. Personnel files are often retained too long after an employee leaves, when they no longer fill legal requirements or have practical reference value. The resulting back-up of old records complicates the ability to handle current ones. If it is believed necessary to retain information beyond five to six years after an employee leaves, a space-saving alternative to total retention is to retain only the employee history card, and/or the final performance appraisal.

Computer lists and reports are a particularly unique security problem. They are large and unwieldy, and include details of many employees in a single report, compounding the damage resulting from their loss. In addition, they are updated weekly or monthly; therefore, there is a rapid build up of old reports and difficulty in recognizing that a theft has occurred.

Security of computer produced material depends largely on filing organization and planned disposal. Computer lists should be shredded or burned under the supervision of a personnel department representative on a weekly or bi-weekly basis, depending on the frequency with which they are issued.

7 TRAINING

The U.S. health system has long been conscious that training is a necessary adjunct to both patient care and research.

Hospitals have traditionally played a large role in the teaching of physicians. But it was not until the technology explosion of the 1950s and 1960s, along with awakening public expectations for better medical care, that serious doubts were voiced concerning our nation's ability to provide the numbers of people and variety of skills health care facilities would need in the 1970s and 1980s. In the year 1900 the number of practicing physicians was equal to all other health workers combined. By 1940 the nonphysician group had increased to a ratio of 5:1. It was estimated at 11:1 in 1960 and 13:1 in 1973. Indications are that by 1980, twenty allied health workers will be needed for every practicing physician.

Technology has spawned a host of unique and highly specialized skills, and the end is not in sight. Almost weekly new jobs are created. Others are combined or eliminated. Still others are retitled to reflect broadened responsibilities.

One perceptible result of all this is that the physician is being viewed more as the senior member of what is essentially a team effort. Younger doctors, in particular, seem to welcome this new opportunity to practice their skills over a wider range of patients. In the years just ahead we may find, for example, the nurse practitioner or physician assistant an altogether acceptable deliverer of health services. Says Dr. Alfred Yankauer, "Both . . . have now been produced and utilized in sufficient numbers to demonstrate unequivocally that as many as 50-75% of the U.S. ambulatory primary care encounters traditionally calling for the 'physician's touch' can be handled alone by a non-physician, working in collaboration or close communication with a physician upon whom he can draw for back-up in those cases which he cannot handle alone."[21]

Our efforts to cope in the late 1960s with what appeared to be an incipient health manpower crisis were not always fruitful. A stupefying variety of privately and publicly financed training schemes were directed toward health-related occupations. Many were ill-defined. Others imparted skills for which no clear demand was evident. Some were categorical, underwriting only the training of the poor, veterans, or minorities—with little foresight to prepare for the despair engendered once the money was spent, the syllabus learned, and the promise of jobs still unmet. Planners often neglected to address employers' absolute as well as seasonal needs until a whole class was ready to graduate. For their part, employers avowed a need for mathematics or chemistry when in truth they meant only arithmetic or weighing and measuring.

Yet many successful training efforts were launched, and a fair number still survive. Perhaps there is an excuse. Who could have foreseen the end of typhoid fever, diphtheria, pulmonary tuberculosis or poliomyelitis, together with their elaborate technologies? Heart disease, genetic catastrophe, cancer, rheumatoid arthritis—these and others may similarly respond to some higher understanding of the disease process. We may then need to shift our manpower again.

Meanwhile, the recent past has taught those who train or finance training a few useful lessons, and it is possible to make some tentative assessments and recommendations.

To begin with, the personnel director knows that training can be expensive, its results hard to measure. He must also understand that trained health manpower is at once his most valuable yet fragile asset. A hospital training program provides a whole environment where gifted people should want to learn, produce, and help cure the ill. Training should thus reflect the continuing internal need for specialized skills and the more elusive goals of good employee relations.

There remains an even larger public policy question, one requiring the personnel director to examine health manpower training as a cooperative rather than a solitary venture. It may be summarized through the following observations and proposals.

1. The creation and maintenance of a trained pool of health manpower is a community-wide problem. The cost of education and training ought to be underwritten—in part at least—by the public which demands and consumes health resources. One-third of our nursing graduates, for example, still come from programs based in hospitals. Most impose severe and unequal burdens on already strained finances.
2. Training should be of uniformly high quality.
3. Skills ought to be readily transferable from one institution to another.
4. Employers should participate in setting trainee selection standards, course content, and by providing teachers.
5. Trained health manpower ought to be available at those times of year when the need is greatest.
6. Class size should be geared to carefully predetermined market needs balanced against maximum economy of training effort.
7. Subjects common to more than one occupation ought to be taught at the same time.
8. Individuals, once trained, should be able to progress within health occupations to the extent of their own abilities.
9. Members of minority groups as well as the unskilled and underskilled should be included in the health system through special training programs. Training ought not be confused with the edification of the young. Age alone should not be a deterrent to the ongoing educative process.
10. Gender-related stereotypes (*e.g.*, female nurses; male physicians) need further examination. Deliberate effort is required to encourage the entrance of women into traditionally male occupations and vice versa. Male/female or black/white wage differentials should be sought out and eliminated.
11. Trained workers deserve to be paid no less than what comparable skills command in nonmedical fields.
12. Equal opportunities, equal pay for equal work, and compliance with affirmative action programs and other federal regulations should be actively encouraged.
13. The needs of employer and employee have basic similarities. Both must gain from resources ex-

pended on training; the patient should ultimately profit most.

Education and training cannot take place in an academic vacuum. Wasted time and expenses inevitably result when neighboring institutions each establish programs to train small numbers of people. By using the facilities of a single hospital for basic instruction, the technicians most localities might need could be trained at an affordable cost. On a larger scale, hospitals have demonstrated the value of regional or centralized facilities. Several hospitals could participate in developing curriculum materials, funding (grants or tuition payments), teachers, surplus equipment, and the like. Local high schools and colleges can provide the needed classroom instruction and, for certain occupations, academic credits required by national certification bodies.[22]

Cooperation offers other advantages. Technical developments can be quickly communicated and shared. Curricula can be shortened, lengthened or altered to fit changing job requirements. Participating institutions could determine the annual supply-demand cycle for skilled people in its broadest perspective and arrange graduation dates to coincide with demonstrated seasonal needs. State employment services have proved most helpful in conducting spot surveys of vacancies. In an eastern city, for example, a one day sampling of those hospitals comprising 40% of the area's bed capacity revealed 10 vacancies for trained histology technicians. Six months later the vacancies for all hospitals (based on the same 40% bed sample) were estimated at 25. Since only enough equipment, money, and teachers were available to train 8 technicians and the specter of sampling error existed, 8 began the six month classroom-laboratory portion of the program. Six months later the 6 who finished training started their clinical affiliations at a time when predictions had proven sufficiently accurate to find places for them in participating hospitals. This approach has been used with success in the training of nursing aides, dental assistants, medical transcribers, orthopedic technicians, and others. Seasonal demand can never be predicated with complete accuracy. It is therefore prudent to train somewhat fewer people than appear to be needed. Training resources can thus be spread over more occupations. Remaining manpower deficits will normally be alleviated by already existing instruction programs and by individuals moving into your area.

Wasted dollars are not the only penalty our educational system's lack of vigilance has wrought. More graduates of many six-month to four-year courses find no jobs awaiting them because educators and hospitals have not developed even the simplest predictive tools

which may make students who would want to switch majors aware of changing manpower demands. The alarming rise in both education and health care costs and the frequent misdirection of training effort make it all the more imperative for institutions to look beyond their own walls and work in concert to develop a series of rational supply-demand equations.

We have, of course, been discussing education and training in its largest sense. Many other alternatives exist. These include the following.

- Formal RN, LPN, x-ray, laboratory and similar training programs leading to licensure or national certification.
- Hospital-paid educational conferences and memberships in national societies for managerial and technical employees.
- Tuition and programs under which the institution reimburses a portion of tuition costs to an employee who has successfully completed previously approved courses. (See Chapter 16 for a sample form.)
- Management development courses and conferences sponsored by state hospital associations, the American Management Association, the Health Law Center, and similar organizations. It is important to reinforce such activities through regular management meetings, newsletters, and objective setting and evaluating conferences between the manager and his seniors.
- In-service training on a continuing basis. These programs have long been employed by nursing departments and range from attendance at grand rounds to demonstrations of body mechanics, first aid procedures and fire safety. The in-service training concept is expandable to almost every other hospital department.
- On-the-job training. It is done now every time a supervisor teaches a new employee how to post a credit, wax a floor, or prepare a salt-free meal. The Hospital Research & Educational Trust (HRET) of the American Hospital Association offers a wide variety of training manuals covering a number of occupations. Professional societies also sell or rent slides, training films and the like, covering their own fields. One or two phone calls or letters could save time and money in locating ready-made training materials.
- Special programs. These include brush-up typing, telephone techniques, Spanish conversation, English as a second language, medical terminology, radiation safety, racial awareness, etc. Once established, those programs lend themselves easily to cooperative ventures among neighboring hospi-

tals. One institution, by inviting others to send employees to its 44-hour medical terminology course, was able to reduce the out-of-pocket cost to $10 per employee trained. The other hospitals reciprocated in kind.

It is imperative that the teaching-learning process must resolve first around objectives. To permit it to focus elsewhere is to risk needlessly scarce resources for uncertain gain. Before embarking on any new training program or taking advantage of an existing one, ask the following questions.

1. Is there a continuing demand for this skill in your hospital? Could the need be caused by low pay or poor supervision? Could it be remedied more cheaply than through a training program?
2. What benefit will the hospital gain from offering this course?
3. What is the estimated cost per person trained? What is the total cost of the program including space?
4. How long should each training cycle last? When should it be repeated?
5. Does the course already exist elsewhere? Would your present tuition assistance program be less costly?
6. Released time, versus on-the-job training, versus after-hours program—which approach is best?
7. What, if any, academic credit can be given to course graduates? With minor changes, can national accrediting standards be met, if such exist?
8. Will vendors (*e.g.*, telephone company, IBM) help underwrite courses using their equipment?
9. Who will develop the curriculum? What materials are already available and may be bought or borrowed?
10. Who will teach the course? Understanding a subject is one thing, being able to teach it is quite another.
11. Can the course be taught better with audiovisual aids? Have you considered movies, slides, tapes, closed circuit television?
12. Does the course lend itself to individual or small group training as well as to larger classes? Conversely, can you train ten students as cheaply as five?
13. Is your training site conducive to learning? Is it convenient, pleasant, and quiet? Learning is difficult. Do not create additional problems.
14. Are department heads and supervisors supportive? What part did they play in curriculum development? Will they make good teachers?
15. Should course attendance be mandatory?
16. What recognition should be given those completing the course—certificate, promotion, pay increase?
17. What effect will the course have on your employee relations image?
18. Could the program be shared with the employees of neighboring hospitals? Could you reciprocate with other institutions and make training less costly for all?

Many institutions have created, equipped and staffed centralized facilities to coordinate training activities. No one person can develop adequate expertise in all fields. The training director's role therefore is one of leadership in:

surveying training needs
stimulating ideas and selecting alternatives
procuring of resources such as money, training equipment and teachers
curriculum development
educating teachers
developing alliances with other hospitals, colleges and government agencies to conduct training on a cooperative basis
preparing training grant applications to foundations and government agencies
evaluating results

Education and training are the responsibility of every manager and supervisor throughout the institution. Under the guidance of the personnel director or training director all should expect to participate actively in the management of change. All must be encouraged to search both internally and externally for the means to create new skills and update old ones. Only in this manner will a sensible strategy of manpower development replace the caprice and waste of the past.[23]

8 DEVELOPING PERSONNEL POLICIES

Personnel policies, as the heart of any personnel program, deserve particular attention if they are to achieve several important objectives. By thoughtful development and communication such policies can:

- Insure to all employees an equitable level of treatment.
- Insure to the hospital the optimum level of cost efficiency in personnel decisions.

- Provide to managers and supervisors valuable supportive guidelines for management action.
- Insure employee confidence in the hospital, minimizing the potential for union organization.
- Insure that the hospital complies with governmental laws and regulations.

8-1 Personnel Policy Subject Matter

There are probably as many opinions as there are hospitals of what is appropriate subject matter for personnel policies. Broad coverage is needed to be in keeping with two current trends that have particular impact on hospital administration.

First, people are increasingly suspect of large institutions and often suspect their employers as well. As employees they want a clear understanding of their rights as well as the rules under which they work. These demands come from a variety of sources on behalf of employees—from state and federal governments, from professional organizations, from labor unions, and from individual employees.

Such demands for information and assurances are reasonable and have encouraged hospitals to review and update programs and policies and to define more equitable employee relations practices.

A second trend affects management practices and policies. The public increasingly demands improved quality and efficiency from hospitals. Since the payroll is the largest single component of hospital expense, policies regarding personnel management and expense are often incorporated as "personnel policy." The personnel policy manual therefore must include an extensive employee relations policy as well as a management policy.

In terms of categories, there are several broad subjects that are generally defined as personnel policy.

1. *Salary Programs and Economic Benefits* involving direct payment to the employee or direct cost to the hospital (policies of salary grades and ranges, shift premium pay, vacation leave, benefits and life insurance).
2. *Noneconomic Benefits and Employee Services* including those whose cost to the hospital is not as visible (employee health services, credit unions, arrangements for tax-deferred annuities or pre-retirement counseling).
3. *Employee Relations Practices* encompassing hospital-wide work rules and employee rights (grievance and disciplinary procedures, meal and rest break provisions, attendance/absenteeism policies).

4. *Major Noneconomic Personnel Programs* which are both hospital and employee oriented (performance appraisal, the employee communications system, employee training and development, and the retirement policy).
5. *Management Oriented Personnel Policies and Procedures* involving control over personal utilization or expense (centralized employment, authorizing new positions, employment of relatives) and; finally,
6. *Statements of Support and Compliance* with laws and regulations involving either the required or voluntary statement of policy in areas such as Equal Employment Opportunity, Affirmative Action, and the Employee Retirement Income Security Act disclosure provisions.

It is important to consider what subject matter is inappropriate. By definition, that which is included as hospital-wide policy limits the options and initiatives of individual managers. In light of this, it is necessary to balance the need for hospital-wide policy with the need to inspire vigorous and innovative management within the various departments.

To achieve this balance, broad policies often define areas reserved to the initiative of department managers. This is particularly important in salary administration, with employee evaluations, promotions, and with grievance and disciplinary actions.

Additionally, problem areas and programs which are truly unique to a department should be managed by that department head in collaboration with the director of personnel. The personnel professional can do more than interpret hospital-wide policy. As an adviser and consultant to department heads and as a representative of the administrator, he can develop departmental policy with a department head and influence the "grass roots" policies and practices of the hospital.

8-2 Approaches to Policy Development

Since the time when all hospital policies were the strict prerogative of the trustees, a more comprehensive system for policy development has evolved, including several possible approaches dependent on needs and subject matter. Two premises have been accepted by many trustees and administrators.

First, many policies have become so complex that they require management specialists including personnel people, fiscal professionals and legal and actuarial consultants, to draft and advise on policy.

The second premise recognizes that a policy's success is as dependent on its acceptability as it is on its technical excellence. Personnel policies particularly have a very personal impact on employees whose response and support (or acquiescence) can significantly influence their long-range success.

Also important to the implementation of a new policy is its degree of acceptability to managers and supervisors. As the first-level interpreters and administrators of policy they influence its success by their own degree of commitment. They are in a position to accurately gauge its strengths and weaknesses and potential for acceptance by employees. Both supervisors and employees should be sold a new policy. More important, both groups can contribute valuable suggestions for improving personnel policy.

Though the nature of personnel policies requires the involvement of many, the professionally trained personnel director is the natural "floor manager." He must: (1) sense where policy change is needed; (2) integrate the ideas of others to complement his own; (3) develop the technical data required to support recommendations; and (4) sell the resulting new or changed policies to the administrators as well as to those who will be affected by the changes. To do this, he must encourage participation of the appropriate groups.

Employee participation is probably the least utilized and most underestimated necessity. Though the opportunities for *formal* participation are limited if actual collective bargaining is to be avoided, contacts with employees should be continuous and ongoing. Small group meetings between employees and personnel professionals, *with and without* supervisors present, effectively indicate that the hospital is seriously interested in the employees' viewpoint on personnel policy. As a continuing process, meetings provide a means of gauging employees' attitudes and the hospital's need for change, particularly towards employee relations policies.

It is possible to encourage employee participation by conducting a nonbinding referendum concerning a choice among several possible benefit improvements. Usually the question is over several possible changes in a single benefit (*e.g.,* additions to health insurance).

Manager and supervisor participation in policy development should be more formalized and extensive. By establishing a standing Personnel Policy Advisory Committee of representative managers and supervisors, this group can be involved in several levels of policy development. By its continuing dialogue with the personnel director it provides a two-way conduit for information and ideas, a "sensing" device to anticipate needed change.

In its role in reviewing and advising on draft policies, it improves their overall quality and provides an indication of the reception they will receive if adopted. An additional benefit is the supervisory development which occurs when supervisors become involved in hospital-wide policy. Their perspectives can be substantially broadened by the experience, and the hospital can evaluate promotable supervisors.

The Personnel Policy Advisory Committee is a practical means of gaining continuous operating level management input and guaranteeing a vigorous pace of policy improvement. In practice, all managers and supervisors should have an opportunity to contribute to the policy review process. This can be done by making sure that supervisors are made aware when a subject is to be reviewed and to invite their comments. Policy review may also be the subject of periodic management meetings.

Technical/Managerial participation in policy development usually focuses on the personnel director and his staff. As the "floor manager" as well as the staff professional he is responsible for the process from the original draft policy to the presentation of the recommendation for administrative approval. It is essential that operating managers at the associate/assistant director level be involved in the most appropriate way that the nature of the policy suggests. Ideally, this should be a one-on-one review with the personnel director. Although associates may not have formal responsibility for such policy, they are keystones to its effective implementation. Their support is essential to its success.

The personnel director is also "floor manager" on economic policies requiring technical expertise for prudent and efficient salary and benefits programs. In these areas, the fiscal director provides valuable counsel and support and should collaborate in the presentation. Participation in economic policy development should be limited to senior associates to insure confidentiality during the preparation stage.

Finally, there is sometimes a need in policy development for *consultant participation*. The hospital must function within the law, and its policy commitments must be prudent. Though the trained personnel professional should be competent in legal and actuarial subjects, he should also be aware when outside support is needed.

Legal and actuarial consultants should be acquainted with the hospital on a continuing basis. Management consultants can be valuable particularly to augment the personnel professional on major program and policy development. Consultants in labor relations, unemployment and workmen's compensation should be frequently called upon. Most consultants will agree that they will provide the technical absolutes, but that the total policy must complement the personality and needs of the individual hospital. In this regard, consultant participation augments rather than replaces the participation of others.

There may be questions as to the relative value of participation versus speed in implementation. The personnel director will find himself in the role of expediter, often establishing a schedule for completion of the policy review and fitting participation within that schedule.

It should be emphasized, however, that this model is designed to move toward more effective policies and a more democratic process and to achieve the success of policies requiring support by large numbers of supervisors and employees. Ideally it should prevent the commitment of the hospital to an impractical or unacceptable policy.

8-3 Communicating New Personnel Policy

The so-called "moment of truth" for a new personnel policy is the time when the change is announced to those who will administer and be affected by it. The best opportunity to communicate, to sell, and to gain support for a new policy is at the time of its introduction, when important impressions are being formed.

Where personnel policy is concerned, there are two important audiences for communications, the managers and supervisors, who are the interpreters and administrators, and the employees to whom the policy applies. Each group has its own information needs and each will have its own momentary anxieties.

Supervisors will want to be familiar with the policy in a personal way if, in fact, it affects them as individuals. In addition they will want to feel comfortable administering the policy. Hence, they will need added background and information on procedures and rules to be sufficiently knowledgeable to answer employee questions.

Employees may respond to the change with exuberance, animosity, or with disinterest, but always with a degree of apprehension. Specifically designed communication approaches for each group are necessary for success.

8-4 The Personnel Policy Manual

The principal and most permanent communicator of policy is the Personnel Policy Manual. Its principal value is as a basic all-inclusive document to insure continuity of policy interpretation. Equally important, it is a guideline and reference for management action and the basis for other communications.

Because of their complicated mission, policy manuals should be attractive, written in a vigorous and straightforward style, and well-organized as an easy reference. The presentation should dictate a smoothly functioning policy.

The manual should be designed as a reference to (1) the philosophical statement or intent of the hospital on a certain subject (Statement of Policy), (2) the resulting rules, regulations, and necessary explanations, and (3) operating procedures to insure that the policy is effectively carried out. Except for the statement of policy, which is basic, the other components will vary dependent on the policy.[24]

The format should serve the needs of the policy. It needs to be flexible rather than rigid. Hence, one policy manual may include a list of rules while another may include, instead, a question and answer format. There might be examples of how the policy will affect an employee (e.g., payment of pension or disability benefits), or a chart to show who is involved and how they are affected (e.g., vacation benefits varying by time and job category).

The Personnel Policy Manual will be used principally by supervisors, managers, and administrators, including the personnel department staff, although it is designed for employees as well as employers. Thus, management should be expected to be fully acquainted with it. It should be the subject of management meetings, and everyone at management levels should be responsible for understanding it.

Additionally, employees should be aware of it and it should be available to them. All new policies should be posted on bulletin boards and distributed to all new employees at their orientation.

Unquestionably the complexity of the Personnel Policy Manual will vary with the size and complexity of the hospital. Large hospitals will tend to have more detailed policies and rules (see Chapter 16 for The Peter Bent Brigham Manual, that of a 2,000 employee teaching hospital).

Smaller hospitals may well have policies that are simpler and fewer in number. In such cases the Personnel Policy Manual may be a major section of a hospital administrative manual.

8-5 Policy Communication

The strategy of introducing new policy includes not only critical timing but also a selection of media based on the size and nature of the audience. Though they will usually be of interest to all supervisors, some policies may interest only a select involved employee group (e.g., management employee salary administration or authorization of new positions). Some will be important to employees' families (e.g., salary and economic benefits), whereas other policies will be of interest principally to employees only (*e.g.*, meal breaks).

Communication to management should precede other publicity and be as comprehensive as possible. Senior associates should receive copies of new policies prior to others and at that time comment or question the director of personnel. A management meeting (with supervisors) should also precede a general announcement at which time a descriptive presentation should be made. Policies and policy summaries should be distributed together with the communication that will be sent to employees. This meeting should precede notice to employees by a day or two to enable managers to resolve any questions they may have.

If it is a major policy change, managers and supervisors should be requested to discuss it with employees in a group setting directly after the employee notification. On major policy matters the administrator should initially notify the employees. For minor policies the personnel director re-enforced by managers informs the employees. The initial contact may take the form of an internal letter, letter in the employee house organ, or a letter to the home if the subject matter is appropriate. An alternative approach for lesser matters is to provide an enclosure to the pay envelope.

In addition, bulletin boards should carry a copy of the new policy and all communication should include two or more telephone numbers to call for further information. These telephones, in the personnel department, should be staffed for a period to accommodate evening and night shift employees. The personnel department should also be available to speak to groups within other departments as requested. This is particularly valuable for policies that are more consecutive than past practice.

The above sequence will, of course, vary with the circumstances and the magnitude of the policy involved. It is, however, important to consider these as basic components in most situations. They include notification to management on a personalized basis followed by employee notification by both administrators and supervisors. Supervisors take a great interest in and are thus involved in the success of the program or policy. Personnel professionals should always be available as communicators and to support operating supervisors. With policy success the communication process should meld the management group more closely together and generate increased confidence by employees in the hospital's employee relations program.

9 COMMUNICATIONS

Effective communications are indispensable to a sound program of employee relations. The goals of such a program can, in fact, only be achieved by means of a continuous and open dialogue between employer and employee. The hospital's attitude toward its employees should be clearly articulated and employees should be encouraged to express their ideas, problems, and aspirations to the hospital.

The personnel professional should be part of the communications function, concerned with the various groups which must be addressed, the mechanisms of communication to be used with each group, and the feedback indicating the relative success of the employee relations programs. In addition, he must be proficient as a writer and publisher, as a speaker and organizer of meetings, and as a counselor and mediator in one-to-one problem solving.

There are at least two distinct groups of people who are important to the achievement of employee relations goals. They are the professional staff, department heads, and supervisors, on one hand, and all remaining employees on the other. Communicating with each requires a delicate nuance of emphasis, using a broad selection of techniques.

9-1 Communicating with the Management Supervisor

No group communicates the attitude of the hospital to employees more influentially than do department managers and supervisors. Their daily personal contact with employees puts them in an out front position to function as "personnel administrators" in the field. They are usually in a position to confront and respond to problems at the work site before small matters become major issues and at a time when they may best be resolved. They hear of and experience both dilemmas and opportunities that call for policy changes and are in position to make or recommend such changes. To assure their effectiveness in this role requires carefully cultivated channels of communication with supervisory management and the personnel and administrative offices.

9-2 Vehicles of Communication

The methods of communication with supervisory management reflect the small and manageable size of the group, its relative homogeneity and the continuous need for two-way give-and-take through the spoken and written word.

9-3 The Personnel Policy Manual is the basic document reflecting employee relations policies of the hospital. It should contain three types of information:

A. The *policy statement* should reflect the general attitude of the hospital toward a subject. It must necessarily be written in broad terms to allow some discretion and flexibility based on the needs of a situation.
B. A supplemental *administrative procedure* is often added to provide more specific instructions when appropriate for processing information or otherwise handling routine incidents covered by the policy.
C. The *supervisor's guidelines* provide additional information to help them administer the policy (*e.g.*, legal basis for policy, results of violations, decision-making authority, supportive details).

9-4 Management Newsletters are an effective means of maintaining communications with supervisors regarding changes or interpretations of policy, about employee relations problems recently resolved, about plans of the hospital affecting supervisors, and for general information about management. Such newsletters should be distributed on a regular basis (often monthly) and may also include supervisory techniques and other developmental literature. As a residual benefit, they serve as a further mark of status to the recipient. Information in this newsletter is generally of permanent value. A section of the Personnel Policy Manual should discuss filing such newsletters.

9-5 Periodic Management Meetings prove a two-way communication with supervisors. Such meetings allow for "comparing notes" between supervisors, discussing common problems, reviewing policies, and making presentations of an instructional or advisory nature by the administrator, personnel director, fiscal director, or others. Management meetings should be hosted by the administrator or personnel director, kept within strict time limits, and managed by the personnel director who is responsible for developing content. Attendance should be strongly encouraged and limited to the supervisory level and up to allow the greatest possible freedom of discussion of management problems.

9-6 The Personnel Policy Advisory Committee should be a standing committee of key managers, providing guidance for the continuous review of personnel policies. In this capacity these people can offer substantial insights on the effectiveness of policy from a perspective very close to the employee.

9-7 Personalized Coaching of supervisors by the professional personnel staff provides guidance to the supervisor in handling specific situations. It is of particular value as a communications link before supervisory mishaps occur in handling disciplinary situations, grievances, and anticipated personnel and job function changes. Its essence is the use of the personnel professional as a somewhat detached counselor in the administration/communication of personnel policy.

9-8 Communicating with Employees

Communication with employees in a health care institution is aimed at those employees who are not yet organized or who are subject to a union organizing campaign. If they are, then the employer is much more limited in his ability to communicate directly and must carefully read the relevant sections in Chapters 3 and 4 of the *Health Care Labor Manual* to insure that he will not be subjected to a charge of unfair labor practices. Once the employer becomes aware of a union organizing drive, all such communications must be carefully scrutinized from a legal standpoint to make certain they do not constitute objectionable conduct which could lead to a bargaining order. We cannot emphasize too strongly the need for a regular pattern of communicating with employees *before* the advent of a union.

The employees as a group are a more complex and diverse audience than the supervisors. Because of the large variety of occupational specialties in a hospital, employee backgrounds tend to be varied. Levels of interest in the hospital and its fortunes also vary substantially based upon the age, sex, pay, and responsibilities of each employee. Traditional communications have thus tended to focus on salaries, benefits, and work rules plus social activities. This trend is changing somewhat as these issues give way to employee demands for more information and participation in both policy and clinical matters. Communication vehicles include a wide variety of written materials plus a number of two-way approaches in groups as well as on a person-to-person basis.

9-9 *Written Communication Vehicles*

1. The *Employee Handbook* has traditionally been the primary publication for employees. Versions vary from the very abbreviated handbook to the one which rivals the Personnel Policy Manual in completeness. A sample outline of a handbook can be found in Chapter 16. The use of a single comprehensive booklet—a personnel policy manual—for employee information is becoming less common as marketplace competition and government regulations of hospital affairs re-

quire more detailed information and often separate publications.

2. *Collective bargaining agreements* are much like the employee handbook mentioned above with at least one important difference. Raymond Fleishman writes, "The collective bargaining agreement is the 'personal manual' for bargaining unit employees and the personnel policy manual is the 'contract' for nonunion employees."[25]

3. *Single subject pamphlets* are being used more frequently with the advent of various insurance benefits. Schedules of in-house training and developmental programs are often in pamphlet form.

4. Many hospitals issue a *quarterly publication*, aimed at both employees and other interested parties (*e.g.*, active medical staff, trustees, benefactors). This provides a broader range of information, but must not be expected to take the place of an internal publication which has a higher concentration of employee-slanted material.

5. *House organs* are published weekly or monthly, and deal strictly with subjects of interest to employees. This publication is particularly well received when it is obviously an unselfish effort by the hospital to communicate with and inform employees. Hence, the important qualities of the house organ are frequency, brevity, content of employee interest, and a lack of propaganda. The quality of presentation is strictly secondary. Often better results are obtained from duplicated typed copy that is simply illustrated than by professionally prepared material that looks like a management presentation.

6. *Letters to employee homes* concerning employee-related topics and employee activities should be periodically sent. These letters update and inform the employee's family about the hospital. Such letters then seem more natural and less inflammatory if they become necessary during a union organizing drive.

7. *Bulletin boards* are used profitably to publicize job openings, one-time letters from the administrator, and pictures of hospital and employee activities.

8. *"I've Got a Question" forms* doubling as an envelope, are part of a program providing direct contact between the employee and the administrator. Response is expedited when anonymous queries are answered on the bulletin board.

9. *The Employee Annual Report* is a modified annual report provided to employees about the hospital's financial and clinical activities.

10. *Fringe Benefit Annual Report* provides an individual annual update on fringe benefits including such items as:
    a. value of employee's pension fund;
    b. vacation accrual;
    c. life and disability insurance coverage;
    d. annual value of hospital paid fringe benefits for the previous year;
    e. summary of other benefits.[26]

Much of written communication is of an informational nature, often publicizing benefits and other programs. Other approaches stress two-way communication which invite employee response in matters of personal interest and in the solving of work-related issues.

9-10 *Two-Way Communication Vehicles*

1. *Employee Discussion Groups* may be scheduled during meal times with luncheon served without charge. Ten to fifteen employees are asked to have lunch (or supper) with the administrator and/or the personnel director. No other members of management are usually present. The objective is to solicit from employees ideas for correcting operations or employee relations problems. It is imperative that the discussion be directed toward issues, not personalities.

2. *Monthly In-service Training* meetings for *all* departments offer problem solving as well as job training opportunity.

3. *"Fact-Fone"* is an approach whereby employees may call a telephone number and (1) hear a prerecorded message about hospital happenings followed by (2) an opportunity to speak onto a tape for an unlimited amount of time to present a problem or idea. Response is either individual or via bulletin board.

4. The *Employee Advocate* is assigned to either the administrator's office or the personnel director's office. His sole responsibility is to represent the employee in problem situations including grievances.

5. An *Employee Committee*, however, formed to recommend or discuss changes in wages, hours, or working conditions on behalf of other employees and themselves, has been found by the NLRB to be a labor organization as defined by Section 2(5) of the Act.[27] Therefore, the health care institution which encourages the formation of such a committee may be subject to Section

8(a)(2) charges of unfair interference with and/or domination of protected concerted activities.[28] A concerted activity does not have to be a union activity to be protected.[29]

Such committee members, when they feel management is unresponsive to their requests, frequently opt to bring in actual unions to reinforce their demands. In many industrial situations, employee committees have been converted into an organizing tool by labor unions.

Additionally, management may discover too late that it has been dealing only with representatives who may not have been truly responsive to the employees' needs, thus lulling the administration into a sense of security which was not realistic.

Therefore, management should communicate with small groups of employees on a rotating basis as well as by those methods outlined above.

9-11 Communication Techniques and Pitfalls

Written communication to employees involves a large volume of material. Rarely will a personnel department have either the expertise or manpower to write and publish all such material. Periodicals are usually best published by the public relations organization with the content decisions being the responsibility of an editorial board which includes the personnel director.

When preparing brochures and manuals which are more permanent in nature, the personnel specialist should assume responsibility for content, again being supported by public relations and outside firms for presentation and publication expertise.

The writing style for virtually all employee communications differs radically from more precise and formal business communications. Employee communications require clarity, brevity, and an informal, personal style. This is best typified by what is seen on television news and in newspapers, probably the two communication styles most familiar to employees.

A common pitfall is reliance only on a single vehicle or on written communications. In fact, no single publication will be attractive enough to be read by all employees. Hence, where there is something important to communicate, a number of media should be involved.

Most important, there is no substitute for personal contact. Every effort should be made by members of the personnel staff to be continuously available outside the department and around the hospital, whether at meetings or through individual contacts, clarifying policy and procedure, investigating problems, and lending credibility to the employee relations program.

NOTES*

1. The National Health Council, Inc., 1740 Broadway, New York, New York, 10019, offers a convenient summary of major health occupations and sources of additional information. The pamphlet entitled "200 Ways to Put Your Talent To Work in the Health Field" is suggested.

2. See Volume II, Chapter 16 for additional examples of personnel department organization charts.

3. See Volume I, Chapter 9 on Equal Employment Opportunity and Volume II, Chapter 16 containing sample log forms.

4. See Chapter 9 for more complete information on civil rights legislation. *See also,* Executive Orders Number 11246 (race, color, religion, national origin) and 11375 (sex) as well as Revised Order Number 4 in the same chapter.

5. For a further discussion of advertising media and techniques, *see* Accetta, *Hospital Employment Can Be Sold,* HOSPITALS, J.A.H.A. (June 1, 1972) p. 73.

6. Much has been written on the subject of testing. See the discussion of testing in Chapter 9 of this manual.

In addition, see C. Rappaports, *Employment Testing: Apropos or No,* HOSPITALS (JAHA) (March 16, 1975). The American Hospital Association has issued a number of papers on federal legislation. See in particular Memorandums 4, 17, 20 and 22 for further information on testing.

7. See Vol. II, Chapter 16.

8. See Vol. II, Chapter 16 for special section entitled "Interviewing Techniques."

9. This section should be read in conjunction with Chapter 9, particularly with the Equal Pay Act discussion.

10. For a detailed discussion of job evaluation techniques using the point system, factor analysis, ranking and grading approaches see L.R. BURGESS, WAGE AND SALARY ADMINISTRATION IN A DYNAMIC ECONOMY (1968).

11. See Chapter 16 for samples of job descriptions.

12. This section should be read in conjunction with the sections of Chapter 9 that deal with sex discrimination and benefits under Title VII and the Equal Pay Act and with the section on benefits under the Age Discrimination Act.

13. 29 U.S.C. § 1001 et seq.

14. See "Social, Recreational, and Holiday Programs," Personnel Policies Forum Survey No. 109, Bureau of National Affairs, Inc., Washington, D.C. 20037, March, 1975.

15. See Warner, *New System for Paid Absences Benefits Hospital, Staff,* HOSPITALS (JAHA) 81 (Jan. 16, 1975).

16. According to articles in NEWSWEEK (January 20, 1975) and the WALL STREET JOURNAL (June 17, 1975), 80% of TRW's 11,300 Systems Group employees have chosen to mix benefits according to individual preferences.

17. See Burrow, *Coinsurance Enhances Benefit Plan,* HOSPITALS, (JAHA) 53 (Feb. 17, 1975).

18. 29 U.S.C. § 1001 et seq.

19. For further discussion of benefits, see S. Babson, Jr., FRINGE BENEFITS (1974).

20. This section should be read in conjunction with the section of Chapter 8 that deals with the recordkeeping requirements of the Fair

*All references to Volumes I and II are to the *Health Care Labor Manual.*

Labor Standards Act and the sections of Chapter 9 that deal with recordkeeping requirements of Title VII and the Age Discrimination Act.

21. Alfred Yankauer, M.D., Professor of Community and Family Medicine, University of Massachusetts Medical School.

22. See note 1, *supra.* The National Health Council, Inc. lists both accrediting agencies and the approximate length of each training program.

23. For a further discussion see H. Gatzke & S. Yenney, *Hospital-wide Education & Training,* HS, *JAHA* 93 (March 1, 1973). *See also* Hospital Continuing Education Project of the Hospital Research and Educational Trust, TRAINING AND CONTINUING EDUCATION: A HANDBOOK FOR HEALTH CARE INSTITUTIONS (1970).

24. The writer of a personnel policy manual might well be guided by including the subject matter of negotiations between an employer and a union. For examples see Chapter 5, pages 5:5, 5:6, 5:17, and 5:18.

25. R. Fleishman, *Living with a Contract,* HOSPITALS (JAHA) 51 (Nov. 16, 1973).

26. See the section on Benefits in this Chapter.

27. Sunrise Manor Nursing Home, 199 N.L.R.B. 1120, 84 L.R.R.M. 1146 (1972).

28. *Id.*

29. Salt River Valley Water Users Assn. v. NLRB, 206 F.2d 325, 32 L.R.R.M. 2548 (9th Cir. 1953).

3. Organization Development

MARK W. DUNDON

INTRODUCTION

Experience with organization development (OD) in health care is limited as it is in most industries; therefore, the term needs to be defined for purposes of this article.

There are a number of definitions and there are variances among them. The most widely accepted is by Beckhard:

Organization Development is an effort planned, organization-wide, and managed from the top to increase organization effectiveness and health through planned interventions in the organization's processes, using behavioral science knowledge.[1]

Personnel Interest

The director of personnel has had a historic concern for the people in the organization, how well they have gotten along, and how effectively they have worked there. Through the director's efforts, fair wage and salary programs have been developed and administered. Policies for fair treatment have been proposed and implemented. Job evaluation and personnel appraisal programs have been instituted, management training programs conducted, and personnel advocacy undertaken. All of these efforts will be enhanced by the OD program.

Need for OD

OD is needed for increased organization effectiveness because of:

1. the advent of new workers with different values
2. the increased size and complexity of the hospital organization
3. the increased external pressure for improved performance
4. the increased rate of change and greater uncertainty about organizational survival
5. the failure of historic methods of dealing with organizational problems
6. the greater expectations on the part of all employees and managers

Today's employees do have different expectations of work and of the organizations in which they are employed. This is pointed out by Harry Levinson in his book, *The Exceptional Executive*:

The organization within which a person works and the leadership which represents the power in that organization are both important aspects of the environment of that person. They define the modes within the organizational structure through which aggression may be expressed and affection obtained or given by promotion, emotion, transfer, reward, assignment, job definition, and other methods of control. The organization and its leadership have an important bearing on how a person feels himself to be as an adult, whether he fulfills the aspirations of his ego ideal, whether he is held in esteem or whether he judges himself a failure.[2]

Added to the fact that employees have increased expectations of the organization in which they work, they also bring with them a set of values that is considerably different from the values held by the managers. The values of today's workers are more personalistic; that is, idealistic, with the emphasis on personal choice and responsibility, with direction coming from within. Today's managers tend to be either formalistic or sociocentric. Formalistic means that they emphasize rationality control and order in their lives. Sociocentric values stress personal growth, human dignity, work satisfaction, and democratic processes, with emphasis on collaboration and group relationships. It is not hard to see that the employee having one set of values, working for a manager with another set, will provide many opportunities for conflict.[3]

Almost every hospital in the country has increased in size and complexity over the last ten or fifteen years. Many of their departments today weren't even dreamed of ten years ago, and the number of specialties that staff these departments only recently have come into existence, along with their schools and accrediting bodies. The integration of these many new specialists adds more sources of conflict for the hospital organization.

External pressures are increasing by leaps and bounds. The Joint Commission on Accreditation of Hospitals is changing its standards continuously. Federal, state, and local governments are revising their regulations and increasing their intervention into the hospital organization. Along with the increased regulation there is a nationwide desire to decrease cost escalation.

The rate of change in society and the world seems to increase exponentially; in the medical field, the technological change is particularly significant to hospitals. Among their other fears are the now fairly common pressures that can force a hospital to go bankrupt or go out of business. This is another stress point for the organization and its members. Up to a few years ago, many managers felt that the old ways were the best ways. Many still feel this way, but history probably will prove this incorrect. If managers were to command employees today, as they might have 50 years ago, they would have instant revolt on their hands. The value conflict alone would be enough to assure this.

Because of these many stresses and strains in the environment in which health care finds itself today, organization development will become imperative if hospitals are to prosper and grow as all of its members, particularly the managers, would want it.

Role of the Personnel Director

Since the personnel function is considered one of the key staff positions in the hospital, the personnel director must have the confidence and respect of the chief executive officer. Because that executive is a key to the success of the operation and must be highly supportive of the interest in maximizing results through the organization's development program, it is essential that the personnel director recognize the executive's role as the primary one in the change process and the personnel head is the main associate in developing and implementing the plan. This article outlines the objectives of an OD program, discusses the OD process, explains the different types of intervention used in implementing action plans, describes the essential elements of a successful OD program, and provides helpful hints for dealing with current problems.

OBJECTIVES OF AN OD PROGRAM

The objectives of an OD program will vary, depending on the specific problems of the organization as developed in the diagnosis phase, but there are a number of recognized goals:

1. To build trust among individuals and groups throughout the organization, and up and down the hierarchy.
2. To create an open problem-solving climate throughout the organization so that problems are confronted and differences clarified, both within and between groups, in contrast to sweeping problems under the rug or smoothing things over.
3. To locate decision-making and problem-solving responsibilities as close to the information sources and the relevant resources as possible, rather than in a particular role or level of the hierarchy.
4. To increase a sense of ownership of organizational goals and objectives among all personnel.
5. To stimulate collaboration between the interdependent persons and interdependent groups in the organization. Where relationships clearly are competitive, such as the contest for limited resources, it is important that competition be

opened and managed so that the hospital can benefit from the advantages of such rivalry and avoid suffering from the destructive consequences of subversive disputation.

6. To increase awareness of group process and its consequences for performance—that is, to help persons become aware of what is happening between and to the group members while they are working on the task, e.g., communications, influence, feeling, leadership styles and struggles, relationships, management of conflict, etc.[4]

It is clear from these objectives that the concern of the program is with the entire organization and its subgroups, and not solely with individual members. Individuals definitely will be affected by the program, both directly and indirectly, but that is not the thrust of the effort.

The top managers, especially those responsible for the OD program, will be interested in measuring and assessing its results. To do this, it is useful to develop a set of end result variables and intervening variables that can be measured to determine the hospital's progress through the efforts of the OD program.

End result variables are items that relate to the outcome of the work of the organization, such as units of service, revenues, costs, net revenues, etc., in accomplishing the primary goals. Intervening variables are those that reflect the current condition of the internal state of the organization, its loyalties, skills, motivation, and capacity for effective interaction, communication, and decision making.[5]

Exhibit 3-1 is an example of a set of end result variables for a hospital that attempts to show measurable items that result from effective day-to-day work. Exhibit 3-2 is an example of intervening variables that would be affected directly by the OD program. The OD effort is aimed at improving the intervening variables, which in turn will enhance the end results. These two sets of variables can be used to educate personnel as to what the organization seeks to become, and as it does so, what the effect will be on the hospital's work.

Now that it is clear what the OD program is trying to accomplish, the OD process is examined next.

Exhibit 3-1 End Result Variables

Employee Orientation
Turnover rates, organizationwide and departmentally, would be low and improving. Absenteeism would be decreasing. The number of disciplinary procedures would be declining. The percentage of internal promotion would be high and rising, and employee attitudes toward the hospital would be excellent.

Patient Orientation
The mortality rate would be low; the infection range would be very low and improving. The number of patient complaints would be negligible, and patients' understanding of their problems, disabilities, or treatment would be very high; patient attitudes toward the hospital would be excellent. Waiting time in the emergency room would be minimal, as it would be for all services. Spiritual and psychological needs of patients would be met very well.

M.D. Orientation
There would be optimal use of professional staff time as demonstrated by good M.D.-R.N. rapport. Normal tissue would be very low and decreasing. The length of stay for patients would be low, compared to the service area; the rate of rehospitalization would be negligible. The M.D. attitude toward the hospital would be excellent. Results of diagnostic procedures would be very rapid and highly accurate. The medical staff would be made up of a good mix of specialties; it would be growing in number and have a high percentage of board-certified M.D.s. There would be few disciplinary problems, few M.D. complaints, and a high level of consultation among medical staff members.

Organization Orientation
Third party attitude toward the hospital would be excellent. Room rates, compared to other hospitals in the service area, would be lower. Staff hours per patient day would be lower. The budgeted revenue and expense would be within ± 1 percent. The percentile on the hospital administrative services report would be optimal, in either the first or fourth quarter. Net revenue would be the maximum allowed in the service area. Public attitude toward the hospital would be excellent and improving.

Source: St. Charles Hospital, Ohio.

Exhibit 3-2 Intervening Variables

Communication

Accurate, clear, and concise information flows horizontally (between and within work groups), as well as vertically (between and among workers, supervisors, and top management).

Decision-Making Practices

Decision making is participative and takes place at the levels having the most accurate and complete information (i.e., the practice is decentralized).

Motivational Conditions

The organization formally (e.g., through promotions and pay increases) and informally (through praise from supervisors) encourages, acknowledges, and rewards high levels of employee performance. The reinforcement develops a climate of self-motivation (desire, not fear).

Human Resources

Employees are used to the utmost of their potential and have opportunities to improve themselves while serving the hospital (in-house education, training, and career advancement). Jobs are structured with respect for the total organization design and individual growth.

Technology/Facilities

The hospital uses state-of-the-art, well-maintained, and/or efficient equipment, resources, and procedures that meet the needs of the community.

Goal Emphasis

Emphasis is placed on employees' attainment of clearly stated, realistic performance goals and standards that are designed to stimulate growth through self-measurement and supervisory evaluation.

Work Facilitation

Supervisors' technical competence facilitates the work of their employees, as do their delegating responsibilities, providing clear explanations of tasks and responsibilities, and exercise of appropriate control over staff.

Satisfaction With Work

Employees feel they are making an optimal individual contribution to the hospital and have a sense of challenge, autonomy, and responsibility without being overburdened with unreasonable amounts of work.

Relations With Fellow Workers

Employees work as a team, cooperate with their coworkers, are loyal to both their work group and the hospital as a whole, and perceive a family atmosphere as existing within the institution.

Influence

The organization and supervisors have influence over employees; employees have influence over their supervisors and work groups; and the hospital as a whole is responsive to influences from the surrounding community.

Source: St. Charles Hospital, Ohio.

AN OD PROCESS

Consultant Entry and Contracting

The first step in the OD process is to involve an external consultant who is a specialist at the very beginning. Few, if any, hospitals have in-house OD skills available and even if they did, the presence of an external consultant still is imperative if the process is to be successful. The consultant's relationship usually begins with an exploratory meeting to discuss the administrator's concern and view of the organization and its problems. The consultant will want to get some idea of what the problem is and whether involvement will help the organization. The expert will assess the openness and frankness of the managers and the organization's readiness for change.

After the initial meeting, the consultant and the chief executive officer will need to establish a psychological contract and set the ground rules and expectations of both parties. The consultant will give the managers an understanding of what is involved in the process and that it will take considerable time to create any significant change. The managers will have to accept the consultant's intervention, agree to participate in the data collection in an open and forthright manner, and be willing to act on the goals that are set by the group, which then will be evaluated as the process proceeds. The consultant will want the managers and, especially, the chief executive officer (CEO) to accept ownership of the organization's problems.

The second part of the psychological contract will be to determine the consultant's role in the change process, including working standards and the expert's responsibilities. The relationship must be voluntary on the part of both the CEO and the consultant and temporary in the sense that it will not go on forever. The consultant's role is to help the client analyze problems and facilitate the various phases of the change process.

The third part of the psychological contract defines the role and responsibilities of the chief executive officer and the personnel manager in the change process.

After a psychological contract has been established, the key participants must agree on how the external consultant is to enter the organization. The usual and most reasonable entry point is at the data collection stage of the action research model, which is described next.

Action Research Model

A hospital is a large and complex organization that requires considerable effort to change. It often is help-ful to use a model to demonstrate the change process to all involved. The action research model (Figure 3-1) consists of four processes:

1. Data collection from members of the organization
2. Feedback to the various groups in the organization
3. Joint action planning based on the feedback
4. Implementation of the action plan

This process is repeated again and again as the program advances toward the goal of a more effective organization.

Data Collection

The first step in the action research model of organization change is the collection of data. Much time, effort, and money must be spent on this phase. The organization may choose to develop its own data collection instrument, with the help of the consultant. Measurement instruments also are available commercially.

Sources of information on predesigned questionnaires are:

Figure 3-1 OD Process—Action Research Model

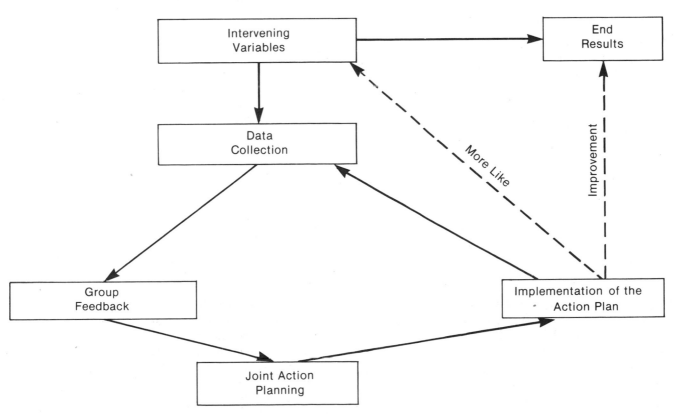

Source: St. Charles Hospital, Ohio.

Instrumentation in Human Relations Training by J. William Pfeiffer and Richard Heslin (1973). University Associates, Box 615, Iowa City, Iowa 52240

Measuring Human Behavior by Dale A. Lake, Matthew B. Miles, and Ralph B. Earle, Jr. (1973). Teachers College Press, Columbia University, 1234 Amsterdam Avenue, New York, N.Y. 10027

Other examples of available questionnaires include:

Profile of Organizational Characteristics by Rensis Likert

Organizational Climate Questionnaire by Litwin and Stringer

The consultant may recommend both kinds of questionnaires since the predesigned form can be used to compare the hospital with similar organizations that have utilized it previously. The internal questionnaire determines the organization's progress from its present state to a more effective entity.

The process of developing the data collection instrument usually begins with representatives of a broad cross-section of the hospital who meet with the consultant to review the issues. The consultant then develops a series of in-depth questions that should reveal the climate and attitude of the entire population of the organization. The questionnaire also should include questions that compare the organization's present position in relation to the intervening variables and, subsequently, track its movement toward its optimal level.

The initial set of questions is reviewed by the original group to make sure it is relevant and is clear and understandable to everyone. When the questionnaire has been approved by the initial group and by top management, it is administered to all members of the organization.

One approach in doing this is to have employees, while on duty, go to a specific site to answer the questions in the presence of the OD consultant. The individuals must have complete confidence that the responses will be confidential and that there will be no possibility that they will be identified. This is a very critical issue because there will be a great deal of fear the first time through this process that must be recognized and dealt with. When an external person controls the information gathering and members of the organization are not allowed access to the individual questionnaires, the employees usually feel secure and, as a result, are open in their responses.

This process usually takes considerable time because of the nature of a hospital, since a few persons on each unit may be absent from their work stations at any one time. Normally, the process requires three to four days, depending on the size of the hospital. The afternoon and night shifts also must have full opportunity to respond.

A second method of data collection is to mail the questionnaires to the employees' homes, with a self-addressed, stamped envelope, requesting that the individuals fill them out and return them by a certain date. The response to this kind of inquiry has been very encouraging and offers considerably less disruption to the organization during its workday. One hospital, St. Charles Hospital in Oregon, Ohio, tried this in 1978 and received a 90 percent response.

There are advantages to both methods of gathering information. When the questionnaire is filled out at the hospital, the advantages are:

1. It is a fast method of gathering information.
2. Employees don't feel inconvenienced in responding because they are being paid to answer.
3. There is an assurance of a reasonable response since most persons won't mind doing this while on duty.

The mailed questionnaire has these advantages:

1. Employees have a greater sense of confidence that no one other than the consultant will see their responses.
2. Employees may take their time in responding.
3. Employees may respond whenever they feel in the mood to do so.
4. The mailed questionnaire is less expensive to administer since there is less organizational disruption.

As the organization does develop and the managers become more skillful with the change process and data collection, the need for the written procedure may be replaced by a direct interviewing process involving three or four general questions that managers can cover in their units. If the direct feedback method is used, it will be necessary to repeat a written questionnaire to be sure that the process is continuing as planned and that there are no breakdowns because of the face-to-face method.

For the direct feedback method of information gathering to be effective, the participants must prepare themselves to discuss their feelings and perceptions with their managers. Exhibit 3-3 presents questions to be handed out in advance that will act as the framework for the meeting. This process of direct feedback should not be attempted until the organiza-

Exhibit 3-3 Preparation Questions for Direct Feedback Session

---

YOUR HOSPITAL 19____ SURVEY PROCESS

Periodically, we feel it is important to get your input on various aspects of your job and Your Hospital. Through your input, we can develop plans to ensure that Your Hospital provides a positive environment for both patients and staff.

The following questions, which deal with a number of issues, are intended to help you think about your job and Your Hospital. The questions may not include all areas of interest to you; therefore, we have provided space below for you to add other points as you wish.

Look over the questions and jot down your thoughts and ideas. No one in management will see what you have written, so please give us your honest response.

Thank you in advance for your effort. Your preparation and participation in the survey process is appreciated.

1. What are your thoughts about the practices or policies within Your Hospital and/or your work group?
2. Describe the way you see communications working in Your Hospital and/or your work group.
3. What are your thoughts about Your Hospital's benefits, salaries, promotions, and continuing educational opportunities?
4. Describe your relationship with your immediate supervisor.
5. What other thoughts and ideas do you have about Your Hospital, your work group, and this feedback process?

Source: St. Charles Hospital, Ohio.

---

tion has had at least two or three complete rounds with the written questionnaire so that both members and managers are comfortable with the OD process.

The consultant also may choose to interview individual members of the organization. This is particularly helpful where there may be hostile individuals who would like to vent their feelings and believe that the existing method does not provide an appropriate opportunity. This also is helpful where, for some reason, a department or individuals choose not to involve themselves in the data collection.

After all the data have been collected, the consultant organizes and summarizes the material. The expert may analyze it for the organization or may collaborate with the chief executive officer to develop specific recommendations for the OD effort.

Group Feedback

There must be a review and comment series of meetings with all employees so that management may have a clear understanding of what they are saying about the organization and so the staff can hear the outcome of the survey. This can be done in several ways that should, and will, change as the organization gets more experience in both the collection and use of data. The first time an organization goes through this process, it could be handled in two ways:

1. The chief executive officer and top assistants could review the data with each unit that has been identified in the questionnaire as a separate entity.
2. The data could be reviewed by the external consultant.

The choice of who is to conduct these feedback sessions will depend on the capabilities of the chief executive officer and top assistants and the severity of the organization's problems. If the problems are very severe and widespread, it probably would be better for the consultant alone to conduct the feedback sessions. The advantages of the latter method are:

1. It is less threatening to the members of the organization.
2. It is faster since the expert already is a trained and skilled interviewer.
3. The consultant's objectivity is difficult for any member of the organization to duplicate.

The advantages of having the chief executive officer and top assistants doing the review are:

1. Those with primary responsibility for the organization get an intimate view of what is going on in the minds of the employees.
2. They obtain information they could get in no other way.
3. The CEO acquires greater comprehension of the organization's problems based on experiences in the group feedback.

Joint Action Planning

Now that all the data have been collected and verified by the feedback sessions, it is time to develop action plans with the members of the organization. These action plans should be considered on three levels:

1. organizationwide
2. departmental
3. individual units where the department is very large, as in nursing service

The action plan should be related to the information gathered through the questionnaires and feedback sessions. The plan needs to relate to the issues brought out that relate to the entire organization. This action plan should be developed by the chief executive officer, top assistants, and the external consultant. If the consultant has been responsible for the group feedback, the expert's role will be obvious in the development of the organizational action plan. The consultant has the information and a feel for the organization's problems that are essential in developing the plan. If the expert did not conduct the group feedback but collected and summarized the written data for management, the consultant still has a good feel for the situation.

The consultant brings a level of expertise to this important stage of the process that rarely is available in the organization. The expert also brings an objectivity and ability to deal with problems at the top that no one else in the organization possesses, especially if the chief executive officer is involved.

After the action plan has been developed, it should be checked out with department heads and supervisors, as well as some of the lower level personnel. Again, this is a good role for the external consultant. The completed action plan should be submitted to the board of trustees for review and approval. This assures the commitment to change at the highest level.

Each department and subunit should develop its own action plan, based on information gathered in the initial step. It is very important at this stage that the plan be documented completely and that all members of the affected group be involved in its development and concur with the action so its results will be positive and helpful in increasing the unit's effectiveness. Each action plan must be submitted to the next higher level of management for review and acceptance, so that the subordinate manager and unit may be held accountable for achieving the agreed-upon results in their action plan.

In developing the plan, each group at every level should select actions that will address the major problems, particularly those it can change in a short time. In the early stages of a change process, it is good for the group to have some success at creating positive changes in day-to-day functions.

Implementation of the Action Plan

Now it is time to implement the action plan. Several OD interventions arise: team building; intergroup problem solving; third party facilitation; consulting pairs, which are commonly agreed-upon types of intervention; plus several less commonly recognized processes such as consultant network, operational planning, objective setting, and organization restructuring.

All of these techniques could be used, some of them simultaneously in different parts of the organization to deal with different problems. The choice of action depends on the problem that surfaced in the diagnostic phase.

Team Building

The most common and widely known technique is building an effective team by:

- Increasing mutual trust among the members of the team so that each one feels free to state views openly without fear of criticism.
- Building mutual support among the team members.
- Improving communications between the members of the team to increase mutual understanding.
- Developing team objectives that can be understood by all members.
- Developing effective ways of dealing with the conflicts that necessarily arise during the team's efforts.
- Increasing utilization of the capabilities of the individual members of the team.
- Increasing personal acceptance of responsibility by each member and greater effort in creating a positive team climate, characterized by openness, supportiveness, and a sense of freedom.[6]

Intergroup Meetings

Intergroup meetings or problem-solving sessions are used to resolve situations where conflict is obvious and debilitating. These meetings may involve different units of the organization, such as pharmacy and nursing service; or line and staff conflicts, such as between the finance department and the laboratory; or groups outside the hospital, such as a medical clinic and the admitting department. The purpose of this action is to focus on the problem and attempt to reduce intergroup conflict.

Third Party Facilitation

This involves the use of a third person who is skilled in the analysis of a particular problem and helping the parties resolve their differences based on the diagnosis and a mutual understanding that this individual would develop.

Consultant Network

A consultant network should be developed that will include both the external expert and a group of internal consultants. The external consultant must develop a close, continuing work relationship with the chief executive officer and the personnel director to help those responsible for the change effort to discern and deal with trends and roadblocks more objectively. The external consultant can be particularly helpful to the chief executive officer in dealing with specific and personal problems that arise. The external consultant also can assist in developing a group of internal consultants. Because the relationship with the external consultant is not permanent, there is a need for internal consultants who have special skills in various types of interventions who can assist one another, other managers, and supervisors. They constitute an expert resource available when the external consultant is not and can assist the organization in continuing the change process after the outside expert has left. The in-house group should be responsible to the director of the change effort—the personnel manager.

Operational Planning and Objective Setting

Operational planning is another developmental technique that can be very effective in moving an organization to a much more effective state. Operational planning is short-range, up to one year in duration. It may deal with specific problems that the organization is experiencing in accomplishing its goals, or it may set objectives to accomplish the goals more effectively. Operational planning is not only organizationwide but also departmental in thrust. It is aimed at the short-term improvement in achieving goals and can be accomplished in two ways.

One way is through a management-by-objectives program, the most common technique in performance improvement. (This technique is discussed in Article 12 of this book.) Another way is by a method called Personal Management Interview (PMI), which is de-

scribed by R. Wayne Boss as a regular private meeting between supervisor and immediate subordinates.[7] This method requires the establishment of objectives for each manager at the beginning of the use of the PMI process. The meetings are held on a regular, frequent basis, usually every two weeks. The format includes a discussion not only of progress in meeting objectives but also of administrative and organizational problems, the training of subordinates in administrative and management skills, and the resolution of interpersonal issues and problems between supervisor and subordinates.

Organization Restructuring

There is another type of intervention that can have significant impact on the effectiveness of the organization: the classical pyramidal organizational structure. This has been around for many years but no longer may be as effective in certain situations and in certain types of organizations. Some of the new structures involve variations on the team approach theme, including *project management*, a type of unit formed to accomplish a specific objective using the resources of multiple departments; it may be assigned to a functional department or to a special project manager. Another type of structure is the *matrix organization*, where multiple project managers control planning, scheduling, costs, and individuals assigned to their project, while line managers exert control in terms of technical direction, training, and compensation. In this type of organization, the worker has two bosses. A third type of structure involves *venture teams*, which are like the matrix teams and frequently are used to meet the demand for a breakthrough in product marketing. This also is a multidisciplinary team, somewhat similar to the matrix team, offering a different approach to the traditional operations in marketing departments. As executives learn how to use the different types of structures, they build more adaptive organization structures so they can respond more effectively to the challenge of change that faces their organizations.[8]

This is not a totally inclusive group of OD interventions, but it represents a reasonably comprehensive list of possibilities that may be used in creating more effective organizations for hospitals. Additional resources are available for interested readers.[9,10]

ESSENTIAL ELEMENTS IN A SUCCESSFUL OD PROGRAM[11]

Since considerable money and effort will be expended by an organization in an OD program, certain elements must be considered before even beginning the effort. If some of these elements are missing, the chances of a successful program are reduced significantly. These elements are:

1. commitment of the chief executive officer
2. cultural preparedness in the organization
3. realistic expectations about the success of the effort
4. internal tension and pain
5. involvement of persons in power positions
6. development of internal resources
7. methods of holding persons accountable
8. a competent consultant
9. a clear psychological contract between the chief executive officer and the consultant
10. technically competent supervisors

Commitment of the Chief Executive Officer

The commitment of the hospital's chief executive officer is absolutely essential to the success of the effort. The commitment must be both to the effort in psychological terms and to the role that the executive must play in the OD effort. As Chris Argyris says in his article, "The CEO's Behavior: Key to Organization Development":

Because of the way most companies are organized, the chief executive officer is the focal point of power and responsibility for managing and renewing organizations. The CEO is, therefore, the key to the success of the organization development programs.[12]

All this is not new, but what has not been spelled out clearly is the what and the why about the chief executive officer that makes this person the key to the success of organization development. The answer is behavior.

The way the chief executive officer actually behaves is crucial to the survival of the organization and renewal activities. It is the CEO's behavior and, subsequently, that of other officers that ultimately does or does not confirm the idea that the organization development is necessarily credible and inexorably linked to the individual's leadership style.

R. Wayne Boss, in his article "The Effects of Leader Absence on a Confrontation Team-Building Design," points out that the absence of the leader from a team-building process may actually result in a regression of the group over a period of time, so it is absolutely essential that the chief executive officer be committed and involved in the change process.[13]

Cultural Preparedness in the Organization

Cultural preparedness includes certain minimal levels of the institution's health that will indicate there is some chance of producing positive results through the organization development effort. These include interpersonal trust among staff members, their willingness to resolve problems and to be held accountable, and their level of psychological health. There must be at least a moderate level of trust, particularly among the managers, so that when the intervention phase begins there will be some possibility of individuals' being open and honest with each other. It may seem obvious, but a willingness to resolve problems is not always present, nor do persons in the various units feel a need to change existing circumstances. Accountability is a necessary part of the cultural preparedness because managers must be willing both to hold others accountable and to be accountable themselves. Psychological health should be present at least at minimal levels because if a person is wounded seriously psychologically, there is no way for that individual to be responsible and participate effectively, especially if confrontation is required.

Realistic Expectations

It must be understood that a great deal of time will be required to correct the problems created over many years. A small organization of several hundred persons can expect to see significant results within one to two years and its management group can experience change within six months.

In larger organizations of a thousand or more employees, the process is much slower. The management group may expect to see results within six months to a year and, the whole organization in three to five years, and the process can take five to eight years to reach everyone.

Outcomes that might be expected include:

- an improvement in overall communications, up and down and across the organization
- improvement in the openness and honesty of that communication
- increased sensitivity on the part of managers toward their employees and toward each other
- increased ability of the managers to effectively deal with interdepartmental conflicts
- increased effectiveness of meetings, producing better results in as much as 25 percent less time

Organizations will experience many other outcomes, depending on their history and problems.

Internal Tension and Pain

It may sound strange to say that there must be pain before there can be effective change, but that is a necessary ingredient for members of the organization feeling a need to change. If pain is not present, it could be a handicap to the successful change effort.

Involvement of Persons in Power Positions

Not only does the chief executive officer need to be involved, so, too, do subordinates and the informal leaders of the organization. If the informal leaders are not somehow involved in the process, the chances of success are extremely limited.

Development of Internal Resources

If an organization change effort is to be successful, there must be a group of internal OD consultants who can continue the effort without the help of the external consultant. Persons inside the organization need to understand the process and its various elements and be skilled at both diagnosis and intervention so that, as problems occur, an in-house expert always is present who can deal skillfully with those issues.

Methods of Holding Persons Accountable

Before an OD effort can be successful, there must be an established means of holding individuals accountable. (See earlier section on operational planning and objective setting.)

A Competent Consultant

External consultants are essential in the change process. They should be expert in organization development and have not only academic credentials but also the experience that qualifies them to help guide the institution. The International Association of Applied Social Scientists, which has an accrediting function for certifying OD practitioners, may be used for reference. The Academy of Management has an OD section that also may be helpful as a reference source.

Clear Psychological Contract

A clear understanding between the external consultant and the chief executive officer is imperative to avoid the danger of misunderstandings that might destroy the effort. There should be an agreement about the role of the consultant, the role of the chief executive officer, and the expectations of both regarding the change program.

Technically Competent Supervisors

The organization's leaders must have high technical competency in their own areas of responsibility as well as high-level ability to become competent in the technical aspects of the change process itself.

Obviously, these critical elements are present in varying degrees in each organization, but before beginning an OD program they must be examined to determine whether the commitment of the time and resources to the effort has any chance of succeeding.

OTHER HELPFUL HINTS

Publicity

One of the least noticed aspects of a change process is communication of the results of the data collection and the action plans. All of the effort put into the organization development program can be lost if there is not a planned program of feedback to members through multiple and numerous communication methods on a continuous basis. The institutional house organ definitely should be used, and it is suggested that a column be developed to report activities of both the entire organization and its subunits on a regular basis. The manager of each area should continuously report back to the entire unit the results of its action plan and what is happening because of the organization development effort. This report should include the efforts and results of both the unit and the organization.

Especially in the early stages of a change process, there will be many questions regarding the policies that are put into effect. These elements usually can be changed fairly easily, have immediate results, and are highly visible. Each time there is a change as a result of the OD effort, that change should be called to the attention of all employees as being a result of the program. Frequently these changes revolve around an employee benefit policy and can have cost implications; therefore, they should be folded into the hospital's budgetary process.

One of the other obvious changes that will be requested involves professional development of the managers. This usually comes from the managers themselves and typically will be part of their action plan that, again, should be reported to the institution as a result of the OD effort.

The point is that even though the top managers are aware of the OD impact on these changes, other persons in the organization may not make the connection at all. Continual reminders of the OD program impact will enhance the results and everyone's commitment to the program.

A Good Consultant

The consultant is critical to the success of the OD program. Not only must the individual be competent technically, there also must be a good rapport between the consultant and those with whom the expert works in the organization. It is imperative that the consultant be compatible with the chief executive officer, personnel director, and other top managers. The consultant will be with the organization for a considerable time and all will be working together very closely. The consultant must be respected not only as a professional but also as a person and genuinely liked by top management and staff. A consultant should not be picked merely because of technical qualifications; the individual should be congenial and an authority from whom a great deal may be learned.

Patience Is a Virtue

Many times it will seem as though the program is going nowhere and is not meeting expectations. Individuals change at different rates, and the greater the need for change, the longer it will take to effect it. Coupled with patience is the need for desire—desire to change the organization to a considerably more effective one than it is now and one that is a peaceful, achieving winner.

CONCLUSION

This all sounds very easy, but it is not. Just discovering what an organization wants to be (intervening variables) is a difficult, time-consuming process. Remember that this effort is going to last from several years to as long as ten years or more in the very large hospital. But a spirited and enterprising organization is an exciting place to be, so it will be well worth the time, effort, and money—and then some.

NOTES

1. R. Beckhard, *Organization Development: Strategies and Models* (Reading, Mass.: Addison-Wesley, 1969), p. 9.
2. Harry Levinson, *The Exceptional Executive: A Psychological Conception* (New York: A Mentor Book, 1968), pp. 42–43.
3. G. H. Varney, *Organization Development for Managers* (Reading, Mass.: Addison-Wesley), p. 6.
4. J. J. Sherwood, "An Introduction to Organization Development," in J. W. Pfeiffer and J. E. Jones, eds., *The 1972 Annual Handbook for Group Facilitators* (San Diego: University Associates, 1972), p. 432.
5. Rensis Likert, *New Patterns of Management* (New York: McGraw-Hill Book Co., 1961), p. 61.
6. Varney, p. 157.
7. Wayne Boss, "Toward Reducing Regression Following a Confrontation Team-Building Session: The Personal Management Review." Prepared for presentation at the International Conference on Work Humanization, Dubrovnik, Yugoslavia, April 1978.
8. R. G. Murdick and J. E. Ross, "People Productivity and Organizational Structure," *Personnel* 49, no. 5 (1973): 32.
9. W. L. French and C. H. Bell, Jr., *Organization Development: Behavior Science Intervention of Organizational Improvement* (Englewood Cliffs, N.J.: Prentice-Hall, Inc., 1973).
10. E. F. Huse, *Organization Development and Change* (St. Paul: West Publishing Co., 1975), p. 11.
11. A majority of this material is from A. Wayne Boss, "Essentials for Successful Organization Development Efforts," *Group & Organization Studies* 4, no. 4 (1979): 496–504.
12. Chris Argyris, "The CEO's Behavior: Key to Organization Development," *Harvard Business Review* 51, no. 2 (1973): 55–64.
13. R. Wayne Boss, "The Effects of Leader Absence on a Confrontation Team-Building Design," *Journal of Applied Behavioral Science* 14, no. 4 (1978): 469–478.

4. The Changing Hospital Personnel Function As Seen by the Executive Recruiting Consultant

JERAD D. BROWDY

The decade of the 80s will see considerable change in the direction of hospital personnel administration. The future should be exceedingly bright for the competent, well-rounded, human resources executive but may be uncertain for the traditional hospital personnel practitioner who has not progressed beyond the employment and recordkeeping stage of personal development or experience.

As executive recruiting consultants engaged by health care institutions throughout the country, we are seeing chief executive officers demonstrate a marked change in attitude toward the personnel function. This has been especially true during the last two years, with an increasing number of enlightened administrators thinking in terms of a broad human resources function directed by a sophisticated professional operating as a key member of the executive group. To appreciate this change in attitude fully, it is necessary to relate what our experiences typically have been.

It has not at all been unusual during the course of recruiting and consulting assignments to discover that personnel directors were not involved in the process. In many instances they were not even aware that the chief executive officer had retained outside assistance. Obviously, there are some situations in which the need for confidentiality is such that only the chief executive officer or a few board members may know that a consulting or recruiting assignment is being undertaken, but in most cases the personnel director should have been an active participant (and should have been the first to recognize the need for consulting advice). Sometimes this noninvolvement was due to the personnel director's lack of credibility in the organization. More often than not, however, this omission was not a matter of the individual. Rather, it was because the administrator did not fully appreciate the importance of the personnel function and did not feel it was necessary for the personnel director to be involved. Frequently, it has been necessary to devote a considerable amount of time and energy to convincing a chief executive officer that the personnel director had to be involved actively in the consulting project.

As more institutions develop corporate organization structures, assistant administrators, directors of nursing, and chief financial officers are having their titles changed to vice president. But all too often this same recognition has not been given personnel executives, who during such reorganizations may actually have had their reporting relationship changed downward. In some executive compensation consulting assignments, the chief executive officer has ranked the personnel director at the same level as department heads rather than at upper management levels.

The personnel department frequently is viewed by hospital management as nothing more than an employment or recordkeeping function. The personnel function often was disjointed, with nursing maintaining its own records, department heads doing their own hiring and even setting their own wage rates. The personnel director may or may not have been a member of the chief executive officer's "inner circle" or management committee, and even if on such a committee, the individual's recommendations may not have been given much weight. All too often, the personnel director was not included in the corporate planning process and did not discover that events were occurring and decisions being made that directly affected employee relations until after the fact. In numerous situations, even the best recommendations made by the personnel director and accepted by the chief executive were overruled or discarded later because of opposition from others in the management group (even though the executive believed the personnel director was right). In some institutions it appeared that the role of the personnel director was "to be seen but not heard."

When undertaking recruiting assignments for hospital personnel directors, chief executives frequently expressed a preconceived bias in which they felt that candidates presented to them in all probability would be the best of the mediocre. This is an unfortunate attitude, but one that has persisted because of the negative experiences so many have had with their personnel function. The reasons for this attitude are really twofold.

Certainly there are executives who do not fully appreciate the importance of the personnel function and would make life difficult for even the best personnel executive. However, much of this negative attitude may be justified.

Obviously, it is unfair to generalize or categorize individuals, because we do come in contact with very competent and well-respected hospital personnel executives. However, an increasing number of hospital personnel directors throughout the country are being terminated for poor performance (or lack of performance). A definite pattern is evolving as to why this is occurring. In the main, the personnel executives in trouble today are noncompetitive and have preferred to maintain a low profile rather than being visible in the organization. They have little understanding of the real world of personnel outside of their own hospital. They do not understand hospital economics as related to personnel. They react to crises after the fact rather than anticipating problems. Their basic technical experience has been primarily in employment and recordkeeping and they only have a perfunctory knowledge of the more sophisticated aspects of personnel. They are afraid to take risks and they cannot "sell" their programs effectively. They avoid confrontation, hoping the issue will disappear. Many view their primary responsibility to be the advocate of the employee rather than a key member of management. They are seen as the last to know what is really happening in the

institution, and others in management have more credibility with the employees. Chief executives are most vehement in their criticism about these last two failings.

If there is any one concern that is almost universally expressed by chief executives it is that hospital personnel directors are not aware of the most recent trends in their own profession. This criticism may be justified because by and large hospital personnel executives whose total experience has been in health care are not aware of the latest developments in the field. For example, the American Society of Personnel Administrators consists of more than 20,000 personnel executives representing business, industry, government, and academia, but a little less than 3 percent of its membership comes from health care. The American Compensation Association has a membership of more than 5,000 compensation specialists yet fewer than 2 percent come from health care. There is virtually nothing in the professional personnel literature that has been written by those in health care. This is directly reflected in the attitude of chief executive officers who feel that hospital personnel executives do not have an understanding of the broader issues necessary to assume an upgraded position in the organization.

It is not the intent of this article to dwell in detail on why the personnel function is changing. Obviously, changes in labor legislation, work attitudes, and the women's movement have created pressures on all employers, hospitals being no exception. As hospitals are faced with cost containment and regulation, however, the necessity to utilize individuals in the most efficient, economical manner without affecting patient care becomes imperative. These factors, then, are primary among those that are forcing administrators to realize their organizations require a highly sophisticated executive who will be involved at the highest levels of the institution (including the board), with emphasis on long-range personnel planning, personnel development, assessment and identification of talent, and changes in managerial and organization structure and behavior.

As more chief executives begin to think in terms of the more sophisticated human resources management function, the position is beginning to be upgraded in the organization hierarchy. However, as this change in thinking occurs, there also is a hardening of executives' attitudes toward personnel directors. In most of our assignments to recruit personnel directors, previous hospital experience was a requirement from which there could be no deviation. Now, an increasing number of executive officers believe that the talent they require cannot be found in health care. This is especially true with respect to positions that are beginning to pay salaries in excess of $40,000. The fact is that while the human resources position is being upgraded in the organization, individuals being selected for this restructured job more often than not may come from outside the health care field. Even more important, the traditional personnel director is being relegated to a secondary position in this new function.

It is disconcerting to hear chief executives say that the better personnel people are to be found outside of the health care field. This is a harsh statement. Industrial personnel executives or those coming from the business sector are not necessarily better than those in the health care field and many of them do not really have the humane qualities necessary to succeed in this field. What is better about them is that they are more aggressive and much more knowledgeable about developments in their profession.

In many respects, hospital personnel administration today is at the level of the industrial field 20 years ago. At that time, many of the industrial personnel executives were similar to the hospital personnel directors who now find themselves having difficulties. Today, however, industrial personnel executives, especially those who have reached a position of prominence in their organization (in most large organizations the chief personnel executive enjoys vice presidential status and is a key member of the management team), have educational backgrounds that may be oriented toward business, finance, marketing, or the behavioral sciences. *They know how to sell their programs and they are not afraid to take risks.* As more of these individuals enter the health care field from private industry, they will make a tremendous impact not only on their own institution but the hospital personnel field in general.

In reviewing experiences with personnel executives (whether or not from health care) who have an excellent record of accomplishment and enjoy the highest degree of credibility in their institutions, a commonality of traits and attributes emerges:

1. They have a high degree of self-confidence and ego strength.
2. They are politically astute, and can quickly identify and work with the real power structure in the organization.
3. They act rather than react to situations and are not afraid to make decisions.
4. They are willing to take risks and take unpopular stands. They will make decisions to solve immediate problems rather than waiting for a slow-moving approval process.
5. They are articulate and possess excellent oral and written communications skills.

6. They will not be coerced or "bullied" by their peers in the organization and will fight for acceptance of their recommendations and for their proper place in the structure.
7. They have extensive experience in the more complex areas of personnel such as compensation, labor relations, management development, organization development, staff planning.
8. They can implement approved programs successfully.
9. They are well respected by their peers in the organization, especially by the directors of nursing and finance.
10. They can successfully develop "pipelines" into the organization and have up-to-date knowledge of what really is going on in the organization. (Many chief executives feel this is the most important talent in a successful personnel director.)
11. They fully understand that the personnel executive's primary responsibility is as a management representative.

In light of the discussion to this point, what then are the implications of this changing perception of the hospital personnel function? For the institution, and particularly the chief executive officer, it means an upgrading of the position in the organization structure not only because of the importance of the function but also because of the demands made by individuals being considered for the job. There already is a great deal of evidence of this. As more chief executives say they want this more aggressive and sophisticated individual, such candidates are demanding as a condition of employment a reporting relationship directly to the chief executive officer or the chief operating officer. The more sophisticated candidates believe, and rightly so, that they must enjoy the same reporting relationship as the directors of nursing and finance. Some chief executives are lowering their sights rather than accept these preconditions, but others (some reluctantly) are accepting them if necessary to attract the right candidate.

If chief executive officers really are serious about recruiting this more aggressive and knowledgeable personnel executive, they will have to be firm in their commitments. This means that, traumatic as it may be, others in hospital management will have to accept as their peer a much more aggressive personnel executive than they probably have worked with in the past. This will cause conflict and some of these aggressive personnel executives may not survive, but those who do will have a marked impact on their institutions—and they certainly will have earned the respect and admiration of their peers.

For the present hospital personnel director, the implications are quite serious. The hard fact is that in the decade of the 80s, many current hospital personnel directors will not survive. Those who do and who prosper are those who can market and sell their programs effectively. Rather than trying to be inconspicuous, they literally will fight for their place in the organization. But even more important, they will recognize that they have not kept abreast of the latest developments and will make a concerted effort to become more actively involved in professional organizations in which there is an exchange of ideas among all types of personnel executives. They will take the lead in developing a more sophisticated human resource function for their organization.

There are exciting opportunities ahead. The rewards, both professional and financial, will be great for those able to rise to the challenge. A new breed of hospital personnel executive is being born. That birth will create trauma and conflict, but ultimately it will result in stronger institutions, better able to survive because of the effective utilization of their most important resource—people.

5. Recruitment, Screening and Selection

NORMAN METZGER

Reprinted with permission from *Personnel Administration in the Health Services Industry*, 2nd. ed., by Norman Metzger, SP Medical & Scientific Books, Division of Spectrum Publications, Inc., New York, © 1979.

Personnel Managers and other department heads must utilize every possible technique to locate, screen and select people they need. If they are going to be successful, they must reexamine their personnel practices. If jobs are not filled, if new and dynamic people are not attracted to a company, the policies must be changed. A company cannot survive without the human resources to keep it alive, vigorous and growing.[1]

Effective recruiting involves a determination of future needs, the clear definition and description of the types of people needed and an evaluation and determination of methods to be used in each particular case. In addition, it includes an investigation of the whole process of demand and supply. The most marked of changes in employment methods over the years has been the establishment of centralized screening and decentralized hiring. When the personnel department receives a requisition, several questions must be answered immediately: What are the specific job requirements for this position? What kind of person must be found to meet these requirements? Where should the department start looking to find an individual who matches these requirements?

RECRUITMENT

Recruitment is a positive mechanism. It involves finding applicants and encouraging potential employees to seek jobs at a specific institution. Before establishing a sound recruitment program, it is important that the sources of personnel are identified. Some of these sources are:

1. Present employees.
2. Employee referrals.
3. Applicants at the gate.
4. Write-ins.
5. Public employment agencies.
6. Private employment agencies.
7. Unions.
8. Retired military personnel.
9. Other retired individuals.
10. Schools and colleges.

Present Employees

Most institutions agree that promotions from within encourage present staff members to be more efficient and, indeed, kindle the spark of motivation present in all employees. The institution is offered a candidate for the position whose record is well-known. By using the mechanisms of transfer and promotion, lower-level jobs become available which the institution may find easier to fill. Careful consideration should be given to the procedure for effecting the fullest possible use of internal sources. This procedure would include:

1. Job posting.
2. Use of personnel records.
3. Skill banks.
4. Reemployment of former employees.

Job posting developed in many institutions through union pressures. It can be as effective in a nonunionized institution as in a unionized one. It is a practice found in many successful enterprises where preference is given to present employees in all opportunities for transfers and promotions. The usual procedure is to post the job on bulletin boards throughout the institution and include a brief description of the requirements. A concomitant instrument in effecting a successful job posting program is a specific personnel policy covering the criteria for promotion and transfers (Exhibit 5-1). In addition, an application for transfer (Exhibit 5-2) is a useful form and should include the supervisor's recommendation regarding the employee's qualifications. The employee's personnel record files can be very effective in determining the past record of an applicant for transfer and promotion. The employee's prior experience can be ascertained by a review of these records. Skill banks have been developed by many institutions to obviate unnecessary recruitment on the outside for skills that are available internally. Information on previous skills of present employees may be developed into computerized rosters from which lists of employees who have a specific skill can be made available at times of recruitment for specific job opportunities. The reemployment of former employees is facilitated by keeping up-to-date lists of employees who have been either laid off or voluntarily terminated. Several institutions have successfully recruited registered nurses by reviewing past records of terminations in the nursing department and communicating with each qualified nurse who voluntarily terminated over the past five years.

It is well to keep in mind the reluctance of supervisors to facilitate transfers or promotions of employees from a job in their department to a higher-rated job in another department. A good employee, both well-motivated and efficient, is a precious commodity which some supervisors feel must be protected and hoarded at all costs. It is important that the institution educate its supervisors to prevent blocking of transfers and promotions for qualified employees. A supervisor who permits and encourages upward mobility will build a well-motivated and efficient work force.

Employee Referrals

Experience has indicated that present employees are an excellent source for referral of qualified applicants for openings in their own institution. It is not surprising that present employees will carefully pre-screen any applicant whom they refer for employment to their institution. They seldom are willing to engender the criticism and embarrassment that may develop from referring an unqualified applicant. There is little question that morale is boosted when employees find that their recommendations are considered and accepted. It also follows that if an employee is dissatisfied with his job, he will not refer his friends or relatives for employment. Again, positions are posted in such a program and announcements of openings are made through the various employee communication vehicles. Some of the more successful nurse recruitment programs have incorporated bonuses for employees who refer nurses for employment. One institution offered $100 for each registered nurse referred by an employee and hired. This method of hiring is relatively inexpensive and can add to the overall good will in the institution. It is important that rejections of candidates referred by present employees are handled in the most careful and considerate manner. Reasons for the rejection should be clearly communicated to both the candidate and his sponsor.

Applicants at the Gate

Probably the largest single source of candidates is those who apply to the institution's employment office without any formal solicitation on the part of the institution. They do not involve any recruitment cost for the institution and often are attracted to applying for positions by the reputation of that institution. Since they are not responding to a specific solicitation, the institution is often faced with applicants for nonexisting positions. It behooves the employer to arrange for brief interviews even if positions are not available in order to generate good will within the community. This is an investment for future recruitment needs.

Write-Ins

A group of applicants similar to those who walk in without solicitation are those who write in without solicitation. Again, prompt and courteous responses to such inquiries are in order. It can be productive to keep a file of such applicants who either walk in or write in and find no positions available. Many employment offices of health care institutions keep up-to-date records of such inquiries. These files are pruned on a regular basis and reviewed when positions do become available.

Exhibit 5-1 In-House Personnel Policy

PERSONNEL POLICY # 6.1

	Issued: 11/1/70
PROMOTIONS AND TRANSFERS - CRITERIA Page 1 of 2	Revised: 6/1/74

The following statements describe the bases upon which employee promotions and transfers are made.

6.11 Definition of Promotion: Promotion is defined as the permanent reassignment of an employee to work at a higher job classification and compensation rate. Promotion occurs when:

    6.111 the employee transfers to a higher position (promotional transfer);

    6.112 the employee's present position is reclassified upward.

    (See also Personnel Policy #7.4, " Promotional Increases," and Personnel Policy #7.6, "Reclassification").

6.12 Definition of Transfer: Transfer is defined as the movement of an employee from one position to another. If the move is to a higher position, it is considered a promotional transfer. Transfers are further defined as:

    6.121 intradepartmental - where the transfer is within the department;

    6.122 interdepartmental - where the transfer is to a different department.

6.13 Criteria for Promotion: Where a promotional vacancy occurs and two or more employees are under consideration, the following factors are considered in selection:

    6.131 For bargaining unit positions, the employee with the greatest classification seniority will be promoted, unless there is an appreciable difference in their ability to do the work. If there is such a difference, the more able employee will be promoted.

    6.132 For non-bargaining unit positions, ability to do the work and classification seniority are considered. Where ability is relatively equal, the senior employee is promoted. The Medical Center is the sole judge of

MOUNT SINAI MEDICAL CENTER

Exhibit 5-1 continued

PERSONNEL POLICY # 6.1

PROMOTIONS AND TRANSFERS - CRITERIA

Issued: 11/1/70

Page 2 of 2   Revised: 6/1/74

---

the ability of an employee to do the work.

(See also Personnel Policy #5.3, "Seniority - Application.")

6.14   Criteria for Transfer: Where a vacancy occurs and two or more employees are considered for a non-promotional transfer to the position, the following factors are used in selection:

6.141   For bargaining unit and non-bargaining unit positions, ability to do the work and classification seniority are considered. Where ability is relatively equal, the senior employee is transferred. The Medical Center is the sole judge of the ability of an employee to do the work. (See also Personnel Policy #5.3, "Seniority-Applications.")

6.142   If it is necessary for a department to transfer one or more employees from among a group of employees performing the same work to (an)other position(s) within or outside the department, the selection is based on operational needs. Individual employee circumstances and seniority are taken into account wherever possible (See also Personnel Policy #5.3, "Seniority - Application." For details concerning pre-layoff transfers, see Personnel Policy #17.14, "Layoff and Recall.") and/or relevant Union Contract.

6.15   Trial Period for Promotions and Transfers: Employees who are permanently transferred or permanently promoted shall be subject to a trial period of two (2) months.

6.151   Permanent employees who do not successfully complete the trial period are eligible for return to their previous positions.

6.152   The supervisor is responsible for the evaluation of the transferees' and promotees' work performance during this trial period. Such evaluation will be communicated to the employee.

MOUNT SINAI MEDICAL CENTER

Exhibit 5-2 Application for Transfer Form

THE MOUNT SINAI MEDICAL CENTER

Posted Position
Referral Application

SECTION I – Completed by Employee

Name _____ Life # _____ Department Name _____

Date Hired _____

Hospital Extension _____ Home Phone _____ Current Position Title _____ Time/Day Available for Interview _____

Interested in position No./Title _____ Posting Location and Date _____

Please provide any information you wish that you consider relevant to your application for the above posted position:

_____

Employee Signature _____ Date _____

SECTION II – Completed by Employee's Current Supervisor

If the above named employee is accepted for another position, we can release him/her from this department on the following date _____ Supervisor's Signature _____

SECTION III – Completed by Supervisor with Posted Vacant Position

Date Applicant Interviewed _____ Accepted for vacant posted position ( ) Date scheduled to start _____

Rejected for vacant posted position ( ) Specify reason _____

_____

Signature _____ Date _____

SECTION IV – Completed by Personnel Department

Date application received in Personnel _____ Date of Personnel interview _____

Date referral scheduled _____ If no referral, specify reason _____

Disposition _____ Date employee notified of disposition _____

Signature of Employment Manager _____ Date _____

Issued 9/77 – Personnel Department

Public Employment Agencies

A wise man once said you do something well and have several sidelines. The same advice might be given to institutions in meeting their recruitment needs. All possible sources should be explored. Since 1933, larger communities throughout the nation have been served by public employment offices that have been valuable sources of applicants for open positions. These public offices have also been charged with the job of administering unemployment compensation benefits. As a result, they have an added interest in discovering job opportunities for those who are out of work. Employment agencies are a key source of applicants. An institution can place an opening with such an agency, either by telephone or in person. Many of these agencies are equipped to do testing that is invaluable to the smaller health services institutions unable to do such testing on their own. Recently the United States Employment Service introduced a new computerized job bank system. This has increased their effectiveness. Of course, *there is no fee charged to either employers or employees for such services.*

Private Employment Agencies

There are approximately 10,000 private employment agencies in the United States. More and more private employment offices specialize in skilled manual and white-collar manpower. These agencies are an excellent source for the recruitment of personnel for higher level positions. Some of the more sophisticated agencies are using data processing techniques which facilitate the matching of employer requirements and applicants in the file. Many institutions develop close relationships with the private agencies based upon their past success in filling jobs for them. *Where the skills sought are in short supply, the employer usually takes the responsibility for the fee.* In the cases of low-level positions and those skills normally in sufficient supply in the labor market, the applicant pays the fee soon after starting on the job. Some agencies are parts of national chains and, therefore, can call upon branch offices in other cities in searching for applicants. This offers a marked advantage in recruitment of highly specialized categories. In selecting an agency, an institution can be guided by the agency's membership in a state or national association that subscribes to certain professional or ethical standards. Pell lists certain recommendations in dealing with private employment agencies.[2]

1. DO:

Learn which employment agencies are best for different types of jobs.
Get to know the staff of the agencies with which a company works.
Learn what special or added services agencies offer.
Communicate with the agency—let them have full job specifications and give them feedback on the results of interviews.
Periodically evaluate the success of the agencies with which you work.
Understand the agencies' fee schedules.

2. DO NOT:

List the same job with too many agencies in the same area.
Accept referrals from agencies on applicants previously referred by other sources.
Refer an applicant sent by an agency in whom there is no interest to another employer.
Accept referrals from an agency without a clear understanding regarding who is to pay the fee and how much it will be.

Unions

Institutions having collective bargaining agreements with unions often have available to them union hiring halls. Some contracts provide for such services as the first contact to be made by the employer before hiring from the outside. Clear language should be provided on the options of the employer in using a union hiring hall. The following is a provision of a collective bargaining agreement for the use of a union hiring hall.

1. The institution shall notify the union employment service of all bargaining unit jobs and training position vacancies and shall afford the service 24 hours from the time of notification to refer an applicant for the vacancy before the institution hires from any other source.

2. Neither the union employment service in referring nor the institution hiring shall discriminate against an applicant because of membership or nonmembership in the union.

3. The cost of operating the employment service shall be borne by the union.

4. The institution retains the right to hire such applicants referred by the employment service as it deems qualified in its sole discretion.

5. The institution retains the right to hire applicants from other sources in the event the em-

ployment service does not refer qualified applicants within such 24-hour period.

6. The institution shall not be required to notify the employment service of any job vacancy which must be filled without delay in order to meet an emergency or to safeguard the health, safety or well-being of patients.

Retired Military Personnel

Retired military personnel offer a potentially excellent recruitment source, as do veterans released from military service. Many of these individuals are highly qualified and possess skills often not found in the civilian population. The military has expended enormous funds in training such individuals and many of these skills are transferable to civilian occupations. Institutions recruiting such personnel do so by advertisements in military publications and referring job openings to separation centers. The Retired Officers Association in Washington, D.C., is a useful agency to contact. *This agency does not charge any fee.*

Other Retired Individuals

More and more institutions have found a pool of qualified, well-motivated individuals made available by early retirement programs in industry and other institutions. Some of these individuals, often in their early fifties, have retired from positions held for 20 and 30 years and now seek to gain employment in new positions. They offer the institution upwards of ten years of productive working time. There are many Forty-Plus clubs in existence in large cities throughout the country which can provide applicants well-qualified for positions which institutions may have available. *There is no charge for such services.* In addition, handicapped workers offer still another source of productive, well-motivated applicants.

Schools and Colleges

Visits to campuses and high schools have produced excellent candidates for positions in the health service industry. Many institutions have developed programs which provide periodic visits to local schools and colleges at which time general information is provided the senior classes as to opportunities available in the institution. Working closely with the school's placement office, a year-round educational program is possible which can attract highly qualified young applicants. These individuals offer a firm educational base for institutional training programs. In developing a program

to recruit graduates of local schools and colleges, it is essential that visits be planned in advance; announcements clearly made to the schools well before the visit; arrangements made for interviewing time and space; and contacts carefully developed with members of the academic community.

RECRUITMENT ADVERTISEMENT

The most widely used recruitment technique is that of placing classified ads. Two major considerations go into the decision to place a help-wanted ad: (1) the media to be used, and (2) the layout or construction of the ad. The media available to the employer include daily newspapers, weekend newspapers, trade publications and specialized newspapers and magazines. A careful analysis must be undertaken as to the audience reached by each of these media. *As with all other recruitment techniques, it is essential to maintain records which will indicate the success of each of the media based upon the type of skill sought.* Many institutions find trade magazines quite effective for the placement of recruitment advertisements for professional and managerial positions. On the other hand, the help-wanted section of the local newspaper produces best results for nonskilled, low-level applicants.

In deciding upon the construction of the ad, cost and potential results must be carefully weighed. Classified ads are used most frequently because of the low cost involved, while display ads, which are larger and more costly, are used for difficult-to-recruit positions. In some cases blind ads are preferred. These are classified or display ads which do not identify the institution. The applicants are directed to a box number which affords the institution the opportunity to review résumés without the need to communicate rejections to those obviously not qualified. When an institution enjoys a good reputation in the community, the blind ad is not as effective as placement of an ad which identifies the institution. Many qualified applicants are drawn to specific institutions solely on their reputation. Yet there are times when blind ads are essential to preserve the confidential nature of the recruitment since the institution may not want to indicate to present employees or to prospective employees its identity. Some ads ask for reply by letter while others direct the applicant to a phone number. Still others list interviewing hours at specific times for those who wish to respond to an ad. In the construction of an attractive ad that will improve the quality of responses, Pell suggests a system he calls AIDA:[3]

1. *Attention*—one must attract attention to the ad. It must be seen to be read. Typeface can attract readers. The headline should be one or two words which have pulling power.
2. *Interest*—once the eye has been attracted to the ad, it is essential to develop interest in the job. Salary and fringe benefits are certainly interest factors. Others are special advantages offered, information about the company and opportunities for the geographic area.
3. *Desire*—amplification of the interest factors plus the extras which the job offers in terms of growth, job satisfaction and personal value help create this desire. Readers are more interested in themselves than anything else. Write the ad to appeal to them, not to satisfy the writer's ego.
4. *Action*—not only must the ad be appealing, but also it should instigate action. Give him the name, the phone number and the time the applicant should call.

In addition to advertising of open positions, many institutions have available special recruitment literature for applicants. This literature is usually distributed at the time of the interview but can be forwarded to an applicant in advance of the interview. It should be graphically appealing and contain pertinent information to attract the qualified applicant to the institution.

Selection

While recruitment is a positive mechanism designed to bring in as many applicants as possible, selection can be considered a negative mechanism. A proper selection program lets only the qualified applicants through the sieve. An attempt is made to appraise qualities the institution feels are indicative of success on the job. This process necessitates the making of a value judgment, a forecast as to which applicants will turn out to be productive employees. As with any forecasting there are tools of the trade:

1. The application blank.
2. The interview.
3. Tests.
4. The reference check.
5. The preemployment physical.

The selection process is made up of various stages which should be designed to permit candidates through each phase at a numerically decreasing rate. Calhoun likens the procedure to an inverted triangle (Figure 5-1).[4]

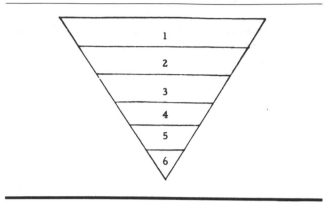

Figure 5-1 The Selection Triangle

Application Forms

The application form plays a simple, yet important role in selection. Its contents can discourage unsuitable applicants and its design can reflect the company's dignity, reduce to a minimum the time needed to fill it out and simplify its review. Its wording and its comprehensiveness affect the efficiency and validity of the selection process.[5]

The application blank must be designed for the specific task it is to perform, namely, to improve the selection of applicants. It can, if properly designed, greatly reduce the time required for the interview which will follow its completion. It should provide definitive indicators which an experienced interviewer can quickly interpret. In the final analysis, its primary objective is that of comparing the applicant's qualifications with the qualifications required for the available job. It is the most widely used personnel selection device. Most application blanks contain the following items:

1. Identifying information:
   a. Name, address, telephone number.
   b. Date of birth, marital status and number of dependents.
   c. Social Security number.
   d. Height, weight and physical characteristics.
2. Education and training:
   a. Record of grade school, high school, technical or trade school, college and graduate school completion.
   b. Special skills developed through other training.
3. Work experience:
   a. Prior positions with dates of employment, salary, duties and reason for leaving.
4. Personal references.

5. Record of service in the armed forces.
6. Hobbies and leisure time interests.

In the construction of an application blank, it is important for the institution to carefully review the appropriate state and federal laws affecting questions in application blanks and employment interviews. Exhibit 5-3 is an example of an all-inclusive application blank.

Three common purposes of the application blank are:[6]

1. Preliminary screening to determine whether or not an interview is needed.
2. An interview aid to provide an outline of basic facts which may be elaborated during the interview.
3. A selection device based on the blank's own merits.

Recent studies indicate that most applicants are relatively honest in reporting work history on application blanks. Although some applicants give advantageously inaccurate replies to reasons for separation, job duties and wages, apparently the implied verification of application facts (which should be clearly stated on the form itself) is a sufficient deterrent to falsification of information. Mandell suggests that the specific application blank which will produce the best results must be designed in relation to the selection methods used and selection ratios which will apply. He states, for example:

1. A brief form will do if the next step in the selection process is an inexpensive written test which will eliminate a large percentage of the applicants.
2. If a résumé is requested first, the scope of its contents should be suggested.
3. A biographical information blank reduces the need for depth in the application form.
4. A general application blank can be supplemented by a check list prepared for each type of work to ensure that the applicant has the necessary qualifications.[7]

In constructing an application blank, the designer should not fail to recognize that some applicants will find varying degrees of difficulty and discomfort in their attempt to complete it. It may be necessary to tailor application blanks to the varying levels of applicants that apply to an institution—for example, one for professional employees, a second for semiskilled employees and a third for nonskilled employees.

Another consideration is the eventual use of the application blank. Some institutions use the blank as a permanent personnel record; therefore, it must include many items otherwise superfluous for selection and placement. Some application blanks are printed on expensive and thick stock which when folded can be inserted into a Cardex file and may be used for wage and salary administration purposes. Usually where such a decision is made, i.e., *to use it as a permanent personnel record application blank,* the cost of such forms for all applicants becomes prohibitive when one considers a normal selection ratio of 10 applicants for one hire. Therefore, if the institution has made a decision to use a permanent personnel record application blank, it may find a *preliminary short-form application* useful. The preliminary short-form application will elicit key information necessary to make an initial screening to determine if the applicant appears to possess the requisite background for the position available. Then, and only then, the permanent application blank may be completed. Although this practice is not uncommon, it is not the most satisfactory procedure. The permanent personnel record should be separated and distinguished from the application blank. Only applicants who are hired should complete permanent records.

THE INTERVIEW

The most valuable single device used in the selection process is the face-to-face interview. The employment interview has the following function and objectives:

Employment interviewing is the open exchange of information between persons of acknowledged unequal status for a mutually agreed upon purpose, conducted in a manner that elicits, clarifies, organizes, or synthesizes the information to affect positively or negatively the attitudes, judgments, actions or opinions of the participants thereby making possible an objective and rational evaluation of the appropriateness of an employee for a specific job.[8]

While application forms are often sketchy, incomplete and at times misleading, the task of evaluating applicants, a most difficult and demanding one, is best accomplished through sound interviewing techniques. Such techniques require complex skills such as psychological sophistication, understanding of the dynamics of human development and familiarity with the kinds of abilities, motivations, interests and personality patterns best suited to specific work situations.[9]

Exhibit 5-3 All-Inclusive Application Blank

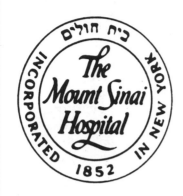

THE MOUNT SINAI MEDICAL CENTER

ONE GUSTAVE L. LEVY PLACE - NEW YORK, N.Y. 10029

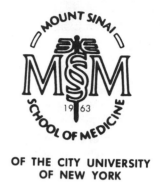

**OF THE CITY UNIVERSITY
OF NEW YORK**

*APPLICATION for
EMPLOYMENT*

RETURN TO: (check one)

☐ MOUNT SINAI SCHOOL OF MEDICINE EMPLOYMENT OFFICE

☐ MOUNT SINAI HOSPITAL EMPLOYMENT OFFICE

☐ MOUNT SINAI HOSPITAL PROFESSIONAL NURSE
RECRUITMENT EMPLOYMENT OFFICE

☐ MOUNT SINAI SERVICES EMPLOYMENT OFFICE

EQUAL EMPLOYMENT OPPORTUNITY THROUGH AFFIRMATIVE ACTION

Exhibit 5-3 continued

THE MOUNT SINAI HOSPITAL AND THE MOUNT SINAI SCHOOL OF MEDICINE OF THE CITY UNIVERSITY OF NEW YORK ARE EQUAL EMPLOYMENT AFFIRMATIVE ACTION EMPLOYERS. PERSONNEL ARE CHOSEN ON THE BASIS OF ABILITY AND QUALIFICATIONS WITHOUT REGARD TO RACE, COLOR, RELIGION, SEX, AGE, NATIONAL ORIGIN, MARITAL STATUS, HANDICAP OR VETERAN STATUS IN COMPLIANCE WITH FEDERAL, STATE, AND MUNICIPAL LAWS.

NAME (PRINT) LAST   FIRST   MIDDLE   DATE   SOC. SEC. NO.   POSITION APPLIED FOR

ADDRESS   CITY   STATE   ZIP CODE   TEL. NO.   ARE YOU 18 YEARS OR OLDER ☐ YES ☐ NO

CITIZEN OF U.S.   ☐ YES   HAVE YOU EVER BEEN EMPLOYED BY MOUNT SINAI- IF YES, INDICATE DATE AND POSITION   IF NOT - PLEASE SPECIFY AGE
☐ YES ☐ NO   IF NOT - DO YOU HAVE LEGAL RIGHT TO WORK IN U.S. ☐ NO   ☐ YES ☐ NO

DO YOU HAVE ANY RELATIVES EMPLOYED BY MOUNT SINAI OTHER THAN SPOUSE
☐ NO ☐ YES
IF YES - LIST NAMES

YOU MAY NOT BE ASSIGNED TO A POSITION WHERE YOU WOULD SUPERVISE OR BE SUPERVISED BY A RELATIVE.

HOW DID YOU LEARN OF MOUNT SINAI
☐ ADVERTISEMENT
☐ OTHER

TYPE OF POSITION
☐ FULL TIME ☐ PART TIME ☐ TEMPORARY
☐ PERMANENT ☐ SUMMER

SHIFTS AVAIL.   HOURS AVAIL.   DAYS AVAIL.   I AGREE TO ROTATE ALL THREE SHIFTS AS REQUIRED

SIGNATURE

DATE OF U.S. MILITARY SERVICE
BRANCH OF U.S. MILITARY SERVICE

WHICH FOREIGN LANGUAGES DO YOU READ AND/OR WRITE AND/OR SPEAK FLUENTLY

SKILLS:

TYPING (SPECIFY) ☐ ELECTRIC ☐ MANUAL ☐ OTHER   W.P.M.
☐ STENO   W.P.M. ☐ DICTAPHONE ☐ MEDICAL TERMINOLOGY

PLEASE LIST OTHER SPECIAL SKILLS:

HAVE YOU EVER BEEN CONVICTED OF A CRIME OR OFFENSE OTHER THAN A MINOR TRAFFIC VIOLATION ☐ YES ☐ NO IF YES, PLEASE EXPLAIN:

WHEN   WHERE   DISPOSITION OF OFFENSE

ARE THERE ANY ARRESTS OR CRIMINAL PROCEEDINGS CURRENTLY PENDING AGAINST YOU ☐ NO ☐ YES - IF YES, PLEASE EXPLAIN -

NEW YORK STATE LAW AGAINST DISCRIMINATION PROHIBITS UNJUSTIFIED DISCRIMINATION ON THE BASIS OF A CRIMINAL CONVICTION RECORD

DO YOU HAVE ANY IMPAIRMENTS, PHYSICAL OR MENTAL, WHICH WILL INTERFERE WITH YOUR ABILITY TO PERFORM THE JOB FOR WHICH YOU ARE APPLYING? PLEASE DESCRIBE. _____

ARE THERE ANY POSITIONS OR TYPES OF POSITIONS FOR WHICH YOU SHOULD NOT BE CONSIDERED OR JOB DUTIES YOU CANNOT PERFORM BECAUSE OF A PHYSICAL OR MENTAL OR MEDICAL DISABILITY. - PLEASE DESCRIBE _____

EDUCATION	NAME OF SCHOOL	ADDRESS	YEARS COMPLETED	DATE LEFT	IF GRAD. DEG./MAJ.	NOT GRAD. - LEVEL COMPLETED NO. of CREDITS
HIGH SCHOOL or highest grade attended						
COLLEGE/ UNIVERSITY						
TECHNICAL or NURSING SCHOOL						
GRADUATE SCHOOL						

PLEASE LIST PROFESSIONAL LICENSES AND/OR CERTIFICATION BELOW:

TYPE	STATE	EXPIRATION DATE	REGISTRATION NUMBER

Exhibit 5-3 continued

THE FOLLOWING SECTION TO BE COMPLETED BY PROFESSIONAL NURSING APPLICANTS ONLY:

SPECIFY BELOW YOUR PREFERRED AREAS OF CLINICAL NURSING | DESIRE HOUSING ☐ YES ☐ NO | I AGREE TO ROTATE ALL THREE SHIFTS
1.   2.   3. | | SIGNATURE

R.N. AND L.P.N.

IF YOU DO NOT HAVE A CURRENT AND VALID N.Y. STATE NURSING LICENSE, HAVE YOU MADE APPLICATION   ☐ NO   ☐ YES   WHEN

TYPE - R.N. L.P.N. OTHER.........	STATE ISSUED	EXPIRATION DATE	REGISTRATION NO.
1			
2			
3			

EMPLOYMENT HISTORY	PLEASE COMPLETE SECTION EVEN IF YOU ATTACHED RESUME. LIST CURRENT OR MOST RECENT POSITION FIRST AND COVER PERIODS OF EMPLOYMENT FOR THE LAST SEVEN (7) YEARS

FROM / TO /	EMPLOYER'S NAME/ADDRESS TEL. NO./SUPERVISOR	POSITION TITLE / JOB DUTIES	REASONS FOR LEAVING
			FINAL SALARY
FROM / TO /			REASONS FOR LEAVING
			FINAL SALARY
FROM / TO /			REASONS FOR LEAVING
			FINAL SALARY

IS ANY ADDITIONAL INFORMATION RELATIVE TO CHANGE IN NAME, USE OF AN ASSUMED NAME OR NICKNAME NECESSARY TO ENABLE A CHECK ON YOUR WORK RECORD? -IF YES- PLEASE EXPLAIN

DO YOU AUTHORIZE US TO CONTACT YOUR PRESENT EMPLOYER FOR REFERENCE PRIOR TO MOUNT SINAI

EMPLOYMENT   ☐ YES   ☐ NO

AUTHORIZED SIGNATURE

IF EMPLOYER IS NO LONGER IN BUSINESS HOW MAY WE CHECK THIS REFERENCE

APPLICANT'S AFFIDAVIT:

I CERTIFY THAT THE INFORMATION CONTAINED IN THIS APPLICATION IS CORRECT TO THE BEST OF MY KNOWLEDGE. I AUTHORIZE INVESTIGATION OF ALL MATTERS CONTAINED IN THIS APPLICATION AND AGREE THAT ANY MISLEADING OR FALSE STATEMENTS WOULD BE CAUSE FOR REJECTION OF THIS APPLICATION OR WOULD BE SUFFICIENT CAUSE FOR DISMISSAL AFTER MY EMPLOYMENT. I UNDERSTAND THAT MY EMPLOYMENT IS CONTINGENT UPON SATISFACTORY COMPLETION OF A PHYSICAL EXAMINATION BY A MOUNT SINAI EMPLOYEE HEALTH SERVICE PHYSICIAN; THE RECEIPT BY MOUNT SINAI OF SATISFACTORY WORK REFERENCES AND MY SATISFACTORY COMPLETION OF THE PROBATIONARY PERIOD OF EMPLOYMENT FOR MY POSITION. I HEREBY AUTHORIZE MY PRESENT/PAST EMPLOYERS TO FURNISH MOUNT SINAI WITH THEIR RECORDS OF SERVICE. I AGREE IF EMPLOYED TO SUPPLY MOUNT SINAI WITH SUCH VERIFICATIONS AS THEY MAY BE PERMITTED BY FEDERAL STATE, AND MUNICIPLE CODES AND REGULATIONS TO REQUEST OF ME AND TO ABIDE BY ALL MOUNT SINAI'S RULES AND REGULATIONS.

_____   _____
DATE   SIGNATURE

Exhibit 5-3 continued

REFERRAL:

DEPARTMENT NAME _____ DEPARTMENT HEAD _____

POSITION _____ REPLACING _____

PERMANENT _____ TEMPORARY: FROM _____   TO _____

RECOMMENDED SALARY _____ PRE-EMPLOYMENT PHYSICAL DATE _____ STARTING DATE _____

(SALARY RECOMMENDATIONS ABOVE MINIMUM MAY NOT BE COMMUNICATED TO APPLICANT UNLESS APPROVED BY PERSONNEL)

ACCEPTED _____ REJECTED   (STATE REASONS BELOW) _____

SIGNATURE _____ DATE _____

DEPARTMENT COMMENTS:

PERSONNEL COMMENTS-CHECK LIST-

The interview has been described as "the conversation with a purpose." There are four objectives of the selection interview:

1. Matching people with jobs.
2. Serving as a means for creating good feeling toward the institution.
3. Dispensing job and institutional information in order to provide the applicant with a factual basis for accepting or rejecting employment if offered.
4. Providing the interviewer with an opportunity for obtaining data relevant to making a sound employment decision, such data not being available from other sources.

The selection of a truly qualified interviewer is essential to the success of the employment program. The successful employment interviewer knows in advance the kinds of information he wishes to obtain. Although he has a plan for the interview, he does not stereotype his interviews. Before asking the applicant into the interviewing room, he will have reviewed all pertinent information such as the job description, the job specification and the application form. He must schedule the interview so that enough time is provided to effectively draw out the applicant and provide information for both parties to the interview to make a sound decision as to employment. Enough time must be scheduled to ensure that maximum success is derived from the interview. In a study made by Mandell, the median length of total interviewing time per applicant among those firms participating was found to be 30 minutes for plant employees, 45 minutes for office employees, 90 minutes for college graduates, two hours for salesmen and engineers and three hours for supervisors and executives.[10]

In the case where a great number of applicants apply for the same position, it is important to conduct a screening rapidly to save the institution's time as well as the applicant's. Yet it is desirable to leave the applicant feeling that his candidacy has been given reasonable consideration. One of the most important steps in expediting the *screening interview* is to plan in advance those elements in a candidate's qualifications which are most crucial in determining his possible suitability for the opening at hand. For example, frequently it is a practice in the screening interview for the interviewer to spend a great deal of time determining the employee's technical qualifications for the job. However, the nature of the position may require the employee to work overtime or to work unusual hours. If the interviewer spends half an hour determining the potential employee's technical knowledge and experience and then finds that he is unwilling to work the required hours, he has wasted valuable time. The screening interview is merely an opportunity to determine in a rather general way whether the employee is qualified and suitable for the job opening. Intensive consideration of his technical qualifications and personality considerations should be left for the later stages of the interview or, if possible, for a second interview which might be called the *placement interview*. Thus, in preplanning for the interview, the interviewer should have isolated those factors which are essential for more thorough consideration of the candidate. For example, a secretarial job specification may have shown that the following qualifications are essential:

Must have at least two years experience. Must be familiar with office routines. Must be able to type 50 words per minute and take shorthand at the rate of 110 words per minute.

Therefore, the primary objective in the screening interview is to put the candidate at ease and determine as rapidly as possible if he or she meets these *basic* requirements. The interviewer may then want to dig more deeply into specific experience, work attitudes and personality factors.

The initial screening interview indicates whether the candidate is generally qualified for the job. The purpose of the placement interview is to determine specifically and in depth whether the candidate meets the detailed requirements of the job and whether his work habits, attitude and personality are compatible for work in the organization. In addition, during the placement interview, the interviewer should cover every item on the application form to ascertain that he understands the candidate's work record and can verify (through questioning, reference checks and personal contacts) the data given by the candidate. Briefly, some of the basic areas to consider in following the application form during the placement interview are as follows.

1. *Work history:* In many instances applicants unintentionally (and occasionally, purposely) leave gaps in their work history or overestimate the length of time spent in a particular job. Sometimes it helps to verify information by asking the specific dates when the applicant started with previous employers and the specific dates he left. All intervening periods between jobs should be accounted for. The exact title or position description of each job should be clearly identified. Determine the specific title the applicant actually carried in the job and the exact, detailed nature of his duties. In each instance the interviewer should find out why the applicant left his previous employer. The in-

terviewer should delve into the applicant's feelings about his previous supervisor and determine what the applicant liked best and least about his previous jobs. Very often attitudes or patterns of behavior are disclosed that are useful in evaluating his suitability for the present opening. For example, the candidate may show that he likes jobs in which he is closely supervised and receives a great deal of instruction. If he is applying for a job requiring independent action and general supervision, it may not be an ideal situation for him.

2. *Educational background:* An individual's feelings and reactions concerning his learning and educational experiences can often yield additional information about his job attitude. The interviewer should determine why the applicant left school (if he did), which subjects he liked best and why, and which subjects he liked least and why. He should check closely any unexplained gaps in educational experience.

3. *Outside activities:* Discussion of educational experiences often leads easily into discussion of other interests, hobbies and off-the-job activities. The interviewer should again apply the open interviewing technique and give the applicant a chance to talk freely about his interests and activities. If the job demands mental alertness, professional skill and curiosity, the interviewer should look particularly for interest in books, periodicals and technical journals. In listening to the applicant talk about his social activities, the interviewer should watch for clues which indicate the applicant's desire to associate with others or his interest in exerting leadership in group situations.[11]

Five Parts of the Interview

The interview logically breaks down into five separate but, in some ways, overlapping phases:

1. Warm-up stage.
2. Getting the applicant to talk stage.
3. The drawing-out stage.
4. Information stage.
5. Forming an opinion stage.

In the *warm-up stage,* the interviewer attempts to develop rapport with the applicant. It is important that the interview be held in uninterrupted privacy in order to develop a closer relationship with the interviewee. Almost all applicants are nervous during the interviewing stage. The obvious need to discuss personal information in an interview mandates complete privacy. There is nothing more disconcerting to an applicant than having his train of thought disturbed by an incoming telephone call or a third party entering the inter-

viewing room and holding a discussion with the interviewer. Informality is an important adjunct to this getting-acquainted stage. Some interviewers use a topic of general social interest to put the applicant at ease. No matter which method is used, the intent is to remove the initial tension experienced by an applicant when he first enters the interviewing room. It is essential that the interviewer set an environment conducive to the flow of relevant information. One authority points out that the interviewer will be more successful in breaking the ice and relaxing the candidate if he gets the candidate talking rather than carries the bulk of the conversation himself. He suggests that if the candidate is tense, the interviewer may want to prolong the small talk; if he appears to be at ease, he may want to shorten it.[12]

The second stage is *starting the applicant talking.* Here the application form can well assist the interviewer in selecting the one good question to trigger the applicant's flow of conversation. For example, an interviewer in observing the prior work record of the applicant may start this stage off by stating, ''I see that you worked at Metropolitan Hospital for three years. Can you tell me about your job and what you did?'' He then permits the applicant to talk and set the pace.

In the *drawing-out stage,* the interviewer attempts to elicit from the applicant answers to questions which were not developed by the applicant when he presented his background. The applicant may have left out details. The interviewer cannot afford to permit such lapses regarding essential information.

In the *informational stage,* the interviewer now presents a picture of the institution and the specific job under discussion. Here he must present to the applicant all pertinent information and answer any questions the applicant may have. This can be a very crucial part of the interview since the questions posed by the applicant may reveal a great deal about his needs, his fears and his aspirations.

In the last stage of the interview, *an opinion must be formed.* This is often done by making notes after the applicant has left the office. Exhibit 5-4 is an example of an applicant evaluation form [to be] completed by interviewers at the end of the interview. Taking notes during the interview is to be discouraged; if absolutely necessary, minimized. It can be very disconcerting and disruptive to the interviewee.

Pitfalls of Interviewing

The key to the successful interview is the interviewer himself. Too often the interviewer falls into one of the many pitfalls producing an ineffective evaluation

Exhibit 5-4 Interviewer Evaluation Form

```
                    APPLICANT EVALUATION FORM FOR INTERVIEWER

Name _____  Job considered for _____

Interviewer_____  Date  _____
------------------------------------------------------------------------------------

INSTRUCTIONS:  Your rating of each factor should be reflected by placing a check ☑ above the position on the
               scale that best reflects your evaluation.

1.  PREVIOUS EXPERIENCE:

    Consider similar job duties, similar working conditions,
    same degree of supervision exercised and/or received.
                                                     Below Average | Average | Above Average

2.  EDUCATION AND TRAINING:

    Consider formal education, major fields of study and
    specialized training received for the available position.
                                                     Below Average | Average | Above Average

3.  MANNER AND APPEARANCE:

    Consider general appearance, speech, nervous mannerisms,
    self-confidence and aggressiveness.
                                                     Below Average | Average | Above Average

4.  EMOTIONAL STABILITY AND MATURITY:

    Consider friction with former supervisors, relationships
    with peers, reasons for leaving job, job stability.  Con-
    sider sense of responsibility, attitude towards work and
    towards family.
                                                     Below Average | Average | Above Average

5.  SUPERVISORY POTENTIAL:

    Consider previous leadership experience.  Consider de-
    gree of aggressiveness, self-confidence.
                                                     Below Average | Average | Above Average


    OVER-ALL RATING FOR SPECIFIC POSITION:

    Consider all the facts you have learned about the        ☐ Above Average
    applicant, how well is he fitted for this job in com-    ☐ Average
    parison with other men doing this work in the firm       ☐ Below Average
    or in comparison with your standards.

ADDITIONAL COMMENTS:



☐ Hire      ☐ Do Not Hire     ☐ Hold Until _____    ☐ Refer to _____
```

of the candidate and a poor result from the interview. Personal bias is not uncommon, be it favorable or unfavorable. The way an applicant dresses, the length of an applicant's hair, his speech mannerisms, his ethnic background—all may affect the interviewer's impression. It is important for the interviewer to be as objective as possible in order to reach a proper evaluation. *Personal bias has no place in the interviewing room.* Most of these biases are illegal as well as improper. The use of pseudoscience and myth, ridiculous at times, pops its ugly head into some interviews. Some people believe that there are criminal types—that certain physical characteristics denote reliability, accuracy, loyalty and honesty. These "natural" judgments of character are completely unreliable and have no place in the interview. Although appearance may be important for certain jobs, it cannot be used as a reliable guide to ascertain personality traits. Another pitfall is the stereotype interview. Interviewers should not allow themselves to fall into a comfortable routine, no matter what problems may be present in a specific interview. Some interviewees require a nondirective approach while others require far more guidance in the interview. The interviewer should be flexible in his approach and be aware of the personality and needs of the interviewee. Still another pitfall is the illusion of previous experience. Too many interviewers believe that in order to succeed at a job, the applicant must have had exactly the same type of experience in the past. This is unsubstantiated by facts.

The interviewer should not show by word or manner that he is critical of anything the applicant says or does. This can destroy his effectiveness. Interruptions by the interviewer should be kept to a minimum as long as the applicant is presenting information relevant to the final decision that must be made. Talking down to or above an applicant should be avoided. The interviewer should be sensitive to his own use of language, keeping in mind the educational and experiential background of the applicant. Inappropriate standards should not be applied since these may be too low or too high for the job. In either case selection based upon such false standards can result in poor placements. By using higher standards overqualified applicants may be hired, leading to turnover and discontentment in the job. By using lower standards applicants may be accepted who will require intensive training and produce a morale problem.

The halo effect is not uncommon in interviews. An interviewer may find something good or something bad in the applicant's background or presentation and, therefore, judge all his credentials on the basis of this one good or bad aspect. The question of note-taking referred to earlier is the subject of much debate among specialists in the field of interviewing. There is no debate over the need for brief notes following the interview, but most practitioners believe that note-taking can inhibit the applicant from presenting a free flow of information. It is best to limit the amount of note-taking by unobtrusively jotting down impressions without giving an indication of censure or concern over the specific information being recorded so as not to embarrass or inhibit the interviewee.

Pell directs the interviewer's attention to the framing of questions. He suggests: *Don't* ask questions that can be answered by "yes" or "no." This stifles information. Instead of asking, "Have you had any experience in budgeting?" say, "Tell me what you have done in budgeting." *Don't* put words in the applicant's mouth. Instead of "You have called on discount stores, haven't you?" ask "What discount stores have you called on?" *Don't* ask questions which are unrelated to your objectives. It might be interesting to follow through on certain tidbits of gossip that the applicant volunteers, but it rarely leads to pertinent information. *Do* ask questions which develop information as to the applicant's *experience* ("What were your responsibilities regarding the purchasing department?"), *knowledge* ("How do you feel about heavy travel?") and *motivation* ("Why do you wish to change jobs now?").[13]

The Successful Interview

To review the ingredients that will increase both the effectiveness of the interview and the chance of a proper placement, the following check list is offered:

1. The goal of interviewing is to match people with available jobs. In order to do that, the interviewer must know what he is looking for and place in juxtaposition information on what the particular applicant can do.
2. Ad hoc interviewing produces ad hoc placements; the successful interview is based upon a plan which although formal is flexible.
3. Tools of the game are necessary in this as well as all management techniques. Therefore, good selection methods must start with the collection of facts such as:
   a. the job specification;
   b. the type of supervisor and style of supervision to be exerted on the successful applicant;
   c. facts about the applicant.
4. The most successful way to preliminarily assemble the facts about the applicant is by use of an application form. This form should be as detailed as necessary and tailor-made to the specific needs of the institution. It is not uncommon to use several types of application forms for the various skill levels in the institution.
5. The key to successful interviewing is sympathetic listening. People talk to people whom they believe will listen to them. It is therefore necessary to ensure maximum privacy, expend uninterrupted attention and display an interest in what the applicant has to say.
6. Criticism has no place in the interviewing room. The interviewer should be receptive to all information offered by the applicant and should not disclose a critical attitude as to its content. The physical environment plays an important role in eliciting maximum information from the candidate and in reducing the tension with which most interviews begin.
7. The successful interviewer is aware of his own prejudices and should try to avoid their influence on judgments he is called upon to make during the selection interview.
8. Skills must be developed in how and when to close the interview, how and when to communicate rejection and how to evaluate the qualifications of candidates for employment.

REFERENCE CHECKS

Almost as prevalent as the application blank in the selection procedure is the use of reference checks. Yet, although a large majority of institutions send out formal reference checks, many do not use the facts presented in response to such requests. It would appear that many institutions request the information to attempt to affect the honesty of the applicant's responses since it is felt that the mere implied suggestion of seeking reference checks will improve the quality of response as to its accuracy. There is, of course, a great deal of skepticism as to the validity of information elicited from reference checks. Certainly most institutions discount letters of reference produced by the applicant and addressed to that universal someone, "To Whom It May Concern." To ensure the accuracy and sincerity of reference checks, they must be private and confidential. The most common technique of sending form letters or form cards to former employers has proved to be less effective than face-to-face interviews or telephone interviews of former employers. It would be an excellent policy for an institution to check the applicant's last employer by telephone, using the letter or card form for other employers.

Reference checks are often completed by personnel departments who have little contact with the applicant in question. To further ensure the validity of the reference, it is imperative to attempt to obtain the reference directly from the applicant's former immediate supervisor. Therefore, requests to former employers should be sent to the attention of the supervisor identified on the application blank.

Another factor which must be considered in attempting to evaluate the effectiveness of reference checks is the general reluctance of most individuals to put into writing anything derogatory about an individual who has worked for them. This is less of a problem in telephone checks and still less in face-to-face interviews with former employers. When more intensive checks of prospective applicants' backgrounds are required, such work can be accomplished through organizations specializing in preemployment background investigations. Some of these organizations are national in character and have resources throughout the country. Their agents make personal visits to former employers and neighbors. Their reports are objective and usually quite reliable.

PREEMPLOYMENT PHYSICALS

Most health service institutions have no problem in accepting the need for physical and health standards that must be established for specific jobs. With the advent of new regulations guaranteeing safety factors, such standards are given prime consideration. The preemployment physical is a useful and important tool in determining the employability of an applicant. Such physicals should be as all-inclusive as possible, but certainly extensive enough to evaluate the physical conditions which appear to be required by the job

specifications. The applicant turned down for physical reasons should be so informed. Such examinations should be given in advance of hire in order to obviate the expense, complexity and embarrassment of terminating a candidate within the first few days of employment on the basis of a physical defect which might affect his ability to do the job and which could have been predetermined.

AFFIRMATIVE ACTION

Affirmative action is a term widely used in the area of recruitment, placement and employee relations in general to describe a policy whereby employers are required to make an extra effort to hire and promote those individuals considered to be in a protected class.[14] Under present law a protected class includes those individuals who have been the subject of past discrimination in hiring and promotion: Blacks, Asian Americans, American Indians, Spanish-surnamed Americans and women.[15] With final interpretations of various aspects of the laws involved in this complex area still pending, at best we can only present an overview of the statutes which affect recruitment, screening, interviewing and final selection of candidates for employment.

Equal employment opportunity is the law of the land, mandated by federal, state and local laws, presidential executive order and court decisions. The effectiveness of these laws has been questioned by those who review statistics which indicate greater levels of unemployment, nonemployment and underemployment for minorities and women. Income levels have been shown to be lower for those groups, and there is indication that a most pervasive discrimination today results from normal, often unintentional and seemingly neutral practices throughout the employment process.

A sample diagram of one type of employment process is provided by the Equal Employment Opportunity Commission (EEOC) (Exhibit 5-5). It indicates several phases where rejection is possible during the employment process. These then are the critical areas of concern in implementing an affirmative action program. The major areas of affirmative action legislation and sources of legal protection under Equal Employment Opportunity guidelines follow.

1. *The Civil Rights Act of 1866.* Following the Civil War, Congress sought to specify that the newly freed Blacks be accorded full equity with white citizens of the United States. The Civil Rights Act of 1866 was initially interpreted as applying only to governmental discrimination. However, subsequent court interpretations have held the Act to include private sector employees.

Exhibit 5-5 The Employment Process

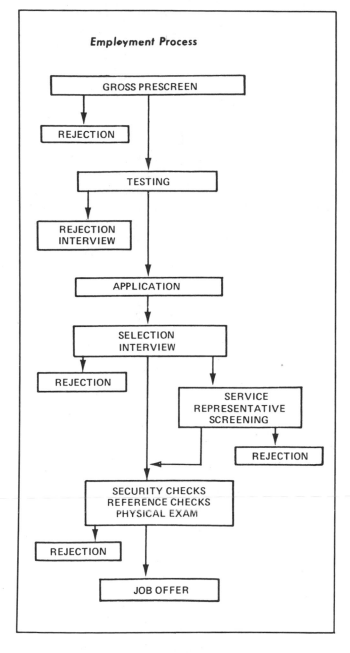

2. *Title VII of the Civil Rights Act of 1964, as amended by the Equal Employment Opportunity Act of 1972.* This Act applies to organizations engaged in industry affecting interstate commerce, employing 15 or more persons, and prohibits job discrimination based on race, color, religion, sex or national origin. The United States Equal Employment Opportunity Commission (EEOC) was created to administer Title VII and to assure equal treatment for all in employment. With the 1972 amendments, the EEOC is empowered to prosecute cases of alleged employment discrimination in federal courts and to order an em-

ployer, if found guilty, to undertake an affirmative action program to correct inequities. Title VII does not explicitly require affirmative action; however, EEOC has been guided by several court decisions which have remedial effects. When a court finds a violation of equal employment law, Title VII provides that it may "order such affirmative action as may be appropriate" for its elimination. As amended, Title VII now covers: (1) all private employers of 15 or more persons; (2) all educational institutions, public and private; (3) state and local governments; (4) public and private employment agencies; (5) labor unions with 15 or more members; and (6) joint labor-management committees for apprenticeship and training. It is Title VII that defines the protected class categories consisting of the groups mentioned above. One major exception to Title VII is the bona fide occupational qualification (BFOQ) which allows an employer to hire employees on the basis of religion, sex or national origin in instances where religion, sex or national origin can be shown to be a bona fide occupational qualification reasonably necessary to the normal operation of the employer's business.[16] The other major exception is "business necessity" which allows the employer to disproportionately reject the members of a protected class as employees if by doing so he fulfills a specific business purpose or necessity that could not be fulfilled by any alternative employment practice. Courts have interpreted "business necessity" very narrowly, requiring overriding evidence that a discriminatory practice is "essential" to safe and efficient operation of the business and a showing of extreme adverse financial impact.

When a charge of discrimination is investigated by EEOC and reasonable cause is found, an attempt at conciliation is made. If this fails, EEOC may go to court to enforce the law. An individual, or an organization on behalf of an individual, who alleges discrimination may sue an employer and/or file a complaint with EEOC.[17]

3. *Executive Order 11246 (as amended by Executive Order 11375).* This order, issued by President Johnson in 1965, requires affirmative action programs by all federal contractors and subcontractors with 50 or more employees and contracts of $50,000 or more. Such employers must have an approved affirmative action program on file with the Office of Federal Contract Compliance Programs (OFCCP). The OFCCP has in turn delegated responsibilities to approximately 16 other executive branch agencies. Specific requirements for such "result oriented" programs are spelled out in Revised Order No. 4 issued by OFCCP and are similar to court interpretations of Title VII require-

ments. In 1970, Order No. 4 specified 177 elements of the written plan and Order No. 14 stipulated how compliance reviews will be held.

Nondiscrimination requires an elimination of all existing discrimination factors whether overt or inadvertent. All employment policies and practices must be examined in order to establish a neutral personnel administration process. Affirmative action goes beyond lack of discrimination. In employment law, affirmative action means taking specific actions in recruitment, hiring and upgrading which are designed to eliminate the present effect of past discrimination. Minorities and women may already be qualified for better jobs, but continuing barriers throughout employment systems may be preventing advancement. The major part of an affirmative action program must be the recognition and removal of these barriers so that minorities and women can compete for jobs on an equal basis. The primary legal obligation of affirmative action is to change employment barriers which discriminate against people. The most important measure of an affirmative action program is its results.

4. *The Equal Pay Act of 1963 as amended by Education Amendments of 1972 (Section 6(d) of the Fair Labor Standards Act).* This Act prohibits discrimination in wages by stipulating that equal pay be provided for men and women performing similar work. This is applicable to all employers having workers subject to a minimum wage under the Fair Labor Standards Act (FLSA). In 1972 this Act was extended beyond employees covered by FLSA to an estimated 15 million additional executive, administrative and professional employees, including academic administrative personnel and teachers in elementary and secondary schools, and to outside salespersons.[18]

5. *The Age Discrimination and Employment Act of 1967 as amended in September 1978.* This Act prohibits employers of 25 or more persons from discriminating because of age against persons who are 40 to 70 years of age in any area of employment. A major change in recruitment advertising has been effected because of the Act. Advertising copy can in no way imply age of a desirable applicant by using such phrases as "Junior Executive," "young," "retired person," "supplement your pension," "recent college graduate."[19]

6. *Vocational Rehabilitation Act of 1973.* This Act requires federal contractors and subcontractors with 50 or more employees and $50,000 or more in contracts to maintain an affirmative action program ensuring the hiring and promotion of qualified handicapped people. Section VII of the Act defines "handicapped individual." Section 503 requires federal contractors to take affirmative action for such individuals. Section 504 forbids discrimination against the handicapped under any program or activity receiving federal financial assistance. The Department of Health, Education and Welfare published the handicapped regulations which implemented Section 504, effective June 3, 1977. Joseph Califano, Secretary of HEW, has said that regulations require "dramatic changes" and may impose "major burdens" on institutions receiving HEW funds.[20] Compliance with the regulations will require a revision of employment practices, provision of special aids and interpreters for handicapped persons and, in many cases, structural alterations to buildings. The statute provides: "No otherwise qualified handicapped individual in the United States . . . shall solely by reason of his handicap be excluded from the participation in, be denied the benefits of, or be subjected to discrimination under any program or activities receiving federally financed assistance."[21]

Included in the definition of handicapped are those suffering from emotional disturbances, alcoholism and drug addiction. Subpart B, Employment Practices, sets out requirements for nondiscrimination in employment of handicapped persons.[22]

7. *Vietnam Era Veterans Readjustment Act of 1974.* This Act requires affirmative action on behalf of disabled veterans and veterans of the Vietnam era by contractors holding federal contracts of $10,000 or more. Section 2014 covers regulations regarding employment of veterans in the federal sector. It is enforced by the Veterans Employment Service of the Department of Labor.

Implementation of Affirmative Action Programs

The mechanism by which an affirmative action program is developed follows.

1. *Workforce analysis.* The institution lists the total number of job incumbents from a protected class in each recognized job title within the organization. The numbers are converted to percentages known as "workforce statistics."

2. *Collection of availability statistics.* The institution must collect statistics covering each job title reflecting the number of available members of the protected class living in the organization's relevant recruitment area. These statistics are obtained from census information and other sources. Relevant recruitment areas, although usually defined by reasonable geographical bounds, can vary for different job titles. In some cases national figures must be used.

3. *Utilization analysis.* The institution compares its workforce statistics with availability statistics to de-

termine which job positions reflect underutilization of protected class members.

4. *Hiring and promotion goals*. The institution should identify areas of underutilization and prepare an affirmative action plan. This plan is kept on the premises and only submitted to the government if a compliance review has been initiated as a result of complaints received by the government. Annually the institution is required to submit an EEO-1 (workforce analysis) form.

5. *Penalties*. In some instances of flagrant underutilization the EEOC may require the organization either through voluntary conciliation agreement or by court order to pay money equal to the estimated losses suffered by the protected class members as a result of the institution's discriminatory hiring and promotion practices. The OFCCP is empowered to order similar cash awards through voluntary conciliation agreements, and in the absence of voluntary agreements to suspend or cancel the organization's contract.[23]

CONCLUSION

First impressions are lasting ones. The individuals responsible for recruitment in a hospital or home have far more responsibility than most administrators assume or are willing to admit. A substantial part of the applicant's impression of the institution is formed at the outset—when he first appears in the employment office. It is therefore essential that all employees assigned to the employment office of the personnel department effectively represent the institution: they must accurately and honestly communicate the hospital's policy and philosophy. In addition, successful recruiting is built upon successful interviewing techniques. A personnel director (employment interviewer) does not have to like people. He simply has to understand them.[24] Understanding people who apply at an institution's employment office encompasses the recognition of "uneasiness" and "concern" that the applicant brings into the interviewing milieu. Full recognition and appreciation must be given to the interview as a two-way communication vehicle: the applicant is given the opportunity—indeed, motivated—to present his full credentials to the interviewer; the institution, through the interviewer, is given the opportunity to present complete information about itself to the interviewee.

The appearance of the personnel office is the first indication of the institution's concern for people. The physical characteristics of all areas of the institution play an important part in molding employee impressions. The investment in a professional employment program is one that pays off in measurable ways to the institution. The cost of recruitment, often excessively high, can be minimized, turnover can be appreciably affected and controlled, and the institution can depend upon a pool of competent and qualified employees.

NOTES

1. Arthur R. Pell, *Recruiting and Selecting Personnel* (New York: Regents Publishing Company, A Division of Simon and Schuster, 1969), Preface.
2. *Ibid.*, p. 42.
3. *Ibid.*, pp. 19–21.
4. Richard P. Calhoun, *Managing Personnel* (New York: Harper & Row, 1966), pp. 147–8.
5. Milton M. Mandell, *Choosing the Right Man for the Job* (New York: American Management Associations, 1964), p. 158.
6. Lipsett, Rodgers, and Kentner, *Personnel Selection and Recruitment* (Boston: Allyn & Bacon, Inc., 1964), p. 42.
7. Mandell, *op. cit.*, p. 186.
8. Dean B. Peskin, *Human Behavior and Employment Interviewing* (New York: American Management Associations, 1971), p. 12.
9. Theodore Hariton, *Interview: The Executive's Guide to Selecting the Right Personnel* (New York: Hastings House Publishers, 1971), p. 11.
10. Milton M. Mandell, *Employment Interview*, No. 47 (New York: American Management Associations, 1961).
11. Material for this part of the chapter developed with the assistance of Dr. Leslie M. Slote, management consultant.
12. Hariton, *op. cit.*, p. 44.
13. Pell, *op. cit.*, p. 104.
14. James W. Higgins, "A Manager's Guide to the Equal Employment Opportunity Laws," *Personnel Journal*, Vol. 55, No. 8 (August, 1976), p. 410.
15. *Ibid.*, p. 407.
16. Eleanor Wagner, "Avoiding Illegal Employment Practices," *Hospitals, J.A.H.A.*, Vol. 49, No. 12 (June 16, 1975), p. 46.
17. For further information on Title VII, write: Office of Public Information, EEOC, 1800 "G" Street, N.W., Washington, D.C. 20506.
18. For information on the Equal Pay Act, write: Wage and Hour Division, Employment Standards Administration, U.S. Department of Labor, Washington, D.C. 20210.
19. *Ibid.*
20. Statements by Joseph Califano, Jr., Secretary of the Department of Health, Education and Welfare, press release (April 29, 1977).
21. 29 *United States Code* @ 794.
22. Regulations Section 84.3(j) (page 22678) and analysis (pp. 22685–7), *Federal Register* (May 4, 1977).
23. The author wishes to acknowledge the research of Mary Louise Creedon, Affirmative Action Coordinator for The Mount Sinai Medical Center, and David Emerson, graduate student in Health Care Administration, Baruch College of the City University of New York.
24. Leonard Berlow, "How to Recruit Military Personnel for Health Areas," *Hospitals, J.A.H.A.*, (July 16, 1969), pp. 80–86.

ADDENDA

Addendum 5-A

EMPLOYMENT AGENCIES: THE REPUTABLE VS. THE QUESTIONABLE*

How do the practices of the new renegade employment agencies compare with those of long-established, reputable personnel firms? *Business Management* consulted Nevin I. Gage, who operates a highly respected employment agency in Stamford, Connecticut. Here's how the two kinds of agencies shape up.

Service	*Reputable Agencies*	*Questionable Agencies*
Recruiting:	Engage in selective recruiting occasionally, and then only to fill the urgent needs of client companies at their specific requests. Most applicants obtained through newspaper advertising.	Do all their recruiting through a large, heavily indoctrinated staff of "counselors." Prospects are called at home between 6 and 8 PM and Saturdays. This builds up reservoir of applicants. No selective recruiting for specific jobs.
Applicant motivation:	Encourage applicants to seek positions commensurate with their highest skills, to set salary requirements at high but realistic levels.	Promise salary advantage to raise recruitment volume. Later, urge applicants to reduce salary demands to assure faster placements.
Résumés:	Always provide personnel managers with résumés whether requested or not. Encourage applicants to prepare detailed résumés in a professional manner. Help them revise their résumés when necessary.	Do not provide personnel managers with résumés if it can be avoided. Insist on blind interviews. Standard pretext: "We are selling you the man, not an employment record."
Screening applicants:	Interview in depth, to be certain that applicant is qualified in every particular for job he is seeking. Give approved tests when need is indicated. Question applicant to determine whether he is emotionally qualified for job and is likely to have a rapport with his prospective employer.	Spend minimum of time to get basic information. No testing by "counselors." Start here to maintain control of applicant and condition him to accept first job offer.
Screening companies:	Study employers' record for fair employment practice. Do not send applicants to companies known to have poor reputations for job security, salaries or benefits.	None.
Placement follow-up:	After a reasonable interval, contact both applicant and his new employer to determine whether both are satisfied.	None.

---

*Taken from an article entitled "Employment Agencies That Will Bilk You," *Business Management* (July 1968), p. 34.

Addendum 5-A continued

Advertising:	Advertise only the existing job, not an imaginary opening so dramatized as to attract applicants.	None, or very little.
Counselors:	Employ only experienced, professional counselors with proved records for placing the right people in the right job.	No previous experience in personnel work is required. Persons with background in selling goods or services are preferred. Persuasive telephone voice is an asset.
Job orders:	Never send an applicant out for an interview unless a specific job order requesting a man with his qualifications has been received.	Rarely match applicants with job orders, except for general job category. Theory is that companies will be satisfied with applicants who approximate job descriptions. Frequently try to "pump in" applicants.
Personnel managers:	Try to understand their problems. Don't demean them by attempts to reach department or division managers.	Regard company personnel managers as inefficient clerks. Try to bypass them whenever possible.
Fees:	Either make firm agreements with client companies so that the latter pay fees, or inform applicants that fees will be chargeable to them.	Tell applicants virtually all fees are company-paid, but have no firm, contractual agreements with companies. Applicants must sign contracts requiring them to pay the fees if they accept jobs and the companies refuse to pay.

Addendum 5-B

PERSONNEL POLICY # 4.7

| ·RECRUITMENT Page 1 | Issued: Revised: |

The responsibility for recruiting and screening applicants for employment rests with the Employment Section. The following statements describe the resources and methods utilized by the Employment staff and the guidelines that must be observed in attracting and referring candidates.

4.71   Employment Advertising: The Employment Section is budgeted and is responsible for the planning and placement of employment ads, selection of media and development of advertising programs.

4.711   Individual departments are not authorized to place employment ads.

4.712   In the interests of economy, a single ad will ordinarily be placed for two or more similar positions vacant at the same time in different departments.

4.713   Although the Employment Section is responsible for the coordination of Medical Center-wide employment advertising, the suggestions of departmental supervisors are welcomed.

4.72   Private Employment Agencies: The Employment Section is responsible for the placement of job orders with private employment agencies and is budgetarily accountable for reimbursable agency fees upon the hiring of referred applicants.

4.721   Individual departments are not authorized to deal directly with private employment agencies.

4.722   The Employment Section determines whether a position is to be recruited through a private agency.

4.723   The Employment Section selects the agency(s) based on such factors as ability to attract and screen qualified applicants, fee schedule, fee payment and refund arrangements, agency advertising practices, etc.

4.724   The Employment Section determines whether an agency fee will be reimbursed by the Institution.

4.725   The Institution will not evade nor abet an applicant or employee in the evasion of a legal obligation to an employment agency.

Addendum 5-C

```
┌─────────────────────────────────────────────────────────────────┐
│                    PERSONNEL POLICY # 4.8                         │
├──────────────────────────────────────┬──────────────────────────┤
│                                      │ Issued:                   │
│        SELECTION AND PLACEMENT       ├──────────────────────────┤
│                             Page 1   │ Revised:                  │
└──────────────────────────────────────┴──────────────────────────┘
```

The Employment Section recruits, screens and refers employment applicants for placement in vacant positions among the Medical Center's various departments. It is the individual department head's responsibility to select for employment the applicants qualified to perform the assigned work. The following statements describe the steps taken in the selection and placement of Institution employees, except professional medical staff, faculty, and social workers.

4.81   Employment Application: Employment applicants are to complete an employment application. Documents relating to age, citizenship, licensure, education, etc., may also be required. (See Personnel Policy #4.1, "Employment Standards"). Applications are screened by an Employment receptionist before an interview is held.

4.82   Employment Interview: Applicants meeting minimum job requirements are interviewed by an Employment interviewer. The interviewer elicits comprehensive information as appropriate.

4.83   Employment Tests: Employment testing is one of several techniques utilized in the selection of applicants. Test results are to be considered together with experience, background references, and the interviewer's evaluation as criteria for selection. Testing procedures are in comformity with Equal Employment Opportunity guidelines.

    4.831   Specialized employment tests given by operating departments are to be reviewed by the Employment Section to assure that test content is germane, administration is consistent and results are equitably applied.

    4.832   Test results, as all other employment information, are to be kept confidential within the Employment Section, and they are not to be disclosed to the applicant.

4.84   Reference Check: The Employment Section routinely checks employment and educational references, wherever possible, before a job offer is made. Reference check results are discussed with the departmental supervisor to assist him in making the selection decision. Unacceptable references generally preclude referral of an applicant to the department.

    4.841   Unacceptable references received after an applicant has begun work are discussed with the departmental supervisor

Addendum 5-C continued

PERSONNEL POLICY # 4.8	
SELECTION AND PLACEMENT Page 2	Issued: Revised:

and, where appropriate, the Employee Relations Section, Security Department or Employee Health Service depending on the nature of the information received.

4.842   Discrepancies between the information on the application and the information obtained in the reference check are discussed directly with the employee. If the employee is unable to reconcile the discrepancies, the matter is brought to the attention of the departmental supervisor and the Employee Relations Section for resolution.

4.843   Reference information is confidential and should not be discussed with anyone, including the applicant except as in 4.842.

4.85   Departmental Interview: The Employment Section will refer to the department the best qualified applicants available. Applicants with less than minimal job requirements will not be referred. Departmental interviewers need not review with the applicant basic information elicited at the initial employment interview but should instead concentrate on assessing the applicant's specialized job qualifications in terms of the specific requirements of the job. The departmental interviewer should review with the applicant the duties, responsibilities and conditions of the position.

4.851   Before an offer is made, the departmental supervisor must confer with the Employment interviewer to discuss the applicant's acceptability, to determine whether additional follow up is required (e.g., references, licensure), to establish an offering salary, and to assure that appropriate pre-employment arrangements have been made. Job offers are made only through the Employment Section. Department supervisors are not authorized to make job offers.

4.86   Pre-employment Physical Examination: Before an applicant is accepted as an employee he must take a pre-employment physical examination and meet the health standards appropriate to his job assignment.

4.87   Licensure: In accordance with legal requirements and professional codes applicable to various professional and paramedical positions, the Institution will require satisfactory evidence of licensure.

6. Management Recruiting

BERNARD J. RYAN

When an organization needs to fill a vacancy it can promote from within or conduct a campaign to locate and attract a competent outsider—a simple enough choice at first blush. There are many benefits associated with internal promotion, as any personnel manager or chief executive officer will point out. Among them are improved morale, reduced turnover because the organization is constantly renewing itself, speed and cost (outside searches can be expensive), little or no training and orientation, little or no loss in momentum, and so on. An often repeated complaint by jobseekers is, "There is no opportunity for advancement because my employer fills vacancies from outside."

The decision to promote from within or to seek outside talent is not always an easy one, particularly if an officer or chief executive is needed. If an institution is launching a new product line or service or is confronted with new or increased regulatory compliance burdens, attracting a competent manager from another company who already possesses the needed knowledge and skills may be the preferable course. Generally, though, a balanced mixture of internal promotion and outside recruiting helps to prevent management inbreeding and yields better long-range results.

ASK FRIENDS FOR SUGGESTIONS

There are several alternatives to pursue in locating executives from outside the organization. One is to inquire among friends and acquaintances—the do-it-yourself approach. This sometimes is a productive method. But it has its limitations and risks. Bankers, accountants, advertising agencies, and lawyers frequently are asked by clients to identify potential candidates; they do, when they can ethically. Being objective about friends can be difficult; working with friends in a business environment can produce some conflicts and complications. The casual hit-or-miss nature of this approach can be time-consuming, troublesome, and expensive in a highly competitive executive market. The fact that an institution is searching for a key executive inevitably becomes known. This information may be exploited by competitors and can disturb employees with unfounded concerns.

ADVERTISING

Another do-it-yourself method is advertising in newspapers and trade journals—historically the most familiar form of recruiting to employers and jobseekers alike. At the entry and lower management levels, advertising can be an effective tool. Judging from the thousands of ads published daily and especially in the Sunday editions of the major newspapers across the country, companies must feel they are getting results to justify the expenditure of such huge amounts of money.

The advertising approach has many limitations, primarily because it mainly reaches only persons actively looking for jobs. But even those who are looking confidentially often will not respond to ads, whether or not the advertiser is identified. In addition, most successful managers do not read advertisements on any regular basis. While it can't be said categorically that advertising is all good or all bad, successful recruiting by this means does depend on luck. At the clerical and lower management levels where the universe of candidates is virtually unlimited, ad response usually is fairly high, so the element of luck is less important. But for key management and senior slots, dependence on advertising is less productive. It does not tap that limited pool of talent: the busy executives who will not take the initiative to read and answer ads. It leaves unanswered the question, "Did we get the best person for the job?"

EMPLOYMENT ORGANIZATIONS AND CONSULTANTS

While the top managements of most large companies are familiar to some degree with the executive recruiting process, the general public, in the main, is confused; and no wonder, with so many different types of organizations involved in the employment process, all claiming to be consultants. Nor is it readily apparent from the names or descriptions adopted by the thousands of organizations in this field just what services they perform.

The various kinds of organizations are employment agencies, executive or career counselors, out-placement consultants, and executive recruiting consultants.

Employment Agencies

These can be identified by the fact that they are licensed for a specific purpose by the state in which they operate. They work for jobseekers and their fees are contingent upon placing these persons in jobs. Usually their fees are paid by the employing companies, but if the company does not, the individual is obligated for the fee. Some states regulate the maximum fees employment agencies can charge. For jobs at lower levels, the agencies provide a very useful service. However, because they must make placements before they are paid, they can't always afford to invest the time to learn about the particular problems and opportunities of institutions or to investigate the best prospects thoroughly. Some agencies follow the practice of duplicating résumés of jobseekers and sending these, unsolicited, to a large number of companies simultaneously in the hope of making a fit with a current opening.

Executive or Career Counselors

These serve the executive seeking another position. Their fees vary widely and are paid, usually in advance, by the individuals seeking employment. Some career counseling firms charge on an hourly basis, others a fixed amount, and some base their fee on a percentage of targeted salary—often 10 percent or more. Their fees are not contingent upon the executive's finding a new job since they cannot be in the position of guaranteeing employment. Many firms require a signed contract that usually states the fee and describes the services to be performed. In addition, they may charge the institution hiring their client a fee as well.

Services can vary widely among career counselors. They often include some type of testing and evaluation, counseling in letter and résumé preparation and distribution, and advice on interviewing and negotiating with prospective employers.

A word of caution to executives contemplating the services of career counselors: be sure to understand fully and in detail what services are to be provided. Insist that they be spelled out clearly in writing and, where practicable, reviewed by an attorney before signing. Trusting the results of the tests also requires caution. Of course, if administered and evaluated by a reputable outside independent organization such as a university, tests can provide very useful and valuable personal data. Investigate the reputation of the firm as well. Admittedly this can be difficult because dissatisfied clients are reluctant or embarrassed to come forward and admit they didn't receive what they expected.

Out-Placement Consultants

These are the newest entry into the employment industry. Clients of these organizations are companies that feel an obligation to provide assistance to terminated employees in finding new jobs. Fees are paid by the client companies. Their services are quite similar to career job counselors, e.g., testing, evaluation, résumé preparation, job searching; the essential difference is in who pays the fee. There are estimated to be hundreds of out-placement consulting firms. Some combine out-placement with career counseling or even recruiting. But out-placement and executive search under the same roof are thought to be a conflict of interest by some and are not condoned by the Association of Executive Recruiting Consultants.

This segment of the employment industry seems to flourish in periods of economic recession when companies are closing plants, cutting back on the work force, or just cleaning house and feel obligated to assist their displaced employees. But this is an add-on of sorts. The day-to-day staple of the out-placement business is assisting the individual executive who no longer is needed (or wanted). Altruism is not the only motive, though; the passage of federal laws barring age discrimination has been a boon to the out-placement business.

The Executive Search Consultant

These are perhaps the least understood catalysts in matching the right person with the right job. This mystique—largely of their own making—surrounding the "headhunters" (a term executive recruiting consultants dislike), what they do, what they do not do, and how they work is giving way gradually as the profession matures. Executive recruiters and employment agencies often are confused, to the recruiter's dismay. Executive recruiting firms work for companies seeking (searching for) executives; they do not represent individuals seeking jobs—that's the province of the employment agency. Their fees are paid by the companies they serve and are not contingent upon the hiring of the candidate(s). Their clients include the usual business organizations, government agencies, hospitals, universities, and trade associations.

The executive recruiting profession has had extensive growth since its beginnings in the late 1940s and early 1950s. Estimates of the number of search firms in existence range to more than 1,200, with annual billings of about $300 million, according to James H. Kennedy, editor of *Consultants News*. At present, only about 60 of these firms are members of the Association of Executive Recruiting Consultants, Inc. (AERC). Founded in 1959, the AERC, composed of the leading firms in the executive recruiting business, formulates and monitors standards of professional conduct for the profession. To qualify for membership, recruiting firms must adhere to a rigid code of ethics. The AERC monitors the professional practices of its member firms and has expelled some for violations of ethics.

Many business organizations have found that professional search consultants are the best means of finding candidates for executive positions. The search process is a team effort between the client and the consultant—the better they work together, the more successful the outcome. The search consultant and management have distinct responsibilities: the search consultant must find the candidates and management is responsible for hiring them. The principal advantages the professional search consultant offers are competency, objectivity, and integrity. Through contacts developed over many years and using carefully maintained files of executives and industries, executive recruiters are able to offer a wider selection of candidates, in less time, at lower costs while maintaining the anonymity of their clients. Their assistance in negotiating the terms of employment often avoids embarrassment to both the client and candidate.

The typical recruiting project begins with a meeting of the appropriate client company management and the search firm. The client should be sure to meet the consultant who will be responsible for conducting the search. In describing the position to the recruiting firm, don't hold back; be as thorough and frank regarding any potential problems as with the opportunities. The more information the search consultant has, the better. Beware of the recruiter with quick solutions; there are no shortcuts to a thorough search. Most recruiters provide their client with a written confirmation covering preliminary specifications, a clear understanding of both parties' responsibilities, and the agreed fee arrangements. The AERC's Code of Ethics and Professional Practice Guidelines makes this a requirement for member firms.

The most time-consuming portion of a thorough search is the identification of prospective candidates. It is here that the search consultant's mettle is tested. This phase consumes many hours of hard, tedious detail work and requires skill, tact, imagination, intuition, patience, and intellectual integrity. When the prospects are identified, the search consultant approaches them directly, in confidence and privacy, acquainting them with the details of the position. But the identity of the client is still withheld, and is revealed only when the searcher and the prospect have determined that there is mutual interest. At least one and sometimes several meetings will occur before a prospective candidate is introduced to the client company. Included in the candidate evaluation process are reference investigations obtained by the consultant from reliable and objective sources with the candidate's prior knowledge and consent. When satisfied that a candidate meets the specifications of the position, the search consultant will prepare an appropriate report of business experience and personal background for presentation to the client.

AN INDUSTRY HERE TO STAY

Professional executive recruiting is here to stay. Thirty-five years ago there were a mere half-dozen or so firms with combined annual billings of about $500,000 to $700,000. Today several of the largest firms claim revenues of $10 million to $15 million each. The recruiting industry has achieved respectability. It no longer is in search of an image.

The professional search consultant is compensated for services provided and cannot guarantee a placement; the client organization has the final hiring responsibility. To undertake a search project where the fee for services is dependent on an "if we produce" basis is unprofessional and not in the best interests of the business community. This type of financial contingency would tend to destroy objectivity and lead to compromise or promotion of the wrong candidate.

The essential difference between the employment agency and the executive recruiting firm is the commitment to invest sufficient time to find and then assist management in selecting a qualified manager for a carefully defined, bona fide need—and be paid for these services.

7. A Brief Look at the Federal Equal Employment Opportunity Laws

BETH ESSIG and MICHAEL H. SINGER

There can be no doubt that the federal equal employment opportunity laws have been the greatest single cause of change in the American workplace during the last 20 years. Although constitutional and statutory antidiscrimination provisions have existed since shortly after the Civil War, it is primarily since the passage of the Civil Rights Act of 1964 that great strides in eliminating discrimination in employment have been made. This analyzes the most important concepts and considerations of equal employment opportunity under federal law.

Simply put, these laws require that employment decisions—such as hiring, promoting, discharging, and the like—be made solely on the basis of the worker's job qualifications or other job-related criteria. To accomplish this, they bar the employer from considering certain general characteristics such as race, national origin, religion, gender, and, to a lesser extent, age. There are some, very limited situations where these factors may be considered. These include rare cases where the person's having a certain characteristic is a "bona fide occupational qualification." In all instances, an employer's primary focus should be on the qualifications, not characteristics, of the individual.

Where impermissible consideration of any of these classes of characteristics is made, discrimination on that basis is said to occur. Thus, refusing to hire blacks may be discrimination on the basis of race and consid-ering only Catholic applicants may create discrimination on the basis of religion.

Whenever dealing with a discrimination problem, the first step is to identify which protected group is involved. It is important to realize that each type of discrimination is wholly separate and involves different factors. In a race discrimination case, data about religion or gender are completely unimportant; the only issues pertain to how persons of different races (white, black, Asiatic, etc.) are treated. Similarly, in a gender discrimination case, the fact that 25 senior citizens were just hired is irrelevant even though it would be very important in an age case.

The federal government takes an active role in the enforcement of the equal employment opportunity laws. Its principle agency is the Equal Employment Opportunity Commission (EEOC), where many discrimination charges are first brought and investigated. The Department of Health and Human Services (HHS) also is involved frequently. Other agencies on the federal, state, and local levels take active part in investigating and enforcing the laws.

The laws designed to protect employee rights also prohibit an employer from retaliating (with discipline, discharge, nonpromotion and the like) against an employee who has filed a charge, even if the employer feels the charge is baseless. Charges of retaliation filed by an employee can be very difficult to defend. A decision to discipline an employee who has filed a charge, whether or not that charge has merit, should be made with great care and with an eye as to whether the action will be supportable by objective documentary evidence.

RACE

Discrimination on the basis of an individual's race is absolutely prohibited. The law does not recognize *any* bona fide occupational qualifications in this area and there are no exceptions. (Most of the developing law concerning race is focused on affirmative action, which is beyond the scope of this article.) Thus, a person's race *never* can be considered in making an employment decision. Obviously, then, it is illegal to refuse to employ or promote persons belonging to a certain race. This is true even if customers or coworkers have a preference for one race or another.

Subtler forms of racial discrimination probably will be more of a problem in a hospital. Certain supervisors may discipline members of one race more harshly than those of another, or promotions and recommendations may reflect a manager's biases. Each such situation is a potential problem with far-reaching impact. A black who is disciplined for just cause may well win a discrimination case if whites or Hispanics were "let off the hook" when they misbehaved. Lenient treatment for one means lenient treatment for all.

NATIONAL ORIGIN

Discrimination on the basis of national origin—the country where the employee or the person's forebearers were born—is prohibited by Title VII of the Civil Rights Act of 1964. Some state and local laws also may offer protection. Of all types of discrimination prohibited by federal law, national origin cases appear to be the ones brought least frequently. This is because there is a certain overlap with race discrimination as, for instance, in charges brought by Hispanics or Orientals.

The few cases that have been pressed show that the basic legal requirements are fundamentally the same as for race. A person born in Italy must be treated the same as one whose grandfather came from Haiti.[1]

The EEOC regulations mention several examples of employment practices that could give rise to discrimination charges: requiring or testing for English, where speaking English is not job related; using a person's surname (or maiden name) as a factor in hiring or promoting; having height or weight requirements that tend to disqualify a person from consideration; considering membership in a lawful organization that promotes a

nationality, or whether the applicant is a citizen of the United States. Citizenship may be considered only if the job involves national security concerns. Ordinarily, this would not apply to a hospital.

As with race, the law seeks to eliminate all considerations except the job-related qualities of the individual employee. It should be noted that here, too, customer or coworker preference cannot be considered legally.

RELIGION

General

Title VII prohibits discrimination against individuals on the basis of their religion. Thus, federal law absolutely prohibits employment decisions based on the fact that the person holds certain religious views. A Jewish health care institution, for example, cannot refuse to employ non-Jews. In consideration of benefits, discipline, and the like, the employee's religion also cannot be a factor.

A more legitimate involvement with employees' religion occurs when their beliefs affect the manner in which they may perform. The most serious concern of the health care industry is in accommodating the Sabbath observer because a hospital must operate seven days a week, 24 hours a day. The wearing of religious dress (e.g., beards or robes), the scheduling of numerous holidays off, the refusal to perform abortions or sterilizations, and the refusal to pay union dues are examples of the kind of legitimate religious practices and beliefs that may pose problems to health care institutions.

Section 701(j), added to Title VII in 1972, requires that employers make "reasonable accommodations" to an employee's or a prospective employee's "religious observance or practice" as long as that accommodation does not work an "undue hardship on the conduct of an employer's business."

Definition of Religious Practice and Belief

The 1972 amendment defines religion to include "all aspects of religious observances and practice, as well as belief." The employee need not be a member of what is commonly viewed as a traditional religious organization. In regulations promulgated in 1979, the EEOC held that a religious belief may be a moral or ethical one as long as it is "sincerely held with the strength of traditional religious views." This definition, which has its roots in the Vietnam era conscientious objector cases, has been generally accepted by the courts. The definition is very subjective and will depend, in large part, on the individual employee's views and the sincerity of the beliefs. From the employer's perspective, an employee's assertion of a religious belief will be very difficult to disprove in a litigation context.

The employee need not have held the particular beliefs for a long period of time. For example, the beliefs and practices of an employee who converts during the term of employment must be reasonably accommodated if that can be done without undue hardship on the employer's business.

Since the statute requires that "all aspects" of religious practice be accommodated, the scope of protected activity is fairly broad. Thus, even the duties of a clergyman or church elder must be reasonably accommodated.

Reasonable Accommodation without Undue Hardship

As explained, once the employee proves that the conduct is motivated by a sincere religious belief, the law requires that employers make reasonable accommodations. Health care administrators should explore every possible alternative before determining that a reasonable accommodation cannot be made. Before attempting to do so, and once it is determined that some kind of accommodation is necessary, it is best to elicit from the employee or prospective employee precisely what potential religious factors might affect the job. During the interviewing process, as discussed later, an employer cannot ask whether a prospective employee has any particular religious needs.

This information will aid in determining whether it is possible to accommodate the individual or what type of accommodations are necessary. For example, some Sabbath observers will work in a medical emergency on the Sabbath while others will not; some individuals will perform abortions necessary to save a mother's life, others will not.

In the 1979 regulations, the EEOC offered suggestions as to what accommodations it considers the law to require in the context of a Sabbath observer:

1. The employer should allow and in fact help the Sabbath observer in finding an employee who is willing to swap shifts.
2. The employer should explore alternative positions within the institution that might be more suited to the needs of the Sabbath observer.
3. The employer should institute a flexible work schedule if possible. (This alternative does not really apply to positions in a health care institution that involve direct patient responsibility because of the necessity of seven-day-a-week scheduling.)

Religious practices other than observance of the Sabbath also must be accommodated if possible. For example, a nurse who refuses to perform an abortion could be offered a transfer to a service that does not perform that procedure. Recent cases indicate that a health care facility will have to allow an employee to wear religious dress if it is not unsanitary and does not pose a safety threat.

The Health Care Amendments to the National Labor Relations Act permit an employee with a religious objection to union dues to pay an equivalent sum to a nonreligious charity.

Undue Hardship

An institution need not make accommodations if they would result in an undue hardship to the organization. Precisely what can be termed as "undue hardship" is unclear. Evidently this is a relative concept dependent, in part, on the size of the organization, the frequency with which the accommodation will have to be made, and the number of employees requiring such action. Clearly, neither the infrequent payment of premium wages nor the temporary payment of premium wages while working out a possible accommodation will be considered undue hardship. It is unclear whether more will be required of an employer.

The Constitutional Issue

The constitutionality of Section 701 has been challenged successfully in a federal court.[2] This challenge was based on the premise that the government requirement that employers make reasonable accommodations to practitioners of certain religions is unconstitutional in that it violates the First Amendment's prohibition against federal involvement in the establishment of religion. Until this question is decided by the Supreme Court, it is the better practice to continue complying with Section 701 and the regulations promulgated in it.

HANDICAP

General

Discrimination on the basis of an employee's handicap is prohibited by The Rehabilitation Act of 1973. In addition, at least 40 states have statutes that protect handicapped employees from discrimination. Two sections of this act are especially critical in the context of the health care industry: 503 and 504.

Section 503 imposes affirmative action obligations on an employer who is a government contractor or subcontractor. (This section is considered in greater depth in Article 8, dealing with the EEOC and affirmative action.)

Section 504 requires employers to make reasonable accommodations to qualified but handicapped employees and prospective employees. Health care institutions that directly or indirectly receive federal funds, own or use federal real property, or have programs financed by the federal government are required to comply with Section 504. A federal court, in what may be an aberration, found that payment of Medicaid or Medicare monies was for services provided and was not federal financial assistance.[3] According to that case, the receipt of such funds alone was found to be insufficient to bring a health care facility within the purview of that section. The court ruled that Section 504 covers only those employers who receive federal funds for the purpose of providing employment. A subsequent decision by a different federal court came to precisely the opposite conclusion.[29] Caution is advised, therefore, until the United States Supreme Court rules on this issue.

Qualified Handicapped Individuals

Health and Human Services, the federal agency primarily responsible for the enforcement of Section 504, defines a handicapped person as one "who has a physical or mental impairment that substantially limits one or more of life's major activities, has a record of such an impairment, or is regarded as having such an impairment." The definition is expansive and protects an individual who is not actually handicapped but is merely perceived as handicapped.

The statute specifically states that only "qualified handicapped individuals" are to receive the special protection. Thus, if a handicap significantly restricts someone's ability to do the job, the individual need not be hired, subject to "reasonable accommodation" principles discussed later. On the other hand, a handicap that does not affect performance may not be considered in making employment decisions.

The key to determining whether a particular handicapped individual is qualified will hinge on whether the handicap is job related. Preemployment testing must evaluate only job-related skills. Care should be taken to avoid tests in which the applicant's impairment or handicap will prevent successful completion of the exam unless the impediment affects a bona fide occupational qualification. For example, a speech impairment should not cause an applicant to flunk a test unless speech is a job-related skill. (Preemployment testing is discussed in more detail in the section on the hiring process later in this article.) The fact that the impairment makes the employer, or coworkers, uncomfortable is no excuse if the person can do the job.

In an important case involving the admission of a hearing-impaired nursing student to a nursing school, the Supreme Court found that although the applicant met the technical requirements for admission, she did not meet what was characterized as the physical requirements (*Southeastern Community College v. Davis,* 1979).[4] Thus, the applicant was qualified for admission if her handicap was overlooked, but the Court determined that her rejection was appropriate because her handicap made her an unsuitable candidate. The Court found that the ability to hear was essential to the clinical phase of the nursing program and critical to patient safety.

Of special interest to the health industry is the fact that drug addiction and alcoholism are included in the definition of "mental impairment" and therefore protected by Section 504. Nonetheless, HHS seems predisposed to permit hospitals to limit the employment of individuals with this type of handicap in positions that involve the dispensing of drugs or that would provide the individual with access to drugs.

Reasonable Accommodations

Even after an employee is found to have a job-related handicap, the employer still is obligated to make "reasonable accommodation without undue hardship" to the operation of the facility.

There are few cases outlining what constitutes a reasonable accommodation without undue hardship. Courts have turned to the analogous area of discrimination on the basis of religion for guidance. HHS will take into account the size and nature of the business, the type and cost of the accommodation, and the composition of the work force in deciding whether or not an accommodation is reasonable. The type of accommodation that will be required for the handicapped has not yet been made clear. In the *Davis* case, the Supreme Court determined that requiring a clinical supervisor to accompany the hearing-impaired nursing student while she performed her clinical duties was beyond what was required by Section 504. On the other hand, cases have required that employers provide blind lawyers with readers, an obviously significant additional cost. If the religious discrimination cases provide a clue, then an employer will not be required to bear more than a *de minimus* cost. Thus, each handicapped employee or prospective employee should be evaluated carefully on an individual basis and a determination should be made whether the handicap can reasonably be accommodated.

During the interview process, prospective employees may not be asked if they are handicapped. If they volunteer the information, it is recommended that the interviewer and prospective employee attempt to work out some type of reasonable accommodation.

The Preemployment Physical

Many states require that hospital employees receive preemployment as well as periodic physical examinations. Although preemployment physicals may not be conducted, a posthire preplacement physical examination can be conducted.

The Self-Evaluation

Every federal agency that distributes financial assistance is charged with promulgating its own regulations to assure compliance with Section 504. The regulations must include an enforcement and hearing mechanism and a requirement that recipients of the aid sign assurances of compliance with the section.

Each recipient also is obligated to notify its employees of their rights under Section 504 and to consult with "interested persons," including the handicapped or those representing such individuals. Section 85.5(b) of the HHS regulations requires that each recipient conduct a self-evaluation of the employer's compliance with Section 504. This self-evaluation must be made with the assistance of handicapped persons or their representatives (in cases involving union members it probably is best to consult with the union) and should detail steps to be taken to remedy problems identified by the self-evaluation plan.

GENDER DISCRIMINATION*

General

Discrimination on the basis of gender in the workplace is prohibited by Title VII of the Civil Rights Act of 1964, The Fair Labor Standards Act (the Equal Pay Act) and, to some extent, the Fifth and Fourteenth Amendments to the Constitution. While this section

discusses only these federal laws, it is important to keep in mind that many states and localities have gender discrimination laws that are more stringent or all-inclusive. For example, a New York City law prohibits certain discrimination based on sexual preference but federal law does not.

Basically, the Federal law says that decisions affecting the hiring, promoting, treatment, and pay of employees (and job applicants) are to be made only by considering the workers' abilities; their gender may not be considered unless it is a *basic* requirement of the job (more on this very narrow exception later). Obviously this means the employer must ignore personal notions ("I prefer men") when hiring or fixing a pay rate. It also requires that preconceived notions ("a woman is too weak" or "a man is too insensitive") must be ignored.

For most purposes, a rule that applies to one gender should apply to the other. If married men are employed, married women must be also. If childless men are employed, so must females be. Commonly held beliefs ("she'll just get pregnant and quit"), which is a dubious hiring formula anyway, cannot be followed legally if the result is not hiring persons of a particular gender. *All employees and prospective employees must be judged simply by their individual abilities and qualifications and treated the same as persons of the other gender.*

In addition, under a separate provision of the law, sexual harassment on the job not only is unsavory, it now is illegal.

Particular Jobs for a Particular Gender

As already stated, in filling any particular slot it is illegal to consider only persons of a particular gender unless "sex . . . is a bona fide occupational qualification reasonably necessary to the normal operation of that particular business."[5] Thus in casting a movie, it obviously is proper to consider only women for the role of Martha Washington. It is not proper to consider only men to be camera*men* because there is nothing about the job that a capable woman cannot do.

In the hospital (and elsewhere), almost every job is like the camera operator's; any qualified person can do it. Thus, a simple, safe rule: *If the position does not involve intimate contact with patients, the employer may never consider the gender of the applicant during the hiring process.*

Some hospital jobs do involve intimate physical contact with patients, however. For professional positions (doctors, nurses, therapists), contact with a patient of the opposite gender is generally accepted. Thus because general nurses traditionally are allowed to function on male wards, it is unlawful to refuse to consider a male nurse for a female floor.[6] At best, the hospital "will have to prove that there is a factual basis for its contention that . . . substantially all men would be unable to perform effectively . . ."[7]

In fact, the only difficult areas involve nonprofessionals who perform such work as abdominal preps or giving baths. Often females (usually nurses or aides) do this work on women, and males (usually orderlies) on men. The question is whether it is permissible to consider men for an aide's position, for example, on the basis that being female is a "bona fide occupational qualification." While there may be times when a hospital will be upheld on this, it will have to prove that the gender-based decision was appropriate. In one case it was improper not to consider a male even though all the patients were female. The judge was not persuaded that a man would be incapable of performing the job, even though there would be intimate contact with women.[8]

In a way, these cases are similar to the airline stewardess case. Airlines used to hire a few men (called pursers) and many women (called stewardesses) to work the cabins. Their basis for hiring mostly women was "customer preference," surveys showing that the majority of both men and women passengers preferred stewardesses. When challenged, the courts ruled that customer preference could not be considered and that it was unlawful to involve an applicant's gender for either type of work.[9] The result was that airlines did away with separate job titles and now have male and female "flight attendants" who are chosen for their ability to do the work, not on the basis of their gender.

In hospitals, too, the safe route is to do away with distinctions and create one job that is filled by both genders. If a particular task requires someone of a particular gender such as a man who will not be prepped by a woman, then the hospital can assign the appropriate person. That type of job assignment is far easier to defend than general, gender-based hiring.

Tests and Requirements

Some job descriptions have size, height, strength, or other requirements that are not per se gender based but tend to disqualify women from consideration. As with other prehiring requirements, these are permissible only if they are job related and can be justified by the employer.[10] The best way to justify any requirement is by a test that meets the federal validity regulation.[11]

Unequal Wages

The law requires that men and women performing substantially similar work receive the same compensation (which means both pay and benefits). This does not mean that every technician, for example, must earn the same salary. Pay differentials still may be based on seniority, merit, or productivity, as long as these are applied fairly to both men and women and are not used as a ruse to violate the intent of the law.

For most jobs in which both men and women are employed, the law merely requires that the same pay formula (starting pay, raises, etc.) apply to both. Thus, the pay formula for all floor nurses should be independent of gender, and a male and female with identical background, tenure, and responsibility should be paid the same. On the other hand, a male nurse who earns less than a female nursing supervisor could not complain, provided the difference is based on the supervisor's different (and greater) responsibilities, not on gender.[12]

In the hospital, most problems have arisen in the gender-based job titles: orderlies and aides, porters and maids. Generally, aides are paid less than orderlies, maids less than porters. The rationale is that in each group the males do more and more demanding work than the women. For example, in some institutions, orderlies catheterize men, but nurses (not aides) do the women. Orderlies help with lifting and traction setups and security, the aides do not.

In most cases on this issue, the courts find that these differences are minor and that the basic job (the bulk of the work, the hours, the conditions, and the stress) are substantially similar. Under those circumstances, the courts have decided it is illegal to pay aides less.

In at least one case, a similar problem was raised because the janitors, a group composed of males, were paid higher than the maids, a group composed entirely of females.[12a] Despite contentions by the hospital that the janitor job was more demanding, the court found the work was substantially the same. Even though the janitors did certain extra work (filled soda machines, ran some light machinery, and carried garbage), the regular and basic parts of the jobs (cleaning) were the same.

A few cases have found (based on the particular jobs in that hospital) that orderlies had enough extra responsibility so that the job could be considered different from the aides' and that they could be paid more. One judge pointed out, however, that the hiring discrimination problem remained because women were not considered for the better (higher paid) position.[12b] In other words, if these are in fact two different jobs, men and women should be considered for each.

Were that done, having separate pay rates for each position would not raise a serious question of gender-based wage discrimination.

Marital Status, Pregnancy, and Children

The law demands that men and women be treated the same with regard to marriage and raising children (pregnancy raises slightly different questions, which are discussed next). Unless a hospital hires only single and childless men, it should forget about requiring women employees to be single or childless.

Some employers believe that mothers make unreliable and easily distracted employees ("they'll be out every time Junior has a cold"). As with any other gender-based rationalization, even if it were true 99 percent of the time (and the authors have no reason to believe it is true at all), it may not be held against any particular applicant. It should be presumed that an otherwise qualified applicant will come to work. How the children are cared for is strictly the employee's concern.

Should a mother have an attendance problem because of a child, care should be taken to treat her the same as men with similar situations. If men have been given time to care for their children, then obviously so must women. But more than that, if there has been a generous absence allowance for men for other reasons, a strict "motherhood" policy will violate the law.

In the EEOC's view, employers are not permitted to refuse to hire, to suspend, or to discharge a woman because of a pregnancy-related condition as long as she can perform "the major functions necessary to do the job."[13] Thus, rules such as those requiring leaves of absence after a certain stage in the pregnancy are not permitted. Similarly, the fact that a pregnant woman is not married may not be a basis for any comment or discipline. In other words, as long as the women are capable of substantially performing, pregnancy cannot be considered by an employer in any employment decision. Further, the fact that a pregnant woman makes coworkers or patients uncomfortable is not sufficient to justify discharge.

Any absences caused by pregnancy-related conditions, including giving birth, must be treated as any other sick or disability absences or leaves. Thus, the same policies for use of vacation time, seniority accrual, and the like must be followed. If jobs are held open for men on medical leaves, they must be held for mothers until they are medically able to return. Also, rules that require a woman to take a certain amount of time off are improper—once she is able to return to work, she may do so. Should a mother desire to remain on leave after she is medically able to return to work, she must be given this time in the same way that men are allowed personal leaves of absence.

Federal law also requires that disability benefits cover pregnancy-related conditions in the same way as other medical conditions. This is covered more fully in Article 2, Part II.

Sexual Harassment

While most persons recognize and accept innocent flirtation, sexual harassment—where an employee is made to choose between giving sexual favors and being disciplined or abused—is not lawful. Current federal regulations (which are in a state of flux and may be expected to change) outlaw harassment when sexual favors are even impliedly part of the job, when punishment or advancement result from the refusal of or accession to sexual demands, or when the harassment amounts to creating a hostile or threatening environment for the unwilling employee. An employer may be sued where a supervisor is guilty of the misconduct and where it ignores a known situation where nonsupervisors are sexually harassing a coworker.

AGE DISCRIMINATION

Discrimination against employees because of their age is prohibited on the federal level by the Age Discrimination in Employment Act of 1967 (the ADEA). The ADEA protects all persons between the ages of 40 and 70 from discrimination on the basis of their age. The ADEA covers hiring, firing, terms of employment, compensation, and fringe benefits. There are limited exceptions to this rule as it applies to fringe benefits, especially in the pension and health insurance areas. Many state and local governments also have laws prohibiting discrimination based on age. These laws often are far broader than the federal and include persons as young as 18 years and up in the protected class.

On the federal level, the responsibility for enforcing the ADEA rests with the EEOC; until July 1979 it had been under the Department of Labor.

The principal thrust of the ADEA is to bar consideration of age in making employment decisions unless the employee or applicant is not within the protected age group. For example, if a 68-year-old woman, rather than a younger person, is laid off, she could complain that she was victimized because of her age. If in fact she was chosen for an age-related reason (such as "she'll retire anyway in two years and Jimmy will be around for 40") she would be right. If she was over 70 (or under 40) she could not complain even if her age was considered in the decision because she would not be in the protected group. Of course, if the employment decision was based on factors other than age (such as the younger person's being more able or her being incapable of still performing), then the decision would be legal even though she was within the protected age group. This, of course, does not mean she cannot file a discrimination charge, but the employer should prevail if the defense is presented properly.

Perhaps the most noticeable effect of the ADEA is that it is unlawful to have a mandatory retirement age below 70.

The Hiring Process

It is unlawful to advertise for a young person to fill a particular position. According to recent EEOC regulations, such phrases as "recent college graduate," "young," or "between the age 25–35," are prohibited by the ADEA. However, asking individuals to state their ages is not prohibited, although the EEOC finds it highly suspect since it will tend to discourage older applicants. The EEOC regulations require that if an employment application requests date of birth or other age-identifying information, the application contain language to the effect that, "The [ADEA] prohibits discrimination on the basis of age with respect to individuals who are at least 40 but less than 70 years of age" (79 CFR 1625.5).

On the other hand, the regulations recognize that an age requirement under certain circumstances may be a bona fide occupational qualification. Courts have upheld a maximum hiring age with the most consistency when they could determine that it was essential for the public health. For example, federal courts have found that bus companies may lawfully refuse to hire anyone over 35. However, there are judicial decisions that go the other way and great care should be taken before a minimum or maximum age requirement is set.

THE HIRING PROCESS

Because a decision as to who should fill a particular job is largely subjective, the ease with which an organization can discriminate during the course of the hiring process is obvious. (The criteria for promotions from within are substantially the same as those for hiring from the outside.) As a result, it is important to proceed through the process with caution and attention to: how the job is advertised, what requirements are established for it, and what questions or tests are used at an interview. It should be borne in mind that every applicant who is not hired can accuse the employer of discrimination. The employer's ability to justify the nonhiring (or nonpromotion) decision will be crucial in avoiding extensive proceedings.

Advertising the Job

There are specific constraints on how a job may be advertised. Notices may not indicate that persons of a particular group are ineligible, except in those very rare cases where there are nondiscriminatory reasons for such ineligibility. For example, the old "Help Wanted-Female" or "Help Wanted-Male" columns no longer are permitted because gender-based hiring is illegal in most situations.

It also is impermissible to use techniques that discourage a certain class of persons from seeking the position. For instance, a notice stating "English Preferred" could discourage Hispanic applicants and would be improper unless English were a bona fide occupational qualification.

Some care should be taken in choosing the publications in which advertisements are run. If they are published only in the "Irish Echo," only whites and Irish would be likely to know of the openings. This will become an invitation for charges of discrimination for reasons of race or national origin by someone outside those groups.

Job Requirements and Prehire Testing

It is natural for an employer to have certain expectations of the individual being hired: experience, strength, a level of education, or whatever. Every such requirement, however, eliminates certain persons from consideration, and often affects more from one group than another. For example, a minimum height rule tends to eliminate more women than men (a "gender discrimination" problem) and more Hispanics and Orientals than others (a "race and/or national origin discrimination" problem). Similar effects may be caused by requiring a high school (or college) degree, demanding the employee speak English, pass a preemployment exam, or a host of other prerequisites.

The law requires that whenever a prerequisite or test has an adverse impact on a specific group protected by the discrimination laws, it must be discarded unless the requirement truly is job related. In other words, there must be a correlation between not meeting the prerequisite and ability to do the job.

Thus, when choosing a worker, employers must focus only on what the job demands, not on characteristics they would like in their work force. So, where demanding a high school diploma may have an adverse effect on blacks, for instance, it cannot be a job prerequisite unless there is a correlation between having a diploma and the ability to do the job. Although it may be that high school graduates are better workers, a generality such as this will never justify an adversely impacting requirement. Of course, at least for certain jobs the reverse might well be true. One preconceived notion is as bad as the next, and both must be ignored. The question must be whether high school graduates are better for the particular job in question.

Often an employer purposely wants an overqualified individual because of an intent to promote that person quickly. It is proper when hiring for one job to require promotion-related capabilities, but only if most persons in that job have quick (within not more than five years) progression. Skills that will be learned at the entry position may not be measured. It also is wise not to measure skills that will be learned in a short, introductory period. Such tests are invalid if they create adverse impact.

An easy trap to fall into, because of a preconceived notion or prejudice, is for the employer to assume that a certain person will fail to meet a requirement and therefore refuse to consider employing that individual without testing. For example, if a certain amount of strength is truly needed for the job, it is permissible to give a test to make sure that the applicant can perform. It is not proper to refuse to consider women (or any other type, for that matter) because of the general idea that they are smaller and thus weaker. Even if, for example, 97 percent of all women should fail the strength test, each female applicant has the right to take that test and be judged on her own individual abilities. Any woman who is refused consideration and who shows she can do the job will have a strong discrimination case. Therefore, whenever there is a legitimate job requirement, it is wise to employ testing procedures to measure each applicant's ability to perform.

The EEOC will assume that any prehire test has an adverse impact if the pass rate for any protected group is less than 80 percent of the rate for the biggest group. In a race case, if 10 out of 15 whites pass, at least eight out of 15 blacks must pass or adverse impact will be presumed. Note that each type of discrimination (race, gender, etc.) is considered separately, so that effects on each race are compared only to one another but not to the effects on a gender or age group.

If there is adverse impact from a test, it does not mean it is invalid, but the employer will have to justify using it by showing (1) that what it measures is job related and (2) that there is no other way to identify qualified applicants that has less adverse impact. The EEOC has established detailed regulations for validating such procedures.[14] If procedures such as testing are used, detailed recordkeeping requirements have been established. Failure to produce these records on request of the EEOC can create a presumption of misconduct.

The Interview

In discrimination law, it is wise to remember that anything the manager asks may be used against that employer. This includes questions in preemployment forms and applications. Questions should not be asked, therefore, about elements that cannot legitimately be considered in the hiring process.

Some improper questions are obvious: What is your religion? What country are your grandparents from? What are you, Puerto Rican? If the person is not hired, the individual might well charge that the answer to such a question was the reason.

Many questions touch only indirectly upon areas that may not be considered in hiring. These also must be avoided. For example, the question "Is that your maiden name?" involves whether a woman is married and also whether her national origin is different from that of her surname. Since marital status and national origin have no legal place in the hiring process, the question only creates trouble.

Obviously, not all such questions can be eliminated. On the other hand, the temptation is not to consider the questions seriously enough. In many instances, an employer may not even care about the specific answer, but is only trying to get a "feel" for the applicant. Unfortunately, the rejected applicant (and potential complainant) may not feel the same way.

PROCEDURE

Whether or not an institution actually discriminates, at some point a disgruntled employee is likely to file a claim of discrimination. Employees may file their claims with a local agency or, if there is no such entity or it has not acted, with the EEOC or, in the case of handicap discrimination, HHS. In addition, employees who have certain types of complaints may take them directly to state or federal court. Any complaint, no matter how frivolous it may seem at first, should be taken seriously and handled with care. At some point a decision will have to be made whether to involve an attorney.

The discussion that follows outlines the prehearing procedure of the EEOC. HHS follows a substantially similar formula, as do many state and local agencies.

An employee who has a claim of discrimination may go to the local office of the EEOC where someone will assist in making out a charge. Once a charge is filed it can be withdrawn only by the complainant and with the consent of the EEOC. The charge must be filed within 300 days of the alleged act of discrimination. Under Title VII of the Civil Rights Act of 1964 §706(c), the EEOC must defer any charge for 60 days to a state or local fair employment agency. The state or local agency is permitted to waive its right to exclusive processing of the claim.

Usually within 10 days of the filing of the charge, the EEOC will assign an investigator to the case and mail a copy of the charge to the employer. Often the charge is accompanied by a long and detailed questionnaire designed to elicit facts surrounding the particular episode as well as general information about the employer's employment practices. The time to respond to the charge is short, but generally can be extended upon request to the examiner. If the examiner is contacted for this or any other purpose, it is useful to relate the employer's view of the case. Up to that point, the representative will have spoken only to the complainant and may have a one-sided view of the facts. An informal discussion may allow the EEOC to begin to see the employer's side.

Immediately upon receipt of the charge, the employer should conduct a thorough investigation of the facts and circumstances surrounding the alleged acts of discrimination. After the investigation, the employer's position should be set forth in a written position paper supported by as much documentary evidence as is available. A clear, concise, and thorough statement submitted by the employer may persuade the EEOC investigator to make a favorable recommendation. It therefore is absolutely critical that all disciplinary action be fully and carefully documented.

The EEOC has broad subpoena powers and during the investigation may request substantial amounts of data or documents or even interviews with employees. It is, of course, recommended that the employer cooperate fully. If a request is particularly burdensome or onerous or if the agency seems to be overreaching, the employer may want to contact the field representative assigned to the case to see if something more satisfactory can be worked out. Someone from management or an attorney may want to be present at all employee interviews, although the EEOC need not grant such a request.

Crucial to defeating a discrimination charge is the ability to show that whatever the employer allegedly did to the complainant was justified, based on all facts surrounding the particular incidents cited. It often is helpful if the employer can show that all employees who engage in similar conduct are treated the same. For example, if a female employee is discharged for habitual absenteeism and charges sex discrimination, documentation that proves that men also are terminated for the same conduct may win the case for the employer.

Statistics for the entire institution might also be helpful—for example, in a race or gender case, statistics indicating the number of blacks promoted or women hired might dissuade an investigator from finding "reasonable cause" to continue to prosecute.

Customarily, the EEOC arranges a formal fact-finding conference before deciding whether or not there is "reasonable cause to believe" that there has been a violation of Title VII. At these conferences there usually is no opportunity for direct questioning or cross-examination by representatives of the employee or employer. Only the EEOC investigator will ask questions. It is essential that in addition to the persons or documents that the EEOC has requested, the employer, with the permission of the investigator, bring whomever and whatever is thought to be important to substantiate the company's (or hospital's) position. It probably is a good idea for the employer to prepare any witnesses beforehand by carefully reviewing with them questions they are likely to be asked.

At the investigation stage, one of the EEOC's aims is to try to negotiate a settlement of the dispute. As early as possible, therefore, the employer should make an estimation as to whether and on what terms it might be advisable to settle. Various facts can contribute to that decision: for example, the employer's perception of chances for success, the downside liability, and the cost of defending an action.

At some point, the EEOC will decide there is or is not "reasonable cause." If "no reasonable cause" is found, then the charge is dropped and the claimant may, if the individual so requests, be given a "right to sue letter." The claimant may then bring an action in court but will have a minimal chance for success.

If "reasonable cause" is found, the EEOC will attempt to obtain voluntary compliance with what it proposes as a conciliation agreement. If voluntary compliance is not forthcoming, the EEOC informs the attorney general and makes a recommendation as to whether the Justice Department should intervene on behalf of the claimant. If the attorney general decides not to process the claim, the employee may request and obtain a right to sue letter and process the claim through the courts. If the Justice Department takes the case, it then processes it through the court system.

CONCLUSION

The rules discussed here may sometimes seem overly restrictive, the complaints burdensome. But the fairness and chance of equal opportunity that these laws seek to bring to the employment area cannot be dismissed easily. As with most areas of the law, the best defense to a discrimination charge is not clever lawyering but actually being in compliance with the regulations.

A coordinated effort by an institution's personnel, supervisory, and legal staffs, with an eye toward basic fairness and common sense, is likely to go far in eliminating excessive complaints and in successfully defending any charges.

NOTES

1. *Lucindo v. Cravath, Swaine & Moore*, 425 F.Supp. 123 (S.D.N.Y. 1977).

2. *Anderson v. General Dynamics*, Convair Aerospace Division, ___ F. Supp. ___ (S.D. Cal. 1980).

2a. U.S. v. Calsron Medical Center, F. Supp. (S.D. N.Y. 1980).

3. *Trageser v. Libbie Rehabilitation Center, Inc.*, 540 F.2d 87 (4th Cir. 1978), *cert. denied* 447 U.S. 947 (1979).

4. *Southeastern Community College v. Davis*, 47 U.S.L.W. 4689 (S. Ct. 1979). This case dealt specifically with admission criteria to academic institutions. It is likely that the principles it sets out will be applied more widely.

5. Title VII § 703(e).

6. *Sibley Memorial Hospital v. Wilson*, 488 F.2d 1388 (D.C. Cir. (1973).

7. *Fesel v. Masonic Home of Delaware, Inc.*, 428 F.Supp. 573 (D. Del. 1977).

8. See *Sibley, supra,* note 6.

9. *Diaz v. Pan Am*, 442 F.2d 385, *cert. denied*, 92 S. Ct. 275.

10. *Dothard v. Rawlinson*, 433 U.S. 321 (1977).

11. *Los Angeles v. Manhart*, 98 S. Ct. 1370 (1976).

12. In one case, female nurses in a public hospital claimed under-payment. Even though they earned the same as other nurses in the vicinity, the charges that they were paid less than male civil servants whose jobs were not substantially similar but who did work of comparable worth to the employer. The court rejected the claim, stating that the law did not compare "worth" of two jobs, but merely looked to see if they were "substantially similar." *Lemons v. Denver*, CA 10, No. 78-1497 (1980). There are indications, however, that the EEOC will continue to push for broader applications of the law, using formulas such as the "worth" of the employees, and that some courts may accept such comparisons. See *Gunther v. County of Washington*, 20 FEP 792 (1979).

12a. *Brenner v. South Davis Community Hospital*, 538 F.2d 859 (10th Cir. 1976).

12b. *Hodgson v. Golden Isles Convalescent Homes, Inc.*, 468 F.2d 1256 (5th Cir. 1972).

13. 29 CFR § 1604.

14. 29 CFR 1606, *et seq.* Ways to show a test is valid are whether it measures skills important to performance (content validity), employee characteristics that have proved as important to performance (construct validity), or whether there exists a statistical correlation between achievement on the test and success in at least some part of the job (criterion-related validity).

8. Equal Employment Opportunity and Affirmative Action Guidelines for Health Care Administrators

MARY LOU CREEDON

INTRODUCTION

Equal employment opportunity is the law. It is mandated by federal, state, and local legislation, presidential executive orders, and specific court decisions.

The primary law is the Civil Rights Act of 1964. Congress provided federal legal enforcement in Title VII of the act, specifically prohibiting discrimination because of race, color, religion, sex, or national origin in all employment practices. The U.S. Equal Employment Opportunity Commission (EEOC) was created to administer Title VII to assure on-the-job equality. This and other federal and state laws expressly forbid overt discrimination against individuals in employment matters.

Administration of these laws confirmed that discriminatory practices were deeply ingrained in society and continued to have a deleterious effect on employment practices, with employers sometimes not conscious of the results of their policies. The courts have held that in order to promote equal employment opportunity, positive affirmative action is required to eliminate the effects of past discrimination, along with result-oriented activities beyond the establishment of neutral, nondiscriminatory merit hiring. The intent of this article is to shed light on the requirements that health care providers must meet to assure equal employment opportunities.

Title VII as amended now covers all private employers of 15 or more persons, all public and private educational institutions, state and local governments, public and private employment agencies, labor unions with 15 or more members, and joint labor-management committees for apprenticeship and training.

Title VII and the EEOC do not explicitly require any specific form of affirmative action nor any written remedial plan. It is the courts that have ordered comprehensive affirmative action. The EEOC was given direct access to the courts in 1972 when the act was passed to greatly strengthen its powers and jurisdiction. It is important to know *what* the courts have identified as discrimination prohibited by law and *what* remedies have been ordered.

In 1965, President Johnson signed Executive Order 11246, which prohibited discrimination in employment by contractors and subcontractors doing business with the federal government. Specific affirmative action guidelines known as Revised Order No. 4 (issued in 1971 and amended in 1977) spell out in detail what is required by federal nonconstruction contractors who have 50 or more employees and contracts totaling $50,000 or more. This is essential reading for any health care provider receiving federal money for treatment, research, or educational programs. Contrary to Title VII and the EEOC, Revised Order No. 4 does require a written affirmative action plan for employers holding federal contracts.

These obligations are being changed constantly by new or strengthening legislation, executive orders, or court interpretations. Jurisdiction has been expanded to include not-for-profit institutions, particularly those receiving large sums of federal money. Hospitals, research centers, and schools of medicine are particularly targeted for compliance reviews. Health care providers or educational institutions must ask themselves whether or not they receive federal monies and, if so, to what extent. If the requirements fit, they must comply with Revised Order No. 4.

THE CIVIL RIGHTS ACT OF 1964

The Civil Rights Act of 1964 is the major law that forbids discrimination in employment because of race, color, religion, sex, or national origin. It is Title VII of this act that specifically makes it unlawful for an employer to discriminate against any employee or applicant for employment. Title VII creates a five-member commission, the Equal Employment Opportunity Commission, with authority to prevent any persons from engaging in "unlawful employment practices"[1] that would result in discrimination. Many other state and federal laws and executive orders also prohibit employment discrimination.[2]

When equal employment laws were enacted, it generally was believed that discrimination took place primarily through conscious, overt actions; therefore, these laws were designed expressly to prohibit such actions. To some degree, overt discriminatory activities have declined, although statistics continue to show underemployment of minorities and women. It often is the normal, neutral employment practices that perpetuate the old ways and present unintentional discrimination. In the words of Supreme Court Chief Justice Warren E. Burger:

Under the (Civil Rights) Act, practices, procedures, . . . neutral on their face, and even neutral in terms of intent, cannot be maintained if they operate to freeze the status quo of prior discriminatory employment practices . . . . Congress directed the thrust of the Act to the consequences of employment practices, not simply the motivation.[3]

The major focus of equal employment laws now is to identify and eliminate systemic discrimination that may result from regular employment processes. The courts have recognized the existence of systemic discrimination and have attempted to rectify it through specific remedial actions. As noted, Title VII does not explicitly require affirmative action; however, it does provide that when a court finds discrimination, it may "order such affirmative action as may be appropriate"

for its elimination. Where a compliance investigation or an employer's self-audit produces a finding of discrimination, the EEOC is guided by remedies and requirements determined by the courts. It is not unusual for the courts to order comprehensive, positive steps, including numerical hiring and promotion goals, to compensate for the effects of past discrimination.

Strengthening amendments known as the Equal Employment Opportunity Act were added to Title VII in 1972, giving the EEOC direct access to the courts. The impact of this expanded jurisdiction has been felt by more employers. An overview of rulings since then indicates that "if a statistical survey shows that minorities and females are not participating in the employer's work force at all levels in reasonable relation to their presence in the population and the labor force, the burden of proof is on the employer to show that this is not the result of discrimination."[4]

The Supreme Court has held that:

What is required . . . is the removal of artificial, arbitrary and unnecessary barriers to employment when the barriers operate invidiously to discriminate on the basis of racial or other impermissible classification.[5]

These "artificial, arbitrary and unnecessary barriers" include recruitment, selection, placement, testing, systems of transfer, promotion, seniority, lines of progression, and other basic terms and conditions of employment.[6]

The most important aspect of the court rulings is that it often is not enough for the employer to open up the hiring system to minorities and women. The employer also may have to restore the economic status of those in an "affected class," i.e., those who have suffered and continue to suffer effects of past discrimination. Under Title VII, back pay may be awarded to an entire "affected class" extending up to two years prior to the date a discrimination charge is filed. This practice is extremely costly to any employer.

In many instances the courts have required that the employment process be altered until specified numbers or percentages of minorities and females have been hired, trained, or promoted into specific job categories. Certain goals must be reached in a timely way, with the courts monitoring progress.

The 1972 act provides that discrimination charges may be filed against an employer by an employee or applicant for employment, by an organization on behalf of the allegedly aggrieved individual(s), or by a member of the EEOC. With these expanded rights, the U.S. Congress established regional litigation centers throughout the United States to provide more rapid and effective court action against employers.

The EEOC investigates job discrimination complaints. When it finds reasonable cause that the complaint may be justified it attempts, through conciliation, to reach an agreement with the employer to eliminate the discrimination. If conciliation fails, EEOC may go directly to the courts. However, voluntary remedial action will avoid the prospect of costly litigation and a sudden interruption of business.

Court rulings have established that if an employer is found to have discriminated, even if there was no conscious intent to do so, affirmative action may be mandated. The courts may outline the specific remedies that employers must follow. The courts have given great weight to statistical employment data.

It is recommended that those who fall under the act conduct a voluntary self-audit to identify any possible discriminatory employment practices, intended or unintended. In the self-audit, a mere statement of non-discrimination will not suffice if the EEOC investigates a complaint. The question the agency will ask is: "How do you know you do not discriminate if you have never undertaken an analysis of your work force," if that be the case.

A voluntary Affirmative Action Program (AAP) should start with (1) the formulation of an all-encompassing policy and statement of commitment, (2) the selection of a prominent hospital official with line authority to administer the program, and (3) careful defining of this person's duties and responsibilities. These three elements should be part of the institution's policy manual.

In responding to an EEOC investigation, it is best not to collect data hastily and run the risk of presenting the results of the hiring policies in an unfavorable light. The present work force should be analyzed to identify jobs, departments, and work units where minorities and women may be underutilized. Underutilization is defined as having fewer minorities or women in a particular job category than would reasonably be expected by their presence in the relevant labor market.[7] If underutilization is found, voluntary goals—with a timetable for achieving these goals—should be established. Investigators are skeptical if a self-audit finds no areas of underutilization. To justify any practice or policy that has a "disparate effect" on groups protected by the law, an employer must demonstrate compelling "business necessity" and that no alternative nondiscriminatory practice can achieve the required purposes.[8]

The next step in achieving voluntary compliance is to develop an outreach program to find minorities and women who qualify or can become qualified. At this juncture it is wise to review job descriptions and hiring criteria to determine whether they do reflect the job as it is to be performed. Energies should be spent on getting minorities and women into upwardly mobile jobs.

The health care institution then should develop systems to monitor and measure progress toward meeting the established goals within the timetable. If the goals are not met on time, it is important to record the obstacles that prevented doing so.

It is necessary to communicate the company's affirmative action policy and commitment both internally and externally and explain how this will be done in the policy manual. All statements of policy and commitment should be updated annually. It is through the dissemination of these statements that the health care institution establishes an image as an EEO employer in the community. During an investigation, it is important that the employer is perceived by employees and the community as being committed to furthering EEO.

Recordkeeping obligations under Title VII are limited to maintaining "records relevant to the determination of whether unlawful employment practices have been or are being committed."[9] Only one form is required, the EEO-1 Employers Information Report, which must be filed annually by all employers of more than 100 persons and all holders of government contracts or subcontracts of more than $10,000.[10]

EXECUTIVE ORDER 11246

As noted earlier, in 1965, one year after passage of the Civil Rights Act, President Johnson issued Executive Order 11246. This aimed at preventing discrimination by employers who do business with the federal government, either as prime contractors or subcontractors. The order did not specifically address sex discrimination, so Executive Order 11375 was issued later to rectify this omission. These orders are administered by the Department of Labor through its Office of Federal Contract Compliance (OFCC).

The orders require written commitments to advance equality in employment in all firms with contracts of more than $50,000 and with 50 or more employees. Hospitals, health care agencies and institutions, and colleges and universities that receive federal grants are included.

Again differing with the EEOC, the executive order includes recordkeeping obligations that are enormous and particularly costly for not-for-profit organizations. Sophisticated data processing systems often are unavailable and manual tabulation of data may be necessary to be in compliance. Health care institutions, colleges, and universities must depend on personnel generalists to perform essentially the same recordkeeping and program planning as is required of profit-making federal contractors. There is no relief under the law for not-for-profit institutions that are federal contractors as a result of receiving federal grants. Medical schools receive millions of dollars in such research grants, and hospitals and ambulatory care centers may receive federal monies for treatment programs.

A key provision of the executive order requires that the contractor develop and disseminate a nondiscrimination policy statement. This should be posted in conspicuous places, available to employees and applicants for employment. It should appear in all solicitations and advertisements for employees placed on behalf of the contractor. All labor unions or representatives of workers should be advised of the contractor's commitments to nondiscrimination and affirmative action. Every purchase order and subcontract must include these provisions so that they also will be binding upon these groups as well as the prime contractor.

Compliance reports may be required, as well as contracting agency access to books, records, and accounts. These compliance reports contain information as to the contractor's practices, policies, programs, and employment statistics and must be in the format designated by the Labor Department.

Should a contractor be found not to be in compliance with these executive orders, the contract may be cancelled or suspended and the contractor may be ruled ineligible for future federal contracts. Other sanctions also may be imposed and specific remedies may be invoked. The Labor Department may publish the names of the contractors that fail to comply, thus causing negative publicity. It may be recommended to the Department of Justice that proceedings be brought against the contractor to enforce these orders. Criminal proceedings can be brought for filing false information.

A specific blueprint for development of an affirmative action program (AAP) is contained in Revised Order No. 4, which spells out in detail the requirements of such a written plan. It is an essential document for persons responsible for developing AAPs for their federal contracting employer. It covers nonconstruction contractors from the for-profit as well as not-for-profit sectors.

Within 120 days of the commencement of the contract, each prime contractor or subcontractor with 50 or more employees or a contract of $50,000 or more must develop a written affirmative action program for each of its establishments. These written programs as well as the good faith effort required to transform them from paper commitments to equal employment opportunity are judged by compliance officers of the OFCC. The most important measure of an AAP is the results it achieves in increasing employment opportunities for minorities and women.

As Revised Order No. 4 states:

An affirmative action program is a set of specific and result oriented procedures to which a contractor commits itself to apply every good faith effort. The objective of those procedures plus such efforts is equal employment opportunity. Procedures without effort to make them work are meaningless; and effort, undirected by specific and meaningful procedures, is inadequate. An acceptable affirmative action program must include an analysis of areas within which the contractor is deficient in the utilization of minority groups and women, and further, goals and timetables to which the contractor's good faith efforts must be directed to correct the deficiencies and, thus to achieve prompt and full utilization of minorities and women, at all levels and in all segments of its workforce where deficiencies exist.[12]

The areas in which employers may be deficient cannot be analyzed unless they know the composition of their work force. The personnel information system must be updated continually so that a sex and ethnic code is attached to each employee's name or identifying number. The affected classes protected under law are blacks, Spanish-surnamed Americans, native Americans, Orientals, and females. The workers must be listed according to job title, ranked from the lowest paid to the highest paid in a department. In each job title the total number of incumbents must be shown as well as the breakdown of how many males and females are in each group. The wage rate or salary range must be given for each job title.

The next step is to arrange the job titles into job groups (one or a group of jobs having similar content, wages, and opportunities). Up-to-date job descriptions and a sound wage and salary system are essential to grouping the jobs correctly. Once the jobs are grouped, they can be analyzed to see whether minorities and women are being underutilized in any unit. All of the following eight factors must be considered for both minorities and women:

1. The minority population of the labor area surrounding the facility.
2. The size of the minority unemployment force in the labor area surrounding the facility.

3. The percentage of the minority work force as compared with the total work force in the immediate labor area.
4. The general availability of minorities having requisite skills in the immediate labor area.
5. The availability of minorities having requisite skills in an area in which the contractor can reasonably recruit.
6. The availability of promotable and transferable minorities within the contractor's organization.
7. The existence of training institutions capable of training persons in the requisite skills.
8. The degree of training that the contractor is reasonably able to undertake to make all job classes available to minorities.

The utilization analysis is the most complicated and time-consuming part of a written AAP. Percentage of underutilization is determined for each of the eight factors.

The AAP must list the specific channels that will be used to disseminate policy. There must be planning meetings with management and supervisors who will be responsible for seeing that the goals are met within the stated time frame. Meetings with union officials are particularly important to gain their full support and cooperation. The most important group that needs to be aware of the employer's commitments are the workers. All communication channels available to employees should be used so that the policy statement is always visible.

Documented periodic review of policies and procedures regarding recruitment, screening, hiring, training, promotion, and transfer must be undertaken to ensure that they do not discriminate. Other personnel actions such as compensation, benefits, layoffs, return to work, tuition reimbursement, and social and recreational programs must be reviewed.

When writing an AAP, the most helpful document is Title 41, Public Contracts and Property Management, Chapter 60-60.9, OFCCP, which is the guideline used by compliance officers when conducting a compliance review. This guideline indicates what specific parts of the AAP will be scrutinized and to what degree.

Not-for-profit organizations will see the immediate need for internal reporting systems that will help identify the need for remedial action and measure the effectiveness of the contractor's programs. Increased staff is necessary to keep up with the increased demands of the regulatory agencies. The government estimates that there are 178 elements that must be contained in an acceptable AAP.

It now is time to set attainable goals. This should not be done without consultation of those directly responsible for hiring, both in the personnel department and at the division, department, and unit levels. Predictions as to expansion, contraction, economic climate, turnover, and other variables in the marketplace should be evaluated before establishing goals, especially timetables for when these goals will be met. If goals are not established, there must be a statement corresponding to the eight factors listed earlier as to why a goal is not necessary. If goals are not met within the timetable, detailed reasons for the lapses must be reported in writing.

The AAP must be updated annually. All supporting data such as rosters, progression line charts, applicant flow charts, and applicant rejection rosters must be made available to OFCCP. All data must contain the sex and ethnic code for each person listed.

The AAP must contain more than the work force analysis, utilization analysis, and goals and timetables.[13] An AAP must be dated correctly and the time period that it reflects must be given. A statement of commitment to EEO and AAP should be signed and dated by the chief executive officer. The person with overall responsibility for implementation of the program should be designated and the duties and responsibilities listed. Ideally, it is a prominent executive with line authority. All internal and external disseminations of the contractor's EEO policy should contain the name and location of the person responsible for implementation.

More compliance reviews are being conducted, especially preaward reviews for grants to medical schools. OFCCP has proposed increasing yearly reporting (beyond the standard EEO-1 now required) in the form of a yearly summary of the contractor's AAP. The stated purpose is to "assist OFCCP in establishing a priority compliance review selection system," not to determine compliance status. It appears that OFCCP will target industries or contractors for review based on the submitted data.[14] There is great opposition to this proposal. Colleges and universities have joined with business and industry in objecting to this new burden and the additional risk it may impose. Contractors are concerned that these AAP summaries will become open to disclosure under the Freedom of Information Act. They are particularly sensitive to having the confidentiality of their AAPs exposed. Heretofore, it has not been necessary to submit an AAP to the government unless the contractor is under compliance review.

9. Job Evaluation through Measures of Occupational Satisfaction

PAULA L. STAMPS

INTRODUCTION

Concern with people's satisfaction with their work has been relegated mostly to the academic domain of occupational sociologists and industrial psychologists, who have focused their efforts primarily upon employees in nonprofessional jobs. This has successfully isolated both the type and content of investigation of people's perceptions about their jobs. The two major motivations for the study of work satisfaction are a humanitarian emphasis and the ever-present intuitive relationship between satisfaction and productivity. The humanitarian focus has strong precedence in American thought, where the ideals of equal opportunity and concern for "common people" influence the public's thinking and, to some degree, the nation's social policy. As a country with a high standard of living, the United States also can afford to invest in such social research. Irrespective of this humanitarian motive, the philosophical premise remains that the satisfied worker will produce more, even though this has not been documented consistently.[1]

Almost all of the American research has retained its emphasis upon the individual employee, rather than analyzing the structure and organization of the work environment itself. Although usually framed in the interest of increasing satisfaction of the employees, much of the interest in job satisfaction really works from the "blame the victim" model, since society concentrates on job satisfaction rather than job evaluation or job redesign and ignores the organizational or structural problems.

This article presents a measurement system that is structured in such a way as to be utilized as a management information tool to provide job evaluation data that can lead to redesign of the work environment for health professionals. The emphasis is on the application of this scale and its utilization as a management information tool. The first section describes very briefly some of the previous attempts at measuring job satisfaction in the health field and notes some of the methodological problems. The next section describes the development of the measurement scale as well as the results of its various administrations. This section is designed so that complete information is available to those who are interested in using this scale. The last section discusses the relationship of this scale to job evaluation and points out the necessity of using the scale to begin an investigation of some of the structural and organizational aspects of work.

STUDIES OF WORK SATISFACTION IN THE U.S.

The study of work satisfaction is a relatively new field of research but one that has changed as a result of changing views of work and its meaning. In the early part of this century, work was seen either as a means of survival or as a moral duty. The rapid growth of industrial organizations during the century's first three decades created an emphasis on maximizing the output of workers and machines and minimizing the investment and expenditures by the organization.[2] In the 1920s, Taylor established his principles of scientific management that tied efficiency to monetary reward, with one of his main assumptions being that job satisfaction would increase as the worker's prosperity increased, which in turn would lead to increased productivity.[2]

Almost all of the subsequent studies have focused on the development of a theory of work satisfaction that is based on the psychological needs of the individual. As a result of this research, three major theories of job satisfaction have evolved: need fulfillment,[3,4,5] social reference group,[3] and the two-factor theory that suggests that satisfaction and dissatisfaction are influenced by totally different factors.[6,7,8,9,10]

Most of the occupational satisfaction studies have had a practical purpose because they are designed as means to increase productivity. Although many aspects of the job and the employee have been investigated, the studies are hard to compare because of the tremendous differences in both methodology and organization they cover. The relationship between satisfaction and productivity that has been implied in almost all occupational satisfaction studies has not stood up well in the light of empirical research.

Brayfield and Crockett note no relationship of satisfaction and job performance in their review;[11] Vroom, analyzing data from 20 studies, found the median correlation between satisfaction and performance to be only .14.[4] Other more recent studies have verified this lack of relationship.[12] A stronger relationship seems to exist between dissatisfaction and both absenteeism and turnover rate, and possibly accidents (although it may be that accidents lead to dissatisfaction), as each is a way of avoiding an unpleasant situation.[4,11,13,14,15,16,17] Both absenteeism and turnover reduce organizational effectiveness and, although both are related to satisfaction, the direction and nature of the relationship is not always as clear as is desired.[18]

It is not easy to measure the level of occupational satisfaction. Most of the difficulty in methodology stems from the survey tools themselves, and different questions yield very different results. For example, two common questions are: "How satisfied are you?" and "If you had to do it again, would you pick the same job?" The results from the latter question indicate a higher level of dissatisfaction than the former question.[19] Lawler and Porter have further demonstrated methodological problems using the simple question, "Are you satisfied?" When given the option "yes or no," the number of satisfied responses was high. However, if the same respondents were allowed to answer "yes" or "no," or "undecided," the incidence of job satisfaction dropped.[19] Problems with the wording of questions and the type of measurement scale used have produced biased responses, thus bringing into question the ability to compare results of the studies.

As might be expected, the methodologies of measuring level of satisfaction have varied from study to study. Some researchers have obtained information leading to quantification of level of satisfaction by personal interviews. Herzberg, for example, interviewed employees about related past work incidents that led to feelings of increased or decreased satisfaction.[7] Others, especially those working in the health field, examined level of satisfaction through personality tests.[20] By far the most common method of collecting data is with some sort of questionnaire. Total scores often have been based on responses to the questionnaire items, most frequently involving an unweighted summation of the individual's numerical responses to the different items for an overall score. Some questionnaires have been given both before and after specific changes were made in the work situation,[21] or as an exit interview for those leaving the job.[22,23] More complicated measurements have compared feelings toward a present occupational situation with a previous one, or what employees perceived their peers to be receiving. Current level of satisfaction is then computed by comparing the difference between the two measurements.[21] Still other studies have examined factors involved in level of satisfaction and have weighted them to combine their importance and the amount of satisfaction with each factor.[24]

Work Satisfaction Studies in the Health Field

In the health care field, nurses have been the employee group most frequently studied. Job satisfaction studies on nurses have used many of the traditional occupational research approaches. Several studies have focused on turnover rate, either by doing a retrospective study of nurses who have left[22] or by giving a questionnaire with a follow-up comparing the replies of nurses who left within the year to those who stayed.[23,25]

The threat of unionization has motivated other analyses.[20] Studies have employed the Herzberg, Hoppock, and Maslow theories to test how their assumptions pertain to the health care field.[13,26] More elaborate designs have correlated results of job satisfaction with personality tests. The hypothesis of such a study is that personality can predict job satisfaction so that prospective employees could be screened with personality tests at employment interviews.[20]

Most of the results of these studies indicate a fairly substantial amount of dissatisfaction with nurses' work roles. The National Commission for the Study of Nursing and Nursing Education found that the shortage of nurses was related not so much to the lack of trained nurses, as to their unwillingness to work within their profession.[27] A 70 percent nationwide turnover rate was correlated with widespread job dissatisfaction. This study also emphasized that the majority of nurses continue to be employed in hospitals even though they experience the least amount of work satisfaction there.

This certainly was underscored by the nursing research survey done by Godfrey, the largest sample of nurses ever studied.[28] The amount of job dissatisfaction in the United States is not restricted to the nursing profession, however. For example, the University of Michigan has completed an eight-year analysis of employee attitudes, surveying 1,500 workers in 1969, 1973, and 1977.[29]

The question as to what causes dissatisfaction is complex but most probably goes beyond the mainly psychological orientations of present research. Satisfaction and dissatisfaction are not absolute, although the psychological theories of motivation tend to treat the former as if it were an absolute quality whose only parameter is the individual. Even when the research reveals an insight into the impact of the organizational structure upon work satisfaction, it tends to be ignored. Communication problems are highlighted in the Godfrey survey, with startling differences in perceptions of staff and administrators.[28] Even though the administrative personnel almost always were portrayed in a negative light, the conclusions were concerned with possible changes only for the nursing staff. The major conclusion of the study seems to be that only individual solutions exist. In fact, there is a need for another way of evaluating satisfaction that analyzes expectations as well as current conditions, then includes the necessary next step to present a methodology for making changes in the work environment. The next section describes an instrument that not only measures level of satisfaction but also provides a way of incorporating these results into the organization.

DEVELOPMENT OF A MEASUREMENT INSTRUMENT

Three objectives need to be met in the development of an instrument to measure level of satisfaction of health professionals. One is the ability to *adequately measure* the complex phenomenon of job satisfaction. The second is the development of a tool simple enough to be *practical* to use. It is not true that these two objectives are mutually exclusive: it is possible to design a measurement instrument that theoretically is sound and also usable in a continuing system. None of the existing questionnaires adequately fulfilled these two objectives. Therefore, it was decided to approach the problem from the direction of attitudinal measurement, which would permit two types of data to be gathered: qualitative assessment of responses to the individual items and a quantitative summary score. The third objective is to create a measurement instrument that is a *management information tool*, one that not only provides insights into the occupational satisfaction of health providers but also allows the creation of information that may lead to structural change in the organization. The best way to obtain information on occupational satisfaction and data for use in a management information system is to combine respondents' perceptions of their current position along with their ideal professional situation or their expectations.

Development of Components

Several important concepts are mentioned repeatedly in connection with level of satisfaction. Although some demographic variables such as age[30,31] and some nonwork factors such as personal life and/or home environment[7,30] are mentioned, by far the most common factors cited are those related to the job situation itself. Of these, several that are reported consistently as being most important are reviewed here:

- *Supervision* includes the general level of independence as well as various models of supervision, such as authoritarian or egalitarian. In general, the relationship of level of satisfaction and types of supervision depends on the type of job, the size of the group of employees, and the amount of independence they desire.[4,21,30]
- The higher the perception of *occupational status*, both to the individual and to the organization, the higher the levels of satisfaction with the job.
- For some, the idea of *security* is related directly to high occupational satisfaction.[7,30,32]
- The amount of *achievement* that the employee perceives possible in the job, along with recognition for these achievements, directly is related to the level of satisfaction.[7,21,32]
- An obviously important factor—the amount of *remuneration* in terms of pay, salary, or wages—

is judged most commonly in relation to other workers in the same situation.[4, 7, 21]

- Types of *interpersonal relations* involved in a work situation usually are related to level of satisfaction and involve the actual work group in both formal and informal contexts.[4, 7, 21] Vroom especially noted that individuals in isolated positions had a higher turnover rate than those in jobs that involved interaction with their fellow workers.[4]

- A commonly noted factor is the concept of *job content* or type of work, which includes the number and type of hours a person is required to work as well as the type of tasks required. Low levels of satisfaction are significantly related to jobs with repetitive kinds of tasks or to those in which the employee has little choice.[4, 21]

After reviewing this literature and talking with both clinical and nonclinical health professionals, six components of occupational satisfaction were selected. These appear most relevant to the health field and include the most important concepts noted in the literature. These six are defined as follows:

1. Pay: dollar remuneration and fringe benefits received for work done.
2. Autonomy: amount of job-related independence, initiative, and freedom either permitted or required in daily work activities.
3. Task requirements: tasks that must be done as a regular part of the job.
4. Organizational requirements: constraints or limits imposed on job activities by the administrative organization.
5. Interaction: opportunities and requirements for both formal and informal social contact during working hours.
6. Job prestige/status: overall importance or significance felt about the job at the personal level and to the organization.

Description of the Measurement Instrument

These components then become the first section of the questionnaire that measures the relative importance of the various aspects or elements of job satisfaction. This section essentially consists of a statement of ideal expectations. It compares the six components of satisfaction in a forced choice among all possible combinations of pairs. That is, the respondents are asked to choose the member of each of 15 pairs (i.e., autonomy or pay; task requirements or autonomy) that is more important to them as a contributor to their own level of satisfaction. The relative importance of each component is weighted by modification of the paired comparisons test described by Edwards.[33] In this procedure, the frequency with which the component is chosen more important is determined, this number is converted into a proportion, the proportion to a Z-statistic, and through two more transformations into a rank on a scale from zero to one, zero being the value arbitrarily assigned to the least important component. These rankings then serve as the weighting to determine both a weighted score for each component and the total score.

The Appendixes contain the complete questionnaire given to the most recent sample of nurses, with Appendix 9-A showing the first part of the questionnaire.

The second section of the measurement instrument is a Likert-type attitude scale that measures current levels of satisfaction for each of the six components (Appendix 9-B). This scale is composed of approximately ten statements per component. The items are arranged randomly throughout the questionnaire so that the respondent does not become aware of the specific component being examined. The response mode is on a seven-point scale with a neutral midpoint. Half of the items within each component are phrased positively and half negatively. In the process of scoring, the negative scores are reversed so that a higher component score denotes a higher level of satisfaction with that component. Each of the six components is treated as a separate dimension of current level of satisfaction. Each component, therefore, yields a separate score; a total score also may be derived from the entire scale. The rankings of level of satisfaction with the components (based on the attitude scores for each component) may then be compared with the rankings of the importance of the components (derived from the scale values of the paired comparisons).

One additional step is then taken in developing an overall score: to produce one score that reflects both importance and actual satisfaction, the average component score is multiplied by its appropriate weighting coefficient, thereby producing weighted component scores. These six scores are summed to produce a single figure, the Index of Work Satisfaction (IWS). This weighted scoring procedure produces a total index that emphasizes the relative importance of the components so that more heavily weighted components have a greater influence on the total score.[34]

Results of Previous Administrations of the Scale

This measurement instrument has been administered in six separate settings over the last six years:

1. Summer 1972 to 246 nurses in a hospital setting.[34]
2. Spring 1974 to 42 staff members (physician, nurses, and support staff of a private free service ambulatory group practice).[35]
3. Summer 1974 to 450 nurses in a hospital setting. [36,37,38]
4. Summer 1975 to 22 physicians and 16 nurses at Ryder Memorial Hospital at Humacao, Puerto Rico.[39]
5. Spring 1978 to 100 hospital nurses.[40]
6. Spring 1979 to 48 registered emergency medical technicians.[41,42]

As might be expected in research such as this, there were several objectives for each study. In all cases there were the dual objectives of developing a measurement scale and providing information to the research site. Three of the studies (2, 4, and 6) included an additional objective of broadening the scale to include other health professionals. In the Puerto Rican study (#4), a cross-cultural research objective was added.

In all studies, the major research objective was that of revising the measurement instrument itself. It was changed significantly as a result of study 3. The revised scale was used in all later studies and statistical comparisons were analyzed from studies 5 and 6. Appendix 9-A contains the most recent revision and factor loadings from studies 3 and 5, both of which were on samples of hospital nurses. This section provides an overview of results from all administrations and a comparison of those results. For more detailed information, the articles specific to each study should be consulted.

Table 9-1 shows the rankings of the ideal or expected components of work satisfaction, that is, the results of the paired comparisons part of the scale. It is interesting to note that in all mainland samples, autonomy is ranked higher than any other component by both hospital and ambulatory nurses, as well as physicians and support staff in the ambulatory setting. For all three samples of hospital nurses, the same three components are ranked highest: autonomy, job status, and pay. For ambulatory care nurses, task require-

Table 9-1 Results of Paired Comparisons of All Studies

HOSPITAL-BASED STUDIES					AMBULATORY STUDIES			
1. Summer 1972	3. Summer 1974	4. Summer 1975 (Puerto Rico)		5. Spring 1978	2. Spring 1974			6. 1979
246 Hospital Nurses	450 Hospital Nurses	Hospital Nurses	Hospital Physicians	100 Hospital Nurses	Nurses	Physicians	Support	48 REMTs at Private Ambulance Company
Autonomy*	Autonomy	Pay	Pay	Autonomy	Autonomy	Autonomy	Autonomy	Professional Status
Job Status	Job Status	Organizational Requirements	Organizational Requirements	Pay	Task Requirements	Job Status	Pay	Doctor-Nurse-REMT-Relationship
Pay	Pay	Status	Task Requirements	Job Status	Pay	Interaction	Job Status	Autonomy
Task Requirements	Task Requirements	Autonomy	Interaction	Task Requirements	Job Status	Pay	Task Requirements	Interaction
Interaction	Interaction	Interaction	Status	Interaction	Interaction	Organizational Requirements	Interaction	Task Requirements
Organizational Requirements	Organizational Requirements	Task Requirements	Autonomy	Organizational Requirements	Organizational Requirements	Task Requirements	Organizational Requirements	Pay
								Administration

*These present descending ranks, i.e., autonomy is viewed as most important and organizational or task requirements as least important.

ments are more important than job status. It is of interest that for the REMTs (registered emergency medical technicians), the most important component was professional status, which probably reflects their professional struggle for recognition from other direct care providers.

Table 9-2 shows level of satisfaction with the current occupational situation. Once again, the similarity of results is striking: job status is the highest level of satisfaction of all mainland nurses and the three components with which they are most satisfied are job status, interaction, and autonomy. It is intriguing to note that, for the small sample size of physicians and support staff in the ambulatory setting, autonomy is the highest ranked as well as the one rated as the most satisfying. The REMTs once again are slightly different in that they are more satisfied with their job status and task requirement than most nurses. For all samples, the level of satisfaction generally is lower for organizational and administrative aspects of their jobs.

Table 9-3 shows two examples of the values on the attitude scale (Adjusted Component Mean and Median

Component Scale) as well as the Index of Work Satisfaction. The Index of Work Satisfaction can be used to produce a weighted total score. This allows for more quantitative assessment and can be used to compare changes over time.

Statistical Analysis and Revision of the Scale

The first complete statistical analysis of the scale used the data gathered as part of study #3, which had a sample of 450 hospital nurses. Within this study, three crucial aspects of the scale itself were analyzed:

1. Validity of previously identified work satisfaction components *and* validity of the individual items.
2. Reliability of the attitude items.
3. Comparison of the technique of a weighted Index of Work Satisfaction to an unweighted total score.

Although the process of scale refinement is a largely theoretical or conceptual issue, it is important to ac-

Table 9-2 Results of Levels of Satisfaction of All Studies

HOSPITAL-BASED STUDIES					AMBULATORY STUDIES		
1. *Summer 1972	*3. Summer 1974*	*4. Summer 1975 (Puerto Rico)*		*5. Spring 1978*	*2. Spring 1974*		
246 Hospital Nurses	*450 Hospital Nurses*	*Hospital Nurses*	*Hospital Physicians*	*100 Hospital Nurses*	*Nurses*	*Physicians*	*Support*
Job Status**	Job Status	Task Requirements	Pay	Job Status	Job Status	Autonomy	Autonomy
Interaction	Interaction	Pay	Task Requirements	Autonomy	Interaction	Organizational Requirements	Interaction
Autonomy	Autonomy	Autonomy	Administration	Interaction	Autonomy	Interaction	Job Status
Organizational Requirements	Task Requirements	Administration	Interaction	Pay	Organizational Requirements	Task Requirements	Task Requirements
Pay	Pay	Interaction	Status	Task Requirements	Task Requirements	Job Status	Organizational Requirements
Task Requirements	Organizational Requirements	Status	Autonomy	Organizational Requirements	Pay	Pay	Pay

*Numbers represent the study numbers contained in Section 4, *Results of Previous Administration*.
**These are ranked in descending order, from highest to lowest.

Table 9-3 Component Scores of the Attitude Scale and Index of Work Satisfaction Scores for Two Studies

Study #5, Spring 1978
HOSPITAL STUDY

Study #2, Spring 1974
AMBULATORY SETTING

Job Satisfaction Component	Adjusted Component Mean*	IWS**	Component	Median Component Score (0-60)	IWS** (0-1)	Component	Median Component Score (0-60)	IWS** (0-1)	Component	Median Component Score (0-60)	IWS** (0-1)
Autonomy	37.72	.63	Job Status	39.17	0.65	Autonomy	50.00	0.83	Autonomy	47.00	0.79
Pay	35.82	.60	Interaction	38.00	0.63	Organizational Requirements	38.33	0.64	Interaction	44.17	0.74
Job Status	48.54	.81	Autonomy	31.67	0.53	Interaction	37.50	0.62	Job Status	39.17	0.65
Task Requirements	23.50	.30	Organizational Requirements	27.50	0.00***	Task Requirements	36.67	0.00***	Task Requirements	35.00	0.58
Interaction	36.97	.62	Task Requirements	26.67	0.44	Interaction	37.50	0.62	Organizational Requirements	34.17	0.00***
Organizational Requirements	23.08	.00***	Pay	21.67	0.36	Pay	29.17	0.49	Pay	15.83	0.26

*As various components had a differing number of questions pertaining to them, the mean value for a component had to be adjusted so that the means could be compared. For example, a mean value of 18.86 for autonomy must be understood with the knowledge that the maximum score for satisfaction with that component is 30.00 (scores are adjusted).
**Index of Work Satisfaction.
***End Point of Scale versus actual value.

knowledge the critical element of precision of measurement. Without a valid measure of occupational satisfaction, the first objective cannot be attained, and if this objective cannot be reached or is not accomplished in a thorough manner, it profoundly jeopardizes the ability to achieve the remaining two objectives. Therefore, the results of the statistical revision of the scale are reviewed here.

Validity

One of the best methods of assessing the validity of a scale is through factor analytic techniques, which provide a valuable and powerful analytic tool. It is not a technique that answers all questions, but it does provide an excellent basis for addressing the complex problem of validity. The method used here was the principal component analysis with a varimax rotation.[43] This produced seven factors that accounted for 59 percent of the variance among the items, with 48 of the original 72 items chosen for inclusion in the revised

questionnaire on the basis of the factor analysis. The factor loadings on each of the items that were retained in the scale are shown in Appendix 9-B.

Although the items did not group into the components exactly as they had been identified originally, the concepts of these new factors are quite similar to the original ones. For example, the items that loaded heavily for the revised pay component all were originally thought to be measuring satisfaction with pay; the interaction component is almost the same, as is the autonomy component. The revised task component contains one former "interaction" item; the original organizational requirements component was renamed to be more specific to administration. It contains items not only from the former "organizational requirements" component, but also one each from the former categories of "task requirements," "autonomy," and "job status." A new and separate factor that arose relates to a specific type of interaction: that between physician and nurse. Although this is an aspect of interaction as defined previously, the responses were distinct to this central type of interaction between two direct care providers. Conversations with the respondents involved in all studies also verified that this is viewed as a special type of interaction that is unique to the health care setting.

This analysis suggests redefining some of the components to the following:

1. Pay: dollar remuneration and fringe benefits received for work done.
2. Autonomy: amount of job-related independence, initiative, and freedom either permitted or required in daily work activities.
3. Task requirements: tasks that must be done as a regular part of the job and the organization of work as it relates to the amount of time allotted to patient care and administrative work.
4. Administration: effect of administration on job procedures, personnel policy, and the amount of staff participation in making these policies.
5. Interaction: opportunities and requirements for both formal and informal social contact during working hours.
6. Professional status: generated feelings toward the profession, the skills, usefulness, and status of the job.
7. Doctor-nurse relationship: amount and type of professional interaction among physicians and nurses.

Internal Reliability

Internal reliability was determined by use of Cronbach coefficient alpha, a random split-half reliability test. Reliability for the 72-item original test was .929; for the 48 items chosen by factor analysis it was .912. This obviously supports the use of the shorter version of the scale.

Table 9-4 shows the intra subscale reliability coefficients for each of the revised components for three studies. In general, those factors with more items have higher scores, but all fall within an acceptable range for reliability.

Correlation of Weighted and Unweighted Total Scores

A weighted total score was developed originally for the instrument to combine the importance of the component with the amount of satisfaction derived from the current occupational situation as shown in Table 9-3. Its use is supported both by Herzberg's and Maslow's theories, which suggest that different components of job satisfaction produce different amounts of

Table 9-4 Intra Subscale Reliability Coefficients

	Study		
Subscale	Study #3 (Original Scale) N=450	Study #5 (Revised Scale) N=100	Study #6 (Revised Scale) N=48
Pay	.846	.880	.830
Organizational Requirements (Administration)	.839	.837	.800
Interaction	.828	.758	.835
Professional Status	.760	.799	.600
Doctor-Nurse Relationship	.700	.791	.712
Task Requirements	.699	.776	.663
Autonomy	.696	.662	.738
Split-half reliability for whole scale, (original 12-item scale: .912)	48 items— .912	48 items— .928	48 items— .900

satisfaction, and by the suggestion that linking incentives to those more important and less satisfied needs leads to greater motivation and higher productivity.[7, 24, 32]

The weighted score method may be criticized, however, because the rank order computations are time consuming and therefore detract from the instrument's use. The arbitrary zero-weighting of the least important component cancels out this component in the final weighted score. Also, it has not been shown conclusively that a weighted score always measures more than an unweighted score. Both scores are rather arbitrary values that represent an attitude, and the seven-point unweighted score may be as sensitive to variation in subjects' responses to different components as a total weighted score.

To determine the difference between a weighted and nonweighted total score, a Kendall's tau correlation statistic was used producing a .86 correlation between the weighted and unweighted total score. This high correlation suggests that the weighted and unweighted scores are similar. One possible explanation for the high correlation is that the score ranges for the fairly homogeneous sample of nurses are not great, which reduces possible differences between weighted and unweighted scores. In addition, the factor analysis suggests that the responses vary by components, with certain factors eliciting stronger responses, thus producing groups of content-related questions. This would suggest that respondents react differently to the different factors, which would appear in an unweighted score. Thus, weighting the components to emphasize their differences may be redundant.

In deciding whether to weight scores, the theoretical question arises: which method of scoring better measures such a concept as an attitude, which is hard to quantify anyway. Certainly, the more practical approach is that of nonweighting, which appears to provide the same information as the weighted score. A negative aspect of not weighting the scores is related to the decision to retain the paired comparisons part of the questionnaire (Appendix 9-A). A decision to use a simple summation might indicate that this part of the scale is unnecessary. However, it must be remembered that the paired comparisons also provide critical information for application of the findings of this scale, which will be discussed later. To eliminate them entirely is not recommended. They can and should be included regardless of whether those data are used to create a weighted score.

Administration of Revised Scale

These statistical analyses produced a revised scale that needed to be administered again. The primary objective of study #5 was to provide that possibility. The results of the paired comparisons of the study are shown in Table 9-1 and of the level of satisfaction in Table 9-2. Table 9-3 shows the Index of Work Satisfaction and scores on the attitude scale. Table 9-4 provides the results of the reliability analysis, and the scale in the Appendix contains the factor loadings for the items from the revised scale. Results from study #6, which also used this revised scale, are included on Tables 9-1, 9-2, and 9-4.

Of primary interest here, of course, are the results of the statistical analysis, since some of the other results of these two administrations were described previously. As can be seen from Table 9-4, the reliability of both the overall scale and the subcomponents has not suffered in any way. The overall reliability of the 48-item scale (.912 and .900) is very comparable to that of the original 72-item scale. This is important because it permits use of a more practical shorter scale without losing any estimates of reliability. As can be seen, the reliability coefficients of each of the subscales vary, but all are clearly within an acceptable range.

The results of the correlation of the weighted and unweighted scores also were similar to the previous statistical analysis. In study #3, this correlation was .86; in study #5, it was .87, and in the last study it was .87.

The factor loadings for items used in studies 3 and 5 can be seen in the scale in Appendix 9-B. While there was not 100 percent agreement between the actual identification of items with factors, both factor analyses are supportive of the overall integrity of the scale, as can be seen by close examination of that scale. Further, in study #3 it was possible to account for 59 percent of the variance with 7 factors; study #5 produced 13 factors that accounted for 70 percent of the variance, and the last study (#6, given to REMTs) accounted for 80 percent of the variance with 16 factors. These results are very supportive of the notion of correctly identifying the components themselves as well as the identification of items that provide a valid and reliable measurement for these aspects of work.

Caveats

Some caveats are in order so that the limitations of this work will not be overlooked. Providing a validated measurement instrument is a lengthy process at best. This process is even more protracted when dual objectives exist, as has been the case in this research. Every one of the six sites involved research while at the same time obtaining information about satisfaction levels of the health professionals needed to change or modify work situations. The advantage of this is clear: this is a measurement device that has been developed in real-life situations, not in simulated or laboratory settings. A successful effort was made to broaden the scale considerably from the initial use of hospital nurses alone. In every setting in which this scale has been used, there has been very positive feedback. It has generated a high level of interest and some 150 persons across the country are using it now in the context of their personnel supervision.

From a research point of view, the similarity of findings and of the statistical results is quite promising. This similarity occurs despite the fact that the scale has varied slightly in each study. In some studies there have been as many as 12 attitude items per component, while in others as few as three items per component have been used. In studies #5 and #6, an uneven number of items per component were used, as can be seen from the scale in the Appendix. Despite this, the reliability (Table 9-4) and validity (Appendix 9-A) are well within the acceptable range.

At this point, however, until further statistical validation can be completed, this measurement instrument must be viewed as a very promising and practical management information tool that still is in the developmental stages. One of the main methodological problems has been assuring an adequate response rate. A varying response rate has existed among the studies, mostly dependent upon the method used to distribute and collect the questionnaire. In study #1 there was a 73 percent response rate using mailed returns. Study #3 also used mailed returns, with a 62 percent response rate. The questionnaires at the ambulatory facility (study #2) were distributed personally, self-administered, and picked up personally. This technique resulted in a 90 percent response. In the Puerto Rican study (#4), a 73 percent response was obtained by the same technique. (It should be noted, of course, that this is the most suspect of all the studies, since this is a cross-cultural setting. Although the author was sure of the translation of the scale, it was not possible to be certain that the same components were equally important in that setting.) Study #6, which also was mailed, had a response rate of 89 percent, which is very high for that technique.

By far the lowest response is that of study #5, in which only 30 percent of the sample returned the questionnaires that were distributed with the paychecks to the collection boxes. This raises two concerns: from a research point of view this is unacceptable, especially since there was heavy dependence on this study for comparison of the statistical results from study #3. From a practical point of view, it is important to look critically at this in order to understand how to avoid such a low response rate in the future. Clearly the value of this to meet the third objective—the development of a management information tool—is worthwhile only if a good response can be obtained.

The reasons for this low response rate were several, most of which were discovered after the fact. One of the key reasons was a miscommunication between the hospital administration and the nursing administration. The nurse administrators were not included in the planning as fully as they should have been. There was too much reliance on the advice of the hospital administrator who suggested, for example, that unlocked collection boxes for the questionnaires be placed in the nursing supervisor's office. This led to many concerns about confidentiality. Confidentiality of responses is an important issue and one that had been dealt with successfully by involving staff nurses as well as their immediate supervisors.

This was the first unionized hospital to be included in the studies, although the impact of unionization per se is hard to determine. Probably more important is the fact that the data collection period took place during the time of union negotiations. It is highly likely that placing the collection boxes in the nursing supervisor's office was not wise during union negotiations.

Some theoretical caveats also must be presented. One problem in adapting theories to a practical use is that theory frequently contains concepts that cannot be put into practice even though they are basic to the theoretical model. For example, the Maslow model of hierarchy of needs suggests that self-actualization is the most important need for many people, yet the work situation is such that many jobs fulfill neither this nor the hypothesized lower level needs. The Herzberg two-factor theory suggests that achievement, recognition, work itself, interpersonal relations, factors in personal life, job security, status, and pay will add more to satisfaction than do company policy and administration, supervision, and working conditions. However, many of these, such as achievement, interpersonal relations, factors in personal life, and status are difficult for management to control or improve. Thus, while a questionnaire that measures these areas is important as it substantiates or disproves a motivation theory, it may have less practical value. This is why management efforts to improve satisfaction often concern what are considered peripheral areas such as personnel policy, working conditions, supervision, or organizational structure. It is critical to be able to measure those areas of an occupation that are theoretically known to be important, but to measure them in such a way as to provide meaningful information to management.

The concept of self-actualization is mentioned repeatedly in the literature but it is difficult to measure. It does not appear as a separate component in this measurement instrument for that reason. Other concepts not included in this questionnaire that perhaps should be are factors inherent in the working environment itself, such as facilities or workspace available. These factors undoubtedly are important and may be as vital as the ones that have been identified in this data collection instrument.

Although the components included are the most important ones, their ranking does not correspond with either Maslow's or Herzberg's suggested hierarchies. Pay, autonomy, and status rank high, as Herzberg would predict. Interaction, while lower in importance, is an area of high on-the-job satisfaction and can be considered a satisfied need. Organizational requirements are less important and less satisfied, as might be predicted. The surprising factor is task requirement, which ranks low both in importance and in satisfaction, although it might be expected that this would be central to job satisfaction.

What seems necessary in the field of job satisfaction is to determine which factors, either job-related or biographical, are most influential and most predictive. This has yet to be done on a definitive basis. Much of the work in the field has been developed for use by management. While such scales are useful because they cover areas that can be measured objectively and improved, they are limited because they ignore other areas of the job and of personal life that are more difficult to assess objectively even though they may be crucial to job satisfaction.

This scale is an improvement because it covers more of the Herzberg or Maslow satisfiers, but these studies suggest the need to develop a more comprehensive scale that includes the use of multiple regression or some other method of determining best predictors of satisfaction. A test could be a good predictor of job satisfaction without including all possible factors, as suggested by Herzberg's theory. In addition, it is necessary to improve measurement of all possible relevant factors so that their relationship to satisfaction can be determined, rather than to continue to measure only the objective aspects of the job. This approach, coupled with further investigations of individual differences in satisfaction and motivation, seems to be the direction necessary to develop a theory on which to base practical measures.

BEYOND JOB SATISFACTION TO JOB EVALUATION

Many persons note that job satisfaction is not directly manipulable and thus is of little practical significance in making recommendations for change. That this is true speaks more to the inability to broaden the definition of "occupational satisfaction" than to imprecise measurement instruments. Most job satisfaction surveys ignore the role of organizational goals and values. These usually are taken as given variables, while the role of the person trying to measure satisfaction is limited to altering motivation and behavior by changing people's attitudes.[44, 45] It is not that there is no information on the impact of organizational attributes on satisfaction. For example, the influence of factors such as degree of centralization of decision making or the method of organization of nursing tasks is asserted frequently.[46, 47, 48] However, only one study has analyzed effectively the impact of factors under the control of management on nurses' job satisfaction. This study employed several structural measures of organizational attributes including the number of beds needed, given the total unit personnel, and the educational composition of the unit.[49] Formal organizational structure deserves more attention in relation to satisfaction levels; Porter and Lawler reviewed studies investigating the relationship between job attitude and behaviors and seven structural properties of organizations, including four properties of subunits in organizations.[19]

In all cases, however, these organizational characteristics are not analyzed as far as their possibility for change or for their potential control by management or administration. The measurement instrument described in this chapter provides data that can identify areas that need to be changed in the work environment. The next step is to identify items that are under the control of the nursing administration and/or the nursing staff and institute changes that seem indicated. This at least will permit a move away from the victim-blaming model of occupational satisfaction and make it possible to address the serious constraints that may exist as a result of the immediate work environment or the larger organization. This clearly involves the giving up of control and redistribution of power within an organization. The implication of this for hospitals, for example, is beyond the usual committees that nurses are invited to join. Rather, it involves spreading out a real decision-making power.

This is an organizational challenge for most health care facilities, since they often are large hierarchical institutions. It should be emphasized that the use of this instrument allows the collection of data that then can be utilized in such a way as to create effective and needed changes. Use of this measurement tool does not ensure success but it clearly initiates a change process. The appropriate use of this scale thus becomes one of an ideological position. Therefore, it is important to present what the author feels are the most important suggestions for ensuring that this scale will be administered successfully in an organization.

Hints to Ensure Success

These suggestions have been gathered as a compilation of six direct experiences of the author in using this scale as well as communication with other investigators and administrators who also are utilizing it.

1. Planning

The most important aspect to ensure successful administration of this scale is the appropriate planning phase. This should involve all levels of personnel in the administrative hierarchy. For example, if nurses in a hospital are to be surveyed, not only should hospital administrators be involved, but nurse administrators, staff nurses, and nurse leadership in any union that exists. Ideally, the use of this scale should arise from a concern to translate often ubiquitous staff dissatisfaction into discrete areas that are amenable to correction. The more involved are all levels in the planning phase, the more successful the venture will be.

In this phase, specific areas of concern may be included. For example, in one hospital a specific area of interest was that of appropriate dress for the nursing staff. In another hospital, the issue of staff nurses' participating on committees was raised. In both cases, specific questions were added to the measurement scale to aid in the decision-making process. This whole measurement process is best viewed as a way of obtaining organized and systematic input from groups often left out.

2. Motivation

Of paramount importance in this process is the *honest* estimation of motivation for using this measurement instrument, so that the potential for manipulation is removed. This scale builds on Maslow's and Herzberg's theories about job satisfaction, where satisfaction with each component can be compared with its importance (paired comparison rank) to indicate which areas of work need improvement.

When a component receives high scores in both importance and satisfaction with the actual job, it can be assumed that the respondents are satisfied with it (job prestige/status and autonomy fit this category). When a component receives high or moderately high importance by paired comparisons but low satisfaction on the questionnaire scores, it may be considered an area in need of improvement (such is the case with the pay component). Where the component has received low ranking in importance, there are several interpretations depending on the on-the-job satisfaction score. If the factor has received high scores on current satisfaction, it can be assumed that the respondents are satisfied with this area (as with interaction). Where both importance and on-the-job satisfaction scores are low, it may be that the factor is relatively unimportant and the respondents expect little satisfaction, or they may feel that satisfaction is unattainable in this area and thus have devalued it. Both task and organization may be interpreted in either of these ways.

While this gives an administrator the desired information about various areas of dissatisfaction, a major source of danger is that it may enable management to manipulate the working environment to the benefit of the administration. This could be done by discovering the relative importance and level of satisfaction of components of work and then linking incentives to some of these while ignoring others.

For example, if pay is a source of dissatisfaction but it is not valued highly, it may be easier to change scheduled work shifts than to deal with possible inequities in salary. This use obviously should be avoided because in the long run it does not contribute to anything but further alienation of providers and administrators. When the scale is used appropriately, it can create channels of communication between various levels of health professionals. It also can make possible specific changes in management and the organization through a comparison of administrative constraints with expectations and satisfactions of the health care providers.

This measurement instrument is designed as an evaluative tool that will provide information about direct care providers that can be used to alter the work environment as needed. For the process to work, there must be a willingness on the part of the administration to redistribute power and on the part of the respondents to represent their perceptions accurately.

3. Adequate Response Rate

It is imperative to try to obtain a 100 percent sample. There is an obvious reason for this: a larger and more representative sample will allow for more elaborate statistical analysis and therefore will make it possible to interpret more subtle changes. A more practical concern is related to the issues discussed previously, however. If the information is to be used as part of a management information system, it is imperative that everybody be represented.

The actual method of distributing the questionnaire will differ, depending on the group of health care providers being surveyed. In a complex organization such as a hospital, questionnaires are distributed best either through unit leaders or through the same system that distributes the paychecks. Retrieving the completed questionnaires is a more complex problem and is related to another critical issue. The use of this data collection instrument triggers an increase in information flow and communication throughout the organization. For this to happen, the respondents must be assured that their responses will remain absolutely confidential. If they are not assured of this, they either may fail to answer the questionnaire, resulting in a low response rate, or will give only those answers that they feel are acceptable. The seriousness with which they respond is influenced by their estimation of the administrator's or manager's respect for their candid opinions. Therefore, it is important that no one who has direct supervisory or administrative authority over the group being surveyed actually handle the questionnaires or be involved in the data analysis unless it is a person the respondents have accepted.

One possibility may be that questionnaires be mailed back in an envelope that is provided. A data collection box that is locked and placed in a nonthreatening place also is a good move. The best strategy is to have the questionnaires picked up personally by someone.

4. Grouped Data

It should be emphasized to all respondents that no individual will be able to be identified, and the questionnaire should be constructed so that this is true. Most organizations want some demographic or organizational characteristics included on the questionnaire. A common desire is to identify certain units that may have particularly high levels of dissatisfaction. In measuring the level of satisfaction of hospital nurses, for example, items such as specialty, unit assignment, educational level, shift worked, and part-time or full-time staff are included. To the extent that these variables produce valuable information and to the extent that individual nurses cannot be recognized, these all obviously add information. However, in a case such as this, the compromise must be in the direction of increasing confidentiality rather than increasing knowledge. Therefore, all possible cross-tabulations of these variables should be arrayed in "dummy tables," with the criteria being that no fewer than seven persons exist in the most narrowly defined category, such as full-time medical surgical RNs on the fifth floor.

5. Interpretation of the Data

After the data analysis, the most important step remains: interpretation of the data. For this purpose, several tables should be prepared. The first is a frequency distribution of the responses to each item, as shown in Table 9-5. This makes qualitative information available immediately and also allows better interpretation of the more quantitative analysis. The second general table that should be developed is shown in Table 9-6, which combines the ranking of the paired comparisons or expectations in comparison with the rankings of the level of satisfaction with these same components in the present job. This table makes possible a summary of these two important parameters. For example, the sample of ambulatory nurses (Table 9-6) shows an immediate discrepancy: nurses value appropriate skill allocations (task requirements) very highly but have a relatively low level of satisfaction with this component. The ambulatory clinic in which this research was conducted used this information to change the nature of the role of the nurses by increasing their responsibilities.

Table 9-5 Frequency Distribution of Responses to Selected Attitude Items for Three Studies

Items	Study #3			Nurses			Study #2 Physicians			Support Staff			Study #5		
	Ag.	Un.	Dis.	Ag.	Un.	Dis.	Ag.	Un.	Dis.	Ag.	Un.	Dis.	Ag.	Un.	Dis.
Pay Component:															
1. My present salary is satisfactory.	57.7	2.8	39.6	0	0	100	50	0	50	25	0	75	70	0	30
2. Considering what other (doctors, nurses, support) make, the pay here is adequate.	66.5	9.3	24.2	20	0	80	29	0	71	20	15	65	60.6	1.0	38.4
3. Even if I could make more money in another situation, I am more satisfied here because of the working conditions.	73.3	5.7	21.0	50	10	40	75	0	25	45	10	45	67.7	4	28.3
Autonomy Component:															
1. I feel that I am supervised more closely than I need to be and certainly more closely than I want to be.	15	2	83	30	0	70	-	-	-	10	10	80	18	2	80
2. A great deal of professional independence is permitted—if not required—of me on my job.	71.2	5.4	23.4	50	0	50	100	0	0	90	5	5	-	-	-
Task:															
1. A lot of what I do each day could be done just as well by someone with less skill and training.	40.3	2.9	56.8	60	10	30	75	0	25	60	5	35	-	-	-
2. There is too much clerical work and paperwork required of personnel here.	80.4	2.8	16.7	40	0	60	12.5	25	62.5	20	40	40	89.9	1	9.1

Table 9-5 continued

	Study #3			Nurses			Study #2 Physicians			Support Staff			Study #5		
	Ag.	Un.	Dis.	Ag.	Un.	Dis.	Ag.	Un.	Dis.	Ag.	Un.	Dis.	Ag.	Un.	Dis.
3. I could deliver much better care if I had more time with each patient.	69.4	7.9	22.7	80	0	20	50	12.5	37.5	58	10.5	31.5	72.8	2	25.3
Interaction: 1. The staff members don't hesitate to help one another when things get in a rush.	82.6	0.7	16.7	90	0	10	29	14	57	79	5	16	42	2	6
2. There is a lot of professional consciousness here; personnel seldom mingle with others of different professions.	10.2	2.5	79.3	70	0	20	12.5	12.5	75	15	15	70	9	3	88
Organization: 1. It is my general impression that most of the staff like the way work is organized and done here.	54.8	5.7	39.4	10	10	80	50	12.5	37.5	35	10	35	48.5	4	47.5
2. In my opinion, this clinic is not organized with the needs of the patient given top priority.	37.1	3.6	59.4	40	10	50	37.5	0	62.5	25	10	65	44.5	3	52.5
3. I have all the voice in planning policies that I want to have.	29.9	7.6	62.4	10	10	80	62.5	0	37.5	37	21	42	19.4	5.1	75.5
Job Status: 1. My particular job doesn't require much skill.	7.5	1.4	91.1	50	0	50	25	0	75	50	0	50	9	3	88
2. I can't help but feel that others don't really appreciate my job and what I have to do.	35.5	4.7	59.9	20	10	70	50	0	50	15	10	75	-	-	-
3. I can't think of many other jobs I'm more capable of doing that are more important to people than being a (nurse, physician, etc.).	78.3	6.5	15.1	80	10	10	100	0	0	70	10.5	10.5	-	-	-

Ag. = Agree
Un. = Unsure
Dis. = Disagree

The third table that may be developed is similar to Table 9-3, which allows for comparison of the actual scores of each subscale as well as calculation of the weighted Index of Work Satisfaction. As was shown earlier, this calculation of the weighted score is necessary only for those who wish to pursue this more quantitative assessment. The author's research indicates that there is a high correlation between the weighted and unweighted scores, so the extra computation may not be necessary.

As was noted, however, this does not mean that the paired comparisons should not be administered: this section provides an important context in which to interpret the findings and it is the inclusion of this part of the scale that enables valuable evaluative information to be passed on. After this scale has been administered to many groups, it may be possible to make generalized statements about relative values of a certain group of health professionals, with the assumption that the rankings of these components are consistent. Until that time, the paired comparisons part of the scale should be given to every group of respondents.

The final set of tables developed are variations of these three: cross-tabulations of all the relevant demographic and organizational variables with the results of the scale, i.e., attitude scale, paired compari-

Table 9-6 Comparison of Levels of Satisfaction with the Paired Comparison Rankings: All Studies

Study 1: Summer, 1972 246 Hospital Nurses		Study 3: Summer, 1974 450 Hospital Nurses		Study 5: Spring 1978 100 Hospital Nurses	
Paired Comparisons	*Level of Satisfaction*	*Paired Comparisons*	*Level of Satisfaction*	*Paired Comparisons*	*Level of Satisfaction*
Autonomy	Job status	Autonomy	Job status	Autonomy	Job status
Job status	Interaction	Job status	Interaction	Pay	Autonomy
Pay	Autonomy	Pay	Autonomy	Job status	Interaction
Task Req.	Org. Req.	Task Req.	Task Req.	Task Req.	Pay
Interaction	Pay	Interaction	Pay	Interaction	Task Req.
Org. Req.	Task Req.	Org. Req.	Org. Req.	Org. Req.	Org. Req.

Study 2: Ambulatory Nurses		Study 2: Ambulatory Physicians		Study 3: Ambulatory Support Staff	
Paired Comparisons	*Level of Satisfaction*	*Paired Comparisons*	*Level of Satisfaction*	*Paired Comparisons*	*Level of Satisfaction*
1. Autonomy	1. Job status	1. Autonomy	1. Autonomy	1. Autonomy	1. Autonomy
2. Task Req.	2. Interaction	2. Job status	2. Org. Req.	2. Pay	2. Interaction
3. Pay	3. Autonomy	3. Interaction	3. Interaction	3. Job status	3. Job status
4. Org. Req.	4. Org. Req.	4. Pay	4. Task Req.	4. Task Req.	4. Task Req.
5. Interaction	5. Task Req.	5. Org. Req.	5. Job Status	5. Interaction	5. Org. Req.
6. Org. Req.	6. Pay	6. Task Req.	6. Pay	6. Org. Req.	6. Pay

Study 6: REMTs	
Paired Comparisons	*Level of Satisfaction*
1. Professional status	1. Professional status
2. Doctor-Nurse-REMT Relationship	2. Task Requirements
3. Autonomy	3. Interaction
4. Interaction	4. Autonomy
5. Task requirements	5. Doctor-Nurse-REMT Relationship
6. Pay	6. Administration
7. Administration	7. Pay

sons, and the Index of Work Satisfaction. These more specific tables will allow extensive analysis of any subgroup that is desired, within the requirements of preserving confidentiality.

6. *Use of the Information*

By far the most important step is this last one and it clearly is related to the second suggestion. The information gained from the administration of this scale should be used in a nonmanipulative way to change the organization so as to better meet the needs of the respondents. If there is no intention to use the results in this way, it is much better not to administer the questionnaire.

The process involved is one that opens up an organization and increases information flow. As such, it builds up certain expectations on the part of the group being studied. If these expectations are not met, the result may very well be a more repressive organization.

A FINAL WORD

If occupational satisfaction is expanded to include not only the adaptation of the individual to the organization but also the designation of work itself, then the results of the survey process can be extremely useful to the organization. For example, if only in one area, that of turnover rate, an effective impact can be demonstrated, that alone probably is worth it. It is true that the turnover rate of nursing personnel in a hospital may take too much attention. It may or may not be an important economic factor, as Price and Mueller comment, although they also say that when the turnover rate exceeds 60 percent, it almost always is an economic loss for the hospital.[50] Other studies note that data from resignation interviews suggest that nursing turnover can be reduced anywhere from 25 percent to 30 percent if the causes of dissatisfaction are eliminated.[51,52,53] Such a reduction obviously could result in higher levels of nursing performance as well as a more satisfied atmosphere within the hospital.

Much of the description of this scale has involved nurses in a hospital setting. However, it should not be overlooked that the scale also has been administered to physicians, nurses, and other direct care professionals in an ambulatory setting as well as to registered emergency medical technicians. The scale is designed to be used for all direct care providers in many types of health care settings. In all cases, the issues being addressed are important and appropriate. It is a rare organization that has a free and easy flow of information and communication. Utilization of this scale often starts that process.

It should be clear that the measurement instrument itself is designed to gather data at the levels of expectations and current level of satisfaction. However, by including both of these levels, the application of the information becomes crucial. The third objective for this research then becomes paramount: that of creating a management information system that includes a clear orientation toward application of the findings to the *organizational* level. Without this third objective, the two other objectives—precise measurement and a practical measurement tool—are meaningless.

NOTES

1. Paula L. Stamps, "Satisfaction of Direct Care Providers," in *Ambulatory Care Systems: Vol. III—Evaluation of Outpatient Facilities* (Lexington, Mass.: D.C. Heath and Co., 1978), pp. 75–106.
2. R. Bendix, *Work and Authority in Industry* (New York: John Wiley & Sons, 1956).
3. Abraham K. Korman, *Industrial and Organizational Psychology* (Englewood Cliffs, N.J.: Prentice-Hall, Inc., 1971).
4. Victor Vroom, *Work and Motivation* (New York: John Wiley & Sons, 1964).
5. Edward E. Lawler and Lyman W. Porter, "The Effect of Performance on Job Satisfaction," *Industrial Relations* 7 (October 1967): 20–30.
6. Frederick Herzberg, *Job Attitudes: Review of Research and Opinion* (Pittsburgh: Psychological Service of Pittsburgh, 1957).
7. Frederick Herzberg, B. Mausner, and B. Snyderman, *The Motivation to Work,* (2d ed.) (New York: John Wiley & Sons, 1959).
8. Robert T. House and Lawrence A. Wigdor, "Herzberg's Dual Factor Theory of Job Satisfaction and Motivation: A Review of the Evidence and Criticism," *Personnel Psychology* 20 (Winter, 1967): 369–384.
9. E. A. Locke, "What Is Job Satisfaction?" *Organizational Behavior and Human Performance* 4 (1969): 309–336.
10. R. Katzell, R. Barret, and T. Parker, "Job Satisfaction, Job Performance, and Situational Characteristics," *Journal of Applied Psychology* 45 (1961): 65–72.
11. A. H. Brayfield and W. H. Crockett, "Employee Attitudes and Employee Performance," *Psychological Bulletin* 52 (1955): 386–424.
12. R. L. Kahn, "The Meaning of Work," in A. Campbell and P. E. Converse, eds., *The Human Meaning of Social Change* (New York: Russell Sage, 1972).
13. B. B. Longest, "Job Satisfaction for R.N.'s in the Hospital Setting," *Journal of Nursing Administration* 4, no. 3 (1974): 46–52.
14. Rensis Likert, "Patterns in Management," in Edwin A. Fleishman and Alan R. Bass, eds., *Studies in Personnel and Industrial Psychology,* 3d ed. (Homewood, Ill.: Dorsey, 1974), pp. 85–115.
15. H. Metzner and F. Mann, "Employee Attitudes and Absences," *Personnel Psychology,* 1953, in Abraham K. Korman, ed., *Industrial and Organizational Psychology* (Englewood Cliffs, N.J.: Prentice-Hall, Inc., 1971).
16. I. C. Ross and A. Zanter, "Need Satisfaction and Employee Turnover," *Personnel Psychology,* 1975, in Victor Vroom, ed., *Motivation and Work* (New York: John Wiley & Sons, 1964), pp. 93–128.
17. L. Porter and R. Steers, "Organizational, Work, and Personnel Factors in Employee Turnover and Absenteeism," *Psychological Bulletin,* 80 (1973): 151–176.
18. Curt Tausky, *Work Organizations: Major Theoretical Perspectives,* 2d ed. (Itasca, Ill.: Peacock, 1978).
19. L. Porter and E. Lawler, *Managerial Attitudes and Performance* (Homewood, Ill.: Richard D. Irwin, Inc., 1968).
20. N. Impartu, "Relationship Between Porter's Need Satisfaction Questionnaire and the Job Description Index," *Journal of Applied Psychology* 56 (October 1972): 397–405.
21. P. C. Smith, L. Kendall, and C. Hulin, *The Measurement of Satisfaction in Work and Retirement* (Chicago: Rand-McNally and Co., 1969), pp. 193–202.
22. S. B. Denman and F. D. Ryder, "Occupational Satisfaction and Dissatisfaction Among Psychiatric Aides," *Hospital and Community Psychology* 22 (April, 1971).
23. G. A. Nichols, "Job Satisfaction and Nurses' Intentions to Remain With or to Leave an Organization," *Nursing Research* 20 (May-June 1971): 218–228.
24. E. Lawler, *Motivation in Work Organizations* (Monterey, Calif.: Brooks/Cole Publishing Co., Inc., 1973).
25. S. Wright, "Turnover and Job Satisfaction," *Hospitals, J.A.H.A.* 31 (October 1957): 47–52.
26. Bernard M. Bass, *Organizational Psychology* (Boston: Allyn & Bacon, Inc., 1965).
27. J. P. Lysaught, *An Abstract for Action.* Report of the National Commission for the Study of Nursing and Nursing Education (New York: McGraw-Hill Book Co., 1973).
28. M. A. Godfrey, "Job Satisfaction—or Should That Be Dissatisfaction? How Nurses Feel About Nursing," *Nursing 78* Part I: 8(4) 89–104; Part II: 8(5) 105–120; Part III: 8(6) 81–95.
29. Boston Globe, Thursday, March 15, 1974, page 43.
30. R. Hoppock, *Job Satisfaction* (New York: Harper and Brothers, 1935).
31. C. Hulin and P. Smith, "A Linear Model of Job Satisfaction," *Journal of Applied Psychology* (1965): 49.

32. Abraham Maslow, *Motivation and Personality* (New York: Harper & Row, 1954).

33. Allen L. Edwards, *Techniques of Attitude Scale Construction* (New York: Appleton-Century-Crofts, Inc., 1957).

34. Eugene B. Piedmont, *Work Satisfaction Among Nursing Service Personnel at Hospital A.* (Amherst, Mass.: University of Massachusetts, Department of Sociology, 1972).

35. Paula L. Stamps, E. B. Piedmont, D. B. Slavitt, and A. M. Haase, "Measurement of Work Satisfaction Among Health Professionals," *Medical Care* 16 (April 1978): 337–352.

36. Dinah B. Slavitt, "Measurement of Job Satisfaction Among Health Care Professionals." M.S. Thesis, University of Massachusetts/Amherst, 1975.

37. Dinah B. Slavitt, Paula L. Stamps, Eugene B. Piedmont, and A. M. Haase, "Nurses' Satisfaction With Their Work Situation," *Nursing Research* 27 (March-April 1978): 114–120.

38. _____ , "Measuring the Levels of Satisfaction of Hospital Nurses," *Hospital and Health Services Administration Journal* 24, no. 3 (Summer 1979), pp. 62–72.

39. G. Ramirez, *Work Satisfaction Among Doctors and Nurses: The Case of an Outpatient Clinic at Humacao; Puerto Rico.* M.S. Thesis, University of Massachusetts/Amherst, 1975.

40. Howard E. Bond, *An Analysis of Job Satisfaction Among Health Care Professionals.* M.S. Thesis, University of Massachusetts/Amherst, 1978.

41. B. Shopnick, *Measurement of Occupational Satisfaction Among Registered Emergency Medical Technicians-Ambulance.* M.S. Thesis, University of Massachusetts/Amherst, 1979.

42. Paula L. Stamps and B. A. Shopnick, "Acceptance of R-Emt's by Nurses and Physicians," paper presented at New Professionals Section, American Public Health Association annual meeting, 1979.

43. N. H. Nie, C. H. Hull, J. G. Jenkins, K. Steinbrenner, and D. H. Bent, *SPSS: Statistical Package for the Social Sciences* (New York: McGraw-Hill Book Co., 1975), pp. 118–121.

44. G. Ramirez, *A Conceptual Analysis of the Framework and Implications of Work Satisfaction Research and Practice.* Ph.D. Dissertation, University of Massachusetts/Amherst, 1980.

45. L. F. Davis and A. B. Cherns, *The Quality of Working Life* (Vols. 1 and 2) (New York: The Free Press, Division of Macmillan Publishing Co., 1975).

46. A. D. Brief, "Turnover Among Hospital Nurses: A Suggested Model," *Journal of Nursing Administration*, October 1976, pp. 12–19.

47. K. L. Ciske, "Primary Nursing: An Organization that Promotes Professional Practice," *Journal of Nursing Administration*, April 1974, pp. 22–25.

48. M. Kramer, *Reality Shock: Why Nurses Leave Nursing* (St. Louis: C.V. Mosby, 1974).

49. F. C. Munson and S. S. Heda, "An Instrument for Measuring Nursing Satisfaction," *Nursing Research* 23 (1974): 159.

50. J. L. Price and C. W. Mueller, "How to Reduce the Turnover of Hospital Nurses," in Norman Metzger, ed., *Handbook of Health Care Human Resources Management* (Rockville, Md., 1981).

51. L. K. Diamond and D. J. Gox, "Turnover Among Hospital Staff Nurses," *Nursing Outlook* 6 (1958): 388.

52. S. D. Saleh, R. D. Lee, and E. P. Prien, "Why Nurses Leave Their Jobs—An Analysis of Female Turnover," *Personnel Administration*, January-February 1965.

53. Veterans Administration, *Survey of Factors Relating to Job Satisfaction Among VA Nurses: 1960 and 1970* (Washington, D.C.: U.S. Government Printing Office, 1973).

Part A of the Questionnaire:
Paired Comparisons*

Listed and briefly defined on this sheet of paper are six terms or factors that are involved in how people feel about their work situation. Each factor has something to do with "work satisfaction." We are interested in determining which of these is most important to you in relation to the others.

Please carefully read the definitions for each factor as given below:

1. *Pay*—Dollar remuneration and fringe benefits received for work done.
2. *Autonomy*—Amount of job-related independence, initiative, and freedom either permitted or required in daily work activities.
3. *Task Requirements*—Tasks that must be done as a regular part of the job.

4. *Organizational Requirements*—Constraints or limits imposed upon job activities by the administrative organization of the hospital.
5. *Interaction*—Opportunities and requirements presented for both formal and informal social contact during working hours.
6. *Job Prestige/Status*—Overall importance or significance felt about the job you perform.

Scoring: These factors are presented in pairs on the questionnaire that you have been given. Only 15 pairs are presented: this is every set of combinations. No pair is repeated or reversed.

For each pair of terms, decide which one is the *more important* for your job satisfaction or morale. Please indicate your choice by checking the line in front of it.

For example: if you feel that PAY (as defined above) is more important than AUTONOMY (as defined above), check the line before PAY.

_____ PAY   OR   _____ AUTONOMY

We realize that it will be difficult to always make choices; however, please do try to select the factor which is more important to you. Please make an effort to answer every item: don't change any of your answers.

---

*For complete information about scoring this scale, contact the author.

1. _____ JOB PRESTIGE/STATUS   or _____ ORGANIZATIONAL REQUIREMENTS
2. _____ PAY   or _____ TASK REQUIREMENTS
3. _____ ORGANIZATIONAL REQUIREMENTS   or _____ INTERACTION
4. _____ TASK REQUIREMENTS   or _____ ORGANIZATIONAL REQUIREMENTS
5. _____ JOB PRESTIGE/STATUS   or _____ TASK REQUIREMENTS
6. _____ PAY   or _____ AUTONOMY
7. _____ JOB PRESTIGE/STATUS   or _____ INTERACTION
8. _____ JOB PRESTIGE/STATUS   or _____ AUTONOMY
9. _____ INTERACTION   or _____ TASK REQUIREMENTS
10. _____ INTERACTION   or _____ PAY
11. _____ AUTONOMY   or _____ TASK REQUIREMENTS
12. _____ ORGANIZATIONAL REQUIREMENTS   or _____ AUTONOMY
13. _____ PAY   or _____ JOB PRESTIGE/STATUS
14. _____ INTERACTION   or _____ AUTONOMY
15. _____ ORGANIZATIONAL REQUIREMENTS   or _____ PAY

Part B of the Questionnaire:

Attitude Scale with Component and Factor Loadings Identified*

The following items represent statements about satisfaction with an occupation. Please respond to each item. It may be very difficult to fit your responses into the seven categories: in that case, select the category that *comes closest* to your response to the statement. It is very important that you give your *honest* opinion. Please do not go back and change any of your answers.

INSTRUCTIONS FOR SCORING. In the far right hand space, please place the number that *most closely* indicates how you feel about each statement. The *left* set of numbers indicates degrees of *Disagreement.* The *right* set of numbers indicates degrees of *Agreement.* The *center* number means "undecided;" please use it as little as possible. *For example,* if you *strongly disagree* with the first item, write 0 in the blank. If you *moderately agree* with the first statement, you would write 5 in the place provided.

REMEMBER: The more strongly you feel about the statement, the further from the center you should circle, with disagreement to the left and agreement to the right.

Factor Loadings			DISAGREE				AGREE			
Study #3	Study #5		Strong	Moderate	Weak		Weak	Moderate	Strong	
594	.70648	1. My present salary is satisfactory. (P)	0	1	2	3	4	5	6	_____
	.54500	2. When I'm at work in this hospital, the time generally goes by quickly. (S)	0	1	2	3	4	5	6	_____

*The components are identified by the following: P = Pay; S = Status; I = Interaction; D/N = Doctor, Nurse Relations; OA = Administration/Organization Req.; T = Task Req.; A = Autonomy.

			DISAGREE			AGREE		

| *Factor Loadings* | | | *Strong* | *Moderate* | *Weak* | *Weak* | *Moderate* | *Strong* | |
Study #3	Study #5								
455	.68570	3. The nursing personnel on my service don't hesitate to pitch in and help one another out when things get in a rush. (I)	0	1	2	3	4	5	6 _____
9135	.76868	4. There is too much clerical and "paper work" required of nursing personnel in this hospital. (T)	0	1	2	3	4	5	6 _____
45	.31201	5. It's my general impression that most of the nursing staff at this hospital really like the way work is organized and done. (O)	0	1	2	3	4	5	6 _____
722	.79148	6. Physicians in general don't cooperate with the nursing staff on my unit. (D-N)	0	1	2	3	4	5	6 _____
905	.427997	7. I feel that I am supervised more closely than I need to be, and more closely than I want to be. (A)	0	1	2	3	4	5	6 _____
059	.64790	8. Excluding myself, it is my impression that a lot of nursing personnel at this hospital are dissatisfied with their pay. (P)	0	1	2	3	4	5	6 _____
994	.70787	9. Even if I could make more money in another hospital nursing situation I am more satisfied here because of the working conditions. (S)	0	1	2	3	4	5	6 _____
145	.59573	10. New employees are not quickly made to "feel at home" on my unit. (I)	0	1	2	3	4	5	6 _____
107	.65467	11. I think I could do a better job if I didn't have so much to do all the time. (T)	0	1	2	3	4	5	6 _____
386	.38666	12. There is a great gap between the administration of this hospital and the daily problems of the nursing service. (O)	0	1	2	3	4	5	6 _____
126	.30354	13. I sometimes feel that I have too many bosses who tell me conflicting things. (A)	0	1	2	3	4	5	6 _____
224	.70285	14. Considering what is expected of nursing service personnel at this hospital, the pay we get is reasonable. (P)	0	1	2	3	4	5	6 _____
163	.51068	15. There is no doubt whatever in my mind that what I do on my job is really important. (S)	0	1	2	3	4	5	6 _____
969	.67363	16. There is a good deal of teamwork and cooperation between various levels of nursing personnel on my service. (I)	0	1	2	3	4	5	6 _____
613	.43905	17. The amount of time I must spend on administration ("paper") work on my service is reasonable and I'm sure that patients don't suffer because of it. (T)	0	1	2	3	4	5	6 _____

			DISAGREE				AGREE			
Factor Loadings			*Strong*	*Moderate*	*Weak*		*Weak*	*Moderate*	*Strong*	
Study #3	Study #5									
675	.58942	18. There are plenty of opportunities for advancement of nursing personnel at this hospital. (O)	0	1	2	3	4	5	6	_____
945	.78187	19. There is a lot of teamwork between nurses and doctors on my unit. (D-N)	0	1	2	3	4	5	6	_____
455	.76729	20. On my service, my supervisors make all the decisions. I have little direct control over my own work. (A)	0	1	2	3	4	5	6	_____
224	.76675	21. The present rate of increase in pay for nursing service personnel at this hospital is not satisfactory. (P)	0	1	2	3	4	5	6	_____
466	.49686	22. I am satisfied with the types of activities that I do on my job. (S)	0	1	2	3	4	5	6	_____
473	.40911	23. The nursing personnel on my service are not as friendly and outgoing as I would like. (I)	0	1	2	3	4	5	6	_____
284	.71761	24. I have plenty of time and opportunity to discuss patient care problems with other nursing service personnel. (T)	0	1	2	3	4	5	6	_____
007	.62752	25. There is ample opportunity for nursing staff to participate in the administrative decision making process. (O)	0	1	2	3	4	5	6	_____
554	.25620	26. It is possible, at this hospital, for some nursing service personnel to get better pay because of "favoritism" or "knowing somebody in the right place." (P)	0	1	2	3	4	5	6	_____
064	.39334	27. What I do on my job doesn't add up to anything really significant. (S)	0	1	2	3	4	5	6	_____
905	.39006	28. There is a lot of "rank consciousness" on my unit. Nursing personnel seldom mingle with others of lower ranks. (I)	0	1	2	3	4	5	6	_____
946	.55440	29. I don't spend as much time as I'd like to taking care of patients directly. (T)	0	1	2	3	4	5	6	_____
2619	.34911	30. There is no doubt that this hospital cares a good deal about the welfare of its employees, nursing personnel included. (O)	0	1	2	3	4	5	6	_____
440	.26543	31. I am sometimes required to do things on my job that are against my better professional nursing judgment. (A)	0	1	2	3	4	5	6	_____
5288	.55584	32. From what I hear from and about nursing service personnel at other hospitals, we at this hospital are being fairly paid. (P)	0	1	2	3	4	5	6	_____
4416	.30516	33. Administrative decisions at this hospital interfere too much with patient care. (O)	0	1	2	3	4	5	6	_____

Factor Loadings			DISAGREE			AGREE			
Study #3	Study #5		Strong	Moderate	Weak	Weak	Moderate	Strong	
5831	.63478	34. It makes me proud to talk to other people about what I do on my job. (S)	0	1	2	3	4	5	6	_____
3655	.36276	35. I have the feeling that this hospital in general—and my service too—is not organized with the needs of patients given top priority. (O)	0	1	2	3	4	5	6	_____
369	.39626	36. The nursing personnel on my service don't often act like "one big happy family." (I)	0	1	2	3	4	5	6	_____
038	.85608	37. I could deliver much better care if I had more time with each patient. (T)	0	1	2	3	4	5	6	_____
557	.63700	38. I'm generally satisfied with the way nursing work is organized and gets done at this hospital. (O)	0	1	2	3	4	5	6	_____
498	.51463	39. Physicians at this hospital generally understand and appreciate what the nursing staff does. (D-N)	0	1	2	3	4	5	6	_____
611	.72132	40. The only way that nursing personnel at this hospital will ever get a decent pay schedule will be to organize and, if necessary, strike. (P)	0	1	2	3	4	5	6	_____
438	.30487	41. If I had the decision to make all over again, I would still go into nursing. (S)	0	1	2	3	4	5	6	_____
213	.42814	42. Nursing personnel at this hospital do a lot of bickering and backbiting. (I)	0	1	2	3	4	5	6	_____
684	.50279	43. I have all the voice in planning policies and procedures for this hospital and my unit that I want. (O)	0	1	2	3	4	5	6	_____
501	.38372	44. Considering the high cost of hospital care, every effort should be made to hold nursing personnel salaries about where they are, or at least not to increase them substantially. (P)	0	1	2	3	4	5	6	_____
691	.41126	45. My particular job really doesn't require much skill or "know-how." (S)	0	1	2	3	4	5	6	_____
7098	.46602	46. The nursing administrators generally consult with the staff on daily problems and procedures. (O)	0	1	2	3	4	5	6	_____
2822	.51267	47. I have the freedom in my work to make important decisions as I see fit, and can count on my supervisors to back me up. (A)	0	1	2	3	4	5	6	_____
3485	.79020	48. An up-grading of pay schedules for nursing personnel is needed at this hospital. (P)	0	1	2	3	4	5	6	_____

10. Job Analysis and Job Descriptions

NORMAN METZGER

Reprinted with permission from *Personnel Administration in the Health Services Industry,* 2d ed., by Norman Metzger, published by SP Medical & Scientific Books, Division of Spectrum Publications, Inc., New York, © 1979.

The need for scientific wage determination in any enterprise, including hospitals and homes, is well-established. Wage rates in the health care industry have risen to unprecedented heights through a spiraling succession of negotiations and pressures, both market and societal. Although wages may not be the key to motivation (and indeed one despairs at the absence of a concomitant rise in efficiency when wages are raised) employee dissatisfaction about wages is quite pronounced in hospitals and homes. This dissatisfaction has two separate causes:

1. Inequities among wage rates paid within classifications and in classifications employees consider similar to their own.
2. Individual or group pressure for higher earning power.

For many years hospitals and homes have been dealing with wages by fiat: an arbitrary order of importance is established and an arbitrary wage structure follows. This method is certainly eroded by group pressures from unions, professional associations and employees with skills which are in short supply. A sounder method of establishing wages is through job evaluation. The central purpose of job evaluation is threefold: to determine the relative worth of the various jobs in the institution; to establish a wage scale which incorporates fair differentials among jobs; and finally, where necessary, to correct pay inequities.

Job evaluation serves three major purposes:

1. Wage rates which will be defensible can be established on a quasi-scientific and logical basis. They are thus removed from the world of conjecture, arbitrariness and subjectiveness.
2. The bane of health care administration, *personalized rates,* will be abolished. Consequently, select pressure groups so prevalent in most hospitals and homes will be neutralized. No longer will the administrator be faced with the problem of misclassifying the secretary to a chief of service who protests that his secretary should receive as much as the secretary to the director of the institution.
3. Job evaluation is a key tool for the administration in attempting to meet competition by establishing a formal wage pattern that will conform with health care wage rates in the area and, in general, with community wage rates.

To fully appreciate and understand the worth of job evaluation, one must consider the entire process from inception to fruition. The components of a job evaluation program include:

1. Job analysis.
2. Job descriptions.
3. Job specifications.
4. Job evaluation.

5. Wage structures.
6. Wage and salary administration.

JOB ANALYSIS

Job analysis is the scientific determination through intensive study and review of the actual nature of a specific job. It involves a study of each of the tasks which make up a job, including the skills, knowledge, abilities and responsibilities required of the worker. Its earliest origins can be traced to the time and motion studies first developed by Frederick W. Taylor in 1881 at the Midvale Steel Company. Taylor's use of analysis was directed toward determining a standard time for production. The purpose of motion study was pointed toward improving the methods of performing jobs. Industrial engineers look to eliminating unnecessary elements of the job and simplifying those that must be done. The industrial engineer conducting a time/motion study approaches it from the point of view of the job operation by observation and timing. He studies the sequence of operations, notes the machines and equipment involved and observes the movements of the worker in detail. His purpose is to improve the sequence, establish standards, simplify the work and conserve effort. Time and motion studies, however, do not provide the most complete answer to wage determination.

Job analysis, on the other hand, merely takes the job *as it is*, describing the duties, responsibilities, working conditions and relationship to other jobs, and does not involve itself with possible changes in the operation. The National Personnel Association in 1922 defined job analysis as "that process which results in establishing component elements of a job and ascertaining the human qualifications necessary for its successful performance." This definition sees job analysis as establishing job elements, which truly is the job of the industrial engineer. A more modern connotation envisions job analysis as reporting what currently exists in a job and *not* establishing job elements. There are basically three steps in the analysis of any job:

1. Identifying the job completely and accurately.
2. Describing the task of the job.
3. Indicating the requirements for its successful performance.

In the first step of job analysis, *identifying the job,* a specific job must be distinguished from every other job in the organization. It must be given a title and its geographic location must be clearly indicated. In describing the duties and responsibilities of the job, one is concerned with such factors as where the work comes from, what the worker does to it and what mental and physical processes are necessary for completion of the job. When the duties and responsibilities of the job are identified, the approximate time that each is performed must be indicated. In analyzing the skill and physical requirements, one must be concerned with mental skills—education, judgment, initiative—and manual skills—dexterity and motor skills. The physical requirements include such factors as standing, sitting, reaching and lifting. The working conditions and job hazards direct attention to the general environment in which the job is performed.

DEFINITION OF TERMS

At the outset, it is necessary to define some of the terms common to the process of job evaluation.

Job: A job is made up of tasks and responsibilities which, when considered as a whole, are regarded as the regular assignment of the individual employee.

Occupation: An occupation is a group of closely related jobs which have many characteristics in common; however, each job of the occupation has its individual characteristics.

Position: Many employees may work at the same job. Each employee is said to be occupied in a position. For example, the job of porter in a hospital may be filled by 50 individuals who occupy 50 positions.

Job description: A job description is a written report including the duties and conditions to be found in a specific job.

Job specification: A job specification is a section of the job description which addresses itself to the personal requirements, skills and physical demands of the job.

USES OF THE JOB ANALYSIS

Job facts are secured through the process of job analysis for many reasons. Some of these end products follow:

Job evaluation: Job analysis and job evaluation are not synonymous. Job evaluation is an end result of a job analysis. It establishes a foundation upon which a plan can be implemented to determine basic wage and salary differentials. These salary differentials are based upon the relative differences in job requirements.

Selection and placement: Job analysis results in job descriptions and specifications which provide an orderly and effective guide for matching applicants to positions in the interviewing procedure. Appropriate tests may be developed as a result of job analysis results. The job specification developed from the job analysis breaks down the job into its various components and, more importantly, details the qualifications necessary for jobholders.

Performance evaluation: Once again the job description developed from the job analysis may be used, this time to quantify specific elements to be measured on the job—standards against which an employee may be rated. These specific criteria for the successful jobholder may be used as a guide for merit rating.

Training: Job analysis can provide detailed information that serves as a basis for the training department's development of curriculum.

Labor relations: Job analysis provides a specific breakdown of duties that can be used to answer grievances regarding the nature of the employee's responsibilities. Job analysis, producing a job description, serves as a means of developing a mutual understanding between the administration, the union and employees regarding the specific duties of each job. It may eliminate or reduce grievances regarding pay differentials if the analysis is used to produce a scientific job evaluation.

Wage and salary survey: Job analysis provides a method of comparing rates of jobs in one institution with those in another.

Organizational analysis: Job analysis can clarify lines of responsibility and authority by a detailed breakdown of each job. It can indicate functional, organizational positioning of jobs.

THE JOB ANALYST

A threshold decision must be made as to who will conduct the job analysis. There are three basic sources from which job analysts may be selected:

1. Employees within the institution.
2. Personnel supplied by consulting firms.
3. Personnel recruited from outside the institution.

Notwithstanding the source from which the job analyst is obtained, he (she) must have the ability to get along with others and be able to maintain an objective point of view. The analyst must write clearly and concisely, analyze and interpret diverse data and, in many instances, work on his own. It is essential that he obtain a high degree of cooperation from employees and supervisors in areas where he will be studying jobs. Upon this degree of cooperation rests the success

of the entire program. It has been said that the only way to learn job analysis is by doing it. Although many college-level courses incorporate the subject of job analysis within the rubric of overall personnel administration, the person involved in the field must receive intensive training as to the organizational structure, its nuances and the personalities involved. It is obvious that choosing an employee presently in the employ of the institution has many advantages. He will know the organization, be familiar with its operating procedures, traditions and mores, and have a good understanding of the personalities involved. He is more likely to be accepted than the outsider who suffers from the suspicions of others as to his ultimate role.

STEPS IN THE DESIGN OF THE PROGRAM

Several steps must be taken to ensure the success of a job analysis program. First, the development of the plan; second, the presentation of the plan to top administration; third, the presentation of the plan to the supervisory group; and finally the presentation of the plan to the nonsupervisory group.

Development of the Plan

Careful planning is the hallmark of the successful job analysis program. The first decision to be made is the method of conducting the analysis. Each of the methods, their advantages and disadvantages, will be discussed later in this article. Marketing is probably the most important aspect to be considered in the planning stage. Obtaining employee and supervisory participation is essential. Methods of presenting the program to the administration, supervision and rank-and-file employees must be carefully developed. The selection of job analysts and their training is still another aspect to be considered in the planning stage.

Presenting the Plan to Top Administration

The acceptance by top administration of the need for and worth of a job analysis program is essential in assuring the success of that program. In order that the top administration may have facts upon which to make its decision with regard to authorizing a job analysis study, a complete presentation covering the various phases of the program and outlining in depth the steps to achieve the desired results must be made. Such a presentation to the director and his immediate staff should include such items as:

1. The nature of job analysis.
2. The main objectives of the program.
3. Why the organization will benefit from such a program.
4. Reference to the experience of other institutions preferably in the same field with such programs.
5. The cost of the programs.
6. Cost savings to be derived from such a program.
7. Who will conduct the program?
8. The methods to be used in assembling the information.

Presenting the Plan to the Supervisory Group

A combination of approaches can be used in presenting the proposed job analysis study to the supervisory group. Some of the more prevalent and successful methods are:

1. Staff meetings.
2. Individual meetings with supervisors.
3. Memoranda from the top administration to the supervisory group.

The combination of any or all of these methods is not unusual. The program will not suffer from over-communication. Full and broad publicity will aid in its acceptance and guarantee its results. To reduce problems that result from suspicions and lack of understanding on the part of the supervisory team, maximum participation of supervisors must be obtained. They must understand the complete method of job analysis and the hoped-for results. This requires an educational program wherein the basic nature and philosophy of a job analysis program are communicated. Strong emphasis should be placed on the benefits to the supervisors from such a program. In general, supervisors will be reluctant to spend the time required to implement a job analysis program unless they first accept and acknowledge that there will be positives for them which develop from such an endeavor. In addition, it is wise to assign to each supervisor a specific responsibility as part of the program. The supervisor himself may be responsible for explaining the procedures to the employees. As described later in this article, the supervisor may well fill out the job analysis questionnaire or aid the employee in completing the form. In either case, it is essential that he be made to feel a part of the program and not an outsider.

Presenting the Plan to the Nonsupervisory Group

The fourth cornerstone in ensuring the success of the plan is the full understanding and cooperation of the employees in the institution. They must understand *why* such a program is necessary and the benefits that will accrue to them from the program. Letters to the employees from the administrator, group meetings with employees, individual interviews with employees and departmental meetings led by supervisors all play a role in obtaining maximum cooperation of the non-supervisory group. It is a well-established principle that employees want to know what is going on and want to participate in effecting change. Any assumption that employees are not interested in an explanation of a new program is an invalid one. The need to feel a part of things is a pervasive one. A program such as this should not be legislated; it should be "sold" to the employees. Communication, once again, is the key to this marketing procedure. In addition, it is best to introduce the job analyst to the employees in advance to facilitate and ease the analyst's job.

TRAINING THE ANALYST

Once the analysts who will conduct the program are selected, various methods or combinations of methods are used to train them. Among these are:

1. A study program involving literature that is widely available.
2. Lectures and conferences during which the analysts are presented the details of *what* they are to do and *how* they are to do it, and a careful review of the forms to be used.
3. Role playing during which the analysts conduct practice interviews, followed by a critique and a refinement of the techniques.

It is important that the analyst understand the advantages to the institution of such a program. He must be instructed in the method of completing the information on a questionnaire, in conducting interviews with supervisors and with employees and in methods of obtaining information through observation.

Not the least of the training essentials is in the area of writing drafts of the data assembled. The style of writing such drafts must be as uniform as possible. It is on the basis of such information that job descriptions are developed. Therefore, a terse, direct style must be employed, and all words that do not impart necessary information to an understanding of the job duties should be omitted.

HOW TO COLLECT THE DATA

There are basically three methods of obtaining information about jobs:

1. The analyst may make use of a questionnaire sent to the job incumbent, who fills it in, has it checked by his supervisor and returns it when completed.[1]
2. The analyst may interview the worker or the supervisor or both to obtain the necessary information.
3. The analyst may collect the data from personal observation.

A discussion of each of these methods follows.

Questionnaire Method

This is the most rapid and economical of the methods. The worker or the supervisor or both complete a questionnaire which covers all phases of the job, its environment and overall responsibilities. The questionnaire is then returned to the job analyst who carefully reviews it for content and completion and edits it in preparation for the writing of a job description. The preparation of the questionnaire is critical to the success of this method. It must be carefully prepared to solicit all the pertinent facts about the job and, therefore, must indeed be universal in application since most job analysis programs include varying and disparate jobs. In the development of a questionnaire, the use of check boxes can reduce to a minimum the writing required of the employee. A closer review of the contents of a job information form and the typical subdivisions of such a questionnaire follow (see Exhibit 10-1):

1. The employee's name, the department, his present position, job classification and date of preparation.
2. Description of duties (job content) with approximate percentage of time applied to each duty. This section calls upon the employee to describe the duties and responsibilities of his position. He is asked to include enough detail and use language that will clearly convey the content and requirements of the position to a person not familiar with the work. He is asked to describe regular ongoing activities and then periodic or occasional duties. He must make estimates of the frequency with which each duty is performed, *e.g.*, daily, weekly, monthly, and approximate percentage of working time normally consumed on each of the duties.
3. The educational requirements of the job. Include the minimum education normally required to perform the work satisfactorily. It does not follow that the incumbent's present educational background coincides with the requirements of the position.
4. Experience requirements. Here the employee is asked to indicate the nature and extent of experience required for an individual with the specified educational background to perform the work satisfactorily. This includes previous experience and necessary break-in time with the present employer.
5. The employee is asked to describe the degree of supervision exercised over his position and guidance available to him in performing his task.
6. The impact of errors. The employee is asked to describe the results of errors possible from improper performance of the work.
7. A description of the responsibility for contacts with others such as employees in his department and in other departments, department heads, medical staff, patients, visitors and outside officials.
8. If his position entails working with confidential data, the employee is asked to describe the nature of the data, the degree of confidentiality and the effects of disclosure. He is asked to describe precautions that must be taken to keep the information secure.
9. Physical demands. Here the employee is asked to describe the physical exertion required to perform the work. How often and with what frequency does the work require standing, walking, lifting, reaching, stooping or pushing.
10. Mental, visual and manual coordination. A description of the aspects of the work that require attention to detail, concentrating on critical procedures, overcoming distraction, coordinating simultaneous operations and exercising manual dexterity.
11. Several sections deal with responsibility for equipment or process, for materials and for safety and welfare of others.
12. Working conditions. The employee is asked to describe the surroundings in which the work is performed and to indicate disagreeable conditions present in the work area, such as heat, cold, dampness, fumes, noise, dust and dirt, and whether exposure is constant, frequent or occasional.
13. Unavoidable hazards. A description of accident and health hazards incident to work even though all possible safeguards are observed.
14. In the case of supervisory jobs, the character of the supervision exerted. The supervisor is asked to describe the degree of responsibility and authority which he applies to other employees.

Exhibit 10-1 Sample Job Information Form

THE MOUNT SINAI HOSPITAL

JOB INFORMATION FORM*

A.   B.

Review Requested By   Date | Department   Section

PURPOSE OF REVIEW: | Current Job Classification

( ) To classify new position. | Position or Functional Title

( ) To ascertain whether job changes | Employee's Name   Employee #
     require reclassification of
     position. | Position

( ) To ascertain whether estab- | Prepared By   Date
     lished classification is
     appropriate. | Approved By   Date

( ) Departmental job audit.

( ) Other: _____

_____

C. JOB CONTENT — Describe the duties and responsibilities of the position. Include enough detail and use language that will clearly convey the content and requirements of the position to a person not familiar with the work. Describe regular, ongoing activities first, then periodic or occasional duties. Indicate the frequency with which each duty is performed, e.g., daily, weekly, monthly, and the approximate percentage of working time normally consumed.

	Frequency	Approximate % of Time
_____		
_____		
_____		
_____		
_____		
_____		
_____		
_____		

*Excerpt

Exhibit 10-1 continued

H. CONTACTS WITH OTHERS — Describe the responsibility to service, deal with or influence other persons.

With Whom?	Individuals Dealt With	Purposes of Contacts	Frequency
( ) Employees in own Department			
( ) Employees in other Departments			
( ) Department Heads			
( ) Administrative Officials			
( ) Medical Staff			
( ) Patients			
( ) Visitors			
( ) Outside Officials			
( ) Others			

I. RESPONSIBILITY FOR CONFIDENTIALITY — If position entails working with confidential data (e.g., medical reports, financial statement, personnel records), describe the nature of data, degree of confidentiality, and effects of disclosure. Describe precautions that must be taken to keep the information secure.

J. PHYSICAL DEMAND — Describe the physical exertion required to perform the work, how often, and with what constancy does the work require standing, walking, lifting, reaching, stooping, pushing, etc.

K. MENTAL, VISUAL AND MANUAL COORDINATION — Describe those aspects of the work that require attention to detail, concentrating on critical procedures, overcoming distraction, coordinating simultaneous operations and exercising manual dexterity.

L. RESPONSIBILITY FOR EQUIPMENT OR PROCESS — Indicate the probable dollar value of careless damage to equipment or loss of time because of incorrect performance of a work process. Describe the situations in which such losses are possible.

M. RESPONSIBILITY FOR MATERIALS — Indicate the probable dollar value of a typical loss due to careless waste or spoilage of material or supplies. Describe the situations in which such losses are possible.
$

N. RESPONSIBILITY FOR SAFETY AND WELFARE OF OTHERS — Describe the extent to which care must be exercised to prevent injury, discomfort, or impairment of health of others. Indicate possible accidents resulting from misuse of equipment, mismanagement of medical care, etc.

O. RESPONSIBILITY FOR WORK OF OTHERS (NONSUPERVISORY POSITIONS ONLY) — Check the statement that most closely describes the employee's responsibility for instructing, guiding, or assisting others in their work.

( ) Responsible solely for own work
( ) Responsible for leading up to ten employees in work group
( ) Responsible for maintaining work flow of more than 25 employees
( ) Responsible for instructing, guiding, or assisting one or two employees
( ) Responsible for maintaining work flow of up to 25 employees

P. WORKING CONDITIONS — Describe surroundings in which work is performed

Indicate disagreeable conditions present in work area, e.g., heat, cold, dampness, fumes, noise, dust, dirt, etc., and whether exposure is constant, frequent, or occasional

Q. UNAVOIDABLE HAZARDS — Describe accident and health hazards incident to work even though all possible safeguards are observed.

Exhibit 10-1 continued

R. SUPERVISION OF OTHERS (SUPERVISORY JOBS ONLY)
Character of Supervision — Listed below are a variety of administrative and supervisory functions. Indicate in the appropriate column the degree of responsibility and authority with which the employee acts in each function. Use the following definitions as a guide:

NA - Not applicable to this position.
1 - Has authority to act only after approval by supervisor.
2 - No authority to act but has responsibility to recommend action and to implement action after approval is received.
3 - Has full authority to act without prior approval but must advise supervisor after action is taken.
4 - Has full authority to act without consulting supervisor before or after action is taken

FUNCTION	NA	1	2	3	4
Plan Work Schedules					
Assign Work to Employees					
Review Completed Work					
Instruct Employees on the Job					
Develop Training Programs					
Determine Standards of Performance					
Appraise Employee Performance					
Reprimand Employees for Failure to Meet Performance Standards					
Discipline Employees for Infraction of Regulations					
Investigate and Resolve Grievance					
Select Applicants for Employment					
Discharge Employees for Unsatisfactory Performance					
Recommend Salary Action					
Grant Time Off					
Authorize Overtime					
Approve Supply Requisitions and Petty Cash Expenses					
Purchase Capital Equipment					
Prepare and Maintain Budget					
Develop and Implement Improved Methods and Procedures					
Direct Patient Care or Action					
Other: Describe:					

Source: Mt. Sinai Hospital, New York, New York.

15. Scope of supervision. Here the supervisor is asked to indicate the number and types of employees directly and indirectly supervised.

Advantages of the Questionnaire Method

The questionnaire method is the most rapid for obtaining information. Time is often a prime consideration, and by using questionnaires distributed to the employees whose jobs are to be described, more jobs can be analyzed than by the interviewing method in the allotted time. It ensures maximum participation of employees since by its very nature a questionnaire can be sent to a large number of employees without the involvement of too much of their own time as well as the time of the administration. It has the distinct advantage of channeling employee thinking regarding their jobs because of the well-planned format of the questionnaire. In the final analysis it is one of the least costly methods of obtaining job information. An adjunct advantage reported by one observer is that problems dealing with cross-divisional responsibilities can be identified and corrected.[2]

It is well to note that all advantages of the questionnaire method stem from the design of the questionnaire. The critical element in the success of this method is the specificity of the questionnaire, and

often institutions have developed separate questionnaires for clerical, technical, professional and service jobs.

Disadvantages of the Questionnaire Method

It is almost impossible to design a questionnaire that will bring forth complete information on all jobs. Because of the varying backgrounds of employees who are asked to fill in questionnaires, terminology is often inconsistent, and therefore interpretation of the questionnaire is difficult at times. Hourly and clerical employees often are ill-equipped to write paragraphs or answer questions that will give the analyst the necessary information to describe the job.[3] This method requires extensive editing of information. Experience with questionnaires indicates that often they must be supplemented by interviews to clarify information and complete responses. Low-level personnel do not take the time to provide extensive, clear and complete information about their job duties. The absence of personal contact minimizes the chances for employee understanding of the program. It has been noted that some employees resent the questionnaire approach and suspect that their job rate might depend on what they write and not on what they do.[4]

Interviewing Method

In obtaining job analysis data, the analyst may interview either the supervisor or the employee involved in doing the job, or both. The analyst usually has a plan or guide to follow in his questioning and can get more complete and accurate information regarding a job in an interview than would usually be obtainable through any other method. The procedure is quite simple. First, the analyst observes the worker on the job while he is performing a complete cycle. He will than ask any questions that arise about any specific part of the operation. The analyst takes notes, often copious in nature, indicating the areas which he has failed to grasp or questions which he may have about a specific aspect of the job. He will then study the information that he has noted to check for continuity of data. He will talk directly with the worker and/or the worker's supervisor. Often it is wise to recheck the worker's comments and the analyst's notes with the supervisor. It is essential that the worker be informed during the interview and observation stage that he must perform his job in the usual manner.

Good interviewing in job analysis is quite similar to effective interviewing in other aspects of personnel work. Of course, the purpose is quite different: securing a patterned or preplanned set of job facts. An important secondary purpose is that of winning the understanding, cooperation and interest of the employees and supervisors interviewed. Patton, Littlefield and Self suggest a guide for job analysts during the interviewing procedure:[5]

1. Introduce yourself; review briefly the purposes of the analysis; give any individualized explanation needed; answer questions.
2. Follow your interview guide or work-sheet form in asking questions, but recognize that the various items of information will not always come out in any set order.
3. Phrase questions clearly and follow through with each until a full understanding is reached.
4. Use a high degree of tact and show interest in anything the employee has to say. Be a careful listener.
5. Avoid making promises or giving expressions of opinion regarding the probable value of the job at this stage and avoid making suggestions as to possible improvements in working methods.
6. Write up the job just as you find it, disregarding both the ability of the employee on the job and any previous notions which you may have had regarding the job. If you think erroneous information has been given, make notes and check later but do not directly question the truth of the interviewee.
7. Assure the employee that you will let him check and verify the description before it is written up in final form.
8. Thank the employee for his cooperation.

Advantages of the Interviewing Method

More than any other method, interviewing permits the analyst to secure complete and accurate information. It obviates the employees having to complete questionnaires at home if their jobs do not provide facilities for work of this nature and also avoids the necessity for employees to describe their work in writing, which is often very difficult for employees with little background in such a skill. The personal touch is a decided asset in explaining the program and winning employee understanding. Editing and standardizing language is minimized since the analyst is carefully trained in writing his observations from the interview. By firsthand interviewing and observation, the analyst is able to accurately reduce the information to the more essential aspects of the job.

Disadvantages of the Interviewing Method

This method requires a great deal of time when a large number of jobs must be analyzed. Therefore, it is relatively expensive because the salaries of both the analyst conducting the interview and the employee (who may well be less productive during that stage) are involved. Because of the time and expense, this method is usually applied to a limited number of employees and does not provide for the broad participation which is the hallmark of the questionnaire method.

Observation Method

This method is quite similar to the interview method except that the analyst only observes the operation and does not question the employee. Rarely used on its own, it is often combined with the interview method or the questionnaire method. During the observation method the analyst makes notes, avoids disturbing the worker and carefully observes the "what, how and why" of the skill involved and the physical demands of the job. He then reviews his notes, attempting to assure continuity of operation. His primary concern is to discern the factual information from judgment or impression. It has been said that the chief characteristic of the scientific method is the requirement that the observer be trained to distinguish what he observes from what he would like to infer. This indeed is the crux of the observation method. Its disadvantage lies in the fact that it would be quite difficult to apply this method for operations that require mental skills to a large degree, as well as to operations which are long-run and, therefore, must be observed over long periods of time.

Observation and Interview: Combined Method

After reviewing the advantages and disadvantages of the observation method and the interview method, it is not difficult to deduce that by combining these two methods most of the disadvantages are minimized and the advantages maximized. The analyst would first obtain as much information as possible by observing the job without disturbing the worker. After reducing his observations to notes, he would interview the supervisor and the worker to supplement facts. This would ensure the assembling of information which could not be obtained by observation and provide the mechanism to verify and augment those facts obtained by observation.

During the observation method the analyst makes notes, avoids disturbing the worker and carefully observes the job as it is being done. He then reviews the notes with the worker and the supervisor to fill in where necessary and to modify impressions which may not be based upon the actual elements of the job.

THE MECHANICS OF JOB ANALYSIS

The following is a typical plan for implementing a job analysis.

1. Visit department head:
   a. Explain the purpose and objectives of the plan.
   b. Discuss the desired method for obtaining the information, *e.g.*, questionnaire, observation, interview.
   c. Make maximum effort to obtain the understanding of the department head and, therefore, his cooperation.
   d. Secure a list of all the jobs in the department by title and the number of employees in each title. (This information can be obtained in advance from the personnel department and verified with the department head.)
2. With the approval of the department head, visit the supervisor and/or assistant supervisor:
   a. Explain the purposes and objectives of the plan.
   b. Obtain an overview of the work of the section.
   c. Discuss the specific job in question with emphasis on the nature of the work and the details of the job.
   d. Obtain recommendations of the most desirable employees to observe during the course of the study on the basis of efficiency and willingness to cooperate with the analyst.
3. Observe employees at work:
   a. Carefully note each operation performed.
   b. Make certain all observable operations have been noted.
   c. Separate judgment or impression from factual information.
   d. Check for specific items to be included in the job analysis schedule.
   e. Report factual data of working conditions, equipment and materials used.
   f. Question the worker about those operations which are not observable and obtain from the worker an estimate of the percentage of time such operations are performed.
   g. Review the notes concerning the job elements with the worker, ask for suggestions and obtain from him an estimate of the percentage of time each operation is performed.
4. Review observations and notes with assistant supervisor and/or supervisor:
   a. Determine if the job has been thoroughly covered.
   b. Obtain estimates of percentage of time for each operation. (Check these estimates against the estimates noted from comments of the employee.)
   c. Obtain information as to the relationship of this job to other jobs in the section.
5. Write the first draft of the analysis in prescribed format.
6. Have department head review and approve the original draft:
   a. Allow all supervisors concerned the opportunity to review and edit the original draft.
   b. Revise draft on the basis of comments, changes and criticisms suggested by the reviewers and obtain written approval of contents before final typing.
   c. Arrange for typing of the completed analysis—one copy to be retained in the analysis file, one copy to be forwarded to the wage and salary administrator, one copy to be forwarded to the personnel director and one copy to be forwarded to the department head.

JOB DESCRIPTIONS

No single instrument is as important to effective wage and salary administration as the job description, yet there is evidence that it receives far less attention than it requires to assure either that it is properly prepared in the first place or that its uses are properly understood or directed.[6]

The process of obtaining job facts through job analysis moves to the next critical step: the writing of a statement of the duties, responsibilities and job conditions. Having completed the task of assembling all the requirements of a specific job, the job analyst has at hand, through a questionnaire, notes from an interview or direct observation, all the pertinent items which make up the regular assignment of an employee on an individual job. Having conducted a job analysis, he has in front of him the following information: the objective of the job, including its basic mission and what it accomplishes; to whom the incumbent reports; how many people he supervises; what levels and types of positions report directly to the incumbent; which areas and operations are included in the position; to what extent the incumbent is responsible for actions and decisions, completely or partially; whether his actions are subject to approval from his supervisor; the extent to which he is responsible for results; the type of planning involved in the job; other units of the institution which are directly affected by this planning; the relationships of the incumbent in the job to other departments within the institution and others outside the institution; the extent and nature of his responsibilities for policy interpretation; the procedures and methods to be followed; and specialized technical information required to handle the job.

The analyst is now prepared to write a job description. *A job description is a listing of the duties and responsibilities of a particular job, written in narrative form.* Its content and style may vary considerably, based upon the end to which it will be used. There is a guideline which may be followed when the description is to be used for the standard purpose of job evaluation, training and/or planning. An effective job description has four basic subdivisions: *"heading," "job summary," "duties performed"* and *"personal requirements."* Patton, Littlefield and Self offer the following principles as a guide to writing effective job descriptions:[7]

1. Arrange duties in logical order. If a definite work cycle exists, duties may be described in chronological order. When the work cycles are irregular, more important duties may be listed first, followed by less important ones.

2. State separate duties clearly and concisely without going into such detail that the description resembles a motion analysis.

3. Begin each sentence in the "duties performed" section with an active, functional verb in the present tense, such as "tests," "performs," "adjusts," etc. For brevity, the subject of each sentence is omitted. It is understood that the job title is the subject.

4. Use quantitative words where possible. Rather than "pushes loaded truck," write "pushes hand truck loaded with 100 to 500 pounds of steel plates."

5. Use specific words where possible. Instead of writing that a patternmaker "makes" patterns, write that he "saws stock to length on circular saw and roughly to width on ripsaw; shapes with woodworking machines and hand tools." Avoid vague words and ambiguous generalizations such as "handles," "assists" and "prepares," unless further information is given which makes the meaning specific. If the words fail to evoke a mental image of the work, rephrase using a more specific verb.

6. State duties as duties; postpone statements of qualifications until the "personal requirements" or "job specification" section.

7. Avoid proprietary names that might make the description obsolete when equipment changes occur. Write "operates automatic electric desk calculator" instead of "operates Friden calculator."

8. Determine or estimate the percentage of total time spent on each activity and indicate whether duties are regular or occasional. The description should not imply that the jobholder spends most of his time at a demanding task when, in actuality, it may be performed only 5 percent of the time. Be sure to define such words as "periodic," "occasional" and "regular."

9. Limit the use of the word "may" with regard to performance of certain duties. Rating committee members will want to know whether the duty is performed or not performed; they are often confused if the description states that the operator "may perform" the duty. Nevertheless, occasions arise when the use of "may" is justified toward the end of the duty section when a "saving clause" broadening the description of duties must be inserted.

Heading

The job in question must be differentiated from all others in the organization. Therefore, the selection of the appropriate title is essential. In addition, concomitant identifying information should be established such as the department in which the job is performed and a job code number. Two helpful sources in job identification are *The Dictionary of Occupational Titles* and *Job Descriptions and Organizational Analysis for Hospitals and Related Health Services,* both published by the United States Department of Labor, Washington, D.C.

The importance of selecting an appropriate job title should not be underestimated. Social behaviorists have pointed out repeatedly the important roles that status and recognition play in the motivation of employees. Not only should the selected title *distinguish* a job from every other job in the organization, it should also be fully *acceptable* to the incumbents. Very often a job may have a master or generic title which encompasses several functional titles. In addition to the master title, any alternate titles by which the job may be known should be listed in the "heading" section. The title, as far as possible, should be similar to one used in the past for that job in that institution. Optimally, it should be one that is commonly used throughout the health care industry. It should be set up in its natural form, not in inverted form: *e.g.*, nursing technician, not technician—nursing. It should be brief and should indicate wherever possible the skill and supervisory levels involved. In addition to the department in which the job is assigned, the date the information is secured should be clearly indicated at the top of the form. This keys the reader into the timeliness of the information. Where possible, the job description heading should include the name of the supervisor responsible for the specific job and the current salary or range for the job. All of this may be contained in the code number, which may be made up as follows: a section for indicating the department, the number(s) for the generic type of job, the number(s) for the skill level and the number(s) for the position.

Job Summary

This section of the job description gives the reader an overall concept of the purpose, nature and extent of the task performed. It is also meant to show how the job differs generally from others in the organization. This is best accomplished by a brief statement which avoids generalities and precedes a detailed presentation of the duties. It aims to give immediate understanding to the reader of the nature of the job without a profusion of details. Otis and Leukart present five points in the writing of an effective "job summary" section:[8]

1. The statement should be as brief as possible and still encompass its purpose.
2. Words should be selected carefully to carry the maximum amount of specific meaning.
3. The statement should differentiate the job from all other jobs accurately enough to be used in classifying workers on the job.
4. The purpose of the job must be clearly stated.
5. The job summary must conform to the what-how-why job analysis formula.

The "job summary" section is not one which encompasses details, duties and responsibilities. It is generalized in nature and has as its avowed purpose the establishment of the uniqueness of the job. It must communicate the *central purpose of the job*.

Duties Performed

This section is a complete description of duties of the job and is often referred to as the *body* of the job description. Each duty must be written in logical work order. This may be done either by describing the duties chronologically or by combining those which are of a similar nature. The decision as to how to present the tasks should be dependent on which method creates the clearest presentation. When writing the "duties performed" section, it is important that the requirements not be based upon the incumbent since he may be overqualified or underqualified for the position. It is essential to state the *minimum* requirements for the *average* incumbent. A succinct, direct style should be used. Each sentence should begin with a functional verb: for example, "transports patients to and from operating or treatment rooms, sets up equipment, instruments and medications for surgeons." It is best to use the present tense to minimize the number of words to be used. The pitfall one finds too often in job descriptions is that they are unnecesssarily protracted. On the other hand, it is essential that each important duty be described. The job analysis material should be reviewed carefully before writing the "job summary" section. Grady offers three important questions which should be answered in the affirmative upon review of the job analysis information:[9]

1. Have you indicated clearly the knowledge and skills required on the job?
2. Have you shown the responsibilities and authority inherent in the job?
3. Have you included a statement of working conditions?

He also makes the following suggestions in writing the "duties performed" section:[10]

1. Start each paragraph with an active verb.
2. Use telegraphic style (complete sentences are not essential, but making sense is).
3. Avoid the use of general words such as "maintains," "checks," "handles," "prepares," "takes care of" *unless* the level of work is further specified.
4. Make plentiful use of "such as" and "by doing" (one or two examples frequently are clearer than several sentences of description).

Personal Requirements

The "personal requirements" section or "job specification" section is concerned primarily with reflecting the skill involved and the physical demands of the job. It is used as the basis and justification of the values which will be assigned to each factor for the purpose of evaluating the job's worth. It is used as well to facilitate selection and placement.

Since the most widely used job evaluation plan is the point-factor method, the specification under this plan would encompass from six to twelve specific factors. The most common factors found in a job specification are those for education, experience, initiative, ingenuity, physical demands, working conditions and unavoidable hazards. The job is then broken down into its requirements paralleling the job factors to be used in evaluating the job. The analyst must determine and describe the extent of each factor in the job. Once again each factor is described in terms of the *minimum* requirement for the *average* incumbent. For example, under the factor "education," a typical specification would include "ability to read or write and speak English, follow directions and make simple arithmetic calculations equivalent to four years of high school education." The specification for experience would include the years of experience necessary to perform the requirements of the position in a satisfactory fashion, *e.g.*, "over seven years of progressive experience as a cook in a hotel, restaurant or hospital." Under the specification for working conditions, the description in a normal situation might read, "Works in a well-lighted kitchen; subject to burns and scalds from hot equipment and foods and injury from falls on slippery floors." Unavoidable hazards are included under the working conditions factor. In some instances specifications may be written separately for unavoidable hazards. All the specifications must be specific and quantitative. Patton, Littlefield and Self suggest several key principles in writing the specification section:[11]

1. Break down the job requirements parallel to the job factors to be used in evaluating the jobs. For each factor selected for use in the job evaluation plan, determine the extent of that requirement in the job being described.
2. Be as specific and quantitative as possible.
3. State the *minimum* requirement for the *average* jobholder. Avoid confusing a jobholder's personal qualifications with the minimum requirements of the job.
4. Distinguish between the job's minimum requirement and the hiring qualifications. A low-level job may require no more than the ability to read, write and do simple arithmetic. Yet the hospital may require all entering employees to possess a high school diploma to ensure their advancement.
5. Check to ensure that every duty corresponds to the requirements.

An effective job specification will go further than a mere mention of personal requirements. It will seek to provide measurements of each of those requirements. Many job specifications contain minimum scores which must be attained on both intelligence and mechanical aptitude tests.[12] The job specification contains substantiating data for each factor to be considered. These substantiating data are measured against the degree descriptions for each factor contained in the wage and salary manual (see Exhibit 10-2).

Updating of Job Description

It is imperative that once the job description for each job is carefully constructed a system be developed for keeping it up to date. It is necessary to change the job description whenever significant changes are introduced into the job requirements. If such changes occur within the responsibilities of existing jobs, a new description must be written. It should be standard operating procedure for the line supervisor to inform the wage and salary manager of any significant changes to the job description and request an audit of the job. As a safeguard, many institutions schedule a periodic audit of all jobs in the organization. Each month the wage and salary section of the personnel department is responsible for auditing a specific number of jobs to update the job descriptions. Whenever a new job is created, there is a need to conduct a job analysis to produce a job description.

Exhibit 10-2 Sample Job Evaluation Form

MOUNT SINAI HOSPITAL   Code No. _____211_____
NEW YORK, NEW YORK   Department(s)_____

Personnel Department   Labor Grade _____9 H_____

JOB EVALUATION SPECIFICATIONS

Job Title __NURSING AUXILIARY__   Class ___A___   Total Points ___180___

	FACTORS	SUBSTANTIATING DATA	Degree	Points
SKILL	EDUCATION	Ability to read and write and speak English, follow written and verbal instructions and use simple arithmetic and equipment.	3	25
	EXPERIENCE	Previous experience in related auxiliary nursing work preferred. On-the-job training yields full productivity in 6 months to 1 year.	2	40
	INITIATIVE AND INGENUITY	Requires ability to work from detailed procedures in performing work. Must use tact and judgment in dealings with patients, nurses and staff. Receives close supervision.	2	25
EFFORT	PHYSICAL DEMAND	Lifts, pushes and carries equipment, wheels portable apparatus; turns, bends, reaches and pulls in handling patients and setting up equipment.	3	15
	MENTAL OR VISUAL DEMAND	Must be mentally and visually alert during surgery and administration of treatments. Requires manual dexterity in setting up equipment and administering treatments.	3	15
RESPONSIBILITY	FOR EQUIPMENT OR PROCESS	Probable damage to equipment or instruments is negligible because of close supervision.	1	5
	FOR MATERIALS	Probable loss of materials and instruments is seldom over $10.00 because of immediate supervision.	1	5
	SAFETY OF OTHERS	Compliance with standard procedures and safety precautions essential in order to prevent accidents or cause further discomfort to patients.	3	15
	WORK OF OTHERS	Responsible for own work only.	1	5
CONDITIONS	WORKING CONDITIONS	Works in operating room and other patient-care surroundings.	3	15
	UNAVOIDABLE HAZARDS	Subject to burns and cuts from instruments, equipment and chemicals, and respiratory ailments from fumes.	3	15
	REMARKS:			

Source: Mt. Sinai Hospital, New York, New York.

This should be done at the outset. In fact, it is advisable to write the job description before an individual is hired for the new position. Brandt makes mention of specific changes which require the careful attention of the wage and salary section and alert them to the need for a revision of the present job description:[13]

1. A change in physical facilities or surroundings which might affect the comfort, fatigue or hazard factors of a job, creating or eliminating the need for protective garments or equipment and/or altering the way in which functions are performed.

2. A technological change might make the job easier or more difficult to perform. It might create or eliminate a need for special knowledge. It might also affect the time needed to perform a particular function so that the employee would be required to operate several machines or processes instead of one or the function might now be combined with other functions in order to fill out the job tour.

3. A change in supervisors might result in a realignment of several jobs into completely new combinations of functions which could entail an increase or decrease of difficulty and/or respon-

sibility of any given job. Some of this restructuring might be a reflection of current interest or of a drive for more efficient use of manpower.

CONCLUSION

The job description has become indispensable to the process of classifying work into management components, for it is one of the important means by which the energy of the organization is unified in constructive channels.[14] Evans points out that "A clear line of demarcation can be drawn between a typical job description program for blue collar workers and that which is customarily found at managerial levels. Many survey respondents stated that they used their managerial position descriptions entirely for purposes unconnected with compensation rates. Rather . . . the principal goal of their program is to improve organization using the job description as a diagnostic tool to uncover defects."[15]

The job description plays an important role in administration as well as in manual positions within the organization. It is more than mere support for the salary program and may be used effectively in meeting performance standards. It has been stated that "when a manager and his subordinate are having an earnest discussion of some plan or decision affecting the subordinate's work, the conversation rests on the assumption that the two men are in fair agreement about the nature of the subordinate's job. . . . If a single answer can be drawn from the detailed research study (presented in the report), into superior-subordinate communication on the managerial level in business, it is this: If one is speaking of the subordinate's specific job—his duties, the requirements he must fulfill in order to do his job well, his intelligent anticipation of future changes in his work, and the obstacles which prevent him from doing as good a job as possible—the answer is that he and his boss do not agree or differ more than they agree in almost every area."[16]

In order to ensure maximum agreement between superiors and subordinates, the administration must provide well-written job descriptions. These descriptions must then be widely publicized and complete agreement as to their content obtained from the supervisor and the incumbents in each job. The descriptions will be used to establish a foundation upon which to build a formal job evaluation plan and to provide an effective and objective guide for intelligent selection and placement as well as detailed information for inaugurating training programs. With proper quantification, the job descriptions will be used as a standard by which employees may be rated.

NOTES

1. Charles W. Brennan, *Wage Administration* (Homewood, Ill.: Richard D. Irwin, Inc., 1963, p. 94.
2. Robert P. Vorhis, "*Collecting Data Through Questionnaires,*" in Milton L. Rock, *Handbook of Wage and Salary Administration* (New York: McGraw-Hill Book Company, 1972), pp. 1–39.
3. *Ibid.*, pp. 1–37.
4. *Idem.*
5. John A. Patton, C. L. Littlefield, and Stanley Allen Self, *Job Evaluation: Text and Cases* (Homewood, Ill.: Richard D. Irwin, Inc., 1964), p. 81.
6. Alfred R. Brandt, "Describing Hourly Jobs," in Rock, *op. cit.*, pp. 1–11.
7. Patton, Littlefield, and Self, pp. 93–4.
8. J. Lester Otis and Richard Leukart, *Job Evaluation* (Englewood Cliffs, N.J.: Prentice-Hall, Inc., 1948), p. 266.
9. Jack Grady, "How to Write a Job Description," *Job Evaluation and Wage Incentives* (New York: Conover-Nast Publications, 1949), pp. 66–7.
10. *Ibid.*, p. 66.
11. Patton, Littlefield, and Self, pp. 94–5.
12. Dale Yoder, *Personnel Principles and Processes* (Englewood Cliffs, N.J.: Prentice-Hall, Inc., 1956), p. 98.
13. Brandt, pp. 1–22.
14. Gordon H. Evans, *Managerial Job Descriptions in Manufacturing* (New York: American Management Associations, 1964), p. 13.
15. *Ibid.*, p. 19.
16. Norman R. S. Maier, L. Richard Hoffman, John J. Hooven, and William H. Read, "*Superior-Subordinate Communications and Management,*" 52 (American Management Associations, 1961), p. 9.

11. An Integrated Approach to Performance Evaluation in the Health Care Field

HOWARD L. SMITH and NORBERT F. ELBERT

Reprinted with permission from *Health Care Management Review*, Vol. 5, No. 1, Winter 1980, published by Aspen Systems Corporation, Germantown, Md., © 1980.

Performance evaluation is a critical responsibility confronting contemporary health care administrators. Increasingly, administrators, nursing directors and supporting supervisors are required to assess individual and organizational performance. In many cases, however, the traditional methods of reviewing performance are proving inadequate or unacceptable.

Several factors are responsible for this failure to attain satisfactory performance appraisal. High levels of education and professionalization germane to health and medical care have stimulated a demand for improved personal performance evaluation. Revised definitions of effective performance that include both cost-effective resource allocation and high-quality patient care have added to the need to achieve more sophisticated methods of evaluation. Finally, ancillary personnel are demanding fair assessments of their performance. The dilemma exemplified by these pressures creates a major problem for all health care administrators.

In resolving the inherent problems of health care performance appraisal, administrators should implement evaluations at three main levels—organizational, departmental and individual. The inadequacies of a disjointed performance evaluation system often reflect an administrator's incapability in achieving a total view of health services. This partial view can be accompanied by personnel dissatisfaction, inequitable reviews and failure to know where a health care institution is headed. Yet with an integrated approach to performance assessment, a foundation is established for comprehensive improvement of the delivery of health care services.

AN INTEGRATED MODEL OF PERFORMANCE EVALUATION

Despite the continuing development of evaluation procedures such as professional standards review organizations (PSROs) and medical audit procedures, integrated performance appraisals still remain to be achieved. Health care administrators will discover that these disjointed evaluative programs are not the sole foundation of a comprehensive system. Instead, they represent incremental elements of what should be an integrated attempt to assess performance.

Whether for a hospital, nursing home or medical clinic, an integrated model of performance evaluation must deal with three levels of evaluation criteria. At the first level are the immediate criteria which represent the critical behaviors of the individual's work task accomplishment, for example, an RN's ability to successfully irrigate a catheter. The second level forms the intermediate criteria for evaluating departmental or subunit performance, for example, nutritious meals from food service. On the third level, referred to as ultimate criteria, are organizational outcomes that reflect the overall effectiveness of the health care institution, such as rehabilitated patients after a minimal length of stay. These three criteria levels are the primary components underlying an integrated model of performance evaluation as seen in Figure 11-1.

According to this model of performance evaluation, individual behavior (task performance, personal growth and job satisfaction) can be appraised through several commonly used measures such as trait ratings, single global ratings, behaviorally anchored rating scales and objectives-oriented ratings. Departmental performance dimensions such as effectiveness, morale, absenteeism, personnel turnover and efficiency are often measured through surveys and other rating schemes. Examples of organizational performance, such as effective patient care and efficient services, can be measured through cost analysis and alliance with evaluative agencies (PSROs). Since situational factors make a universal health care performance model unattainable, an integrated program of performance evaluation should attempt to include variables relevant to the specific setting, yet representative of (and coordinated through) the immediate, intermediate and ultimate criteria levels.

In moving from operational levels toward the top administrative positions of a health care organization, performance criteria become less objective and, consequently, subject to greater measurement error. As evaluation progresses from individual performance to organizational levels, the specificity of goals tends to decrease, making them difficult to measure. For example, it is easier to evaluate whether a medical records supervisor has performed adequately (maintained precise records) than to assess if the group practice clinic employing the medical records supervisor has actually delivered medically acceptable care.

ORGANIZATIONAL PERFORMANCE EVALUATION

Three basic evaluation criteria can be used in assessing the performance of health care facilities: effective patient care, efficient resource utilization and return on investment. These criteria must be developed for proper appraisal of health care outcomes.

Figure 11-1 An Integrated Model of Performance Evaluation for the Health Care Setting

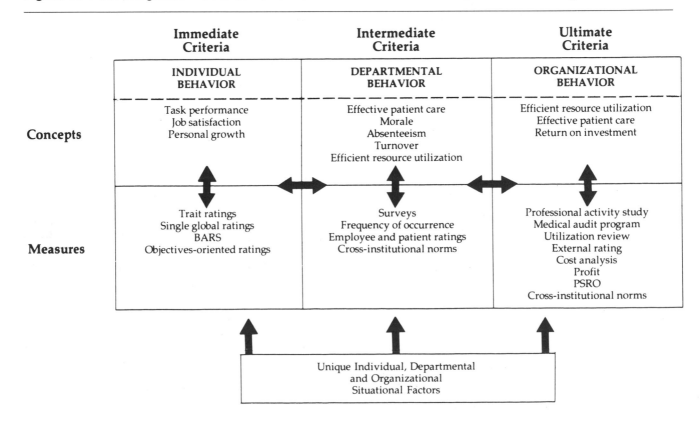

Source: Reprinted with permission from J. M. Ivancevich, A. D. Szilagyi, and M. M. Wallace, *Organizational Behavior and Performance,* Goodyear Publishing Co., Inc., Santa Monica, Calif., p. 422, © 1977.

Effective Patient Care

A primary criterion of organizational performance in the health care field is effective patient care—the maintenance, partial rehabilitation or cure of a patient's physical or mental health. Fortunately, many new methods have been created for measuring effective patient care in the health services sector. However, the rapid transitions in quality assessment have also brought some confusion in attaining a single clear interpretation.[1]

Peer review through the PSRO is one method that attempts to evaluate, among other processes and outcomes, patient care. Professional standards review organizations apparently can contribute to improved care as well as enhance physician and other health care professional learning.[2-4] Professional standards review organizations and quality assurance programs have been successfully developed in many areas of health care including hospitals, nursing departments and long-term care facilities.[5-10] Definitions of what constitutes effectiveness will continue to change as health care professionals develop a better knowledge of what comprises patient welfare. While most models of effective care are susceptible to criticism regarding their lack of comprehensiveness, efforts continue to further the advanced measurement and evaluation of patient care.

Efficient Resource Utilization

Organizational efficiency and cost containment are important aspects of efficient resource utilization for the modern health care administrator. Although quality care will likely remain primary compared to the necessity to contain costs, many PSRO and utilization review programs are serving as monitors on both quality and cost of service.[11,12] Some hospitals have achieved good results in creating cost-containment programs that increase efficiency with little adverse impact on patients.[13,14] These trends will probably be repeated for other private and public health care facilities in the future.

Health care administrators must recognize the environmental factors that affect internal attempts at efficient performance. Some examples of the diverse elements include changing health and epidemiologic trends, attitudes of health consumers, personnel values toward work, federal and state legislation and technological imperatives for the highest quality of patient care. The extremely large number of external factors affecting health care organizations do not help an administrator who is striving toward evaluation and control of performance efficiencies. Nonetheless, these factors can be neither delegated nor ignored.

Return on Investment

A third criterion of organizational performance is return on investment. Profitability, the essence of organizational survival, is inexorably linked to efficient performance and quality care. Successful health care organizations with a strong motivation to achieve resource efficiency are also capable of providing an adequate return for invested resources (profitability broadly defined). The concept of return on resources should not be limited solely to proprietary health care facilities as profitability concepts may be extended to nonprofit organizations as well. Functioning under the not-for-profit category does not mean that health care organizations can ignore return on organizational resources. Inadequate recognition of return on investment will result in serious long-run organizational maladies that could eventually jeopardize survival.

As seen above, the first level of criteria in an integrated performance evaluation model for health care facilities centers on organizational factors. Health care administrators may be reluctant to measure organizational performance because of the difficulties in measuring goals and concepts such as efficiency, effective patient care or return on investment. Consequently, they should be cautious regarding over-allocating a disproportionate amount of time and effort in appraising departmental and individual performance.

DEPARTMENTAL PERFORMANCE EVALUATION

Generally, objectivity in judging departmental criteria is improved over judging organizational criteria because only internal outcomes are typically measured, such as employee morale, absenteeism, turnover, departmental effectiveness and efficiency.

Morale

Employee morale is a significant indicator of departmental performance. It shows the extent to which individuals' needs are satisfied within their total job situation. For example, morale involves the degree to which nursing aides in long-term care facilities feel that their personal aspirations are fulfilled in addition to organizational goals. Taken in this context, a department supervisor must view the morale-building process as a function of individual needs as well as job satisfaction. The degree to which these personal needs and satisfactions can be used to attain higher morale depends on the types of tasks and jobs the department is responsible for completing.

Although the tasks required of maintenance personnel may not satisfy status needs in a manner comparable to the tasks completed by nursing or social services personnel, department supervisors are responsible for maintaining high employee morale for all. The social stigma attached to tasks, the salary/wage level or even the difference between salaried and hourly wage personnel are all primary reasons for the health care organization's failure to fulfill individual needs, thereby resulting in low morale. Administrators and supervisors can improve morale in many cases through better organizational behavior methods such as motivation, goal setting, leadership or job enrichment.[15]

Absenteeism

The monetary cost and effect on patient care resulting from nursing personnel absenteeism increasingly underscore the importance of absenteeism as a criterion of departmental performance. As a result, there seems to be a growing acceptance among some health care administrators of the value of survey and interview methods for assessing departmental morale. Morale may also be measured by departmental records concerning employee turnover and absenteeism. An evaluation of morale levels will typically reveal inverse relationships between morale and absenteeism as well as between morale and turnover. As morale increases, absenteeism and turnover should decrease.

Employee Turnover

Excessive employee turnover within a given department may be indicative of poor management practices (salary administration or supervision practices) within the department. It may also be caused by the inability to fulfill individual needs. A survey of morale for department personnel may reveal reasons for such dissatisfaction. Organizational development processes such as training and education, participatory goal setting, job enrichment or job enlargement may be needed to reduce turnover, increase morale and therefore contribute to overall increased departmental effectiveness.[16]

Health care organization and health consumer alike experience the tyranny of employee turnover. From the institution's perspective, turnover is very expensive, especially for hospitals, whenever skilled profes-

sionals are terminating employment.[17, 18] Health consumers, such as long-term care facility residents, can be confused or dissatisfied by the constant influx of new personnel. Health care administrators should maintain programs of surveillance on employee turnover.[19]

Effective Patient Care

The contribution a department makes in terms of quality patient care is an essential evaluation component regardless of the service of the department. For many health care facilities, such as hospitals and nursing homes, nursing departments or units are increasingly developing quality assurance programs in meeting the challenge of promoting patient care.[20-28] Nonetheless, administrators should attempt to evaluate the contribution made by nonmedical departments toward patient care. For example, in nursing homes the quality of food may be an important determinant in rehabilitation, or in medical clinics a pharmacy that correctly dispenses medications with a personal touch may create greater patient satisfaction. These ancillary departments are vital components of the total health care organization.

Patient evaluation of department-related services can, in some instances, prove to be a valuable asset in performance evaluation. Hospitals sometimes accomplish this by asking the outgoing patient questions that are designed to elicit information about the care received. This may be measured by either a survey-feedback approach or interviews.

Interviews can be conducted by a nurse, social worker or person with whom the patient will not be inhibited in answering questions. Any attempts to approach patients must be done judiciously in order not to infringe on privacy or health processes. For maximum effectiveness, the patient evaluation data that are gathered must be carefully integrated with other internal evaluation data.

Efficient Resource Use

The efficient use of resources by departments in health services institutions can be measured through several methods. Zero-base budgeting, for example, analyzes how well a department has achieved its purpose while adhering to established budgetary constraints. The cost efficiency of each department can also be compared with cost indices from historical norms of performance (as well as other institutional standards) to determine departmental ability to meet the challenge of rising costs and stable budgets. Cost-efficiency analysis must account for the amount of incremental effectiveness achieved in relation to resources allocated toward departmental goals. The analysis must also consider broader organizational priorities that may weaken departmental priorities. A reordering of goals and objectives may be needed, not only to examine the status of health care goals, but also to examine the role of departmental and individual goals within the organization.

INDIVIDUAL PERFORMANCE EVALUATION

Individual performance appraisal is most neglected by supervisors and administrators, perhaps because they misunderstand the purpose behind evaluation.[29] Lack of training in evaluative skills also contributes to this dilemma.[30]

Health care administrators should recognize that the assignment of responsibility to personnel for the completion of delegated tasks makes the individual performance evaluation both possible and necessary. In the case of the medical technician, evaluation is possible because the appraisal process identifies the relevant dimensions of the task for which the employee is responsible, for example, drawing and analyzing blood samples. Assignment of responsibility makes evaluation necessary because health care effectiveness depends equally on valid performance at the individual level as well as the departmental and organizational levels.

From the health care administrator's perspective, individual evaluation represents a positive process for influencing the motivation of employees.[31] If personnel perceive that improved performance results in increased compensation or benefits, their efforts will usually be more pronounced. The evaluation process should be the key that reinforces the belief that effective behavior leads to desired results. Performance appraisal can also provide feedback to employees on their performance, thereby increasing knowledge about themselves.

The individual performance evaluation may present a basic conflict between administrators and employees. The health care organization, in order to be more effective, needs comprehensive data on the nature of the employee's ability and performance. Employees may attempt to perform well only on those measures that determine rewards while ignoring those behaviors that go unrecognized. As an illustration, a nursing aide or orderly may concentrate on changing linen and straightening rooms (which is observable and usually rewarded) while neglecting personal interactions with the patient (which is difficult to observe and therefore seldom rewarded). Consequently, the methods of measurement used by administrators are probably the single most important determinant of success in the individual evaluation process.

Trait Methods of Measurement

Although there are basically four types of measurement methods, the most frequently used appraisal method involves traditional trait ratings.[32] Personality and performance traits such as creativity, responsibility and loyalty are easily observed. The major problem with their use is that they do not adequately reflect behavior and are therefore likely to promote suppressed hostilities or defensiveness by staff personnel.

Nursing personnel have traditionally been evaluated by this method.[33] When confronted with a comment by nursing supervisors such as "You need to demonstrate more responsibility on the job," nurses typically react to refute the statement by pointing out the times they have behaved in a responsible manner. Simply telling staff that they have been rated low on a trait does not explain how they should change their behavior.

In addition to employee defensiveness, the problem of interrater agreement may be encountered. Different supervisors may not agree on the proper definition of each behavioral trait being measured. As a result, raters confuse the evaluation with their own inconsistencies and personal idiosyncrasies concerning effective performance.

Global Perceptions

Some health care organizations rely on a second method of individual performance appraisal using a single rating for all individual performances. In these cases, administrators simply request one rating of overall performance for an individual. For example, when a nursing supervisor is evaluating three nurses, one may be rated excellent, another rated average and the third rated poor in performance. Global ratings offer a number of advantages: (1) an employee's relative standing is established compared to all employees, (2) they ensure that a variety of employee behaviors are included, (3) supervisors typically are willing and capable of making the ratings and (4) the ratings are useful when determining pay and promotion decisions. For all their good points, however, single global ratings do not provide definitive feedback when counseling is needed. They can produce defensiveness when a particular ranking is not justified in the opinion of the staff member.

Behaviorally Anchored Rating Scales

A third method of individual evaluation that has only recently been introduced involves behaviorally anchored rating scales (BARS). The BARS system measures employee effectiveness through specific behaviors anchored to a scale that ranges from ineffective to effective performance. The development of BARS is a time-consuming process requiring, as a prerequisite, a large number of employees who perform reasonably similar tasks. It has received some use in nursing departments—an application that is aided by the size of nursing departments and the ability to identify nursing skills.[34]

A sample of the employees, along with their supervisors, generates a list of task dimensions and associated critical behaviors. A second sample of employees and supervisors then proceeds to "retranslate" the critical behaviors by matching them to the task dimensions. The result is a thorough job analysis that reveals specific items of effective behavior as judged by the personnel and supervisors most familiar with the task itself.

The BARS system of evaluation has proven to be more acceptable than either traditional trait ratings or single global ratings in the areas of acceptability by supervisor and subordinate, counseling and clarification of the nature of the job. For salary and reward determinations BARS and single global scales have equivalent effectiveness. The only negative drawback to BARS is the requirement of similar job tasks, but this is not a problem in large health care organizations.

Objectives-Oriented Methods

The fourth type of measurement procedure involves objectives-oriented ratings such as management by objectives (MBO). The MBO system typically involves administrator-employee development of specific objectives and agreement on how these objectives are to be measured. For example, a medical records supervisor may discuss with a medical records clerk the goals (more readable entries and more correct filing) that the clerk will seek to achieve in the next six months. The primary advantage of MBO lies in eliciting employee participation which may ultimately produce greater commitment for the attainment of specific goals. Objectives-oriented techniques are particularly attractive in overcoming the weaknesses of the BARS approach.

The basic weakness of the MBO system is encountered in jobs that do not consist of easily measurable attributes that are therefore difficult to appraise objec-

tively. Even so, many hospitals and medical centers are implementing MBO programs with apparent success.[35-38]

An ideal solution to the problem of developing a good individual performance evaluation system in the health care field would be the simultaneous implementation of BARS and MBO systems. Behaviorally anchored rating scales can provide performance measures for largely behaviorally oriented positions that are difficult to objectify (health social work or special needs education). Behaviorally anchored rating scales can also be used to determine the suitability of objectives for each individual. The MBO system would act as an effective deterrent to the problems of lack of developmental feedback. The integration of BARS and MBO in an evaluation system would also offer the following advantages: (1) it would allow the employee's fullest level of participation in the evaluation process, (2) it should facilitate the development of objective measures and (3) it can assist administrators and personnel when setting moderately difficult goals.

The above solution represents an ideal model that many health care administrators should strive to achieve. However, as so often occurs, the ideal is never realized. An alternative would be the operation of two somewhat separate appraisal systems: one to handle extrinsic rewards such as pay and bonuses, the other for development training and intrinsic motivation purposes. When separated by time, and when the developmental sessions are held after the reward decisions have been made, constructive employee development can take place without pay and promotion considerations lurking in the background.

ACHIEVING INTEGRATED PERFORMANCE EVALUATION

Health care administrators must recognize the need to apply integrated models of performance appraisal in their organizations. Equal concentration should be placed on organizational, departmental and individual evaluation. None of these assessment categories should be sacrificed at the expense of the others. Emphasis must be given to developing more advanced individual performance evaluation programs in the health care context in view of current trends to concentrate on broader performance issues.

The achievement of integrated performance evaluation in health care organizations is found in commitment from administrators. They are responsible for developing detailed evaluative programs as well as a health philosophical commitment by personnel. The appraisal programs must be interrelated at individual, departmental and organizational levels. The procedures and expectations from the review process must be communicated with absolute clarity. Furthermore, personnel must be convinced that, as people, they are an important part of the larger evaluation process. Their concerns must be equally addressed as must those of the health care organization. A performance evaluation program constructed on this philosophical foundation will establish a framework for improved performance, *i.e.,* better patient care with increased operational efficiency, by satisfied health care professionals.

Only by viewing health care facilities as extremely complex, dynamic organizations can administrators best engage in a system of performance evaluation which considers the relevant situational factors of the health care environment. Recognition of variables which must be considered in establishing goals at all levels of the organization is of the utmost importance. Evaluation criteria must be realistic, while at the same time enhancing organizational growth and development. Alignment of individual, departmental and organizational goals is the preferred end product of overall health care performance evaluation. This requires a continuous effort on the part of management. The health care administrator must be aware that the integrated development of performance criteria begins at the organizational level, moves to the departmental level and culminates at the individual appraisal session.

NOTES

1. W. J. McNerney, "The Quandary of Quality Assessment," *New England Journal of Medicine* 295, 27 (December 30, 1976): 1505–1511.

2. R. Dorsey and F. Sullivan, "PSRO: Advantages, Risks and Potential Pitfalls," *American Journal of Psychiatry* 132, no. 8 (August 1975): 832–836.

3. L. Eddy and L. Westbrock, "Multidisciplinary Retrospective: Patient Care Audit," *American Journal of Nursing* 75, no. 6 (June 1975): 961–963.

4. W. F. Jesse et al., "PSRO: An Educational Force for Improving Quality of Care," *New England Journal of Medicine* 292, no. 7 (March 27, 1975): 668–671.

5. A. J. Altieri et al., "Developing Quality Long-Term Care," *Geriatrics* 32, no. 7 (July 1977): 126–142.

6. S. T. Hegyvary and R. K. Dieter Haussmann, "Monitoring Nursing Care Quality," *Journal of Nursing Administration* 6, no. 9 (November 1976): 3–9.

7. R. K. Chow, "Development of a Patient Appraisal and Care Evaluation System for Long-Term Care," *Journal of Long-Term Care Administration* 5, no. 2 (Summer 1077): 21–27.

8. L. C. Dennis, R. E. Burke, and K. M. Garber, "Quality Evaluation System: An Approach for Patient Assessment," *Journal of Long-Term Care Administration* 5, no. 2 (Summer 1977): 28–51.

9. K. A. Kahn et al., "A Multidisciplinary Approach to Assessing the Quality of Care in Long-Term Facilities," *Gerontologist* 17, no. 1 (1977): 61–65.

10. G. E. Molloy, "Quality Assurance and the Survey Process," *Journal of Long-Term Care Administration* 5, no. 2 (Summer 1977): 1–20.

11. R. Kahan and R. G. Tobin, "Utilization Review Can Be a Tool for Improvement," *Hospitals, JAHA* 52, no. 6 (March 16, 1978): 89–94.

12. P. Schwenn, "Bed Utilization Improved Under Program's Three Review Phases," *Hospitals, JAHA* 50, no. 18 (September 16, 1976): 76–78.

13. L. Swearingen, "Staff's All-Out, Ongoing Efforts Help Hospital Fight Inflation," *Hospitals, JAHA* 51, no. 18 (September 16, 1977): 125–128.

14. J. Thueson, "Hospital's Programs and Progress in Cost Containment Reported," *Hospitals, JAHA* 51, no. 18 (September 16, 1977): 131–138.

15. R. G. Holloway, "Management Can Reverse Declining Employee Work Attitudes," *Hospitals, JAHA* 50, no. 20 (October 16, 1976): 71–75.

16. C. Pence and M. Kunsa, "Management Structure Review Results in Program Consolidation," *Hospitals, JAHA* 52, no. 5 (March 1, 1978): 58–61.

17. A. Levenstein, "The Tragedy of Turnover," *Supervisor Nurse* 8, no. 2 (February 1975): 74–75.

18. H. L. Smith and L. E. Watkins, "Containing Hospital Manpower-Turnover Costs: A Model for Action," *Health Services Manager* 11, no. 10 (October 1978): 1–3.

19. _____ , "Managing Manpower Turnover Costs," *Personnel Administrator* 23, no. 4 (1978): 46–49.

20. D. Block, "Evaluation of Nursing in Terms of Process and Outcome," *Nursing Research* 24, no. 4 (July-August 1975): 256–263.

21. D. A. Billie and J. Jurkovic, "Nursing Process Audit: The Style Is Individual," *Nursing Administration Quarterly* 1, no. 3 (Spring 1977): 77–84.

22. A. Davis, "Development of a Blueprint for a Quality Assurance Program," *Supervisor Nurse* 8, no. 2 (February 1977): 17–28.

23. H. Gassett, "Q for Q—Quest for Quality Assurance," *Supervisor Nurse* 8, no. 2 (February 1977): 29–35.

24. P. L. Glasson, "The Struggle for Total Quality," *Supervisor Nurse* 8, no. 2 (February 1977): 36–40.

25. S. T. Hegyvary and R. K. Dieter Haussmann, "Monitoring Nursing Care Quality," *Journal of Nursing Administration* 5, no. 5 (June 1975): 17–26.

26. _____ , "Correlates of the Quality of Nursing Care," *Journal of Nursing Administration* 6, no. 9 (November 1976): 22–27.

27. _____ , "The Relationship of Nursing Process and Patient Outcomes," *Journal of Nursing Administration* 6, no. 9 (November 1976): 18–21.

28. _____ , "Nursing Professional Review," *Journal of Nursing Administration* 6, no. 9 (November 1976): 12–17.

29. R. Kennedy and A. B. Vose, "Preparing the Nurse Manager to Assume New Accountabilities," *Hospitals, JAHA* 51, no. 1 (January 1, 1978): 66–69.

30. P. Fairley, "Performance Appraisals—Key to Your Employee's Growth," *Hospital Financial Management* 7, no. 9 (September 1977): 32.

31. S. Peterfreund, "Employees Must Have Sense of Freedom, Worth," *Hospitals, JAHA* 50, no. 16 (August 16, 1976): 60–62.

32. L. W. Porter, E. E. Lawler, and J. R. Hackman, *Behavior in Organizations* (New York: McGraw-Hill Book Co., 1975), pp. 326–331.

33. L. Wiley, "Job Evaluations: Giving and Getting Them with Less of a Hassle," *Nursing* 5, no. 11 (November 1975): 75–80.

34. A. Marriner, "Evaluation of Personnel," *Supervisor Nurse* 7, no. 5 (May 1976): 36–39.

35. L. P. Haar and J. R. Hicks, "Performance Appraisal: Derivation of Effective Assessment Tools," *Journal of Nursing Administration* 6, no. 7 (September 1976): 20–29.

36. A. J. Hinton and M. M. Markowich, "Supervisor, Employee Participate in Goal-Oriented Appraisals," *Hospitals, JAHA* 50, no. 1 (January 1, 1976): 97–101.

37. R. K. Murray, "Management by Objectives: Useful in Establishing a Merit Appraisal System," *Health Services Manager* 10, no. 2 (February 1977): 1–5.

38. M. L. Riordan, "Patient Care Management in Action: One Center's Experience," *Hospitals, JAHA* 51, no. 1 (January 1, 1978): 70–76.

12. Management by Objectives

THEODORE W. KESSLER

INTRODUCTION

The management of organizations inherently must focus on results or output related to expressed goals or some implicit purpose for the effort. The trend in progressive organizations has been to organize the major endeavors into a systematic framework to assure an optimum utilization of human resources, effective integration, and timely monitoring of progress.

At the start it should be made clear that this article deals with a concept and process, not labels. Management by objectives (MBO) has been the most universal label in the lexicon of management jargon; however, others such as goal setting, work planning, performance standards, etc., have surfaced. Debates have centered on the definition of an objective vs. a goal, often obscuring the issue. As a practical matter, let it be assumed that all of the terms relate to essentially the same subject and merely differ in form, emphasis, or application. How these distinctions can be incorporated in a structure designed to meet the specific needs of a health care organization will be described later.

The contemporary state of the art perhaps can be traced back to Peter F. Drucker's, *The Practice of Management,*[1] which inspired many executives to view their role differently because he brought a new perspective to the process of managing. Since then many other notable practitioners such as George S. Ordiorne, Marion Kellogg, Walter Mahler, and Glenn Varney, to name a few, have contributed conceptual applications, developed workable processes, and created new understanding for enlightened managers committed to improved performance.

Over the last several decades, operating in scenarios running the gamut of economic and social change, MBO has had its ups and downs. At one extreme it was extolled as a panacea for what ailed organizations; at the other extreme, it was maligned or distorted as a manipulative scheme intended to exploit subordinates.

In more recent years, further misconceptions appeared with the increased interest in participative management styles, OD (organization development), and the like. Some were asking if MBO was compatible with various management philosophies and leadership styles. The evidence to date suggests that an effective application of MBO depends primarily on the sensible adherence to a few basic principles applied realistically to the management setting and circumstances. Autocratic styles of managing can use MBO effectively; so can participative forms of management. For other reasons, participative styles of management may foster a climate that enhances involvement, commitment, and innovation as worthwhile attributes of the MBO process.

PRINCIPLES

The following principles should be the basis for developing a framework for use in applying an MBO process in a specific setting. They generally will be relevant to any results-oriented organization that is dedicated to improvement, realistic about its capabilities, and consistent or predictable in its behavior.

- *Simplicity:* Paperwork, forms, and reports must be kept to a bare minimum as they are not ends but means. Many MBO efforts die under the weight of paper generated by well-intentioned managers who apply a bureaucratic approach.
- *Planning:* The fundamental up-front requirement is the ability and willingness to plan the work. The sequence, priorities, time frames, and integration for increasingly demanding and complex settings make skilled planning essential.
- *Integrity:* Participants in the process rely on each other. Relationships built on trust and openness tend to avoid the ''Catch 22'' situations and exploitive behaviors that undermine the process.
- *Sharing:* An exchange of knowledge and information about the work will facilitate mutual understanding, support, and subsequent feedback.
- *Ownership:* Commitment to results and effective execution of the process is a function of perceived accountability. Staff MBO ''czars'' have limited success because the process often is imposed on managers rather than embraced by them as an effective tool and skill inherent in their leadership role.
- *Outputs:* It is essential to control outputs, not activity. Output is value added to the outcome and helps focus the effort applied to essential work.
- *Rewards:* Accomplishment is a self-fulfilling gratification enhanced by the recognition of others. Motivation is stimulated as personal growth leads to added value, as reflected in the compensation worth of the individual.
- *Continuity:* The process should be viewed as a continuing cycle capable of refinements for more complex needs as the participants develop their skills.

These principles are essential to the integrity of the MBO concept and process. They form the framework and checkpoint for effectively introducing the concept and managing the process. Regardless of the managing style, work is accomplished through a team effort. Most typically, a ''one-on-one'' (manager and subordinate) arrangement is the team for a specific element of work. This implies a cooperative, effective working relationship and a mutual interdependence requiring periodic assessment to assure its viability. The participants can use these principles as a frame of reference

to determine how the process is being applied and agree as necessary on modifications to assure the intended result.

Underlying the principles are the definitions that describe them:[2]

- Business objectives: These are set forth in an open-ended statement that indicates the long-term direction, broad aims, and the common purposes for which all employees are to work.
- Business assumptions: These constitute a statement of conditions that are expected to occur or prevail during a forward business cycle. The assumptions, together with other known factors, constitute the prime guidelines for planning by each operating component.
- Goals: These form a statement of a result to be achieved within a specified time period.
- Work plans: These provide a detailed listing of actions to be taken, by time schedule, to produce an end result identified in a goal.
- Milestones: These form a system for charting work to be completed, showing starting time, interim points, and completion dates.
- Work reviews: These occur in sessions involving two or more persons who examine the plans, progress, barriers, and alternatives for achieving a pre-determined result.
- Accomplishment summary: This consists of a self-prepared listing of significant results achieved during a designated time period.

PROCESS

The process can be described as a systematic flow of events, interactions, and transactions on a face-to-face basis. The dialogue should lead to formulation of plans, understanding of expected results, negotiated resources, and challenging commitments.

The question of where it all begins is the usual dilemma in starting the process. Some advocate a top-down process to maximize control and direction while others suggest a bottom-up route to stimulate interest, use the best talents of the participants, and motivate subordinates to be creative and committed.

Experience suggests that some flexibility is desirable but within a framework of objectives and strategic or operational direction developed by top management of the organizational component involved. This does not preclude appropriate input throughout the organization in developing this framework. An integral part of this process also requires a statement of business assumptions, including available resources, so that planning is done within that context.

Concerns are expressed about the relative value, importance, and difficulty of the goals and their usefulness to the enterprise and importance to the individual(s) responsible for the outcome. Managers must seek a reasonable balance and equity among participating peers, not unlike compensation considerations, yet avoid stifling natural desires of some to undertake exceptional challenges compatible with the needs of the organization. For the most part, goals are set in the context of the scope of the position and should be consistent with the basis for the function as currently perceived.

Although it is possible for a manager to evolve the process with a subtle transition, it generally is more effective to set the stage by determining what significant changes in the way the organization now operates will require an action plan. It may involve assessing managerial style, values and norms, autonomy, tempo, and other characteristics. As pointed out earlier, it is not necessary to reshape the whole organization as a precondition to using MBO, but it should be determined what can be conducive to the process and what may become dysfunctional.

An explanation and preferably a dialogue with the participants outlining initial expectations and their roles in the process will help assure understanding and, it is to be hoped, support from those involved.

Assuming a top-down process for illustrating the essential steps, the manager should be prepared to share the objectives, direction, and/or key goal areas with subordinates, and should provide relevant assumptions. The manager then requests subordinates to draft appropriate goals supportive of overall objectives, work, or action plans with time frames and measurements to track progress and completion. A one-on-one review is scheduled to negotiate appropriateness and resources, develop understanding, and establish mutual commitments. Documentation at this point should reflect essentially the outcome of the review and approval.

Depending on the nature of the goals and work plans such as the complexity, urgency, and integration with others, follow-up progress reviews should be scheduled to assure early identification of problems and required modifications. As goals and work plans are completed or modified, the process is recycled. At any given point the record reflects past contributions or accomplishments, progress to date on current plans, and future commitments negotiated mutually. A useful byproduct is that this information provides a significant input to formal performance appraisals that are designed to summarize performance periodically and let the individuals know where they stand. Obviously, the MBO process provides earlier feedback and tends to minimize discrepant assessments later.

The heart of the process is a well-defined goal stated as a result to be achieved within a specified time period deemed to be worthy of the efforts, difficult but attainable, essential to the organization, and involving a commitment to do it. A well-thought-out, logical, and realistic plan of action designed to produce the desired result plus free exchange in a dialogue involving understanding, support, and sharing of information are the ingredients that foster growth, trust, and competency when effective coaching skills are practiced.

From another perspective,[3] there are three important requirements:

1. Self-commitment: Employees are not ordered to do something, nor simply handed a set of goals, nor treated as puppets. Rather, individuals commit themselves to accomplishing the goals and work plans.
2. Self-analysis: Individuals perform work related to the commitments and, when there is a variance, they are the first to know and act accordingly.
3. Self-motivation or self-discipline: Individuals have a strong desire to succeed, to accomplish. Negative variances from the intended result are a challenge.

These three requirements add up to self-supervision. An effective manager is one who can get above-average results from average people. This requires getting subordinates to supervise themselves. It is evident that the process has a logical flow, incorporates behavioral research findings and principles, offers flexibility to match a range of skill levels, and, above all, can be relevant and meaningful to participants seeking performance improvement.

APPLICATIONS

The MBO concept has been used in numerous settings by those who found old ways ineffective, those who tended to be experiment minded, and those who were inclined to research the state of the art or current practices in their organization and felt obliged to pursue the conclusions of that research.

To illustrate several applications and approaches in significantly different settings, the following examples cover a broad spectrum. The first deals with a major corporation[4] noted for its long-standing contributions in human resource management. The General Electric

Company addressed the concept of MBO by focusing on a work planning and review process based on certain internal research projects indicating significant opportunities for improved performance and working relationships. The simplicity of the process offers a wide range of applications. The following describes how the process is structured and applied.

How Work Planning and Review Was Developed

To get work done, some form of work planning always is going on. All supervisors give task and work instructions to their subordinates and have some sort of system to check the work to make sure it is being done properly. Nearly every subordinate at some time or other will ask questions about work assignments or offer suggestions to the supervisor. Most supervisors and subordinates spend a fair amount of time together in the normal course of daily work and can discuss job duties and job tasks. However, few supervisors make optimum managerial use of time spent with subordinates because of certain difficulties inherent in the supervisor-subordinate relationship, because of operating problems, pressure of business, and crash programs; and because of the well-known problems in communication.

At the same time, most subordinates want to do a good job. Most of them often feel they do not understand fully what the boss wants. They want a better feel for how they are doing. Almost every subordinate wants to have feelings of accomplishment, interesting work, and additional responsibility. They want to be able to offer suggestions upward and to have them weighed carefully, even though they may not be accepted. In other words, supervisors want to do a better job of managing and subordinates want to improve their own work performance. The question is, "How do we set up conditions whereby people can be helped to do a better job?"

Initially, GE had hoped that its performance appraisal process would help. Research indicated that it did not. The biggest problem was found to be the self-conflicting role of the supervisor as both a counselor and a judge. Because performance appraisal was tied so closely to subsequent salary action, the supervisor was being forced to play the role of judge with regard to salary action, while at the same time and in the same place was expected to play the role of a helper in terms of advising employees on how to improve work performance. These two roles are incompatible. For this reason, in the new approach, they were separated. The next step was to ask, "How is it possible to provide a climate in which managers can act as helpers to improve work performance?" The answer was work planning and review.

What Is Work Planning and Review?

The work planning and review process consists of periodic meetings between subordinate and supervisor. The meetings are oriented toward the daily work and result in mutual planning of the job, a review of progress, and mutual solving of problems that arise in the course of getting it done. The process does not involve formal ratings; rather, it provides the basis for the employee and manager to sit down informally, discuss the job to be done, and then (1) agree on a plan and (2) review progress.

The process was designed to take advantage of known principles that relate to certain conditions necessary for subordinate motivation and job growth. They are not exhaustive but do include the essential ingredients that must be present for best personnel utilization. The three basic motivational principles are:

1. An employee needs to know what is expected on the job.
2. An employee needs to know what individual progress is being made.
3. An employee needs to be able to obtain assistance when and as needed.

Figure 12-1 shows how these principles apply to the job. The next step is to explore how the work planning and review process fits these principles.

An Employee Must Know What Is Expected On the Job

- Work performance is improved appreciably when the employee knows what results are expected. Work planning and review sessions provide the individual with information as to the results expected, the methods by which they will be measured, the priorities, and the resources available.
- Work performance is improved appreciably when the employee knows it is possible to influence the expected results. The process is sufficiently flexible to permit the individual to have some say about the results expected, the methods by which they will be measured, and the priorities. The degree of influence the employee exercises will vary according to the situation.

Figure 12-1 Work Planning and Review Diagrammed

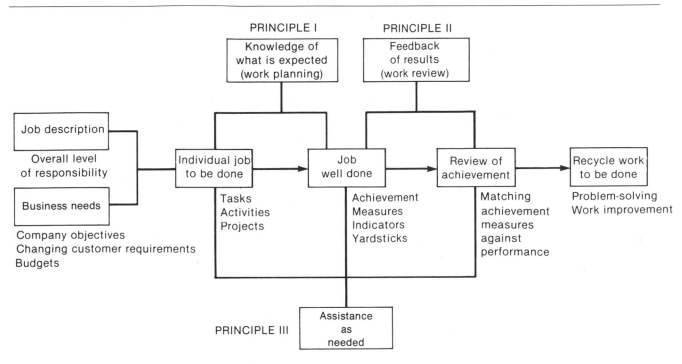

Source: Increasing Management Effectiveness through Work Planning, General Electric Company, Aircraft Engine Division, Cincinnati, Ohio.

An Employee Needs to Know What Individual Progress Is Being Made

This is the most important (and basic) of the three principles. Learning (job improvement) takes place most effectively when employees have the opportunity to compare their performance (successes as well as problems) against agreed-upon measures. There are several important corollaries to this principle:

- Knowledge of results must be as precise and specific as possible. Work planning develops specific, measurable goals. Work review allows the subordinate and manager to review results against the goals.
- Knowledge of results must be as immediate and relevant as possible. The flexibility of the process enables the supervisor to have review sessions when most appropriate, and the discussion can be limited to only those items of performance that are relevant to the current situation or have just been completed.
- Knowledge of results that comes from the individuals' own observations is more effective than that obtained from someone else. When the goal measurements have been made specific, em-

ployees can evaluate their own progress more objectively. In addition, the supervisor can use the flexibility of the process to encourage this.

In summary, the work planning and review process is designed specifically to give knowledge of results that is objective, timely, and flexible enough to permit self-assessment. Either the subordinate or the supervisor can schedule a review session when either feels it is most appropriate, thus allowing for immediate knowledge of results.

An Employee Must Be Able To Obtain Assistance When Needed

To improve job performance, the employee must be able to obtain assistance, coaching, and guidance as needed:

- The employee must feel free to request assistance when necessary. Employees will ask for help only when they are not "punished" for such an action—for example, when this is not seen as an admission of weakness or as ultimately resulting in criticism.

- The supervisor must feel free to offer assistance as necessary. At times, every supervisor sees a need to help a subordinate. This may come in the form of pointing out mistakes, suggesting a different approach, or in any one of a number of ways. To be most effective, this must be done in a constructive rather than threatening fashion. The supervisor must avoid causing a defensive reaction that would only reduce the employee's effectiveness.
- The supervisor must act as a helper rather than a judge in order to establish this climate. In work planning and review sessions, the emphasis shifts from the judging implicit in appraisals to concentration on accomplishing mutually acceptable goals. The emphasis moves from the weaknesses of the subordinate to a job-centered operations approach. A climate is established for the employee to receive assistance when and as needed. Work planning and review is a process that establishes a climate of mutual cooperation. Instead of stressing or accumulating past mistakes or successes to justify a salary action, employee and supervisor should use the review sessions as opportunities to learn how to improve future work performance. Instead of dealing in subjective opinions, praise, or criticism, they should jointly search for better measurements of mutually acceptable goals. The subordinate becomes a partner rather than a defendant.

How Is Work Planning Done?

Experience with the work planning and review cycle has demonstrated that supervisors typically go through a process of experimentation before they settle on a method that is most effective for themselves and their subordinates. Because concentration is on the basic concept rather than on any particular technique, such experimentation is encouraged. In other words, the specific technique should not transcend the basic purpose: improving work performance. To this end, supervisors are encouraged to experiment and modify the process so they can do their own best job of applying the three basic motivational principles.

However, discussions with supervisors applying the concept indicate that some simple do's and don'ts considerably shorten the process of experimentation. As Figure 12-1 illustrates, the first motivational principle requires developing mutual understanding between employee and supervisor as to what is expected. This consists of two closely related parts: (1) outlining the job to be done and (2) outlining achievement measures

or yardsticks to determine when a job has been done well.

The Job to Be Done

The job to be done stems from two different but related sources: the job description and the organizational needs. The job description usually changes infrequently. It summarizes the overall responsibility of the position and of the individual. On the other hand, organization needs are changing constantly. This is reflected in the changing tasks individuals must do.

Supervisors have a twofold responsibility in defining the job to be done: (1) They must be sure that specific tasks and projects contribute to stated needs. (2) They also must make certain that supervisor and subordinate develop the fullest possible understanding about the job to be done. One good method of increasing understanding is to have the subordinate prepare a list of suggested goals and commitments before the planning session; then in the session the two can discuss the goals and make whatever changes may be necessary to reflect the supervisor's ideas.

Some Do's and Don'ts in Outlining the Job to Be Done

Do:
- Ensure supervisor-subordinate agreement on major plans and tasks.
- Make plans specific rather than general.
- Relate work plans to business needs.
- Change work plans to conform with changing business needs.
- Have subordinates develop their own work plans when capable.
- Keep it as informal as is practicable; jot down work plans rather than have multiple carbons made.

Don't:
- Try to set work goals too far in advance.
- Make activities, responsibilities, or tasks too broad.
- Become overinvolved in completing forms; instead, concentrate on mutual understanding.
- Be inflexible about changing work plans in response to need.

The Job Well Done

Identification of the specific goals, tasks, or activities is only the first part of implementing the principle of "knowledge of what is expected." The second part is to develop achievement measures or success criteria.

These measures help both parties to determine when a job is done well and to outline areas where improvement seems needed. They must be outlined in advance so that both participants can agree with them. Developing achievement measures is easier said than done. They must be designed carefully to answer the question for supervisor and subordinate, "How will we both know whether the job has been done well?"

The yardsticks, or success measures, should be specific to the task and should be as objective as possible. However, good judgmental, subjective measurements are better than poor objective measures. Time deadlines, of course, are one type of measurement, but they should be used alone only when they are the sole factor of job success. If subordinates develop their own work plans, they should develop the results measures at the same time.

Do:
- Be sure the measures cover the whole project.
- Make certain that achievement criteria are spelled out clearly before the employee starts the task.
- Make sure that supervisor and subordinate agree on the yardsticks before the job is started.
- Make measures as specific as possible.
- Make measures as objective as possible.
- Be willing to change measures if the task or conditions change.
- Approach from a positive, rather than negative, direction.
- Identify factors that can be used to improve job performance.

Don't:
- Use time deadlines only; they are only part of a job well done.
- Develop the measures as a way of "trapping" the subordinate.
- Make the yardsticks too broad or general.
- Become overinvolved in completing forms; instead, concentrate on mutual understanding of what is expected.

In summary, the steps in work planning are:

1. Have the employee develop a set of work goals and measurements; supervisors who wish to do this alone may omit this step.
2. Schedule a planning session.
3. Ensure that supervisor and subordinate come to a mutual agreement during the planning discussion on tasks, due dates, and measurements of achievement.

4. Write down the finally agreed-upon goals and yardsticks after the planning session; the supervisor then should keep one copy and give the other to the employee.

A COMMUNITY HOSPITAL EXAMPLE

Large profit-making corporations can use such a process, but can it work in small, nonprofit type organizations such as a community hospital? An application in such a setting is illustrated by the goal-setting process employed by St. Charles Hospital in Toledo, Ohio. This is a medium-sized Catholic community hospital involved in an organizational development (OD) program over several years. The goal-setting process is viewed as an integral part of the OD activities and congruent with their basic principles and values.

Over the last several years various refinements in the process evolved. Changes were designed to encourage more ownership and commitment to the goals, simplify the paperwork, provide better linkage of individual objectives to key goal areas developed by top management, and focus more attention on results to be achieved rather than having fuzzy work plans or outcomes. More complex goals involving an integrated effort with other functions were developed as the skill and confidence level of managers improved.

The current process begins with an annual planning meeting by top management of the hospital to identify broad major categories of prime interest and high priority for the coming year. From this, more detailed identification of related goals in each category is completed with accountability assigned to a specified member of top management. Budgeted resources are reviewed to confirm allocation or adjustments. This process recently resulted in six broad categories and, subsequently, 46 specific goals for the hospital.

The six key goal areas are patient services, organizational development, education, physical plant, external affairs, and operational issues. Examples of specific goals in the patient services area are the "development of a program for nursing regarding role and duty to monitor quality of care," and "research feasibility of nurse practitioners and physician assistants to define role, assess feasibility, and determine training needed." Under organization development, a goal specifies "identification of two unproductive norms evident in employee behavior as focus for management skill training." The operational issues cover a wide variety of matters such as a goal to "research and evaluate a new hospitalwide telephone system" and "develop an orientation program for new physicians added to the medical staff."

Department heads in collaboration with their respective division heads select goals applicable to their functional area. Goals requiring integration with functional interfaces are planned jointly, with a series of subgoals and work plans developed accordingly. In addition, intradepartment goals and plans are developed based on the need and priority as perceived at that level. For example, a goal to revise certain internal scheduling routines for a department to improve efficiency could be of major importance to the department but not impact others directly. In effect, department heads have the responsibility to strike a balance between stated hospital goals where they have a participatory role and their own departmental objectives within the framework of allocated resources.

Goals and work plans are reviewed by division heads (top management team) to assure proper application of criteria for a well-stated goal, logical and complete work plans to achieve the result, including time frames and accountability, and appropriate measurements of progress, completion, and how well done.

Communications with all members of management on the final plans is done through group meetings to share the composite result. Other sharing techniques can be developed so long as adequate information is conveyed to those impacted, where coordinated efforts are required, and when a general overview of the coming year's work stimulates support and commitment from the total organization. Further communication usually takes place throughout all levels of the organization consistent with a participating style of management. Periodic reviews of progress or modification are necessary to maintain momentum, awareness, and commitment. Exhibit 12-1 formats a goal and structures key information in a concise manner. Exhibits 12-2 and 12-3 are examples of typical goals developed by individuals in collaboration with their manager, with notations for each progress review completed.

MBO usually has been associated with annual planning efforts; however, practitioners such as George S. Odiorne have suggested a variety of other applications: discipline by objectives, career development, zero-base budgeting, performance appraisal systems, and compensation programs.[5] The fundamentals of the process are inherent in the modern-day world of work with innovative managers.

FINAL TIPS

Executives engage in a variety of activities, actions, and techniques as they practice the art of managing.

Since an MBO process can be basic to the manager's repertoire and philosophy of managing, it may be helpful to examine some observations of this system in action. Odiorne makes an astute observation regarding the "Activity Trap."[6] This deals with how well-defined, worthwhile goals become blurred as everyone gets busy in activity that becomes an end in itself. The real danger is that the harder people run, the farther behind they get. It's all too easy to agree with the boss on activity to be maintained or started, but more difficult for common understanding and agreement on the desired results. Individuals are susceptible to losing sight of why they are doing what they are doing. The manager needs to focus on output rather than activity per se and periodically examine what *really* is going on, rather than assume all is well because previously stated intentions were good.

Harry Levinson, viewing MBO from a psychological perspective, points up the risk of engaging in a "con job" on the subordinate for what is intended to be a "negotiation."[7] The manager then is well on the road to manipulating and exploiting the subordinate. The process eventually will fail in that climate. Goals must be reasonably achievable and may stretch the employee's capabilities; however, understanding and support are essential for recognizing conditions beyond the individual's control.

Quantifiable goals allow useful measurement and should be used where possible, but good subjective measures are better than poor quantifiable ones. Once a goal is agreed on—that is, a statement of the outcome or result—the focus should shift to how it will be accomplished. The work planning aspect offers flexibility for subordinates to influence and shape the plans consistent with methods and approaches most effective for them. The manager guides and coaches to help assure success without usurping the subordinates' role.

Leaders at the top of a health care institution should determine first that they have an appropriate organization structure and have done the necessary strategic planning before engaging in MBO. In addition, they should ask themselves, "Are we doing the right things?" and "Are we doing it right?" This self-examination serves as a point of departure when the leader begins to energize the organization into action with MBO.

In the final analysis, each manager, regardless of the setting in a hospital or business enterprise, must determine the mission, the roles of various participants, and how most effectively to marshal resources to achieve the desired results. Hospital management is increasingly using proved techniques and concepts from the industrial sector and adapting them as neces-

Exhibit 12-1 Sample Form for Planning Goals

ST. CHARLES HOSPITAL
GOAL PLANNER—1980

_____   _____
              Name   Department

GOAL (include existing status and expected outcomes—see criteria on back).

_____

_____

_____

_____

Identify hospital goal area if appropriate   _____

TIME FRAME: Start _____ Completion _____

INDIVIDUAL ACCOUNTABLE FOR RESULT   _____

ACTION STEPS	WHO	START	COMP.	REVIEW DATE(S)

GOAL REVIEW

Criteria for a Good Goal

- You must be able to control outcome.
- You must be able to exceed goal.
- You must be able to measure goal achievement.
- You must have a monitoring system.
- You must be flexible.

Exhibit 12-2 Progress Report on Goals—I

ST. CHARLES HOSPITAL
GOAL PLANNER—1980

Kate Bernhart

Name

Communications

Department

GOAL (include existing status and expected outcomes—see criteria on back).

Evaluate/recommend new in-house telephone system. Presently have OBT 608 PBS, 24 remaining station lines and frequent call back alarms indicating overload. Expected outcome to implement new technically updated system for future growth and reduce rising costs.

Identify hospital goal area if appropriate   Operational issue #14

TIME FRAME: Start 9/01/79   Completion 8/80

INDIVIDUAL ACCOUNTABLE FOR RESULT Kate Bernhart

ACTION STEPS	WHO	START	COMP.	REVIEW DATE(S)
1. *Define requirements*	KB	1/80	1/80	
—research characteristics and features of new system				
—current site survey		1/80	3/80	3/80 *done*
—identify standards such as service grade, user requirements, cost control, etc.		2/80	4/80	
—summarize equipment and user needs		3/80	4/80	4/80 *done*
—determine need for outside consultant		3/80	5/80	5/80 *done*
2. *Prepare request for proposal*	KB			
—develop specifications		4/80	6/80	
—qualify vendors		5/80	6/80	
—initiate 3 R.F.P.'s including telephone co.		5/80	6/80	6/80
3. *Evaluate proposals*	KB	6/80	8/80	8/80
—comparative analysis				
—develop selection criteria				
—identify trade off considerations				
4. *Presentation to management staff*	KB	8/80	9/80	9/80
—determine financial consideration such as lease/buy, cash flow, etc.				
—prepare presentation material				
—recommend system and alternative option				

expand search

Exhibit 12-3 Progress Report on Goals—II

ST. CHARLES HOSPITAL
GOAL PLANNER—1980

John Angus   H.R.D.
_____   _____
Name   Department

GOAL (include existing status and expected outcomes—see criteria on back).

To put all employees' educational activities on the computer. Presently manual system. All records in
H.R.D., not readily accessible to managers.

Identify hospital goal area if appropriate _____

TIME FRAME: Start April 1, 1980   Completion December 31, 1980

INDIVIDUAL ACCOUNTABLE FOR RESULT John Angus

ACTION STEPS	WHO	START	COMP.	REVIEW DATE(S)
1. Contact Marlene Forsythe to discuss computer application for employee continuing education records. Including programs within and outside St. Charles and any certificates or registries obtained.	J.A.	Apr. 1	Apr. 30	Apr. 30
2. Investigate possible linkage of employee educational records to be part of Personnel Data System for cost/benefit justification.	J.A.	Apr. 1	Apr. 30	Apr. 30
3. If appropriate, take necessary actions to ready records for computer input. —financial needs (CRT) —formulate/design existing record system to be easily recorded in	J.A.	May 15	Sept. 15	July 15
4. Install CRT in H.R.D. office for input.	J.A.	May 15	Sept. 30	
5. Final decision on actual date for transfer of educational records from manual to computerized system.	J.A. & M.F.	Sept. 15	Sept. 30	Sept. 30

sary. MBO, properly applied, is a fundamental step forward for any progressive institution.

NOTES

1. Peter F. Drucker, *The Practice of Management* (New York: Harper & Row, 1954).

2. Aircraft Engine Division, *Increasing Management Effectiveness through Work Planning* (New York: General Electric Co., 1968), p. 4.

3. Walter Mahler, *The Meaning of Management by Objectives,* (Mahler and Associates, 1970), p. 3.

4. Aircraft Engine Division, *Increasing Management Effectiveness,* p. 4.

5. George S. Odiorne, *Special Management Reports,* ''Dynamics of MBA'' (MBO Inc., 1976–1978), passim.

6. _____ , ''Activity Trap,'' (University of Massachusetts, December 1976), passim.

7. Harry Levinson, *The Levinson Letter* (March 1, 1979).

13. Management by Expectations

LAWRENCE C. BASSETT

Employee performance appraisal has a generally poor reputation. Personal interviews, discussions with hundreds of managers at all organizational levels, and a review of writings on the subject in a variety of professional and business journals indicate that only a small percentage of those responsible for appraising the performance of subordinates enter the process with willingness or a generally positive attitude. Even when appraisal is carried out regularly, it usually is done as a ritual and, although this usually is concealed, unwillingly. There has to be a better way.

The underlying causes for the negative attitude (and consequently less-than-desired results) can be traced to the method by which most appraisals are conducted. Although sophisticated approaches are used sometimes, the most frequently applied methodology involves the completion of an appraisal form followed by a discussion, usually inadequately prepared, in which the supervisor attempts to justify the evaluation. The employee may have an opportunity to have comments or responses noted on the record, and there may be a section in which improvements in performance are targeted for achievement before the next review. However, unless supervisors are well trained in interview techniques, the process tends to fail to accomplish its goals of improved performance, satisfied

employees who know where they stand, and the establishment of accurate, objective measurements.

While there are variations on this theme, efforts to improve the process often focus on improving the rating form. ("If only we had a better form, appraisals would be better" is the cry.) Some forms are better than others, but experienced professionals rarely, if ever, find a form that is clearly and consistently successful or enjoys anything near universal acceptance by employees. Even with a better-than-average form and well-trained supervisors, there are difficulties that negate the potential benefits of the process because the appraisal interview, a key part of the process, too often becomes a confrontation from which both parties leave with negative feelings and frustration. Obvious exceptions occur when a supervisor has nothing but good things to say and accompanies an entirely positive interview with an increase in salary, or when a supervisor merely avoids discussing anything unpleasant.

Even a form carefully developed by the employees who are being rated does not reduce the difficulties when they do not accept the evaluation as accurate. Charges that the evaluations are subjective lead to clashes of opinions that most supervisors find distasteful since they impact negatively on the friendly working relationship they want to maintain.

Those familiar with the appraisal process realize that other emotional problems must be overcome. Many supervisors feel it is difficult to sit in judgment and find

Note: In this article all exhibits are grouped at the end.

the task of criticizing distasteful, particularly if they themselves resist criticism leveled against them. Moreover, when resistance to criticism is expressed openly, it generates the kind of unpleasant exchange that can weaken the employee-supervisor relationship, so that honest appraisals become the exception rather than the rule. In addition, most institutions have supervisors, usually those untrained as managers, or those who recently have been promoted out of the ranks, who are so concerned with being admired by their subordinates that they avoid the appraisal process at all costs. They prefer to win popularity contests as a way of bolstering their confidence. Even when the institution enforces compliance with appraisal policies, and forms are completed and interviews carried out as mandated, the effort can be superficial and a meaningless ritual.

The health care field has other characteristics that further impede successful appraisal. Most supervisors are not highly trained in their management functions so the underlying causes for failure during the interview are exacerbated. Furthermore, many supervisors, including head nurses, have 24-hour responsibility and must evaluate employees on different shifts. Because of the many disciplines present in the health care setting, there is the need, as well, to rate the performance of employees doing jobs or practicing skills little understood by those to whom they report.

MANAGEMENT BY OBJECTIVES

These problems have been a longtime concern. Much work has been done by employee relations specialists and behavioral scientists, particularly during the last several decades. However, while some promising results spring up occasionally, most problems have essentially remained. When management by objectives made its appearance on the appraisal scene, it was and still is heralded by many managers as the best and most effective approach yet. In many respects it works well, but it has important limitations.

MBO attempts to establish objective and measurable yardsticks by setting specific goals upon which employee and supervisor agree. Performance, when measured, becomes a factor of how well the objectives have been achieved. The key element, which is the mutual agreement, in many cases proves to be only tacit agreement rather than genuine conviction that a goal is realistic and achievable. Even when salary increases are tied to the accomplishment of objectives, many of the emotional ingredients take hold and the program is in danger of losing steam after a few years.

Only in sophisticated organizations has MBO proved successful as a continuing process.

Perhaps the most important deficiency of MBO is that it concentrates on somewhat long-range goals and objectives without fully considering either *normal* day-to-day activities or behavioral considerations that are not tied directly to the goal but that are desired by the organization. In addition, MBO does not lend itself well to the bulk of the jobs in the nonexempt categories or at the lower levels of an organization. It is primarily a tool for use in executive-type appraisal.

MANAGEMENT BY EXPECTATIONS

What is needed is an approach that deals effectively with emotional factors, establishes objective measuring mechanisms, assures employee acceptance, and can be used for all levels of jobs while achieving almost universal success. Management by expectations (MBE), implemented and tested in a variety of organizational settings, gives such a promise.

Essentially, MBE is the identification of end results than can be associated with the proper, successful performance of any given activity or function. It is a word picture of what should happen when an assignment or behavior is carried out appropriately. This in itself is not entirely new, but how agreement on these end results is determined and the manner in which the standards are used is the key behind the use of MBE. A look at what the concept is and how it's applied provides an understanding of why it works.

It is a normal part of the thought process for immediate judgments to be made on what is being observed or addressed. Judgments that someone is *slow* or *lacks initiative,* that something is *neat* or *messy,* reflect in part the observer's personal thought associations based upon past experiences and learning. Conclusions are reflections of what the observer perceives subjectively based on comparisons with the desired mental picture. Difficulty arises when the observer's associations of what is *good* or *bad* are different from the associations held by another. When applied to specific job situations, opinions (mental associations) of what constitutes the desired end results are referred to as *standards.*

For example, the length of time to perform a given treatment, carry out a certain test, process an insurance claim, or transcribe dictation is based on an unspoken and unwritten association in the mind of the supervisor and the employee as to what the time-work volume should be. When a supervisor's judgment (associations) are different from the employee's, problems arise. The supervisor may feel the employee is slow, since the association of volume of work in a time period has not been achieved, while the employee feels the supervisor is expecting too much, because the subordinate's association calls for a lower volume of work in the same time period. Likewise, what constitutes (or is associated with) high-quality work may become individualized judgments based on the experiences, background, training, and outlook of those involved.

Consequently, all other things being equal, those who are considered the poorest workers may not be the least capable; it may be more that their standards (associations with fast or good performance) are lower than the supervisor's. Conversely, individuals considered good workers may not be more capable but their standards, or associations, are higher than those of the evaluator.

Agreement and Acceptance

MBE is a process by which the associations expressed as expectations by all parties involved are developed and identified so there is agreement and acceptance of the criteria against which performance or behavior will be measured. What makes MBE particularly desirable is that it is applicable to the full range of jobs, from production-oriented functions to intangible executive and administrative positions. In addition, when employees understand it, they accept it since they are involved in some critical ways.

When standards are set, the question of whether they will be supported depends on the attitude of employees. Frequently, clear standards do not exist since much of a job may be either intangible or nonspecific in nature and since written guidelines are unavailable. Dietary supervisors want food served that is pleasing to the eye as well as the taste; housekeepers want clean rooms. Practical ways of establishing such personalized standards are illusive. MBE addresses this by bringing to the surface the perceptions and mind pictures of the employees performing the work so that standards in the form of descriptions of the desired end results can be developed and formalized.

MBE uses employees by employing another truth: an individual performing a given job or function in most cases is the one most familiar with the detail and nuances of that activity. Managers who supervise an activity they once performed suffer a loss of familiarity with details or lack knowledge of recent changes. Consequently, the individual performing a function is the person best able to identify the standards. In addition, when there is a need to evaluate the performance or behavior of someone performing an unfamiliar activity, which is common where an administrator has responsibility over a variety of operating departments, the need to involve the job incumbent is mandatory. There is no dispute over whether a supervisor has the authority and responsibility to set standards, but this does not mean an employee cannot be an integral part of the process. In MBE this involvement is one of the principal reasons why the process works and the standards are accepted by all parties.

Concern that employees entrusted with helping to set standards may make things easy for themselves is not warranted. Essentially, most people enjoy a challenge and to at least some degree are competitive by nature. An essential to the success of MBE is the fact that most individuals also are competitive with themselves. By bringing out this self-competitive spirit, supervisors find that employees tend to establish standards higher than they will accept from others. In fact, MBE shows that there are many times when supervisors, in an attempt to avoid standards the employees cannot achieve, will reduce the level of expectations put forth by subordinates. Motivated employees frequently set unrealistically high expectations.

An additional factor that ensures the success of MBE is the involvement of employee groups. People are social creatures. They enjoy being with others and benefit from the comfort, support, and presence of peers. Even loners usually have friends and benefit from being part of a team. MBE provides the opportunity for the establishment of expectations through a group activity. This builds further support for the results and, as an important byproduct, for the acceptance of a high standard since most members of a group want to be perceived as achievers and will adopt the highest of whatever standards are placed before them.

The group process results in uniform standards useful during orientation and training of new employees. They will accept standards set by peers even though demands may be placed on them that are greater than may have been acceptable in previous employments.

Versatility: Concept, Not Procedures

That MBE is the application of a concept rather than a set of procedures gives it versatility. Since it involves a word picture, it becomes practical to set standards on any assignment or communication when it is clear what is being sought or needed at the completion of the activity. Telling someone what to do does not always achieve the desired outcome, whereas letting someone know what end results are anticipated gives them the freedom to do what will achieve those results. Just as important, it becomes possible for the employees to evaluate how well their work was performed, since they can measure outcomes in terms of whether the end results were achieved. Evaluation then becomes immediate and self-administering.

To managers, the most satisfying part of the process occurs after standards are established, for when MBE is practiced, the role of the supervisor turns from criticizer to coach. Since the employees have helped identify the procedural and behavioral results expected of them, it becomes possible for the workers to conduct self-evaluations. Those experienced in the use of self-appraisal find that most employees are remarkably honest. Only when a worker is deliberately or unintentionally self-deceptive need the supervisor carry out the traditional "heavy" part of the appraisal. Thus, with agreement attained more easily and objectively, managers can concentrate on how improvement can be achieved (a cooperative effort), rather than what has to be improved (a more threatening process).

With the process complete, attention can be turned to the appropriate appraisal form, though it quickly becomes apparent that the form is merely a record of what has occurred and in itself no longer is a key element. The form, instead of being the foundation of the appraisal system, is only a handy tool, and while care still is needed in its design, it no longer has its traditionally vital importance. In fact, experience with MBE shows that effective appraisal is possible even without a formal appraisal form.

The use of expectations as a device in management goal setting and appraisal in itself is not novel. What will be different to most managers is the coordinated effort to establish and sustain the continuing process as part of everyday organizational life.

To summarize MBE is to identify its key components:

- Outcomes expressed in word pictures clearly define target standards, thus removing or reducing subjectivity and confusion.
- Expectations are individualized to specific functions or jobs and thus are tailored directly to the personalities of those involved and to the work environment.
- Those involved have a chance to participate and reveal personal values and standards, thus leading to a participative process within realistic guidelines. MBE as a group process strengthens interpersonal relationships and leads to objective standards accepted by the entire group.
- MBE is competitive, but competition principally is between an employee and self, the most acceptable and nonthreatening form of competition.

- Employees set standards that they would resist if established by others. Their involvement in the setting of standards assures criteria for good performance that they support and that are tailored to the job.
- MBE focuses on expectations that result from proper performance or behavior rather than from technique, thus permitting objective evaluations of the performance of those carrying out functions not undertaken by the evaluator.
- Individuals can measure and trace their own progress based upon their knowledge of the expected outcomes. They can evaluate both the quality and quantity of their work.
- MBE deals with the job or assignment in total and can address behavioral and personality characteristics that have an impact on job performance, as opposed to the rating of personality traits incidental to job requirements.
- The supervisor's role in MBE is more that of a counselor and helper than that of a criticizer, thus strengthening the relationship and contributing to better communications and better performance.

INSTALLING AN MBE PROGRAM

MBE can be implemented within a short time, but developing standards and introducing a new approach to performance appraisal is not something to be rushed into without planning and the training of managers. As with any newly introduced procedure, managers have periods of uncertainty, but encouragement leads to a quick mastery of the various applications of the concept. Success breeds success, and managers should soon be building upon their own experiences and be able to carry out MBE with minimal guidance.

Although tailored to the characteristics of the organization, the procedures adopted should include some of the following basic steps, using employees performing the jobs whenever possible.

MBE As an Appraisal Tool

1. Develop Job Descriptions or Lists of Job Functions As the Basis for Establishing Expectations

The functions performed by an employee need to be identified if word pictures are to be made of the end results expected to be visible when the work is carried out properly. If an up-to-date job description is available, it becomes the best tool to use, but its absence should not preclude an employee's listing the various functions normally performed. (A side advantage of using job descriptions is that each time one is reviewed, it is updated, thus precluding time-consuming periodic rewriting.)

2. *Identify the Key Elements in the Job*

Every job is made of components, but some parts consistently must be carried out properly if performance is to be considered generally acceptable. (Dispensing medications is an example. A nurse cannot be considered satisfactory even if errors are occasional.) Obviously, it is desirable that every part of a job be done properly, but it is not wise to average good and bad points. In other words, to avoid overall evaluations that do not properly balance the more important aspects of the job against the less important, the identifying of key components is a help. This assures that evaluations reflect the relative importance of functions. Invariably, employees who perform the job identify the key components more critically than do their supervisors.

3. *Develop Word Pictures to Describe the Expectations Associated with the Successful Carrying Out of Each Function*

Using a group process whenever possible, each function should be addressed individually. A list of end results that can be expected if the function is carried out properly should be developed. The expectation, or word picture, can be general or very specific, depending upon the characteristics of the job. (See Exhibit 13-1, which illustrates expectations developed by licensed practical nurses.)

4. *Develop a Written Format That Matches the Duties in the Job Description (or List of Functions) with the Expectations*

The specific form in which expectations are coupled with the function can be tailored to the preferences of those involved. When job descriptions are used, expectations can follow right after the function being addressed. In other cases, expectations can be placed on the reverse side of the job description or on a separate page. (Placing the expectations im-mediately below the function can be effective, but the amount of paper generated may be greater than if the expectations were maintained separately. Exhibit 13-2 illustrates the use of a nursing assistant job description, followed by expectations.)

5. *Ensure Agreement on the Key Elements and Expectations*

While the competitiveness brought out during the process of identifying expectations can produce high standards, it is necessary for employee and supervisor to agree. When agreement is achieved, the formal benchmarks against which appraisals will be measured also fall into place. If there is disagreement, discussions should focus on the differences in order to reach a consensus. As a general rule, supervisors would be prudent to adopt the expectations established by their employees even if they seem disappointing to the manager. Insisting upon standards not supported by employees can lead to merely the appearance of agreement, and to negative consequences.

6. *Develop a System of Evaluation*

When standards have been developed, evaluation should start with employee self-appraisal. In actuality, self-appraisal on a continuous basis without supervisory input is possible when employees have copies of the expectations they helped develop. Such informal self-appraisals provide an employee with a sense of direction. Periodically, depending upon the nature of the organization, the supervisor should review the scores. Reviews may be made on specific dates, e.g., the employee's anniversary, at the conclusion of the orientation period, etc.

7. *Develop Scoring Symbols*

When evaluating performance against expectations, a scoring system can be established that reflects the level of accomplishment. One scoring system used by some hospitals that avoids "schoolish" terminology or traditional categorizing follows:

Evaluate each expectation with one of the following symbols:

O Performance surpasses expectations for the function. Performance in that function is clearly outstanding.

G Performance is good. The expectation is met fully.

S Performance is affected by special circumstances in that expectations may be met at minimal levels but that general improvement is needed if performance is to be considered good. *S* also may indicate there is a satisfactory reason why the expectation is not met fully, such as the individual's being a new employee, newly assigned duties, or unavoidable factors. *S* indicates that progress is attainable and anticipated.

B Performance is below expectations and improvement is necessary before it will be considered satisfactory.

In some organizations, employees have developed a symbol to be used between good and outstanding. It has been found that in general this is not necessary. In addition, a special symbol (such as an asterisk after the expectation) indicates where improvement is possible, even if the expectation is being met or exceeded. When used, this is a developmental and motivational device.

8. Determine Final Scores

Supervisors should review the employees' scores and note differences, which if the MBE process has been carried out properly will be minimal in most cases. Using expectations matched to job functions should result in evaluations that consistently satisfy both parties. Where differences exist, the employee should be requested to illustrate how the expectations were met. Similarly, supervisors should be prepared with specifics to indicate why their evaluation differed.

9. Determine an Overall Score

An overall evaluation should be made based upon achieving the key expectations. When most of the key expectations have received *O*

scores, an overall score of outstanding might be in order.

10. Develop Remedial and Development Plans

Where improvement is desirable or needed, a plan of action should be developed with the supervisor taking a leading part. Leaving employees to their own devices will not bring the positive results that usually occur when there is a team effort.

11. Tie In Performance Appraisals with Salary Increases

Performance appraisal is carried out best independent of salary increases in order to focus upon performance characteristics. Even if appraisal is to be used as part of a merit program, it should be done up to two months earlier, followed by a review of the scores at the time the supervisor is making a recommendation. Various formulas, allocating dollar amounts or percentages, can be designed to fit the organization's budget and employee relations practices. This becomes practical where there is experience with the MBE process.

Specific procedures will vary with the institution, but the individual in charge of the employee relations function generally is the coordinator of the program.

MBE is not a panacea, nor will it cure every organizational ill. Work always will be needed to improve the techniques of certain supervisors and to find answers where the process doesn't bring about the results desired. However, it is effective and practical. It answers most questions asked by skeptical supervisors, and in practice it works. In time, it will be refined within each organization that employs it. But the level of sophistication to which it can be developed is great, and its adaptability to almost every setting assures that once the concept is understood and mastered, it will become one of a supervisor's most useful and effective management skills.

Exhibit 13-1 Expectations Developed by Licensed Practical Nurses Working in a Group

1. On all occasions patients are approached in a courteous, friendly manner and their rights and dignities are respected.

2. Employees maintain the same professional demeanor when caring for an unconscious or nonoriented patient as when caring for a conscious patient.

3. Knowledge is exhibited of where to obtain necessary supplies and equipment (and correct method for charging for them) to perform procedures; safe and economical use is practiced.

4. Good body mechanics and correct methods of moving, lifting, and transporting patients are practiced.

5. Policies and procedures are understood and performed as outlined in the procedure manual.

6. Assistance and advice are sought from a registered nurse whenever the employee has any doubts concerning the performance of the procedure.

7. Patients are clean, dry, and comfortable, with the call bell in reach and the unit in order after completion of a procedure.

Exhibit 13-2 Nursing Assistant Job Description and Expectations

MAIN DUTIES: (Routine Supervision)
Self Ratings

PERFORMS CLERICAL DUTIES SUCH AS RECORDING OF INTAKE AND OUTPUT, AND CHARTING OF VITAL SIGNS.

Expectations:

1. Information on worksheets is recorded accurately, legibly, and promptly.

2. There is full knowledge of the normal ranges of vital signs. Any variations are reported to the nurse responsible for the patient.

3. There is understanding of the individual patient's limits of intake. Normal amounts of output and variations are reported to the nurse responsible for the patients.

PASSES TRAYS TO PATIENTS AT MEALTIME, FEEDING PATIENTS AS NECESSARY. PASSES OUT BETWEEN-MEAL NOURISHMENTS.

Expectations:

1. The patient is prepared for meals, is comfortable in bed or chair, and is washed prior to meal.

2. Trays are delivered courteously, and food is prepared as necessary in an unhurried manner.

3. The dignity of patients is respected and there is courtesy while the patient is being fed.

4. Fluid intakes are charted as necessary at the completion of the meal.

5. Dietary aides are assisted in the collecting of trays promptly after patients have eaten.

MAINTAINS SAFE, CLEAN, ORDERLY WORK AREA AND WORK PRACTICES.

Expectations:

1. The patients' units are kept in order, i.e., soiled linens properly disposed of, waste materials discarded in appropriate areas and containers, patient's personal items neatly arranged within reach of patient, surfaces of unit furniture wiped clean, etc.

2. Ward clerks are asked to contact housekeeping department for large spills requiring floor to be mopped.

3. Assignment sheet is checked regularly for assigned tasks in kitchen or utility room. Counter surfaces are clean, neat, and in order.

Exhibit 13-3 Expectations of Performance As Developed by Housekeeping Employees

1. Employee is at work station ready to work at scheduled time.
2. Work is performed so that there is pride in the results.
3. Objects in high and difficult-to-reach locations (television sets, corners, etc.) are cleaned as well and as thoroughly as other areas.
4. Employee has a reputation for cooperation and for being a good team player (with other workers and supervisors).
5. Employee always is well groomed and has a high standard of personal hygiene.
6. Employee arrives at work with a good mental attitude for whatever is assigned.
7. Employee is properly and neatly dressed in a clean uniform when on the job.
8. Work is performed and fill-in for others is carried out willingly and without complaint.
9. Other workers are given the respect and cooperation that the individual expects to receive.
10. Employee's voice level and behavior are considerate of patient needs.
11. Employee always appears pleasant and in good nature.
12. Employee is supportive of fellow workers and positive of what is said about others.
13. Absences from work areas always are reported or cleared in advance.
14. Equipment, facilities, and work area always are clean and in order.
15. The department head is aware in advance when employee may be late or absent from work.

Exhibit 13-4 Purchasing Director Job Expectations for Performance Review (Samples)

1. All vendor lists and catalogs are accessible and current, and when possible are cross-referenced for use by others.
2. Reports on vendor interviews and changing pricing and other conditions are maintained.
3. Criteria for delivery of ordered materials are maintained and audited periodically. Expediting of purchased materials is done automatically according to a schedule either by the Director of Purchasing or someone delegated.
4. Quality and quantity of materials purchased meet the needs of the departments, including agreement upon substitution when necessary.
5. Department heads and others feel they are up to date and have confidence in the Purchasing Director concerning new equipment processes, etc., that may be available.
6. Audits of competitive bids and other purchases show the hospital prices to be within budget and, where discernible, the lowest possible for the quantity and quality purchased.
7. Inventories of materials, particularly those used frequently, are maintained properly so that shortages or depletions are incurred infrequently, if ever.
8. Discounts and other special pricing arrangements are obtained whenever practical or possible.

Exhibit 13-5 Sample Employee Performance Review Guide

_____ Hospital

Name _____ Position _____

Completed by _____ Date _____

If you prefer, indicate the answers to questions 1 & 2 on the job description, which then should be attached.

1. What parts of the job (if any,) clearly *exceed* expectations for good performance?

_____

_____

_____

_____

2. What parts of the job (if any,) are performed *below* what should be expected for good performance?

_____

_____

_____

_____

3. Place an asterisk next to any of the items indicated in questions 1 & 2 that are key elements of the job, in that their acceptable performance is mandatory.

4. How does total performance compare with:

    6 months ago   ( ) the same   ( ) better*   ( ) not as good*

    1 year ago   ( ) the same   ( ) better*   ( ) not as good*

5. How does current performance compare with overall expectations?

    ( ) O: Performance surpasses expectations for the function.*

    ( ) G: Performance is good and fully meets expectations.

    ( ) S: Special situation: Performance may be below expectations but with satisfactory reason such as new employee, new duties, unavoidable factors, etc. Progress is attainable and anticipated.*

    ( ) B: Below expectations: Improvement is necessary before function is performed satisfactorily.*

6. During past 6 months, how many different times was person absent? _____ Total days? _____

7. During past 6 months, how many different times was person late? _____

*Use reverse side to give explanations, illustrations, and employee comments.

_____

*COMMENTS FROM REVERSE SIDE

(Include explanations, plans for improvement, and any unresolved points discussed with employees. Attach additional sheets if necessary, and if employee wishes to write additional comments.)

ACTION RECOMMENDED

▫ Step increase recommended   ▫ Extend probation _____ months

▫ Delay step increase 3 months   ▫ Probation completed satisfactorily

▫ Step increase denied   ▫ Performance review only: No actions

▫ Placed on probation

Reviewed by: _____ Date: _____

Date copy given to employee: _____

Employee signature _____

14. Performance Salary Increase Program

RALPH A. ANTHENIEN

This material describes a Performance Salary Increase program for salaried exempt and nonexempt personnel covering more than 3,800 employees in the Kaiser-Permanente Medical Care Program (KPMCP). This package was developed for use by all supervisors and is provided to all other salaried employees for their orientation to this program. It is reprinted from a booklet distributed to all new salaried employees upon hiring.

This merit pay program fulfills a variety of needs, including:

- It provides for individual salary increases.
- It involves the supervisor in determining the salary increase.
- It provides consistent salary increase guidelines throughout the organization.
- It provides for a continuing performance appraisal program.
- It outlines performance standards for salaried employees.

It must be noted that an effective application of this program requires a sound job evaluation and classification system as well as compensating individuals reasonably well with respect to the outside market. The requirements become more apparent when the reader reviews the *Pay for Performance* section, which is the heart of any merit pay program.

The material covers the responsibilities of each party, the necessary forms, the procedural aspects of the program, and the philosophy and conceptual aspects of a pay-for-performance system.

INTRODUCTION

Our salary increase program for salaried employees was developed over twenty years ago to fit the Kaiser-Permanente Medical Care Program's needs and requirements at that time.

Since that time, our organization, as well as the hospital-medical industry generally, has changed significantly. The impact of compensation in a tight labor market, inflation, governmental regulations and employee relations actions such as labor negotiations has an even more significant relationship today to our salaried employees and "management" group. The Kaiser-Permanente Medical Care Program continues to need to achieve its maximum return for its salary expenditures as well as to motivate employees to achieve their best.

The following paragraphs outline the basic purposes of the salaried performance increase program which has been designed and modified over the years to more effectively meet our requirements:

A. *Key Objectives*

The key objectives of this program are that it (a) provides for individual salary increases based on the employee's performance, (b) provides the supervisor with the opportunity and responsibility to determine how much an increase to give and (c) provides consistent guidelines throughout the program to compensate individuals with similar performance levels in the same manner.

This program, in addition to emphasizing the supervisor's responsibility, emphasizes the evaluation of the employee's performance, the granting of salary increases relating to that performance, and the two-way communication of this assessment and recommended action between the individual employee and his/her supervisor.

B. *Operating Requirements (Budget)*

Salary administration recommendations and required management approvals with respect to the annual operating requirements (budget) will be accomplished in approximately October of each year for timely consideration in the medical care program's budget and forecasting decisions.

The approved salary administration operating requirement will provide a cost ceiling for management but will not be communicated to individual departments or units.

The Employee Relations Department, Salaried Compensation section, will develop an annual salary increase guide (Grid Chart) within the management approved limitations, to control overall salary increase costs and to insure consistency throughout the medical care program. The salary increase guides will permit individual entities, departments, facilities and supervisors the flexibility to grant salary increases in accordance with their own circumstances, and in line with our objectives, (but without a specific budgetary limitation).

C. *Salaried Wage Structures*

The Employee Relations Department will develop exempt and nonexempt salary structures for required management approvals in approximately November of each year. The salary schedule will be developed whenever possible to provide the Kaiser-Permanente Medical Care Program with the optimum ability to attract, retain, and motivate competent employees.

D. *Scheduled Review Dates*

Individual supervisors will plan for the salary increases and assess the performance and performance levels for their employees at least on an annual basis. Supervisors should also consider other factors as, (a) The Salary Increase Guide, (b) date of last increase, (c) relationship to bargaining group employees and their forthcoming adjustments, (d) internal or competitive salary inequities, and (e) other pertinent points that will assist in achieving sound salary administration.

E. *Other Salary Administration Procedures*

New Employees – New employees should be reviewed for possible salary increases six months from date of hire if they were hired at or below the 25th percentile of their grade range. In any event, they should receive a performance appraisal within six months of hire.

Recommendations should be received from the salaried compensation section with respect to the treatment of transfers, organizational promotions, current reclassifications and salary inequities (red circle, green circle). Such salary administration procedures are normally part of the overall salary administration program and in many cases are already covered under regional policies, procedures, or guidelines.

OBJECTIVES

In addition to providing KPMCP with the opportunity to ATTRACT QUALIFIED INDIVIDUALS, our total compensation program must also provide the opportunity to:

1. RETAIN COMPETENT EMPLOYEES
2. MOTIVATE EMPLOYEES TO ACHIEVE MAXIMUM CAPABILITY

The salary increase program is designed to improve our opportunity to retain and motivate employee performance by more effectively achieving the following objectives of our PERFORMANCE SALARY INCREASE PROGRAM:

1. Attain maximum utilization of salary increase expenditure.
2. Individualize performance salary increases.
3. Grant salary increases based on performance as related to KPMCP requirements.

4. Increase immediate supervisors' effective participation in planning and recommending performance salary increases.
5. Attain *effective* understanding between supervisors and employees pertaining to salary increases, performance, responsibilities, organizational relationships, and objectives.
6. Maintain salary expenditure within KPMCP operating requirements.

KEY ELEMENTS

Planning

- Establish Overall Expenditure Needs and Guides
- Preliminary Performance Rating
- Salary Increase Guide
- Salary Increase Planning

Action

- Individual Performance Evaluation
- Specific Recommendations
- Employee Communication

Appraisal

- Continual Review of Program's Effectiveness

PRIMARY RESPONSIBILITIES

Supervisor

- Preliminary Performance Rating
- Salary Increase Planning
- Individual Performance Evaluation
- Specific Recommendations
- Employee Communication

Regional Management

- Establish Overall Expenditure Guides
- Approve Salary Planning

Employee Relations

- Recommend Overall Expenditure Needs
- Establish Annual Salary Increase Guide
- Review Salary Planning and Increases
- Coordinate Flow of Program
- Insure consistency and control of program are maintained
- Review Program Effectiveness

PROCEDURES

A. Salary Planning

1. *Employee Relations* communicates program to supervisors of salaried employees.
    a. Distribute and review performance salary increase booklet through the Personnel Managers.
2. *Employee Relations* develops annual salary increase guide and prepares salary increase planning forms.
    a. Prepares annual increase guide based upon estimate of regional rating distribution and approved budgetary constraints.
    b. Orders, reviews, and prepares computerized salary increase planning forms.
    c. Collects, develops, and reviews estimated increases for other groups of employees such as Local 250, Local 29, CNA, etc.
    d. Develops and obtains primary approval for salary and wage structures.
3. *Employee Relations, Department Managers* and *Facility Managers* develop projected salary increases for forthcoming calendar year.
    a. Plan salary increases for employees based on preliminary performance rating, employee salary range quartile, date of last increase, and annual salary increase guides.
    b. Indicate on planning form the next projected salary increase(s) for the coming calendar year.
    c. Obtain approvals from appropriate department manager, facility managers and entity heads as required.
4. *Employee Relations* consolidates salary actions by entity and location and obtains necessary approvals and makes adjustments in plan as required.

B. Salary Actions during Year

1. *Employee Relations* notifies supervisors prior to planned salary action.
    a. Thirty days prior to tentative increase date, forward to supervisor (via location Personnel Director) a salaried employee evaluation form together with a transmittal letter and completed NPA [Notice of Personnel Action] based upon the "planned" action.

Exhibit 14-1 Flow Chart of Procedures for Forecasted Performance Increases and Growth Promotions

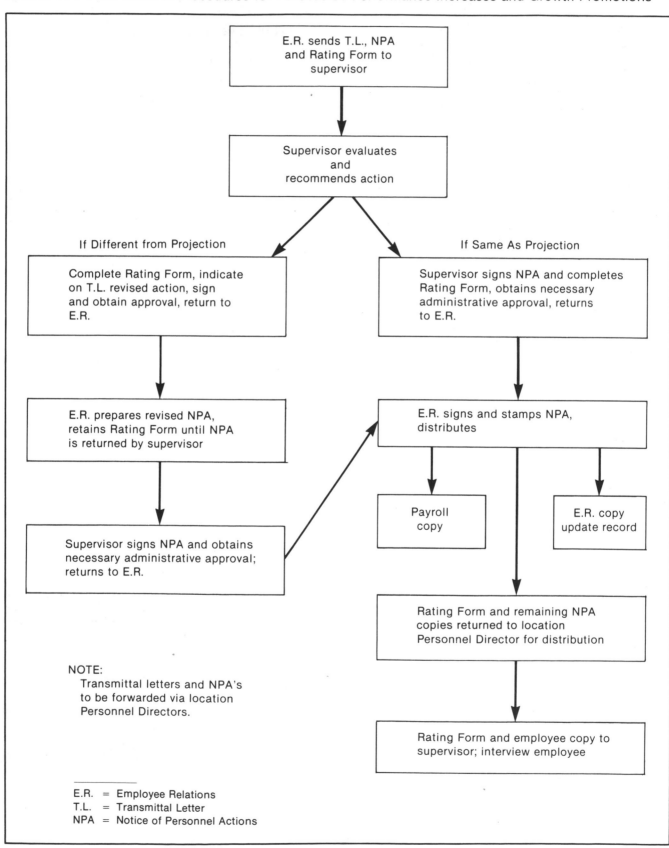

NOTE:
Transmittal letters and NPA's
to be forwarded via location
Personnel Directors.

E.R. = Employee Relations
T.L. = Transmittal Letter
NPA = Notice of Personnel Actions

Exhibit 14-2 Covering Memo on Performance Review

INTER-OFFICE MEMORANDUM

To   Date

At

                                               From

Copies To

                             sample   At

Subject   PERFORMANCE REVIEW

Attached is a Performance Evaluation Form (#04366) to be utilized with the Performance Salary Increase Program and a completed NPA based upon your planned action.

You should appraise the above employee's performance in relation to the position's responsibilities as reflected in the position description. Complete the Performance Evaluation Form, and determine whether or not your forecasted salary action is currently appropriate. Your decision should be based upon your current appraisal of the employee's performance.

If the planned action is still appropriate, sign the NPA, obtain your Department Head's signature and return it with the completed Performance Evaluation Form to Employee Relations. Employee Relations will return the appropriate copy(s) of the NPA and the Performance Evaluation Form to you. You should *then* inform the employee of the salary increase and review his performance with him.

If the forecasted salary action is no longer appropriate either in date or amount, indicate the recommended change below, obtain required approval, and return this letter with the completed Performance Evaluation Form and the *unsigned* NPA to Employee Relations. A revised Notice of Personnel Action (if required) will be sent to you.

Upon receipt of the signed NPA, Employee Relations will return the appropriate copy(s) and the Performance Evaluation Form for your discussion with the employee.

You *must* submit a completed Performance Evaluation Form before the NPA will be forwarded to Payroll for processing.

If you have any questions or problems with the above, please call Employee Relations, extensions 6131, 6172, 6115, or 6130.

Revised Date_____

Amount _____

Percentage _____

_____

Supervisor Approval

_____

Executive Approval

(For forecast changes)

Exhibit 14-3 Sample NPA (Notice of Personnel Action)

NOTICE OF PERSONNEL ACTION

KAISER-PERMANENTE
MEDICAL CARE PROGRAM

CURRENT		SEQ	RUN DATE	CHANGE TO	☐ NEW HIRE ☐ TERM / LOA ☐ RE-HIRE ☐ CHANGE	DATE PREPARED

REG

ENT	EMPL NO	INITIALS	LAST NAME	EFFECTIVE DATE	1 B	ENT	EMPL NO	INITIALS	LAST NAME	EFFECTIVE DATE

LOC	DEPT	EXPENSE	MARITAL STATUS	SEX	HIRE IN EEO	HOME PHONE NUMBER	LOC	DEPT	EXPENSE	MARITAL STATUS	SEX	HIRE IN EEO	HOME PHONE NUMBER

FIRST NAME	M.R. NUMBER	SOCIAL SECURITY NO	1 C	FIRST NAME	M R NUMBER	SOCIAL SECURITY NO

STREET ADDRESS	STREET ADDRESS

CITY	STATE	ZIP	1 D	CITY	STATE	ZIP

CURRENT STATUS

CURRENT STATUS

JOB CODE	JOB TITLE	JOB CODE	JOB TITLE

EMPL CAT	EMPL STATUS	GRADE	STEP	SCHED SHIFT	SCHED HRS	SPEC DIFF RATE	1 F	EMPL CAT	EMPL STATUS	GRADE	STEP	SCHED SHIFT	SCHED HRS	SPEC DIFF RATE

REASON	BASE RATE MONTHLY	HOURLY	SHIFT RATE CODE	SCHED SHIFT RATE	SHORT HR RATE	REASON	BASE RATE MONTHLY	HOURLY	SHIFT RATE CODE	SCHED SHIFT RATE	SHORT HR RATE

DATES

DATES

ORIGINAL HIRE	CONTINUOUS SERVICE	SICK LEAVE	BIRTH	1 G	ORIGINAL HIRE	CONTINUOUS SERVICE	SICK LEAVE	BIRTH

VACATION	IN POSITION	LEAVE OF ABSENCE RETURN	TERMINATION DATE	REASON	VACATION	IN POSITION	LEAVE OF ABSENCE RETURN	TERMINATION DATE	REASON

PAYROLL

PAYROLL

FED WITH EXEMP	FICA SDI	STATE WITH EX	CITY WITH EX	FEDERAL DOLLARS	STATE DOLLARS	INCR HRS	INCR DATE	1 H	FED WITH EXEMP	FICA SDI	STATE WITH EX	CITY WITH EX	FEDERAL DOLLARS	STATE DOLLARS	INCR HRS	INCR DATE

ENT	LOC	DEPT	EMPL NO.	LAST NAME & INITIALS

REMARKS:

Sample "NPA"

PREPARED BY	SUPERVISOR	PERSONNEL	ADMINISTRATION

94615 (REV. 9/77)

PAYROLL

Exhibit 14-4 Sample Performance Evaluation Form

PERFORMANCE EVALUATION — SALARIED PERSONNEL

EMPLOYEE   POSITION TITLE

ENTITY   LOCATION   DEPARTMENT   TYPE OF PERFORMANCE EVALUATION

☐ Interim   ☐ 6 Mo's. Evaluation   ☐ Annual

Key Performance Factors complete where appropriate	Relative Factor Weight	RATING					Key Performance Factors complete where appropriate	Relative Factor Weight	RATING				
		5	4	3	2	1			5	4	3	2	1
Job Knowledge							Oral Communication						
Judgement and Decisions							Written Communication						
Plan and Organize Work							Human Relations						
Management of Resources							Quantity of Work						
Adaptability to Stress							Quality of Work						

Overall Performance Rating	− 5 +	− 4 +	− 3 +	− 2 +	− 1 +
	Unsatisfactory	Meets Min. Requirements	Meets Requirements	Exceeds Requirements	Outstanding

COMMENTS

1. COMMENT ON ACHIEVEMENT OF SPECIFIC GOALS AND OBJECTIVES

SEE ATTACHMENT ☐

2. COMMENT ON SPECIFIC SIGNIFICANT CONTRIBUTIONS EMPLOYEE HAS MADE

SEE ATTACHMENT ☐

3. SPECIFIC AREAS WHERE IMPROVEMENT IS NEEDED

SEE ATTACHMENT ☐

4. MANDATORY COMPLETION FOR LINE MANAGERS AND SUPERVISORS · COMMENT ON SPECIFIC CONTRIBUTIONS MADE IN EQUAL EMPLOYMENT/AFFIRMATIVE ACTION INCLUDING ACHIEVEMENT OF GOALS AND OBJECTIVES.

SEE ATTACHMENT ☐

FOR PERSONNEL **OTHER THAN** LINE MANAGERS AND SUPERVISORS:

☐ Deficient in Support of   ☐ Supports   ☐ Exceptional Support of Organizational AAP/EEO Goals and Objectives

RECOMMENDED ACTION IN VIEW OF PERFORMANCE RATING

SIGNATURE OF RATING SUPERVISOR	DATE / /	SIGNATURE OF REVIEWING SUPERVISOR	DATE / /

DATE EVALUATION DISCUSSED WITH EMPLOYEE   EMPLOYEE SIGNATURE   Date: / /

NOTE: SALARY INCREASES SHOULD NOT BE DISCUSSED WITH EMPLOYEE UNTIL APPROVAL.

94366 (REV. 9-78)   **DISTRIBUTION:** WHITE = PERSONNEL • CANARY = EMPLOYEE COPY • PINK = EMPLOYEE RELATIONS GOLDENROD = AUXILLARY COPY

Exhibit 14-5 Reverse Side of Personnel Evaluation Form

INSTRUCTIONS

REVIEW FREQUENCY: . . . . For new employees, no later than six months after employment. For all other employees, at least once every 12 months, unless a significant change warrants a supplementary review.

RESPONSIBILITY: . . . . You as immediate supervisor are responsible for reviewing each of your subordinates.

PERFORMANCE STANDARDS: . . . . . . You should evaluate the employee's actual performance results as related to the position responsibility and requirements for the period under review.

Do not be influenced by prior evaluations, length of service, experience or education.

You should evaluate an employee on each factor against standard performance for the position.

RELATIVE FACTOR WEIGHTS: . . . . . . The ten factors will vary in importance for different positions. The relative factor weights are to distinquish the significant from the less important factors for the particular job when determining an appropriate overall performance evaluation. You should assign these factor weights after evaluating all individual factors. Do not attempt to be overly precise, a broad indication will suffice. If any factor is not applicable to the position being evaluated, so indicate in box.

PERFORMANCE INTERVIEW: . . . . . . After completing the Performance Evaluation, and after obtaining the necessary signatures and approvals, you must route the evaluation and any planned salary adjustment actions through the Regional Employee Relations Department **before you discuss** this evaluation with the employee. This discussion should then inform an employee of his overall and specific performance as well as pointing our where and how improvements can be made. This discussion should provide an opportunity to the employee to comment about his work relationships and progress.

FOR FURTHER DETAILS, CONSULT THE PERFORMANCE EVALUATION GUIDE

94366 (REV. 9-78) REVERSE

Exhibit 14-6 Continuation of Performance Evaluation Form

NOTE: ATTACH TO PERFORMANCE EVALUATION FORM

PERFORMANCE EVALUATION ATTACHMENT — SALARIED PERSONNEL

EMPLOYEE			POSITION TITLE		
ENTITY	LOCATION	DEPARTMENT	PAGE NO.	TOTAL PAGES	DATE

INDICATE WHICH SECTION OF PERFORMANCE EVALUATION BEING CONTINUED:

Sample Continuation Sheet

SIGNATURE OF RATING SUPERVISOR	DATE	SIGNATURE OF REVIEWING SUPERVISOR	DATE
DATE EVALUATION DISCUSSED WITH EMPLOYEE	EMPLOYEE SIGNATURE		Date:

94367 (11-78)   **DISTRIBUTION:** WHITE = PERSONNEL • CANARY = EMPLOYEE COPY • PINK = EMPLOYEE RELATIONS
GOLDENROD = AUXILLARY COPY

b. If the completed employee performance evaluation form and NPA or transmittal letter are not returned by tentative increase date, a reminder is sent to the supervisor for action with a copy to the facility administrator.

2. *Supervisor/Department Head*
   a. Completes salaried performance evaluation form. Determine if planned salary action is still appropriate. If so, sign NPA, obtain your supervisor's approval and signature. Return all forms to Employee Relations.
   b. If planned salary action is no longer appropriate, indicate change and sign in space provided on transmittal letter. Obtain your supervisor's approval and *return* the transmittal letter, NPA, and completed performance evaluation form to Employee Relations.

3. *Employee Relations*
   a. If signed NPA is received, approve notice of personnel action and distribute copies to:

      1. Payroll - for further processing.
      2. Local Personnel Office for distribution to:

         a. Supervisor - for announcement of increase
         b. Department head
         c. Personnel files

   b. Return salaried performance evaluation form with appropriate copy(s) of Notice of Personnel Action to supervisor (via location Personnel Director) for discussion with employee.
   c. If change is indicated on original transmittal letter, review for conformance with policy.

      1. If recommendation is not in conformance with policy, consult with supervisor/department head to resolve differences between recommendation and established policy.
      2. Obtain entity head approval for forecast changes as may be appropriate.
      3. Forward new transmittal letter and revised NPA to the supervisor (via location Personnel Director) based on revised information.

PAY FOR PERFORMANCE

A. Introduction

In order for a merit salary increase program to work effectively, all participants must have an understanding of *how* the program functions as well as *why* it is structured as it is.

B. The Salary Increase Guide Chart

In our merit salary increase program, the two key factors which determine the percentage amount of an individual's annual salary increase are:

1. the employee's salary range quartile before salary increase, and
2. the employee's overall performance rating.

In our program, a Salary Increase Guide Chart is prepared by Employee Relations each year, and this Guide Chart specifies the salary increase percentage available for each combination of employee performance and employee salary range quartile.

By salary range quartile, we mean the position of a specific salary in relation to the whole salary range for that particular grade. We say that a salary between the salary range minimum and the 25th percentile is in the 4th quartile; that a salary between the 25th percentile and the midpoint of the grade is in the 3rd quartile; and so on. As an example, our exempt grade 13 currently has a minimum salary of $1465/mo., a 25th percentile of $1610/mo., and a midpoint of $1750/mo.; therefore, a salary of $1525/mo. is in the *4th quartile* of grade 13, and a salary of $1700/mo. is in the *3rd quartile*. The importance of the salary range quartile will be apparent as you look at Exhibit 14-6a shown on page 213.

As you can see, for any particular salary range quartile, the Salary Increase Guide Chart is constructed so that the available salary increase percentage *increases* as performance level *increases*. For example, the bottom row in the above example represents salary range quartile 4, and we can see that an employee whose salary prior to increase is in the fourth quartile will be eligible to receive an increase of 6.5 percent—7.5 percent if his performance is "Meets Requirements;" 8.5 percent—9.5 percent if performance is "Exceeds Requirements;" and 10.5 percent—11.5 percent if performance is viewed as "Outstanding." This same concept holds true for any particular salary range quartile—that is, *the salary increase percentage increases as performance level increases*.

Exhibit 14-6a Salary Increase Guide Chart

5 UNSATISFACTORY	4 MEETS MIN. REQUIREMENTS	3 MEETS REQUIREMENTS	2 EXCEEDS REQUIREMENTS	1 OUTSTANDING	SALARY RANGE QUARTILE
"NO INCREASE" AREA			2.5—3.5%	4.5—6.5%	1 75th
		2.5—3.5%	4.5—5.5%	6.5—7.5%	PERCENTILE 2 MID-
	2.5—3.5%	4.5—5.5%	6.5—7.5%	8.5—9.5%	POINT 3 25th
	4.5—5.5%	6.5—7.5%	8.5—9.5%	10.5—11.5%	PERCENTILE 4 GRADE

(diagonal label: SAMPLE ONLY)

*NEW-HIRE REVIEW	4.0%	5.0%	6.0%	7.0%

*Applies only to those whose starting salary does not exceed the 25th percentile of their grade.

Exhibit 14-7 Sample Guide for Salary Increases

SAMPLE ONLY

Salary Increase Guide

Unsatisfactory 5	Meets Minimum Requirements 4	Meets Requirements 3	Exceeds Requirements 2	Outstanding 1
No increase	No increase	No increase	No increase	7.0%-8.0%
No increase	No increase	No increase	6.0%-8.5%	8.5%-10.5%
No increase	No increase	5.0%-7.5%	7.5%-10.0%	10.0%-12.0%
No increase	3.0%-4.0%	7.0%-9.0%	9.0%-12.0%	12.0%-14.0%

You will also notice that, for any particular performance level, the Salary Increase Guide Chart is constructed so that the salary increase percentage *decreases* as salary range quartile *increases*. In other words, of all employees who are rated as "Exceeds Requirements," for example, larger percentage increases are available to those at lower pay levels than at higher pay levels. (The reason for this will be explained later.) Thus, referring to the example Salary Increase Guide Chart, we see that an "Exceeds Requirements" employee whose salary is in the 4th quartile can receive an increase of 8.5 percent—9.5 percent, while an "Exceeds Requirements" employee whose salary is in the second quartile can receive an increase of 4.5 percent—5.5 percent. Thus, the second major feature of the Salary Increase Guide Chart is that the salary increase percentage *decreases* as salary level within range *increases*.

Now, let's look at the reasoning behind the construction of the Salary Increase Guide Chart in the manner just described. Why, for example, do we want the Salary Increase Guide Chart to provide for larger percentage pay increases for higher levels of performance? The answer is almost intuitive . . . we want our employees to be *motivated* to perform as well as their abilities will permit, and we feel that the lure of potentially larger pay increases for higher quality job performance will serve as a motivator for each employee to do his best. Looking at it from another point of view, what's to motivate an employee to try harder and perform his work better if doing so will have little or no effect on his salary increase? The point is that we believe that the opportunity to earn greater salary increases for better work performance will tend to encourage our employees to perform as well as they can.

On the other hand, the reason the Guide Chart provides for smaller pay increases at higher pay levels within a given salary range is a little more subtle and requires more explanation. The key to understanding this concept is to understand the significance we attach to the various points within a salary grade range—particularly the minimum, the midpoint, and the maximum. Regardless of which salary grade we are talking about, each of these reference points has the same conceptual significance.

The most significant point within any salary grade range is the MIDPOINT, because the midpoint is intended to represent the competitive average rate of pay for work of the level of complexity represented by the grade in question. This means that we would normally expect a fully qualified employee whose work performance is at least as good as the average in the marketplace to be paid a salary in the vicinity of the midpoint rate. Naturally, there can be a wide dispersion of actual employee salaries within any salary range, and not all employees will be paid at or near the midpoint salary.

To the extent that we pay salaries which are significantly less than the grade midpoint salary, what justifications are there to do so? One which may be obvious is the degree of experience an employee has in his position: it is unlikely that someone fairly new to his position can perform *all* aspects of his work in a fully satisfactory manner, at least initially. He justifiably should not earn the same pay level as a fully qualified and experienced employee at the same grade level, because he is still learning some aspects of his job, and he probably requires more supervisor guidance than the fully qualified employee. Thus, relative inexperience in the position is one rationale for paying less than the grade midpoint.

A less pleasant rationale for paying at a rate significantly less than the grade midpoint salary is poor employee performance. If an employee does not produce at the level reasonably expected for workers of similar experience at his grade level, he logically should be paid less than norm performers, if he is to be retained at all.

Without there being some agreed-upon lower limits, the preceding raises the question of just how much less than the midpoint salary can we justifiably pay someone to account for his lack of experience or his poor performance. The answer, of course, is the salary range MINIMUM. In fact, the MINIMUM is essentially defined to mean the lowest salary we would pay to anyone worthy of holding the job in question. In effect, it represents the pay rate for the least experienced candidate we would consider for the position, or the pay rate for the lowest level of performance we would tolerate from an incumbent in the position.

What about salary rates which exceed the grade midpoint . . . what is our justification for paying anyone a rate which exceeds the midpoint? The most acceptable rationale for paying such "premium" salaries is that the employees who command such salaries are notably better performers than the average of all workers who perform such work. In such cases, management feels that the additional quality and effort produced by very good performers is worth additional dollars, and that, by virtue of their high level performance, these employees deserve to be paid higher than the average for other employees at their grade levels.

How much higher than the midpoint rate is management willing to pay an employee for being an exceptional performer? The answer is the salary range MAXIMUM, which is as far above the midpoint as the minimum is below it. The MAXIMUM represents the highest premium management is willing to pay for *exceptional* work performance at any grade level.

Now that we understand the significance of the minimum, midpoint, and maximum, we are in a better position to understand why at any performance level the Salary Increase Guide Chart provides for relatively large pay increases for lower-paid employees and relatively smaller increases for highly-paid employees (i.e., those who are paid more than the grade midpoint). With limited budget resources available for all salary increases, we have to allocate these resources in the most cost-effective manner, and this is done on essentially a "worst first" basis. For example, if we have two "Outstanding" employees, one of whom is paid in the 4th quartile while the other is paid well above the midpoint, we want to reduce the difference between these two employees' pay levels. To the extent that we have an "outstanding" employee paid less than the midpoint we should feel conceptually uncomfortable, because a "Meets Requirement" employee should be able to attain a midpoint-level salary, given enough time in position. Thus, we want to accelerate the growth in salary level of the low-paid "Outstanding" employee in order to get his pay up and beyond the midpoint where, theoretically, it belongs. On the other hand, once an employee's pay exceeds the grade midpoint, he is already being paid a premium salary, and we want to slow down the rate at which he is pulling away from the midpoint. This treatment satisfies our conceptual sense of "rightness," and it allows us to distribute our limited salary increase funds in the most cost-effective manner.

C. The Performance Evaluation

We have already pointed out that *employee performance* is the *key variable* in determining the percentage amount of salary increase in a merit salary increase program. Obviously, then it is crucially important that we have a mutual understanding of the performance evaluation process, and that we have a common understanding of the meaning of performance terms such as "Outstanding," "Meets Requirements," and so on. Let us first look at the matter of performance level definitions, and then we can comment on the process of conducting a performance evaluation on any particular employee.

Performance Levels: The Concept of Normal Distribution

If we look at the work performance of a large enough group of employees, we would expect to see a wide range of quality in performance: a very few employees

may be very poor performers who are unsuited for the work they are paid to perform; a few others may be inexperienced and therefore not yet quite up to performing at the level expected of experienced workers; a substantial number of employees would likely be performing at the level one would expect from fully competent and experienced employees; a few others may have demonstrated an ability to perform all job requirements in the expected manner, as well as to perform at greater than the expected level for significant job duties; and, a relatively small number of employees may perform virtually all job duties in a truly exemplary manner.

We call this kind of distribution of performance a *normal distribution*. In statistics, a normal distribution means that, for whatever feature we are measuring, we expect most of our sample to be concentrated around the average, with relatively fewer and fewer samples to be found as we move farther and farther from the average in either direction. In the case at hand, this means that we would expect to see the bulk of our employees performing at a "Meets Requirements" level, with substantially fewer employees performing at "Meets Minimum Requirements" or "Exceeds Requirements," and a very few performing at an "Unsatisfactory" or an "Outstanding" level. The statistical characteristics of a normal distribution, if applied to our entire spectrum of work performance, suggest that we should expect to see the following percentages of our employees rated at each of the five performance levels:

Outstanding	2.5%
Exceeds Requirements	13.5%
Meets Requirements	68%
Meets Minimum Requirements	13.5%
Unsatisfactory	2.5%
	100%

However, we feel that the process of employee selection substantially reduces the likelihood that we would place employees in positions where their performance would be "Unsatisfactory" or "Meets Minimum Requirements;" in fact, we select employees with the expectation that they will "Meet Requirements," with the hope that some will evidence a higher level of performance and that only a very few will not meet expectations. Thus, we take the selection process into account in modifying our normal distribution of work performance, and the following represents our expectation of a more reasonable distribution of work performance:

Outstanding	5%
Exceeds Requirements	35%
Meets Requirements	55%
Meets Minimum Requirements	5%
Unsatisfactory	—
	100%

This means that, if we selected 100 workers and compared their work performances, we would expect 5% to be rated "Outstanding," 35% to be rated "Exceeds Requirements," and so on. Please note that our zero expectation of "unsatisfactory" performance does not mean that we'll never have someone whose performance is "Unsatisfactory" . . . it simply means that it should happen so rarely that it's not worth assigning an expectation number to it.

Performance Levels: What Do the Terms Mean?

We have all had experiences which suggest that a word or a group of words may have a different meaning to us than they do to someone else . . . your definition of a word such as "Outstanding" may differ from your friend's opinion of what "Outstanding" implies. Therefore, we want to describe as clearly as possible what we want each of our performance level designations to mean to all of you who will be involved in the merit program, either as a rater of others or as one whose performance is being rated. Let us begin with the pinnacle.

1. OUTSTANDING: (5%) This signifies the very best performance we can possibly expect of any employee in any given position. An outstanding employee has *mastered* every element of the assigned position and is performing at a level well beyond that normally expected of the vast majority of experienced workers with similar duties. The employee demonstrates personal *initiative* and an *innovative* flair in accepting new assignments, and he/she can be depended upon to consistently achieve high quality results. Employees rated at this level should be considered *prime* candidates for promotion, and their work record should be brought to the attention of top management.

POSSIBLE SYNONYMS: Exceptional, unique, superlative.

2. EXCEEDS REQUIREMENTS: (35%) This designation applies to workers whose performance is *clearly* and substantially above required performance, and which occasionally excels. The employee exhibits *complete* job knowledge and an ability to use that knowledge to adapt to changes in the work environment, usually with a minimum of supervisory guidance. He/she demonstrates special abilities, above those normally required for competent performance, in important aspects of the work; and he/she evidences no troublesome performance deficiencies in any element of the work. Continued performance at this level suggests that the employee is a good candidate for promotion.

POSSIBLE SYNONYMS: Commendable, noteworthy.

3. MEETS REQUIREMENTS: (55%) This designation applies to the substantial majority of employees who, on balance, perform at or somewhat above the required level; it encompasses good to very good performance. Employees at this performance level may exhibit some particular strengths and perhaps some areas of weakness in performance of job duties, but typically, the strengths more than offset the weaknesses. Job knowledge is fairly complete and is not a factor which significantly limits successful job performance.

POSSIBLE SYNONYMS: Competent, proficient, normal.

4. MEETS MINIMUM REQUIRE-MENTS: (5%)

A. As applied to fairly new incumbents, this designation implies that the only apparent barrier to attaining fully competent performance is the lack of some important pieces of job knowledge, which in most cases will be gained through on-the-job experience.

B. As applied to an experienced employee, the first evaluation at this level is a warning signal. It signifies that the employee makes too many errors or otherwise simply fails to perform some important aspects of the job in a manner that can be reasonably expected for someone of his or her experience and knowledge.

POSSIBLE SYNONYMS: Not quite sufficient, needs improvement.

5. UNSATISFAC-TORY:

This designation applies to employees who fail to meet the minimum acceptable standards of performance with respect to assigned duties, responsibilities, or conduct a *significant* portion of the work time, for whatever reason. Employees at this performance level should be considered for reassignment to a lower level position, if possible; otherwise, termination is the final alternative.

POSSIBLE SYNONYMS: Unacceptable, deficient.

D. The Performance Review Process

Up to this point, what you have read in these pages is primarily oriented toward your technical understanding of the merit salary increase program. However, it is important to keep in mind that the major purpose of such a program is the motivation of our employees to perform as well as they can and to encourage their personal development. Determining the amount of a salary increase is *not* an end in itself . . . rather, it is a means to an end.

It is the performance review (or "interview") which provides supervisors with an opportunity to sit down with each of their employees to discuss each one's job responsibilities, performance, and progress. These performance interviews are among the most important of all supervisory duties, because discussions of this sort should encourage the employee to continue doing the things he does well, and they help the employee to understand which features of his work performance need to be improved.

This latter point deserves special emphasis. Most of us would probably enjoy a discussion with a subordinate when the subject matter is the employee's strong points; but, we would probably feel a natural reluctance toward discussing the employee's weaker points because of the *assumed* negative connotations of such a discussion.

SOME WORDS OF CAUTION

One feature of the merit salary increase program which hasn't been discussed is its role as a cost control mechanism. Most of us are aware that top management makes budget allocations each year for items such as new facilities and equipment, expansion of services, renovations, and so on; but we may not be accustomed to thinking of salary costs as a budgeted item, when in fact they must be. The Salary Increase Guide Chart is a key mechanism which can be used to insure that salary adjustment costs are held within *approved budget limitations*.

It's important for you to have some understanding of how this works. Each year, the Employee Relations Department will prepare a Salary Increase Guide Chart which will allocate salary increase expenditures as outlined in the preceding pages, but we can expect to see variations from year to year in the Guide Chart depending for the most part upon economic circumstances. Three factors are taken into account in developing the annual Guide Chart: management's approved salary increase budget percentage; the distribution of actual employee salaries within the salary ranges; and the *expected distribution of employee performance ratings*.

Please note that the first two of these three factors are knowns, while the latter one is estimated. It is this very fact which makes it so important that supervisors and managers are aware of what we consider to be a reasonable distribution of employee performance ratings (i.e., up to 5% "Outstanding;" up to 35% "Exceeds Requirements," and so on), because we use the *expected distribution* as though it were a known in constructing the Guide Chart.

To the extent that performance raters tend to exceed the expected distribution of performance ratings, we will tend to overspend the salary increase budget. Some organizations which use a merit salary increase program prevent the problem of overspending because of excessively high performance ratings by using the concept of *forced performance distributions*.

Under the forced distribution concept, management allocates a predetermined number of each performance level rating to each manager. For example, if a manager has 20 salaried employees whose performance he rates, he is permitted to have two (10%) rated as "Outstanding," five (25%) rated as "Exceeds Requirements," twelve (60%) rated as "Meets Requirements," etc. This approach virtually guarantees that the salary budget will not be exceeded.

We consider the use of a forced distribution system as something to be used only if supervisors and managers demonstrate an inability to keep their performance ratings within statistical reason. Rather, we prefer to educate performance raters on the mechanics of the program and what it is intended to accomplish, and we hope that doing so will produce results that are in line with management expectations.

E. The Performance Evaluation Form

The performance appraisal is used to determine an employee's overall performance level for purposes of performance increases and/or an employee's satisfactory development in his position. In view of these uses, it is *essential* that performance ratings be based on objective and work related factors having direct impact on such performance. A distinct effort should be made not to distort ratings of work performance by estimates of potential or by personal biases. Each individual must be rated against the requirements of the position (via the position description or position content questionnaire) during the review period indicated.

The ten principal factors shown on the performance evaluation form [Exhibit 14-4] may only be relative in varying degrees and some may not be appropriate in every case. These factors are *not* what the employee is being measured on. He or she is being measured against the requirements, responsibilities, and accountabilities shown on the position description and the ten factors have been formulated as those basic factors which are useful in *discussing* poor, accept-

able, or outstanding performance. It may be, other, unlisted factors are important elements in the position and should, therefore, be included in the narrative section of the evaluation.

There are many factors, however, which are *not* job related, are extraneous and will not be used, considered, or referred to in the evaluation process. They include:

1. Time in position/time in company.
2. Time before retirement
3. Age
4. Race
5. Color
6. Sex
7. National origin
8. Handicap
9. Veteran status
10. Religion
11. Physical appearance
12. Marital status
13. Relationship to others (Relatives, associations, etc.)

Also, it is important to only consider the performance level experienced during the evaluation period in question. The level of performance experienced during previous periods should not influence the current assessments. Naturally, it would be permissible to denote *improvement* or *deterioration* as compared to previous periods.

The following questions may be asked in preparing an evaluation of each factor:

1. *Job Knowledge*
   What has this individual done to actually demonstrate depth, currency, or breadth of job knowledge in the performance of duties?
2. *Judgement and Decisions*
   Does this person think clearly and develop correct and logical conclusions? Report on how this person grasps, analyzes, and presents workable solutions to problems.
3. *Plan and Organize Work*
   Does this person look beyond immediate job requirements? How well does he/she anticipate critical events?
4. *Management of Resources*
   Does this individual "manage" to achieve optimum economy through effective utilization of personnel and material? Consider the balance between minimum cost and false economy to the ultimate expense of the project or objective.

5. *Adaptability to Stress*

   What is the effect of stress on this person's performance? Does he/she work as well or better under adverse conditions? In difficult situations, heavy workloads and pressures, does his/her work deteriorate?

6. *Oral Communication*

   How well has this person been able to present ideas orally?

7. *Written Communication*

   How well has this person been able to present ideas in writing?

8. *Human Relations*

   How does this person work with and relate to others? How does this person demonstrate his/her support of the company's Equal Opportunities and Affirmative Action programs?

9. *Quantity*

   How does the volume of work compare to your expectations of all things such as interruptions, special projects, etc. considered? You must, of course, balance quantity of work with quality of work considered next. Standard output will vary for different kinds and levels of positions, and in each instance the supervisor should refer to the position description in determining a reasonable standard.

10. *Quality*

    How accurate, presentable, or reliable is the work of this individual? Does it need more or less checking? Does it meet organizational standards, policies, and procedures? How consistent was the quality of his work under varying conditions? Is the work complete and thorough? Again, this factor must be balanced with quantity.

In evaluating the "Level of Performance" for each factor, compare the employee's accomplishments of his job objectives with the "Standards of Performance" reflected in [Exhibit 14-8]. These standards of performance are to be used as guidelines for evaluating the employee, and are not to be construed as the all-inclusive ideal. Rather they establish certain minimum requirements for a specific performance level. An "Outstanding" rating for any factor also presupposes that the employee meets all the criteria for "Exceeds Requirements" and "Meets Requirements" for that factor. These "standards" are *not to be used* or *paraphrased* as specific examples in the narrative sections of the evaluation form. They are simply standards by which the evaluator can judge which performance ratings are supported by the specific accomplishments of the employee.

The determination of the *overall performance level* of the employee constitutes the core of the review, and requires careful attention. It represents the supervisor's judgement as to the employee's overall performance of the *position's* responsibilities and requirements. In determining the overall evaluation, consideration must be given the *relative weighting* of the ten key performance factors and the level of performance noted for each factor. In this way, a "weighted average" composite level can be determined for the overall performance level. You can refer to an earlier part of this section for a narrative description of each performance level to assist in this determination.

Please feel free to contact your local Personnel Manager for assistance or contact any staff member in the Employee Relations Compensation Section.

In completing the narrative sections of the evaluation form, be *specific* and give illustrative examples of accomplishments that occurred during the review period. Feel free to use Attachments for additional space. (Exhibit 14-6 may be used for this purpose.)

The following questions may be posed when collecting data for completion of these sections:

1. *"Comment on Achievement of Specific Goals and Objectives"*

   Review of an employee's performance, factor by factor, the objectives and goals established for this individual's areas, and in reviewing the job description or position content questionnaire will provide a supervisor with data in which to complete this section. Also comment on the extent to which the employee has accomplished the objectives assigned to him/her . . . formally or informally. Note significant departures from program and schedule for objectives and give reasons.

2. *"Comment on Specific Significant Contributions Employee Has Made"*

   Indicate the most significant contribution the employee has made to his unit, the department, or the organization during the review period. Give *specific* examples in which to support the performance levels given in the first section and note those areas which deserve special praise or attention.

3. *"Specific Areas Where Improvement Is Needed"*

   This review may discover areas in which the employees should/must improve. One factor may be below standard, or, if improved, would greatly enhance his/her effectiveness. These areas noted should also include *what* is being done or should be done to improve them.

Exhibit 14-8 Standards for Evaluating Salaried Employees' Performance

SALARIED PERFORMANCE STANDARDS
(To be used with Performance Evaluation Form # 94366)

Performance Factors	(5) Unsatisfactory	(4) Meets Minimum Requirements (Needs Improvement)	(3) Meets Requirements	(2) Exceeds Requirements	(1) Outstanding
		Standards:	Standards:	Standards:	Standards:
1. Job Knowledge (Depth, currency, breadth)	• Has serious gaps in technical and professional knowledge • Knows only most rudimentary phase of job • Lack of knowledge affects productivity • Requires abnormal amount of checking	• Technical and professional knowledge is inadequate for the job • Must be assigned only routine duties and monitored regularly • Requires close supervision	• Demonstrates adequate technical and professional knowledge required for the job • Searches out facts and arrives at sound solutions to problems • Broad knowledge of related jobs and functions • Conversant with significant job-related developments	• Possesses keen insight and the ability to evolve it into practical solutions • Keeps informed of important developments in related fields • Can handle difficult situations effectively • Broad knowledge of related missions • Rarely requires guidance or assistance	• Possesses superb technical and professional knowledge • Sufficiently well versed in his/her job to discuss and implement improved methods resulting in savings in manpower or material • Maintains and increases professional and technical knowledge • Actively pursues new ideas and developments and their relation to the overall mission • Recognized authority in his or her field
2. Judgement and Decisions (Consistent, accurate, effective)	• Reluctant to make decisions on his or her own • Decisions are usually not reliable • Declines to accept responsibility for decisions	• Usually makes sound routine decisions • Tends to procrastinate on necessary decisions • Reluctant to evaluate factors before arriving at decisions	• Seeks out all available data before arriving at decisions • Consistently provides accurate decisions • Accepts responsibility for decisions and learns from incorrect judgements • Provides effective decisions by clear and logical thinking	• An exceptionally sound, logical thinker • Does not hesitate to make required decisions • Decisions are consistently correct • Opinions and judgement are often solicited by others	• Keen, analytical thinker • Makes accurate decisions under intense pressure • Extremely effective in exercising logic in broad areas of responsibility
3. Plan and Organize Work (Timely and creative)	• Fails to plan ahead • Disorganized and usually unprepared • Objectives are not met on time	• Scheduling and organizational efforts normally fail • Encounters difficulty with tasks other than routine • Finished products are usually behind schedule	• Careful, effective planner • Anticipates and solves problems • Effectively balances resources • Finished products are consistently submitted on time	• Plans beyond requirements of present job • Plans coincide with related activities • Is flexible and able to adjust priorities • Frequently called on to organize complex tasks	• Able to anticipate critical events and makes prior provisions to deal with them • Plans encompass all feasible contingencies • Extremely effective in utilization of resources
4. Management of Resources (Manpower and material)	• Wastes or misuses resources • No system established for accounting of material • Causes delay for others by mismanagement	• Accomplishes conservation of material on a sporadic basis • Squanders resources to get job done	• Uses minimum material with good results • Establishes controls to ensure that manpower and material are accounted for and conserved • Develops and uses cost-effective methods	• Excellent results accomplished at minimum cost • Consistently suggests methods of conserving resources • Skillfully uses cost-effectiveness studies	• Extremely effective in use of material • Consistently seeks and projects ways of using existing equipment • Is often assigned to difficult and important projects where limited resources are a significant factor
5. Adaptability to Stress (Stable, dependable) flexible	• Panics in new situation • Tendency to shirk difficult situations • Reaction is unpredictable	• Prefers to work on routine tasks • Jumps to erroneous conclusions in new situations • Hesitates to become involved in new situations	• Flexible and open to new ideas • Willingly seeks assistance in difficult situations • Provides reliable decisions under pressure • Consistently displays calm and controlled behavior	• Readily adapts to fluctuations and changing priorities • Consistently performs well in difficult situations • Anticipates changes and is prepared to react accordingly	• Responds quickly and effectively to crises • Systematically succeeds where others fail • Consistently provides outstanding leadership and guidance under difficult and stressful conditions

Exhibit 14-8 continued

Performance Factors	(5) Unsatisfactory	(4) Meets Minimum Requirements (Needs Improvement)	(3) Meets Requirements	(2) Exceeds Requirements	(1) Outstanding
	Standards:	Standards:	Standards:	Standards:	Standards:
6. Oral Communication (Clear, concise, confident)	• Does not convey ideas clearly and concisely • Has limited vocabulary • Cannot express thoughts in a logical sequence	• Only occasionally able to verbally convey useful information • Briefings and discussions frequently exhibit a lack of confidence	• Gives direct and understandable responses to questions • Gives briefings which are organized and well presented	• Very articulate in a wide range of difficult communications situations • Puts extra effort into conversing well • Capable of persuading an audience	• Delivers concise, well-organized presentations • Is often called on to present and explain difficult and complex subjects • Can sway a hostile audience to his or her point of view
7. Written Communication (Clear, concise, organized)	• Written communications are inadequate due to errors in vocabulary, spelling and grammer • Communications often raise doubt as to exact meaning • Others must continually seek clarification or correct errors	• Clarity of written communications is inconsistent • Only occasionally able to convey a cogent idea • Extensive editing and correcting is usually required before communications can be dispatched	• Writing is clear and concise • Written instructions and reports are readily understandable • Written communications are consistently well organized and grammatically correct	• Written reports can be easily followed by all readers • Communications are succinct and concise, containing only those words necessary to express an idea	• Able to describe complex or technical concepts so well that even the casual reader can readily comprehend the idea • Is consistently chosen for the most important and difficult writing assignments • Is frequently asked to edit the written correspondence of others
8. Human Relations	• Openly and knowingly practices discrimination • Uses racial epithets or sexual slurs maliciously • Is deliberately hostile to minorities or members of the opposite sex • Does not show any consideration or concern for others	• Displays very limited sensitivity to equal opportunity policies • Treats minorities or members of the opposite sex markedly different than other personnel • Employs inflammatory or derogatory terms toward minorities or members of the opposite sex • Tends to lack concern for peers and subordinates	• Treats all personnel fairly and equitably • Voluntarily participates in activities in support of equal opportunity • Shows concern and is sensitive to needs of others	• Demonstrates exceptional skill in working with others and eliciting their cooperation • Establishes and enthusiastically maintains standards of equal opportunity • Encourages practice of equal opportunity and treatment in all activities • Displays a high degree of sensitivity and concern for others	• Demonstrates clearly superior ability to work with others and to elicit their cooperation • Displays extreme sensitivity and a deep concern in all dealings with peers and subordinates • Is extremely effective in solving human relations problems - solutions always reflect fair and equal treatment
9. Quantity	• Assignments and tasks are often not completed on a timely basis • Completes assignments in a sporadic basis and overall completion rate is unsatisfactory • Often wastes time in completion of non-essential tasks or duties while higher priority items await attention • Does not meet time limits or expectations on a frequent basis • Does not adjust pace to meet work demands	• Does not complete all required work in a timely basis • Does not always anticipate work flow or adjust to peak and slack periods of work • Works sporadically, and at times unable to adjust work level to demand • Often does not establish or meet deadlines in completion of long projects. Therefore, is not often able to take corrective action in order to meet deadlines	• Completes all required work assignments on time • Able to anticipate work flow and accomodate for peak periods and slack periods • Works at a steady pace generating a normal amount of output in a satisfactory manner • Establishes time targets to insure work is progressing as planned and takes necessary corrective action to meet deadlines	• Completes all required, in addition to "extra" work assignments, in a most timely manner • Assists others frequently in completion of their assignments • Frequently volunteers and completes additional work or projects • Able to forecast work peak loads and arrange and adjust pace to easily accomodate extra assignments as necessary • Consistently meets all deadlines while often completing more than expected or required	• All work is completed at a fast pace and is consistently completed early • Continually assists others in the completion of their assignments • Continually volunteers for additional assignments and projects and meets deadlines with ease • Easily adjusts to changing workloads and completes all assignments as required
10. Quality	• Frequent errors are made and validity of completed work must be frequently checked for accuracy • Completed work does not often meet expectations or does not meet standards, policies or procedures • Other staff members must frequently assist employee in the adequate completion of work assignments • Completed work must often be redone, or reassigned in order to meet acceptable standards	• Most work completed is accurate but mistakes or inaccuracies are discovered. Some work completed does not meet expectations or does not adhere to policies or standards • Employee does not always spot check work in order to discover and take corrective action and errors or problems • Work needs frequent follow-up to insure accuracy, objectives and expectations are met	• Work completed is accurate, adheres to policies and procedures and is acceptable in all respects • Employee conducts periodic spot audits to insure that work meets standards • Meets expectations in work assignments. Work is completed and rarely needs follow-up	• Work completed is always accurate and thoroughly checked for completeness. Needs little, if any, supervisory review for accuracy • Work produced exceeds normal expectation and adheres to all standards of quality, policies and procedures • Work is extremely presentable and exhibits those qualities of professionalism and is clearly superior to the "normal" work expected	• Regardless of situation, always completes work assignments with clearly exceptional accuracy, and serves as a "model" for high quality work • Acts as a resource person for others in the completion of accurate work • Work always exceeds standards, meeting policies, procedures and expectations and is thoroughly checked prior to submission. Needs no follow-up or checking for accuracy • Works consistently brings praise as to the degree of accuracy, understandability and remark `results

4. *"Comments on Specific Contributions Made in Equal Employment/Affirmative Action Including Achievement of Goals and Objectives"*
This section *must* be completed for all those individuals who supervise others or have the effective recommendation to hire, fire, or change status of others. The accomplishment and progress on the affirmative action goals and in the support of the affirmative action program should be reviewed in this section. *Specific* data and accomplishments must be noted in this section and in any required attachments.

Those employees who have no supervisory or line authority need only have an assessment on their "support" of organizational goals and objectives. However, any employee that is rated "Deficient in Support Of" these goals must have the specifics outlined in an attachment.

The remaining portions of the form should be completed as outlined. When the form is returned by Employee Relations, a discussion should be held with the employee and copies of this assessment provided to him. The employee should sign the file copies to indicate that he was provided an opportunity to review this assessment with his supervisors.

THE PERFORMANCE REVIEW AND EMPLOYEE COMMUNICATION

Performance evaluation without communication is less than half the job.

After completion of the performance evaluation, the supervisor must review and discuss the results of the evaluation in detail with the employee. The interview itself and information shared during the interview is far more important than the evaluation form used.

It is suggested that prior to the interview, the individual should draw up his accomplishments against predetermined goals. If goals were not established for the appraisal period, he/she should be asked to list major accomplishments in terms of responsibilities in order of importance.

Purpose:

The objectives of the performance appraisal interview are threefold:

1. *Establish/Clarify Mutual Goals between The Managers and Their Subordinates*
Provides an opportunity for supervisor and subordinate to *clarify* and establish their mutual expectations. The supervisor should explain to their employees what is expected of them and how their performance and achievements are to be measured. Employees must also have ample opportunity to discuss and review their own ambitions, goals and expectations. An *effective, two-way* communication must be established in order to avoid basic misconceptions or misunderstandings and in order to establish a sound foundation for improved working relationships.
2. *Identify Both Individual Accomplishments and To Identify Strengths and Weaknesses*
Provides employees with feedback as to the level of their performance and acknowledges and recognizes special areas of achievements. While most subordinates receive some indications of how they are doing on a continuous basis – a complete discussion of all aspects is of significant importance. This evaluation also allows supervisors a chance to point out to their subordinates areas in which they need to improve *and* suggestions as to how to go about it. This can easily be the most fruitful aspect of the performance review and supervisors should take full advantage of it.
3. *Provide an Opportunity for Planning Career Development*
From information received during the appraisal interview, the employee receives valuable information for planning his/her own career — information about new administrative techniques, improved human relations skills and understanding, and a better understanding of the skills required at higher level positions. The interview can provide a highly motivating tool for continuous self-development. Most development programs fail because the individual does not clearly recognize the specific needs for development. An individual must be plainly aware of his needs for development, for without such knowledge, training and development appear superfluous or irrelevant.

Discussion

In planning and conducting performance discussions, the following points are provided as guides:

1. The interview should proceed in private and in a relaxed atmosphere; an effort should be made to put the employee at ease.
2. The purpose of performance evaluation and discussion should be carefully explained, along with a brief description of how the evaluations were determined.
3. For effective communication to take place, the employee should be given a chance to talk also. The employee should be encouraged to express his thoughts for effective communication to occur.
4. In discussing an employee's problem or improvement points, supervisors should stress a plan of action for improving them. Bear in mind that any plan of action for improvement or development should start with the employee's agreement and commitment.
5. Supervisors should refrain from making promises they may not be able to keep. Salary increases or promotions *should never be* announced unless and *until* they have been *finally approved* by the Employee Relations Department.
6. Before concluding the discussion, the supervisor should briefly summarize the main points. Many points may have been discussed, and unless properly put into perspective, major issues may be overshadowed by insignificant comments.

Performance Appraisal Counseling Checklist

Attached is a checklist which supervisors may find helpful in preparing for a performance appraisal interview/discussion.

PERFORMANCE APPRAISAL COUNSELING CHECKLIST

This list of critical requirements should be used in planning performance appraisal counseling sessions. The use of the appropriate items on this list and *specific* examples of work accomplished during the evaluation period will aid supervisors in conducting an effective performance evaluation with their subordinates.

During your counseling session make certain that these areas are thoroughly discussed:

1. Typical level of performance of assigned duties.
2. Achievements deserving special note.
3. Minor deficiencies.
4. Serious deficiencies.
5. Plans for training and education.
6. Future assignments/Career planning.

The following functional areas may also be discussed as appropriate:

A. Proficiency in Completing Assigned Responsibilities
1. Possessing fundamental training.
2. Improving effectiveness.
3. Keeping well informed in profession/specialty.
4. Applying training and information.
5. Showing ingenuity in profession/career.
6. Handling related assignments.

B. Proficiency in Supervising Personnel
7. Matching personnel with the job.
8. Delegating authority.
9. Providing instructions.
10. Insuring comprehension.
11. Providing reasons and explanations.
12. Supporting authorized actions.
13. Encouraging ideas.
14. Developing teamwork.
15. Setting a good example.
16. Assisting subordinates.
17. Evaluating subordinates.
18. Looking out for subordinates.

C. Proficiency in Planning, Directing Action
19. Managing resources (cost conservation).
20. Resolving problems.
21. Making use of experience.
22. Long-range planning.
23. Taking prompt action.
24. Suspending judgement.
25. Making proper decisions.
26. Retaining facts.

D. Acceptance of Organizational Responsibility

27. Complying with policies and directives.
28. Accepting organizational procedures.
29. Subordinating personal interests.
30. Cooperating with associates.
31. Showing loyalty.
32. Taking responsibilities for subordinates.

E. Acceptance of Personal Responsibility

33. Attending to responsibilities.
34. Attending to details.
35. Assignments completed on time.
36. Being fair and scrupulous.

37. Adapting to the job.
38. Participating in community/professional activities.

F. Proficiency in Handling Administrative Details

39. Understanding instructions.
40. Scheduling work.
41. Obtaining information from records.
42. Checking accuracy of work.
43. Writing letters and reports.
44. Obtaining cooperation.
45. Presenting finished work.
46. Keeping others informed.

15. Performance Appraisal in Health Organizations

GARY S. LEVITZ

Managers in health organizations, as in any industrial entity, strive to keep their operations within a budget. Health managers, in contrast to those in other industrial sectors, often are more constrained and influenced by external pressures and regulations that press for cost containment and efficiency. As a result, if health organizations are to be competitive, they must develop and adopt new methods of management and apply successful industrial techniques to improve performance. With the effective transfer of this knowledge, health organizations, through the integration of industrial models, can become both more efficient and more aware of the effectiveness of their activities on a day-to-day basis. However, many areas of industrial management practice have been ignored by executives of health care institutions.

One such technique that has not attracted as much attention in the health field as in other industrial areas is employee performance appraisal. This is one field that holds great opportunity for effective health management. Through the design, implementation, and maintenance of an employee performance appraisal system, both individual and organizational performance may be monitored and improved, with the end result being a more efficient and effective institution.

The need to monitor the activities of the health care organization and its personnel is clear. Salaries and wages may be as high as 60 percent to 70 percent of the total operating costs of the average hospital. This makes it clear that a linkage exists between the successful operation of the organization and the effective and efficient performance of its employees. The institution's direct and indirect costs of turnover, absenteeism, and job withdrawal provide additional reasons to develop an employee appraisal system. Finally, a good performance evaluation system can help the organization attract and retain high performers. It is in this context that the design and implementation of strategies that the health manager may adopt are considered.

Too often, performance appraisal systems in health organizations rely primarily on tenure as a major, if not sole, criterion for determining wages. Administrators need to understand the influences a performance system may have on employee turnover and absenteeism and its link to productivity improvement and measurement. Based on this understanding, administrators may begin to apply motivational and developmental principles to the design and implementation of a performance appraisal system. The key to good design is to encourage performance based on developmental principles rather than to rely on traditional methods that are based on judgments—or no judgment at all, as when tenure is a criterion.

Administrators may not take the time to learn about new ways of motivating employees unless they are convinced that the new principles will, indeed, result in a return greater than current methods are producing. Such is the case with performance appraisal. Many organizations have adopted a haphazard approach of

225

applying the appraisal process to one or two departments, leaving the rest to rely on traditional methods. The end result is not a system but an approach that, in fact, may be detrimental to the overall organizational performance. This will be due, in large part, to the conflict and disagreement on goals. The challenge to health management is to study the benefits of a performance appraisal system and to integrate it into its operation on an organizationwide basis with a long-term commitment.

Performance appraisal in health organizations provides the focus for this article. The first section of the article presents arguments for the implementation of an employee appraisal system. This is followed by a discussion of the purposes of performance evaluation and its contribution to management control. There are many approaches to performance appraisal and some of them are presented in the next section. Some implementations of these programs have met with overwhelming success; this and the possible reasons for some of the failures are discussed next. The benefits of adopting management by objectives (MBO) in the health care institution, its contribution to improving organizational effectiveness, and its many definitions follow. Appraising employee performance in MBO and the process of goal setting are discussed. The final sections highlight applications of MBO in health organizations, discuss the importance of implementing and maintaining the system, analyze recent applications in the health care field, and conclude with guidelines for establishing an MBO program.

REASONS FOR IMPLEMENTING AN APPRAISAL SYSTEM

The development and monitoring of a performance appraisal system should become a key part of management's responsibility for several reasons:

- Evaluation of employees is a critical management task. Management needs to be able to make administrative decisions that reflect changes in employees' status, such as actions on merit raises, bonuses, promotions, transfers, and release.
- Management needs to have up-to-date information on the performance of individual units and departments. Through the measurement of individual performance, management can obtain information on the larger units of which the particular employee is a part.
- Performance appraisal programs provide information to managers on the skills and abilities of individual employees. This information helps to validate the organization's selection procedures and

provide an evaluation of an employee's participation in training programs.
- The system provides information on the quality of managers' supervision.
- The accomplishment of these procedures provides information for analyzing the role of management in bringing about changes in the performance and subsequent development of employees.

A meaningful employee appraisal system may aid the organization by helping individuals identify areas for change, improvement, and development. It also may provide supervisors with information on the quality of the direction they provide. If this is to be accomplished, the manager must adopt the role of a counselor rather than judge. The manager then can assist individuals in increasing their abilities through a helping relationship, rather than through the traditional superior/subordinate posture. However, if a manager is to adopt a new practice, time must be available during which the new procedures can be implemented slowly. In large part, this gradual implementation may be necessary to counter resistance to new techniques. The development of an employee appraisal system provides a new dimension of managerial control that can have benefits beyond those provided by current systems.

It is very important that the manager be certain that the employees' activities are not random but are predictable and contributing to the accomplishment of the organization's goals. Most organizations attempt to assure that there is appropriate behavior through a recruitment process that screens individuals and places those with given abilities and skills at the appropriate job level. In this process, management attempts to identify potentially successful performers prior to their employment by comparing them with the characteristics of employees currently performing the same types of jobs well. Various prehiring approaches are used, among them aptitude tests, achievement tests, interviews, collection of biographical information, and licensure. Organizations also provide training and development programs in cases where they are committed to the development of particular employees.

It would appear that if these activities were carried out successfully at a basic level, a performance evaluation system would be unnecessary. Unfortunately, this is not the case. Performance evaluation, in and of itself, can contribute significantly to the success of other areas through identification of individuals who are performing at different levels: some whose performance is unacceptable, others whose performance is exemplary and worthy of recognition. The identification of the different levels of competence may help those involved in the selection process to pinpoint employees who would benefit from a training and development program. The benefits of a performance evaluation and appraisal program appear to be substantial from a management perspective. However, an effective system also can contribute indirectly to increased levels of job performance and satisfaction.

Cummings and Schwab[1] discuss the impact of performance appraisal on important managerial and individual outcomes. Performance evaluation, in their perspective, is a managerial technique for improving organizational operation and individual satisfaction through the effective linking of performance and rewards. Management can affect employee self-images through the definition of criteria it identifies as important in the appraisal system. An effective system attempts to maximize personal and organizational goals. Individuals take the path they perceive as a way to achieve their own objectives through the accomplishment of organizational goals. A good appraisal system provides individuals with the opportunity to achieve both.

The performance appraisal system provides information for organizational control and maintenance through the measurement of effectiveness and efficiency of individuals and units. It also can increase satisfaction and performance, as has been indicated. The information it generates can be useful in identifying individuals for reward and/or further training. When used properly, the system should be both evaluative and developmental for employees and the organization at the same time. Yet too many managers view performance appraisal as being solely evaluative. When managers adopt such a perspective, employees tend to view such systems more as disciplinary than as helpful.

PURPOSES OF PERFORMANCE EVALUATION

Cummings and Schwab offer a framework for an analysis of the different approaches to performance evaluation.[2] The system is best for the organization and makes its greatest positive contribution in the areas of job satisfaction and productivity when it is viewed and operated as a developmental program. The time orientation focuses on future performance rather than on a critique by management of past performance. A developmental system improves performance through self-learning and personal growth whereas a judgmental system attempts to improve employee performance through changing personnel and the reward system. A key aspect of a developmental program is

the means by which it achieves its objectives. Specifically, a developmental system includes both a goal-setting process and developmental programs (one of which is management by objectives, which is discussed in detail later in this article). Judgmental programs attempt to measure past performance and use a variety of techniques such as rating scales, rankings, and comparisons (also discussed in this article).

The operation of these two distinctly different types of systems has implications for the way in which the rater is viewed by the employees. In the developmental system, the rater is viewed as a counselor or a guide, and the rater views the role as providing encouragement to the employee in the process of self-development. The evaluative system places the rater in the role of an evaluator, one who must judge the value of the employee's previous performance. As a result, the individual being rated in an evaluative system usually is passive or defensive of previous performance. In the developmental system, however, the individual is actively involved in the learning process and in plans for future gains in job performance.

This discussion highlights the fact that all managers are involved in performance appraisal, whether or not it is systematized and whether or not it is judgmental or developmental. The argument being advanced in this article is that all managers should be involved in an organizationwide formal appraisal system and that it should be developmental in nature and focus. The role of performance appraisal in any organization, and in health organizations in particular, is becoming more crucial to the institution's effectiveness. Information that is a byproduct of such a system also may provide links to other areas that are crucial to the appropriate functioning of management.

APPROACHES TO PERFORMANCE APPRAISAL

Performance appraisal systems produce many benefits and, as a result, many programs are in use.[3, 4] There are four general categories of approaches involved in the development of a system:[5]

1. comparative procedures
2. absolute standards
3. direct indexes
4. management by objectives

Each of the first three is described briefly in the following section; the fourth area receives greater attention, providing a major focus of this article.

Comparative Procedures

In this type of evaluation, an appraisal is made by comparing an employee against others on the criterion of interest. There are four procedures by which these comparisons generally may be made.

Straight Ranking

The evaluator considers all of the employees to be appraised and identifies the best performer, second best, and so on to the very weakest.

Alternative Ranking

The evaluator is given an alphabetical list of employees and identifies the best and weakest individuals. These individuals are removed from the list and placed on a separate ranking sheet. The process is then repeated starting with the original list.

Paired Comparison

One employee at a time is compared with every other one. An individual's final ranking is determined by the number of times that person is chosen over the others.

Forced Distribution

The evaluator is forced to assign a certain proportion of the unit's employees to each of several categories on each criterion. The evaluator may be forced to appraise 10 percent of the subordinates as lowest on a factor, 20 percent as below average, 40 percent average, 20 percent above average, and 10 percent highest.

Absolute Standards

When systems using absolute standards are used, there are significant differences from the comparative procedures just described. Systems using absolute standards evaluate individuals against written standards rather than against other employees and measure several factors of global performance rather than a single dimension. Some of the procedures that use absolute standards follow.

Critical Incidents

The evaluator is expected to record positive and negative incidents that relate specifically to activities required for successful completion of a job.

Weighted Checklists

The first step is to identify and assign a weight to each of the tasks to be evaluated. The evaluator then is given a checklist of statements on employee performance and the scores are summed.

Forced Choice

The evaluator is forced to choose the item that is most descriptive of an employee from a cluster of items.

Graphic Rating Scale

The graphic rating scale is perhaps the most widely used performance evaluation procedure. Presented with several statements about employee characteristics or performance, the evaluator checks a point along a scale that represents the assessment of the individual on that characteristic. The scale categories can reflect any of a number of dimensions ranging from below average to above average, or unsatisfactory to outstanding. The individual is evaluated by checking the appropriate box along the dimension being scaled. Excellent examples of this method are provided by Guion.[6]

Behaviorally Anchored Rating Scales (BARS)

The process of developing a behaviorally anchored rating scale (BARS) system of evaluation is similar to the development of critical incidents. This process is used to construct the rating scale applied in a BARS system of evaluation. Specifically, characteristics that contribute to successful job performance are identified and then reduced to a manageable number of dimensions. Judges (managers) then are asked to describe critical incidents that apply to the behavioral dimensions. These reviewers then place a scale value next to the critical incidents. After pilot testing, a value on a BARS is developed that is job related, and specific incidents on the rating scale are used. The employee's evaluation is determined by summing the scores across all categories. The use of BARS represents movement away from a judgmental approach to evaluation and is directed toward the accomplishment of evaluations that are developmental in nature.[7, 8, 9, 10]

Direct Indexes

Through the use of direct indexes, it is possible to obtain information on performance without engaging in an evaluative process. This means that it is not necessary for superiors to assess employee performance. There are two methods of direct index appraisal.

Measures of Productivity

Measures can be developed that quantify some elements of output, such as gross sales or quality of product produced. In the health sector, measures of occupancy or visits or services produced may be used. Such measures are useful when an individual has substantial control in producing a particular output or when groups are being evaluated to appraise the effectiveness of supervision. In other situations, however, they should not be applied.

Measures of Withdrawal

Measures of turnover and absenteeism can provide direct information on productivity and indirect information in such areas as job satisfaction and employee morale.

Management by Objectives (MBO)

Management by objectives is a method directed toward a result-based development program involving the establishment of goals (or objectives) by the use of superior-subordinate conferences. MBO goes beyond an evaluation technique and usually is integrated with other institutional maintenance and control programs that may include such functions as training, motivation, planning, and organizational development. Briefly, the MBO program involves:

1. defining employee goals and establishing a realistic time period for their accomplishment
2. determining how the accomplishment of these goals will be measured
3. coming to an agreement on these two factors, with the superior playing a supportive role and helping the subordinate to accomplish goals.
4. performing a self-appraisal prior to the goal-setting meeting with the employee's superior
5. discussing the appraisal with the supervisor and setting new goals

MBO programs are becoming increasingly popular.[11] In large part this may be because an MBO program contributes to the development of employees and in some part because, when implemented properly, it can contribute to and influence the organization's planning process.

Many of the *Fortune 500* industrial firms responding to a survey indicated that they had MBO type programs in operation.[12] The popularity of MBO stems from a variety of reasons. An effective program results in decisions being made on employees and their performance based on the outcome of their efforts rather than on personality traits. In other programs, personal biases and prejudices may influence raters, resulting in conflict and high levels of dissatisfaction. MBO programs also may force, or at least encourage, administrators to implement effective planning operations and management information and control systems. A properly implemented program also can result in a system that is not difficult for superior or subordinates to operate. This system can provide information for decisions about promotions and compensation. The main benefit is derived from the fact that as the organization moves away from an evaluative approach, it creates an environment in which the appraisal system may be used to help individual employees develop and reach their potential.

With this benefit in mind, MBO had been adopted by many organizations in various economic sectors. Yet before such programs can be successful, there may be obstacles that must be overcome. Otherwise, MBO may be less effective than if there had been adequate preparation through training and study of the organizational climate or if the institution's members had been willing to be more open.

Traditional MBO programs are result oriented. They may focus attention away from how results are achieved so that it is difficult to correct performances. Comparisons with subordinates are difficult in this system because of the individual goal-setting process. However, when the program is understood by the participants, and training is provided, MBO may be developed to correspond with larger organizational goals. Furthermore, once top and middle level management is involved and committed to its operation, there is an excellent opportunity for success.[13, 14]

WHY PERFORMANCE EVALUATION SYSTEMS SOMETIMES FAIL

A performance evaluation system such as MBO is part of and contributes to good management planning and control measures. Any health organization that strives to be effective and efficient needs formal mechanisms through which its activities may be monitored. As an example, the personnel function needs to direct its activity toward the monitoring of employee performance in addition to its traditional tasks of employee selection and recruitment. Yet it is important that this activity not occur independently of the other functions of management. In cases where performance appraisal is not integrated throughout the organization, the system is likely to be doomed to fail. Through an analysis of the reasons why performance evaluation systems may fail, the characteristics of well-designed programs may be identified.

Performance evaluation systems may fail for a variety of reasons, but it appears that the major factors may be classified under two categories:

1. systems that fail because they are not part of the larger personnel and management systems
2. systems that fail because of operational problems.

Although this article focuses later on one particular system (management by objectives), the reasons for failure of appraisal systems are discussed first because they are applicable to the development of an effective performance appraisal system based on management by objectives.

One reason systems fail is that they are not part of the personnel programs or that the personnel operation is not a part of the overall management system. Specifically, the personnel functions should include recruitment and selection, assignment of employees to specific jobs and tasks, training and development, on-the-job monitoring and control, and performance evaluation. This last phase, or responsibility, often is delegated to supervisors who are not given any training in techniques or methods. As a result, evaluation often takes place through the use of scaling procedures such as those outlined earlier. It is important that the personnel department contribute to the entire organization its expertise in the area of performance evaluation and develop a system that contributes to the other functions of management through a developmental evaluation procedure. For this to be accomplished, the tasks of staffing, leadership, and motivation must be viewed as a responsibility of the entire management team.

A second reason for systems failure is operational problems. Performance evaluation systems are based on the development and measurement of standards. Very often, these standards are not made operational properly or have no bearing on the performance of the job. The characteristics of well-written standards are described by Latham and Locke.[15] These standards also may not be linked adequately to a compensation system. Criteria should be developed that contribute to guiding individual behavior through a linkage to compensation if appropriate behavior and results are to be achieved. A very common operational problem is

the result of inadequate training of the evaluator. All too often the evaluator, when faced with forms or procedures that are judgmental, may turn to favoritism as the easy solution. The result is that individuals are judged on how well they are liked rather than on how well they are performing.

These problems are not without consequence. If a program is forced on an organization and its members and if its procedures are not fair, equitable, and understood, further implementation surely will result in low morale and dissatisfaction among the employees involved.

When judgmental approaches such as scaling are used, it is possible for some biases to affect the ratings independent of the effects of favoritism. Some of these factors are:

1. Halo effect: the rater assigns the same value to each factor being rated for a particular employee based on the knowledge of only one characteristic.
2. Meaning of evaluation standards: words such as satisfactory and excellent may mean different things to different evaluators.
3. Rating toward the mean: some evaluators may rate all their subordinates within a narrow range of values, regardless of true differences in performance.
4. Timing: some evaluators may be overly influenced by recent events instead of relying on the intended time frame.
5. Bias: an evaluator's biases, such as toward the sex or family situations of the persons being evaluated, can influence the overall evaluation.

It is possible to minimize the effects of these rating errors if:

1. the criteria focus on a single job activity
2. performance is observed regularly
3. terms are defined clearly or are eliminated if no clear definition is possible; words may mean different things to different people, such as "average" or "satisfactory"
4. raters are trained and do not have to evaluate large groups of subordinates
5. the evaluation criteria are stated clearly and are meaningful to the task being performed[16, 17]

The basic conclusion from this is that evaluation must be part of an organization's continuing management function. Successful performance appraisal programs are those that have a high degree of supervisor and subordinate participation and support and give the individual employees criteria for evaluation that are linked to the performance of their jobs. As part of the organization's commitment to the system, the person doing the ranking or engaging in an evaluation discussion must be trained properly in the methods and objectives of the evaluation procedures. With an adequate management information system, this can contribute to the successful operation of a performance appraisal program.

As noted earlier, one method that is becoming increasingly more popular but, with its popularity, less understood is management by objectives (MBO). In the following section MBO programs are discussed in a fashion that highlights their usefulness as a method of performance evaluation that links the personnel function to the organization's overall objectives.

REASONS TO ADOPT MBO

The term management by objectives (MBO) was used first by Peter F. Drucker in 1954.[18] Drucker made the point that in this system, each manager should have clear objectives that are identified with and support those of upper management. Individuals thus can acquire an understanding of their own objectives, their manager's, and the organization's.

Since publication of his book, many authors have supported or expanded on this concept. Douglas McGregor advocated MBO as a method to encourage the discussion of employee strengths and potential, making the superior more of a counselor than a judge.[19] Whereas Drucker first viewed MBO as a method of integrating the activities of an organization, McGregor began to apply it as a performance appraisal technique. More recently, the MBO approach has been advocated as an appraisal technique that should be linked to management's strategic planning functions. The development of MBO to its current position has been a gradual process. Today it is advocated as a managerial task.[20, 21, 22, 23, 24, 25]

MBO is associated with the organizational processes of planning, organizing, staffing, leading, and controlling. When used in another fashion, an MBO program can be used to bring about organizational change. It is important that the institution have stability in the intraorganizational environment and be open to and tolerant of self-evaluation (which of course a full-fledged MBO program would necessitate).

Definitions of MBO

Although there are numerous definitions of MBO programs, some of which are discussed later, there are some common elements:[26]

1. goal setting
2. involvement of managers in participation in the formulation of personal goals and methods to accomplish these goals
3. periodic reviews of progress toward the accomplishment of these goals
4. evaluation of performance
5. self-appraisal
6. feedback and evaluation
7. suggestions for development and training

The MBO process may be viewed as a cycle of events that includes planning, setting objectives and goals, negotiation, performance, review of performance, and evaluation and feedback.

Raia, in another approach, looks at MBO as a series of phases consisting of four central elements:[27]

1. goal setting
2. action planning
3. self-control
4. periodic reviews

George S. Odiorne, a frequent author on management by objectives, defines MBO as a

process whereby the superior and subordinate managers of an organization jointly identify its common goals, define each individual's major areas of responsibility in terms of the results expected of him, and use these measures as guides for operating the unit and assessing the contribution of each of its members.[28]

McConkie addressed the issue of definitional problems through the identification of 39 authors who had multiple citations or publications on MBO.[29] He then identified the common elements of their descriptions and definitions of how performance appraisal should be conducted under MBO. McConkie found that almost complete agreement existed on three items specific to goal setting in MBO programs. These items indicate that goals and objectives:

1. should be specific
2. should be defined in terms of measurable results
3. should be reflective of both individual and organizational perspectives

More than 80 percent of the authorities agreed that periodic goal reviews facilitated effective MBO; 70 percent agreed that a specific time period for goal accomplishment should be included as part of the goal, and 68 percent felt that wherever possible, the indicator of the results should be quantifiable, or at least verifiable.

Linking MBO to performance appraisal, it appears that an effective system that provides a setting for managers and subordinates to establish objectives against which performance is measured provides better data for management than do traditional methods. Using these concepts, McConkie concluded that MBO could be defined as

a managerial process whereby organizational purposes are diagnosed and met by joining superiors and subordinates in the pursuit of mutually agreed upon goals and objectives, which are specific, measurable, time bounded, and joined to an action plan; progress and goal attainment are measured and monitored in appraisal sessions which center on mutually determined objective standards of performance.

The key areas of management involvement that contribute to the success of such programs relate to administration's commitment to and understanding of their features. While many management teams may pay lip service to their involvement in the MBO process, there are several structural and operational systems that signify to the other members of the institution that management is, indeed, committed to a successful program. These programs and procedures are very important during the implementation phase and also during the continuing process of evaluating performance through objectives.

THE MBO APPRAISAL SYSTEM

Migliore describes a framework for the implementation of an MBO program that is based on identifying purposes, objectives, and desired results, and evaluating performance in achieving them in a nine-step process:[30]

1. defining the organization's purpose and reason for being
2. monitoring the environment in which it operates
3. assessing the organization's strengths and weaknesses realistically
4. making assumptions about unpredictable future events
5. prescribing written, specific, and measurable objectives in principal result areas that contribute to the organization's purpose
6. developing strategies on how to use available resources to meet objectives
7. making long-range and short-range plans to meet objectives
8. appraising performance constantly to determine whether it is meeting the desired pace and remaining consistent with the defined purposes
9. reevaluating purpose, environment, strengths, weaknesses, and assumptions before setting objectives for the next performance year

This system clearly reflects an interest in matching the program to organizational goals. However, it is difficult to bring together organizational units in a fashion that takes advantage of or recognizes the fact that interdependencies may exist.[31]

Health care institutions present one such problem. Health organizations, whether they be hospitals or ambulatory care entities or long-term care facilities or programs, bring together persons from different disciplines to perform specific functions that contribute to the quality and efficiency of production of patient treatment or service. Yet the successful treatment program, in terms of both health outcome and costs, generally requires a high degree of coordination and activity among these individuals in different departments. These persons, by definition, have different training, backgrounds, and appreciation of what tasks need to be performed and their appropriate order. Therefore, it is extremely important that the program be linked to a total management perspective so that individual objectives are developed in the context of the contributions of other departments and other individuals. Of course, the context of the general overriding purposes of the organization must be considered in such a review.

Organizations do not run themselves. It is the role of management to provide direction and purpose. Through the work of the individual employees, the organization may either accomplish its objectives or fall short. It thus is essential that its objectives be related to and understood by the employees. An MBO program makes this procedure a part of the objective-setting process, separating it from the individual goal-setting process.

During this process, the individual employee and the superior decide on goals (or objectives) that should be accomplished within a specified period. Objectives such as the ones outlined during this process are developmental and, according to Carroll and Tosi, can contribute to accomplishing the following:[32]

1. They document expectations in the superior-subordinate relationship as to what is to be done and the level of attainment for the period specified by the goal.

2. They provide members with a firmer base for developing and integrating plans and personal and departmental activity.
3. They serve as the basis for feedback and evaluation of the subordinate's performance.
4. They provide for coordination and timing of individual and unit activities.
5. They draw attention to the need for the control of key organizational functions.
6. They provide a basis for work-related rewards as opposed to personality-based systems.
7. They emphasize change, improvement, and growth of the organization and the individual.

THE PROCESS OF GOAL SETTING

The implementation of an MBO program relies heavily on a successful process of goal setting at the organizational level and its subsequent linkage to similar actions at the department and individual levels. There is some difficulty in making a hard-and-fast decision as to how much subordinate participation should occur during these stages. In general, it is impossible to specify precisely how much participation should occur because of variances in organizations and management styles. There is a range of opinion, however, on just how much participation is appropriate. Some feel that having the subordinates set their own objectives through participatory goal setting is more effective than having a superior do so. Arguments may be advanced for each of these extremes, but in practice it appears that a position somewhere in the middle may be most appropriate.

Subordinates, when involved in determining their own objectives, may be more committed to these goals. On the other hand, the superior may have the best idea of what the institution is trying to achieve and how the individual may contribute best to the accomplishment of these organizational objectives. The method of goal setting used will depend on the characteristics of management and of the individuals involved, and most likely will fall between the extremes. There is much disagreement on this issue, however, so some of the findings on participatory goal setting and its impact on performance are reviewed next.

The linkage between MBO and goal setting and its subsequent impact on employee performance have been receiving a great deal of study.[33, 34, 35, 36, 37] The goal setting process, in practice, is implemented quite differently among MBO programs. Chacko, et al., list six dimensions of MBO in which the goal-setting process may vary:[38]

1. in the degree of participation or involvement in the process on the part of the person whose goals are at issue
2. in the degree of difficulty of the goals that are set individually
3. in the degree of specificity of the goals that are set initially
4. in the levels of goal achievement elicited and the degree to which such information is fed back to the performer
5. in the degree of difficulty of the goals that are set subsequently
6. in the degree of specificity of the goals that are set subsequently

Differences along these dimensions exist because, in large part, there is not universal agreement on the nature and content of a successful goal-setting process. Recent analysis of the impact of participatory goal setting on performance is based on the 1968 work of Locke.[39] He advances the hypothesis that conscious goals regulate behavior. Recent reviews of research indicate that difficult objectives rather than less difficult goals generally are associated with better performance.[40, 41]

Locke's theory predicts that significant improvements in performance will occur when participative goal setting is used over situations in which superiors assign goals to the individual. A number of analyses of goal-setting programs have been performed since Locke's theory was advanced; unfortunately, the evidence is not conclusive that one method of goal setting is better than another. While some work seems to support the theory,[42,43,44,45,46] other analyses indicate that it does not hold in practice.[47,48] In light of these seemingly contradictory findings, some authors have attempted to account for other factors.

One interpretation centers on the contribution of attribution theory.[49] This work suggests that individuals attribute performance outcomes to internal or personal factors, indicating that these persons' perceptions of the causes of performance outcomes may have a greater and more direct influence on satisfaction than participation in goal setting.

In another study examining the role of feedback, Kim and Hamner found that goal setting alone enhanced performance without a formal knowledge of a results program, supporting Locke's theory of goal setting.[50] However, they found that when evaluative and nonevaluative feedback were added to a goal setting program, performance generally was improved over a group that participated in goal setting only.

Although there may be some contrasting evidence on goal setting, it does appear that there is value in conferences with employees to discuss their progress toward their goals and objectives. This is a major characteristic of MBO programs. However, there is not too much agreement on how frequently these meetings should occur. Early authors on MBO advocated that objectives and goals be reviewed every six months.[51,52] At least one author recommends review every six months and resetting goals every year.[53] Most of the recent literature recommends that there be flexibility and that periodic reviews be used.[54]

Feedback is an important part of any performance evaluation system. Through participatory goal setting and feedback, the employee will have relevant information on which to improve performance. Yet many employees are hesitant to participate in feedback or evaluation sessions because they are evaluative, rather than developmental in purpose. Successful evaluation interviews can occur in an environment where (1) there is adequate training for both the evaluator and the individual on the purpose of the program, (2) criteria are fair, (3) the evaluator is not biased, (4) both parties to the interview are prepared, and (5) the interview focuses in some part on future objectives.

MBO IN HEALTH ORGANIZATIONS

Many MBO programs do not succeed because they have failed to recognize that "it is not sufficient to delineate an objective in one portion of the health system while not fully integrating other parts of the system that are concerned with that objective."[55] An MBO system of appraisal should reflect the interdependency of organizational units. For example, one paper described how a system review using an MBO framework could be linked to hospital cost containment programs.[56] It is important that systems of performance appraisal, of which MBO is one, reflect an interest in other areas of management; it also is important that health managers understand that there are many benefits that can accrue from performance appraisal.

To date, not many individuals in health settings embrace performance appraisal. This often is used as an argument against such programs. As members of professional groups, in addition to being members of the organizations in which they work, employees often feel that evaluation should be performed by peers and not necessarily linked to the structure and operation of the management of the entire institution. Clearly, while much of this feeling may be justified and result from many years of professional training, there still needs to be some way for the management of the

health institution to appraise employees and get an understanding of the effectiveness of the organization.

In this context, it is important to develop a system that will contribute to individual growth and development. The use of subjective or trait evaluations, forcing choices on numerical scales, or the marking of checklists do not, in and of themselves, contribute to the type of evaluation to which health care employees would respond. These employees are not saying that they will not submit to an evaluation; they are saying that any evaluation in which they participate should provide them with an opportunity to develop their professional skills to greater levels so that they may make greater contributions to the organization.

The evaluation system must be linked directly to the performance of job-related activities. When developing an MBO program, it is necessary to establish standards of performance. Much has been accomplished in establishing standards for hospital service departments such as central supply and housekeeping. As an example, Neese describes how MBO can be implemented in the hospital business office.[57]

However, there is little literature describing a meaningful managerial performance appraisal system for departments related to patient care such as radiology or pathology that takes into account the fact that they are interrelated with other departments. In developing standards for these departments it is necessary to measure service in some way that is acceptable to both physicians and nurses.[58] The key to the development of successful standards is the full participation of all relevant employees. Such a procedure is described by Malesko.[59]

One technique of value in the development of objectives is the job analysis. Through job analysis at the departmental level, two steps may be accomplished:

1. The organizational and departmental goals and their interrelationship may be discussed and identified.
2. The manager will list specifications and responsibilities for the job. This position description helps to outline the responsibilities to be discussed in the later steps of the goal-setting procedure.

The job analysis is a procedure for obtaining detailed information about the duties involved in each position and the qualifications employees should have to hold those posts. Next, a job description is developed that includes information on duties, working conditions, supervision received, etc. A job specification also is developed that covers the qualifications a prospective or current employee should have to be considered for the position. At the same time these procedures are being accomplished, a job evaluation may be performed. When a dollar value is attached to the work, the job evaluation relates that value to other jobs in the organization. The job analysis provides information that is useful for personnel planning, recruitment and retention of employees, compensation, training, and, of interest here, performance appraisal.

An effective performance evaluation system should be based on an inspection of skills and performance, not on the employee's personal attributes. The job analysis procedures also may lead to the development of objective criteria, which should be used in a performance evaluation. These criteria should be selected on the basis of their reflection of both the quality and quantity of the work performed. They also should measure elements over which an employee may have influence and should be measured over a meaningful period of time.[60]

In the development of these work standards, it is important for health organizations, in particular, to remember that output will differ among hospitals and within hospital departments. Using sound management techniques and procedures, the standards developed should reflect the unique characteristics of the community, organization, department, and, possibly, the individuals under study. Health institutions may vary the amount of an output produced as a result of random fluctuations or because of variation due to the day of the week or season of the year. Personnel skills, mixes, and scheduling also influence the validity of the standards. In general, it should be remembered that the standards that are developed should result from a review of the organization's current activities and future plans that are understandable by all personnel.

There is some discussion as to how precisely an individual's goals and responsibilities should be stated. This issue has been discussed in the context of continuing responsibilities. Schoderbek and Plambeck have developed an argument for identifying and setting performance standards for the continuing functions of a job.[61] Specifically, if goals and objectives of a job are stated and used for performance evaluation, then employees will react and devote most of their time to these objectives. This will result in a lessening of the importance of the administrative aspects of a job despite the fact that these may be of greater importance than the specified objectives. In a later study it was found that continuing responsibilities may not be included adequately in the evaluation process, although employees surveyed felt that it was an important part of their jobs.[62] In the development of objectives, these duties and responsibilities should be included. Another

approach is linking behaviorally anchored rating scales (BARS) to MBO programs.

Many of these problems may be addressed if there is an adequate assessment of the organizational goals, mission, and purpose. Such an evaluation should be viewed as an essential component of the implementation of an MBO program. Through this goal setting at the organizational level, a health care institution can accomplish at least four tasks:

1. It can establish an organizational definition of its current goals.
2. It can make an assessment as to whether or not it is acceptable to maintain the organizational status quo for the short term.
3. It can, if the answer to that point is not acceptable, set new short-range goals for the specified time period.
4. It can identify the optional courses available and make choices among them.

This evaluation should be linked to subsequent analyses at other organizational levels. The objective of these sequential evaluations is to ensure that objectives and goals correspond at different levels in the organization.[63]

APPLICATION OF MBO TO HEALTH ORGANIZATIONS

If MBO programs are to be successful in health organizations, managers must be flexible and willing to make modifications in what otherwise might appear to be a system of prescribed procedures. MBO should not be viewed as a rigid system, for there are a number of ways to make it work.[64] There are situations where tailor-made approaches have been successful. White, for example, found that an MBO program could be implemented effectively in a public health care facility.[65] He also concluded that techniques such as goal setting and participative management improve employee satisfaction and performance.

A 1976 study found that 41 percent of those surveyed were using a formal MBO program and another 33 percent indicated that they would be soon.[66] Of the hospitals that were using MBO, 93 percent felt that it made at least some improvement in performance effectiveness. Other successful implementations of MBO programs in health organizations have been reported.[67, 68, 69, 70, 71] Cain and Luchsinger describe how an MBO program may be applied to nursing departments.[72] In an interesting application, Cannon relates how MBO was used to manage a five-year contract.[73]

MBO can be applied effectively in health organizations where there is an integrated management approach and a motivation to have the system work.[74, 75] This motivation should be based on an interest in the development of employees and in rewarding those who are effective and efficient performers. Mobley studied the relationship between managers' evaluations of MBO and the extent to which goal attainment was related to their merit compensation. He found that managers who judged MBO programs to be successful felt that the program was indeed related to merit compensation.[76]

Another advantage of such a method is the type of information provided by the MBO system and its linkages to other managerial systems. It is possible to gain better control over day-to-day management practice through integrated reporting systems.[77] MBO programs also may result in a feeling of greater communication and involvement in decision making among an organization's members.[78] An MBO program, when combined with others such as job enrichment, may enhance both productivity and work satisfaction.[79, 80]

Despite the numerous examples of successful applications of MBO to health organizations, there still is significant resistance. Some possible explanations for this resistance:

1. MBO is seen as difficult to adapt to patient care departments.
2. Too much time is spent in setting objectives.
3. Management and employee goals sometimes are different.
4. Job descriptions may not fit.
5. Superiors may not be willing to formally evaluate their peers.
6. The purposes and objectives of the program for the organization and for the individual are not well understood.

GUIDELINES FOR IMPLEMENTING MBO

Before a program is begun, management should be aware of the total process of performance evaluation through objectives. Through this discovery process, management and employees can understand the level of commitment needed and the length of time required for a successful program. A number of guidelines, such as the following, can provide a useful overview of the MBO program:

1. Management and employees should be committed to and in support of the MBO program. It may be necessary to perform a survey to determine how open the organization's climate is.
2. All individuals involved in the process should develop an understanding of the purpose and objectives of the program.
3. Management and other personnel should meet to develop common goals.
4. Department objectives should be developed that are consistent with those of the health organization.
5. Job descriptions should be written in result-oriented form with statements on the measurement of satisfactory performance.
6. Subordinate-superior goal setting should occur at regular meetings.
7. Clear, valid, and measurable objectives for the individual need to be set and agreed upon.
8. Superiors should be trained in evaluation methods, developmental methods, and performance interviewing.
9. Feedback sessions should be scheduled based on individual needs and should be developmental in nature.
10. Employees should view the MBO program as being linked to the reward system.
11. Continual monitoring of the system should occur through a linkage with other management functions.

The benefits that accrue from the operation of an MBO program suggest that it is worthwhile for the management team to invest the time, effort, and energy in the development, implementation, and maintenance of such a system. Some advantages that may result from a successful program include:

- improved planning and direction of activities toward the accomplishment of organizational goals
- the linking of institutional management functions to control systems through the development of appropriate work standards
- a reduction in role conflict
- a better understanding of how performance is linked to rewards
- increased employee satisfaction through the use of objective criteria
- the career development of personnel

Through an understanding of the total MBO program and its linkage to performance appraisal, compensation, and other management functions, the performance of health workers may be controlled better.

Performance appraisal through MBO is an important method for maintaining an effective and efficient health organization.

NOTES

1. L.L. Cummings and D.P. Schwab, *Performance in Organizations: Determinants and Appraisal* (Glenview, Ill: Scott, Foresman and Company, 1973).

2. Ibid.

3. Andrew Baggaley, "A Scheme for Classifying Rating Methods," *Personnel Psychology,* Summer 1974, pp. 139–144.

4. William F. Glueck, "Performance Evaluation and Promotion," in William F. Glueck, ed., *Personnel: A Diagnostic Approach* (Dallas: Business Publications, 1978), pp. 283–334.

5. Cummings and Schwab, op. cit.

6. Robert M. Guion, *Personnel Testing* (New York: McGraw-Hill Book Co., 1965).

7. J. P. Campbell, M. D. Dunnette, R. D. Arvey, and L. W. Hellervik, "The Development and Evaluation of Behaviorally Based Rating Scales," *Journal of Applied Psychology,* February 1973, pp. 15–22.

8. M. R. Blood, "Spin-offs from Behavioral Expectation Scale Procedures," *Journal of Applied Psychology,* August 1974, pp. 513–515.

9. S. Zedeck and H. T. Baker, "Nursing Performance as Measured by Behavioral Expectation Scales: A Multitrait-Multirater Analysis," *Organizational Behavior and Human Performance,* June 1972, pp. 457–66.

10. D. P. Schwab, H. G. Henneman, III, and T. A. Decotiis, "Behaviorally Anchored Rating Scales: A Review of the Literature," *Personnel Psychology,* Winter 1975, pp. 549–562.

11. G. P. Latham and G. A. Yukl, "A Review of Research on the Application of Goal Setting in Organizations," *Academy of Management Journal* 18 (1975): 824-845.

12. J. Singular, "Has MBO Failed?" *MBA,* October 1975, pp. 47–50.

13. J. M. Ivancevich, "Different Goal Setting Treatments and Their Effects on Performance and Job Satisfaction," *Academy of Management Journal,* 20 (1977): 406–416.

14. J. M. Ivancevich, J. H. Donnelly, Jr., and J. L. Gibson, "Evaluating MBO: The Challenges Ahead," *Management by Objectives,* Winter 1976, pp. 15–24.

15. G. Latham and E. Locke, "Goal Setting—A Motivational Technique That Works," *Organizational Dynamics,* Autumn 1979, pp. 68–80.

16. H. J. Bernardin and C. S. Walter, "The Effects of Rater Training and Diary Keeping on Psychometric Error in Ratings," *Journal of Applied Psychology,* February 1977, pp. 64–69.

17. R. G. Burnaska and T. D. Hollman, "An Empirical Comparison of the Relative Effects of Rater Response Bias on Three Rating Scale Formats," *Journal of Applied Psychology,* June 1974, pp. 307–312.

18. Peter F. Drucker, *The Practice of Management* (New York: Harper & Row, 1954).

19. Douglas McGregor, *The Human Side of Enterprise* (New York: McGraw-Hill Book Co., 1960).

20. S. Carroll and H. L. Tosi, Jr., "Goal Characteristics and Personality Factors in a Management by Objectives Program," *Administrative Science Quarterly* 15 (1970): 295–305.

21. George S. Odiorne, *Management by Objectives: A System of Managerial Leadership* (New York: Pitman, 1965).

22. P. Mali, *Managing Objectives* (New York: John Wiley & Sons, Inc., 1972).

23. Arthur X. Deegan, III, *Management by Objectives for Hospitals* (Germantown, Md.: Aspen Systems Corporation, 1977).

24. R. Henry Migliore, "The Use of Long Range Planning/MBO for Hospital Administrators," *Health Care Management Review* 4, no. 3 (Summer 1979): 23–28.

25. A. P. Raia, *Managing by Objectives* (Glenview, Ill.: Scott, Foresman and Co., 1974).

26. Dallas T. DeFee, "Management by Objectives: When and How Does It Work?" *Personnel Journal,* January 1977, pp. 37–39, 42.

27. Raia, *Managing.*

28. Odiorne, *Management by Objectives.*

29. Mark L. McConkie, "A Clarification of the Goal Setting and Appraisal Processes in MBO," *Academy of Management Review* 4, no. 1 (1979): 1–12.

30. Migliore, "The Use of Long-Range Planning."

31. George S. Odiorne, "Management by Objectives: Antidote to Future Shock," *Journal of Nursing Administration* 5 (February 1975): 27-30.

32. Stephen J. Carroll and H. L. Tosi, Jr., *Management by Objectives* (New York: Macmillan Publishing Co., Inc., 1973).

33. H. L. Tosi, Jr., H. J. Hunter, R. Chesser, J. R. Tarter, and S. Carroll, "How Real Are Changes Induced by Management by Objectives?" *Administrative Science Quarterly* 21 (1976): 276–306.

34. George S. Odiorne, "The Politics of Implementing MBO," *Business Horizons,* June 1974.

35. Carroll and Tosi, "Goal Characteristics."

36. J. M. Ivancevich, "A Longitudinal Assessment of MBO," *Administrative Science Quarterly,* 17 (1973): 126-138.

37. Ivancevich, "Different Goal Setting Treatments."

38. Thomas Chacko, T. H. Stone, and A. P. Brief, "Participation in Goal-Setting Programs: An Attribution Analysis," *Academy of Management Review* 4, no. 3 (1979): 433–438.

39. E. A. Locke, "Toward a Theory of Task Motivation and Incentives," *Organizational Behavior and Human Performance* 3 (1968): 157–189.

40. G. P. Latham and G. A. Yukl, "Effects of Assigned and Participative Goal Setting on Performance and Satisfaction," *Journal of Applied Psychology* 61 (1976): 166–171.

41. R. M. Steers and L. W. Porter, "The Role of Task-Goal Attributes in Employee Performance," *Psychological Bulletin* 81 (1974): 434–452.

42. G. P. Latham and G. A. Yukl, "Assigned Versus Participative Goal-Setting with Educated and Uneducated Wood Workers," *Journal of Applied Psychology* 60 (1975): 299–302.

43. Latham and Yukl, "Effects of Assigned and Participative Goal Setting."

44. J. M. Ivancevich, "Changes in Performance in an MBO Program," *Administrative Science Quarterly* 19 (1974): 563–574.

45. G. P. Latham and J. J. Baldes, "The Practical Significance of Locke's Theory of Goal Setting," *Journal of Applied Psychology,* 60 (1975): 122–124.

46. G. P. Latham and S. B. Kinne, "Improving Job Performance Through Training in Goal Setting," *Journal of Applied Psychology* 59 (1974): 187–191.

47. Carroll and Tosi, "Goal Characteristics."

48. R. M. Steers, "Task-Goal Attributes, in-achievement, and Supervisory Performance," *Organizational Behavior and Human Performance* 13 (1975): 392–402.

49. Chacko, *et al.,* "Participation in Goal-Setting."

50. J. S. Kim and W. C. Hamner, "Effect of Performance Feedback and Goal Setting on Productivity and Satisfaction in an Organizational Setting," *Journal of Applied Psychology* 61 (1976): 48–57.

51. Drucker, *Management.*

52. Douglas McGregor, "An Uneasy Look at Performance Appraisal," *Harvard Business Review,* 35 (May-June 1957): 89-94.

53. R.E. Lahti, "Management by Objectives," *College and University Bulletin* 51 (July 1971): 31–33.

54. McConkie, "A Clarification."

55. Arthur Gerstenfeld, "MBO Revisited: Focus on Health Systems," *Health Care Management Review* 2, no. 4 (Fall 1977): 51–57.

56. Gordon Dodson and Don C. Dodson, "An MBO Approach to Cost Containment in Health Organizations," *Journal of Health and Human Resources Administration*, November 1978, pp. 150–176.

57. Linda Neese, "MBO in the Hospital Business Office," *Health Services Manager* 11, no. 6 (June 1978): 3–5, 10.

58. John Charnock, "Can Hospitals be Managed by Objectives?," *Journal of General Management* 2, no. 2 (Winter 1975): 36–47.

59. Stephen Malesko, "Developing Work Standards for Hospitals," *Management Controls*, November 1974, pp. 239–245.

60. Latham and Locke, "Goal Setting."

61. Peter P. Schoderbek and Don Plambeck, "The Missing Link in Management by Objectives—Continuing Responsibilities," *Public Personnel Management* 7, no. 6 (January-February 1978): 19–25.

62. Tom Kuffel, Peter P. Schoderbek, and Donald L. Plambeck, "The Role of Continuing Responsibilities: Some Empirical Results," *Public Personnel Management* 8, no. 7 (January-February 1979): 26–31.

63. Howard L. Smith and Norbert F. Elbert, "An Integrated Approach to Performance Evaluation in the Health Care Field," *Health Care Management Review*, Winter 1978, pp. 59–67.

64. George L. Morrisey, "How to Implement MBO in Your Organizational Unit," *Training and Development Journal* 31 (April 1977): 8–10, 13.

65. Donald D. White, "Effects of a Management by Objectives System in a Public Health Care Facility," *Journal of Business Research* 2, no. 3 (July 1974): 290–302.

66. Fred Luthans and Jerry L. Sellentin, "MBO in Hospitals: A Step Towards Accountability," *Personnel Administrator*, October 1976, pp. 42–45.

67. L. P. Harr and J. R. Hicks, "Performance Appraisal: Derivation of Effective Assessment Tools," *Journal of Nursing Administration* 6, no. 7 (September 1976): 20–29.

68. A. J. Hinton and M. M. Markowich, "Supervisor, Employee Participation in Goal-Oriented Appraisals," *Hospitals, JAHA* 50, no. 1 (January 1, 1976): 97–101.

69. M. L. Riordan, "Patient Care Management in Action: One Center's Experience," *Hospitals, JAHA* 52, no. 1 (January 1, 1978): 70–76.

70. Gerstenfeld, "MBO Revisited."

71. R. K. Murray, "Management by Objectives: Useful in Establishing a Merit Appraisal System," *Health Services Manager* 10, no. 2 (February 1977): 105.

72. Cindy Cain and V. Luchsinger, "Management by Objectives: Applications to Nursing," *Journal of Nursing Administration*, 8 (January 1978): 35–38.

73. JoAnn Cannon, "Using MBO in Managing Contracts," *Health Care Management Review* 3, no. 1 (Winter 1978): 41–51.

74. Herbert H. Hand and H. Thomas Hollingsworth, "Tailoring MBO to Hospitals," *Business Horizons*, February 1975, pp. 45–52.

75. Deegan, *Management by Objectives for Hospitals*.

76. W. H. Mobley, "The Link Between MBO and Merit Compensation," *Personnel Journal* 53, no. 6 (June 1974): 423–427.

77. Stanley L. Sokolik, "Feedback and Control—The Hollow in MBO Practice," *Human Resources Management*, Winter 1978, pp. 23–28.

78. Cecelia Golightly, "MBO and Performance Appraisal," *The Journal of Nursing Administration* 9, no. 9 (September 1979): 11–20.

79. Denis D. Umstot, "MBO and Job Enrichment: How to Have Your Cake and Eat It Too," *Management Review*, February 1977, pp. 21–26.

80. Rensis Likert and M. Scott Fisher, "MBGO: Putting Some Team Spirit into MBO," *Personnel*, 54 (January-February 1977): 40–47.

16. Communications

NORMAN METZGER

Reprinted with permission from *Personnel Administration in the Health Services Industry*,
2d ed., by Norman Metzger, published by SP Medical & Scientific Books, Division of
Spectrum Publications, Inc., New York, © 1979.

Effective cooperation in large teams requires purposive communication—that certain ideas must be shared among all teammates, and that informal communications cannot be depended on to achieve these results. Some essential ideas may not be communicated, while others may be circulated and modified in possibly erroneous form. Unplanned communication may have been adequate when working teams were small, when the whole team worked—and perhaps lived—in the home of the master craftsman, but such unplanned procedure cannot be depended on when teams include thousands of team members who may be scattered among the maze of divisions, departments, plants and buildings.[1]

Communication is the exchange—upward, downward, laterally—of information and ideas. To be successful it must result in a common understanding between all who are part of the communication network. Much of what the administrator or supervisor does in some way resembles what the subordinate does. The key difference between the manager and the worker is that the manager must get work done *through* other people. This can only be accomplished by means of sound communication. Communication is neither an appendage nor an afterthought in the organization's life-style. It is the cornerstone of organizational life and existence. Within the complex organizational patterns of the modern health services institution, it is clear that communication programs must be developed on a sophisticated level with the prime goal of optimizing understanding and effecting maximum cooperation of all levels of staff. Of course, it is a *sine qua non* that communication grows best in a climate of trust and confidence. An administration that does one thing and says another cannot in the final analysis expect communications, whether formal or informal, to be effective. Still another organizational life-style which is counterproductive to effective communications is referred to as "playing it close to the vest." Some institutions believe that employees should be told as little as possible and that information should be disseminated only on a "need-to-know" basis. In a survey among industrial workers conducted in the early 1950's (see Exhibit 16–1), employees indicated that "feeling in on things" was one of the major needs not fulfilled by their management. Rounding out the three most important needs expressed by these workers was "full appreciation of work done" and "sympathetic help on personal problems."[2] It is readily seen from this study that the three major needs expressed by workers dealt with the communication patterns—too often guarded, meager or neglected—of the institution.

Drucker urges upon all institutions an improvement in general employee communications. "To measure work against objectives requires information. . . . Management must try to convey this information—not because the worker wants it, but because the best in-

Exhibit 16-1 What Do Workers Want Most?

The average foreman says that good wages, job security, and promotion are his workers' basic desires.

Workers rate full appreciation of work done, feeling "in" on things, and sympathetic help on personal problems as their chief wants. But foremen say these are the least of their workers' job goals.

These are the findings of a spot survey conducted by *Foreman Facts* in 24 industrial plants. Foremen were asked to rank the 10 key factors listed below in the order of their importance to workers. Then workers in the same plant were asked to do the same. When the two lists were matched these were the results:

JOB GOAL	Ranked by Workers	Ranked by Foremen
Full appreciation of work done	1st	8th
Feeling "in" on things	2nd	10th
Sympathetic help on personal problems	3rd	9th
Job security	4th	2nd
Good wages	5th	1st
"Work that keeps you interested"	6th	5th
Promotion and growth in company	7th	3rd
Personal loyalty to workers	8th	6th
Good working conditions	9th	4th
Tactful disciplining	10th	7th

Source: Reprinted with permission from *Foreman Facts,* Vol. 9, No. 21 (Newark, N.J.: Labor Relations Institute), 1952.

terest of the enterprise demands that he have it. The great mass of employees may never be reached even with the best of efforts, but only by trying to get information to every worker can management hope to reach the small group that in every plant, office or store leads public opinion and molds common attitudes."[3]

PLANNING COMMUNICATION

The planning of communication is essential to producing the resultant optimum objectives. It is inconceivable to think of any form of interpersonal relationship and activity which is not dependent upon communication. One study found that the typical executive spends about 75 percent of his time communicating and about 75 percent of this time communicating in individual face-to-face situations.[4] Too often, even though the parties are speaking the same language, understanding escapes either one or the other. Merrihue suggests the following essential steps in the planning of communication:[5]

1. Know your objective. What is it that you intend to accomplish by this communication? The sharper the focus, the better the result.

2. Identify your audience. It is necessary to know who you are communicating with in order to select the proper language and the proper media.
3. Determine your medium (or media). The method of communication will often determine the success of the communication. A decision must be made on how best to communicate the message.
4. Tailor the communication to fit the relationship between sender and receiver. The key to this element of effective communication is the relationship climate. Is it one of fear or confidence?
5. Establish a mutuality of interest. Empathy, the ability to see the other person's point of view, is a priceless ingredient of effective communication.
6. Watch your timing. This is critical to the effectiveness of the communication. It is important to decide who should receive the communication first.
7. Measure results. Has the desired response occurred?

ESSENTIALS OF GOOD COMMUNICATION

It is a well-established principle that there is a positive relationship between good supervisory communication and effective performance. There are basic rules which are the cornerstone of successful communications:

1. Before communicating, clarify the idea in your mind. Too often we tend to communicate with undefined ideas and unclear objectives.
2. Examine the *real* objective of the communication. It is important to establish at the outset the goal or central reason for the communication.
3. Adapt the language of the communication and the setting to the specific situation. It is essential that the proper words be selected with regard to the intelligence and background of experience of the receiver. The total physical and human setting must be considered in planning for effective communications. This includes a sense of timing and, of course, the physical setting which must afford both participants privacy, if necessary.
4. It is often not what you communicate but how you communicate that will affect results. It is imperative that the sender be sensitive to the importance of his tone of voice, expression and, of course, as mentioned before, his language.
5. Communication should be precise, brief and clear in presenting facts. Unnecessary words complicate communications. All facts should be stated in as objective terms as possible, avoiding abstractions and, whenever possible, providing illustrations.
6. Follow up communications. It is important to measure results to see how effective the communication was and, of course, learn from the mistakes of ineffective communicating.

LISTENING: THE KEY TO GOOD COMMUNICATION

Sitting *up* and listening is half (at least) of the process of communication. Developing the art of listening requires in most cases relearning and unlearning bad habits developed over the years. Most of us do not know how to listen. We are often guilty of listening for facts or listening intelligently for the verbal statement alone when the art of listening is the discerning of ideas. Our biases also enter into our listening habits. It is not unusual for certain words—rhetoric—to prejudice our appreciation and understanding. We may well not like the way a speaker "looks" or not like his voice and, therefore, pay little attention to or discount what he has to say. Some of the prevalent and counterproductive listening habits follow:

1. Talking too much. It is obvious that if one talks too much, one cannot have enough time to listen.
   a. Do you spend too much time explaining or defending your own position, thereby neglecting a careful evaluation of the other individual's position?
   b. Are you so intent on framing the answer to a question which has yet to be fully communicated to you that indeed you stop listening in the midst of someone's communication?
   c. Are you often puzzled about what the other individual really meant?

   All of these actions require a reassessment of our "talking" and "listening" habits. The key to these problems is in disciplining oneself to ask questions and wait—remaining silent—for enough time to pass for the other individual to communicate to you. It requires a disciplined approach to listening by appreciating the power of silence.

2. Asking leading questions. One of the most common pitfalls of communication is framing questions in such a way that the "right answer" is obtained.
   a. Are you receiving only the answers you were secretly wishing for?
   b. Are you receiving only limited responses which are guarded?

   In order to obtain the true responses of people to whom you are communicating, it would be best to outline the important areas in which questions should be asked and to frame the questions so that they are "open-ended." This will leave the other individual free to answer in any way and in as elaborate a fashion as he chooses.

3. Selecting the wrong time and the wrong place to communicate.
   a. Is your communication hasty and does it reflect your desire to hurry it?
   b. Do you have one foot out the door and only one ear unlocked when communicating?
   c. Do you communicate in public when the subject cries for a private audience?
   d. Are the phones ringing? Do people come barging in? Are you constantly distracted when in the midst of communication?
   e. Do you communicate too soon or too late?

   It is best to plan your communication time so that a full discussion can be had and the listener and speaker can give full attention to the discussion. It is also best to communicate in an atmosphere without distractions. It is important to be sensitive to the dignity of the listener; therefore, certain communications must be held in private and the listener should not be embarrassed in the presence of his peers.

A special study by the United Hospital Fund of New York lists underlying principles of effective employee-management communication:[6]

1. Communication should not be regarded as a tool or "helping" aspect of the organization, but as the essence of organized activity and the basic process out of which all other functions derive.
2. Communications should be subjected to accepted management principles of analyzing, planning, coordinating and evaluating.
3. Organizational communication should be thought of as directional—upward, downward or horizontally from the sender. Each direction poses different technical and psychological problems which must be solved if communication is to be successful.
4. Ineffective communication within an organizational system can mean wasted time and resources and, therefore, can result in lower productivity and higher costs than necessary.
5. It may be important to change an individual's attitudes—so that he will be motivated to apply the principles and skills he has learned.
6. Although most communication is verbal, communication in a variety of nonverbal ways should be recognized: through gestures, facial expressions, body postures and movements, tone of voice and dress. Most of all we communicate by our actions.
7. People generally hear, read, observe and choose to understand only those parts of the message that relate to their own interests, desires and needs.
8. Our choice is not between communicating or not communicating, but between communicating effectively or ineffectively, between contributing or not contributing to reach the goals of the organization.
9. Repetition is important in communication. Many people miss a message the first time around.
10. Feedback is a critical element in communication. There must be a way for the sender to observe the effect of his message on the receiver's behavior.
11. The greatest barrier to communication probably lies in the area of human relationships.
12. Communication does not occur merely because the message is *sent;* it must also be *received* with reasonable fidelity.

13. The administrator should think not only of solving "communication" problems per se, but also of solving specific organizational problems by consciously applying specific communication techniques.

INSULATED CHIEF ADMINISTRATORS

McMurry points out that many institutions, in spite of the expenditure of huge sums for communications programs, have top administrators who are totally—or almost totally—insulated from what is actually taking place in their own institution. It has been found that much of the information which reaches the chief executive is often incomplete and biased. This is not fortuitous, but rather reflects a temperamental disposition on the part of the chief executive which filters down the line and makes obvious that he (the chief administrator) is not able to accept and assimilate information which happens to conflict with his own values and predictions. There is a great deal of inaccuracy of information transmitted up the line. Add to this the many communication barriers and one would suspect a carefully designed attempt to filter information that reaches the chief administrator. According to McMurry, there are many reasons for this:[7]

1. No subordinate wishes to have his superior learn of anything he interprets to be actually or potentially discreditable to him. He therefore screens information and colors communication.
2. Subordinates soon learn what their supervisor desires to hear. The subordinate's personal anxieties, hostilities, aspirations and system of beliefs and values must inevitably shape and color his interpretation and acceptance of what he has learned and is expected to transmit.
3. Subordinates are often desirous of impressing their superior with the superiority of *their* contribution to the institution and, by the same token, of the inadequacies of the contribution of their rivals.

A chief administrator who wishes to obtain accurate information must develop an organizational style permeated by trust and confidence which will invite a free flow and exchange of information up and down the line.

FACTORS THAT INFLUENCE MEANING

Merrihue states that how much and how accurately meaning is conveyed in communication depends on a number of factors and lists the following:[8]

1. *The functional relationship between the sender and the receiver*. Very often they differ sharply in their policy thinking and their sense of values.
2. *The positional relationship between sender and receiver*. Is it that of an old-timer authoritatively instructing the newcomer? Is it that of a president speaking to a workman?
3. *The group membership relationship*. Is it that of management speaking to management or a member of a union which is overtly hostile to management?
4. *Differences in heredity and prior environment*. Are the backgrounds of sender and receiver relatively homogeneous? If not, meaning will be difficult to convey. Status in life powerfully shapes ideas and attitudes.
5. *Differences in formal education*. What is the capacity of the audience to understand and comprehend the message?
6. *Past experience*. What has been the quality of the human relationships between sender and receiver?
7. *Emotions*. The current emotional state of the sender and receiver can determine whether the correct meaning is exchanged or whether all meaning will be blocked by an insurmountable barrier.
8. *Misunderstanding of words (and the vagaries of semantics)*. Words alone do not convey meaning. Only people can convey meaning through their use of words.

Communication has been likened to a radio set. First, you must select the station. The radio must be tuned for sending and the receiver must be tuned for reception. Selecting the station or the best wave length is critical. There are many messages involved in normal conversation, and often what the speaker means to say and what he actually says differ; in addition, what the other person hears is not always what the other person thinks he hears. In order to maximize communication skills and communicate what you intend to communicate, Odiorne offers a number of principles:[9]

1. Before sending a message, clarify your intentions.
2. In shaping your intentions into language or "code," be certain it is couched in a language or code that the receiver will be able to manage with facility.
3. In transmitting, make certain that all of the media which exist as a channel of communication between the sender and the receiver are being exploited or at least sufficiently exploited so that

the major portion of the message has a possibility of getting through to the receiver.
4. One of the basic requirements of good communication is that the sender have in his mind an accurate image of the receiver and of his decoded capacity.
5. This, of course, requires that he have an image of the receiver himself, his interests, endowments and attitudes toward the sender and the environment in which the message is taking place.
6. Good communications require that there be some interchange, back and forth, between the sender and the receiver in order that the normal, natural inconsistencies and lack of clarity between the sender and receiver in any message be made clear.

COMMUNICATION MEDIA

Hospitals and homes primarily make use of four methods of communication: meetings and conferences, hospital/home or departmental letters, written memoranda and bulletin boards.

Meetings and Conferences

Probably the most widely used method of communication is through meetings and conferences. A critical point in such vehicles is the ability for two-way communication. Conferences usually fall into a didactic pattern with all messages going one way. A conference that provides for discussion and encourages normal give-and-take can be most effective in the communication network. The truly effective conference involves a group of people pooling ideas and experiences. It is well to appreciate that the most effective conference develops from the acceptance of certain preconditions:

1. The meeting is called for a definite purpose, clearly understood by the chairman and participants.
2. The size of the group is limited.
3. Attention is given to the proper grouping of employee levels for the purpose clearly understood (see precondition 1, above).
4. The conference is of a definite length, and time of starting and ending is invariable.
5. A conference room should be large enough and comfortable enough.
6. Advance materials should be distributed to avoid time-consuming activities while the conference is on.

Hospital/Home or Departmental Letters

Letters sent from the institution or a department of the institution to employees are usually used in special circumstances. The announcement of long-range plans or of proposed changes are suitable subjects for such letters. To be successful they should be brief and careful attention directed to the language. This method was judged as one of the three most effective methods of communication in a survey of administrators.[10] Such letters are also used to welcome new employees, announce changes in employee wage scales and fringe benefits and in circumstances where the administrator or department head wishes to address a general appreciation to all employees. The cardinal rule here is that the institution should use such letters only when they have something of the utmost importance to communicate. Letters are probably the most personal of the communication vehicles. Most experts would agree that style is as important as content. Brevity, simplicity and a straightforward approach are all attributes of sound written communications. It is best to test the letter out on key administrators or supervisors before distributing it to employees. Careful attention should be directed toward common errors in written communications (see Exhibit 16-2).

Written Memoranda

Included in this category are the memoranda used between departments, between executives and between levels of employees. This form of communication has the advantage of permanence and verifiableness. It is often used to ensure follow-through between levels of supervision. The largest single criticism of this form of communication is that of wasted time and material: messages contained in memoranda can often be communicated, more effectively, by telephone. It is well to keep in mind that the written memo loses the most important attributes of oral communication—

intonations and facial expressions. Brevity should be the hallmark of this form of communication. If action is required, such action should be clearly indicated along with the requested timing. Memoranda with hidden agenda are inappropriate. Directness and specificity are key ingredients of effective written memoranda. It is best to keep a copy of a memorandum that you have initiated, and good practice to send copies of your memoranda to any individual mentioned therein who may be affected by what you have communicated.

Bulletin Boards

Bulletin boards are an effective communication vehicle for formal announcements. They are most effective when they are able to attract employees by constant changes and careful control of content including prompt removal of out-of-date material. To obtain maximum efficiency from the use of bulletin boards, they should be placed near an entrance or exit, in locker rooms or in the departments themselves. Most institutions that make excellent use of bulletin boards agree that each department should have its own bulletin board. Two-section boards have been found to be the most efficient. One side is used for routine notices to the department while the other section is used for news items, special features, posters and general announcements of a personal nature. The use of posters is an effective and attractive way of getting the institution's message across. Posters may be used in formal series. Here again, constant change is necessary to keep the employee's attention. It is well to date all notices, first with the posting date and second with the date for removal.

POLICY AND EMPLOYEE MANUALS

An essential ingredient of a total communication network is the preparation and distribution of a personnel policy manual and an employee manual. Sound personnel administration encourages and facilitates the employee's optimum contribution toward an understanding of the objectives of the institution. The purpose of the personnel policy manual is to provide administrative and supervisory staff members with a complete documentary on the institution's personnel administration so that the policies and procedures approved by the institution's board may be applied equitably, consistently and with authority. Personnel policies should be designed to promote the mutual understanding, respect and cooperation necessary to maximize the delivery of services in the institution. Exhibit 16-3 is a table of contents for a personnel pol-

---

Exhibit 16-2 Ingredients of Ineffective Written Communication

1. Subtle messages.
2. Limited interest subjects.
3. Rambling style.
4. Pedantic language.
5. Patronizing tone.
6. Incomplete explanation.
7. "Oversell."

Exhibit 16-3 Table of Contents of a Personnel Manual

```
                    PERSONNEL   POLICY   #1.0
   ┌──────────────────────────────────────────┬──────────────┐
   │   INTRODUCTION            Page 2          │ Issued:      │
   │                                           │ Revised:     │
   └──────────────────────────────────────────┴──────────────┘
```

<u>Organization</u>

This manual is organized for convenient reference as follows:

Section 1	INTRODUCTION
Section 2	GENERAL PERSONNEL POLICY
Section 3	ORGANIZATION OF THE PERSONNEL FUNCTION
Section 4	EMPLOYMENT
Section 5	SENIORITY
Section 6	PROMOTIONS AND TRANSFERS
Section 7	COMPENSATION
Section 8	HOURS OF WORK AND TIME OFF
Section 9	EMPLOYEE BENEFITS, SERVICES AND ACTIVITIES
Section 10	PERSONNEL COMMUNICATIONS
Section 11	EMPLOYEE RECOGNITION
Section 12	TRAINING AND DEVELOPMENT
Section 13	EMPLOYEE PERFORMANCE REVIEW
Section 14	EMPLOYEE COUNSELING
Section 15	GRIEVANCE PROCEDURE
Section 16	DISCIPLINARY ACTION
Section 17	TERMINATION
Section 18	EMPLOYEE PUBLIC RELATIONS
Section 19	LABOR RELATIONS
Section 20	HEALTH, SAFETY, AND SECURITY

MOUNT SINAI MEDICAL CENTER

Source: Mt. Sinai Hospital, New York, New York.

icy manual. The institution must develop specific policies in the areas of employment, placement, promotions, compensation, benefits, training, counseling, disciplining, labor relations and many other facets of personnel administration.

The following are general statements contained in the introduction to a personnel policy manual.

Employment: The institution will use every reasonable means available to recruit the most capable employees for the positions to be filled. In compliance with civil rights legislation, and more importantly in observance of the institution's well-established tradition of fairness, equal opportunity will be given to applicants of all races, religions, national origins, cultural backgrounds, age groups, sexes and personal persuasions. Selection is based solely on the applicant's demonstrable ability and qualifications for the job.

Placement: The institution will make every effort to place employees in positions best suited to their abilities and career objectives.

Promotions: The institution will encourage employees to acquire the capabilities requisite for advancement. Equal opportunity will be given to all applicants for promotion. Candidates for promotion will be given preference over outside employment applicants wherever possible. Selection is based on the candidate's demonstrable ability and qualifications for the job. Where the ability of two or more candidates is relatively equal, the more senior employee is selected for promotion.

Compensation: The institution will maintain salaries competitive with those prevailing for comparable jobs in the health care institutions in our area. An equitable compensation structure will be maintained for the institution's numerous jobs based on relative responsibility, knowledge and skill requirements, working conditions and other characteristics. Employees not covered by collective bargaining agreements requiring fixed wages and increments will be given increases based upon individual performance.

Hours of Work: The institution renders around-the-clock service every day of the year. The scheduling of departmental work hours is based on the operational requirements of the institution. Employees will be assigned hours and shifts consistent with departmental needs and, insofar as possible, with individual preferences. Hours will be changed only with appropriate notice to affected employees.

Employee Benefits, Services and Activities: The institution will provide employee benefits, in the form of insurance coverage, pension program, etc., at least comparable to those offered in health services institutions in our area. Services such as employee health service, food service, group purchasing and personal counseling will be made available to improve the employee's working conditions and to assist in the fulfillment of his personal needs. The institution will also promote, support or maintain various programs of recreational or community activities to enhance the employee's leisure.

Training and Development: The institution will afford its employees every reasonable opportunity for advancement through increased knowledge, education, training and experience. Programs will be maintained for employee orientation, on-the-job training, upgrading training, tuition aid and supervisory and administrative development. Where appropriate the institution will provide educational assistance and training opportunities to members of the community.

Employee Performance Review: The institution will maintain programs for the systematic review of employee performance. Such reviews are to take place on a regular, periodic basis and the results of the reviews communicated to the employees. Supervisors are to supplement the formal reviews by keeping employees informed about their current performance progress.

Grievance Procedure: The institution will maintain a formal grievance procedure culminating in binding arbitration for the resolution of employee grievances. Every effort will be made to resolve grievances informally or at the lowest possible step of the procedure. No employee shall be discriminated against for having lodged a grievance.

Employee Discipline: The institution will pursue a policy of enlightened discipline, the primary objective of which is correction, not punishment. Supervisors are encouraged to administer disciplinary action that is equitable and in keeping with the offense; consistent with prior actions and with actions in other departments; progressively sterner after repeated offenses; and designed to persuade the offending employee to improve. Discharge is to be resorted to only if the offense is extreme or after every possible remedial effort has been made.

In a study, the following observations were made as to policy manuals used in hospitals.[11]

1. Very few manuals were readable. Generally they were verbose and poorly organized. Few manuals provided for easy replacement of old pages with revised ones; few had complete indices.
2. Administrators generally had no feedback on manuals—no way of knowing whether a policy or procedure had been read, understood or acted upon.
3. It is expensive and time-consuming to do a completely new manual, but one can be prepared and issued in installments.
4. Most administrators in hospitals and businesses who did not have policy or procedure manuals mentioned both the importance of such manuals and their lack of time to do them.
5. When policies and procedures have been generally understood and agreed upon, management may feel that there is no need for these policies and procedures to be written down.

Policy is a guide to action against which the administrator and the supervisor can measure their immediate, routine decisions that are often made under time pressure. Personnel policy is a simplification and logic-bringing instrument which assists in problem-solving and decision-making.[12]

The employee handbook is an offshoot of the personnel policy and procedure manual. It is more informal than its parent. Its intent is to explain as clearly as possible the policies and rules and general information of the institution. Many employee manuals are broken down into sections. The manual starts off with a welcome letter from the institution's chief executive. A section, "Getting Started," includes the organization's selection policy and deals with such varied subjects, necessary for proper induction of the new employee, as explanation of the probationary period, employee identification system and hours of work. Another section deals with compensation: how employees are paid, shift differentials, overtime practices and time records. Still another deals with important elements of "on the job" seniority, promotions and transfers and grievance procedure. A section, often quite large, will be set aside for time off. This will include an explanation of the institution's policies on holidays, vacations, sick leave, etc. The fringe benefit program is explained in another section. The obligations of the employee will be included in a separate section covering rules and regulations and general guidelines for cooperation. Employee manuals are often illustrated. Every attempt should be made to make them readable and understandable.

ASSESSING EMPLOYEE PERFORMANCE

The immediate supervisor or department head should evaluate the employee's performance at the end of the probationary period and at least once every year. The evaluation should be made in writing and discussed with the employee. Each performance review form is made a part of the employee's permanent employment record.

In considering employees for promotions or annual salary increases, supervisors should evaluate many factors such as skill, knowledge, seniority, dependability and interest in the work. Performance reviews play a decisive role in increasing career opportunities at the institution.[13]

It does not matter at which organization level an employee is: he (she) wants to know where he (she) has been, where he (she) is now and where he (she) is going. Every member of an organization wants to know exactly what the organization and, specifically, his boss expect him to do; how his performance will be measured; what his boss thinks of him; which areas need improvement; and how to move up in the organi-

zation. It is immaterial how well-adjusted an administrator is: almost all abhor the necessity to criticize a subordinate's work. Not only is it easier not to say anything, it is (paradoxically) even easier to terminate a subordinate's employment than to do the distasteful work of improving his performance. Crosby, in full recognition of the problem involved in assessing employee performance, stated, "Although most people agree with the general concept and purpose of formal employee performance appraisal programs, some express reservations regarding their usefulness and benefits. In some instances personal experience has caused people to doubt the validity of such programs. In other instances developing and implementing employee performance appraisal programs has resulted in disappointment. Unfortunately, these misgivings are used all too often as justification for total inaction in a personnel program that could help improve employee productivity, job satisfaction, compensation, stability and morale. A properly planned, developed and implemented employee performance appraisal program should preclude the possibility of failure and should prove most beneficial as a tool by which management can motivate its employees."[14]

Much of the controversy surrounding the evaluation process springs from the justification or lack of justification for the program. The key question here is: What will the program accomplish? There is little difference of opinion on the fact that with or without a formal program, administration will analyze and always has analyzed the performance of its employees. The appraisal function is a fundamental human act. Merrihue states, "The supervisor who obtains the best from his employees is the one who creates the best atmosphere or climate of approval within which his work group operates. He accomplishes this through the following methods:

1. He develops performance standards for his employees and sets them high to stretch the employees.
2. He measures performance against these standards.
3. He constantly commends above-par performance.
4. He always lets employees know when they have performed below par."[15]

It is clear from this description that the essential justification for employee assessment is *achievement*, personal and institutional. Mayfield insists that every supervisor should appraise his subordinates periodically and communicate his evaluation.[16] On the other hand, Odiorne writes, "I can see only mechanical policing methods to create and enforce the strictures of a deadening conformity. Individuality based on the capacity of each free man to express himself as a human being is not a value to be eradicated lightly and it should be cherished."[17]

Unfortunately the writers on both sides of the argument tend to deal lightly with the aspect of appraisal programs as part of an overall communication program. Is the appraisal program a means to conformity? Is it the basis for remedial action? Is it the yardstick to judge the next salary increment? Otherwise astute observers of the management scene have conjured up a phantasmagoria in the field of appraisals. They look at the mechanism too closely. One could find very little argument with their positions critical of the scales and ranking mechanisms, the list of personality traits, the impossible rush toward the arena of empirical judgment. On the other hand, one should not become enmeshed in the shortcomings of the means and lose sight of the worth of the ends. An appraisal program should aim at reinforcing performance by a systematic assessment of observable work achievements rather than intangible personality traits. It should be a tool for a plan for progress, not for conformity and not for criticism.

WHAT IS PERFORMANCE ASSESSMENT?

Performance assessment is a method of evaluating an employee's work performance on the job to which he is assigned. Other names for this method include merit rating, employee evaluation, performance review, performance rating, efficiency rating, personnel progress reports, employee rating and man rating. Wherever these names occur, they all mean the same thing: evaluating the employee's work performance. *Job evaluation* seeks to rate the value of the job with no regard to the performer; conversely, *performance assessment* or *merit rating* rates the person who actually performs the job.

WHY PERFORMANCE ASSESSMENT?

The assessment of employee performance is an essential management tool in evaluating employees for purposes of promotion, transfer, training needs and wage determination; in addition, it functions as a communication vehicle to bolster employee motivation and reduce counterproductive differences in conceptions of duties, priorities and accomplishments between the superior and the subordinate. Some administrators consider the employee performance review as a once-a-year administrative chore—a routine obligation that must be discharged in order to satisfy the personnel department. They consider the completion of the review form a tedious task and the conduct of the interview a superficial personnel ritual. Indeed, they find the communication of the results of the assessment embarrassing, distressing and without any redeeming virtues. More enlightened administrators view the assessment process as a golden opportunity to reinforce their relationship with the employee. They see it as a mechanism to provide support and guidance to the employee to ensure improved performance and development.

The primary purpose of the performance assessment is to *help the employee improve his job performance by:*

1. Developing and obtaining acceptance by the employee of the specific standards against which his performance will be measured.
2. Evaluating the employee's performance in terms of these standards.
3. Developing and following a plan of action to help him overcome obstacles to his development and to strengthen his capabilities.
4. Soliciting his reactions, resolving differences and reaching a mutual understanding of the implications of the review.
5. Offering constructive suggestions and tangible assistance to the employee toward his development.

In the final analysis, the question of whether an institution shall or shall not rate the people who work for it is an academic one. An institution has no real choice in this matter. Management *must* evaluate the performance of all employees. Judgments *must* be made and the only consideration is *how* to make them. Unquestionably an appraisal program can supply a yardstick to measure employees accurately. But who is to weigh the factors? Who, for instance, is to determine the factors that could accurately measure employee performance? It is the personnel director's responsibility to develop such a yardstick in consultation with representatives of the line administration. A program must be developed which will rate employees on the basis of an organized and systematic format which has as its cornerstone methodology incorporating common standards of judgment which can be applied uniformly by all raters. This is an essential ingredient since many performance assessment programs fall short of their mark because the factors being rated are interpreted quite differently by the different raters. Standardization of terms is a key to the successful assessment program.

RATING SYSTEMS

Performance assessment may be completed by one of several techniques.

1. *Assessment interview:* Here the supervisor meets with the employee and discusses the employee's performance, offering an opportunity for response.
2. *Rating scales:* These scales are the graphic or multiple steps which require checking of an appropriate point along a scale of value.
3. *Employee comparison systems:* These systems do not require the use of an absolute standard; rather, the rater is asked to compare the individual employee with other employees being evaluated.
4. *Checklists:* This method provides an opportunity for the rater to indicate the employee's performance by entering checks in the various spaces provided (see Exhibit 16-4).

The last three methods involve the use of a formal rating system and may be augmented by a personal

Exhibit 16-4 Checklist for Employee Performance

THE MOUNT SINAI HOSPITAL
SUPERVISORY ANNUAL REVIEW

NAME_____ TITLE _____ CLASS_____

LIFE NO. _____ DEPARTMENT_____

ADMINISTRATOR _____ TOTAL POINTS _____GROUP_____

DATE ISSUED_____ DATE DUE _____

INSTRUCTIONS—Read Carefully

Each employee's ability and fitness in his PRESENT occupation or for promotion may be appraised with a reasonable degree of accuracy and uniformity through this rating report. The rating requires the appraisal of an employee in terms of his ACTUAL PERFORMANCE. It is essential, therefore, that snap judgment be replaced by careful analysis. Please follow these instructions carefully:

1. Use your own independent judgment.
2. Disregard your general impression of the employee and concentrate on one factor at a time.
3. Study carefully the definitions given for each trait and the specifications for each degree.
4. When rating an employee, call to mind instances that are typical of his work and way of acting. Do not be influenced by UNUSUAL CASES which are not typical.
5. Make your rating with the utmost care and thought; be sure that it represents a fair and square opinion. DO NOT ALLOW PERSONAL FEELINGS TO GOVERN YOUR RATING.

6. After you have rated the employee on all six traits, write under the heading "General Comments" on the back any additional information about the employee which you feel has not been covered by the rating report, but which is essential to a fair appraisal.
7. Read all four specifications for Trait No. 1. After you have determined which specification most nearly fits the employee, place an X in the left square over it. If he does not quite measure up to the specification but is definitely better than the specification for the next lower degree, place in the right square. Repeat for each trait.

	TRAIT	S-1	S-2	S-3	S-4	S-5	S-6	S-7	S-8
1	**CONTROL** THIS TRAIT APPRAISES THE SUPERVISOR'S ABILITY TO CONTROL HIS OPERATIONS. REDUCE COSTS, AND INCREASE AND IMPROVE SERVICE.	☐	☐ THE SUPERVISOR HAS EXCELLENT CONTROLS AND CHECKS ON HIS OPERATIONS COSTS AND ON PERFORMANCE OF HIS SUBORDINATES, RESULTING IN EFFICIENT AND TIMELY SERVICES.	☐ THE SUPERVISOR MAINTAINS CONTROLS OVER HIS OPERATIONS, COSTS AND PERFORMANCE OF SUBORDINATES AND MANAGES TO PROVIDE ADEQUATE SERVICE UNDER UNUSUAL CIRCUMSTANCES.	☐	☐ THE SUPERVISOR MAINTAINS SOME CONTROLS OVER HIS OPERATIONS, COSTS AND PERFORMANCE OF SUBORDINATES BUT NEEDS OCCASIONAL CHECKING FROM ABOVE TO INSURE EFFICIENT SERVICE.	☐	☐ THE SUPERVISOR FAILS TO MAINTAIN ADEQUATE CONTROLS WHICH OFTEN RESULTS IN POOR OR IMPROPER SERVICE AND EXCESSIVE COSTS.	☐
2	**COOPERATION** THIS TRAIT APPRAISES THE INDIVIDUAL'S WILLINGNESS TO WORK HARMONIOUSLY WITH OTHERS TOWARD THE ACCOMPLISHMENT OF COMMON DUTIES AND COORDINATION OF VARIOUS ACTIVITIES.	☐	☐ THE INDIVIDUAL IS EXCEPTIONALLY COOPERATIVE AND GOES OUT OF HIS WAY TO COOPERATE AND COORDINATES HIS ACTIVITIES WITH OTHERS WITHOUT SACRIFICING STANDARDS OR POLICIES.	☐ THE INDIVIDUAL IS COOPERATIVE AND WORKS HARMONIOUSLY WITH OTHER PEOPLE AND IS WILLING TO HELP OUT OTHER DEPARTMENTS.	☐	☐ THE INDIVIDUAL IS NOT EXCEPTIONALLY COOPERATIVE UNTIL THE NEED IS GREAT AND OCCASIONALLY INDULGES IN OBSTRUCTIVE ARGUMENTS.	☐	☐ THE INDIVIDUAL IS OFTEN DIFFICULT TO DEAL WITH, THINKS OF OWN DEPARTMENT OR UNIT ONLY AND IS OBSTRUCTIVE.	☐
3	**METHODS** THIS TRAIT APPRAISES THE ABILITY OF THE SUPERVISOR TO DEVELOP AND INSTALL NEW METHODS AND PROCEDURES.	☐	☐ THE SUPERVISOR HAS A BRILLIANT AND KEEN MIND FOR DEVELOPING MORE EFFECTIVE METHODS AND PROCEDURES, AND HAS AN EAGERNESS TO LEARN AND APPLY KNOWLEDGE.	☐ THE SUPERVISOR IS QUICK TO GRASP NEW IDEAS AND METHODS AND DEVELOPS HIS SHARE OF NEW METHODS AND PROCEDURES.	☐	☐ THE SUPERVISOR LEARNS NEW METHODS AND PROCEDURES SATISFACTORILY. SELDOM DEVELOPS MORE EFFECTIVE METHODS OR PROCEDURES ON OWN.	☐	☐ THE SUPERVISOR LEARNS NEW METHODS AND PROCEDURES ONLY BY EXCESSIVE REPETITION, AND NEEDS CONSTANT GUIDANCE IN IMPROVING OPERATIONS.	☐
4	**PERSONNEL DEVELOPMENT** THIS TRAIT APPRAISES THE INDIVIDUAL'S FACULTY FOR SELECTING THE RIGHT PERSONNEL TO FIT JOB REQUIREMENTS, TRAIN SUBORDINATES, AND AROUSE THEIR INTEREST AND AMBITION.	☐	☐ THE INDIVIDUAL HAS A KEEN ABILITY TO SELECT AND DEVELOP KEY SUBORDINATES AND IS AN OUTSTANDING TRAINER AND COUNSELLOR.	☐ THE INDIVIDUAL APPRAISES PERSONNEL RATHER ACCURATELY AND DOES A GOOD JOB OF TRAINING AND COUNSELLING.	☐	☐ THE INDIVIDUAL IS A FAIR JUDGE OF PEOPLE AND JOB REQUIREMENTS, BUT SOMETIMES DOES NOT DO A GOOD JOB OF TRAINING AND COUNSELLING.	☐	☐ THE INDIVIDUAL IS A POOR JUDGE OF PEOPLE AND JOB REQUIREMENTS AND HAS POOR TRAINING ABILITY.	☐
5	**PLANNING AND ORGANIZING** THIS TRAIT APPRAISES THE INDIVIDUAL'S ABILITY TO ORGANIZE, PLAN AND DELEGATE THE WORK FOR WHICH HE IS RESPONSIBLE.	☐	☐ THE SUPERVISOR DOES FIRST THINGS FIRST, CORRECTLY EVALUATES WHAT CAN AND SHOULD BE DELEGATED AND SHIFTS AUTHORITY AS WELL AS RESPONSIBILITY WISELY AND EFFECTIVELY.	☐ THE SUPERVISOR GETS THINGS DONE, IS SUCCESSFUL IN APPORTIONING WORK LOAD, USUALLY ATTEMPTS TO DELEGATE RESPONSIBILITY AND AUTHORITY TO QUALIFIED SUBORDINATES.	☐	☐ THE SUPERVISOR ORDINARILY GETS THINGS DONE BUT OFTEN FAILS TO RECOGNIZE ABILITY IN OTHERS AND DELEGATE AUTHORITY AND RESPONSIBILITY.	☐	☐ THE SUPERVISOR FREQUENTLY LACKS TIME FOR IMPORTANT MATTERS, IS CONFUSED WITH DETAILS, AND ATTEMPTS TO DO IT ALL HIMSELF.	☐
6	**RESPONSIBILITY** THIS TRAIT APPRAISES THE INITIATIVE OF THE SUPERVISOR TO ASSUME RESPONSIBILITY IN KEEPING WITH GOOD JUDGMENT.	☐	☐ THE SUPERVISOR IS ANXIOUS TO ASSUME MORE THAN HIS SHARE OF RESPONSIBILITIES IN KEEPING WITH GOOD JUDGMENT AND COMMON SENSE.	☐ THE SUPERVISOR ASSUMES RESPONSIBILITY IN KEEPING WITH GOOD JUDGMENT.	☐	☐ THE SUPERVISOR ASSUMES RESPONSIBILITY ONLY ON MATTERS IN WHICH HE IS WELL VERSED.	☐	☐ THE SUPERVISOR SELDOM ASSUMES RESPONSIBILITY OR ELSE ASSUMES RESPONSIBILITY WITHOUT THE NECESSARY QUALIFICATIONS.	☐

Source: Mt. Sinai Hospital, New York, New York.

interview between the rater and the rated after the assessment is made. The *interview method* involves a face-to-face interview between the employee and the person rating him and it is usually accompanied by a formal report of the discussion. The *rating scale method* provides for the employee to be rated against some "standard" that is defined or otherwise described on a scale. It is the most widely used method. Typically these scales are made up of five or more traits or characteristics. The most common characteristics are productivity, quality, job knowledge, versatility, dependability, initiative, appearance, personal relations and cooperation with management. In selecting the traits to be included on a performance evaluation form, there are certain basic considerations. One should choose traits that are:

1. Specific rather than general.
2. Definable in terms to be understood by all raters.
3. Common to as many employees as possible.
4. Observable in the day-to-day performance of employees.
5. Clearly distinguished from other traits.

The American Hospital Association, in its pamphlet *Employee Performance Appraisal Programs,* offers the following definition for these most common elements in a rating scale:[18]

1. *Productivity:* (How much work is done consistently by the employee?) This element refers to the amount of productive work done by a given employee over a period of time. Depending upon the nature of the job, the output can be measured by the number of pieces produced (uniforms ironed, letters written, clinical laboratory determinations made), or it can be based on other measures (both good and bad) of quantity.
2. **Quality:* (How accurate, neat, or complete is the employee's work?) This element refers to the relative merit ("goodness" or "badness") of the employee's work. It refers to wastage; the effective use of supplies, equipment, and materials; and the meeting of specified acceptable standards. It should not be confused with job knowledge, which is concerned with understanding, nor with productivity, which refers to the quantity of production.
3. *Job knowledge:* (How well does the employee understand his job assignment?) This element refers to the employee's job know-how. It refers to whether he has the neces-

sary skills for his job and whether he can recognize defects in his work. It attempts to show if he knows how to meet the duties of his job, whether or not he acts accordingly.
4. *Versatility:* (Does the employee demonstrate ability to perform a variety of tasks?) This element refers to the mental and physical flexibility and adjustment necessary for satisfactory performance on a variety of jobs. It refers to the ability to change easily from one task to another.
5. *Dependability:* (How faithful is the employee in reporting to work and staying at his assigned work?) This element refers to the consistency with which an employee applies himself to his work, not to the amount of output or the quality of his work. It attempts to measure whether he works continuously. It refers to his attendance and punctuality; whether he remains at his job or wanders about; and whether he wastes time, loafs, or works in spurts.
6. *Initiative:* (How well does the employee begin an assignment without direction?) This element refers to the employee's willingness and ability to initiate tasks; to recognize the best way of doing them; and to follow up when necessary, with minimal supervision and direction.
7. *Appearance:* (Does the employee's personal appearance meet the standards for the job?) This element refers to the employee's personal grooming, attire, physical bearing, and taste. An employee's attire usually is dictated by the nature of his work, which should be considered in evaluating this element.
8. *Personal relationships:* (How well does the employee relate to fellow employees?) This element refers to the general pattern of social conduct demonstrated by the employee at his job. It refers to how well he gets along with fellow employees and may be related to such diverse areas as health, alcohol, family, and finances. Because this element represents a broad judgment of personality deviations from established norms, evaluators should rate it cautiously.
9. *Cooperation with management:* (Does the employee accept assignments and suggestions willingly?) This element refers to the employee's willingness to follow orders. It is related to his ability and desire to work with his supervisors as a team and to whether he resists or actively supports approved

changes. It should not be confused with passive acceptance of orders or mere verbal "yessing" of supervisors to gain favor.

Frequently words or phrases are placed at various locations underneath the line of a rating scale for each trait to indicate different degrees of the trait. From three to five "levels" of the trait are usually so characterized including the two at the extremes. Points are assigned to various degrees of each trait together with a total point range for the trait. By adding together the points that the employee receives on each trait, a single point value—a total score—is deduced.

In employee comparison systems of performance assessment, the relative performance of various employees in a group is compared one against another. This method is sometimes referred to as the "Army Rating Scale." In such man-to-man comparisons, individual characteristics, rather than whole-man rating, are used. Each characteristic is described by five gradations. The high man and the low man are scored, and their names are put in appropriate positions on the scale. All other employees are compared with the names at the top and bottom of each trait to arrive at a rating. It is difficult to apply this method to the non-military establishment since it is necessary for each rater to develop his own scale.

A modification of this method is described by Henry and Sparks. They discuss "alternation" ranking reports of present performance as a dependable method of assessing executive potential. The names of a group of employees known to several supervisors are listed on a form. Each supervisor selects the one whose present performance he considers *highest* and the one he considers *lowest*. Then he continues down the list to select the *next highest, next lowest,* until all are rated. He selects alternately until all names listed have been ranked. No specific guide of factors to be considered is used. Each ranker makes his own definition of what will put one man higher or lower than others on the list.[19]

Other types of employee comparisons seek to place all employees in a group in the order of relative performance, with best performance at the top and worst performance at the bottom. Some seek to force the distribution of any group of employees being rated into the lowest, 10 percent; the next lowest, 20 percent; the middle, 40 percent; the next, 20 percent; and the highest, 10 percent.

The check list type of rating offers a number of traits, and the rater merely checks the statements that best fit his assessment of the individual being rated. The list may be constructed with questions, statements, phrases or words which describe the manner in which an employee might perform on the job. The choice of statements is the key to the success of this plan; too often they are permeated with platitudes. Berkshire and Highland describe a variation on the check list technique: the forced-choice performance rating. This method offers a series of blocks of two or more behavior descriptions which appear to the rater to be approximately similar or equal in their level of favorableness or unfavorableness. Yet in studies conducted, certain replies are associated with certain levels of performance. An example of a block of behaviors descriptions used for rating training skills follows:

1. Patient with slow learners.
2. Lectures with confidence.
3. Keeps interest and attention of class.
4. Acquaints classes with objectives for each lesson in advance.

A block of unfavorable items is:

1. Does not answer all questions to the satisfaction of students.
2. Does not use proper voice volume.
3. Supporting details are not relevant.

Prior studies have indicated that certain items can determine the differences between poor and good teachers while others have very little to do with the performance or relative success of the teacher.[20]

DEVELOPING PERSONNEL ASSESSMENT PROCEDURE

The key to designing a merit rating system is an evaluation of organizational needs. The system must be tailor-made to meet the needs of the organization. The steps in establishing a merit rating system include:

1. The determination of the traits to be rated. Usually the institution's administrative group will select traits which are specifically related to performance on the job.
2. Traits must be carefully defined so that each individual delegated the responsibility of assessing performance understands their meaning.
3. The traits selected must be broken down into "degrees" or "levels," and each degree, in turn, must be carefully defined.
4. The traits and degrees within the traits must be weighted. This process assigns point values to each trait which reflects the influence of that trait

on the rating as a whole. The point values for degrees within each trait are established similarly by determining the amount of points for each degree of the trait.

5. The actual conducting of the rating. The employee's immediate supervisor should be responsible for the assessment of the employee's performance. This assessment should be reviewed by the department head and agreement arrived at between both levels of administration. Most successful assessment plans include the discussion of the rating with the employee once the assessment has been completed. Such assessment conferences include a frank discussion of the employee's accomplishments and weaknesses. The appraisal interview involves the interaction of two people, each with his own purpose, knowledge, viewpoints and attitudes. While these differences may be difficult to reconcile, a well-managed assessment interview can help to determine goals and mutually acceptable standards. Both parties can then identify the problems that hinder achievement of their goals and arrive at workable solutions.

A constructive assessment interview is a very valuable management technique. It does, however, require the application of considerable skill, thought and effort. Workers want to know how they stand with their supervisors and it has been found that the whole assessment program is fruitless without a face-to-face communication of results, expectations and plans for improvement.

ADMINISTRATIVE APPRAISAL

The assessment of employee performance does not stop with the blue-collar worker. Administrative appraisal is necessary to strengthen administrative performance by developing a clear-cut mutual agreement on work objectives, plans, and personal and institutional goals. Too often a discomforting situation develops by the absence of sharing the organization's total objectives by the chief executive with his immediate subordinates. The Mount Sinai Hospital, New York City, has developed an administrative appraisal program which incorporates three phases directed toward the final goal of sharing total objectives:

1. The personal appraisal.
2. The peer appraisal.
3. The supervisor appraisal.

A personal appraisal form is given to the executive whose performance is to be evaluated. The executive is asked to outline his job, describing the objectives, responsibilities and duties of the position as he understands them. He is then asked to list the phases of his work that he performs well and those he performs only adequately, and to make specific suggestions as to how he can improve. The narrative form of appraisal includes a statement on what he needs for improvement from his supervisor, from his fellow workers, from the organization and from himself. The executive is then asked to look back on the past year and describe what he considers were his chief accomplishments; to look to the future and describe the areas that he thinks he could profitably develop from the viewpoint of his personal goals and the institution's needs; and to list the changes he would suggest to accomplish such development. Concurrent with his self-evaluation, the executive's supervisor has selected one or two of the executive's peers and asked them to measure the effectiveness of his performance—specifically, to tell how well he functions regarding the needs of their department and how he strengthened or weakened their own efforts to perform effectively. They are asked to outline the executive's principal strengths and weaknesses. This peer appraisal is confidential and is shared only with the administrator's supervisor. It does not become part of the administrator's file. Finally, upon receiving the peer appraisal and the self-appraisal forms, the administrator's superior is asked to complete a two-part supervisor appraisal form based on the assumption that performance improves with coaching and self-development.

The first part of the form lists various phases of the administrator's responsibility: professional knowledge, willingness to assume responsibility, planning, controlling work flow and expenditures, and accomplishment. Here the supervisor is asked to measure the administrator's problem-solving abilities, report writing, meeting of deadlines; his organizational development and relations with the staff; his staff development and communications with subordinates and superiors. In each of these categories the supervisor is asked to identify which of four statements presented to him most accurately reflects the administrator's actual performance and then to support each of his ratings by briefly setting forth instances during the past year that demonstrate the administrator's performance in these areas. The second part asks the supervisor key questions about the administrator to be answered in narrative form. Among the questions are: What are his main strengths? In what respects is he least effective? What actions are you taking to help him improve his performance? Can you suggest any training or experience that will assist him in his development? This form then serves as the basis of the appraisal interview which is conducted in complete privacy. The interview aims not at criticism, but at improvement of performance through recognition of an administrator's strengths and weaknesses. The final step is to get mutual commitment to the goals of the institution. The self-appraisal section of this institution's administrative appraisal program is patterned after Douglas McGregor's suggestion that each subordinate should establish for himself short-range performance goals and ways in which he can improve his efficiency and that of his department.[21] (See Addendum F to this article for forms used in the appraisal program.)

PITFALLS OF RATING

In making ratings there are several pitfalls which should be avoided:

1. Do not let your rating on one factor or your overall impression of the employee influence your rating of other factors.
2. Length of service or job classification should not affect the rating.
3. Do not let your personal bias enter into the ratings.
4. Do not be swayed by previous ratings.
5. Do not give the same rating on all factors (halo effect). There are wide differences in an individual with respect to the various factors. He might contribute very sound ideas and rate high in professional capability and still not meet schedules.
6. Do not rate on vague impressions.
7. Do not rate "sympathetically." If there are special circumstances, note them on an appropriate catchall section of the form.
8. Do not hesitate to go on record with your true opinion.

Ratings wherever possible should be made from accurate data or from observation. Ratings should be based on employee performance during the entire period being reviewed. The rater should be careful not to emphasize recent happenings or isolated dramatic happenings which are not characteristic performances. If an employee has had more than one supervisor during the rating period, each supervisor should complete a separate rating form. A composite rating can then be determined by the present supervisor. In the assessment interview, it is imperative that it be conducted in private. The employee should be permitted to read the review form, and an explanation of the supervisor's appraisal of the employee in terms of the requirements of the job— not in terms of the personal characteristics of the employee—should follow. Where possible, reference should be made to the position description or job outline. The employee's reactions should be solicited. The supervisor should listen attentively and actively. Criticism should be constructive and an emphasis placed on improvements to be made rather than on past failures. Unfavorable comparisons with other employees have no place in the assessment interview. If an employee's performance is deficient, it must be improved. He must be apprised of this fact. He must be told where he stands and agreement arrived at on future goals. The final step is the summary of the appraisal including the employee's strengths, areas for improvement, plans for effecting such improvement, assistance available to him and mutual commitment to the goals to be achieved during the coming review period.

CONCLUSION

The performance evaluation of health care employees is practical and necessary to ensure understanding and to obtain optimal agreement between worker and supervisor on the goals of the institution and the progress (or lack thereof) of the employee in reaching institutional and personal goals. A typical evaluation plan will be conducted as follows:

1. Rate employees in your department on one factor at a time.
2. Select the employee who excels in this one factor and give your rating.
3. Select the employee who should receive the lowest rating on that factor, and give your rating.
4. Consider the remaining employees, one at a time, and by comparison (forced choice) with the highest- and lowest-rated employees, determine the proper rating.
5. After rating all the employees in the group on one factor, follow the same procedure for each of the other factors.
6. After rating on all factors, review each form, taking into consideration the complete picture.
7. Ratings should be made from accurate data whenever possible, or from observation.
8. The rating should be based on the employee's performance during the entire period being reviewed. The rater should be careful not to overemphasize recent happenings or isolated dramatic happenings which are not characteristic performances.

Some change must be legislated if it is to be both permanent and positive. To ensure purposeful change, employee understanding must be obtained. This understanding includes the discovery of things the employee will both like and dislike: if change is to be effected, the worker must learn about both.

Communication is the focal point in a sound employee relations program. Studies in human behavior indicate a clear and urgent need for employees to know what is expected of them and where they stand in the organization. The development of formal communication programs is critical to successful administration. Too often employees of health care facilities, other than the medical staff, are the "invisible people." Medical staff and administration—that is, top administration—make decisions which are autocratically imposed upon the rest of the organization. Without appropriate participation and maximum communication, an organization may well fall below its expected goals. The hallmark of a sound communication program in a health care institution is the development and distribution of a personnel policy manual. Policies, plans and goals should be developed and communicated through various vehicles: conferences, meetings, face-to-face discussions. An organization that develops an atmosphere which facilitates and, indeed, encourages upward and downward communication will ensure its own success. Communication is not the responsibility of one department, i.e., the personnel department. It is not a "single-shot" program. Every member of the management team must be a good communicator. The supervisor's chief responsibility is getting the work done *through* other people. In order to accomplish this, a supervisor must be trained in the art of communication. This includes an appreciation of the importance of listening as an integral part of the entire process.

Finally, it is well to repeat: that communication grows best in a climate of trust and confidence is a *sine qua non*. An administration that does one thing and says another cannot in the final analysis expect communications, whether formal or informal, to be effective.

NOTES

1. Dale Yoder, *Personnel Principles and Policies* (Englewood Cliffs, N.J.: Prentice-Hall, Inc., 1956), pp. 381–2.

2. *Foreman Facts* (Newark, N.J.: Labor Relations Institute, Newark, N.J., Vol. 9, no. 21, 1952): 2.

3. Peter Drucker, *The Practice of Management* (New York: Harper and Bros., 1954), pp. 306–7.

4. C. S. Goetzinger and M. A. Valentine, "Communication Channels, Media, Directional Flow and Attitudes in an Academic Community," *Journal of Communication* (March 1961), pp. 23–6.

5. Willard V. Merrihue, *Managing by Communication* (New York: McGraw-Hill Book Co., Inc., 1960), pp. 23–4.

6. *Improving Employee-Management Communication in Hospitals: A Special Study in Management Practices and Problems* (New York: United Hospital Fund, Training Research and Special Studies Division, 1965), pp. 1–3 to 1–4.

7. Robert N. McMurry, "Clear Communications for Chief Executives" (special report published by *Harvard Business Review*, 1965), pp. 1–15.

8. Merrihue, pp. 18–20.

9. George S. Odiorne, *Personnel Policy: Issues and Practices* (Columbus, Ohio, Charles F. Merrill Books. Inc., 1963), p. 103.

10. *Improving Employee-Management Communication in Hospitals*, p. 2–1.

11. *Ibid.*, p. 2–7.

12. Odiorne, p. 4.

13. Statement in *Personnel Policy Manual*, The Mount Sinai Hospital, New York City.

14. Edwin L. Crosby, M.D., Preface, *Employee Performance Appraisal Programs: Guidelines for Their Development and Implementation* (Chicago: American Hospital Association, 1971).

15. Merrihue, p. 122.

16. Harold Mayfield, "In Defense of Performance Appraisal," *Harvard Business Review*, 38, no. 2 (March-April, 1960): 81–7.

17. Ordiorne, "What's Wrong with Appraisal Systems?" *op. cit.*, p. 79.

18. Employee Performance Appraisal Programs, *op. cit.*, pp. 7–8.

19. Edwin R. Henry and C. Paul Sparks, "Fueling Organizational Change at Jersey Standard," in *The Failure of Success*, Alfred J. Marrow, ed. (New York: AMACOM, A Division of American Management Associations, 1972), p. 296.

20. J. R. Berkshire and R. W. Highland, "Forced-Choice Performance Rating: A Methodological Study," *Personnel Psychology* 6 (1953): 355–78.

21. Douglas McGregor, "An Uneasy Look at Performance Appraisal," *Harvard Business Review* 35, no. 3 (May-June, 1957): 89.

Addendum A Sample Personnel Policy

```
                    PERSONNEL   POLICY   #1.0
```

INTRODUCTION*	Issued:
Page 1	Revised:

Purpose

Every medical center has four fundamental and interrelated responsibilities to its patients, to the community it serves, to its students, and to its employees.

A medical center can effectively discharge its responsibilities to its patients, to its students and to its community only through the capable, harmonious, coordinated and efficient efforts of its employees. Sound personnel administration encourages and facilitates the employees' optimum contribution toward the objectives of the institution.

It is the purpose of this manual to provide administrative and supervisory staff members with a complete documentary on Institution personnel admin- istration so that the policies and procedures contained herein may be applied equitably, consistently and with authority.

Application

If the observance of a policy or procedure results in a dispute or problem, or if the reader is uncertain of specific steps that must be taken, it is urged that the cognizant personnel administrator be consulted for assistance or interpretation. Compensation matters should be referred to the Wage and Salary Manager. Training matters should be referred to the Training and Development Manager. Employment matters should be referred to the Employ- ment Manager. Benefit matters should be referred to the Benefits Manager. Employee and labor relations matters should be referred to the Employee Relations Manager. Matters having a broad or emergent impact on the admin- istration of the Medical Center should be referred to the Vice President for Personnel or one of his assistants.

Changes and Additions

From time to time the contents of this manual will be revised or supple- mented to reflect changed or new policies and procedures. Additional pages will be issued whenever such changes take place. The reader is urged to insert these pages as they are received so that this manual may be maintained as an up-to-date reference.

*Excerpts

Addendum A continued

PERSONNEL POLICY #2.0 — Page 1

GENERAL PERSONNEL POLICY	Issued:
	Revised:

The policies in this manual define the responsibilities of the institution's administrative and supervisory staff in relation to the employees of the Medical Center. These policies are designed to promote the mutual understanding, respect and cooperation necessary to enhance medical care, education and research.

The following personnel policy statements embrace a progressive employee relations philosophy to be shared and applied to the administrative and supervisory staff. They also provide the rationale for the specific policies and procedures outlined in the remainder of this manual.

2.1 Employment: The Institution will use every reasonable means available to recruit the most capable employees for the positions to be filled. In compliance with civil rights legislation, and more importantly, in observance of the Medical Center's well established tradition of fairness, equal opportunity will be given to applicants of all races, religions, national origins, cultural backgrounds, age groups, sexes and personal persuasions. Selection is based solely on the applicant's demonstrable ability and qualifications for the job.

2.2 Placement: The Institution will make every effort to place employees in positions best suited to their abilities and career objectives.

2.3 Promotions: The Institution will encourage employees to acquire the capabilities requisite for advancement. Equal opportunity (as in 2.1) will be given to all applicants for promotion. Candidates for promotion will be given preference over outside employment applicants whenever possible. Selection is based on the candidate's demonstrable ability and qualifications for the job. Where ability of two or more candidates is relatively equal, the most senior employee is selected for promotion.

2.4 Compensation: The Institution will maintain salaries competitive with those prevailing for comparable jobs in health care institutions in the Greater New York Area. An equitable compensation structure will be maintained for the Center's numerous jobs based on relative responsibility, knowledge and skill requirements, working conditions and other job characteristics. Employees not covered by collective bargaining agreements requiring fixed wages and increments will be given increases based upon individual performance.

PERSONNEL POLICY #2.0 — Page 2

GENERAL PERSONNEL POLICY	Issued:
	Revised:

2.5 Hours of Work: ' The Institution renders service around the clock, every day of the year. The scheduling of departmental work hours is based on the operational requirements of the Medical Center. Employees will be assigned hours and shifts consistent with departmental needs, and, insofar as possible, with individual preferences. Hours will be changed only with appropriate notice to affected employees.

2.6 Time Off: The Institution will provide time off — in the form of vacation, holidays, sick leave, special leaves, and rest periods — to give employees adequate opportunity for leisure, recuperation, civic duties and personal activities. The amount of time off and compensation therefor, will be comparable with prevailing practices in health care institutions in the Greater New York Area.

2.7 Employee Benefits, Services and Activities: The Institution will provide employee benefits — in the form of insurance coverage, pension programs, etc. — at least comparable to those offered in the Greater New York health care community. Services, such as Employee Health Service, Food Service, Group Purchasing, and Personal Counseling, will be made available to improve the employee's working conditions and to assist in the fulfillment of his/her personal needs. The Institution will also promote, support or maintain various programs of recreational or community activities to enhance the employee's leisure.

2.8 Personnel Communications: The Institution will make every effort to communicate openly, promptly and accurately with supervisors and employees at every level. A keen responsiveness to improved communications will be encouraged.

2.9 Employee Recognition: The Institution will recognize each employee's individuality and dignity. Supervisory staff are to regard employees not as mere instruments of production or service, but as human beings with human feelings, human needs and human motivations. The Institution will maintain programs to recognize outstanding performance and long service. Supervisory staff are encouraged to recognize and reward outstanding employees not only through formal channels, but also in their personal interaction with these employees.

2.10 Training and Development: The Institution will afford its employees every reasonable opportunity for advancement through increased knowledge, education, training and experience. Programs will be maintained for employee orientation, on-the-job training, upgrading training, tuition aid, supervisory and administrative development.

Addendum A continued

PERSONNEL POLICY #2.0

| GENERAL PERSONNEL POLICY | Page 3 | Issued: |
| | | Revised: |

Where appropriate, the Institution will provide educational assistance and training opportunities to members of the community.

2.11 Employee Performance Review: The Institution will maintain programs for the systematic review of employee performance. Such reviews are to take place on a regular, periodic basis and the results of the reviews communicated to the employees. Supervisors are to supplement the formal reviews by keeping employees informed about their current performance progress.

2.12 Employee Counseling: The Institution will maintain an Employee Counseling program to assist employees in dealing with personal, financial, legal and medical problems that may or may not affect their employment. Any information divulged by an employee in his or her use of this service will be kept in the strictest confidence.

2.13 Grievance Procedure: The Institution will maintain a formal grievance procedure, culminating in binding arbitration, for the resolution of employee grievances. Every effort will be made to resolve grievances informally or at the lowest possible step in the procedure. No employee shall be discriminated against for having lodged a grievance.

2.14 Employee Discipline: The Institution will pursue a policy of enlightened discipline the primary objective of which is correction, not punishment. Supervisors are encouraged to administer disciplinary action that is: equitable and in keeping with the offense; consistent with prior actions and with actions in other departments; progressively sterner after repeated offenses; and designed to persuade the offending employee to improve. Discharge is to be resorted to only if the offense is extreme or after every possible remedial effort has been made.

2.15 Employee-Public Relations: The Institution will encourage the development of courteous, tactful and considerate behavior among the employees so that their dealings with patients and the public will reflect a regard for human values as well as a respect for technical standards.

2.16 Labor Relations: The Institution will honor the right of employees to organize for purposes of collective bargaining and will abide by all legal requirements in this connection. The same labor standards will be observed for unorganized as for bargaining unit employees. The Institution will join with other health care institutions for

PERSONNEL POLICY #2.0

| GENERAL PERSONNEL POLICY | Page 4 | Issued: |
| | | Revised: |

purposes of joint collective bargaining when it is in the best interests of the Medical Center and the Industry. Administrative and supervisory staff should be fully conversant with the terms of our collective bargaining agreements and are to consult with the Employee Relations staff whenever a contract application or interpretation is uncertain. The Institution will observe all provisions of its collective bargaining agreements and expects the same from the employees and their representatives.

2.17 Safety: The Institution will maintain working conditions that are free of hazards to the health and safety of employees, patients and the public. To this end, a continuous safety program will be maintained with the active participation of employees, supervisors and administrative staff from various units of the Medical Center.

2.18 Security: The Institution will maintain security measures and provide the staff and facilities necessary to safeguard the property and personal safety of employees, patients and the public.

2.19 Health: The Institution will make every possible effort to promote the health of its employees by: maintaining an Employee Health Service; making available to employees its outpatient and inpatient services; providing medical and hospitalization insurance, as well as legally required insurance protection.

Source: Mt. Sinai Hospital, New York, New York.

Addendum B Grievance Procedure Policy

PERSONNEL POLICY #15.2	Page 1	Issued:
		Revised:
GRIEVANCE PROCEDURE BARGAINING UNIT		

15.2 Grievance Defined:

A grievance is defined as any dispute or complaint arising between an employee and the Medical Center

   15.21 Grievance Procedure

   15.211 Step 1: Within a reasonable time (except as provided in the Collective Bargaining Agreement Article XXVIII, Discharge and Penalties), an employee having a grievance and/or the employee's Union delegate or other representatives shall take it up with his/her immediate supervisor. The Institution shall give its answer to the employee and/or the employee's Union representative within five (5) working days after the presentation of the grievance in Step 1.

   15.212 Step 2: If the grievance is not settled in Step 1, the grievance may, within five (5) working days after the answer in Step 1, be presented in Step 2. When grievances are presented in Step 2, they shall be reduced to writing, signed by the grievant and his or her Union representative, and presented to the grievant's department head or his or her designee. A grievance so presented in Step 2 shall be answered by the Institution in writing within five (5) working days after its presentation.

   15.213 Step 3: If the grievance is not settled in Step 2, the grievance may, within five (5) working days after the answer in Step 2, be presented in Step 3. A grievance shall be presented in this step to the Personnel Director or Administrator of the Institution, or his designee; and he or his designee shall render a decision in writing within five (5) working days after the presentation of the grievance in this step.

   15.22 Specified time limits are exclusive of Saturdays, Sundays and holidays.

PERSONNEL POLICY #15.1	Page 1	Issued:
		Revised:
GRIEVANCE PROCEDURE NONBARGAINING UNIT		

15.1 Grievance Defined:

A grievance is defined as any dispute or complaint arising between an employee and the Medical Center.

   15.11 Grievance Procedure

   15.111 Step 1: The employee should take up the problem with his or her supervisor within a reasonable time. The employee will receive an answer within five (5) working days.

   15.112 Step 2: If the grievance is not settled in Step 1, the grievance may, within five (5) working days after the answer in Step 1, be presented to the department head or his/her designee. The grievance, at this time, shall be reduced to writing and signed by the grievant. As in Step 1, the employee shall receive a written answer within five (5) working days.

   15.113 Step 3: If the grievance is not settled in Step 2, the employee may present it to the Personnel Director or his designee. The employee will receive a written answer within five (5) working days.

   15.12 The nonunion employee may have another nonunion Medical Center employee represent him at any of the grievance procedure steps if he so desires.

   15.13 Should the grievance still remain unresolved after completion of Step 3, it may be referred by either the employee or the Medical Center to an outside arbitrator for an impartial and binding decision.

   15.14 Specified time limits are exclusive of Saturdays, Sundays and holidays.

   15.15 The costs of the arbitrator will be borne equally by the parties.

Addendum B continued

PERSONNEL POLICY #15.2

| GRIEVANCE PROCEDURE BARGAINING UNIT | Page 2 | Issued: |
| | | Revisec: |

15.23   Should the grievance still remain unresolved after completion of Step 3, it may be referred by the Medical Center to an outside arbitrator for an impartial and binding decision.

15.24   The costs of the arbitrator will be borne by the parties.

THE MOUNT SINAI HOSPITAL
NEW YORK

PERSONNEL COPY

GRIEVANCE FORM

NAME OF EMPLOYEE _____ LIFE NO. _____

DEPARTMENT _____ DATE OF HIRE _____

JOB TITLE _____ DATE SUBMITTED _____

COMPLETE DETAILS OF GRIEVANCE: (INCLUDE SECTION OF AGREEMENT VIOLATED)

_____

_____

_____

_____

_____

(USE REVERSE SIDE IF NECESSARY)

REMEDY REQUESTED _____

EMPLOYEE _____
    (SIGNATURE)

◄◄◄ TIME LIMITS ►►►

DISPOSITION — STEP 1:

SUPERVISOR _____ DATE COMMUNICATED _____
  (SIGNATURE)

ACCEPTED: _____ APPEALED _____
STEWARD

5 WORKING DAYS

DISPOSITION — STEP 2:

DEPT. HEAD _____ DATE COMMUNICATED _____
  (SIGNATURE)

ACCEPTED: _____ APPEALED _____
STEWARD

5 WORKING DAYS

DISPOSITION — STEP 3:

PERSONNEL DIRECTOR _____ DATE COMMUNICATED _____
  (SIGNATURE)

ACCEPTED: _____ APPEALED _____
CHIEF STEWARD

5 WORKING DAYS

Source: Mt. Sinai Hospital, New York, New York.

Addendum C Communication Checklist

DO YOU KNOW HOW TO LISTEN

Listener's Quiz

When taking part in an interview or group conference do you:

	Usually	Sometimes	Seldom
1. Prepare yourself physically by sitting facing the speaker, and making sure that you can hear?	_____	_____	_____
2. Watch the speaker as well as listen to him or her?	_____	_____	_____
3. Decide from the speaker's appearance and delivery whether or not what he or she has to say is worthwhile?	_____	_____	_____
4. Listen primarily for ideas and underlying feelings?	_____	_____	_____
5. Determine your own bias, if any, and try to allow for it?	_____	_____	_____
6. Keep your mind on what the speaker is saying?	_____	_____	_____
7. Interrupt immediately if you hear a statement you feel is wrong?	_____	_____	_____
8. Make sure before answering that your've taken in the other person's point of view?	_____	_____	_____
9. Try to have the last word?	_____	_____	_____
10. Make a conscious effort to evaluate the logic and credibility of what you hear?	_____	_____	_____

Source: Mt. Sinai Hospital, New York, New York.

Addendum D Communication Program

COMMUNICATIONS MATERIALS
FOR A HOSPITAL*

Prepared by Albert N. Webster

October 25, 1966

*Reprinted with permission of the author.

GENERAL OBJECTIVES OF A COMMUNICATION PROGRAM

Communications with employees of the hospital shall support and be guided by the following objectives. These are designed with the intent of developing and then maintaining employee understanding and acceptance of overall hospital goals and motives, so that as a result employees will voluntarily contribute to the maximum extent of their individual capacities, and will cooperate as a group with the administration's steps to assure the success of the hospital.

1. To demonstrate the administration's concern and interest in employees as individuals—in their personal welfare and security.

2. To develop a concept in employees that each one's work is of importance to the overall accomplishments of the hospital.

3. To give employees an understanding and appreciation of hospital objectives, problems and results; to keep them informed as much as possible on matters that affect them; and to point out that their security is based on the sound, continuing and economical operations of the hospital, so that it can serve patients 24 hours a day and provide medical facilities for doctors at a cost patients can afford to pay, thus providing jobs, job opportunity and advancement of employee welfare.

4. To develop better understanding of management's role in the conduct of successful operations and the contribution of community resources in providing materials, machinery and jobs.

5. To develop and maintain employee confidence in the competence, alertness and long-range effectiveness of the administration, so that employees will have respect for (if not agreement with) the administration's operating objectives, programs and plans.

6. To convince employees of the sincerity of the administration's motives toward them, and the integrity and credibility of its policies and pronouncements. As related to union recognition and collective bargaining, to demonstrate to employees that the administration's position and goals are based on the balanced best interests of both the employees and the hospital.

7. To build mutual understanding, respect and confidence among employees at all levels and between organizational units.

8. To promote among employees the maximum possible regard for the hospital as an institution serving the interests of people and making an important contribution to the well-being of the community, and thus to evoke in employees a feeling of pride in the hospital as a good corporate citizen.

Addendum D continued

COMMUNICATION IS—

Behavior.............Speech, writing, action, nonaction, handshake, scowl, smile, silence

that results.............Must actually happen, tested by feedback

in an exchange.............Mutual, send and received, listened to

of meaning.............For both parties, related to needs and/or interests of both

that produces action.............Ranging from work or other desired accomplishment to mere response (agreement, disagreement, yes-but)

SPECIFIC OBJECTIVES FOR COMMUNICATIONS AT A HOSPITAL

1. To keep employees informed of current status of operations and conditions of the hospital

Maintain program of information to employees regarding patient census, services rendered, areas served; point out changes over past years and evidence of growth;

Discuss increasing costs, hospital's success in meeting them, changes in methods, and how it keeps up with new developments.

2. To gain acceptance by employees of the following objectives of the hospital

To make continuously available to the community the best possible care of the sick and injured;

To employ a sufficient staff of qualified, satisfied employees to provide the services required;

To protect the interests of employees as to salaries, hours, benefits, working conditions, fair treatment, considerate supervision, job security, personal growth, and to do so without regard to race, creed or color;

To so manage the hospital that employees will regard it as a good place to work.

3. To develop on the employee's part better understanding of his/her job, and the requirements and standards of performance expected from him/her

Develop and utilize organization charts, job descriptions, performance standards and performance appraisals, and discuss them with employees.

4. To give employees recognition for good performance

Assure salary administration based on performance;

Addendum D continued

COMMUNICATIONS IN A HOSPITAL

The following communications have been listed by participants in Supervisory Development Programs conducted in hospitals. The list should be completed by the addition of communications used or needed in the particular department.

Columns are provided to evaluate each communication. Mark in each column:

1. More than adequate

2. Adequate

3. Needs improvement

The columns are for:

A. Manner—the kind, method, timeliness.

B. Substance—the quantity, quality, accuracy, etc., of the message or meaning being accumulated.

C. Feedback—the presence of an exchange between sender and receiver, opportunity to make contributions, talk back, disagree, ask questions, clarify.

"Counsel" employees for good performance as well as to discipline for poor performance;

Arrange public personal recognition where warranted.

5. To give employees advance information on new services, procedures, operations, policies, etc.

Explain the meaning of and reason for those management actions that affect their job or interests as employees.

6. To obtain reactions, suggestions and viewpoint of subordinate employees; to pinpoint problem areas

Assure "feedback" of what employees are thinking, proper functioning of grievance procedure, and exit interviews;

Encourage and take appropriate action with respect to employees' comments and suggestions.

7. To demonstrate that the hospital's approach to employees relations problems

Aims to deal with employees firmly but with fairness;

Will seek solutions to problems in terms of maintaining a proper balance of the interests of patients, employees, doctors and the community;

Will seek answers from all interests involved so as to assure the continued operation of the hospital on a sound financial basis.

8. To correct, answer or otherwise counteract inaccurate or misleading statements by union leaders, or distortions by them of management's statements or actions

Monitor, catalog and evaluate misleading statements;

Answer, correct, counteract or, by anticipation, offset the more damaging or significant statements;

Select time (usually immediate), media and tone of communications most appropriate to give employees the facts, and develop understanding of hospital's intentions.

9. To improve communication skills of supervisors, managers and administration

Define responsibility to communicate;

Train by actual practice.

Addendum D continued

MANAGEMENT RESPONSIBILITY FOR COMMUNICATIONS

Every member of management and supervision is responsible for communicating effectively with employees under his/her supervision, for ascertaining their reactions and opinions, and for communicating fully on pertinent matters with his/her superior and fellow supervisors.

Specifically, this charge imposes the following obligations on each manager and supervisor:

1. To give each subordinate an understanding of the work he/she is doing, the services he/she provides, and the reasons for the various demands made upon him/her in his/her day-to-day job.

2. When so authorized, to inform subordinate staff members promptly and authoritatively of all hospital policies and practices, regulations, objectives and plans, reasons, problems, successes and failures, and any other information concerning the hospital that affects their work, their individual status, and their attitude toward the hospital.

3. To seek out and use all opportunities to pass along hospital information and viewpoint, to be aware of reactions, ideas and viewpoints of subordinates, and to report information to immediate superiors, as appropriate.

4. To train and counsel subordinate supervisors in the use of effective communications and to facilitate the proper discharge of the responsibility for communications at succeeding lower levels.

5. To share information and experience across department lines as appropriate, and by so doing, to facilitate cooperation and coordination of joint activities.

It shall be the responsibility of members of upper management levels to specify in all management job descriptions the incumbent's duty to pass on information to subordinates; to appraise the overall performance of a subordinate member on the basis, among other factors, of his/her success as a communicator; and, finally, to demonstrate by their own actions that communicating is an inherent part of day-to-day management responsibility and thus set a pattern for those supervisors working under them.

It shall be the responsibility of the originator of a communication to determine, with appropriate staff advice as indicated, how widely the information is to be disseminated among employees. He or she shall indicate this in writing on the communication itself, for the guidance and instruction of those at lower management levels who will receive the communication and be responsible for passing it on.

	A Manner	B Substance	C Feedback
Oral, face-to-face or telephone			
Supervisor-employee			
Between departments			
Between employees in department			
Taking reports (nursing)			
Orientation			
Interviews:			
Hiring			
Appraisals			
Counseling			
Disciplinary			
Exit			
Public address system			
Training			
With patients			
With doctors			
Grievance procedure			
Expressions of attitude			
Social-recreational			
Grapevine			
Memoranda and other written media			
From administration			
From staff personnel			
From department head			
Job descriptions			
Policy manual			
Employees' handbook			
House organ			
Library			
Professional publications			
Procedure manuals			
Suggestion system			
Bulletin boards			
Patient orders			
Work forms (requisitions, orders, etc.)			
Reports			
Financial Statements			
Tickler system			
Letters to employee			
Surveys			
Meetings			
Administrative conference			
Department heads			

Addendum D continued

	A	B	C
	Manner	Substance	Feedback
Meetings (continued)			
Within department			
All employees			
Special groups (head nurse, etc.)			
In service education			
Supervisory development program			
Trustees			
Ward conferences			
Open house			
Committees			
Inspections			
Medical staff			
Interdepartmental committees			
Departmental committees			
Safety			
Employee council			
Outside sources			
Medical forum			
Professional and technical associations			
Community organizations			
Vendors			
Schools-career programs			
Hospital speakers bureau			

Source: Mt. Sinai Hospital, New York, New York.

Addendum E Sample Performance Review

THE MOUNT SINAI MEDICAL CENTER

EMPLOYEE PERFORMANCE REVIEW

Name: _____   Life # _____

Position
Title: _____

Department: _____

Date of
Review: _____

Date of
Hire: _____

Type of
Review:

☐ Annual   ☐ Promotion   ☐ Other: _____

☐ Probationary   ☐ Transfer

INSTRUCTIONS

1. Print or type all information requested.

2. Read through entire Review form so that you are thoroughly familiar with appraisal factors and questions.

3. Complete all applicable sections. Please be concise.

4. Write your evaluation comments just below the questions. If more space is required, please use a separate sheet of paper and number the comments according to the original format.

5. It is recommended that you dictate or write out your evaluation first and then have it typed on the attached form for retention in the Records Section of the Personnel Department.

6. The Appraisal Factors are as follows:

I.	Job Knowledge	VI.	Initiative
II.	Quantity of Work	VII.	Organizing Ability
III.	Quality of Work	VIII.	Development and Training
IV.	Job Attitude	IX.	Supervisory Ability
V.	Judgment		

FACTORS FOR APPRAISAL:

I.   JOB KNOWLEDGE (Extent of employee's job information and comprehension)

A.   Does employee's performance evidence sufficient basic training and experience for the job?
_____

B.   What type and/or how much additional training and/or experience is required for successful performance?
_____

II. QUANTITY OF WORK (output volume, speed and consistency of output)

A.   Describe employee's work performance volume and its impact on overall work quantity.
_____

III. QUALITY OF WORK (accuracy, thoroughness, frequency of errors)

A.   How well does this employee do work requiring thoroughness, follow-up and detail?
_____

IV. JOB ATTITUDE (interest, motivation, enthusiasm and general willingness to perform)

A.   Describe employee's relationships with colleagues, subordinates, supervisors, patients and visitors.
_____

B.   Is employee's job attitude consistent?
_____

V.   JUDGMENT (extent to which decisions and actions are based on sound reasoning)

A.   What types of decisions is employee expected to make?
How effectively has this part of job responsibility been met?
_____

Addendum E continued

B. How well does employee respond to crisis, pressure or emergencies? _____

C. What are areas of improvement here and what steps are you and the employee taking? _____

VI. INITIATIVE (creativity of ideas and actions, extent to which employee is a "self-starter" in meeting goals)

A. Give instances where employee has shown initiative. What were the results? _____

B. Does employee evidence initiative after a problem is defined or often before a problem even exists? Give example of either or both if applicable. _____

C. Is employee's initiative expressed in areas not related to immediate job or primarily to job setting and requirements? Please give examples. _____

VII. ORGANIZING ABILITY (effectiveness in planning and performing work systematically)

A. Is time effectively used in performing tasks? _____

B. How well does employee plan work? Priorities? _____

C. Is employee capable of organizing activities of others in addition to his own? Has this happened? Please give an example. _____

VIII. DEVELOPMENT AND TRAINING

A. In order of importance, state performance characteristics which need improvement.

1. _____
2. _____
3. _____

B. What specific steps are you and the employee taking to improve overall job performance? _____

C. Is/Has this employee (been) involved in any formal training or related program outside of work? If so, what is subject matter? How is employee doing? _____

IX. SUPERVISORY ABILITY

A. How well does employee supervise and/or train staff under direction? _____

B. How might employee be rated overall by his subordinates? Peers? _____

RATING:

- [ ] Substantially Below Standard
- [ ] Below Standard
- [ ] Acceptable
- [ ] Above Average
- [ ] Consistently Effective
- [ ] Exceptional

_____ Employee's Signature

_____ Supervisor's Signature

_____ Department Head or Administrative Signature

EMPLOYEE COMMENTS: _____

Addendum F Sample Administrative Appraisal Plan

THE MOUNT SINAI HOSPITAL

ADMINISTRATIVE APPRAISAL PROGRAM*

Name: _____

Present Position: _____

Date of Hire: _____

CONTENTS

Section I — Introduction
        II — Preliminary Instructions
       III — Supervisor Appraisal Form No. P-134A
        IV — The Appraisal Interview
         V — Personal Appraisal Form No. P-134 B
        VI — Peer Appraisal Form No. P-134 C

*Excerpt

SECTION I — INTRODUCTION

The program is divided into three parts:

1. The Personal Appraisal Form No. P-134 B, is completed by the administrator whose performance is to be appraised.

   Optimum performance is a mutual goal for the organization and the individual. The primary responsibility for initiating administrative development is left where it belongs—with the individual. Much of the friction which develops in a work situation occurs because there is no clear-cut, mutual agreement about work objectives. This part of the Administrative Appraisal Program gives the individual an opportunity to express his understanding and interpretation of what his job entails, and how well he can meet its requirements.

2. The Peer Appraisal Form No. P-134 C, is completed by two colleagues of the administrator (to be selected by the supervisor). Here the individual's performance is appraised by his peers in terms of his contribution to the team effort. Emphasis is on what he does, and whether his performance strengthens or weakens his colleague's efforts to perform effectively.

3. The Supervisor Appraisal Form No. P-134 A, is the part of the Administrative Appraisal Program which should be of most assistance to the supervisor in helping the administrator in his self-development efforts. The supervisor will have the benefit of both the Personal and the Peer Appraisal Forms to assist him in his evaluation.

SECTION II
PRELIMINARY INSTRUCTIONS

Prior to his appraisal of an administrator's performance, the supervisor must accomplish the following:

(a) Administrative Appraisal Program Booklet

    Complete the blanks on Page 1 of the Administrative Appraisal Program Booklet by entering the administrator's name, present position and date of hire.

(b) Personal Appraisal Form

    Complete the blanks on the cover sheet of the Personal Appraisal Form. In addition to the information required in (a) above, this cover sheet should indicate the day, date, time and location set for the Appraisal Interview. The interview should be scheduled to take place 5 or 6 weeks after the date of issue of the Personal Appraisal Form.

(c) Peer Appraisal Form

    The two persons who are to complete the Peer Appraisal Forms should be selected on the basis of interrelated responsibilities and close working association with the appraisee-administrator. An administrator's peers are probably best equipped to evaluate his performance realistically. A careful choice is imperative.

(d) Supervisor Appraisal Form

    When the Personal Appraisal and Peer Appraisal Forms have been returned to the supervisor, he should study them carefully, for they will aid him in his own evaluation. He should then complete the Supervisor Appraisal Form, and prepare for the Appraisal Interview. (See Section IV)

Addendum F continued

SECTION III

SUPERVISOR APPRAISAL FORM No. P-134 A
Instructions

1. Review the entire form before you begin the appraisal.

2. Base your assessments on actual performance in the present job. In considering each quality, think over the results obtained.

3. Be on your guard against the common pitfalls in rating:

   (a) Treat each quality separately. Avoid a "halo" effect.
   (b) Do not permit your personal liking for the individual to influence your rating.
   (c) Avoid the tendency to rate those who hold more important jobs higher than those in less important jobs.
   (d) Avoid this "central" tendency (avoiding the extremes of the scale) by using very high or very low ratings where the appraisee's performance actually warrants such ratings.
   (e) Be sure that your ratings do not reflect an undue bias toward the extremes of the scale.

4. Rate performance during the past year. The appraisal program is based on the assumption that performance improves with coaching and self-development.

5. In each category place an X next to the phrase which most accurately describes the administrator's performance.

PART ONE

A. Professional/Specialist Knowledge

Consider the extent of his professional/specialist knowledge and ability to apply it in his work situation.

On the basis of his actual performance, indicate which of the following statements is most accurate:

☐ 1. His professional/specialist knowledge enables him to solve most problems satisfactorily;

☐ 2. His professional/specialist knowledge is adequate but he often cannot apply it.

☐ 3. His lack of knowledge frequently makes him unable to cope with technical problems;

☐ 4. Both his professional/specialist knowledge and his ability to apply it are of a high order.

Briefly state instances which have occurred during the past twelve months which illustrate the extent of his professional/specialist knowledge and his ability to apply it. Alternatively, give general comments supporting your rating.

B. Willingness to Assume Responsibility

Consider whether he has shown willingness to take on additional and more responsible duties. On the basis of his actual performance, indicate which of the following statements is most accurate.

☐ 1. Generally accepts and discharges responsibilities willingly and follows through to conclusion;

☐ 2. Seeks additional responsibility and authority. Concludes projects well.

Section IV

THE APPRAISAL INTERVIEW

At the risk of being redundant, we repeat here that the Administrative Appraisal Program aims, not at criticism, but at improvement of performance through recognition of an administrator's strengths and weaknesses. A sincere acceptance of this philosophy is a primary and essential step in achieving our objective.

The Appraisal Interview should be conducted in complete privacy — including privacy from unexpected visitors, telephone calls or other interruptions. A friendly informal atmosphere should be established. For this purpose, an interview off the Hospital premises might be helpful. It should be made clear to the appraisee that the purpose of the interview is not to criticize, but to reach agreement on plans for improved performance.

There will probably be areas in which the appraiser's evaluation will agree with the administrator's Personal Appraisal. These should be discussed first, and only then should the points of variance be introduced. At all times, the appraisee should be the central figure in the interview. He should be permitted ample opportunity to explain or justify his opinion, and be assured that his reactions are of prime importance. The supervisor should listen and evaluate, recognizing that his own prejudices could have influenced his judgment.

Every interview involves the interaction of two people, each with his own purposes, knowledge, viewpoint and attitude. While these differences may be difficult to reconcile, a well managed interview can help determine goals and set standards which are mutually acceptable. Both parties may then identify problems which hinder achievement of their goals and arrive at workable solutions. A constructive interview is a valuable management technique which requires the application of considerable skill, thought, and effort.

Addendum F continued

THE MOUNT SINAI HOSPITAL

ADMINISTRATIVE APPRAISAL PROGRAM

Section V

PERSONAL APPRAISAL FORM No. P-134 B

Name: _____

Present Position: _____

Date of Hire: _____

Supervisory Appraisal Schedule: Day: _____

Date: _____

Time: _____

Location: _____

By: _____

Optimum performance is a common goal for the Hospital and the individual. In order to strengthen administrative performance, it is essential that a clear-cut mutual agreement be reached as to individual work objectives and plans for their attainment.

As a key member of the administrative staff, your performance has marked effect upon the successful operation of the hospital. Therefore, within a few weeks, your supervisor will discuss with you his evaluation of your performance over the past year.

At the time of your appraisal interview, you should be prepared to discuss your job and what it entails as YOU see it, and to give your own evaluation of your performance. This form has been designed to give you the opportunity to discuss your job in specifics rather than generalities. It is hoped that, thereby, you can be assisted not only to set realistic goals, but to achieve them. Your administrative development is primarily your own responsibility.

To be completed by _____ To be returned to
                        date

HOW WOULD YOU RATE YOUR PERFORMANCE OVER THE PAST YEAR

(Check appropriate point anywhere along scale)

low................................ high

A. Ability to plan for specific goals .... [ ]

B. Ability to determine suitable course of action .... [ ]

C. Ability to organize for orderly accomplishment................................. [ ]

D. Ability to motivate others.................. [ ]

E. Ability to get along with others.............. [ ]

F. Ability to control people and situations effectively............................ [ ]

G. Ability to select and train personnel......... [ ]

H. Ability to delegate authority and responsibility successfully................... [ ]

I. Ability to follow through until required end result is achieved.................... [ ]

Addendum G Nursing Evaluation Form

THE MOUNT SINAI HOSPITAL
NEW YORK

PERSONNEL EVALUATION FORM
NURSING PROFESSIONAL PERSONNEL

Name: _____
Life No.: _____
Supervisor: _____
Date of Employment: _____
Date of Termination: _____

Position: _____
Assignment: _____
Evaluated By: _____
Type of Evaluation:

( ) Annual   ( ) Probationary
( ) Reference   ( ) Termination
( ) Promotion

OVERALL EVALUATION (Check appropriate point on scale)

Superior	Above Average	Average (satisfactory)	Fair	Poor (unsatisfactory)

Explanation:

Superior   - Outstanding nurse, sets excellent example to associates and auxiliary personnel; recognized as responsible professional.

Above Average - Maintains high standards, displays initiative.

Average   - Performs at satisfactory level, minimum initiative but can be depended upon to follow instructions.

Fair   - Seldom displays initiative, performs at minimal level, seldom does more than is required. Needs follow-up.

Poor   - Unsatisfactory performance, requires frequent follow-up.

SUMMARY

Give a concise but complete summary of nurse's attitude, personal qualifications, relationship with patients and professional acumen. Please note any points of significance not adequately covered in factor ratings.

PRINCIPLE STRENGTHS: _____
_____
_____
_____
_____
_____

AREAS TO BE IMPROVED: _____
_____
_____

ADDITIONAL COMMENTS: _____
_____
_____

		Check point of rating

I   RELATIONSHIP WITH PATIENTS

Evaluate employee's ability to develop rapport with visitors, family, and understand the needs of patient:

0.	Little or no interest in patient; often cold and abrupt	-0
1.	Detached, but not unpleasant	-1
2.	Displays awareness and sensitivity to patients problems and needs	-2
3.	Exceptional interest in patient; patient-orientated; engenders good will	-3

II RELATIONSHIPS WITH OTHERS

Consider cooperation with peers, success in building and maintaining respect and loyalty of subordinates, and attitude towards supervisor:

0.	Displays lack of regard for associates	-0
1.	Usually cooperative, but not always tactful	-1
2.	Meets other half-way, is respected by associates	-2
3.	Engenders good-will, displays and earns loyalty and regard. Consistently builds good relationships.	-3

III PROFESSIONAL CAPABILITY

Evaluate the employee's application of nursing principles and bedside nursing techniques:

0.	Below acceptable standards for present assignment	-0
1.	Minimum ability, fair technique	-1
2.	Carries out assignments with care and accuracy	-2
3.	Superior capability, expert on job	-3

IV GROWTH POTENTIAL

Consider participation in professional organizations and interest in furthering education:

0.	Will not or cannot accept more responsibility	-0
1.	Accepts responsibility, shows interest in growth	-1
2.	Versatile, ambitious; displays ability for increased responsibility	-2

V   ATTITUDE TOWARDS HOSPITAL

0.	Does not reflect understanding and appreciation of Hospital's objectives	-0
1.	Loyal employee; accepts supervision	-1
2.	Extremely "Hospital-Oriented" resulting in high morale of associates	-2

VI PERSONAL QUALIFICATIONS

Consider appearance, vitality, grooming and personal hygiene:

0.	Unkempt, slovenly	-0
1.	Neat, fit and applies principles of personal hygiene	-1
2.	Superior appearance and grooming	-2

Addendum G continued

DEFINITION OF TRAITS

I. RELATIONSHIP WITH PATIENTS

An important aspect of a nurse's job is her/his ability to develop rapport and understanding with the patient.

    A. Consider her/his approach to the patient's well-being.

    B. Consider her/his attitude towards family and visitors.

    C. Does she/he display understanding of basic physical, emotional and spiritual needs of patient?

    D. Is she/he flexible in dealing with the differences in patients due to economic levels, emotional stability, and medical histories?

    E. Does she/he show a sincere concern for people?

As a nurse who is pleasant to patients, but somewhat detached, should be rated near the middle of the scale.

II. RELATIONSHIP WITH OTHERS

Consider this factor as a measurement of the employee's demonstrated ability to work harmoniously with others.

The employee who is reasonably pleasant, cooperates when asked, causes no friction but does not increase the spirit of the group, is about average and should be rated near the middle of the scale. To be rated at the top of the scale, the employee should be an individual who goes out of her/his way to cooperate, thus stimulating willingness and cooperation on the part of others.

III. PROFESSIONAL CAPABILITY

We are concerned here with the nurse's performance; her/his application of nursing principles.

    A. Consider her/his ability to organize and complete assignments.

    B. Consider the degree of care necessary in carrying out procedures.

    C. Consider care of equipment.

    D. Does she/he exercise sound judgment in dealing with problems of patients?

    E. Does she display depth of understanding of techniques and details?

The employee who is satisfactory, no more or less than acceptable, should be rated in the middle of the scale.

IV. GROWTH POTENTIAL

We are measuring the nurse's demonstrated ability to accept additional responsibility and diversified assignments.

    A. This factor is also measured in displayed interest in inservice programs, professional organizations and further education.

An employee who accepts the responsibilities of her/his assignments, no more or less, should be rated in the middle of the scale.

V. ATTITUDE TOWARDS HOSPITAL

Morale and, in turn, effectivity are greatly affected by the employee's motivation. Closely tied-in with the nurse's motiviation is her/his attitude toward the Hospital.

The nurse who readily accepts supervision, understands and is sympathetic to the administration's goals and purposes should be rated in the middle of the scale.

VI. PERSONAL QUALIFICATIONS

We are concerned here with the nurse's appearance and grooming.

    A. Are her/his uniforms clean, neat and well-fitted?

    B. Does she/he maintain good posture?

    C. Application of good principles of personal hygiene?

A nurse who is always well-groomed and sets an example for others should be rated near the top of the scale.

17. Personnel Department's Role in Enhancing Effective Communication within an Organization

EARL J. MOTZER

Communication is the process by which all human interaction takes place. This process determines the climate of an organization. When gaps occur, or when communication fails, problems arise.

PROBLEM IDENTIFICATION

The first role of the personnel department in enhancing effective communications within an organization is to identify the nature and seriousness of communication problems. Some of the more common ones are:

- Insufficient communication from top management to lower level management.
- Lack of two-way communication between departments at all levels.
- Poor communication between supervisors on different shifts in the same department.
- Failure of management to listen to problems and ideas of subordinates.
- Poor communication between staff departments and line management.
- Insufficient information given to employees.

Techniques for identification of these problems include personal interviews, surveys, observations, analysis of problems, and discussions in meetings.

PROGRAMS AND TECHNIQUES

The second role of the personnel department is to provide programs and techniques to improve communications. The main criteria for deciding on a particular program or technique are:

1. Which will get the best understanding on the part of senders and receivers?
2. Which will transmit accurate information at the right time?
3. Which is the most cost-effective?

Downward communication techniques include small employee meetings, employee publications, supervisors' meetings, employee mass meetings, letters to employee homes, pay inserts, bulletin boards, posters, open houses or tours, public address systems, advertisements in local press, radio and television, videotape programs, cassette recordings, memos to all employees, and closed circuit television.

Upward communication techniques include formal inquiries or discussion with employees, first-level supervisors, formal attitude surveys, grievance or complaint procedures, counselling, exit interviews, union representation, formal meetings, suggestion systems, the grapevine, gripe boxes, question and answer columns in employee publications, open door policies, and feedback procedures.

SUPERVISORY TRAINING

The third role of the personnel department is to assist in training supervisors to communicate effectively on the job. The content of this training program should be based on the needs of the specific organization so that supervisors can gain better insight into the communication process, recognize and better understand the importance of nonverbal communication, and become more aware of communication barriers and how to deal with them effectively so they will be better equipped to design training program content.

COMMUNICATIONS PROCESS

Communication involves the transmission (formally and/or informally) of a message (meaning, sentiment, affection, and/or idea) from a sender to a receiver (upward, downward, or lateral). The sender must be alert not only to the individual's own knowledge, experience, and attitude about the message content itself but to that of the receiver as well. Someone who knows very little about a subject or who has had little or no experience with it may not communicate as well. If the sender has a negative attitude about the subject, unless the person is careful to conceal it, the receiver may become aware of and perhaps share in the negativism. In the employment setting, the subordinate may tend to mimic the actions of the superior that are most beneficial to him. If the boss presents a new policy or procedure in the wrong way, the employee may react in the same manner.

TRANSMISSION

The transmission of a message may be in writing, verbal, symbolic, and/or nonverbal. The importance of nonverbal communication often is overlooked. The actions of the sender can give a message to the receiver that does not complement what is intended. The lack of eye contact, poor posture, inappropriate clothing, certain types of facial expression, and signs of nervousness can imply lack of interest, poor attitude, or raise questions as to the credibility of the presentation.

Sensory organs also can play an important part in the effective transmission of a message; the more organs that are involved, the better the chance for comprehension. Senders should attempt to use audiovisual materials when giving oral presentations and should distribute handouts at the conclusion so that receivers can refer to them later for better recall and reinforcement.

STUMBLING BLOCKS

There are many common stumbling blocks to effective communication. Having an understanding of them enables the sender to plan how they can be overcome. Sometimes the sender mistakes form for substance and gets so carried away with delivery techniques that the person forgets to concentrate on the message itself.

Some tend to oversimplify or become too intellectual in approach. They fail to assess adequately their own and the receivers' knowledge and experience. Others tend to talk more than listen and forget that everyone is born with two ears and one mouth and that they should be used in that proportion.

Some receivers prematurely evaluate a presentation, or they daydream, or they permit prejudices to interfere. Knowledge of this fact can help the sender to overcome the impediment. Research indicates that less than half of the message will be retained over a period of time, so proper presentation planning, including the use of more than one transmission mode and sensory organ, is essential.

Communication is most complete where trust and confidence are present. The supervisor who is known to keep promises, to report facts honestly, and to listen sincerely does not have to fall back on phony good fellowship. In the long run, employees are influenced not by what management says, but by what it does. Nobody is fooled when a hitherto unsocial boss suddenly says good morning or asks about an ailing wife because the superior was told to do it in a human relations course or manual. The supervisor who levels with employees, who listens to their problems, and who is genuinely concerned about them can exercise effective leadership even though the person sometimes may forget to say good morning.

Words can have double meaning and it is wise for the sender to explain the main points with examples, or to have a disinterested person review the presentation for clarity. Here are two instances of miscommunication:

1. The lady of the house cautioned the new maid, "Now when you wait on the guests at dinner, I want you to be careful not to spill anything." "Don't worry," said the maid, "I won't say a word."
2. "I hope you thoroughly understand the importance of punctuation," the employer told a newly hired typist. The stenographer said, "Oh, yes, indeed, I always get to work on time."

Another stumbling block to avoid is the use by managers of what are called killer phrases such as: "We've never done it before," "Why change—it's working OK," "The boss will never buy it," and "Our institution is different." Employees tend to find their enthusiasm stifled when their suggestions meet such a response.

TWO-WAY COMMUNICATION

Real communication moves freely in both directions. This is well accepted as theory. In practice, however, managers devote far more attention to telling, informing, and commanding than they do to listening, asking, and interpreting. Thus, even while communicating aggressively, they may fail to tell workers what the employees want or need to know.

To learn whether or not employees really get the message, the supervisor must stimulate them to express their ideas and to ask questions, and then must give careful consideration to any problems that may arise. The problems at times may seem trivial but, if unanswered, they constitute a barrier to understanding and to action.

Communication can be one-way or two-way in nature. One-way communication is easy, fast, and orderly, but questionable as to accuracy because the receiver is not permitted to ask questions to make sure the message is understood. In contrast, two-way communication is slow and possibly frustrating because of the interchange between the sender and the receiver, but it does tend to be more accurate. Two-way communication also makes the receiver feel more involved in the outcome.

Good listening is a very important role for the receiver to maximize comprehension. Some helpful techniques are to look and act interested, put the sender at ease, and empathize with the individual. Asking questions is recommended to clarify points made but the sender should go easy on argument and criticism, be patient, and resist letting tempers flare.

RUMORS

Rumors travel on the grapevine only when a story has importance to both the sender and the receiver and when the true facts are shrouded in some kind of ambiguity. The best way for management to counter them is to follow up with accurate information on a timely basis.

TEN COMMANDMENTS

Harold Koontz's and Cyril O'Donnell's ten commandments of good communication provide an appropriate summary:[1]

1. Clarify ideas before communicating—make sure you know and understand what you are going to say and how best you are going to say it.
2. Examine the true purpose of each communication—make sure it is necessary and that you will be accomplishing what you want to.
3. Consider the total physical and human setting—determine the knowledge and experience of the receiver on the subject so that the best presentation can be developed.
4. Consult with others when appropriate—a technique some people find successful is to have colleagues in another discipline read important reports before they are submitted. They are surprised how people who seemingly know nothing about a particular technical subject can find loopholes in the written words.
5. Be mindful of overtones—your tone of voice and choice of language can affect comprehension.
6. Convey something of value—take into consideration what the receiver wants to hear.
7. Follow up—make certain that every communication has feedback so that complete understanding and appropriate action result.
8. Communicate for the future as well as the present—be consistent with long-range interests and goals.
9. Support communication with action—managers' "do as I say, not as I do" approach has no place in the business world.
10. Seek to understand as well as to be understood—listen carefully to determine the receivers' reaction to the message so that appropriate follow-up can be made.

The personnel department's role in enhancing effective communication in an organization is both important and difficult. A problem can be dealt with effectively when it is identified if there is an understanding of the communication process itself, recognition of the importance of nonverbal communication, and knowledge of how to cope positively with communication barriers. These factors can be of great assistance in providing programs and techniques for solution.

NOTE

1. Harold Koontz and Cyril O'Donnell, *Management: A Book of Readings* (New York: McGraw-Hill Book Co., 1972).

RECOMMENDED READINGS

Beach, Dale S. *Personnel: The Management of People at Work.* New York: Macmillan Publishing Company, 1975.

Clevenger, Theodore Jr., and Matthews, Jack. *The Speech Communication Process.* Glenview, Ill.: Scott, Foresman and Company, 1971.

Davis, Keith. *Human Behavior at Work.* New York: McGraw-Hill Book Co., 1972.

Hicks, Herbert. *The Management of Organization: A Systems and Human Resources Approach.* New York: McGraw-Hill Book Co., 1972.

Schneider, Arnold E., Donaghy, William C., and Newman, Pamela Jane. *Organizational Communication.* New York: McGraw-Hill Book Co., 1975.

18. Training

HENRY C. LaPARO

To meet their societal goals of providing quality patient care in a cost-effective manner, health care organizations and hospitals, in particular, need to create work environments that facilitate the development and use of human resources. The quality of patient care depends almost entirely on the knowledge, skills, and attitudes of the staff delivering it. Hospitals also are labor intensive organizations where human resource expenses are the major component in the operating cost structure.

After scanning across the spectrum of human resource programming, it becomes evident that employee training provides the most direct route for improving the performance and upgrading the qualifications of hospital staff. Training can be a bottom line activity, when the program's objectives serve as the basis for its design as well as for evaluating its operational impact.

However, training's potential for improving employee performance and operational effectiveness can be realized only when line managers view it as an integral part of their own responsibilities rather than a function or activity performed "in vacuo" by an education or personnel department.

WHAT IS TRAINING?

The term training as used in this article is defined in its broadest sense and encompasses the entire range of planned or programmed learning experiences and methods that can be used to facilitate employees in acquiring new knowledge, skills, and/or attitudes, as well as achieving predetermined behavior changes.

For the purist who still insists on the finer nuances that distinguish between "training," "development," and "education," concessions are made on these definitions. Dr. Leonard Nadler, in his book *Developing Human Resources*, defines *training* as "those activities which are designed to improve human performance on the job the employee is presently doing or is being hired to do."[1] *Development* he defines as preparing employees to "move with the organization as it develops, changes and grows."[2] *Education* involves development activities that "are designed to improve the overall competence of the employee in a specified direction and beyond the job now held."[3]

THE HOSPITAL TRAINER

The need to make managers at all levels more acutely aware of their training responsibilities and opportunities is rapidly restructuring the role of the hospital trainer and also is changing the position's job qualifications. Providing line managers with the support, guidance, and encouragement needed to initiate employee training activities requires trainers who are skilled in:

- internal consulting
- employee training program designing
- program administration

It is hoped that this article will be helpful to hospital trainers in assessing and expanding their competencies in these three areas.

Internal Consulting

To promote and gain the active involvement of line managers in employee training activities, a majority of hospital trainers' time and effort must be devoted to the activities encompassed in their internal consultant role. To function effectively as internal consultants, hospital trainers must be proficient in:

- analyzing the causes of job performance problems
- communicating
  —listening
  —questioning
  —writing
  —organizing ideas
- analyzing cost/benefit factors in training
- applying learning theory to the design of instructional systems
- being sensitive to the feelings of others and responding appropriately to those feelings

The conscientious application of these internal consulting skills produces a trainer who gets results by guiding and supporting the active involvement of line managers in training their employees. Such trainers intuitively recognize that their ideas and recommendations are being weighed and evaluated continually by line managers who not only are result oriented but who more importantly have precious few discretionary resources to allocate to any new activity. This is particularly true if it is an activity such as employee training that, because it is new, many department heads feel they can defer without penalty almost indefinitely.

The extremely tight financial situation in hospitals today is making it more difficult to get budgetary approval for new training programs, even when a rigorous cost/benefit analysis indicates that on a long-term basis they have the potential to recoup their costs many times over. This lack of dollars internally has provided an incentive for hospitals to seek external funding and/or resources to support training programs. Government agencies, foundations, jointly administered management/union training and upgrading funds, and both secondary and postsecondary schools are possible sources for funding and other resources (e.g., instructors, training materials, audiovisual equipment).

In the process of obtaining and allocating this external support for the program, the trainer creates an internal network of managers, instructors, and employees/students, all of whom have a common interest, namely, employee training. This network can be invaluable to trainers, as a base for developing support for future efforts because as their job expands to encompass the new role of fund raiser or proposal generator they will:

- gain quick direct or indirect access to existing internal learning resources (inservice staff, classrooms, laboratory space, audiovisual facilities) that otherwise might not be available or be available only on a very limited basis
- facilitate their own professional and career development
- establish formal and informal links with other hospital staff members in a wide variety of functions, as well as in the community that the hospital serves.

There has been a significant increase in both the quality and quantity of employee training programs in the health care sector over the last five years. A key factor in this growth has been the fact that hospital managers at all levels are beginning to experience positive operational paybacks from training programs. And, to cite an adage proved by time, "nothing succeeds like success." Even relatively small institutions have a wide assortment of employee training activities running the gamut from voluntary evening high school equivalency preparatory classes through two-year full-time accredited allied health programs. Hospital administrators also are showing markedly increased interest in supervisory and management training. More and more, administrators are viewing training not only as a means of cultivating or creating a climate conducive to needed organizational and operational changes, but also as a primary vehicle for achieving those changes.

Designing Employee Training Programs

Employee training programs fall into two broad areas: those with formats stressing individual learning, and those with formats emphasizing group learning. A representative sampling of programs in both areas, commonly found in health care institutions, shows these lineups:

Individual Learning	Group Learning
On-the-job training	Courses
Clinical training	Workshops
Internship	Conferences
Coaching by immediate supervisor	Grand rounds
Job rotation	Project teams
Programmed instruction	Behavior modeling

Without question, the most widely used and abused training activity in a hospital is on-the-job training. The vast majority of employees, regardless of their organizational level or prior preparation, acquire a significant portion of their job knowledge and skill at work. This on-the-job learning can be either programmed and effective or unprogrammed and ineffective.

A statement often found on the office wall of hospital trainers reads: "Every organization pays for a training program whether it has one or not." The phrase clearly communicates the idea that many hidden costs are incurred because of poorly organized on-the-job training. However, it falls short by not drawing attention to how the lack of proper training causes a wide array of operating problems. The importance of proper training often comes to the fore only when an employee's lack of knowledge or skills is instrumental in causing or contributing to a cataclysmic event.

Employees in a health care setting provide services and perform tasks that often are life sustaining. A lack of job competency or laxity in their performance not only is ethically inexcusable, it also can result in a malpractice suit against the employee and/or the hospital.

Well-planned and well-executed training programs ensure that employees are prepared adequately to carry out their job assignments. However, many other factors in the work setting can nullify the benefits of sound training. Factors that can undermine training as well as impact negatively on an employee's job performance include:

- indifferent supervision
- inappropriate and ill-conceived work systems and procedures
- poorly maintained equipment and facilities
- inadequate staffing

Inexperienced hospital trainers often get involved in launching programs designed to solve these types of problems. This happens because, unfortunately, too many view training as a universal panacea for almost any operating problem. Further, some line managers desiring to defer or sidestep an operating problem calling for a hardheaded but uncomfortable decision have been known to use training as a foil to muddy the waters. These managers generally view training as a convenient way of buying the time they need to address the real cause of their operating problem more comfortably.

To prevent being drawn into these no-win situations, it is absolutely essential that hospital trainers systematically analyze and assess training needs. The disciplined use of a systems approach in designing programs is a key factor in ensuring that training becomes the solution of first choice only when the root cause of an operating problem can be traced directly back to a lack of job knowledge and/or skill on the part of the employee(s).

A SYSTEMS APPROACH TO TRAINING

The value, as well as the necessity, of systematically approaching the job of designing and conducting employee training cannot be overemphasized. First, a systematic approach forces a rigorous and substantial effort in the all-important planning phase when training needs are identified and defined. Second, it focuses attention on those difficult but necessary logistical considerations that all too often spell the difference between success and failure in a training program. Specifically, a systems approach requires and emphasizes:

- an assessment of instructional needs
- the specification of behavioral objectives
- an instructional design tailored to meet specific objectives
- an evaluation design that quantitatively and in some cases qualitatively:
  - verifies the degree to which learning objectives have been met
  - determines the operational value of the training to the hospital.

In selecting a system design for assessing, developing, implementing, and evaluating the program, the trainer should determine first what, if any, management systems already are in use in the hospital. For instance, if a system approach such as project management is in use, the trainer can save considerable time and effort by using it as the prime vehicle for systematically assessing training needs and carrying out programs.

The logic of using an existing system such as project management becomes quite evident when its major phases are compared with the main activities required in the design and implementation of a training program. Exhibit 18-1 illustrates how easily the major phases of project management can be adopted to serve as a frame of reference for the activities that must take place in developing and conducting employee training programs. Using an existing system also eliminates the need to invest the time and effort ordinarily required to install one specifically designed for planning and implementing training programs.

Figures 18-1, 18-2, and 18-3 illustrate how project management can be used to provide a framework for planning and producing training courses. These schematics track the nature and sequencing of the activities involved in assessing training needs, defining learning objectives, developing course content, deciding on instructional methods, preparing instructional materials, and identifying and selecting instructors and students. The two other phases of project management—implementation and postimplementation review (which are not shown)—serve as vehicles for planning activities involved in (1) carrying out or conducting the course and (2) evaluating the course in terms of participant reaction and operational impact.

Perhaps the main benefit inherent in using a systems approach for planning programs is that it promotes the involvement and commitment of hospital managers, at all levels, in employee training activities. It accomplishes this by creating a climate, as well as an information base, that enables the hospital trainer to:

- review with administrators and department heads the projected benefits, risks, and costs of proposed training programs

Exhibit 18-1 Comparison of Two Types of Programs

Project Management Phases	Training Design Requirements
Formation	Training needs assessed
Preliminary definition and design	Training needs translated into learning objectives
Detailed definition and design	Instructional delivery system designed
Implementation	Training conducted
Postimplementation review	Training evaluated and employee transferred to job

- promote the active involvement of hospital managers not only in the planning but more importantly in the development and implementation of training programs.

ASSESSING TRAINING NEEDS

The keystone in the design of a program is the accurate identification and articulation of the training need(s). A number of methods are used to gather the data or information needed to zero in on or identify

Figure 18-1 Formation Phase (Assess Training Needs)

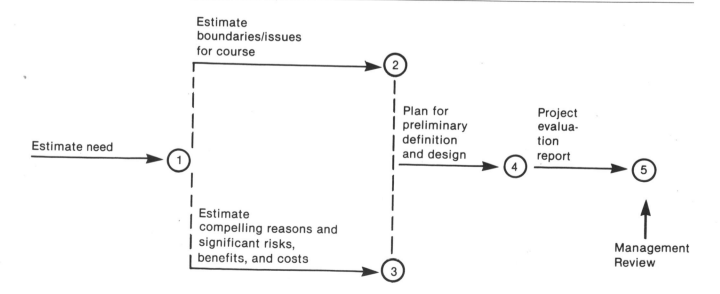

Figure 18-2 Preliminary Definition and Design Phase (Translating Training Needs into Learning Objectives)

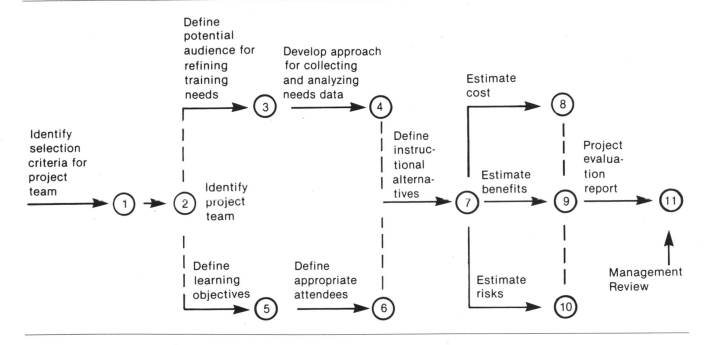

these needs: training needs survey, functional audits, interviews with employees, observation, written and performance tests, and analysis of operating problems. All of these methods are useful and will provide valid results when applied properly and appropriately. Essentially, they all attempt to answer either of two questions:

1. What don't employees know or do that they should know or do?
2. What are employees doing that they shouldn't be doing?

Defining the essential knowledge, skill, or in some cases attitudes needed by employees is the initial step in designing a training program. The design can be facilitated further by refining needs into more precise learning or behavioral objectives. To be useful, behavioral objectives should involve three major elements:

1. Performance: what will the learner be able to do?
2. Conditions: under what conditions (if any) should the learner be able to perform?
3. Criterion: what is considered acceptable performance?

There are essentially two approaches in identifying and articulating potential training needs: the first focuses on the individual employee; the second considers organizational or hospitalwide training requirements.

Individual Training Needs

The simplest and most direct way of assessing an employee's training needs is to compare the requirements of the job with the individual's qualifications. This approach can be used with new employees as well as those already on the payroll. This formula illustrates such an approach:

Job Requirements (Minus) Job Qualifications = TRAINING NEEDS

Discounting technological and administrative changes, at least in the short term, and assuming that there are up-to-date job descriptions and job specifications, it has been found that a major control point for reducing training needs or requirements is in the hiring and selection of new employees. The extra time and effort expended in recruiting and selecting well-qualified persons will more than pay for itself by substantially reducing their training needs.

A formal employee appraisal system is an excellent way of periodically and systematically focusing on the job performance and qualifications of individual employees. Appraisal systems can be prime sources for the type of information needed to identify their training needs. These needs can be defined readily in terms of

Figure 18-3 Detail Definition and Design Phase (Design Instructional Delivery System)

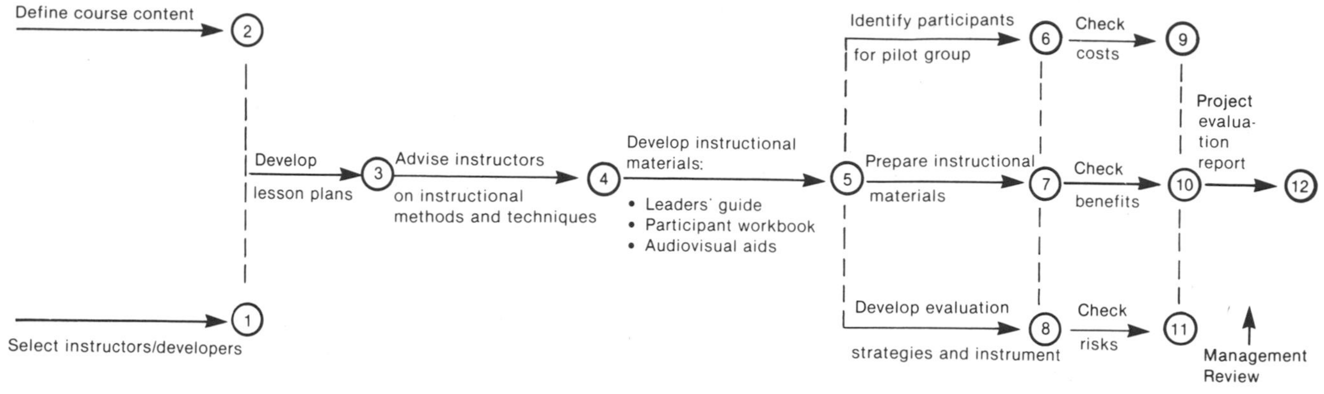

the knowledge and skills required by the employees to perform either their present jobs or to prepare for promotional opportunities.

Figure 18-4 is another way of illustrating training needs (or lack of needs). If the employee in Category I is to become productive, the job qualifications must be expanded to correspond to the job requirements. On the other hand, the employee in Category II whose job qualifications are in excess of present requirements needs either better utilization in the job or reassignment to a more responsible one.

Largely because clearcut standards are lacking, it is not uncommon for the performance of employees in the same job classification to vary widely. For example, as illustrated in Exhibit 18-2, 50 nurse aides are ranked on the basis of their job performance, with No. 1 being the best worker and No. 50 the poorest. What are some of the implications of being the best as opposed to the poorest worker?

First, when it comes to work assignments, the following scenario usually takes place:

No. 1: not only will be given more work to do but also will be assigned the more difficult tasks
No. 50: will be assigned lesser and easier tasks

Second, as far as the tangible reward system or pay and promotion are concerned, the situation usually looks like this:

Pay: a single job rate is much more common than merit pay.
Promotion: few, if any, promotional opportunities exist for nurse aides.

Essentially, what has developed and is continuing to evolve in many work settings is a system dedicated to

rewarding the incompetent and indifferent employee at the expense of the competent and conscientious one. Granted, there always will be some degree of variability in the performance of different individuals in the same job or occupation. However, in fairness to all employees, this variance must be kept to a minimum. This requires establishing job performance standards and ensuring that they are understood by employees and closely monitored by supervisors. If an employee's job performance is below standard, the initial step is to determine whether or not the person has the necessary knowledge and skill to perform the assigned tasks. If the employee is deficient in either job knowledge or skills, training is needed.

However, as happens in many cases, employees do have the necessary job knowledge and skills but their performance still remains below the acceptable standard. These types of situations strongly indicate a real and immediate need for supervisory training.

Organizational Training Needs

The increased participation of hospital administrators and department heads in the design and implementation of programs has significantly sharpened the training needs assessment picture and has increased materially the number of programs geared toward bringing about the operational changes and/or improvements. As might be expected, this has resulted in a shift in emphasis in evaluating training programs. The prime concern no longer is the reaction of program participants to the instructor, instructional setting, and teaching materials; rather, the major focus now is on measuring to what extent anticipated changes in job performance were achieved.

A byproduct of the direct involvement of management has been a much more stringent review of re-

Figure 18-4 Training vs. Utilization Problem

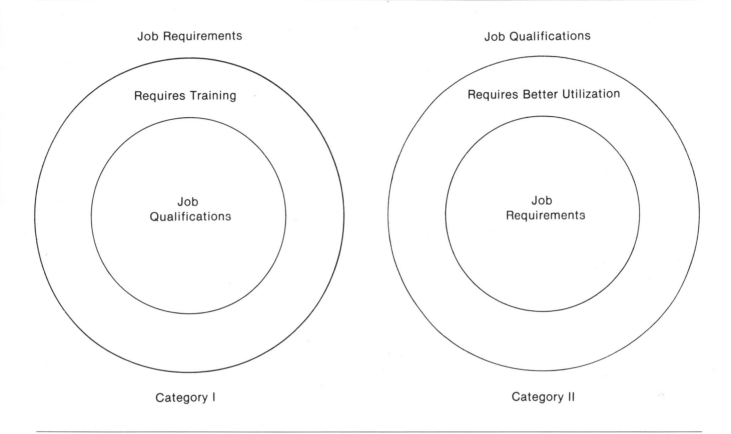

Category I — Job Requirements / Requires Training / Job Qualifications

Category II — Job Qualifications / Requires Better Utilization / Job Requirements

quests for training expenditures. Few hospital administrators are willing to approve monies for training on the general premise that "it's the thing to do." Instead, they are judging the merits of proposed programs on the basis of anticipated operational improvements. In the interest of cost effectiveness, in-house staff members are playing a much more active role in developing and conducting training programs.

This trend toward training based on operational needs, almost to the exclusion of generalized learning programs, is changing the pattern of hospital programs. There has been an increase in allied health training programs, as well as a significant growth in supervisory and management training. The latter are being targeted to increase the competency or skills of hospital managers in very specific areas (e.g., discipline and grievance handling, budgeting and sources of revenue, management of human resources, interviewing skills, handling the troubled employee, problem solving and decision making, time management, conducting effective meetings, and report writing).

Two departments that can provide excellent data for ascertaining organizational training needs are quality assurance and long-range planning. Quality assurance compiles the type of concrete operational data that can be invaluable in precisely identifying short-term training needs. Long-range planning can provide insight into potential or long-term needs based on the hospital's strategic plans.

Exhibit 18-2 Job Performance Rankings Vis-à-Vis Pay/Promotion

Job Performance Ranking	Pay/Promotion
Nurse Aide 1	
Nurse Aide 2	
Nurse Aide 3	
•	
•	Essentially
•	the same
•	for all 50
•	
Nurse Aide 48	
Nurse Aide 49	
Nurse Aide 50	

Setting Priorities for Training Needs

Once training needs have been identified, the question arises as to which ones should be addressed first. This decision, in reality, rests on several factors:

- the priority assigned by administration
  - support for training from top management starts by being responsive to the suggestions and requests of top management
- the estimated cost-effectiveness of the training
  - the cost of the training generally must be less than that of the problem it's designed to solve
- the number and/or organizational level of the employee(s) needing training
  - meeting the training needs of a key administrator can have a much greater organizational impact than a skills training program for a group of hourly employees.

A major dilemma of hospital training directors is how to maintain a balance between available resources and needed courses. Ironically, it is doing what should be done that often upsets this delicate balance. The aware and conscientious training director, by responding on a timely basis to high-priority training needs, particularly new ones, often is forced to reassign resources already allocated to existing programs. The net result is that both new and existing programs are shortchanged and, literally, failure is programmed into both of them.

The most viable solution to being responsive to new high-priority training is to rely on the project management or systems approach cited earlier. It provides an excellent vehicle for surfacing for management's review and decision—not only the merits of the proposed training program but also the resources needed to support it.

INSTRUCTIONAL METHODS

Another important factor in designing employee training is selecting appropriate learning or instructional methods. Based on the experience of many trainers in a wide variety of settings, it's now evident that learner-centered instructional methods are more effective than the more traditional teacher-centered methods. The adult learner wants and needs to be involved actively in the learning process. It is not difficult for employees to be just passive listeners or watchers. This is particularly true of younger workers, most of whom are products of an educational system that has begun to emphasize and organize around the needs of the individual student.

A wide variety of methods are used with adult learners, such as role playing, buzz groups, case studies, brainstorming, and programmed instruction. The choice of method is based on a variety of considerations, including cost, number of participants, employees' educational level and backgrounds, time frame for developing and conducting the program, and the level and type of instructional resources available.

One of the most active practitioners and scholars in the field of adult education is Malcolm Knowles, whose life study is andragogy, or the science of adult learning. He and his contemporaries have contributed a great deal of information and insight into ways and means of facilitating adult learning. At the end of this chapter is a listing of readings dealing with organizing and implementing adult learning.

On-the-Job Training

As mentioned earlier, most hospital employees receive OJT (on-the-job training). During World War II, the War Manpower Commission developed an extremely useful approach to on-the-job training. The two major elements in this approach, which also is referred to as the JIT or Job Instruction Training, are: how to get ready to instruct, and the four-step method of instruction. Exhibit 18-3 is a JIT checklist for planning job instruction. Following it is a detailed explanation of the JIT four-step method of job instruction.

Step 1: Preparing the Employees

Put them at ease. New employees, particularly, are anxious to prove themselves. As a consequence, they often are tense, apprehensive, or frightened. A friendly attitude on the instructor's part, coupled with a conversational approach focusing on the employees' interests and accomplishments, can go a long way toward helping them relax. This approach provides some insight into their ability to learn.

State the job and find out what they already know about it. Give the employees an overview of the particular operation and point out how their particular job fits into the total picture. Ask specific questions about the job and about the employees' prior knowledge and experience. Since instruction begins where their knowledge ends, repeating what they already know is a waste of the instructor's time and theirs.

Get them interested in learning the job. All employees have some type of personal stake in their jobs. It may be an opportunity to do what they enjoy doing; it may be a feeling of personal involvement or

Exhibit 18-3 Planning Checklist for Job Instruction

Have a timetable
How much skill is the employee expected to have?
By what date?

Break down the job
What are the important steps?
What are the key points? (Safety always is a key point.)

Have everything ready
Is the right equipment available?
What materials and supplies are needed?

Have the work place properly arranged
How should the employees keep their workplace?
In any particular order?

---

achievement; it may be more money, the basic need to earn a living; or it may be a combination of all of these motivating factors. Associating the need to learn with their personal stake in the job is a powerful motivating device.

Place them in the correct position. Position the learners so they can both see and hear the demonstration. It may be advisable, in some cases, to have the employee look over the instructor's shoulder to view the demonstration.

Step 2: Presenting the Operation

Tell, show, and illustrate one important step at a time. Introduce the employee to a task by running through it a few times and explaining in general terms what's being done and what's being accomplished. After the overview of the task, break it down into its component steps. The data developed in the task analysis provide the framework for showing and should be geared to the individual learner's ability. Evaluate progress after each step in the instruction process.

Step 3: Trying Out Performance

Have them do the job; correct errors. At this point, employees get to feel what it's like to do the task the instructor has been describing and showing to them. Have them perform the task and encourage them to describe the main steps. If they start to deviate from the proper procedure, get them back on the track with a friendly word or hint. Should they make an error, stop them and explain the proper way before proceeding. As would be expected, it is better to prevent errors than to correct them, particularly if the mistakes could result in improper patient care, loss of materials, or damage to equipment. In correcting errors, the instructor must be sure not to create an impression of being critical because the employees are not letter perfect.

Have them explain each key point as they do the job again. When employees develop a feel for the task to a point where they can perform it without undue strain, have them run through it and explain the key points as they go along.

Make sure they understand. The degree to which an employee understands a job can be determined best through questioning. Such questions should be specific rather than open ended. The type of questions that can quickly get to the root of an employee's understanding and insight into a job are:

Why do you . . . ?
What would happen if . . . ?
What should you do next?

Continue until the instructor knows they know. Before putting the employees on their own, the instructor must be satisfied that they can perform the task properly. They reach this point through repeated practice under close observation, so that their errors are picked up and corrected or eliminated. When an employee repeatedly makes the same error, it might be well to involve the individual in analyzing the cause of the mistake and evaluating the benefits of using the correct method.

Step 4: Following Up

Put them on their own; designate the individual to whom they go for help. Check with the employees frequently, not so much to inspect their work, but rather to let them know the instructor is sincerely interested in their progress. Encourage the learners to think about their job and to ask any questions they may have. Make it quite clear by attitude that such questions are an indication of their interest in the job.

Taper off extra coaching and close follow-up. As the learner's job proficiency increases, the need for close supervision and observation tapers off. However, a hallmark of the good supervisor is a clear understanding of the performance and output levels of subordinates. When a dip in performance or output occurs, coaching is in order.

PROGRAM ADMINISTRATION

Staff departments run the gamut from those providing well-defined and readily identifiable support services (purchasing, finance, security) to those offering support services that still are broadly defined and, more importantly, not too well understood by other staff members (e.g., long-range planning, quality assurance, training, etc.). This being the case, a prime responsibility of the training director is carving out a mission for the training function in conjunction with administration and department heads.

ORGANIZATIONAL CONSIDERATIONS

Much has been written about the organizational placement of the training function in a hospital. The most comprehensive analysis was the 1977 *Hospital-wide Education and Training Study* done by Lovett and Munk under the aegis of the Hospital Research and Educational Trust. A more recent guide on the organization and administration of the hospital's education system is *The Education Function in Hospitals,* published in 1978 by the American Society for Health Manpower Education and Training. It suggests that:

A comprehensive educational system is a product of various functions, beginning with the establishment of educational philosophy and concomitant policy that accurately reflects the needs of the institution and the individuals it serves. As a catalyst in the formulation of such philosophy and policy, the educator provides the educational input and information needed for the institution to address its commitments to and development of the following areas:

- educational and clinical affiliations at secondary, undergraduate and graduate levels
- staff education and training, including preservice and inservice training, staff and management development and training, employee educational counseling, and continuing education
- hospital-based patient education
- community health education
- resource coordination of media, library and learning resources, and information centers.

Whenever feasible, these areas should be centrally coordinated and administered to affect accountability, reduce duplication and fragmentation of effort, control expense, and ensure the educational soundness of programs and activities.[4]

The potential activities and resources listed vis-à-vis those actually encompassed by the hospital's training or education department are a function of:

- the CEO's philosophy
- the creativity and aggressiveness of the training director
- the organizational placement of the training function
- the geographical location of the hospital.
- the length of time the training function has existed in the hospital.

The *sine qua non* of a viable and productive hospitalwide training department is a director who can establish and maintain a working "client" relationship with all levels of hospital management. A policy statement clearly and concisely setting forth the mission of the training department and the services it provides can be very helpful in promoting and facilitating such relationships.

The scope and nature of the training director's job is changing. Its boundaries of responsibility now are beginning to encompass:

- patient and community health education
- the centralization and coordination of knowledge-related hospital activities such as library, audiovisual or media facilities, and health information centers
- liaison with outside agencies and organizations involved in accrediting, funding, and monitoring the performance of hospital-based educational programs.

It also is important to ensure that all hospital employees are informed of the services and programs provided by the training department, particularly when they are eligible to participate. This information can be communicated to employees through bulletin boards, special program announcements, annual or seasonal program brochures, and feature articles in hospital publications.

CONCLUSION

If the immediate past is any indication of the future, the 1980s will witness a substantial growth in the programming of, as well as resources allocated to, hospital training departments. The major forces spurring this growth will be: technological advancements; Equal Employment Opportunity legislation; a growing interest in continuing education on the part of health professionals; the necessity for more comprehensive clinical or vocational training, particularly in the allied health occupations; the requirement for more and better patient and community health education; upgrading of managerial systems and managerial skills; the establishment of performance appraisal systems to monitor and utilize the energies and talents of hospital employees more effectively at all levels; the increasing emphasis on employee training activities in the standards of the Joint Commission on Accreditation of Hospitals; and organized labor's growing interest and involvement in employee training.

During the 80s, the major thrust of the training department will be to provide support and guidance to line managers in the development of learning systems that are an integral part of the work operation. The trainer will be the prime facilitator in establishing the teaching-learning links that will be forged between hospital managers, at all levels, and their immediate employees.

In the future, the results of hospital training activities will be gauged in terms of humanistic, as well as operational, outcomes. Admittedly, much still needs to be done in defining and measuring humanistic outcomes, but progress is being made.

Prof. Francis Gramlich of Dartmouth is among those who have given dimension and meaning to humanistic outcomes. He suggests that an employee's career growth and development can be described as moving from

- dependence to independence
- self-centeredness to cooperation
- subjective to objective thinking
- control by others to self-control.

It is to be hoped that during the 80s, human resource professionals will develop a more definitive system for measuring the results of their efforts. When this happens, the human element in the work equation not only will receive the attention it deserves, but more importantly it may even replace the cost element as the key factor in the managerial decision-making process in hospitals. Why not? People are the major cost element in hospitals.

NOTES

1. Leonard Nadler, *Developing Human Resources* (Houston: Gulf Publishing Co., 1977), p. 40.

2. *Ibid.*, p. 88.
3. *Ibid.*, p. 60.
4. American Society for Health Manpower Education and Training, *The Education Function in Hospitals* (Chicago: American Hospital Association, 1978).

RECOMMENDED READINGS

American Society for Health Manpower Education and Training. *The Education Function in Hospitals.* Chicago: American Hospital Association, 1978.

Broadwell, Martin M. *The Supervisor As an Instructor: A Guide For Classroom Training,* 3d ed. Reading, Mass.: Addison-Wesley Publishing Co., 1978.

Craig, Robert L., et al. *Training and Development Handbook: A Guide To Human Resource Development,* 2d ed. New York: McGraw-Hill Book Co., 1976.

Diekelmann, Nancy L., and Knopke, Harold J. *Approaches to Teaching in the Health Sciences.* Reading, Mass.: Addison-Wesley Publishing Co., 1973.

Dunkel, Patty L. *Curriculum for Educators in Health Care Institutions* (Proceedings and recommendations of an invitational conference). Chicago: Hospital Research and Educational Trust, 1977.

Kirkpatrick, Donald L. *A Practical Guide For Supervisory Training and Development.* Reading, Mass.: Addison-Wesley Publishing Co., 1971.

—————. *Evaluating Training Programs: A Collection of Articles From the Journal of the American Society for Training and Development.* Madison, Wisconsin: American Society for Training Directors, 1975.

Knowles, Malcolm S. *The Adult Learner: A Neglected Species,* 2d ed. Houston: Gulf Publishing Co., 1978.

Laird, Dugan, *Approaches to Training and Development.* Reading, Mass.: Addison-Wesley Publishing Co., 1978.

Lippitt, Gordon, and Taylor, Bernard, eds. *Management Development and Training Handbook.* London, New York: McGraw-Hill Book Co., 1975.

Lippitt, Gordon L., and Lippitt, Ronald. *The Consulting Process in Action.* La Jolla, Calif.: University Associates Press, 1978.

Lovett, Marc, and Munk, Robert J. *Hospitalwide Education and Training.* Chicago: Hospital Research and Educational Trust, 1977.

Mager, Robert F. *Goal Analysis.* Belmont, Calif.: Fearon Publishers, 1972.

—————. *Preparing Instructional Objectives,* 2d ed. Belmont, Calif.: Fearon Publishers, 1975.

McLagan, Patricia A. *Helping Others Learn.* Reading, Mass.: Addison-Wesley Publishing Co., 1978.

Nadler, Leonard. *Developing Human Resources.* Houston: Gulf Publishing Co., 1970.

Odiorne, George S. *Training by Objectives: An Economic Approach to Training.* New York: Macmillan Publishing Co., 1970.

Pfeiffer, J. William, and Jones, John E. *Reference Guide to Handbooks of Instructional Experiences for Human Relations Training and the Annual Handbook For Group Facilitators (1972-1977).* La Jolla, Calif.: University Associates Press, 1977.

Schechter, Daniel S. *Agenda for Continuing Education (A Challenge to Health Care Institutions).* Chicago: Hospital Research and Educational Trust, 1974.

19. Staff Development: Training and Continuing Education

JOHN E. BAER

The objective of education and training in the health care industry: skills once developed by employees must be updated constantly to keep abreast of rapidly moving society and changes in technology.

Developing a well-trained work force is one of the most important responsibilities of an organization. From top executive to first-line supervisor, from professional staff member to unskilled worker, from volunteer to board member, every health care facility must accept the obligation for training and developing its employees and executives.[1] This principle is so vital to the progress of every organization that most large, successful companies spell it out as a matter of policy and devote countless staff hours to training their personnel.

The results institutions achieve in productivity, cost savings, quality, safety, morale, and improved systems are proportionate to the quality of training their employees receive when they begin work and while they are on the job.

In reviewing the success of any organization, it is essential to evaluate the effectiveness of its management and professional staff. Today large corporations recognize that the most critical restriction on their growth and expansion is qualified management personnel. A strong management, coupled with dedicated and competent professional and nonprofessional staff, often will be the ingredient a health care facility needs to ensure its viability. There is now, and will continue to be, a shortage of strong, resourceful, and imaginative administrators, department heads, and supervisors in health care facilities. When these organizations fail to develop individuals for management roles, they limit their chances to increase productivity, to keep down high payroll expenses (through better staffing), to develop sound management systems, to maintain high morale, and most importantly to ensure quality patient care.

The quality of health care depends, to a large degree, on the knowledge, skills, standards of behavior, and activities of practicing health care employees. The emergence of new knowledge and technology, as well as continuing social changes, make an effective staff development program necessary to assist professional personnel to maintain and improve competency in practice.

The major expense of any health care institution is the payroll for those who provide the care.[2] The rising costs of salaries and benefits constitute a major investment. The careful management of this investment will be a necessity for the foreseeable future. Health care administrators will not be able to afford the luxury of underutilizing their greatest resource—the people who work for them. The motivation and skills of those persons will determine, to a great degree, the future quality and cost of health care that will contribute indirectly to the public and government pressures on managers of health care systems. Consequently, health care facilities that do not devote time to staff development programs are shortsighted and will tend to have a weaker and less effective workforce.

OBJECTIVES OF ORIENTATION

Skills once developed by employees must be updated constantly to keep them abreast of advancing society and technology. Therefore, it is most critical that all personnel receive the best in continuing and related education. The creation of a separate education and training department not only is desirable but is necessary to facilitate equitable and pertinent education programs.

The objectives of the education and training department may help in understanding the potential scope and possibilities of such a function. The department should:

1. Coordinate the total education program for the health care facility.
2. Assess educational needs of the employees and the institution and develop sound education programs to meet those needs.
3. Foster a climate in which staff members identify their own learning needs and seek opportunities to meet them.
4. Design, conduct, and evaluate staff development programs and patient education programs that facilitate the attainment of standards of care established in the agency.
5. Assist staff members to acquire the knowledge and skills necessary to fulfill their role expectations.
6. Assist staff personnel to maintain, improve, and update their competency in the provision of health care.
7. Assist in the introduction and orderly adaptation to change in ways that are conducive to the achievement of the institution's goals.
8. Identify, evaluate, and cooperate with internal as well as with outside educational resources to promote and develop programs of basic and continuing education.

FUNCTION OF EDUCATION

The health care facility's education system should be characterized by a coordinated, comprehensive network of programs and activities encompassing physicians, employees, patients, volunteers, board of trustees, and the community at large. Planning of the educational activity should be based on needs analysis, including attitudinal and organizational climate surveys when appropriate. Implementation of the activities should reflect the use of appropriate educational technology and methodology to increase knowledge, skills, and competencies and produce measurable change.

To accomplish this, the education system should be organized on an institutionwide basis so that the needs and resources of the entire organization can be taken into account and activities will not be duplicated or fragmented. Institutionwide education means that all institution-based education is coordinated by a central education and training department with clearly defined responsibility and accountability. The educational activities that would fall under this department include:

- staff education and training, including orientation, preservice and inservice training, and continuing education
- management and supervisory development
- trustee development
- educational and clinical affiliations at secondary, undergraduate, and graduate levels
- patient education
- resource coordination
- community health education

Ideally, other activities such as continuing medical education, inservice nursing education, coordination of audiovisual activities, supervision of a medical illustrator, and the administrative responsibility for the institution's library services should be included as well.

Staff Education and Training

The educator helps in quality control of patient care through educational programming. This should evolve from a process of careful needs assessment, cost identification, selection of appropriate methodologies and format, and evaluation and documentation of results and costs.

The line manager and the director of education and training share the responsibility for maintaining two-way communication on training needs and job competencies. The line manager should provide input into the education department and seek assistance from it in solving performance problems. The educator can help determine if training is needed and provide learning experiences to eliminate skill deficiencies. However, the line manager, with assistance through training from the education director, is responsible for continued application of on-the-job learning. The educator must provide feedback both to the line manager and to the administration regarding the continuing impact of the facility's educational system.

Management and Supervisory Development

The first step in preparing persons to be effective managers and supervisors is to be aware that management is a unique discipline requiring specific skills. A successful health care manager must understand the philosophy, goals, and objectives of the entire organization, as well as the standards and routines that exist in the individual's department. Working in harmony with the administration, the manager becomes a part of the team that will implement management's philosophy and ensure the successful completion of the organization's goals and objectives.

Effective management requires good communication. Communication is the nerve center of any health care facility. Effectiveness is impaired when the necessary information on which to base decisions is not available. Managers and supervisors occupy a unique position as far as communication is concerned. Orders, rules, standards, policies, procedures, and standards of behavior all must be communicated to the employees. Since first-line supervisors have the greatest direct contact with employees, the burden falls most heavily on their shoulders to see that the workers understand what is expected of them.

It is being realized more and more that the skills needed for good management have very little to do with the technical function of the specialized area. The higher a person climbs in the management ranks, the greater the shift of priority from technical skills to management skills. Although the supervisor may require a fair amount of technical skills, the ability to manage successfully is more dependent on executive skills.

Of all the skills necessary to become a successful manager, people skills are the most crucial. Given a high degree of technical and creative ability, managers still will fail if they cannot relate to and communicate with people. Health care facilities would be wise to invest both time and money in strengthening their managers' skills in interviewing; employee discipline, development, and motivation; performance appraisal; communications; problem solving; grievance handling; and team building.

Of course, emphasis also should be given to developing management skills in setting objectives, long-range and short-range planning, organizing and controlling work flow, initiating action, time management, delegation, evaluating results, decision making, and redirecting action.

One commonly accepted definition of management is "the art of getting things done through people." To expect supervisors who have not been trained in the techniques of supervision to accomplish this is as absurd as expecting a purchasing agent, a comptroller, or an executive director to function successfully as an operating room nurse, an x-ray technician, or a bacteriology technician. It rarely can be done. Health care facilities must allocate time and resources to the hiring and development of their most loyal and devoted personnel: their managers and supervisors.[3] Building a management team will pay off in dividends many times over.

Trustee Development

When an individual accepts a seat on a health facility governing board, the person automatically assumes certain duties, responsibilities, and liabilities. No board member can hope to function effectively until these factors are understood clearly. The Joint Commission on Accreditation of Hospitals specifically states that the potential effectiveness of the governing body is influenced in part by a program of orientation and continuing education specifically designed for the board members. Although trustee development remains the primary responsibility of the chief executive officer and the trustees themselves, the education and training department can offer its resources. As part of this effort, it can assist in planning and organizing programs, arranging for and developing resources, and evaluating effectiveness.

Educational and Clinical Affiliation

Establishing clinical affiliations with educational institutions should be a function in which the training department participates. Serving as a liaison with those entities, this department can ensure that the benefits derived by the institution are proportionate to the services and facilities it provides.

In addition, by working with the facility's staff, the training department can make recommendations to educational institutions regarding the competencies that will be needed to meet the growing demands of hospital or nursing home employment. The health care facility, as employer, must have a direct link with the institutions training its employees. The education department should be the conduit through which those institutions can check the quality and relevance of their programs. Important information on supply and demand can be estimated and documented, as well.

Patient and Community Health Education

Health education has two aspects: (1) the education of a specific patient or group of patients in how to manage their disease, and (2) the education of patients, employees, and members of the community in how to maintain their health (preventive medicine). The American Hospital Association has stated that: "Hospitals and other health care institutions, as focal points of community care, have an obligation to promote, organize, implement and evaluate health education programs."[4]

Although much of the teaching responsibility, especially for specific patient education, rests with the health care team and/or a specially trained health educator, the facility would benefit greatly by having patient and health education activities coordinated by a department that could help identify needs, exchange information, reduce costs through shared resources, ensure quality, and evaluate effectiveness.

Resource Coordination

All of these activities demand that appropriate teaching aids and educational materials be available to educators, managers, supervisors, professional practitioners, and patients. An education and training department that consistently takes the pulse of the institution's needs is in the best position to determine what resources are required to meet those needs and coordinate with the facility's library services.

ISSUES RELATING TO EDUCATION

Historically, health care facilities are only beginning to develop education and training departments. In 1970, the American Hospital Association recognized the importance of institutional-based staff development programs when it established ASHET, the American Society for Health Manpower Education & Training. As of 1980, the ASHET membership approached 1,800, with 33 affiliated chapters. ASHET was formed following a six-year study of the educational needs of hospitals by the Hospital Research and Educational Trust (HRET), funded by the W. K. Kellogg Foundation. In October 1979, the AHA *Special Survey on Selected Hospital Topics* identified 3,071 hospitalwide education and training departments. In all, 5,663 hospitals responded to the survey. Of those responding, 1,413 or 25.0 percent engaged in some

form of preparatory educational activities, 1,211 or 21.4 percent in graduate education, 5,025 or 88.7 percent offered some degree of inservice training, 4,062 or 71.7 percent provided continuing education, and 3,120 or 55.10 percent conducted nonpatient community health education. It should be noted that these statistics frequently represented single-department efforts.

Focusing on the 3,071 institutions that indicated having hospitalwide education and training departments, the hospital activities listed in Table 19-1 were identified as the responsibility of the departments named.

Based on these figures, it would appear as though many of the institutions that reported they operated hospitalwide education and training departments more accurately might be said to have nursing inservice education departments; otherwise, management and supervisory development, support and clerical staff training, and technical training might be expected to be offered more frequently.

Centralized vs. Decentralized Activities

When determining how to organize an education and training program, the institution must evaluate the benefits of centralizing or decentralizing the function. In general, there appear to be far more advantages to centralization.

Table 19-1 Education and Training Responsibilities

Activity	Percentage of Departments Directing This Activity
Audiovisual services	79.6%
Community health education	46.5
Continuing medical education	45.6
Educational counseling	27.9
Graduate medical education	12.9
Lab, radiology, and other technical staff training	32.1
Management and supervisory development	55.4
Nursing inservice training	89.0
Patient education	68.5
Preparatory allied health education programs	26.1
Support and clerical staff training	44.8
Trustee development	11.2

Source: Reprinted with permission from American Hospital Association *Special Survey on Selected Hospital Topics,* © 1979.

The major advantages of a centralized department include:

- a clearly defined accountability for education and training throughout the institution
- a centralized educational budget and its monitoring and control
- cost-effectiveness through more efficient and economical use of staff hours, equipment, and materials by avoiding duplication of programs and purchases, and diversion of instructional personnel time into noneducational activities
- institutionwide needs assessment activities to establish education and training priorities
- central control of educational resources and facilities (class/conference rooms, audiovisual equipment/materials, training aids) thus providing greater availability and use
- assurance that all educational programs are evaluated consistently with regard to improving/upgrading employee performance
- provision of a centralized system for maintaining training records for each program and each employee in compliance with accreditation requirements
- provision of a coordinating base for community-sponsored programs held at the health care facility
- equal career mobility opportunities for employees in educational reimbursement, scholarships, and grant availability.

The advantages to a decentralized system include:

- a more secure department head and/or supervisor who may wish to have greater involvement in the design and content of educational programs
- greater control at the departmental level over the hours that training activities will take place involving departmental employees.

Needs Assessment

It is of critical importance that the department assess educational needs of employees and the institution and that it develop sound programs to meet these needs. The needs assessment process is to the education and training department as the institutional budget is to the finance department. It serves as a planning tool and a road map against which to chart its progress.

In determining training needs, a variety of criteria can be used. They fall into two general categories: real needs and perceived needs. Real needs are identified through:

1. the specifics of job descriptions
2. information in policy and procedure manuals
3. the results of formal grievances
4. job site observations
5. requirements of quality assurance programs
6. the results of incident/accident reports
7. the mission, goals, and objectives of the institution
8. turnover records
9. attendance records
10. the results of performance evaluations
11. equipment and supply records
12. financial reports

Perceived needs are identified through:

1. formal interviews with staff, patients/families, the community at large, volunteers, physicians, and trustees
2. group discussions
3. questionnaires and surveys
4. suggestion systems
5. informal grievances
6. exit interviews
7. management and/or employee committees

Regardless of what method is used, it is crucial to involve a representative number of persons in the institution in order to achieve a balanced consideration of topics that truly have the highest priority.

Evaluation

Program evaluation is an extremely important component of the overall education effort. An evaluation of how good any given program is and how well it accomplishes its objectives must be built into its operation. The evaluation can take several forms:

- employees can be given a pretest and a posttest to determine what they may have learned in terms of skills or knowledge
- the education and training department can work closely with line managers to monitor to what extent classroom concepts have been implemented in the work setting
- employee attitude questionnaires can be completed to record worker perceptions of the programs.

The value of a program is perhaps best determined by measurable results. Consequently, criteria against which to judge its success or failure include such indicators as turnover records, incident/accident reports, performance appraisals, quality assurance results, attendance records, grievances, equipment and supply records, and financial records.

In any case, it is essential to determine how successful a program is in relationship to the effort exerted by the education and training department and in terms of the time allocated by those who attended.

Onsite/Outside Programs

In designing programs, it is essential to determine the degree to which monies will be allocated for education and training both at the health care facility and off the premises. Generally, a facility can expose many more staff persons to a program when it establishes a full-time service. Following a needs assessment study, custom-designed programs can be offered to address issues of greatest importance to the institution.

On occasion, it may be more cost-effective or desirable to bring in outside resources to supplement the in-house educators. Outside programs tend to be more expensive and may not be as pertinent to the institution's needs. On the other hand, if a health care facility is contemplating the establishment of a new clinical program or the implementation of a new management system but does not have sufficient information to determine whether or not to proceed, an outside conference could be most beneficial. Further, outside programs enhance learning by removing personnel from the pressures of the work environment and often give the participants a fresh perspective and new ideas. They also create opportunities for staff members to establish informal relationships with other professional colleagues. These relationships often initiate continuing communications with others who share the same professional interests, concerns, and operational problems.[5]

Facility/Consultant Instructors

For organizations that can afford at least a full-time educator, it is preferable to identify an individual who will be onsite and responsive to the needs of the institution. If the health care facility carefully selects a director of education and training, that individual should be able to design and teach a large number of programs throughout the year. An onsite educator has the advantage of working closely with the line managers and knows the organization structure and climate.

Naturally, many organizational arrangements can be established in an education and training department. The most desirable is to have the department report directly to a senior member of the administration. By establishing this type of relationship, the education and training chief can participate more easily in senior management inner cabinet meetings that allow the director to identify the institution's most pressing needs. An additional advantage of an independent department is that it can better supervise other institutionwide activities such as library, audiovisual services, and medical illustration services and classroom and conference room assignment. This type of organizational arrangement is particularly conducive to the movement toward human resource management being embraced by an increasing number of health care institutions.

The health care facility should consider consulting services in three situations:

1. They can be helpful in supplementing the resources of the onsite educator(s), particularly in situations where technical knowledge is required.
2. It may seem desirable to drive home a point by bringing in so-called experts. Outside consultants often are perceived to be *the* authority. Consequently, employees tend to be more receptive and responsive to consultants' espousal of a principle or to their approach.
3. If the health care facility cannot establish one or more full-time positions, it would have to hire consulting services to begin onsite training programs. Under this arrangement, the institution can conduct periodic management and development programs, clinical programs, and staff motivational programs at a much lower cost than it would allocate to a full-time position and to the institutional overhead that accompanies the creation of such a department.

Benefits

The benefits of establishing an education and training department include:

- developing and strengthening internal management skills
- assisting professional staff members to stay abreast of new knowledge and technological advances that impact upon their performance
- promoting high-quality patient care
- maintaining and improving personnel competency in all job categories
- helping to increase productivity
- maintaining high employee morale
- helping reduce staff turnover
- inspiring staff behavioral changes conducive to the achievement of the institution's goals

- assisting administration, through staff education, to overcome operational problems
- providing a convenient resource to assist staff professionals to acquire needed continuing education credits in order to maintain professional licensure
- coordinating programs that satisfy accreditation requirements
- serving as a central depository for staff training and development documents
- serving as a liaison with outside education-affiliated programs
- functioning as a catalyst for staff, patient, and community educational programs

Costs

Although there is a significant financial investment and an allocation of employee time away from the job in establishing and maintaining an effective education and training program, these expenses will be offset by better management, improved productivity, improved communication and internal systems, lower personnel turnover, and other intangibles.[6] Nonetheless, it is essential that administration and the director of education and training develop ways to assess the return on investment of the training dollar.

At present, there is little definitive information regarding the funds being allocated to education and training departments. However, as part of the October 1979 AHA *Special Survey on Selected Hospital Topics,* hospitals were asked "What percentage of your institution's total operating budget supports the 'overall' educational activities?" There was a high rate of nonresponses—almost 41 percent. However, the answers that were received are shown in Table 19-2. Clearly, the figures are inconclusive. What can be

said, however, is that either hospitals do not know how much they are allocating to education and training or for some reason do not wish to divulge this information.

Shared Services

Shared services are particularly effective where budgets are tight, educational resources are limited, and where there is a group of health care facilities in reasonably close proximity to take advantage of these services. Increasingly, institutions are sharing educational services via telecommunications. Through a shared service concept, audiovisual equipment and training aids can be used by a number of institutions. In many geographic areas of the country, technical and functional educators are few and far between. Under such circumstances, virtually any degree of shared or cooperative activity will result in a qualitative upgrading of individual health care facilities.

There are, of course, some negatives to consider in a shared service arrangement. Institutions may give up a degree of autonomy, employees may be required to participate in programs outside their facility rather than in the convenience of their own geographic setting, and participating institutions must establish equitable working arrangements.

In 1978, an innovative and cost-saving shared service program in continuing education was instituted for hospitals in the New York metropolitan area by The Center to Promote Health Care Studies, Inc., of Scarsdale, N.Y. Under this arrangement, participating hospitals contracted to send employees to six one-day workshops at a cost far less than if the same program was not part of this shared service.

SCH Health Care System of Houston and The Center to Promote Health Care Studies, Inc., both re-

Table 19-2 Hospital Budgeting for Education and Training

Hospitals Reporting on Survey		*Percentage of Total Operating Budget Allocated to Education and Training Activities*							
	5,663	*0%*	*1%*	*2%*	*3%*	*4%*	*5–10%*	*11% & over*	*Nonresponsive to this question*
Number reporting to this question	5,663	2,358	336	162	90	307	43	58	2,309
Percentage of hospitals that responded to the survey	100%	41.6%	5.9%	2.9%	1.6%	5.4%	.8%	1.0%	40.8%

Source: Reprinted with permission from American Hospital Association *Special Survey on Selected Hospital Topics,* © 1979.

ported that in shared service arrangements, health care administrators and their staffs were virtually unanimous in wanting management development programs, naming basic supervisory management topics as their first priority.

CONCLUSION

Because of an increasingly aging population, an emphasis on health promotion, and the seeming inevitability of some form of national health insurance, the demand for health services will increase over succeeding decades. With this increased demand, and with the development of new technologies, there is a crucial need to keep professional health personnel informed of developments in patient care. Similarly, given the complexity of the health care organization, it is essential that management and supervisor skills be upgraded.

Health care facilities must recognize that their major expense is payroll for the people who provide care. The rising costs of salaries and benefits constitute their major investment. The careful management of this investment will be a necessity for the foreseeable future. Consequently, health care institutions must ensure that the knowledge, skills, standards of behavior, and activities of practicing health professionals and those who supervise them are reinforced through staff development programs. Institutions that do not devote time, money, and commitment to staff development programs are shortsighted and will tend to have a weaker and less effective work force.

DEFINITION OF TERMS

Education and Training Department: the department providing staff development programs including orientation, preservice and inservice training, continuing education, upgrading and enrichment education, and, in some institutions, patient and community health education, continuing medical education, and development programs for volunteers and trustees.

Staff development: the total process that includes formal and informal learning opportunities. The focus of the process is on assisting individuals to perform competently in fulfillment of role expectations in an organization. Resources both in and outside the institution are used. The primary goal of a staff development program is to provide opportunities for employed personnel to acquire further knowledge and skills and to learn behavior that will enable them to perform their assigned functions safely and effectively in providing health care for patients and community residents.

Preservice education: educational activities that occur prior to an employee's assuming work responsibilities. It may include general or job-specific orientation in the form of classroom or individualized instruction.

Orientation: the means by which new staff members are introduced to the philosophy, goals, policies, procedures, role expectations, physical facilities, and special services in a specific work setting.

Inservice education: educational activities that are specific to an employee's assigned responsibility, with the primary purpose of meeting organizational goals outlined in job descriptions, policy and procedure manuals, and so forth.

Continuing education: educational activities that are designed primarily to improve and update the knowledge and skills and/or to influence behavior of the individual learner, with the primary purpose of meeting the developmental needs of these individuals.

Upgrading education: educational activities whose primary aim is to prepare employees for additional and often more difficult work responsibilities.

Enrichment education: educational activities aimed at the personal growth and development of individual employees irrespective of their responsibilities.

Health education: education aimed at specific individuals or groups (patients, families, employees, community groups) to assist them to maintain or improve their health status.[7]

Continuing medical education: an instructional or training program, generally provided by the employing institution, that is designed to increase the competence or formal education of the medical staff.

Director of Education and Training: a person with a background in adult education, the behavioral sciences, and/or management who directs the activities of the staff of the Education and Training Department.

NOTES

1. This principle has been espoused repeatedly by the American Hospital Association through a series of "Education, Training" and "Human Resources" policy statements and guideline position papers.

2. In 1978, payroll and employee benefit costs represented slightly more than 60 percent of total operating expenses for all U.S. hospitals. Total operating expenses amounted to $70,927,000,000 and payroll and employee benefit expenses to $42,574,000,000 according

to the *1979 Edition, American Hospital Association Guide to the Health Care Field*.

3. A number of medical centers recently have established assessment centers for supervisors. When a supervisory job is available, the potential candidates may be sent through the assessment center procedure. They are observed and assessed while they work on group decision making and on individual supervisory exercises. Frequently, the common characteristics that are identified through this process include skills in planning, organizing, controlling, problem solving, leadership, communications, and human relations.

4. Statement on the *Role Responsibility of Hospitals and Other Health Care Institutions in Personal and Community Health Education* (Chicago: American Hospital Association, 1974).

5. The AHA policy statement titled *Health Manpower Education and Training: Role and Responsibility of Hospitals and Other Health Care Agencies* (1974) discusses this issue from additional perspectives.

6. An excellent analysis of how one hospital examined its internal education costs can be found in the published proceedings of the eighth annual meeting and conference of the American Society for Health Manpower Education and Training (ASHET), New Orleans, 1978. The specific paper is titled "Improving Hospital Education by Studying Basic Cost Estimate," by James F. M. Campbell, director of inservice education at Little Company of Mary Hospital in Evergreen Park, Ill. The other materials in the ASHET written proceeding titled "Papers on Cost Containment Through Hospital-Based Education" also are recommended reading.

7. The American Hospital Association, in its *Policy Statement on Provision of Health Service* (1977), states that the health care delivery system "must be oriented to the maintenance of personal good health and to the prevention of illness rather than being primarily oriented to the treatment of illness after it becomes acute."

In its *Policy and Statement on The Hospital's Responsibility for Health Promotion* (1979) the AHA states: "Hospitals have a responsibility to take a leadership role in helping ensure good health of their communities." It adds that "the hospital should consider developing and participating in communitywide health, educational, and informational activities to actively encourage responsible decisions about health, as well as responsible use of health services by its community."

20. Training and Personnel Development in the Health Care Industry

FRANCES HOFFMAN HACKBART and PATRICIA VUNDERINK

INTRODUCTION

Training and personnel development in the health care industry is a topic of growing concern. Very little literature on training functions exists that applies specifically to the health care setting. This article draws together training sources from various fields and overlays them with a focus on specific health care problems. The article provides a general overview of training and development processes and offers examples of how they operate in the health care setting.

There are several reasons why training and personnel development are becoming more important in health care institutions. One major reason is the rapidly accelerating technology in the health sciences. As equipment and procedures become more complex, technicians and other employees must be retrained on a continuing basis. The technical expertise required today may be outdated in three years and obsolete in five. The employees who perform the procedures or operate the equipment are valuable individuals who will have acquired all the background nuts-and-bolts knowledge about the workplace. Far better to retrain these proved individuals than to replace them with freshly-trained but unproved employees.

Another major reason is the growing acceptance of a humanistic style of management that emphasizes the value of the individual worker. This philosophy increases employee awareness and expectations with regard to the job. The result is a double pressure—on one side, management feels compelled to help employees grow and develop in the job, while on the other side, workers expect this kind of assistance from their employers. Both are pressing for training and development programs to attain their goals.

WHAT IS IT?

There are two basic types of training and development activities in health care settings: orientation and staff development.

Orientation

An initial orientation to the health care institution is essential for all employees, and particularly important for those who have never worked in such a facility. The larger the institution, the more imperative it becomes for employees to have an introduction to their workplace.

A thorough orientation should accomplish a variety of things. It should give the employee a sense of belonging and an appreciation of organizational goals and values. Information on the institution's philosophy and general principles regarding patient care help to inculcate these values. Orientation also should acquaint the new employee with certain basics regarding the workplace, including the following:

- benefits
- payroll procedures
- physical layout of the facility
- location of eating, locker, and restroom facilities
- essentials of health and safety precautions
- organizational structure
- introduction to supervisor(s) and coworkers
- introduction to job description and responsibilities
- instruction in specific duties with which the employee is not already familiar

Staff Development

After the employee has been working for a period of time, training deficits may be noticed or changes in procedures may require new knowledge and skills. Staff development activities deal with these training deficits in a number of ways:

- Classes may be organized to provide exposure to new knowledge for large numbers of workers. For example, a new testing system may be devised for urine samples. All lab technicians must be made aware of the new system and how it works. Classes can be scheduled so that large groups of technicians may be informed at one time.
- Individuals who have unique training deficits may be tutored. For example, a ward clerk may have very poor communication skills when dealing with patients. The clerk may be given individual instruction and practice to improve performance.
- Small working units may share nonproductive attitudes or common skills deficits. These may be dealt with in a combination of small group meetings and on-the-job practice. For example, the persons responsible for registration of new patients may be filling out insurance forms incorrectly. A group meeting describing the proper procedure and providing a practice session could be followed by periodic checks of on-the-job performance. If mistakes continue, further group meetings and practice may be required.
- Individuals or groups may require training for new skills. For instance, a new type of IV tubing might be purchased that requires new setup techniques. All nurses would have to be trained in this new skill through demonstrations and practice sessions.

These are just a few examples of the broad range of topics covered by staff development activities.

WHY DO IT?

The health care industry is highly labor intensive.[1] As such, it requires careful attention to, and development of, its human resources. The industry is one of accelerating technology where constant upgrading and retraining is necessary in order to provide patients with the best possible care. In addition, pressures are exerted by government and regulatory agencies requiring that standards be met. Such influences include the Joint Commission for Accreditation of Hospitals, federal Medicare and Medicaid laws, and state continuing education requirements for relicensure of certain professionals.

Cost-effectiveness is of major concern in the decision to institute training and development programs. It is simply cheaper, in most cases, to retrain than to replace. An experienced employee has heightened abilities in many aspects of a job, as well as having built some loyalty to the organization. As patient care increasingly requires highly trained technicians, the value of the seasoned, retrained employee increases.

A cost-benefit analysis can demonstrate in quantifiable terms how training efforts can pay for themselves in situations where skills deficits exist and must be corrected.[2,3] The procedure for such an analysis, as outlined by Laird, is as follows: ". . . first determine the unit (of output). The second step is to determine the cost of that unit. The third step is to multiply the cost-per-unit by the number of defective units."[4] Finally, the cost per unit must be compared to the cost of training to determine if any benefit accrues from training.

For example, a fictitious "Memorial" Hospital uses the carbon copies of the nursing medication record to bill patients for medications they receive. The carbon copies are not always readable to clerks who enter the items on the patients' bills in the business office. It is estimated that 30 unreadable bills are submitted each week. If nurses who fill out the medication records are taught how to do so with maximum clarity for the clerks, it is projected that the unreadable records could be reduced to zero. Here is how costly this uncorrected problem can be:

Step 1: The unit of output is one medication record.

Step 2: The cost of one unreadable item includes the following elements:

a. The time of the clerk who checks the medication record and must return it to the nurse for clarification, estimated at 10 minutes per record, at a salary of $3.50 per hour, equals $0.58 per record.

b. The time of the nurse who clarifies the document, estimated at 15 minutes per record, at a salary of $7.50 per hour, equals $1.88 per record.

c. The time of the clerk who must revise the patient's bill and send an amended bill to the third party payer, estimated at 30 minutes per record, at a salary of $3.50 per hour, equals $1.75 per record.

Step 3: The cost per unit for the elements listed in Step 2 is $4.21. At 30 units per week, 1,560 unreadable medication records are submitted each year for a total expense of $6,567.60.

Step 4: The cost of training the nurses to prepare records clearly includes the following elements:

a. The time of trainers, estimated at three hours of preparation time and three hours of presentation time (three one-hour sessions) at an hourly rate of $8.00 equals $48.

b. The time of the nurses attending the training, estimated at one hour each for 400 nurses at an average hourly rate of $7.50, equals $3,000.

c. The materials and time involved in creating handouts for the training sessions, estimated at $50. To control the problem on a continuing basis, the information in the training program may be incorporated in existing orientation programs at no additional cost to the institution.

The cost of continuing errors is $6,567.60. The cost of training to prevent the problem is $3,098. Clearly, it is worthwhile to present the program to the nurses.

A key factor in deciding whether or not to institute training programs is the psychological impact such training has on employees. There is the clear message to employees that they have value and that the institution chooses to invest in them. The end result is improved performance or understanding—the goal of any training or development activity. Both of these are motivating factors, and motivated workers generally are more productive.

WHO GETS IT AND WHEN?

Orientation, as stated earlier, is required of all new employees immediately upon arrival on the job. It may be provided on several levels: hospitalwide, departmentwide, and/or job-specific. Depending on the size of the institution, one, two, or all three levels of orientation may be required.

Staff development is provided as needed. Usually, needs become obvious. For instance, procedures were being done incorrectly in irrigating patient catheters and the rate of bladder infections in patients was soaring in one ward. Training for this ward's nurses was arranged quickly to solve the problem. Or a new piece of equipment was purchased for dietary and instruction in its operation was required for any employee expected to use it. Or a medical secretary had consistent problems transcribing doctors' notes and was provided tutoring in medical terminology. Each of these situations arose as a problem involving the need for skill improvement or skill acquisition.

A second type of problem is motivational or attitudinal. Most commonly, this applies to an individual and requires a personal, one-to-one training/counseling approach by a supervisor or trainer. For example, a receptionist may be rude to incoming patients. The individual may be counselled on the reasons for the rudeness and may be taught methods of speaking and expression that will convey politeness to patients.

HOW IS IT DONE?

In the last decade, systematic efforts to design instruction have come to be identified as the systems approach. The emerging discipline of instructional design and technology has become familiar to management in health care institutions as well as in business and industry, military operations, and educational institutions. The design of instructional systems involves a body of knowledge called educational technology. Although this term is commonly associated with computers and other media hardware used for instruction, the growing tendency is to define educational technology as the process of planning, developing, implementing, controlling, and evaluating instructional systems.

The emphasis on *planned learning* is the central thrust of the systems approach. Learning must be planned rather than accidental or undirected so that all employees will approach the goal of making optimal use of their talents in the organization.

Underlying the concept of instructional design are some basic assumptions that require certain elements:

1. Instructional planning should be for the *individual* employee. Organizationwide changes in opinions and capabilities or the diffusion of information or attitudes are desirable; however, instructional systems are designed to enable individuals to develop to their fullest potential.

2. Instructional design has short-range as well as long-range phases. Training in health care set-

tings must take into consideration both types of planning. For example, when a new computer system is installed for use by medical staff, all current staff members must be provided training in operating it. However, provision also must be made for training all future staff members.

3. Systematically designed instruction can greatly aid human development. Some humanists argue that learning situations provided by the organization should provide only a ''nurturing environment.'' A stronger case can be made for sound, planned, and well-directed learning providing the optimal environment for ensuring equal opportunities for the use of individual talents to the greatest potential.

4. Training in health care settings must be based on sound principles of adult learning processes.

Newer Learning Theories

Some of the principles of how people learn have particular relevance to the instructional design process. The principles discussed here relate most specifically to events under the control of the trainer or to the characteristics of adult learners. Some of these principles have been around for some time, and while they remain valid, they take on a renewed significance in light of modern instructional design theory.

New theories suggest that several internal events are important for successful learning. Motivation of the learner, attitudes of confidence in learning, (which sometimes includes the idea of ''self-concept'') and use of individual learning styles (concrete vs. abstract, reflective vs. active) are preconditions for the instruction to be designed. For instance, a young man may be hired as a custodian. He needs the job in order to continue going to school (motivation), he has held similar jobs in the past with success (confidence), and he has learned concrete skills in school and on previous jobs (use of a learning style). This young man should prove successful in learning his new job duties. Newer theories deal with activating and channeling these internal states of the learner.

Other conditions that must be considered are the factual information needed in the learning situation, the individual's problem-solving skills, and the strategies for learning the person already possesses.

Factual information must be communicated to learners in any training setting. However, the acquisition of factual information in and of itself appears to be a dubious goal of an organizational training program. It is the problem-solving skills that must serve as the building blocks for instruction. Effective workers must have the problem-solving abilities and strategies to deal with daily situations away from the training setting.

Orienting Training to the Adult Learner

It is important, when developing programs of any kind for employees, that the trainer orient materials to the learners as adults. There are three essential aspects of the adult learner that should be considered:[5]

1. Adults have varying levels of knowledge and expertise because of different levels of experience. The instructor must assess the employees' knowledge and experience with regard to the training to be provided.[6] Then appropriate instruction can be given with the assurance that any gaps in background knowledge or skills are being filled, but that time is not wasted on material already familiar to the employees.

2. Adults tend to be oriented to the concrete and useful. ''Instructional activities should be task oriented and include active participation by the learner. Adults should experience success in completing the activity and should be able to demonstrate the skill in new situations.''[7] Generally, instruction is job-specific and task oriented so there should not be many problems in achieving this goal. In addition, virtually all new skills *must* be learned for proper job performance, so success is essential in the learning and completing of an activity.

3. Finally, the motivation of the adult learner is important. ''Adults are motivated to learn as they experience needs and interests that learning will satisfy.''[8] In most staff development situations, such felt needs will have arisen and will have prompted the training session(s). Adequate performance on the job is linked to the vital economic question of whether the employee does or does not continue to work. This fact alone provides a degree of motivation in staff training that is not present in other adult learning situations.

Steps in Instructional System Development

The development of an instructional system of any length uses a combination of systematic thinking, theory, facts from evaluation studies, and recycling. Whether for a single session or an entire training program, instructional system development consists of the same series of steps. The following eight steps are derived from several sources:

1. identification and analysis of problems or needs
2. identification of goals, objectives, and performance standards
3. identification of alternative solutions
4. development and design of the program
5. plan for trainee assessment procedures
6. field test, selection, and upgrading of trainers, and selection of trainees
7. measurement and evaluation
8. operational installation

In general, these steps take place in the order shown; however, in practice, elements of feedback and "feedforward" relationships exist. The cyclical, or iterative, characteristic of instructional system design is one of the major strengths of the method because the system returns to problem identification as a direct result of evaluation. In this way the instructional system is in a constant state of evaluation. This approach provides a basis for an accountability system and provides a means by which programs can furnish evidence to administrators of the extent to which training objectives have been attained.

Identification and Analysis

Determining the need for training is a crucial initial step in the system. The existence of the organization depends upon having some type of "output." In the case of the health care institution, the output takes the form of a service, namely, quality patient care. To obtain the necessary output, there must be "inputs." Health care institutions are largely dependent upon the inputs of technology and of people. To perform tasks properly, workers need to master and apply the unique technology pertaining to these tasks. At this point, training and education programs enter the picture. Often, health care organizations cannot hire people who at the time of employment are totally skilled in the unique requirements of their jobs. These institutions need subsystems called "training, education, and development," to help people master their tasks. The subsystems are concerned with changing workers into employees who can perform their assigned tasks in the way the organization wants them done, according to some predetermined standard.

This phase of the process provides information necessary to design the entire program. Problem and need analysis and identification should proceed on three levels: organizational, job, and person.

Organizational Analysis. This phase begins with an examination of the organization's goals. Training and educational programs that are in conflict with those goals are apt to result in confused and dissatisfied em-

ployees. Difficulties arise when training programs and work environments promote different, conflicting values. Requiring upper-level personnel to express their goals will ensure a more successful program and provide a basis for determining whether the system has achieved its objectives.

Organizational analysis also includes a determination of the staffing and physical resources available. Such an analysis requires a sensitivity to the institution's philosophy and its impact on the perceptions employees have of their working conditions. The organizational climate for leadership, motivation, accidents, or turnover must be understood in order to comprehend the behavior of individuals.

Additional indications of training needs and problems at the organizational level are as follows:

1. New or expanded facilities often mean new hiring.
2. New or expanded services often result in a need for employees to learn new technologies and procedures.
3. New equipment creates a need, especially if large numbers of employees are involved.
4. Changes in standards or policies can create a need for individuals to express their feelings about the shifts and to understand the reasons for them.
5. Trends, key requests, and key reports all provide good data for identifying training needs and problems. These communications indicate future plans, changing priorities, problem areas, successes, and failures.

When some indication of a training need arises, more formal procedures for data collection through surveys and interviews can be undertaken. Asking supervisors to outline their training needs is a less fruitful procedure than focusing on the visible behaviors of employees. According to Laird, the two most useful questions in the analysis of organizational training and educational needs are:

1. What are your people doing that they shouldn't be doing?
2. What aren't your people doing that they should be doing?[9]

Job Analysis.[10] A job analysis is essential to determine performance standards for the skills, knowledge, and attitudes needed to perform the task successfully. This analysis begins with a task description, which is a statement of activities performed on the job and the conditions under which the work is performed. The task description addresses the job, not the worker.

The next phase is to specify the tasks required, determine their importance to job performance, and describe in detail the steps necessary to carry out each important task. Task importance often is measured in terms of three criteria:

1. frequency of performance
2. importance of activity in terms of possible consequences of incorrect or incapable performance
3. learning difficulty

Person Analysis. This phase is designed to identify training or educational needs for one person or a small population. The major source of information is the performance appraisal. These appraisals are complex and interact with the information obtained throughout the entire analysis of training and educational needs.

Identification of Goals, Objectives, and Performance Standards

Goals, objectives, and standards serve as sources of feedback, providing important information to supervisors and workers about task performance. The importance of this instructional design phase cannot be stressed too highly. Goal setting as a motivational technique was discussed by Latham and Locke.[11] From their research, it was determined that it did not matter so much *how* the goal was set, but *that* the goal was set. Best performance results were obtained when:

1. The goal was specific rather than vague.
2. There was a time limit on performance.
3. The goal was challenging yet reachable.
4. Supervisors ensured that workers accepted and remained committed to goals.
5. Workers perceived the goals to be fair and reasonable.
6. Employees were given adequate resources— money, equipment, time, and support—for job performance.

Feedback about employee progress toward goals and standards set by the organization is not a sufficient condition for improved performance, but it is a necessary condition.

A complete discussion of how to develop instructional goals, objectives, and performance standards is beyond the scope of this article.[12] However, the work of Gagne[13] has particular relevance in expanding the discussion of instructional design phases in health care settings and is analyzed briefly here.

The instructional systems design process views learning in terms of human capabilities. Gagne posits five different sets of acquired human capabilities: motor skills, verbal information, intellectual skills, cognitive strategies, and attitudes. These are defined further in terms of observable behaviors or human performances. A system of classification, or a taxonomy, of human behavior is important to instructional designers because it enables the trainer to provide and arrange the essential conditions for learning each type of capability. In other words, it allows the proper selection of instructional techniques, methods, and evaluation procedures for each type of learning.

The task of instructional planning consists of assigning performance objectives to the five categories of human capabilities:

Motor Skills

Simple sequences of motor responses, or motor chains, frequently are combined into more complex performances called motor skills. Job performance often consists of interweaving these skills with other kinds of capabilities. The execution of a bodily movement is accomplished best by repeated practice, with provision for ''part skills'' and their integration into the exercise to produce the desired outcome.

Verbal Information

Facts, generalizations, or organized bodies of meaningful knowledge are important to human learning. Information may be needed for an individual to continue learning about a topic or job. Future learning will be more efficient if previous information has been learned well and retained. Much of the information learned may be useful throughout a person's life or career. Information is usually presented to the learner in the form of oral communication or visual presentation.

Intellectual Skills

Intellectual skills serve as the building blocks for instruction and are the capabilities that make individuals competent. This domain includes the learning of rules, concepts, discriminations, and problem solving.

Cognitive Strategies

A cognitive strategy is a special kind of intellectual skill. It is an internally organized skill that governs the learner's own behavior and represents various abilities the individual uses to attend, learn, remember, and think. The designing of instruction in this domain consists of providing the learner with novel problems with unspecified solutions.

Attitudes

Attitudes are complex human states that affect behavior toward people, things, and events. Many writers believe that there are cognitive aspects to attitudes. An attitude is an internal state inferred from observations of the individual's behavior; it is not the behavior itself. The learning of attitudes and the ways of changing them are complex matters. Much evidence exists to show that attitude learning or attitude change is not done entirely through the use of persuasive communications. Two methods for learning in the affective domain are (1) arranging contingencies of reinforcement (behavior modification) and (2) human modeling. A human model must be someone the learner respects and with whom the person can identify.

Skill in describing human behavior and learning capabilities is essential for trainers in organizations. In addition, training specialists must know how to define performance standards. The definition of performance standards often is a joint effort, with both supervisors and trainers playing key roles. Not every organization has established standards. Some have them in an informal sense. However, without some degree of specificity in defining performance standards, it is difficult to make a strong case that the worker is not performing properly. Some questions useful in the process of defining performance standards are:

1. What do you envision your workers doing when the job is performed properly?
2. What things would you like to see them doing— but don't?
3. What things do you specifically praise when you see them performing well?
4. What things do you tell them to avoid doing?
5. What things do you ask them to be sure to do in the future?

The answers to each of these questions provides important material for beginning the process of making performance criteria more specific.

Identification of Alternative Solutions

Training and education in an organization are appropriate solutions when employees lack knowledge or skills. However, when employees can do their work but don't, alternative solutions must be explored. It is at this point in the instructional design process that other human resource development procedures must

be investigated. Feedback mechanisms, contingency management, MBO techniques, job engineering, organization development—all provide possible solutions to problems originally thought to be training issues.

If it is determined that training and education problems do indeed exist, the organization must determine whether programs should be conducted inside or outside the institution.

Some alternative inside solutions other than formal training sessions might include:

- existing in-house programs
- self-study materials
- special assignments
- field trips
- coaching
- bringing in outside trainers

Development and Design of the Program

Decisions must be made for the following aspects of the instructional system:

1. planning the nature of the materials for study
2. identifying the nature of the activities the worker is to perform
3. specifying the role of the trainer(s)
4. scheduling group activities and the instructional methods to be used
5. assessing learner performance

The specific characteristics of instruction may vary among objectives representing different domains or types of learning outcomes, the nature of the individuals, and the characteristics of the assumed learning environment. The fundamental criterion in selecting any instructional method should be its appropriateness toward the achievement of the desired learning outcome.

At this stage in any discussion of instructional systems, learning methods usually are dealt with at length. Complete analysis of the various methodologies are given in the bibliography at the end of this article. One of the best discussions of current instructional methods appropriate for adult learners in training and educational programs in organizational settings is given by Laird in his book *Approaches to Training and Development*.[14] Although not everyone concerned with human resource development in an organization need be intimately familiar with the various methodologies, there must be a knowledge of some principles involved in the selection of instructional modes. Some critical components or principles of selection of training methodologies include:

- There must be a thorough recognition and analysis of the task or job skills and the types of learning outcomes (verbal information, intellectual skill, cognitive strategy, or attitude) to be achieved.
- Jobs or tasks may require learning outcomes in several domains; therefore, components of the tasks or skills must be identified.
- The total learning situation must be carefully sequenced so that essential steps necessary for building more complex skills are not neglected.
- The selection of training methodologies emanates from the types of learning outcomes desired. For example, a lecture or a film is designed to impart verbal information. Problem-solving skills require other types of combinations of training methodologies such as in-basket exercises, role plays, games, simulations, or programmed instruction.
- Training methodologies that make the individuals be passive participants violate sound principles of learning. Provision must be made for their performance of the desired learning outcomes. In other words, learning by observation is hardly as effective as learning through action.
- The decision about selection of training methods is multidimensional. It reflects the learning objectives, the nature of the learners (particularly adult learners), the characteristics of the organization, and the budget available.

Plan for Trainee Assessment Procedures

Careful attention to instructional design procedures in the early stages of the development of the training system will pay important dividends at this stage. Appropriate assessment of trainee progress toward the desired learning outcomes is based upon observations—both formal and informal—of learner behaviors. A plan for assessing whether participants' exposure to the training has changed their performance in any significant way should be developed before implementing the program.

Knowledge of sound principles of learning measurement and evaluation is essential in this design stage. Most assessment of learner performance in organizational settings consists of using object-referenced tests employing a performance standard as the criterion. With a pretest/posttest design, progress by employees toward desired learning outcomes can best be used to evaluate both learner achievement and the effects of the training and educational program.

Field Test, Selection, and Upgrading of Trainers, and Selection of Trainees

In practice, small portions of the instructional system are tried out on some individual learners. The designer analyzes learned responses in order to detect weaknesses in the program. Methods and materials may be revised. There usually is a need to train the instructors by conducting workshops or by arranging for them to see demonstrations of program procedures.

The selection of trainees includes stressing the reasons for enrollment in the program. Enrollment should not be viewed as punitive but a way to learn to do a job well. In addition, the reallocation and rescheduling of the workload must be done to accommodate the time devoted to training and educational activities.

Measurement and Evaluation

Studies of the effectiveness of the instructional system as a whole are important at this phase. The state of evaluation of training in organizations leaves much to be desired. For economic, political, and psychological reasons, evaluation of training programs creates a myriad of defensive reactions. Evaluation is not a particularly glamorous activity and not nearly as exciting as initiating a new training program. Training specialists often stress what people think about their programs more than they stress how effective those programs are in achieving instructional objectives.

The systems approach to the development of organizational training and education programs emphasizes an orderly, planned development of the method. As a consequence, evaluation planning is involved in all phases of the instructional design process.

Evaluation of training programs involves collecting information about reactions to, as well as results of, training. Measuring the attitudes of participants indicates the acceptance of the program. Reaction evaluation is used extensively in organizational training programs because it is relatively simple to administer. However, it tells little about the effectiveness of the program.

The evaluation of learning and behavior change back on the job is difficult and time consuming. The observing, recording, and measuring of job performance changes according to performance standards requires a rather high level of sophistication in tests and measurement.

The results of careful evaluation of the effects of training and educational programs can help determine the contribution these activities make to improve decision making, reduced employer turnover, compensation costs, and grievances. For the organization, the bottom line is improved patient care.

Operational Installation

This phase in the instructional system design has been anticipated throughout the discussion. Many practical matters such as room scheduling and materials storage must be taken care of at this point.

The design of an instructional system is a large undertaking. A major advantage of this systems approach is that it provides for a planned rather than haphazard way of designing learning programs. It also makes provisions for knowing when learning outcomes have been achieved and, therefore, makes it possible to assess the effects of training programs on the contribution toward organizational goals and objectives.

EXAMPLES OF SYSTEM DESIGN

The following examples provide clarification for the novice in instructional system design. They are intended to further understanding of how the method actually operates in the health care setting.

Fire Safety Training

Need Determined

Safety is an overriding concern in health care institutions where so many patients are incapable of helping themselves in emergencies. Fire is one of the most dangerous of such emergencies. Consequently, there is an obvious need for fire safety training for all employees in any health care facility.

Objectives Constructed

The most important requirements in fire safety training are that patients be moved to safety when necessary, that the fire be reported, and that it be contained and extinguished. The objectives for the program would thus be:

1. To list criteria for deciding whether a patient must be moved.
2. To demonstrate methods of moving patients in emergency situations.
3. To list the steps in reporting a fire.
4. To demonstrate methods of containing and/or extinguishing a fire.

Activities Developed

Appropriate activities for achieving the four objectives can be extrapolated from the objectives themselves.

1. Criteria for assessing whether or not a patient must be moved should be listed for employees, explained, and then memorized.
2. Methods of moving patients should be demonstrated to employees and then practiced.
3. Employees should be given a written and/or verbal list of the steps involved in reporting a fire. These should be explained and memorized.
4. Employees should be provided with demonstrations of various means of containing and extinguishing fires. These methods should then be practiced by everyone.

Evaluation Provided

During the training sessions, evaluation may be provided by the instructor's observation of employees as they demonstrate techniques of fighting fires and of moving patients. Written tests may be given to ascertain whether employees have, indeed, memorized the steps for reporting a fire and the criteria for deciding whether patients must be moved. Subsequent to the training sessions, employees may be asked to demonstrate their fire safety skills and knowledge by their supervisors, to assure that these are kept current. For employees whose skills need improvement or whose knowledge is not complete, retraining sessions may be scheduled. At this point, the whole procedure as outlined above would be repeated.

Child Abuse Reporting

Need Determined

Frequently new laws will necessitate training efforts for some or all employees on a hospital staff. This was the case in the enactment of the law requiring medical personnel to report all suspected cases of child abuse with which they came in contact. Here the need is determined by the imposition of a new regulation.

Objectives Constructed

The central concerns of the child abuse reporting law are the designation of what constitutes child abuse and the legal responsibility of medical personnel to report that abuse. Thus the objectives for a training session on the new law for medical personnel might be:

1. to list the signs of abuse most frequently encountered in abused children
2. to list the tests most likely to indicate child abuse in suspected cases
3. to demonstrate techniques for eliciting information from an abusing parent/guardian in a suspected child abuse case
4. to list social agencies in the hospital's immediate areas to which child abuse cases should be referred
5. to list the steps involved in reporting a child abuse case to the proper authorities in the state

Activities Developed

Again, activities appropriate for achieving these results can be developed directly from the objectives themselves.

1. Provide medical personnel with a list and description of the signs of child abuse; discuss these signs, and have staff memorize them.
2. List and discuss tests likely to indicate child abuse and have personnel memorize these.
3. Institute role playing between the instructor (in the part of the abusing parent) and medical personnel to provide experience in the kinds of communications required in such emotionally charged situations.
4. List and describe relevant social agencies and have personnel memorize them.
5. List and discuss steps for reporting child abuse and have staff memorize them.

In cases such as reporting child abuse, the ability to find the information quickly when the need arises may be a more practical approach than the memorization of information about reporting and social service agencies.

Evaluation Provided

During discussion, the trainer can evaluate to some degree the depth of understanding acquired by medical personnel. A written test at the end of the information sessions will reveal whether personnel actually understand what signs to look for in child abuse victims, what tests are required, and where information may be found on steps for reporting cases and for referring families in such situations. The role playing during the training sessions will provide the trainer with a good idea as to the ability of personnel to elicit information from abusing parents/guardians.

Medical Terminology

Need Determined

Doctors may be getting consistently poor transcription of their notes from their secretaries. The problem seems to be that the secretaries do not know medical terminology and so misspell words, frequently leading to confusion regarding the patient's condition. A trainer constructs a quick test to find out if the secretaries have any understanding of the components of medical terms they are expected to work with on a daily basis. The test demonstrates inadequate knowledge.

Objectives Constructed

The need exists for the secretaries to better understand the terms with which they deal every day. To provide the greatest transfer of learning to their everyday working situations, the trainer decides to deal with words in terms of their component parts: root words, prefixes, and suffixes. Some objectives for this group of training sessions might then be:

1. to identify the major body systems on a diagram of the human body
2. to list the major root words connected with each body system
3. to deduce the meaning of a word when provided with a list of prefixes, suffixes, and root words
4. to correctly spell nine out of ten medical terms as dictated on a recording machine by a doctor from the usual case notes.

Clearly, many variations on these objectives also could be included to assure competency of the secretaries in the spelling and understanding of medical terms.

Activities Developed

A variety of approaches may be used in teaching medical terminology:

1. Distribute diagrams of the human body and have secretaries label each body system as it is described and discussed by the trainer.
2. List the major root words associated with each system of the body as it is described. Discuss each root word and have secretaries memorize the major ones with which they will deal most often.
3. Provide secretaries with listings of prefixes, suffixes, and root words. Discuss and explain all

components, then provide secretaries with lists of words composed of these elements and have the secretaries deduce the meanings of the words.

4. Have secretaries practice transcribing dictation that includes words common to their areas of work. This kind of practice can be done until a designated level of competence is achieved—in this case, 90 percent accuracy.

Evaluation Provided

This case most closely parallels the usual classroom situation familiar from school days. Some of the same classroom techniques for evaluation are very appropriate here:

1. A blank diagram of the human body may be given to secretaries and they may be asked to fill in the major body systems.
2. The root words most common to their work may be listed and secretaries asked to define them; or vice versa, definitions may be given and root words requested.
3. A listing of unfamiliar words may be provided to secretaries along with listings of prefixes, suffixes, and root words. They then may be asked to decipher the meanings of these words, with repeated exercises and tests until a given level of competency is reached.
4. A dictated tape could be used for transcription as a test in the same way that it was used for practice purposes during the training sessions.

SUMMARY

Training and personnel development is growing in importance in the health care field. As technology brings changes and as government and accrediting agencies increase regulations, personnel require training in an increasing number of areas. For these and other reasons, it is important for health care administrators to be aware of the training needs in their institutions and to have some understanding of the processes involved in planning for training.

NOTES

1. Nicholas D. Richie, "Health Planning—An Overview," *American Journal of Health Planning*, April 1978, p. 39.
2. Dugan Laird, *Approaches to Training and Development* (Reading, Mass.: Addison-Wesley Publishing Company, 1978), pp. 218–222.
3. James G. Cullen, Stephen A. Sawzin, Gary R. Sisson, and Richard A. Swanson, "Cost Effectiveness: A Model for Assessing the Training Investment," *Training and Development Journal*, January 1978, pp. 24–29. This also contains formats for assessing training costs.
4. Laird, p. 219.
5. Adapted from Malcolm Knowles, *The Adult Learner: A Neglected Species* (Houston: Gulf Publishing Co., 1973), p. 31.
6. John R. Verduin, Jr., Harry G. Miller, and Charles E. Greer, *Adults Teaching Adults* (Austin, Texas: Learning Concepts, 1977), p. 49.
7. Verduin, p. 16.
8. Knowles, p. 31.
9. Laird, p. 54.
10. U.S. Department of Labor, Manpower Administration, *Handbook for Analyzing Jobs* (Washington, D.C.: U.S. Government Printing Office, 1972). This presents a more technical discussion of the task analysis process.
11. Gary P. Latham and Edwin Locke, "Goal-Setting—A Motivational Technique That Works," *Organizational Dynamics*, Autumn 1979, pp. 68–80.
12. The reader is referred to any of the training and education books listed in this article's bibliography.
13. Robert M. Gagne and Leslie J. Briggs, *Principles of Instructional Design* (New York: Holt, Rinehart and Winston, Inc., 1974), *passim*.
14. Laird, *passim*.

BIBLIOGRAPHY

Craig, Robert L., ed. *Training and Development Handbook.* New York: McGraw-Hill Book Co., 1976.

Cullen, James G.; Sawzin, Stephen A.; Sisson, Gary R.; and Swanson, Richard A. "Cost Effectiveness: A Model for Assessing the Training Investment." *Training and Development Journal*, January 1978, pp. 24–29.

Davis, Larry Nolan. *Planning, Conducting, and Evaluating Workshops.* Austin, Texas: Learning Concepts, 1974.

Gagne, Robert M., and Briggs, Leslie J. *Principles of Instructional Design.* New York: Holt, Rinehart and Winston, Inc., 1974.

Goldstein, Irwin I. *Training: Program Development and Evaluation.* Monterey, Calif.: Brooks/Cole Publishing Co., 1974.

Hinrichs, John R. "Personnel Training," in Marvin D. Dunnette, ed., *Handbook of Industrial/Organizational Psychology.* Chicago: Rand McNally, 1976.

Knowles, Malcolm. *The Adult Learner: A Neglected Species.* Houston: Gulf Publishing Co., 1973.

Laird, Dugan. *Approaches to Training and Development.* Reading, Mass.: Addison-Wesley Publishing Co., 1978.

Latham, Gary P., and Locke, Edwin. "Goal Setting—A Motivational Technique That Works." *Organizational Dynamics*, Autumn 1979, pp. 68–80.

Mager, Robert F. *Measuring Instructional Intent, or, Got a Match?* Belmont, Calif.: Fearon Publishers, 1973.

—————. *Preparing Instructional Objectives.* Belmont, Calif.: Fearon Publishers, 1962.

Maynard, H. B., editor-in-chief. *Handbook of Business Administration.* New York: McGraw-Hill Book Co., 1970.

McLagen, Patricia A. *Helping Others Learn.* Reading, Mass.: Addison-Wesley Publishing Co., 1978.

Metzger, Norman. *Personnel Administration in the Health Services Industry.* Holliswood, N.Y.: Spectrum Publications, Inc., 1975.

Richie, Nicholas D. "Health Planning—An Overview." *American Journal of Health Planning*, April 1978, pp. 36–42.

Schein, Edgar H. *Organizational Psychology*. Englewood Cliffs, N.J.: Prentice-Hall, Inc., 1970.

Schneier, Craig, and Beatty, Richard. *Personnel Administration Today: Readings and Commentary*. Reading, Mass.: Addison-Wesley Publishing Co., 1978.

Schwaller, Anthony E. "The Need for Education/Training Programs in Industry." *Phi Delta Kappan,* January 1980, pp. 322–323.

Smith, Reginald L. "Those Aren't People Anymore . . . They Are Mere Bodies Moving By Me." *Hospital Topics,* November-December 1979, pp. 14–15.

U.S. Department of Labor, Manpower Administration. *Handbook for Analyzing Jobs*. Washington, D.C.: U.S. Government Printing Office, 1972.

Verduin, John R., Jr.; Miller, Harry G.; and Greer, Charles E. *Adults Teaching Adults*. Austin, Texas: Learning Concepts, 1977.

Woodington, Donald. "Some Impressions of the Evaluation of Training in Industry." *Phi Delta Kappan,* January 1980, pp. 326–328.

21. Theories of Motivation Applied to Health Care Personnel Management

ARTHUR P. BRIEF

This article provides an overview of contemporary theories of employee motivation and demonstrates how they may be applied to the management of health care personnel. The article consists of four major sections: (1) The importance of employee motivation as a determinant of the overall effectiveness of health institutions is highlighted. (2) The linkages between employee performance and outcomes are discussed as a principal source of motivation. (3) The employee's self-image is assessed as a motivational source. (4) Prescriptions for influencing the motivation of health care personnel are presented.

FOUR DETERMINANTS OF MOTIVATION

It is important first to specify what is meant by the term motivation. This can be accomplished best by examining four categories of factors that are known to be key determinants (or predictors) of employee performance:

1. facilitating and inhibiting factors *not* under the control of the worker
2. the individual's aptitude and skill levels
3. the degree to which the person understands what to do on the job and how to do it
4. the employee's level of motivation.[1]

Facilitating and inhibiting factors not under the control of employees may include such factors as the technology they rely on in performing their jobs and the demand for the services they provide. For instance, the performance levels of laboratory technicians obviously are controlled in part by the speed and accuracy of the equipment they use as well as the numbers and types of tests requested. At least in the short run, most technicians have little, if any, control over the technology they use or the demand for their services. However, it is clear that these are two elements that do influence their productivity.

The case in favor of the second category of factors, aptitudes and skills, is a simple one. The greater the degree of congruence between the aptitudes and skills required to perform a given job and the aptitudes and skills actually possessed by the incumbent, the higher the level of performance. The health care manager largely exerts influence over aptitudes and skills through control of the organization's selection, placement, and training functions. These functions are dealt with elsewhere in this volume.

The third category involves employees' role conceptions or how they view what is expected of them on their jobs. More precisely, role conceptions concern the degree to which employees understand the objectives of their jobs and how to meet those goals. Two major obstacles to acquiring this understanding are role conflict and role ambiguity.[2] Role conflict occurs in a variety of forms and generally refers to the lack of consistency in the demands on the employee. Role ambiguity, on the other hand, simply refers to lack of clarity in the communication of these demands to the worker. An example of role conflict would be where a staff nurse receives competing requests from the charge nurse and an attending physician; an example of role ambiguity would be that a physician's request is confusing or the nurse does not understand how to execute the doctor's instructions. Levels of role conflict and role ambiguity or, more generally, the level of understanding an employee possesses about the job, are in the control, in part, of the health care manager. The basic responsibilities of management include directing the activities of subordinates, providing feedback to them on their task accomplishments or failures, and buffering them from others' demands. The extent to which the health care manager successfully fulfills these responsibilities determines subordinates' level of understanding.

Finally, employee motivation, the topic of interest here, is a principal determinant of performance. Basically, motivation explains the direction, amplitude, and persistence of an employee's efforts, holding constant the effects of constraints operating in the work environment, the individual's aptitudes and skills and understanding of the job. Thus, motivation is concerned with three choices made by the employee: (1) the choice to *initiate* effort, (2) the choice to expend a certain *amount* of effort, and (3) the choice to *persist* in expending that effort over a period of time.[1] This view of motivation implies that employees make *decisions* about their efforts—where to apply them, how much, and for how long. Influencing this decision-making process is the subject of the rest of the article. The role of employee motivation in determining the health care worker's performance level is summarized in Figure 21-1.[3]

MOTIVATION AND ORGANIZATIONAL EFFECTIVENESS

Organizational effectiveness generally is an elusive concept. Therefore, for purposes of this article, the effectiveness of a health care organization is viewed simply, as the degree to which an institution provides optimal health services to a given population group in a cost-efficient manner.[4, 5, 6, 7, 8, 9, 10, 11] Even with this simple view of effectiveness, it can be seen that the health care manager must be concerned with the ability of the institution (1) to adapt to its environment and remain flexible, (2) to provide certain levels of health care defined in terms of both quantity and quality, (3) to maintain the necessary work force defined in terms of both numbers and mix of skills and abilities, (4) to be profitable and/or to contain costs, and (5) to acquire necessary fiscal resources.

Figure 21-1 Predictors of Employee Performance

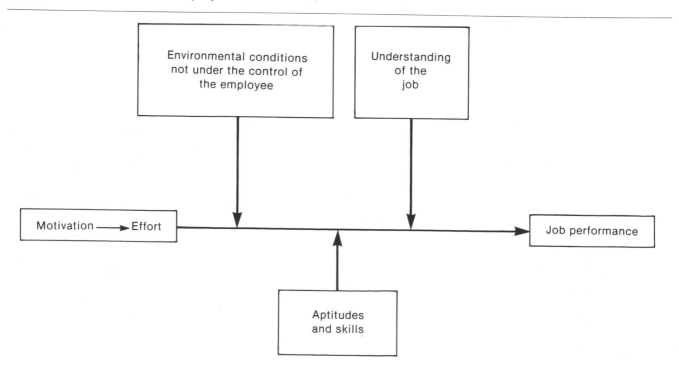

Each of these facets of effectiveness shares at least two characteristics. First, each facet is related to each other facet. In other words, if the health care manager fails to obtain results on any one of the five points, organizational effectiveness at least in the long run also will suffer in terms of each of the other points. Second, attainment of effectiveness requires that people in the organization successfully perform their assigned roles. Thus, employees' job performance levels are a major determinant of overall organizational effectiveness. As noted earlier, motivation through its impact on the direction, amplitude, and persistence of employees' efforts is, in turn, a major determinant of individuals' performance. These relationships are depicted in Figure 21-2.

It is important to specify more clearly what is meant by employee performance. Generally, the level of an individual's job performance is defined in terms of the degree to which the employee successfully carries out the duties and responsibilities assigned to the person's organizational role. Of course, it is assumed that the assigned functions are consistent with attaining the institution's goals. Further, and possibly more importantly, it is assumed throughout the rest of this article that health care managers can and do accurately assess their subordinates' performances.

An adequate treatment of the performance appraisal process clearly is beyond the scope of this article.[12] Nevertheless, the importance and potential tenuous nature of the assumptions regarding the health care manager's measurement of employee performance cannot be understated. Any successful attempt at increasing levels of motivation requires that managers know the goals they want their employees to achieve and gauge whether in fact these individuals have reached these goals. Without such specification of goals and subsequent measurement of their attainment, it is pertinent to ask: "Motivation for what purpose?"

THE CONSEQUENCES OF JOB PERFORMANCE

A principal source of motivation involves the capacity of people to represent future consequences of their behavior in thought.[13, 14] This cognitive capacity is what allows employees to make choices about the application of their efforts. Many different theoretical models are concerned with the links between behavior and consequences or, in the current case, between employee performance and the outcomes that this performance accrues to the individual. For example, Vroom[15] in his expectancy theory of motivation recognizes that one determinant of the force to perform (i.e., motivation) is the perceived association between performing at a given level and subsequently obtaining a given outcome.[16, 17, 18, 19] Vroom labels these types of associations instrumentalities.

According to Vroom, instrumentalities can take values ranging from -1, indicating the employee's belief that attainment of the outcome is certain without performing at the specified level, to $+1$, indicating that performance at that level is believed to be a necessary and sufficient condition for achieving the result. Assuming that the objective is highly desired by the employee, motivation is maximized when the instrumentality for the outcome is at $+1$ the case when the employee is certain that performing at the specified level will lead to attaining a highly attractive result.

Figure 21-2 Motivation and Effectiveness of the Health Care Organization

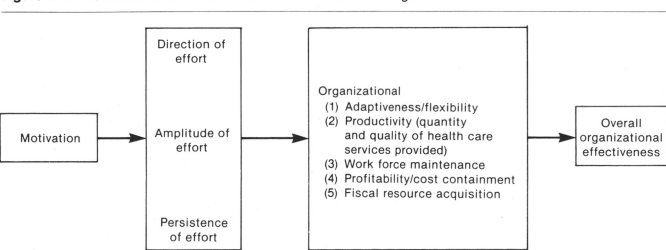

Conversely, assuming that the outcome is highly undesirable, motivation is maximized when the instrumentality is −1—the case when the employee is certain that performing at the specified level will avoid attainment of the highly unattractive result.

Thus far, several important points have been made that warrant reiteration: (1) how employees perceive the relationship between their performance and the outcomes they can attain will influence their motivation; (2) outcomes may either be desirable or undesirable from the employee's perspective; and (3) motivation is maximized when performance is seen by the employee as a means of obtaining a desirable outcome or avoiding an undesirable outcome.

THOUGHT PROCESSES AND PERFORMANCE

All of these points relate to the thought processes of employees—how they perceive performance outcome linkages in their work environments, what results they find desirable or undesirable in those environments, and, ultimately, what choices they make in applying their efforts. Each of these aspects of employees' thought processes is elaborated upon briefly.

First, perceived performance-outcome linkages (and not necessarily those actually in place in the work environment) have the most direct impact on motivation. This recognizes that people react to their environments based upon how they perceive those environments and that there may not be a one-to-one correspondence between these perceptions and objective reality. For example, a health organization may have an explicit policy of basing pay increments at least in part on how well employees do their jobs; however, a sizable number of the employees may not perceive any meaningful level of association between their performance and their pay raises. These employees would report instrumentality values for pay near zero. Thus, it is important that health care managers not only formulate appropriate policies linking performance to various outcomes but that they also ensure these policies are communicated effectively to the employees upon whom they impact.

Second, health care managers must recognize that it is employees' desire or attraction to a given outcome that is important to their motivation, not the manager's degree of attraction to the result. For instance, a manager generally may view promotions as highly desirable; however, a particular nurse may want to avoid promotion from staff to charge nurse for a variety of reasons, including the fear of breaking close friendship ties with peers. Thus, health care managers must con-sider how employees differ in terms of the results they feel to be desirable or undesirable. Even though considerable research has been conducted on these individual differences, further analysis is beyond the scope of the article.[20] It may be important to note, however, that it is the nature and composition of an employee's need structure that largely determines the desirability of an outcome.[21,22,23] Results judged by the individual to be important sources of need satisfaction are the ones that are most desirable.

Also relevant to the topic of outcome desirability is the explicit recognition that employees view some results as undesirable. Recalling the case in which motivation is maximized is when the employee sees performance as a means of avoiding an undesirable outcome, it might be presumed that the health care manager should behave in a punitive fashion toward individuals not reaching a specified performance level. This would be a false presumption for at least two reasons: (1) punishment tends to produce only public compliance and (2) it may reduce the manager's ability to reinforce (i.e., reward) the employee positively.

The first reason suggests that a punitive managerial style works only when the employee is fearful of being detected and punished (e.g., verbally abused by the supervisor) for performing below standard. Thus, the manager must maintain a constant vigilance and be willing and capable of following through on any threats. In many instances, these conditions simply are not met. The second reason suggests that employees continually abused by their supervisors will not find occasional kind words from their punitive managers to be meaningful; therefore, these managers in effect have reduced their reward power.[24,25]

For these reasons, the recommended route to maximizing motivation is for the health care manager to implement policies that allow employees to acquire desired outcomes contingent upon their reaching or exceeding specified performance levels. As will be discussed later, these desired outcomes (i.e., rewards) can be classified as either extrinsic or intrinsic.

The final aspect of the employees' performance-outcome thought processes is, again, recognition that individuals make conscious choices about the application of their efforts. This recognition indicates that employees' behavior is not random and that they attempt to maximize their gains (or utility) under the constraints of the conditions prevailing in their environments. Employees, therefore, probably are viewed by health care managers as rational decision makers. This implies that employees should be dealt with in an overt rather than a covert manner. Thus, necessary information should be provided to employees about the health organization's reward policies to produce efficient decision making; information also should be sought from them about the contents of those policies in an attempt to ensure they are formulated effectively. For instance, managers should seek out information from their employees regarding the desirability of various results before incorporating them in the organization's reward structure.

EXTRINSIC AND INTRINSIC REWARDS

The following paragraphs discuss two types of rewards previously identified—extrinsic and intrinsic—to provide further input into the design of effective reward systems.

Extrinsic Rewards

Employee motivation literature contains several competing views of what in fact are and are not extrinsic rewards.[26] Here, extrinsic rewards are viewed narrowly as desirable work outcomes that are "in the direct control of the health care manager."[27] The quoted clause implies that the manager is actively involved in delivering the reward to the employee (e.g., recommending a pay raise or a promotion). It is not possible to provide a firm listing of extrinsic rewards because as will be shown later some fall into a gray area between extrinsic and intrinsic. Nevertheless, the following extrinsic rewards are representative of those commonly found in health care organizations: pay, promotion, security, praise, warmth, and attractive work assignments. Based upon what has been said, these rewards acquire motivational properties when they are delivered to the employee contingent upon the individual's reaching or exceeding a specified performance level.

If managers want to establish a positive relationship, for example, between their friendship overtures toward their employees (i.e., warmth) and their performance, the managers should behave warmly toward a given individual, depending upon that worker's job performance. This, obviously, is a tough-minded posture for the health care manager; but a supervisor who attempts to befriend all subordinates regardless of their performance should not necessarily expect that friendship to be repaid with better work. It is not recommended that the warm, personable manager begin behaving coldly toward low performing employees; rather, this supervisor should readjust expectations as to the performance outcomes of such behaviors.

The important point is that extrinsic rewards acquire motivational properties if they are delivered contingent upon high levels of performance and withheld in the face of poor performance. This leads to the re-

wards' acquiring motivational properties; it also tends to lead to the following favorable circumstances: (1) employees generally are more satisfied with the levels of the rewards they receive; and (2) dissatisfaction is concentrated among low performing workers and, therefore, voluntary turnovers (quits) are more likely to occur among such individuals.[28]

The probable reason for the former occurrence is that the rewards have been equitably distributed in proportion to the employee's contributions to the health care organization,[29, 30] so the individual associates such treatment positively with job satisfaction.[31,32,33,34] In regards to the latter consequence of delivering extrinsic rewards contingent upon performance, the simple reason why low performers are more dissatisfied than high performers is that they receive fewer extrinsic rewards.

Intrinsic Rewards

Intrinsic rewards are desirable work outcomes that are principally in control of the employee. In other words, the employee is the agent of delivery. Intrinsic rewards may be tangible or intangible. Examples of intangible intrinsic rewards include positive self-evaluation and other forms of self-satisfying thoughts (e.g., feelings of accomplishment and personal growth and development, or satisfaction from helping and serving others).

It may appear that health care managers exert no influence over the delivery of intrinsic rewards. On the contrary, they can influence their availability as well as the performance standards that employees rely upon in determining whether or not their work merits self-reward. Before elaborating on the influences of the manager, it is important to specify the three conditions that define a self-rewarding event. According to Bandura,[13] the three conditions are:

1. Employees have established performance standards to determine the occasions on which their behaviors warrant self-reward.
2. Rewards are freely available for the employees' taking.
3. Even though rewards are freely available, employees reward themselves contingent upon achieving the standards they have established.

Examples of self-rewarding events abound in health care organizations. For instance, the nurse clinician who has determined how many patients must be seen each morning, after meeting that goal provides a self-reward with a coffee break. This nurse can choose freely when to take a break but withholds the reward (i.e., a cup of coffee—a tangible intrinsic reward) until the self-decreed performance goal has been achieved. Another example involves a technician who has just completed assisting in administering a series of x-rays that were quite uncomfortable for the patient. Based upon feedback from the patient, the technician is aware of being quite successful in helping the individual cope with the discomfort and therefore issues a self-reward with positive self-evaluative thoughts such as "I'm pretty pleased with myself for helping that patient through the procedure with a minimum of discomfort."

MANAGERIAL INFLUENCES

Now that the conditions defining a self-rewarding event have been specified, the role of health care managers in influencing the occurrence of such events can be described. Managers have some discretion over the structure (or contents) of their employees' jobs. That job content determines in part the availability of intrinsic rewards.[20] For example, one dimension for describing job content is autonomy—the degree of discretion the incumbent exercises over how and when the work activities are performed. An employee in a job characterized by a low degree of autonomy is likely to find fewer intrinsic rewards available. Take the case of the nurse clinician whose self-reward was a cup of coffee contingent upon the number of patients seen. If this person had been working on a fixed schedule with a coffee break set for 10:15, the intrinsic reward would not have been available.

More generally, a position characterized as "enriched" is likely to afford its occupant a greater array of intrinsic rewards than a more routine, simplified, and repetitive job.[35] An enriched job also is characterized by a high level of variety as well as by activities that the incumbent regards as important and that produce results with which the employee can identify.[36] Examples of enriched jobs in health care organizations include hospital nursing jobs designed around a primary care structure rather than a team or functional structure. A primary care orientation allows nurses more autonomy, the opportunity to utilize a greater variety of skills, responsibility for performing a greater number of activities that have a direct impact on a patient, and an end product (i.e., the health status of a patient) to which the nurse can relate more readily. Thus, nursing administrators wishing to maximize the availability of intrinsic rewards to the nurses they supervise would opt for a primary care structure over a team or function structure. In sum, health care mana-

gers can influence the occurrence of self-rewarding events by designing their subordinates' jobs so as to make necessary intrinsic rewards available more freely.

Merely enriching a job, however, will not necessarily lead to an employee's exhibiting higher levels of performance. The individual first must adopt personal performance standards congruent with the attainment of the health institution's goals and provide self-rewards only when those standards have been met. As noted, managers also can exert influence over the occurrence of these two additional conditions.

First, they can prescribe performance standards and extrinsically reward only employees attaining those levels. This process of differentially rewarding employees is likely to lead to their adopting performance standards congruent with those of the manager.[14,37,38] As argued earlier, it is imperative, therefore, that health care managers link the extrinsic rewards with the employees' performance levels.

A second way managers can influence performance standards is by serving as an appropriate role model from which their employees can learn the desired standards.[13] This simply means that managers who publicly self-reward themselves only when they clearly have achieved performance levels congruent with the goals of the organization are likely to induce their employees to adopt similar standards. This is particularly true if the manager is well liked by the subordinates.

As depicted in Figure 21-3, the health care manager's control over intrinsic sources of employee motivation is indeed less direct than over extrinsic sources. Nevertheless, both forms of performance-outcome linkages are important determinants of motivation; therefore, neither of them should be ignored in the design of the institution's reward systems.

SELF-IMAGE AS A MOTIVATION FACTOR

The previous section dealt with employee expectations regarding performance-outcome linkages as a source of motivation. The motivation source considered next concerns employees' expectations about personal mastery of the tasks comprising their jobs. These task relevant self-images (or self-efficacy expectations)[37] involve employees' conviction that they can perform their jobs at the level required to produce expected rewards. Task relevant self-image also is viewed here as employees' expectations regarding their ability to perform at a satisfactory level.[16,39,40]

Figure 21-3 Performance-Outcome Linkages and Employee Motivation

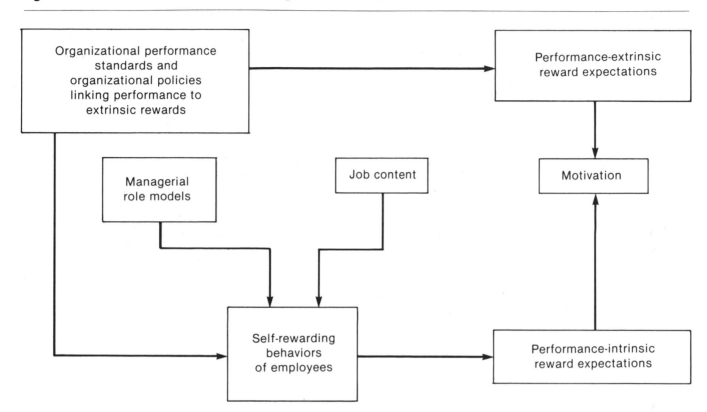

Employees' task relevant self-images at least initially influence their choices of activities and settings and, subsequently, their levels of effort and persistence. For example, a physician who does not feel able to perform a particular surgical technique successfully will not be motivated to do so and, therefore, will not choose to attempt to master it. A visiting nurse finds it necessary to visit a patient that the nurse feels unable to cope with on an interpersonal level; therefore, when the visit occurs, the nurse does not try very hard to please that patient and attempts to move on to the next one as soon as possible. Thus, health care managers interested in maximizing the motivation levels of their subordinates must concern themselves with their employees' task relevant self-images.

There are at least five major sources of information employees rely upon in assessing their task relevant self-images (i.e., levels of personal mastery).[37] As will be shown, each of these sources can be influenced by the manager to varying degrees.

Performance Accomplishments

The first and most important informational source is the employees' evaluation of their performance accomplishments. The task relevant self-images of employees who see themselves succeed on their jobs improve, while the self-images of those who fail worsen. This is particularly true if the failures occur early in the process of learning the job. Health care managers therefore should be very sensitive to the self-images of newly hired employees and others recently assigned to new tasks.

This suggests that when employees are breaking in to new jobs, their learning environments should be structured so that they experience early task successes. Performance standards should not be set so low, however, that employees attribute their successes exclusively to the ease of the task.[41, 42, 43] Rather, the task should be sufficiently difficult to allow employees to feel a sense of accomplishment. More generally, they should be provided with the feedback necessary to allow them to judge their levels of performance more accurately.[44, 45]

Vicarious Experiences

A second source of self-image information is vicarious experiences. Essentially, this refers to the learning that occurs from observing others perform a job. This type of learning, as noted in the previous section, can be called modeling. In this type of situation, employees persuade themselves that if others can master a task, they too should be able to achieve at least minimal competency. More learning generally takes place when the others whose behaviors are observed (i.e., role models) are well liked by the employees and exhibit similar aptitude levels.

Thus, health care managers attempting to influence the task relevant self-images of their employees vicariously should make available role models who are likable and whose current performance levels are attainable by most other workers. This implies that persons assigned to training, coaching, and other model roles need not themselves be superstar performers; rather, their performance levels should approximate what is attainable by the typical employee.

Verbal Persuasion

Verbal persuasion is a third source of self-image relevant information. Frequently, in seeking to improve employees' task relevant self-images, a health care manager will try to convince these individuals that they can master tasks that previously had overwhelmed them. The success of this motivational strategy is dependent upon the self-assuredness of the manager as well as how credible, prestigious, trustworthy, and knowledgeable the supervisor is in the eyes of subordinates.

Logical Verification

A fourth influence on task relevant self-images is logical verification. This is based on the fact that employees derive new knowledge from things they already know. In particular, if employees know they have mastered tasks identical or similar to those required in a new job assignment, they will infer that they also can master this new position. Thus, employees' self-images in regard to their ability to perform the new assignment are enhanced positively.

Health care managers can help their employees maintain and improve their task relevant self-images (a) by progressively assigning them to new tasks that involve minimal differences from those mastered previously and (b) by pointing out the similarities between tasks currently mastered and those being assigned. An alternative to this strategy is to assign employees to new tasks with which they have no familiarity. Clearly, the recommended approach of incremental change is more desirable than assignment to positions radically different from previous ones.

Emotional Arousal

A final major source of task relevant self-image information is the emotional arousal elicited in employees in response to their task environments. It is not uncommon for employees to become tense and anxious (for a variety of reasons) when requested to work at new tasks or to carry out previously learned tasks at higher levels; if they attribute this arousal to personal deficiencies, it is likely their self-images will be damaged. This lowered self-image may lead to even more tension and anxiety, thus causing an escalation in the damage inflicted.[46]

This set of circumstances involving employees' potential emotional reactions to their jobs should not be ignored by the health care manager. The supervisor should be sensitive to the employees' emotional states and how they relate to motivation. Pragmatically, this implies that managers should assist their employees in attributing the causes of their emotional arousal to sources other than their lack of ability (assuming, of course, the employee actually possesses the abilities required by the task).

Emotional arousal in response to task environments can be attributed to three sources other than ability: luck, task difficulty, and effort.[47] In other words, employees may feel uptight about their expected performance on a task because (1) they do not think they possess the necessary abilities, (2) they think chance or fate is the principal determinant of success, (3) they think the task is exceedingly difficult, or (4) they think they will be unable to exert the effort necessary to succeed.

If in fact luck or difficulty are judged to be major influences on task performance, the manager should point this out to help ensure that employees are attributing causes appropriately. If the employees' role is structured so that they are unlikely to put forth the necessary effort, this too should be recognized and dealt with. In total, employees' attributions regarding their experienced tensions and anxieties are difficult for the manager to influence. Essentially what is suggested is sensitivity and candor.

Figure 21-4 summarizes the informational sources of task relevant self-image. Not all five of the sources are equally powerful. The employees' own performance accomplishments are the most potent source of task relevant self-image. Nevertheless, the health care manager does have available several avenues for influencing employees' self-images and, in turn, their levels of motivation. Given the demonstrated centrality of employee motivation in determining the health institution's effectiveness, none of these alternative avenues of influence should be ignored.

Figure 21-4 Task Relevant Self-Image and Employee Motivation

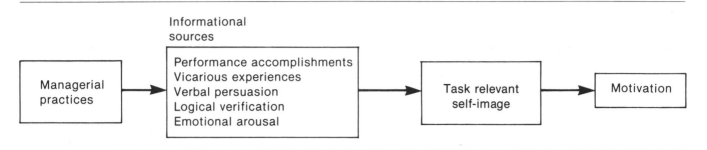

RECOMMENDATIONS

This article has presented various postulates derived with several theories of motivation and their applicability to the management of health care organizations noted. The purpose of this section is merely to summarize briefly many of the prescriptions for motivation previously discussed.

1. *Managers should make sure that all employees thoroughly understand the performance objectives they are expected to achieve.* These objectives should be stated in as specific terms as possible and set at a high enough level to be challenging but not so high as to discourage the employees.[45, 48, 49]

2. *All employees' performances in terms of the degree to which they have attained the objectives specified above should be evaluated periodically and those analyses fed back to the individuals.* Even though the activities recommended in these first two points are likely themselves to have a positive impact on employee motivation, they are viewed here as the necessary prerequisites that must be met prior to implementing any of the other prescriptions to be offered.

3. *Organizational policies should be implemented that allow employees who have attained the objectives specified above to acquire the extrinsic rewards they desire.* The rewards to be covered by organizational policies include those whose distribution typically is governed by formal statements of policy (e.g., pay increases and promotions). The following prescription refers to rewards whose distribution typically is not formalized (e.g., recognition from supervisors and assignment to desirable tasks).

4. *Managers should adhere informally to the intent of these reward policies by attempting to discriminate between high and lower performers in allocating the other extrinsic rewards within the* supervisors' control not governed by formally stated policies.

5. *Managers should attempt to structure the jobs occupied by subordinates in a manner to make intrinsic rewards freely available.*

6. *Managers should attempt to reward themselves in public only when they clearly have achieved performance levels congruent with the goals of the organization.* The previous two prescriptions, enriching the jobs of employees and serving as an appropriate role model, represent some of the managerial activities associated with encouraging self-rewarding behaviors among subordinates contingent upon their attaining specified performance objectives.

7. *In the case of employees breaking into new task assignments, performance objectives initially should be set low enough to allow the subordinates to experience success but not set so low as to encourage them to view the tasks as easy.*

8. *Persons designated as coaches, trainers, and other role models should be interpersonally competent and should not exhibit aptitude levels far beyond the employees they are assigned to assist.*

9. *In the case of employees breaking into new task assignments, the task initially selected should approximate those already learned, and these similarities should be pointed out.*

10. *If managers identify reasons other than an employee's ability that may lead to the individual's failure on a task, these reasons should be communicated clearly to the person and, if possible, the performance obstacles should be removed.* The previous prescriptions all pertain to enhancing employees' task relevant self-images.

11. *Finally, managers must be willing to experiment and take risks when it comes to trying out new motivational strategies.*[50] A dominant characteristic of successful managers is flexibility. This last prescription reflects the need for health care managers to be somewhat adventurous in

selecting alternative strategies for improving the operation of their units. This risky posture, however, must be tempered by the willingness of the manager (1) to thoroughly investigate alternatives prior to adopting them, (2) to evaluate the effectiveness of the alternatives implemented, and (3) in the face of failure, to try something different.

SUMMARY

As depicted in Figure 21-5, the basic theoretical premise of this article has been: Employee motivation is a function of the individuals' expected (1) reward consequences of their work performance, and (2) mastery level of their job. Simply put, motivation is maximized when employees feel that performing at a high level will lead to the attainment of desired rewards and they are able to perform at that level.

Several managerial prescriptions were offered that should lead to increases in these performance-reward expectations and feelings of personal mastery. Given the goals of health care organizations in society and the links between employee motivation and the level of organizational goal attainment, adherence to the prescriptions offered not only makes good management sense; the prescriptions provide one way health care managers can enhance the impact of their activities on the quality of life experienced by the clients of their organizations.

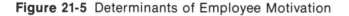

NOTES

1. J. P. Campbell and R. D. Pritchard, ''Motivation Theory in Industrial and Organizational Psychology,'' in M. D. Dunnette, ed., *Handbook of Industrial and Organizational Psychology* (Chicago: Rand-McNally, 1976).

2. A. P. Brief, R. Schuler, and M. Van Sell, *Managing Job Stress* (Boston: Little, Brown & Co., forthcoming). This provides a complete discussion of role conflict and role ambiguity.

3. L. W. Porter and E. E. Lawler, *Managerial Attitudes and Performance* (Homewood, Ill.: Irwin-Dorsey, 1968). This includes a further discussion of performance.

4. A. Etzioni, *Modern Organizations* (Englewood Cliffs, N.J.: Prentice-Hall, Inc., 1964).

5. B. S. Georgopoulos, *Organizational Research on Health Institutions* (Ann Arbor, Mich.: Institute for Social Research, 1972).

6. ———, *Hospital Organization Research* (Philadelphia: W. B. Saunders Co., 1975).

7. B. S. Georgopoulos and A. S. Tannenbaum, ''A Study of Organizational Effectiveness,'' *American Sociological Review* 22 (1957): 534-540.

8. A. K. Kovner, ''The Hospital Administrator and Organizational Effectiveness,'' in B. S. Georgopoulos, ed., *Organization Research on Health Institutions* (Ann Arbor, Mich.: Institute for Social Research, 1972).

9. J. L. Price, *Organizational Effectiveness: An Inventory of Propositions* (Homewood, Ill.: Irwin, 1968).

Figure 21-5 Determinants of Employee Motivation

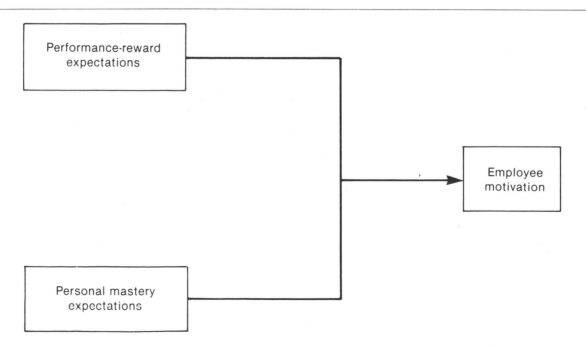

10. R. M. Steers, *Organizational Effectiveness: A Behavioral View* (Santa Monica, Calif.: Goodyear Publishing Co., 1977).

11. E. Yuchtman and S. E. Seashore, "A System Resource Approach to Organizational Effectiveness," *American Sociological Review* 32 (1967): 891–903.

12. L. L. Cummings and D. P. Schwab, *Performance in Organizations* (Glenview, Ill.: Scott, Foresman and Co., 1973). This work includes an introductory discussion on the performance appraisal process.

13. A. Bandura, "Self-Reinforcement: Theoretical and Methodological Considerations," *Behaviorism* 4 (1976): 135–155.

14. R. C. Bolles, "Reinforcement, Expectancy and Learning," *Psychological Review* 79 (1972): 394–409.

15. V. H. Vroom, *Work and Motivation* (New York: John Wiley & Sons, Inc., 1964).

16. H. G. Henaman and D. P. Schwab, "Evaluation of Research on Expectancy Theory Predictions of Employee Performance," *Psychological Bulletin* 78 (1972): 1–9.

17. T. R. Mitchell, "Expectancy Models of Job Satisfaction, Occupational Preferences and Effort: A Theoretical Methodological and Empirical Appraisal," *Psychological Bulletin* 81 (1974): 1096–1112.

18. T. R. Mitchell and A. Biglan, "Instrumentality Theories: Current Uses in Psychology," *Psychological Bulletin* 76 (1971): 432–454.

19. M. A. Wahba and R. S. House, "Expectancy Theory in Work and Motivation: Some Logical and Methodological Issues," *Human Relations* 27 (1974): 121–147.

20. R. J. Aldag and A. P. Brief, *Task Design and Employee Motivation* (Glenview, Ill.: Scott, Foresman and Co., 1979). This book provides a complete discussion of the relationships between job content and employee motivations.

21. C. P. Alderfer, *Existence, Relatedness and Growth: Human Needs in Organizational Settings* (New York: The Free Press, 1972).

22. ——————, "A Critique of Salancik and Pfeffer's Examination of Need-Satisfaction Theories," *Administrative Science Quarterly* 22 (1977): 658–669.

23. G. R. Salancik and J. Pfeffer, "An Examination of Need-Satisfaction Models of Job Attitudes," *Administrative Science Quarterly* 22 (1977): 427–456.

24. W. C. Hamner, "Reinforcement Theory and Contingency Management in Organizational Settings," in H. Tosi and W. Hamner, eds., *Organizational Behavior and Management: A Contingency Approach* (St. Clair Press, 1974).

25. F. Luthans and R. Kreitner, *Organizational Behavior Modification* (Glenview, Ill.: Scott, Foresman and Co., 1975). This work includes a discussion of punishment and reinforcement theory.

26. L. Dyer and D. P. Parker, "Classifying Outcomes in Work Motivation Research: An Examination of the Intrinsic-Extrinsic Dichotomy," *Journal of Applied Psychology*, 1975, pp. 455–458.

27. A. P. Brief and R. J. Aldag, "The Intrinsic-Extrinsic Dichotomy: Towards Conceptual Clarity," *Academy of Management Review* 2 (1977): 496–499. This article offers a more precise definition of such work outcomes.

28. E. E. Lawler, *Pay and Organizational Effectiveness: A Psychological View* (New York: McGraw-Hill Book Co., 1971).

29. G. S. Leventhal, "The Distribution of Rewards and Resources in Groups and Organizations," in L. Berkowitz and E. Walster, eds., *Advances in Experimental Psychology*, Vol. 9 (New York: Academic Press, 1976).

30. ——————, "What Should Be Done With Equity Theory? New Approach to the Study of Fairness in Social Relationships," in K. Gergen and M. Greenberg, eds., *Social Exchange Theory* (New York: John Wiley & Sons, Inc., 1977).

31. J. S. Adams, "Toward an Understanding of Inequity," *Journal of Abnormal and Social Psychology* 67 (1963): 422–436.

32. ——————, "Inequity in Social Exchange," in L. Berkowitz, ed., *Advances in Experimental Social Psychology,* Vol. 2 (New York: Academic Press, 1965).

33. J. S. Adams and S. Freedman, "Equity Theory Revisited: Comments and Annotated Bibliography," in L. Berkowitz and E. Walster, eds., *Advances in Experimental Social Psychology*, Vol. 9 (New York: Academic Press, 1976).

34. E. Walster, C. Walster, and E. Berscheid, *Equity: Theory and Research* (Boston: Allyn & Bacon, Inc., 1978).

35. A. P. Brief and R. J. Aldag, "The 'Self' in Work Organizations: A Conceptual Analysis," Unpublished manuscript. Iowa City, Iowa: The University of Iowa, 1979.

36. J. R. Hackman and G. R. Oldham, "Development of the Job Diagnostic Survey," *Journal of Applied Psychology* 60 (1975): 159–170.

37. A. Bandura, *Social Learning Theory* (Englewood Cliffs, N.J.: Prentice-Hall, Inc., 1977).

38. ——————, "The Self System in Reciprocal Determinism," *American Psychologist* 33 (1978): 344–358.

39. A. K. Korman, "Toward a Hypothesis of Work Behavior," *Journal of Applied Psychology,* 54 (1970): 31–41.

40. ——————, "Hypothesis of Work Behavior Revisited and an Extension," *Academy of Management Review* 1 (1976): 50–63.

41. J. D. Bem, "Self-Perception: The Dependent Variable of Human Performance," *Organizational Behavior and Human Performance* 2 (1976): 105–121. This article includes a discussion of attribution theory.

42. E. E. Jones and K. E. Davis, "From Acts to Dispositions: The Attribution Process in Person Perception," in L. Berkowitz, ed., *Advances in Experimental Social Psychology,* Vol. 2 (New York: Academic Press, 1965). This chapter includes a discussion of attribution theory.

43. H. H. Kelley, "Attribution Theory in Social Psychology," in D. Levine, ed., *Nebraska Symposium on Motivation* (Lincoln, Neb.: University of Nebraska Press, 1967).

44. D. R. Ilgen, C. D. Fisher, and M. S. Taylor, "Consequences of Individual Feedback on Behavior in Organizations," *Journal of Applied Psychology* 64 (1979): 349–372.

45. E. A. Locke, N. Cartledge, and Koeppel, "The Motivational Effects of Knowledge of Results: A Goal Setting Phenomenon," *Psychological Bulletin* 70 (1968): 474–485.

46. I. G. Sarason, "Anxiety and Self-Preoccupation," in I. G. Sarason and C. D. Speilberger, eds., *Stress and Anxiety,* Vol. 2 (Washington, D.C.: Hemisphere Press, 1976).

47. B. Weiner, *Theories of Motivation: From Mechanism to Cognition* (Chicago: Markham Publishing Co., 1972).

48. G. P. Latham and G. A. Yukl, "A Review of Research on the Application of Goal Setting in Organizations," *Academy of Management Journal* 18 (1975): 824–825. This also discusses motivational implications of goal setting.

49. E. A. Locke, "Toward a Theory of Task Motivation and Incentives," *Organizational Behavior and Human Performance* 3 (1968): 157–189. This incorporates a discussion of feedback, as well as the motivational implications of goal setting.

50. B. M. Staw, "The Experimenting Organization: Problems and Prospects," in B. Staw, ed., *Psychological Foundations of Organizational Behavior* (Santa Monica, Calif.: Goodyear Publishing Co., 1977).

22. A Profile of Leadership and Motivation within a Closed Hospital Climate

STEVEN H. APPELBAUM

Reprinted with permission from *Health Care Management Review,* Vol. 3, No. 1, Winter 1978, Aspen Systems Corporation, Germantown, Md. © 1978.

Individual growth among hospital employees can only be recognized and realized when trainees begin to make meaningful, rational decisions in complex hospital situations; a resistive administrative climate stifles individual development. Yet, protectiveness is often exhibited in hospitals, making learning and working less satisfying, less meaningful, and resulting in aborted goals.

To determine the supervisors' readiness for a management development program, a study of leadership styles and motivations was conducted to examine the current climate within a 300-bed northeastern hospital.

TOOLS FOR SOLVING PROBLEMS

The program was intended to provide the participants with tools to be used within their domains of responsibility so they would be able to understand their administrative role, need to communicate, leadership, decision making, problem solving, motivation and management of change-conflict. The tools also provided better understanding of women's roles in the management process and the management by objectives system. An added objective of the program was to develop team-building skills most essential in an interdependent structure and dynamic climate representative of a hospital.

It was most important to determine whether the supervisory personnel felt they were capable of applying new theories and practices in solving real problems within the hospital. This capability was dependent upon these individuals' perceiving the administrative climate in the hospital as being open, supportive, trusting and rewarding. If the trainees perceived the climate to be closed, then developmental failure would intensify fear and anxiety.

SUPERVISORY STYLES

The styles of 90 supervisors were examined in order to gain some insight into the managerial philosophies of hospital supervisors. A McGregor X-Y questionnaire was administered to the 90 trainees in order to determine how they perceived themselves in relation to the job of managing human resources.[1]

McGregor's concern for developing the professional manager implied that any growth in this direction must begin with an examination of the perceptions of the manager concerning the nature of individuals. The starting point is a set of fundamental beliefs or assumptions about what people are like. To illustrate two differing views, two theoretical constructs on human nature were developed in relation to work: Theory X and Theory Y—names chosen arbitrarily as neutral designations.

Theory X

Theory X is identified as management's conventional conception of harnessing human energy to organizational requirements. It assumes:

- Average humans have an inherent dislike of work, and will avoid it if they can.
- Because of their dislike of work, average humans must be coerced, controlled, directed or threatened with punishment to get them to put forth adequate effort toward the achievement of organizational objectives.
- Average humans prefer to be directed, wish to avoid responsibility, have relatively little ambition and want security above all.

These assumptions about human nature form, in very large measure, the rationale for management's approach to developing organizational structures, policies and practices.

Hard vs. Soft Management

Hard, or strong, management is characterized by its use of coercion and threat of punishment to obtain the behavior it desires from its people. Tight controls and close supervision are seen as natural accompaniments.

Soft, or weak, management is exemplified in management's conception of its job as one of satisfying people's demands, being extremely permissive and generally trying to keep harmony in the organization.

The hard approach is seen as producing restricted production output, antagonism ("force breeds counterforce"), militant unionism and subtle but effective undermining of management's objectives.

Soft management is envisioned as resulting in management's abdication of its responsibilities, producing harmonious but ineffective employees—an indolent work force that continually expects more but gives less and less.

Both hard and soft management are irrelevant because they either ignore or misinterpret the findings of behavioral research, particularly in the area of human motivation. Direction and control, whether accomplished through the hard or soft approach, are held to be inadequate for the motivation of people whose needs are primarily social and egoistic.

Theory X has been the traditionally accepted mode of thinking about productivity and motivation, because management has confused *consequences* with cause and effect. Theory X neither explains human nature nor describes it; instead, Theory X assumptions merely demonstrate what happens to people and production as a consequence of management's adoption of this philosophy.

Theory Y

Theory Y is the embodiment of a set of assumptions about people that are quite different from those of traditional management philosophy. These assumptions include:

- The expenditure of physical and mental effort in work is as natural as play or rest.
- External control and the threat of punishment are not the only means of getting people to work toward the organization's objectives. People will exercise self-direction and self-control toward achieving objectives to which they are committed.
- Commitment to objectives is a function of the rewards associated with their achievement (esteem and self-actualization, for example).
- Average people learn, under proper conditions, not only to accept but to seek responsibility.
- Most people are capable of a relatively high degree of imagination, ingenuity and creativity in solving organizational problems.
- Under the conditions of contemporary industrial life, the average person's intellectual potentialities are utilized only partially.

Clearly, the assumptions in Theory Y are optimistic and humanistic. They also reflect an unlimited potential for personal and organizational growth. While Theory X represents a static and somewhat pessimistic view of human nature, Theory Y emerges as dynamic and amenable to the changing nature of organizations and individuals.

Management Must Take Responsibility

If people behave toward their work in the manner that Theory X assumes, the organization is at fault, not the employees, because people are not basically lazy, indifferent, uncooperative or uncreative. The "negative" behavior of Theory X is one fundamentally *created* by management through its excessive degree of control. If people behave in such a way as to validate the assumptions under Theory X, management uses the behavior (in a circular reasoning process) to rationalize ineffective performance. Under Theory Y, management must be ingenious enough to tap the hidden potential of its work force through the development of the inherent need of people to be self-motivated and self-controlled.

Control—External vs. Internal

Central to any discussion of the two theories is the matter of control. Under Theory X, control is *externally* imposed upon the individual by management's supervision and atmosphere of constraint. Under Theory Y, the emphasis is on self-control or *internally* controlled employees. Theory Y implies that, within a climate of trust and respect, employees are capable of putting forth willing effort and are capable of controlling their work habits. This point, carried a step further, leads to the principle of *integration*, or the theory that the individuals' needs (for meaningful work, personal freedom, esteem and creative expression, implicit under Theory Y) can best be met by directing their energies toward the organization's goals. The creation of this meshing assumes that the organization can be significantly more effective if it recognizes human needs and makes adjustments to meet these needs.

Study Results

Ninety supervisory personnel participated in the X-Y study. On a total scale of from 1X to 20X, 60, or 67 percent, had a range of scores which fell between 2X and 13X with the mean score at 7X. The "X" scale corresponds to the Theory X philosophy just described (see Figure 22-1).

On a scale of from 1Y to 20Y, 30, or 33 percent, of the supervisors fell between 1Y and 10Y with the mean score at 3Y. The average score recorded on the McGregor X-Y scale was a 5X. This indicates that supervisors are not truly sensitized and committed to the philosophy of Theory Y, but endorse a more rigid posture in actualizing goals within the institution.

LEADERSHIP BEHAVIOR

Leadership behavior should occupy an equal position between two major variables: consideration and

structure. Most hospital supervisors, however, put greater emphasis upon the need to initiate structure, demonstrating inflexibility and a high degree of scheduling and criticizing.

Structure

While the main focal point of the study was consideration, it was essential to describe structure as measured by the Ohio State Leadership Scale developed by Stogdill and designed to measure the behavior patterns of supervisory and management personnel on both leadership dimensions.[2]

Structure reflects the extent to which supervisors exhibit the behavior of leaders in organizing and defining the relationships between themselves and the group, defining interactions among group members, establishing ways of getting the job done, scheduling and criticizing. A high score on the Ohio State Leadership Scale in this dimension describes supervisors who play very active roles in directing group activities through planning, supplying data, trying out new ideas and others. A low score characterizes managers who are likely to be inactive in giving direction in these ways.

Consideration

Consideration reflects the extent to which managers exhibit behavior indicative of mutual trust, respect, friendship and a positive human relationship toward group or departmental members. A high score on this dimension indicates a climate of good rapport and two-way communication, while a low score indicates an impersonal posture taken by a manager. Both structure and consideration are behaviors which are relatively independent but not necessarily incompatible.

Consideration is not actually a leadership trait, but describes the behavior of leaders in certain situations in an empirical question that is still virtually unanswered. The general norms developed by the Ohio State Leadership Study suggested an average score on consideration to be 44 and an average score for structure to be 40. The higher score for consideration occupies a relationship to the McGregor Scale in which a "Y" emphasis is considered to be more effective and satisfying than the traditional "X" philosophy.

The average score recorded at the hospital for consideration was 45 (one unit more than the norm), but the average score for initiating structure was 46—one unit more than the consideration score but six units higher than the norms developed at Ohio State. This score corroborates the average "X" on the McGregor

Figure 22-1 The X-Y Scale

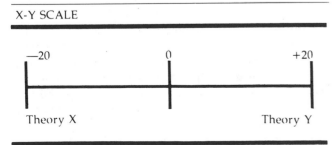

X-Y SCALE

—20   0   +20

Theory X   Theory Y

Scale—a further indication of low sensitivity to a Theory Y philosophy.

MOTIVATION AND NEEDS

The Need Hierarchy

There are five basic need systems according to Maslow, which can account for most of human behavior.[3] These needs are arranged in a hierarchy ranging from the most primitive and immature (with respect to the type of behaviors they promote) to the most civilized and mature. Progression through this need hierarchy by a person may be thought of as roughly equivalent to climbing the rungs of a ladder, one at a time, where awareness of the next highest rung (and, consequently, the experiencing of a need to step up on it) is a function of having successfully negotiated the lower rung. Thus, the natural progression from need to need is thought to occur only to the extent that each lower need has, in turn, received adequate satisfaction.

Should satisfaction for a given need be blocked or unduly delayed, the individual will not develop any awareness of any higher need in the hierarchy; the lower the level at which this impairment occurs, the more primitive and immature are the behaviors employed likely to be. By the same token, should a need level eventually be negotiated after rather severe and prolonged deprivation, individuals may continue to be preoccupied with this need because it has never been—at least in their minds—completely or adequately satisfied; that is, they may become hypersensitive to that particular need.

Preoccupation with such lower need levels may predispose a person to revert back to those levels periodically, especially when higher order needs are blocked. This is a partial explanation of the classic response to frustration which is called regression, the adoption of less mature patterns of behavior under stressful conditions.

Unsatisfied Needs Affect Motivation

The strength of a given need is directly proportionate to its lack of satisfaction. Unsatisfied needs are strong sources of motivation, and satisfied needs yield little motivation. Similarly, since it is the unsatisfied needs which make their presence felt, it will be these which determine the goals with which individuals are likely to be preoccupied and the goal-serving behaviors which they will employ. The significance of unsatisfied needs in the job setting, therefore, lies in the type of goals and goal-related behaviors which the

needs evoke and the relevance of these, in turn, for the organization's program.

The Effect of Environment

There appears to be natural progression upward through the need hierarchy. When people become fixated at a lower level of motivation it is very likely because of constraints in their environment. One implication of this facet of motivation is that managers may be able to decide consciously whether they will function as a source of constraint or as a facilitator of higher level motives in their relationships. Too often, organizations and their representatives erect barriers to the natural progression and development, and either force people to regress to lower levels of motivation then they actually desire or arrest their development to such an extent that they learn to function at a level—typically low—which they perceive as appropriate if they are to remain in the organization. This suggests that the influence of the organization, and especially that of managers, may be as great or greater than that of an individual's personal makeup.

Job Structuring

In many respects, supervisors may be thought of as mediators of need satisfactions in the hospital; that is, they are the individuals who are likely to structure an employee's work in a particular way so that it lends itself to the use of certain behaviors which may be instrumental in attaining satisfaction of that person's needs. This means that the manner in which supervisors structure the work of their personnel has important implications for both the type of needs they will experience in their work and the likelihood that they will find satisfaction on the job.

The structuring of a job entails an analysis of the skills and needs of the worker, in addition to the more direct requirements of the job objectives per se, if truly high and constructive levels of employee motivation are to characterize their performance.

Management of Motives

Whether job designs will be rigid and concerned only with the nature of the end product, or whether they will also serve to create opportunities for the expression of employee needs is very much under the control of the supervisor. By the same token, supervisors' orientation to the whole issue of job design—

whether they view it as a task with little latitude or as one of flexibility—will be significantly influenced by their personal "theory" of what makes people tick and how to motivate others. The nature of the job design—what it allows in the way of opportunities for need satisfaction—and the supervisors' personal theories about what motivates their employees are the two critical issues underlying the management of motives. It is these that will determine the extent to which a supervisor's employees will behave in mature and constructive ways in doing their work.

Should supervisors misread the needs of their employees and focus on inappropriate or irrelevant needs, their management will not have its desired effect. They will miss the target and find that their attempts to stimulate others have very little impact or, worse, unpredictable effects which create tension and a lack of cooperation.

EMPLOYEE NEEDS

Basic Needs

This need system reflects an individual's concern with comfort, strain avoidance, pleasant working conditions and environmental supports. There may be a preoccupation with monetary rewards under this need, to the extent that they serve the achievement of comfort and material possessions in one's private or family affairs.

To the extent that employees are most motivated and stimulated by this need system, they are really concerned with issues that are peripheral to the work they are doing. That is, any job that serves this need is acceptable, and the nature of the work itself is relatively unimportant. When managers focus on this need system and emphasize it most in the management of others, they are acting on an assumption that people work primarily for monetary rewards and are concerned primarily with comfort, avoidance of fatigue and the like. They will try to motivate others by offering wage increases, better working conditions, more leisure time, longer breaks and administrative supports. In effect, they will try to motivate their employees to perform more effectively by emphasizing issues which are really unrelated to the nature of the work at hand.

The normal need strength is average at 48, but the supervisory personnel at the hospital had an average of 51, which indicates their basic needs are a bit higher than the norm and somewhat more unfilled, forcing the overemphasis of this need (see Table 22-1).

Table 22-1 Comparison of Hospital Employee Needs and Maslow's Scale of Normative Values

Motivational Need	Need Strength Range		Average Need Strength	
	Normal	Hospital	Normal	Hospital
Basic	38-58	25-66	48	51
Safety	37-56	20-76	46	56
Belonging	43-63	34-98	54	60
Ego-status	64-84	44-89	75	65
Self-actualization	70-89	35-110	80	71

Safety

This need system reflects an individual's concern with security and predictability. There is a need for order and assurance that one's job is secure and not subject to drastic change. In addition, there is a preoccupation with fringe benefits of a protective nature, such as health insurance, worker compensation and retirement income.

Individuals who are motivated by this kind of need system are those who value the job primarily as a defense against deprivation and loss of basic creature comfort satisfactions. Again, this need system involves issues which are peripheral to the work itself, and any job which affords safety, security and long-range protections coupled with order and predictability will suffice.

If this is the salient need of the employees and managers focus on this need system in their management, managers will find that the employees respond in kind. That is, they will tend to meet the provisions of rules, regulations, job security, fringe benefits and employee protections with fairly conforming and standardized performances. Little innovation or flexibility will be evidenced, risk taking will be avoided and employees will behave as good organization people.

While the normal high range for safety is 56, the high range at the hospital was 76, which corresponded to the high average score of 56 as compared with the normal need strength of 46 (Table 22-1). The personnel indicated a serious lack of trust for the administration. They appeared to be preoccupied with security and motivated only to maintain what they are familiar with rather than developing positive, effective, alternative administrative strategies. Limited innovation and risk taking can be expected until this need is fulfilled.

Belonging and Affiliation

This need system reflects an individual's concern with social relationships and a preoccupation with being an accepted member of the work group or of the organizational family. When this need is the primary source of motivation, individuals value their work as an opportunity for finding and establishing warm interpersonal relationships. Jobs which afford opportunities for a good deal of interaction with one's colleagues and bring one in contact with compatible people are likely to be valued, irrespective of their content.

Managers who identify this need system as the one of primary importance are likely to act in a particularly supportive and permissive way, while placing a good deal of emphasis on the activities of informal groups, extracurricular activities, such as organized sports programs and company picnics. The scale may frequently be tipped in favor of employees' personal and interpersonal objectives, if this will insure harmony and mutual acceptance. If such a need system is in fact the major source of motivation among one's employees, managerial emphasis of the need will lead to a fairly high level of employee satisfaction and loyalty, but this may be accompanied by a performance decrement since the individuals' attention may be diverted from work to social relationships—apparently with supervisory approval. At the same time, emphasis on this need system may often promote dependency and deter one's willingness to take dependent action or to risk alienation from the group, particularly where performance issues are concerned.

While the normal high range is 63 with regard to the need to belong, the hospital supervisors had an actual high of 98 which was abnormally out of range and this also corresponded to the high average score of 60 as compared with the normal need strength of 54. This need system of belongingness also relates to the last need system of security; the greater the need for safety, the greater the need to belong and be accepted as fulfillment. Work will give them this fulfillment but they are being forced to be overly supportive and permissive due to the current climate of uncertainty.

Ego-Status

This need system reflects an individual's concern with achieving special status in the work group or within the organization. As such, it reflects a desire for recognition and for opportunities to demonstrate special competence; it is oriented essentially toward enhancement of the ego. It is the first need system discussed which is closely related to the nature of the work and dependent upon aspects of the job itself for satisfaction. Work which affords the opportunity to display those skills which individuals feel are important and in which they feel they are most competent will be valued as a means toward need satisfaction.

Managers who focus on this need system in their attempts to motivate others tend to emphasize public reward and recognition for services type systems. To the extent that this need system is the dominant source of motivation among employees, a manager may promote both high morale and high performance rates by affording job designs which capitalize on the individual's need to excel, coupled with effective means of providing status-serving rewards.

The normal low range score for ego is at the level of 64, but the actual low score recorded for the hospital personnel was 44, which also corresponded to the low average score of 65 as compared with the normal need strength of 75. The respondents were not experiencing ego fulfillment with their work and appeared not to be optimally motivated to improve their intrinsic value which was being inhibited by the increasing concern to fulfill safety needs and belongingness. When this need is unfulfilled, individuals will only seek to maintain their positions and not seek additional objectives, due to the high risk and uncertainty experienced and associated with failure and negative reward systems.

Self-Actualization

This need system reflects individuals' concern with testing their own potential, and involves a preoccupation with challenging opportunities and chances to be creative. The nature of the work is particularly critical to this need system, since in order for this source of motivation to be satisfied and continue to operate, the job must allow a good deal of fate control, freedom of expression and opportunities for experimentation. In effect, this need system, when it is dominant, motivates individuals to channel their most creative and constructive skills into their work.

Managers who focus primarily on this need system recognize that every job has areas within it which allow experimentation and innovation. When managers appropriately emphasize this need system, they are likely to find that both job satisfaction and performance surpass their expectations, for individual employees become partners in the enterprise as they seek to satisfy their own needs for expression and testing of potentials. Managers who emphasize this system are likely to use techniques for making work more meaningful; they may employ involvement strategies in planning job designs, make special assignments that capitalize on an individual's unique skills, or provide generous latitudes to the employee group in fashioning work procedures and plans for implementation.

The normal low range score for self-actualization is at the level of 70, but the actual low score recorded for the supervisors was 35 (extremely low), which also corresponded to the low average score of 71 as compared with the normal need strength of 80.

Self-actualization is experienced when a supervisor "becomes everything he or she is capable of being." Many supervisors at the hospital will not attempt to self-actualize because their ego-status is much too low to risk this need fulfillment. Also, the previous low scores recorded on belonging and security account for the reluctance and trepidation felt by the supervisors. This leads to a protective climate and makes working less satisfying, less meaningful and results in aborted goals and objectives.

The redesign of jobs is an essential component in rectifying this situation which is temporary and can be corrected via future commitments on the part of top administration and a supportive climate where risk taking and creativity are encouraged and rewarded.

EMPLOYEE MOTIVATION AFFECTS LEADERSHIP

Maintenance Seekers

Those needs falling in the lower two and a half levels of the Maslow hierarchy (viz, basic, safety and to a degree belongingness) are concerned with issues that are peripheral to the work. They involve a preoccupation with environmental factors and, rather than acting as sources of either true motivation or job satisfaction for an individual, they essentially concern hygienic aspects of the work.

When lower level needs are adequately satisfied, the work environment is clean in a psychological sense and does not interfere or compete with the job at hand. Satisfaction of such lower needs, however, will not bring about job satisfaction or increase work motivation. It simply alleviates dissatisfaction and frees individuals to become motivated if their work is rich enough in opportunities.

Attention to these lower need systems by management is primarily a maintenance function which, if performed adequately, may prevent dissatisfactions. While there are some individuals who derive their major orientations from these levels of needs, they are few in number. Those who do may be thought of primarily as maintenance seekers who will contribute little of a constructive nature to the hospital until they have been raised higher in the hierarchy of experienced needs. This is one of the functions of supervisors as they seek to motivate their employees.

Motivation Seekers

The need for rewarding interpersonal relationships, opportunities to demonstrate special competence, and challenging enterprises which promote personal growth are the real sources of motivation in the work setting. Jobs can be designed in such a way as to provide opportunities for the satisfaction of such needs and, consequently, for the expression of those goal-directed behaviors which the hospital deems as truly motivated. Individuals with such higher level needs—and these far outnumber those at lower levels in the hierarchy—are thought of as motivation seekers.

To the extent that motivation seekers can find in their jobs attributes which afford and promote need satisfactions, they will tend to be motivated in a work sense and to experience job satisfaction. Supervisors who emphasize higher level needs help create motivation seekers and at the same time provide outlets for motivated behavior on the part of individuals who already operate at such higher levels. Supervisors mediate opportunities; they may either create barriers and frustrations for employees, or they may promote growth and create channels within the work for the expression of motivation-seeking behaviors. Figure 22-2 presents a profile of the need strengths of hospital and "normal" employees.

JOB SATISFACTION AFFECTS HOSPITAL GOALS

The need pattern and motivation of the hospital supervisors surveyed was at variance with normative behavior. The respondents' basic needs—the need for security and the need for belonging—were all greater than the normal range, which reflects their urgent concern with the climate of the hospital and changes being proposed and actualized by the current administration.

The needs usually associated with growth and development, namely ego-status and self-actualization, were both low, further reinforcing the fact that these individuals will not risk or invest in the hospital until they are more secure, supported and included in decisions affecting their jobs and personal careers.

A resistive administrative climate discourages risk taking and creativity. Learning via management train-

Figure 22-2 Profile of Hospital Employee Needs and Maslow's Scale of Normative Values

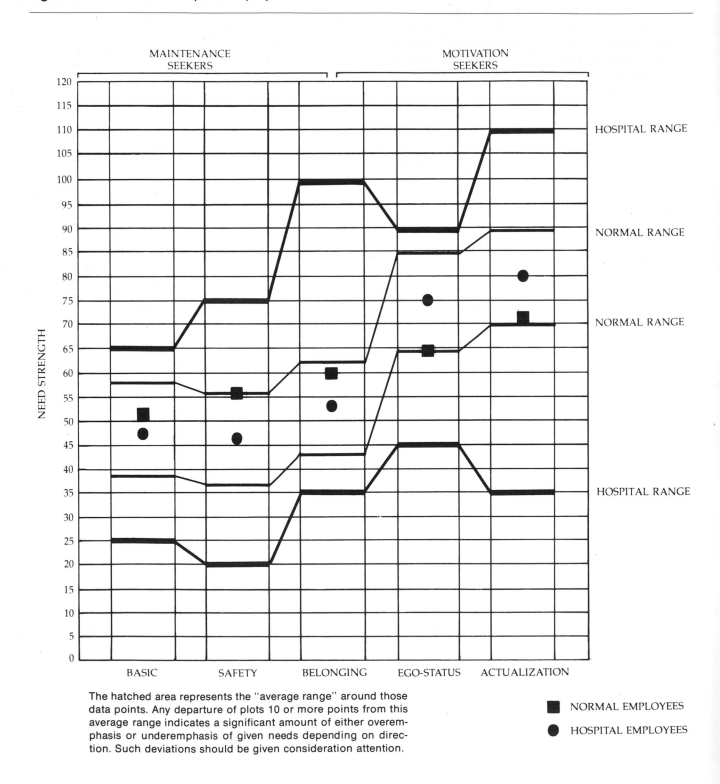

The hatched area represents the "average range" around those data points. Any departure of plots 10 or more points from this average range indicates a significant amount of either overemphasis or underemphasis of given needs depending on direction. Such deviations should be given consideration attention.

■ NORMAL EMPLOYEES

● HOSPITAL EMPLOYEES

ing and development will be stifled among employees who are overly concerned with meeting the basic needs, maintaining structure and functioning within a Theory X climate. If top administration indicates that the management development program is a current goal, then the best of efforts will be diluted within a closed climate.

NOTES

1. D. McGregor, *The Human Side of Enterprise* (New York: McGraw-Hill Book Co., 1960).

2. R. M. Stogdill and A. E. Coons, *Leadership Behavior: Its Description and Measurement* (Columbus, Ohio: Bureau of Business Research, Ohio State University, 1957).

3. A. H. Maslow, *Motivation and Personality* (New York: Harper & Row, 1954).

SUGGESTED READINGS

Fleishman, E. A., Harris, F. F., and Burtt, H. E. *Leadership and Supervision in Industry* (Columbus, Ohio: Bureau of Educational Research, Ohio State University, 1955).

Halpin, A. W. *Theory and Research in Administration* (New York: Macmillan Co., 1966).

23. Antecedents of Employee Satisfaction in a Hospital Environment

STEPHEN E. BECHTOLD,
ANDREW D. SZILAGYI, Jr., and HENRY P. SIMS, Jr.

Reprinted with permission from *Health Care Management Review*, Vol. 5, No. 1, Winter 1980, Aspen Systems Corporation, Germantown, Md. © 1980.

The human resources used in operating a modern hospital represent a growing concern to hospital administrators; health care costs have been rising rapidly and hospital wages represent approximately 55 percent of total hospital operating costs.[1] Employee satisfaction may thus be important both because of its possible relationship to turnover and absence rates[2] and because of its potential impact upon employee productivity.[3] Furthermore, human lives are highly dependent upon the performance quality of the hospital worker, and it is almost a truism that when employees are satisfied with work conditions they also tend to respond with performance of higher quality.[4]

Past research usually dealt with the relationship of satisfaction to such dependent measures. This kind of research undoubtedly played a key role in illustrating the importance of employee satisfaction. The research study upon which this article is based—conducted from 1973 to 1976 at the Indiana University Medical Center in Indianapolis—investigated various dimensions of employees' jobs as they relate to satisfaction at various occupational levels in a hospital environment.

HISTORICAL DEVELOPMENT OF JOB DESIGN

The historical development of job design has progressed through three stages: (1) the degree of job specialization, (2) management's response to worker reactions and (3) the contemporary approaches.[5] This historical development is explained in Figure 23-1.

Phase one saw the emphasis of job design on the increasing specialization of jobs. Before industrialization, the industrial base of most countries focused on the independent shop owner, craftsperson or entrepreneur. In these operations, a few people (or even one person) were responsible for the design, manufacture and sale of a whole product or service. The work proceeded generally at a casual pace, with fairly unstructured tasks and responsibilities.

As industrialization continued, there was a shift toward division of labor and job specialization. Another development was the introduction of scientific management principles, characterized by an increased emphasis on the division of labor, and intense levels of job specialization.

During phase two there was a growing awareness of employee reactions to jobs. The high level of job specialization promoted by the scientific management approach created a number of problems centering on the individual employee's morale and behavior. Low satisfaction, high absenteeism and turnover were partially attributed to the boredom created by the highly specialized, routine nature of the individual employee's work. An early management response to this situation was the techniques of "job rotation" and "job enlargement." These techniques, which generally focused on either rotating individuals between different

Figure 23-1 Historical Development of Job Design

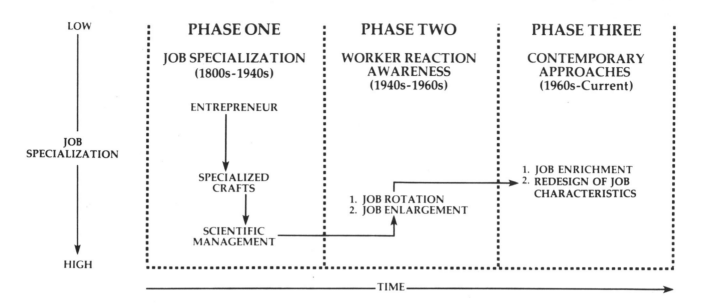

jobs or giving workers more to do, were only stopgap measures toward solving the worker reaction problem.

Phase three involves the contemporary approaches to job design. In each of the various methods within this phase, there is an acknowledgment that improvement in the jobs of workers can come only at the expense of job specialization and through changes in the content, functions, relationships and feedback of the work. One contemporary approach is the redesign of job characteristics. This approach focuses on the key job characteristic dimensions of content, functions and relationships. These job design dimensions are illustrated in Figure 23-2.

Job content includes those aspects that define the general nature of the task. These aspects represent a primary influence on a worker's attitudes toward the work itself. Among the aspects are the job characteristics of (1) variety, (2) autonomy and (3) task identity (i.e., doing the whole job or just a part of it). Job functions are the requirements, methods and work output involved in each job. This factor includes (1) job responsibilities, (2) authority, (3) information flow, (4) work methods, (5) coordination requirements and (6) work output. Relationships involve the interpersonal component of the individual's job: (1) the extent to which interaction or dealing with other individuals or

groups is required and (2) on-the-job friendship opportunities. The final factor involves feedback from the outcomes from the job which generally originates from two sources: (1) direct feedback from doing the task and (2) feedback from other individuals, such as superiors, peers or subordinates.

REDESIGN OF JOB CHARACTERISTICS

Behavioral scientists have suggested for some time that individuals may experience higher-order need satisfaction when they learn that, as a result of their own efforts, they have accomplished something that they believe is personally meaningful. This implies that work satisfaction results from performing a worthwhile task. It has been noted that—

Effective work redesign, then, does not rely on changing attitudes first by trying for example, to induce the worker to care more about the work outcomes, as in zero-defect programs. Instead the strategy is to change the behavior itself, and to change it so that the employee gradually acquires a positive attitude about his work, the organization, and himself.[6]

Figure 23-2 A Framework for Job Design

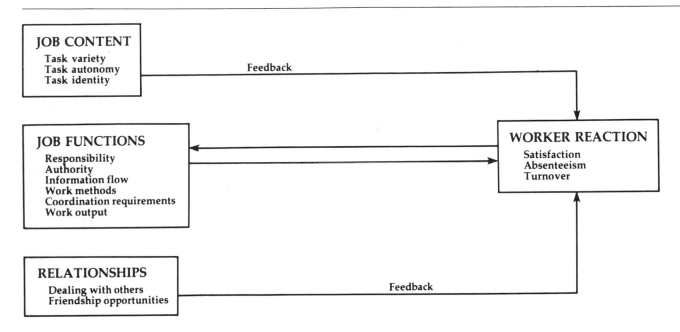

Job redesign effects behavioral change through development of the following dimensions.[7]

1. *The jobs should allow workers to feel personally responsible for a meaningful portion of their work.* A job is meaningful to individuals when they feel that work accomplishment is the result of their effort and control so that they feel personally responsible for whatever successes or failures may result. One way of putting this dimension into operation is through *job autonomy*. Increased autonomy may provide the latitude that the employees require to modify their work behavior.

2. *The job should involve doing something that is intrinsically meaningful to or otherwise experienced as worthwhile by the individual.* There are at least two ways in which jobs can be made more meaningful or worthwhile. First, individuals' jobs can focus on an entire unit rather than just a portion of it. For example, a bank teller may be responsible for satisfying all of a customer's needs—such as checking, savings, loan payments and utility bills—rather than being limited to savings account deposits and withdrawals. Behavioral scientists term this dimension *task identity*, which refers to the "wholeness" of the task. Second is to initiate behavioral change through requirements for development of a variety of skills and abilities in order to accomplish a goal (i.e., *task variety*).

3. *The job should provide feedback about what is accomplished.* Knowledge of one's task performance is a requirement for higher-order need satisfaction. If an employee is working on a job that is meaningful and worthwhile and for which he or she is held personally responsible, satisfaction of higher-order needs will not be obtained unless some form of *task feedback* is provided. Feedback may originate either from doing the task itself or from other individuals (e.g., the supervisor, coworkers or patients).

Task variety, identity, significance, autonomy and feedback have been termed "core" dimensions because they relate directly to the attainment of personal satisfaction from the work itself.[8] In addition, the job characteristics of dealing with others and of friendship opportunities have been found to be positively related to work satisfaction.[9]

CURRENT STATUS OF JOB REDESIGN

Following some early reported successes, job enrichment or job redesign was rapidly implemented in numerous organizational settings.[10] It has recently been estimated, however, that at least half of all job redesign projects are complete failures.[11] Essays which question whether job redesign really works have begun to surface.[12] Reports on the failure of specific projects are beginning to appear.[13] Furthermore, some of the results of successful projects are being explained away.[14]

In short, the manager who is concerned with whether to implement a job enrichment program is faced with a controversial body of literature. This problem is perhaps compounded for the hospital manager since the majority of reports on job redesign have been from industrial implementations.

THE RESEARCH

The study reported here was conducted at a large midwestern university medical center. The services provided at this center included general patient care facilities as well as the major components of research and education. Because of the wide variance in skills and educational requirements, this research setting offered an unusually rich research environment.

The data for the study were collected by means of a questionnaire which was completed during normal working hours in seminar facilities on the premises of the medical center. Questionnaires were collected from 1,161 employees, approximately 80 percent of whom were female.

In order to classify the respondents into occupational categories to test the relationships, the medical center used its own job classification system. This system resulted in the following sample breakdown: 53 *administrative* employees (53 assistant and associate department heads and program coordinators); 249 *professional* employees (134 registered nurses, 93 therapists and 22 medical technologists); 132 *technical* employees (72 licensed practical nurses and 60 laboratory technicians); 227 *clerical* employees; and 272 *service* employees (226 food and building service workers and 46 nurses aides).

MEASUREMENT OF THE VARIABLES

Two distinct sets of variables were measured for this study: job characteristics and work satisfaction. For each variable in the study, employees were asked to respond to a set of questions which assessed the employee's perception of the level of the variable. The following variables were measured by the Job Characteristic Inventory:[15] (1) *Variety*—The degree to which the job requires employees to perform a wide range of operations in their work and the extent to which the job requires use of a broad range of equipment and

procedures. (2) *Autonomy*—The extent to which employees make individual decisions with respect to scheduling, equipment and work procedures. (3) *Task Identity*—The extent to which employees do an entire or integral piece of work. (4) *Feedback*—The extent to which an employee receives information concerning job performance. (5) *Dealing with Others*—The extent to which the job *requires* interaction with others. (6) *Friendship Opportunities*—The degree to which the job allows the employee to establish informal relationships with other employees. (7) *Job Scope*—The average of the employees' responses to the six job characteristic measures. (8) *Job Satisfaction*—The degree to which individual desires, expectations and needs are fulfilled by employment. The "Job Description Inventory" (JDI)[16] was the instrument used to measure the individual's job satisfaction in five areas related to the job: the work itself, supervision, pay, coworkers and the opportunities for promotion. However, only satisfaction with the work itself is reported in this paper.

JOB CHARACTERISTICS ANALYSIS

Each of the job characteristics in this study was measured on a five-point scale (5 is high and 1 is low). Table 23-1 displays the results of an analysis of variance (ANOVA) on each of the six job characteristics by occupational group. In general, job characteristics are distinctly lower for low level occupational groups. In addition, all differences in job characteristics levels due to occupational group are statistically significant. The major exception to this general pattern is task identity where all groups reported high mean levels. In addition, feedback for the administrative group is lower than for any other occupational group.

In order to make the analysis as concise as possible, a summary job characteristic variable (job scope) was introduced. The job scope variable supports the conclusion that there is a positive relationship between occupational level and scope of the job's work content.

Table 23-1 also shows mean work satisfaction levels by occupational group. (Work satisfaction appears to increase with increasing occupational level.)

JOB CHARACTERISTICS—WORK SATISFACTION RELATIONSHIPS

The relationship between job scope and work satisfaction for the total sample is shown in Figure 23-3. This relationship was statistically analyzed through the

Table 23-1 Mean Values of Studied Variables by Occupational Group

(Maximum Score = 5; Minimum Score = 1)

VARIABLE	ADMINISTRATIVE (N = 47)	PROFESSIONAL (N = 213)	TECHNICAL (N = 107)	CLERICAL (N = 197)	SERVICE (N = 120)	STATISTICAL SIGNIFICANCE
Variety	3.47	3.20	2.96	2.73	2.65	p < .001
Autonomy	3.94	3.80	3.64	3.82	3.52	p < .007
Task identity	4.02	4.09	4.10	4.06	3.72	p < .007
Feedback	2.53	2.92	3.31	3.05	3.03	p < .001
Dealing with others	4.68	4.43	4.28	3.74	3.77	p < .005
Friendships	3.83	3.75	3.65	3.52	3.39	p < .001
Job Scope	3.83	3.74	3.69	3.47	3.33	p < .001
Satisfaction with work	4.09	3.85	3.70	3.37	2.84	p < .001

use of a breakdown[17] analysis which examines the means of the dependent variable in direct relationship to the means of the independent variable. The process first computes a mean level of the dependent variable (work satisfaction) for all employees with a high level of the independent variable (job scope). The process continues until a mean has been computed for every level of the independent variable. Finally, differences in the dependent variable means are tested for significance. The results indicate the presence of a strong positive relationship between job scope and work satisfaction.

In order to refine the possible conclusions of this study, this same analysis procedure was used for the administrative, professional and service groups. The analyses of the job scope-work satisfaction relationship for the technical and clerical groups are not reported here because the results were quite consistent with total sample results. Results for the administrative, professional and service groups are displayed in

Figure 23-3 Satisfaction with Work by Job Scope for the Total Sample

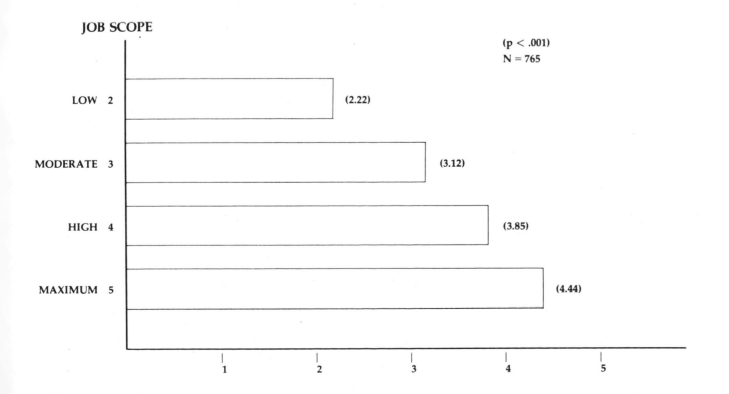

Figures 23-4, 23-5 and 23-6, respectively. The results for the administrative groups were not significant—possibly the result of the small sample size. The employees in the administrative group do appear to have fairly high levels of work satisfaction regardless of the perceived level of job scope. The results indicate a strong relationship between job scope and work satisfaction for both the professional and service group.

DISCUSSION OF RESULTS

The results of this study indicate that job characteristics (i.e., job scope) and work satisfaction were all generally higher for higher occupational levels. This result implies that higher levels of job scope would be associated with higher levels of job satisfaction.

The analysis of the job scope-work satisfaction relationship for each occupational group revealed that the level of work satisfaction was generally dependent upon the level of job scope, but was also dependent upon the occupational level of the employee. It should be noted that space prevented the presentation of results on work satisfaction for each employee level by each job characteristic. These analyses generally showed results which were consistent with the analyses by the summary measure of job scope, with variety and feedback being indicated as the two most important variables. This set of results can be summarized by noting that there was usually a positive relationship between job scope and work satisfaction but that the average level of satisfaction was usually higher for higher occupational levels. This is probably indicative of the fact that there are other elements in higher level jobs (e.g., status, pay, environment) which are satisfying to the employee but which are not contained in the job characteristic measures of this study—dimensions which apparently show their effect on work satisfaction through the crude summary measure of occupational level. These other factors appear to be most strongly reflected in the administrative level, where there was a moderate positive relationship between job scope and work satisfaction.

The other results were noteworthy: (1) The relationship between job scope and work satisfaction was very strong in the professional group and indicated that the major source of satisfaction for these employees was the work itself. (2) Employees in the lowest occupational level (service group) apparently experienced a higher degree of work satisfaction when their jobs had higher levels of job scope. Whether lower level employees can be positively influenced by enriched jobs has been the subject of recent debate.[18] Blue-collar workers have been found to rank order pay and job security higher than interesting work. [Note: The controversy is based, in part, upon a reexamination (see Note 14) of the data reported in "Survey of Working Conditions, November 1970," prepared for U.S. Department of Labor by the Survey Research Center of

---

Figure 23-4 Satisfaction with Work by Job Scope for the Administrative Group

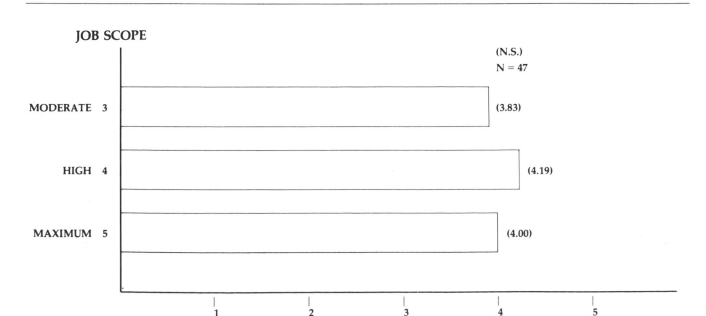

Figure 23-5 Satisfaction with Work by Job Scope for the Professional Group

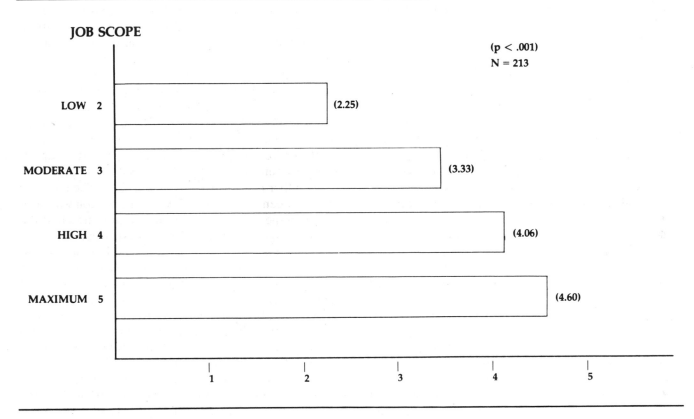

Figure 23-6 Satisfaction with Work by Job Scope for the Service Group

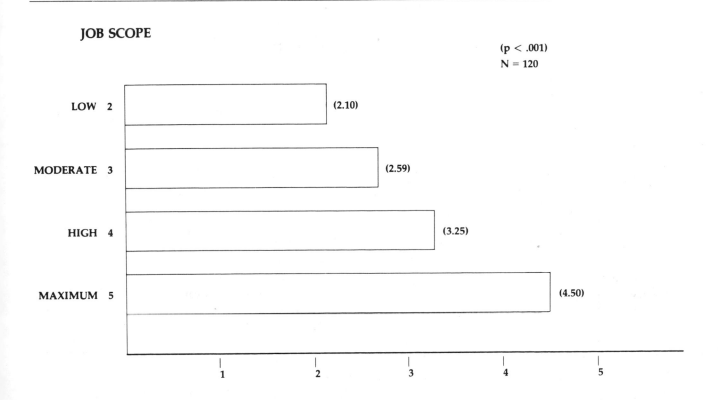

the University of Michigan, Washington, D.C.: Government Printing Office, 1971.] These findings are inconsistent with the results of this study which support the conclusion that jobs with higher levels of job characteristics were more satisfying to lower level employees of this hospital. Other studies, however, have reported results consistent with the results of this study.[19] Such inconsistencies suggest that the job redesign of lower level jobs should not be categorically dismissed. It may be that these differences were a result of differences in the characteristics of the individuals rather than the level of the current job. It should be noted that the studies in which results were inconsistent with those of this study for lower level jobs were not conducted in hospitals.

IMPLICATIONS FOR HOSPITAL MANAGEMENT

The results of this study suggest that jobs with higher levels of job characteristics (job scope) are effective in improving work satisfaction for the majority of hospital employees. In particular, the special importance of the "job itself" has been established as an important and major segment of work satisfaction for professional employees. Furthermore, job scope may influence the satisfaction of employees in the lowest occupational levels.

Like many approaches from the behavioral sciences that propose to solve some worker-related problems, redesigning jobs may not work for all organizations and may also result in a number of negative consequences. Analyses of past job redesign projects that were regarded as failures[20] have resulted in the identification of at least six problem areas that may have a negative impact on job redesign programs.[21]

1. There is an absence of diagnosis before jobs are redesigned.
2. The work itself remains unchanged.
3. There is a failure to consider unexpected side effects on areas related to jobs which are modified.
4. Programs are rarely evaluated.
5. There is a lack of training on the part of management, consultants, and union officers in the implementation of job redesign.
6. The traditional bureaucratic practice creeps into the process of redesigning jobs.

A number of points have been identified for successful implementation of job redesign projects.[22] These points can perhaps be best understood through examination of two major phases of the job redesign process: diagnosis and implementation.

DIAGNOSIS

A careful diagnosis is one of the most important phases of successful job redesign. It has been concluded that to be successful, the diagnosis should be based on theory.[23] While several theories have been used, the *use of a theory* to guide the work design appears to be more important than *which theory is used* because it aids in setting objectives, identifying needed data, learning and evaluation.[24] Regardless of the theory used, the key considerations by which the diagnosis should be guided are (1) the target jobs, (2) the employees involved and (3) the organizational climate.

The Job Itself

Job redesign projects rarely encompass the entire organization. Initially, the projects are usually experimental in nature. Furthermore, it is usually neither feasible nor desirable to modify all jobs within an organization. Thus, it is important at the beginning to assess how changes in targeted jobs can be integrated into the context of the total organizational system. While it may be desirable to improve the employee's job characteristics, some undesirable effects on other facets of the organization (e.g., the information flow, coordination and teamwork requirements) may also occur.

Some jobs may be as good as they can be—it may be impossible to further enrich them. For instance, obtaining meaningful change in a target job may not be possible given current technological feasibility or the capital expenditure required may be so great as to preclude its consideration. Further enrichment of a job may make the job too complex, producing anxiety in the employee. The influence of unions and professionally accepted norms on the content of an employee's job must also be considered. The degree of latitude for change must be accounted for in advance.

The Individuals Whose Jobs Will Change

Are the individuals whose jobs will change ready for the change? One important question in this phase of the diagnosis is an assessment of the extent to which employees are satisfied with current pay, promotion opportunities and job security. Maslow's need hierarchy suggests that lower-level needs must be adequately satisfied before employees will be receptive to enriched jobs tailored to satisfy higher-order needs.[25] If these lower needs are not satisfied, the employees may be more concerned with tangential issues—such as working conditions—than with the job itself. Unfortunately, many managers apparently tend to overestimate their employees' degree of satisfaction of lower-level needs.[26] In addition, employees will naturally be concerned about the effects of job modification upon these lower-level needs.

Whether the employees in question really want their jobs enriched may have a significant impact on the success of job redesign. Considerable evidence indicating that many workers are well satisfied with routine and repetitive jobs has been accumulated.[27] Such employees may seek fulfillment of higher-order needs through outside activities and organizations. On the other hand, some employees may never be satisfied with their work unless the job allows them to satisfy higher-order needs. Consequently, it has been stated that:

> What we need, then, are ways of running organizations that recognize the importance of treating people differently and placing them in environments and work situations that fit their unique needs, skills, and abilities.[28]

Some precautions have been noted in this regard.[29] Managers would be faced with a monumental task if every job was specifically tailored to the individual worker involved. Therefore, it has been recommended that only the two broad categories of higher-order and lower-order needs should be considered.[30] Because individual needs are dynamic it may be necessary to consider continuing evaluation of employee needs. One measure which has indicated potential for individual assessment is growth-need strength. It has been found that employees who are high on growth-need strength tend to react positively to jobs which are high on the core dimensions, while employees who are low on growth-need strength may react negatively to such jobs.[31] Another difficulty may involve the heterogeneity of the workers' needs in a functional work area which requires a homogeneous type of job design. This kind of situation presents a perplexing problem to management. The prime consideration here is the capability of individuals who are not well matched to their jobs to move into the right type of job within the organization.

Another important question is whether the employees are technically competent to handle an enriched job. It has been noted that managers tend to overestimate the technical competence of their employees.[32] Job redesign which goes beyond the em-

ployee's level of competence may result in dissatisfaction, absenteeism, turnover and low quality work outputs.

Organizational Climate

An extremely important part of the diagnosis phase is an accurate assessment of the willingness of all management levels to make a sincere and firm commitment to the job redesign project. Since each work redesign project tends to involve somewhat different technological, organizational and environmental constraints and conditions, unexpected problems always seem to surface. In some cases the chaos may be more apparent than real; nevertheless, many projects fail because management and union officials are not prepared to deal with these situations. Without the proper motivation and training of these persons most projects are doomed to failure.

There is often a considerable degree of pressure on lower level managers to make job enrichment programs successful. As a result, these managers may be inclined to make programs appear successful when they are actually failures. Since there is no guaranteed methodology for work redesign which works well for all organizations, it has been noted that—

> top management needs to create an organizational climate in which the evaluation is viewed as an occasion for learning rather than for criticizing the performance of those who actually install the changes.[33]

Thus, it is extremely important to assess the degree to which the individual managers can achieve a learning environment.

The organization as a whole may have to adopt some new ways of operating. Here again, the commitment of top management is crucial. For example, continued inputs from work study people or extremely detailed job descriptions may cause a great deal of resentment toward management which could easily handicap an otherwise successful project. A work redesign project calls for organizational policies that are tuned to the problems of employees in a new work environment as opposed to traditional organizational practices.

IMPLICATIONS FOR IMPLEMENTATION

While it is beyond the scope and purpose of this article to discuss the detailed methods of job redesign, there are several important general considerations for managers and union officials involved in a job redesign project. Among these are obtaining commitment, evaluation, and anticipation of problems.

Obtaining Commitment

The degree of commitment by management and union leaders should be explicitly specified in advance. Especially important here is the decision on when or under what circumstances the project will be terminated. This implies that the goals of the project and the criteria for evaluation have also been specified in detail. Obtaining the favorable commitment of employees whose jobs will be affected is also an important step. The key is to plan the changes of the work redesign project on a theory-based diagnosis which is understood by all employees who will be affected. This approach is more likely to avoid the eruption of irrelevant problems and gain support and positive contributions on job changes from employees. It may also improve the chances of obtaining an objective evaluation of the project.

Evaluation

A continuing evaluation of the project is needed for several reasons. First, it is necessary to determine whether the desired job changes and employee satisfaction are being realized. Further, it is important to assess the stability of the changes once they are achieved. Another important variable is the rate of change in the target job. (Change which is too rapid may cause unnecessary anxiety in employees.) Continuing evaluation is also needed to determine whether jobs are being changed in undesirable ways and to assess whether termination of the project is required. Finally, periodic evaluation may lead to the early diagnosis of problems which, if left untended, could result in the project's failure.

Anticipation of Problems

The development of contingency plans in advance—to anticipate potential problems—can often make the difference between successful and unsuccessful projects. Although there is no way to anticipate all problems in advance, there are some problems that tend to recur through different projects.[34] For example, providing more autonomy can result in significant changes in the timing and amount of an employee's demand for equipment or other resources. It should be anticipated that supervisors may have difficulty defining their roles during the change process. Adequate consideration should be given to the effects of the

project on employees' pay under the various possible project outcomes. Standard methods of wage administration may be unacceptable. Knowledge that management is concerned with and willing to deal with these problems helps to maintain employee support.

Although the results of job redesign projects have been mixed, none of the reported studies has dealt with a hospital. This study has provided some support for the conclusion that job characteristics are important variables for employee work satisfaction in a hospital environment. Finally, an in-depth analysis of the literature tends to support a conclusion that most unsuccessful projects resulted from poorly administered implementation rather than from the inability of job redesign to produce positive results.

NOTES

1. C. K. Scoville, "Human Resources Development: Emerging Asset for Hospital Management." *Hospital and Health Service Administration* 26 (Winter 1977): 24.

2. L. W. Porter and R. M. Steers, "Organizational, Work, and Personal Factors in Turnover and Absenteeism," Technical Report No. 11 (Irvine, Calif.: University of California, Graduate School of Business Administration, 1972).

3. R. Jacobs and T. Solomon, "Strategies for Enhancing the Prediction of Job Performance from Job Satisfaction." *Journal of Applied Psychology* 62, no. 4 (1977): 417–421.

4. J. R. Hackman and E. E. Lawler, "Employee Reactions to Job Characteristics." *Journal of Applied Psychology Monograph* 55 (1971): 259–286.

5. J. M. Ivancevich, A. D. Szilagyi, and M. J. Wallace, *Organizational Behavior and Performance* (Santa Monica, Calif.: Goodyear Publishing Co., Inc., 1977), pp. 142–144.

6. J. R. Hackman, "Is Job Enrichment Just a Fad?" *Harvard Business Review* 53, no. 5 (September-October 1975): 137.

7. E. E. Lawler, *Motivation in Work Organizations.*

8. Hackman and Lawler. "Employee Reactions."

9. Ibid.

10. R. N. Ford, *Motivation Through the Work Itself* (New York: American Management Associations, 1969).

11. J. R. Hackman, "On the Coming Demise of Job Enrichment," Technical Report No. 9 (New Haven, Conn.: Yale University, Department of Administrative Sciences, 1974).

12. B. E. Calame, "Wary Labor Eyes Job Enrichment," *The Wall Street Journal,* February 26, 1973, p. 12.

13. E. E. Lawler, J. R. Hackman, and S. Kaufman, "Effects of Job Redesign: A Field Experiment." *Journal of Applied Social Psychology,* 58, no. 3 (1973): 49–62.

14. W. Gomberg, "Job Satisfaction: Sorting Out the Nonsense," *AFL-CIO American Federationist,* June 1973, pp. 14–19.

15. H. P. Sims, A. D. Szilagyi, and R. T. Keller, "The Measurement of Job Characteristics," *Academy of Management Journal* 19 (1976): 195–212.

16. P. C. Smith, L. M. Kendall, and C. L. Hulin, *The Measurement of Satisfaction in Work and Retirement* (Chicago: Rand McNally, 1969).

17. N. H. Nie, et al., *Statistical Package for the Social Sciences* 2d ed. (New York: McGraw-Hill Book Co., 1975), pp. 249–275.

18. M. Fein, "Job Enrichment: A Reevaluation," *Sloan Management Review* (Winter 1974): 69–88.

19. L. W. Porter and E. F. Stone, "Job Scope and Job Satisfaction: A Study of Urban Workers," Technical Report No. 22 (Irvine, Calif.: University of California, Graduate School of Business Administration, 1973): 1–23.

20. L. L. Frank and J. R. Hackman, "A Failure of Job Enrichment: The Case of the Change That Wasn't," *Journal of Applied Behavioral Science* (1975): 413–436.

21. Hackman, "Is Job Enrichment Just a Fad?" pp. 130–133.

22. Ibid., pp. 134–137.

23. J. R. Hackman, et al., "A New Strategy for Job Enrichment," *California Management Review* 17 (1975): 57–70.

24. Hackman, "Is Job Enrichment Just a Fad?" pp. 129–138.

25. A. H. Maslow, *Motivation and Personality* (New York: Harper & Row, 1954).

26. Hackman, "Is Job Enrichment Just a Fad?"

27. E. E. Lawler, "For a More Effective Organization, Match the Job to the Man," *Organizational Dynamics* (Summer 1974): 19–29.

28. Ibid.

29. Ivancevich, Szilagyi, and Wallace, *Organizational Behavior,* pp. 158–159.

30. Ibid.

31. Hackman and Lawler, "Employee Reactions."

32. Hackman, "Is Job Enrichment Just a Fad?"

33. Ibid., p. 137.

34. Ibid., pp. 129–138.

24. Employee Incentives

PAT N. GRONER

Reprinted from *Topics in Health Care Financing,* Vol. 3, No. 3, Spring 1977 "Cost Containment: Part I,"
Aspen Systems Corporation, Germantown, Md., © 1977.

INTRODUCING INCENTIVES

The thought of introducing incentives into hospitals isn't new; people have toyed with the idea for years. But—except for a handful who perceived that hospital employees have motivations similar to other workers—most health care leaders shunned the prospect. The typical reaction was that ". . . hospitals deal with people, not 'things'; one should not systematize the relationships between patients and staff."

However, there have been a few mavericks who have felt that at least part of the nation's struggles to control health care costs could be won by introducing well-conceived incentive methods, backed by a viable quality assurance factor. Our hospital has been one of these; now, with more than a decade's experience, results support the philosophy. This is the story.

Background

Baptist Hospital, at Pensacola, Florida, is typical of hundreds of other U.S. hospitals. It opened in 1951 with 95 beds, enjoyed modest success, and expanded five times prior to 1963, when it enlarged to 325 beds. Today, it has 500 beds.

From the beginning, the hospital's management had to scratch for money. To remain solvent, the management zeroed in on cost controls, and the word 'incentive' became part of our operating vocabulary. Sick leave and retirement plans were written to include incentive features; our suggestions plan has a reward scale up to $5,000, another incentive; and from Day One, management utilized hospitalwide employee meetings to communicate, keeping personnel appraised of plans and needs.

Operation began when the 48-hour week for service departments was an area standard. However, it wasn't long before shorter schedules were an objective. To reduce the work week 10 percent without a commensurate drop in pay would have produced a negative result. We approached the goal with a different strategy.

Six months before our target date, we told department heads they could go to a 44-hour week as soon as they could reach the target performance without added staff.

On the average, departments met the objective in less than a month. Those who say "Why hadn't this been tried before?" must recognize that the hours situation was like so many other things: "We had always done it this way, so this way must be the right way."

Later, we used the same method when all departments moved from 44 down to 40 hours per week and a similar approach in placing one department on a 45-hour week (nine hours per day) instead of increasing staff, then letting the departmental personnel work into a 40-hour schedule for the same weekly pay. Management didn't tell staff *how* to do it; instead, people were challenged to find ways to work more effectively—and they did, by eliminating make-work, scheduling more carefully, working smarter. Everyone profited.

However, as was pointed out at the time, this sort of action is possible with universal benefit only when productivity per person goes up. People need an incentive to want to do better. As our country learned in the 1970s, increasing payments without commensurate productivity means inflation. It's a hard lesson.

That lesson, incidentally, was illustrated several ways in the early 1960s, lending emphasis to the productivity experiments. The first was the acceptance of statistical results published by Hospital Administrative Services. HAS figures gave hospitals a benchmark for judging their performance. From the first, HAS was Baptist's cup of tea. Those statistics helped reinforce what our Assistant Administrator John Schill and I strongly believed: generally speaking, the hospital's best departments statistically were also the best in terms of service.

In 1951, when our hospital opened, rates and charges were below state and national averages; local wage scales paralleled charges. Gradually, with economies of size and experience, we maintained our relative position charges-wise, but succeeded in boosting salaries until they approached the state average, although they remained 15 to 18 percent below the national mean.

Growth and Expansion

Then came the day when completion was in sight for the expansion of 1963–64, with a modest 30-bed increase but thousands of square feet of working areas and new services.

What does the average department head do when his institution undergoes such growth? The time-honored response has been to budget additional staffing, and we were no different. John Schill was responsible for non-professional services and, as a student of management, had a sixth sense for this kind of detail. Looking at the Department of Laundry, he developed some interesting deductions.

The Department of Laundry, whose equipment and location were only five years old, was running 30 percent better than comparable hospitals by HAS statistics. However, there were interesting sidelights. Each month, Baptist's laundry was charging 80 hours of overtime to do its work. Linen production varied, with high totals on Mondays (to catch up for weekend days when the department was idle), dipping to a low point on Fridays. There was modest downtime, and supply utilization and linen damage were tangible, although still below average.

Probing these details, Schill asked these questions: *What would happen in our new situation if we got these people to really work smarter? Could we avoid hiring more people if we had an incentive to make the present operators more conscientious?*

He posed the question to supervisor Arthur Bellamy: Bellamy wasn't sure. *Incentive* was a new word for these people. Explaining such a system might be hard.

"Suppose," pressed Schill, "that by doing this we could add 10 or 15 percent to their paychecks? Think they'd understand that?" Bellamy replied: "Let's see what they say!"

The formula developed looked acceptable, if a little unorthodox. An employee meeting was arranged and the plan was outlined in elementary terms, following this outline:

1. The Laundry had been producing quality results.
2. Based upon comparisons, the volume of work was above average.
3. Because of machine downtime, there was a lot of overtime.
4. Supplies used (bleach, detergent, allied chemicals) were inconsistent: sometimes appropriate, in other periods unrealistically high.
5. The expansion would mean about 10 percent more laundering.

Said Schill: "My figures tell me that we could do that work within a regular shift if we eliminate machine downtime, and we could save money by using supplies more carefully."

Then he made his proposal.

"If you're willing, I'd like to see if we can take care of this volume with our same crew. If we can, we'll take the money new people would have been paid and put it in a pot along with supply savings, and share *half* of it with you . . . if you can produce the linen with acceptable quality."

As proposed to the ten members of the department, the hospital was prepared to share with them the saving of Manhours and Payroll, plus half of any supply economies realized, using the immediate past as a base period. Any dollars that had to be paid out as overtime would be deducted from the amount available for sharing.

There were lots of questions. People wanted to know how much they might receive as extra earnings and what would happen if the plan didn't work, or if they didn't feel they could do the work at the faster pace. Schill put his answers in terms they could understand.

Incentive Checks: A Way of Life

The employees agreed, and the test began. Those basic entry level people quickly displayed that they had some industrial engineering talents of their own! New techniques crept into their procedures; a new sense of teamwork emerged. Machine malfunctions diminished and supply usage settled into a flat curve. Production for the enlarged hospital was achieved, with virtually no overtime. Employees who then were earning about $225 per month began receiving incentive checks from 35 to 40 dollars per month. (And remember, these were 1965 dollars.) Equally significant, the people found a new joy in achievement, and in short order spread their story to friends in other departments. Another plus was the byplay in the monthly review meetings.

Schill decided that these meetings would be the appropriate time to distribute the separate incentive checks, printed on different stock and presented in a different setting. The supervisor went over the month's results, showing where the savings came from and covering special incidents that affected results.

Of course, there were problems. Most stemmed from a data base that was inadequate. That need caused Schill and me to look carefully at all future formulas, for without solid historical data it's impossible to develop a valid program. Recently, that need caused the hospital to take a new and more professional turn, as the reader will discover.

Incentive checks became a way of life in Laundry, and employees in other departments began asking "How can we get in on this?"

That was just what John Schill and I were hoping would happen.

In the succeeding five years, one department at a time introduced incentives. First came those whose potential was greatest, where statistical histories disclosed opportunities for improvement, and where the work involved easily measurable quantities (procedures per manhour in Laboratory or Radiology, square feet of space per manhour in Housekeeping, procedures per day in EEG). Departments with less tangible factors (Maintenance, Business Office and Nursing) came more slowly and were more difficult to develop. But in virtually all departments, it ultimately was possible to create a workable formula. By 1970, when John Schill left us to enter private business, we had achieved these results:

1. Employees were earning—and receiving—substantial incentive payments resulting from cost reductions in manhours and supplies.
2. Quality was maintained or improved.
3. Savings made it possible for the hospital to provide lower charges to patients.
4. Morale was high, because employees had an effective input into their earnings.

Subsequent to 1970, we encountered several detours: Schill's departure, a major building program, a change in the community health care atmosphere which demanded management attention and a challenge of the plan by the Internal Revenue Service. All now have been overcome (IRS has fully approved the plan). Thus, in 1975–76, we determined to place a new, more sophisticated emphasis on our incentive plan, assisted by a consulting team from MEDICUS, whose industrial engineers reshaped our do-it-yourself concepts to provide a method now being introduced.

IMPLEMENTATION OF PRODUCTIVITY INCENTIVES

When Baptist emerged from the diversions which had slowed the program from 1970 to 1974, it was apparent we had moved into a new era of employee sophistication, a period when inflation and governmental pressures demanded that we revise the formula methodology. Fortunately, the hospital had assistance from management engineering specialists from MEDICUS Systems, James Hicks and Ernest Williamson, who in two years revised the design without sacrificing the original approaches. Emphasis remained upon the premise that incentives could benefit patient, employees, institution, and public by controlling costs and bolstering quality.

The design incorporated three separate programs to measure achievement, labeled Manpower Utilization, Supply Utilization and Quality Assurance. Each became the comparison of actual levels of performance against established standards. Once comparisons were made for all departments, measures of efficiency and quality with which hospital services were being rendered could be established.

Two of the programs measured efficiency. Manpower and Supply Utilization programs compared performance against established standards. Total dollars saved were to be channeled to a pool from which monies for employee incentive award checks would be drawn. Forty percent of the monies would be equally distributed to all employees. Sixty percent would remain in individual departmental pools and distributed to members there. Also created were performance ratings for each department. These were to provide feedback on efficiency.

Manpower and Supply programs were to encourage personnel cost consciousness.

The third program, however, provided a new, built-in essential. Labeled "The Quality Assurance Program," this plan was intended (1) to assure that there *is* quality improvement, (2) to monitor the degree of that improvement, and (3) to provide for implementation of substantially greater improvements in the quality of care.

The Total Plan

The three programs constitute a total incentive plan to focus on efficiency and quality. And here is a cardinal point: engineers and management recognize that it is important to the hospital, patient and employee that efficiency be improved and maintained. It is of greater importance that quality of patient care not be jeopardized by use of employee incentive plans. The goal in the hospital is to insure that quality *and* efficiency are improved and maintained.

Looking back over this hospital's history of work with incentives, most people involved believe they have found a tool that benefits everyone. It isn't necessarily an easy tool to use—but then, what is?

Manpower Utilization Program

The Manpower Utilization Program compares actual levels of manpower usage to specified standard levels of usage. *Standard* refers to the time determined as necessary for a qualified worker to complete a defined amount of work of specified quality while working at a normal pace under capable supervision and experiencing normal fatigue and delays. Standards for each department were based on engineering methods, past history, national comparisons, and detailed interviews.

Each standard was expressed as a specified number of worked manhours for an appropriate workload unit, with *manhour* as a unit for measuring work equivalent to one man working 60 minutes or two men working for 30 minutes, or some similar combination. *Workload* became the measure for defining level of work or production, such as Manhours Per Patient Day or Manhours Per Procedure.

In the new plan, two standard levels were established for each department, Reward Level and Target Level. Reward Level became the standard of performance established by management as acceptable and at which point, based upon a quarterly average, manpower utilization incentive rewards begin. The Target Level is a 10 percent higher, or more productive goal. The Target Level is designed as the standard of personnel performance which reflects the work pace of a motivated worker with sufficient skill and capability, performing a specified assignment with the benefit of capable supervision.

Both Target Level and Reward Level were expressed in terms of Manhours Per Workload Unit. Included were all productive time, regular worked hours plus overtime worked. *Paid hours* became time for which the employee would be paid (worked hours, sick hours, vacation and holiday hours, etc.). Time included in Paid Hours but not actual worked hours was labeled as *other hours.* Two other classifications in the Manpower Utilization Program were *earned hours* and *saved hours,* the first (Earned Hours) being hours necessary to complete a specified level of workload by working at the pace defined by the Reward Level. Saved Hours became the difference between Earned Hours and Worked Hours (Earned minus Worked equals Saved).

Baptist surveyed 107 cost centers and developed 73 departmental standards, with several departments made up of more than one cost center.

Once cost centers were aligned with the departments and workload units were defined, collection of historical data such as Numbers of Procedures, Pounds of Laundry or Patient Days were ascertained for twelve months, using 29 data sources such as: Labor Distribution Reports, Patient Revenue Usage and Statistical Report, the Census Summary Report, Analysis of Hospital Services/Medical Statistical Report . . . and many others.

Historical data determined actual levels of performance of the prior twelve (12) months for the building of standards.

With analysis of historical trends completed, operations for each department were reviewed. In departments where definable procedures were performed, time requirements for these procedures were determined. Example: in Radiology, 124 different procedures were identified. By timing those frequently performed procedures and obtaining best estimates of time requirements for those less frequently performed, a set of time requirements was established for all procedures. Times were compared to predetermined time standards available from other similar studies. In Radiology, for example, requirements expressed in minutes spent actually performing the procedures provided this set of standards:

Procedure	Minutes
Chest, PA only	5.0
Rib, Bilateral	14.0
Lumbosacral Spine	12.0
Humerus	9.0
IVP	60.0
GI and GE	22.0
Nephrotomogram	95.0

Once time requirements were determined, a standard could be established, reviewed, analyzed and compared with other standards and historical trends for accuracy; it was then fine tuned into a measurement of desired performance, the Target Level. A Reward Level was charted ten percent looser than the Target Level, providing an acceptable level at which incentive pay could commence.

As it was possible to specify Target and Reward Levels, it was possible by knowing actual Manhours and Workload in a period to calculate the Actual Level of performance. The *actual level,* or Productivity Index, is that ratio of Manhours to Workload actually observed in a particular period. The Actual Level is expressed in the same terms as the Target and Reward Levels.

In the plan, two major manpower utilization calculations are made during or at the end of each quarter. One is determination of the Performance or Departmental Rating, the ratio of standard (or Target) time to actual time, expressed as a percentage in Table 24-1.

The other calculation became determination of dollars saved due to efficient use of manpower, achieved by multiplying Saved Hours by the Average Hourly Wage Index for that department. The *average hourly wage index* represents the average hourly wage of persons calculated from Payroll records by dividing Total Regular Dollar Earnings by the Total Regular Hours Worked. This wage index is calculated at the beginning of the quarter and its value is applied to Saved Hours each month to determine dollar savings from manpower efficiencies.

Example: A Medical Nursing Unit's quarterly manpower performance. Productivity Indices, or levels of performance, are measured in terms of Manhours Per Patient Day (MH/PD). Assume that the established

---

Table 24-1 Percentage Performance Rating

$$\text{Percentage Performance Rating} = \frac{\text{Target Level}}{\text{Actual Level}} \times 100$$

manpower standards for this department were as follows:

> Target Level: 4.05 MH/PD
> Reward Level: 4.46 MH/PD

Note that the Reward Level was set 10 percent looser than Target (Target 4.05 + 0.41 = Reward 4.46), allowing for .41 Manhours more Per Patient Day than the 4.05 Manhours Per Patient Day specified by the Target Level.

Assurance Census Summary Report disclosed 1,300 Patient Days on the Unit for the first month of the period, and that Payroll records showed hours as follows:

> Regular   5,200 Hours
> Overtime   200 Hours
> Sick and Other   56 Hours

Manhours equal Worked Hours which equal Regular Hours Plus Overtime Hours: therefore, Manhours were 5,400 (5,200 Regular plus 200 Overtime).

Knowing actual Manhours and actual Patient Days, calculate the Actual Level or Actual Productivity Index:

Actual Level =

$$4.15 \text{ Manhours Per Patient Day} = \frac{5,400 \text{ Manhours}}{1,300 \text{ Patient Days}}$$

At this point, the following factors are known:

> Target Level   4.05 MH/PD
> Reward Level   4.46 MH/PD
> Actual Level   4.15 MH/PD
>   5,400 Manhours
>   1,300 Patient Days

The Nursing Unit has not reached the maximum effective level of performance specified by the Target Level, but the department has displayed a degree of efficiency by surpassing the Reward Level. The exact efficiency or Percentage Performance Rating is calculated by comparing Actual to Target, by the following calculation:

Percentage Performance Rating =

$$\frac{4.05 \text{ Target}}{4.15 \text{ Actual}} \times 100 = 97.6$$

To calculate savings in hours represented by this level of efficiency, one must know Earned Hours and Worked Hours. Worked Hours were 5,400. Earned Hours are determined by multiplying the Reward Level times actual Patient Days:

Earned Hours = 5,798 Hours =

4.46 Reward MH/PD × 1,300 Patient Days

Saved Hours = 398 Hours =

(5,798 Earned Hours = 5,400 Worked Hours)

Assuming that the Average Hourly Wage Index is $4.00, 398 Saved Hours represent $1,592.00 Saved Dollars (398 Saved Hours × $4.00 Per Hour).

The procedure is summarized in Table 24-2. Suppose that in the following month, Worked Hours equaled 5,550 and Patient Days 1,200. These same calculations would yield the results indicated in Table 24-2, Part B. The final month of the quarter, the department performed above both Reward and Target Levels, with the results indicated in Table 24-2, Part C.

The department performed at 101.3 percent efficiency surpassing the Target Level. Occasionally a department might perform at levels better than Target; however, consistent performance at these levels implies that some major factor has changed, suggesting a revision of the standard.

A similar process is followed for each department each quarter. Calculations of Performance Ratings and Dollars Saved are performed monthly. Monthly and each quarter reports specifying Performance Ratings by department are distributed to management personnel for review. Dollars Saved are totaled, and quarterly these Total Dollars Saved are allocated to the Manpower Utilization Pool. A similar pool is generated by the hospitalwide savings on supplies. Quarterly, the two-year program savings totals are added, to provide a disposable dollar figure representing dollars saved from efficient utilization of manhours and controlled use of supplies. The pool arrangement provides a hospitalwide enjoyment of results, thus engendering cooperation. The individual departmental allocations continue to pinpoint results at the point of realization. Table 24-3 suggests how this would work at the close of a typical quarter.

Supply Utilization Program

Revised Supply Utilization focuses on efficient use of material items throughout the institution, comparing historical usage rates with current ones to determine if usage has increased or decreased. When the change is

Table 24-2 Sample Calculation of Percentage Performance Rating

Part A:	Worked Hours = 5,400 MH	
	Patient Days = 1,300	
	Target Level	4.05 MH/PD
	Reward Level	4.46 MH/PD
	Worked Hours	5,400 MH
	Patient Days	1,300 PD
	Actual Level	4.15 MH/PD
	Earned Hours	5,798 MH
	Worked Hours	5,400 MH
	Saved Hours	398 MH
	Avg. Hourly Wage Index	$4.00 MH
	Dollars Saved	$1,592
	Performance Rating	97.6%
Part B:	Worked Hours = 5,550 MH	
	Patient Days = 1,200	
	Target Level	4.05 MH/PD
	Reward Level	4.46 MH/PD
	Worked Hours	5,550 MH
	Patient Days	1,220 PD
	Actual Level	4.55 MH/PD
	Earned Hours	5,441 MH
	Worked Hours	5,550 MH
	Saved Hours	(109) MH
	Avg. Hourly Wage Index	$4.00 MH
	Dollars Saved	$(436)
	Performance Rating	89.0%
Part C:	Worked Hours = 5,200 MH	
	Patient Days = 1,300	
	Target Level	4.05 MH/PD
	Reward Level	4.46 MH/PD
	Worked Hours	5,200 MH
	Patient Days	1,300 PD
	Actual Level	4.00 MH/PD
	Earned Hours	5,798 MH
	Worked Hours	5,200 MH
	Saved Hours	598 MH
	Avg. Hourly Wage Index	$4.00 MH
	Dollars Saved	$2,392
	Performance Rating	101.3%

determined and the cost of the item is known, a dollar value is assigned to the savings.

Many parameters must be isolated to determine impact on resultant costs. If unit costs and demand factors remained constant, effected cost savings for improved utilization of supplies could be determined with acceptable reliability. Then a simple comparison of the Supply and Expense account for each department from quarter to quarter would indicate savings associated with improved utilization. However, this is seldom the case in the health care industry.

Table 24-3 Points of Realization

Department X		Department Y	Pool	
$150	Per Person Saving above Reward Level	$60	Supply Utilization	$10
− 45	30% to Manpower Utilization Pool	− 18	Manpower Utilization	20
$105		$42	Per Person Pool Distribution	$30
30	Pool Distribution	30		
$135	Per Person Share	$72		

Supply utilization must provide a method for determining utilization and realistic standards for evaluations of usage. Since many factors can significantly affect demand (technology changes, patient requirements, vendor policies), a 12-month historical usage rate for each item was established and adjusted into an item standard. Quarterly reviews of influencing factors were applied to utilization rates. Because of high fluctuation for many inventory items, only those items which had been on inventory for at least twelve months were considered. Here the quarter's usage rate for each item was to be compared against the standard usage to minimize non-representative and misleading usage figures. Three-month average usage rates should be indicative of true supply utilization.

There are several ways to evaluate such savings, but the average cost of the quantity of each item in inventory was selected. The hospital's inventory control system generated this average cost statistic for each measured item.

The Supply Utilization Program developed around an existing Materials Management System which utilizes a computer service and a program which automatically maintains quantities of stock items issued and which computes usage rates. The computer was further programmed to perform calculations required to illustrate savings from usage statistics. Manpower Utilization Program comparisons of actual levels against standards were established to the Supply Utilization Program comparisons. Standards used consider the prior 12-month average usage rates for each supply.

This quarterly *historical usage rate* is calculated for each supply rate and becomes the standard against which future usage rates are compared. However, Historical Usage Rates are developed each quarter and can be used to monitor the validity of the initially established standard; if for obvious reasons the usage rate should differ from the preestablished standard, a new Standard Usage Rate can be established. The Historical Usage Weight is calculated in Table 24-4.

Both the Historical Usage Rate and the Standard Usage Rate are expressed in terms of Units of Issue per 1,000 Weighted Patient Units. Typical usage rates might appear as 4.0 Pounds Per Month Per 1,000 Weighted Patient Units, or .025 Dozen Per Month Per 1,000 Weighted Patient Units, or 1.20 Boxes Per Month Per 1,000 Weighted Patient Units. *Weighted patient units* refer to the sum of patient days for Inpatient Services and the units of Outpatient Services which is theoretically equivalent to inpatient days. This was calculated from census summaries and revenue reports in Table 24-5.

Table 24-4 Historical Usage Rate

Historical Usage Rate =	Total Number of Units Issued, Previous Twelve Months
	Total Weighted Patient Units, Previous Twelve Months
Standard Usage Rate =	Adjusted Historical Usage Rate

Table 24-5 Weighted Patient Units

Inpatient Units	= No. Inpatient Days
Inpatient Charges ($) Per Patient	= Inpatient Charges ($) / No. Inpatient Days
Outpatient Units	− Total Outpatient Charges ($) / Inpatient Charge ($) Per Patient Day
Weighted Patient Units	= No. Inpatient Units No. Outpatient Units

The *current usage rate* was calculated monthly for items with Historical Usage Rates. The Current Usage Rate calculation was similar to that for the historical rate, except that only the number of units issued and the weighted patient units for that specific month were considered. The calculation of the Current Usage Rate is contained in Table 24-6.

Another calculation factor is the *average cost per unit*, the issue value for a stocked item, e.g., $.025 Per Dozen or $.122 Per Pound.

The calculation of supply utilization involves determination of Standard Cost and Actual Cost. Since both costs are based on the Average Cost Per Unit, the effects on inflating supply costs are negligible. *Standard cost* is the cost of using a particular item at the Standard Usage Rate at the current patient load, calculated as in Table 24-7. Actual cost is calculated similarly, as Table 24-8 illustrates.

The difference between Standard Cost and Actual Cost represents Dollars Saved (or not saved) in utilization. Total Dollars Saved allocated to the Supply Utilization Pool is the net savings for an entire quarter. By using quarterly usage rates, sharp monthly fluctuations are avoided, and a true saving is obtained.

Calculations are performed by data processing equipment and the summary printout is reviewed monthly to verify that dollars saved are savings effected by efficiency instead of changes in policy or procedure.

Each quarter calculations are performed for each item in stock or related items introduced. Total Dollars Saved (the Supply Utilization Pool) is combined with the Manpower Utilization Pool, representing Dollars Saved from the efficient use of manpower and supplies.

Quality Assurance Program

The Quality Assurance Program is a specialized element which experience taught Baptist Hospital is essential to maintenance of professional integrity in a hospital incentive plan. To measure the degree of care quality, this program compares actual departmental performance with specified criteria. This required a high degree of philosophical analysis; after each study, authors defined the purposes of this new factor this way:

1. Quality Assurance is to periodically calculate an index or grading of the quality of performance in each department.
2. It also is to document areas of activity where improvements in quality are warranted or desirable.

The objective: to insure that increasing efficiencies in manpower and supply utilization do not cause unacceptable decreases in care quality.

Viewing the health care institution as a system, three components common to systems can be described: *inputs* to the system, the *processes* of the system and *outputs* from the system. Inputs enter in the form of patients, professional, technical and administrative personnel, facilities, and materials. These are processed in the system to improve the condition of the patient and produce a recovered patient as an output. Quality assurance has traditionally concerned itself with attainment of objectives in the processing of the inputs. These objectives are converted into standards against which performance is measured. This type of quality assurance program measures the process of the system and frequently utilizes statistical sampling plans to determine whether or not the process is in control. This approach was chosen for Baptist's Quality Assurance Program.

Table 24-6 Current Usage Rate

$$\text{Current Usage Rate} = \frac{\text{Total Number of Units Issued, Current Month}}{\substack{\text{Weighted Sum of Patient Days} \\ \text{and Outpatient Units,} \\ \text{Current Month}}}$$

Table 24-7 Standard Cost

Standard Number
  Units Issued = Standard Usage Rate
       × Current 1,000 Patient Units
Standard Cost = Standard Number Units Issued
       × Average Cost Per Unit

Table 24-8 Actual Cost

Current Number
  Units Issued = Current Usage Rate
       × Current 1,000 Patient Units
Actual Cost = Current Number Units Issued
       × Actual Cost Per Unit

Three steps were employed in developing instruments for each department:

1. Identification of departmental primary goals and objectives;
2. Identification of factors indicative of the level of achievement for each objective;
3. Definition of minimally acceptable levels for each factor.

Although each tool for measuring quality in individual departments is unique, the process for administering the Quality Assurance Program is the same for all.

1. The process begins with periodic inspection of the department's activities to determine the level of achievement for each factor specified, using the tool for that department. The inspector also notes those aspects which are unacceptable.
2. Each factor is rated as to degree of acceptability or non-acceptability. Ratings or gradings are recorded and appropriately weighted, and the sum of weighted ratings generates an overall index. This represents a percentage of the total possible score and is referred to as the Departmental Quality Index.
3. After all results are tabulated, a report is generated which shows the Quality Index and which enumerates areas of weakness and possible areas for improvement.

One example of a typical tool is this figure used in the Quality Assurance Program for Pharmacy. This evaluation report would be completed by the evaluator utilizing guidelines for each attribute provided in an evaluation manual. For example, the first attribute on the report is "Expiration Date." Acceptance criteria is as follows: "Randomly select ten dated items from the Pharmacy shelves or the refrigerator in the Pharmacy. Reject if the expiration is exceeded on any item." The evaluator then notes that expiration dates on the items were acceptable or not acceptable. Similarly, each attribute is evaluated and the result recorded. A total is taken of "acceptable" responses; reasons for unacceptable ratings are also indicated. The Quality Rating is then calculated as in Table 24-9.

Table 24-9 Quality Rating

$$\text{Quality Rating} = \frac{\text{Number Acceptable}}{\text{Number Acceptable and Number Not Acceptable}} \times 100$$

Table 24-10 Quality Index

$$\text{Quality Index} = \frac{\text{Total Number Acceptable}}{\text{Total Number Acceptable and Total Number Not Acceptable}} \times 100$$

Table 24-11 Sample Attribute Rating

Attributes	Acceptable	Not Acceptable
1. Expiration Dates	X	
2. Pricing	X	
3. Narcotic Count	X	
4. Brewer Pre-pack		X
5. Credits		X
6. STAT Orders	X	
7. Labels	X	
8. Brewer Carts		X
	5	3

Several evaluations are made on each department during each quarter, and accumulated into a Quality Index for the quarter, calculated as in Table 24-10. Suppose the attributes in the chart were rated as in Table 24-11. The Quality Rating for this evaluation would be calculated as follows:

$$\text{Quality Rating} = \frac{5}{5+3} \times 100 = 62.5$$

If eight other evaluations were made in the quarter and the total number of Acceptable ratings was 49, and the total number of Not Acceptable ratings was 15, then quarterly index would be:

$$\text{Quality Index} = \frac{49}{49+15} \times 100 = 76.6$$

This would be compared with indices for previous quarters.

WHAT DID WE ACHIEVE?

Perhaps the best way to present clearly and concisely the results achieved through Baptist Hospital's productivity-incentive program is through the use of tables and statistics. Thus, the following depict these accomplishments in the following perspectives:

1. Selected Indicators. These reflect performance and cost saving changes percentagewise in eight departments.
2. Befores and Afters. These tables give specific dollar and activity results in most departments.
3. Hospital Totals. These tables compare Baptist Hospital's performance with comparable Florida and United States groupings, specifically the trends following implementation of productivity-incentives.
4. Hospital Administrative Services. This table presents HAS data for the final quarters of 1964 and 1974, demonstrating a 10-year comparative pattern during which productivity-incentive plans were operational from seven to nine years.

Note that departments included in these comparisons vary. Missing in all four groupings are Electro-encephalography (a one-person department) and the coffee shop (difficult to portray); Electrodiagnostics is not classified in HAS data; Pharmacy, and perhaps other departments, may not be relative in some comparisons.

SELECTED INDICATORS

The percentage indicators in Table 24-12 reflect a consistent pattern of manhour reductions, supply savings and salary increases resulting from productivity-incentives, for the first 12 months immediately following departmental inception.

Befores and Afters

The "before and after" comparisons comprising Table 24-13 demonstrate the improvement experienced with the introduction of productivity-incentive plans. In each instance, the 12-month periods immediately preceding and following implementation are presented. It is the sum of these improvements and the continued relative progress in subsequent years that contributed so significantly to the results depicted throughout this article.

Nursing

The Productivity-Incentive Program in Nursing went into effect in May of 1965. While all indicators reflected good results, the rather dramatic drop in linen costs was particularly significant. This and subsequent years' experience (1967–68 fiscal year reported $15,636 in linen replacement cost) supported the contention that Nursing could control linen loss.

Table 24-12 Selected Indicators

	Up	Down
Laundry Manhours		4.5%
Laundry Volume	13.9%	
Laundry Supplies		27.8%
Average Laundry Salary	18.5%	
Housekeeping Manhours		11.1%
Housekeeping Supplies		12.9%
Average Housekeeping Salary	15.2%	
Laboratory Manhours		4.6%
Laboratory Supplies		3.3%
Laboratory Procedures	3.2%	
Average Laboratory Salary	9.3%	
Nursing Manhours		6.0%
Linen Replacement and Loss		56.5%
Nursing Supplies		7.1%
Average Nursing Salary	11.2%	
Radiology Manhours		5.4%
Radiology Supplies		8.6%
Radiology Procedures		1.8%
Average Radiology Salary	12.1%	
Dietary Manhours		2.4%
Food	3.0%	
Dietary Supplies		24.2%
Meals	1.4%	
Average Dietary Salary	10.3%	
Electrodiagnostics Manhours		18.1%
Electrodiagnostics Supplies		.3%
Electrodiagnostics Procedures		.4%
Average Electrodiagnostics Salary	28.6%	
Medical Records Manhours		11.1%
Medical Records Supplies		18.8%
Average Medical Records Salary	18.2%	

Laboratory

August of 1966 was the month in which a formula was implemented in the General Laboratory. The experience in this department followed that of earlier applications. [Note: The inconsistencies among hospitals in counting laboratory procedures lead to a wide variation in HAS reports. This makes these and other laboratory comparisons between hospitals quite difficult.]

Laundry

In 1964, Laundry productivity averaged 42 pounds of linen per manhour. With a 10 percent increase in capacity, a comparable volume increase was achieved with reduced manhours achieving an almost immediate 20 percent productivity increase as reflected below.

Surgery

Ironically, no productivity element was included in the original plan for Surgery. This superior department

Table 24-13 Before-and-After Comparisons by Department

| | NURSING | |
	1965–66 (12 Months Before)	1966–67 (12 Months After)
Average Census	269	267
Average Paid Hours Per Pay Period	27,385	26,696
Excluding INU and ICCU	26,835	25,232
Linen Replacement	$ 24,724	$ 10,767
Supplies	$ 120,277	$ 111,681
Drugs	$ 168,668	$ 156,006

| | LABORATORY | |
	1965–66 (12 Months Before)	1966–67 (12 Months After)
Procedures	164,131	169,434
Manhours	54,189	51,705
Salaries	$ 121,748	$ 126,991
Supplies*	$ 44,104	$ 42,637
Cost Per Procedure	$1.01	$1.00

*The supply expense, as shown, includes certain procedures performed in outside laboratories.

| | LAUNDRY | |
	1964 (12 Months Before)	1965 (12 Months After)
Pounds of Linen	1,372,565	1,563,819
Manhours	25,897	24,738
Salaries	$ 32,177	$ 35,662
Supplies	$ 11,121	$ 8,027
Pay Per Hour	$1.24	$1.47
Cost Per Pound	3.15¢	2.79¢

| | SURGERY | |
	1964 (12 Months Before)	1965 (12 Months After)
Operations	7,969	8,055
Salaries	$ 112,881	$ 136,458
Supplies	$ 91,734	$ 85,522

| | HOUSEKEEPING | |
| | Fiscal Years | |
	1965	1966
Manhours	110,885	98,565
Salaries	$ 124,663	$ 127,265
Supplies	$ 22,984	$ 20,029
Pay Per Manhour	$1.12	$1.29

| | RADIOLOGY | |
	1965 (Calendar Year Before)	1966 (Calendar Year After)
Procedures	24,598	23,496
Manhours	27,540	26,063
Salaries	$ 62,578	$ 58,960
Supplies	$ 53,998	$ 49,332
Cost Per X-ray	$4.74	$4.61

Table 24-13 continued

DIETARY

| | Fiscal Years | | | |
	1965	1966	1967	1968
Meals	369,346	359,087	364,285	370,116
Manhours	123,909	121,319	120,828	118,521
Salaries	$133,525	$141,497	$155,591	$183,577
Supplies	$ 40,445	$ 41,588	$ 31,582	$ 24,850
Food	$128,994	$130,023	$134,736	$143,088
Pay Per Manhour	$1.08	$1.17	$1.29	$1.54

ELECTRODIAGNOSTICS

	June 1965–May 1966 (12 Months Before)	June 1966–May 1967 (12 Months After)
Procedures	7,626	7,289
Manhours	8,996	7,366
Salaries	$ 12,622	$ 13,233
Supplies	$ 5,067	$ 4,905
Cost Per Procedure	$2.32	$2.49
Pay Per Hour	$1.40	$1.80

MEDICAL RECORDS

	1965–66 (Fiscal Year)	1966–67 (Fiscal Year)	1967–68 (Fiscal Year)
Paid Manhours	19,492	18,791	16,648
Salaries	$36,645	$38,276	$40,012
Supplies	$12,105	$13,459	$10,921
Salary Per Manhour	$1.88	$2.03	$2.40

was 25–30 percent above HAS medians in what was felt to be a rather sophisticated surgical environment for a 325-bed hospital. The goal was supply cost reduction and its five–ten percent improvement set the stage for similar experience in the professional departments which followed.

Housekeeping

A plan was placed into operation in the Housekeeping Department January 1, 1966. A concerted effort on supply reduction in 1965 had already created a saving of $5,756 the previous year. Thus, 1966 supply savings were $8,711 below 1964, or approximately 30 percent.

Radiology

The Productivity-Incentive Plan in Radiology was initiated January 1, 1966. Note that the number of x-rays dropped from the previous calendar year thus making it more difficult to achieve productivity increases and supply savings.

Dietary

A Productivity-Incentive Plan was introduced into Dietary in 1966. The two prime factors in the formula were manhours and non-food supply costs, and there was a stabilization of these costs consistent with results in other departments. This program has proven to be extremely successful, based on results over a ten-year period.

Electrodiagnosis

In early 1966, pulmonary function studies were transferred from this department to the newly created Pulmonary Laboratory. This resulted in a decline in procedures creating, as in Radiology, a difficult situation in which to improve productivity. Nonetheless, productivity did improve from .85 procedures per manhour to .99 procedures per manhour . . . 1.65 percent.

Medical Records

Medical Records began its Productivity-Incentive Program on April 1, 1967. A new and improved central dictation system had been installed in 1966, which led to a substantial volume increase in dictation. The three fiscal years covering these events are depicted.

Hospital Totals

Costs Per Patient Day

Table 24-14 indicates a slower rate of increase in costs per patient day for Baptist Hospital since implementation of productivity-incentive plans. The disparity is not as great as indicated because of the qualifications cited. Furthermore, Baptist enjoyed a steady annual volume increase beginning in 1969, which promotes increased productivity and cost control.

Costs Per Admission

Table 24-15 indicates a slower rate of increase in costs per admission since implementation of productivity-incentive plans.

Average Annual Salaries

The productivity-incentive program can be solely credited with raising salaries of Baptist Hospital personnel from below state and national levels prior to 1965 to above in the years to follow (Table 24-16). The decline in recent years can be attributed to (a) substantial staff increases of short tenure personnel as patient volume expanded and (b) the status quo of the productivity-incentive program forced by the IRS issue referred to in the main text.

Table 24-14 Cost Per Patient Day

Year	Baptist	Florida*	Difference	United States*	Difference
1963	$31.61	$ 39.16	$ 7.55	$ 39.87	$ 8.26
1964	33.41	41.48	8.07	42.47	9.06
1965	36.11	44.11	8.00	45.40	9.29
1966	42.45	47.98	5.53	48.94	6.49
1967	45.62	53.69	8.07	54.99	9.37
1968	51.56	60.11	8.55	62.18	10.62
1969	54.49	67.77	13.28	71.07	16.58
1970	61.05	78.51	17.46	81.80	20.75
1971	70.31	91.20	20.89	93.84	23.53
1972	72.52	99.82	27.30	105.13	32.61
1973	76.15	110.16	34.01	114.43	38.25
1974	83.12	129.37	46.25	127.33	44.31

*Non-governmental, voluntary non-profit, short-term general and other special hospitals, AHA Guide Issues.

Table 24-15 Costs Per Admission

Year	Baptist	Florida*	Difference	United States*	Difference
1963	$186	$270	$ 84	$ 303	$117
1964	202	286	84	324	122
1965	220	304	84	350	130
1966	267	350	83	386	119
1967	298	412	114	452	154
1968	341	481	140	525	184
1969	410	550	140	597	187
1970	479	614	135	676	197
1971	530	693	163	760	230
1972	561	747	186	840	279
1973	614	815	201	908	294
1974	652	979	327	1,005	353

*Non-governmental, voluntary non-profit, short-term general and other special hospitals, AHA Guide Issues.

Payroll As a Percentage of Total Expense

Table 24-17, companion table to Table 24-16, reflects the very significant increase in employee salaries as a percent of the operating expense dollar (and consequent decrease in supply and other expense) that accompanied the implementation of Baptist Hospital's productivity-incentive programs. Note the relative improvement from a five percent deficit as compared to Florida hospitals in 1963 and a ten percent excess in 1966. This 15 percent total gain in relation to Florida hospitals was matched identically when compared to the national category.

Other Expenses

In the preview it was noted that Baptist Hospital "had to scratch hard for financial integrity" from the date of its opening in 1951. Hence, supplies and other expenses traditionally were kept under relatively tight control. In addition to this traditional element, we believe the following have been key contributors to these results:

- The productivity-incentive programs. Please note that other expense during the program's developing years (1966–69) increased only $3.88 per day at Baptist while hospitals in Florida increased $8.68 and U.S. hospitals experienced a $10.07 climb. From these base years, the disparity continued to grow.
- Lower expenses for construction, land acquisition, utilities, and some other supplies and services.

(See Tables 24-18 and 24-19).

Table 24-16 Average Annual Salary

Year	Baptist	Florida*	Difference	United States*	Difference
1963	$3,111	$3,167	$− 56	$3,667	$−556
1964	3,342	3,402	− 60	3,861	−519
1965	3,638	3,511	+128	4,044	−406
1966	4,156	3,659	+497	4,113	+ 43
1967	4,517	4,152	+365	4,510	+ 7
1968	5,140	4,479	+661	4,937	+203
1969	5,322	4,984	+338	5,396	− 74
1970	5,955	5,536	+419	6,013	− 58
1971	6,445	6,156	+389	6,629	−184
1972	6,664	6,402	+262	7,119	−455
1973	6,655	6,586	+ 69	7,454	−799
1974	6,995	7,249	−254	7,865	−870

*Non-governmental, voluntary non-profit, short-term general and other special hospitals, AHA Guide Issues.

Table 24-17 Payroll As a Percent of Total Expense

Year	Baptist	Florida*	Difference	United States*	Difference
1963	51%	56%	− 5%	62%	−11%
1964	58%	55%	+ 3%	62%	− 4%
1965	62%	57%	+ 5%	62%	—
1966	65%	55%	+10%	61%	+ 4%
1967	63%	56%	+ 7%	60%	+ 3%
1968	65%	56%	+ 9%	60%	+ 5%
1969	62%	55%	+ 7%	59%	+ 3%
1970	63%	56%	+ 7%	59%	+ 4%
1971	60%	55%	+ 5%	58%	+ 2%
1972	60%	53%	+ 7%	57%	+ 3%
1973	60%	52%	+ 8%	56%	+ 4%
1974	60%	51%	+ 9%	55%	+ 5%

*Non-governmental, voluntary non-profit, short-term general and other special hospitals, AHA Guide Issues.

Table 24-18 Other Expense Per Patient Day

Year	Baptist	Florida*	Difference	United States*	Difference
1963	$11.87	$17.44	$− 5.57	$15.36	$− 3.39
1964	12.18	18.51	− 6.33	16.33	− 4.15
1965	13.21	19.01	− 5.80	17.46	− 4.25
1966	16.58	21.68	− 5.10	18.97	− 2.39
1967	16.89	23.70	− 6.71	21.89	− 5.00
1968	18.27	26.32	− 8.05	25.04	− 6.77
1969	20.46	30.36	− 9.90	29.04	− 8.58
1970	22.85	34.91	−12.06	33.65	−10.80
1971	28.38	41.31	−12.97	39.13	−10.75
1972	29.33	47.08	−17.75	45.22	−15.89
1973	30.63	53.18	−22.55	50.29	−19.66
1974	33.62	63.51	−29.89	57.55	−23.93

*Determined by subtracting payroll expense from total expense in AHA Guide Issue and dividing by patient days. Non-governmental, voluntary non-profit, short-term general and other special hospitals reported.

Table 24-19 Hospital Administrative Services Indicators

	Baptist	Florida	Difference	National	Difference
Laundry . . . Pounds of Linen Per Manhour					
1964	3,968	—	—	3,454	514
1974	7,385	4,844	2,541	4,544	2,841
Laboratory . . . Procedures Per Manhour					
1964	328	—	—	311	17
1974	1,380	686	694	547	833
Surgery[1] . . . Manhours Per Operation/Visit					
1964	748	—	—	950	202
1974	925	1,123	198	1,058	133
Nursing[2] . . . Manhours Per Patient Day					
1964	592	—	—	558	(34)
1974	512	710	198	552	40
Radiology[1] . . . Procedures Per Manhour/Manhour Per Procedure					
1964	84	—	—	87	(03)
1974	98	143	45	130	32
Food Service . . . Meals Per Manhour					
1964	286	—	—	339	(43)
1974	402	345	57	343	59
Medical Records[2] . . . Manhours Per Bed/Manhours Per Discharge					
1964	385	—	—	673	288
1974	136	205	69	222	86
Pharmacy[1] . . . Manhours Per Bed/Line Items Per Manhour					
1964	110	0	0	283	173
1974	1,747	988	759	1,054	693

[1]Productivity indicator changed 1969.
[2]Productivity indicator changed 1970.

IN RETROSPECT . . . PITFALLS TO AVOID

Anticipating the new version of our program, there have been opportunities to reflect upon lessons learned. Those reflections include discussions with leaders in other hospitals who've attempted our methods. Since everyone profits from the mistakes of others, we'll illustrate the pitfalls we discovered. In reading this, remember: hospitals are unique; no single method applies uniformly. (That's why Southerners eat the tops of the turnip, while Yankees throw away the greens and eat the roots!)

There are a great many principles that might be considered; I have chosen just five pitfall points because they are prominent in our program.

1. You've Got to Be a Believer!

This is fundamental! Productivity-incentives are not a game; they're part of management tactics, a part of a person's economic philosophy; either he believes in incentives or he doesn't. Over the years, I've found many who do not believe that incentives will work in hospitals. They feel the technique is foreign to the hospital environment; or they believe that the plan may work in some hospitals, but not their's. They may see possibilities in some departments, but not in others. If these question marks are present, my advice is: STOP! Incentives will succeed only if people at the top are believers. They've got to be willing to make a personal commitment, with energy and will power to see it through.

2. Productivity-Incentives Are No Substitute for Good Supervision

In the late 1960's, as we began holding seminars to explain the incentives plan, several hospital people envisioned incentives as a substitute for supervision. They reasoned: "By having the financial carrot in front of people, they'll work better, and overcome the built-in problems that some supervisors can't seem to control. Incentives will help prevent absenteeism, tardiness, scheduling arguments, and the like. Instead of fighting the problem of weak supervision, we'll install incentives!"

That won't work.

Incentives will help make good supervisors better, but they are not a crutch, and certainly will not replace the application of sound supervisory actions.

Incentives, per se, will not solve problems of weakness in staff. Peter Drucker repeats a phrase over and over in his books, which to me is so important. He says: "Build upon strengths!" That's true in this program.

3. Your People Have to Have Faith in You

Back in 1964, when we first contemplated our plan, we talked a lot about how to begin. After all, we had shallow data; there were no hospital precedents. The employees had never even heard of such programs. We knew we were going to make errors and have to make corrections. John Schill put the point well when he said: "If people trust us, and have faith, it'll work. If not, the whole thing's not worth fooling with."

He was so right! A plan of this kind must operate on a base of mutual trust. The hospital leadership has got to be able to tell its story to people in department after department and know that what they say will fall on receptive ears. There must be a track record that illustrates mutual trust. Without this, the plan has little hope. If that faith is lacking . . . then you have some other homework to do.

4. Productivity Incentives Are for the Cost Conscious

I have said a lot about cost consciousness, and I don't want to whip a dead horse. But the point bears repeating. Many hospitals have been operated without the kind of cost consciousness that identifies the successful private business. That's not an indictment of administration; it's a reflection on the times, in which government policy often encourages hospitals to be efficient.

Now that picture *is* changing. That's why I believe incentives are moving into a rosier spotlight. But before your hospital takes the critical first step, be sure your management staff has gotten the message that you intend to concentrate on cost control. Make sure they know you mean it, that this program is not some kind of smoke screen.

Incentives require a different management attitude. If your staff is not oriented to a cost control philosophy, STOP! No group can make incentives a motivational factor without cost control as basic policy.

5. Don't Try to Build Rome in a Day

It is not easy to install incentives, and certainly not in all areas simultaneously; in some cases it required us months to make an orderly introduction of plans, beginning with departments where implementation indicated greatest possibility of success.

We moved a step at a time; there was soon pressure to act with greater dispatch, but management declined.

The new method ultimately developed by the MEDICUS men, Jim Hicks and Ernest Williamson, enables hospitals to move more quickly. However, I would caution against this. There is no certain timetable, for circumstances vary with the hospital. Our hospital began in the Laundry because there were reasons to do so; others have found Housekeeping or Dietary more receptive initial targets. The main consideration is to find a place where there is a real chance for success.

The First Step Must Be Sure . . .

There are other pitfalls, I'm sure, but these five are to me the most significant. At the outset, *you* must be a believer; incentives are a motivator, not a replacement for good supervision. Those who will work with incentives must have faith in the people who direct the plan; incentives are for those who are truly cost conscious, and they must be installed in an orderly progression so they can be assimilated into the overall operation.

25. Some Thoughts on Job Satisfaction and Retention

TINA FILOROMO and DOLORES ZIFF

Reprinted from *Nurse Recruitment: Strategies for Success,* Tina Filoromo and Dolores Ziff, Chapter 25, pp. 137 through 156 inclusive, Aspen Systems Corporation, Rockville, Md., © 1980.

COSTS OF TURNOVER

Discussing turnover in an article in *Supervisor Nurse,* Aaron Levenstein comments:

Variety may be the spice of life, and there may be a great deal of interest in seeing new faces and strange places. That may be the aesthetic side of labor turnover—constant changes in the people you work with and who work with you—but it surely destroys efficiency and produces mounting costs. Personnel people in all types of activity have been concerned with the problem for decades. Nowhere has it been more serious than in hospitals.[1]

The cost of turnover in hospitals is astronomical. These costs include recruiting the replacement, orienting the new employee (costs for orientation range anywhere from $1,200 to $5,000, depending on the length and content of the program), the expense of decreased productivity during the orientation period (costs of decreased productivity also include the cost of overtime for experienced employees to fill in), and the expense of closer supervision during the break-in period. There is no doubt that a good nurse recruitment program will look long and hard at nurse turnover and work to keep it at a minimum.

CAUSES OF TURNOVER

When you begin to deal with the question of turnover, one of your first steps must be to find out where the separations are occurring. Narrowing the problem down to one area or to one group of personnel may help in evaluating it.

In his article, Levenstein ponders turnover and its causes:

Compensation, of course, is a critical factor in all situations. However, in recent years, hospital wages and salaries have improved over the dismal levels of the post-World War II era. In the case of nurses, studies have uncovered the reasons for frequent movement from job to job.

The National Commission for the Study of Nursing and Nursing Education reports that in 1970 nurses were among the most turnover-prone groups in the country; among staff nurses, the figure was 70%.

Joanne Comi McCloskey, writing in the *American Journal of Nursing,* recently pointed out that this figure is positively alarming when compared with the 18% turnover rate among women teachers in public schools. In one very important respect, turnover among nurses is just like turnover in business; younger people and relative newcomers on the job are more likely to leave than veterans. Ms. McCloskey's figures show that

363

"nurses who were 18 to 25 years old left jobs on an average of 1.4 years sooner than nurses aged 26 to 35. Turnover was particularly high for new graduates of one year or less. These nurses tended to leave jobs in the first six months."

Significantly, her data showed that neither the nurse's marital status, her husband's income, her educational background, her compensation nor her professional specialty had much to do with her susceptibility to job-leaving.

McCloskey's studies further showed that even though salary and fringe benefits may have attracted a nurse to take a job, it was the psychological rewards or internal satisfaction that kept the employee on that job and stimulated good performance.[2]

In a recent article in *Psychology Today,* Daniel Yankelovich ventures an explanation of the psychological rewards of employment:

A variety of studies have demonstrated that psychological well-being is a complex structure. Among its chief building blocks are: a sense of self-esteem and conviction of one's worth as an individual; a clear-cut sense of identity; the ability to believe that one's actions make sense to others as well as to oneself; a set of concrete goals and values; feelings of potency and efficacy; enough stimulation to avoid boredom; a feeling that one's world is reasonably stable; and an overall sense of meaning and coherence in one's life.[3]

In the fall of 1978, the American Hospital Association sponsored a "Symposium on Issues and Trends in Nurse Recruitment." A basic conclusion reached at this symposium was that retention is more of a problem than recruitment. Suggestions for increasing retention of new graduates were:

- make student training more realistic,
- recruit early in the school year on college campuses,
- make certain what you promise a student is a reality at your institution,
- provide strong and meaningful orientation and continuing education.[4]

G. David Hughes, who teaches in the School of Business Administration at the University of North Carolina (Chapel Hill), claims that recruiting is only 25 percent of the problem. He feels that most of the effort should be directed toward retention. It may be cheaper to retain nurses than to recruit and train new nurses continuously, he concludes.

At the request of a particular hospital, Dr. Hughes conducted a study to determine if marketing can help hospitals to recruit and retain nurses. He began with four critical questions that needed answers before he could proceed with his evaluation. The questions were:

1. What personal needs do nurses (customers) wish to fulfill in choosing among hospitals (brands)? How important are these needs to nurses?
2. What sources of information do nurses use when choosing a hospital (brand) as a place to work?
3. Do the attitudes of present nurses (customers) within the several nursing services (market segments) indicate problems that may produce a high turnover rate (low brand loyalty)?
4. What job (brand) benefits should be added to attract new nurses (customers) and retain the present ones?

To obtain the answers to these questions, Dr. Hughes interviewed hospital administrators, house staff, supervisors, and nurses at the hospital in question, and three other hospitals in the adjacent county. These interviews helped to refine the definition of the problems and to identify items that needed to be included in the questionnaire that would be used.

Next, using a list supplied by the state board of nursing, Dr. Hughes mailed his questionnaire to 300 nurses. The response rate was 65 percent. A detailed analysis of the responses shows the four critical questions to be answered as follows:

What Needs Do Nurses Wish to Fulfill?

Respondents were asked to assign a weight to the criteria that were used when selecting a hospital. The 12 criteria and their weights are shown in Table 1 [25-1]. The focused-group interviews generated a longer list which was then reduced by the client and the researcher. These weights reveal that the most important criterion was the fact that the spouse was in the area. This finding suggests that nurse recruiters will want to work with the personnel offices of local companies and graduate school admission officers to identify nurses whose spouses will be moving into the area.

The second most important dimension, and more important than pay, was the desire to be assigned to the service of one's choice. Closely related to this dimension, and only slightly less important than pay, was the desire to have responsibility that is consistent with training.

Table 25-1 Weights Assigned to Criteria

Criteria	Number of Respondents*	Average Weight
1. Workload	59	8.1
2. Opportunity for university courses	57	5.8
3. Teaching hospital	57	6.1
4. Research hospital	22	4.4
5. Pay	81	11.3
6. Fringe benefits	72	7.6
7. Assigned to the service of my choice	84	14.2
8. Social life	26	6.1
9. Spouse working/studying in the area	42	16.2
10. Reputation of the hospital	66	5.2
11. Responsibility consistent with my training	74	10.4
12. Modern equipment	50	4.6
Total		100.0

*Ninety of the respondents worked at the client hospital.

Source: G. David Hughes, "Can Marketing Help Recruit and Retain Nurses?" *Health Care Management Review* 4, no. 3, Aspen Systems Corporation, Germantown, Md., (Summer 1979): 62. Reprinted by permission.

Table 25-2 Percent of Nurses Choosing Information Sources

Information	Percent
Family, friends	8
Other nurses	4
Nursing school counselors	0
Nursing school teachers	3
My own personal feelings	49
Professional journals	0
Convenience of location	22
Hospital recruiter	3
Employment agency	0
Radio, TV advertising	0
Newspaper advertising	1
Direct mail advertising	0
Other	10

Source: G. David Hughes, "Can Marketing Help Recruit and Retain Nurses?" *Health Care Management Review* 4, no. 3, Aspen Systems Corporation, Germantown, Md., (Summer 1979): 63. Reprinted by permission.

The career dimensions of the job are clearly important to the nurse during the *selection* of a hospital. They are also important considerations for *staying* with the hospital, as will be seen later. These findings are important for recruitment, placing and training nurses.

What Sources of Information Do Nurses Use When Choosing a Hospital?

Answers to this question become important when the nurse recruiter is planning a recruitment campaign. Which media should be used? Should there be an open house for graduating nurses? Should teachers and counselors be kept informed because they are influential? Table 2 [25-2] shows the percentage of nurses in the client hospital choosing various information sources as the most influential when selecting a hospital as a place to work. As can be seen, the source "My own personal feelings" dominated the information sources. This suggests that an open house or a tour of some kind is extremely important to the recruiting process.

What Are the Problems That Produce Nurse Turnover?

Potential turnover problems may be identified by measuring the attitudes of nurses toward job attributes. Attitudes toward 36 attributes were measured. These situations had been identified as potential problem areas during the focused-group discussions. For simplicity, only three of the services and 18 of the attributes are reported in Table 3 [25-3].

A comparison of the percent of favorable responses for all of the services in the hospital with the percentages for these three services identified problems. For example, a comparison of the percentages for service 1 with the average for the hospital revealed that there were problems in the dimensions of clarity of responsibility, task consistency with training, advance knowledge of schedules, effectiveness of the orientation program, management/leadership, patient care versus research and teaching, and communication problems with supervisors. It comes as no surprise, therefore, that only 14 percent of the respondents in this department reported at least a 0.60 probability of recommending the client hospital as a place to work. In contrast, 83 percent of the respondents in service 3 would make such a recommendation.

Table 25-3 Percent of Favorable Attitudes toward Specific Services (the Higher the Number, the More Favorable the Response)

| *Hospital* | *Services*** | | |
*Attitude**	*Average*	*1*	*2*	*3*
Staff nurse/intern responsibility clear	73	86	50	92
Tasks consistent with training	73	57	33	75
Schedule known in advance	78	43	50	100
Orientation program effective	86	57	100	83
Clinical supervision effective	66	29	67	75
Good management of personnel by RNs	59	14	67	58
Good nurse team leadership	76	29	83	83
Care more important than research	57	14	33	75
Care more important than teaching	48	29	33	42
RN part of a team effort	79	57	50	75
Nurse leadership effective	67	29	83	75
Good in-service education	89	71	100	100
Good attitudes between:				
RN/residents	82	71	67	75
RN/physicians	66	57	50	42
RN/LPNs	71	43	83	75
Good communication between:				
RN/physicians	60	71	50	42
RN/LPNs	74	43	83	58
RN/housekeeping	43	57	50	42
Probability of recommending as place to work (0.60 or greater)	66	14	67	83

*The questionnaire gave a fuller description of 36 attributes that were to be evaluated. These descriptions will generally be unique to each hospital.

**Percent of client hospital nurses scoring attitudes four through six and scoring probabilities 60 through 100. (A scale value of six was most favorable.) Services are not identified to preserve confidentiality. A total of nine services were examined.

Source: G. David Hughes, "Can Marketing Help Recruit and Retain Nurses?" *Health Care Management Review* 4, no. 3, Aspen Systems Corporation, Germantown, Md., (Summer 1979): 64. Reprinted by permission.

The training program for service 1 was greatly expanded. Furthermore, a team approach was used when staffing this service.

Which of the 36 attributes are the most important in the minds of the nurses? To answer this question an attitude model was built using multiple regression. This technique identified four variables that were statistically significant in contributing to the probability of the client hospital being recommended as a place to work. These variables were RN/intern responsibility, the relationship between patient care and research, communications between RN and housekeeping, and the feeling of being part of team effort. These four variables accounted for 47 percent of the variance in the probability of recommending the hospital as a place to work.

Attitude models may be used to predict the effect of administrative action. In this case, an improvement of 0.5 scale point along each of these dimensions would change the probability of recommending the hospital as a place to work from 0.66 to 0.77. These models are simple to construct, but they are powerful because they locate precisely those areas that require immediate attention. (Here an SPSS step-regression was used. Variables entered at a probability of 0.05 or less. The coefficients were 0.72, 0.53 and 0.46 respectively. Numbers must be multiplied by 0.1 to transform scale values into probabilities.)

What Job Benefits Should Be Added to Attract and Retain Nurses?

Many job benefits that seemed to have the potential of reducing turnover were identified during the focused-group interviews. The research problem was to measure the importance of these benefits in terms that could be communicated readily to a hospital administrator. Frequently used scales, such as the semantic differential or the Likert scale, do not translate into the budget language of an administrator. There was a need to transform the nurses' perception of benefits into dollar terms.

Several existing scaling techniques were considered, tested and rejected for a variety of technical and practical reasons. Finally, a unique application of a 1927 technique was used. One version of Thurstone's case V requires the respondent to rank order preferences. The nursing questionnaire listed 13 job benefits and monthly pay increases of $10 and $40.

Respondents were asked to rank these 15 benefits. The frequencies of these rankings were then transformed into a monetary value using a computer routine. The result was the magnitude of pay increase that would be required to make the nurse indifferent between the increase in pay and the improved job environment. In economics this job concept is known as indifference theory.

The results of this analysis, which appear in Table 4 [25-4], have several important implications for the hospital administrator. First, it is important to learn that the top four benefits were social psychological, not physical benefits such as equipment or environment. The attitudinal model discussed above also identified the benefit, "feeling part of a team," as an important need. It is clear that recruiting and training methods should focus on this personal need. Second, the monetary values form the basis for establishing priorities when developing means to meet these needs.

The monthly individual values in the first column in Table 4 [25-4] may be translated into annual benefits by multiplying first by 12 to attain a yearly figure and then by the average number of nurses to determine the total for the hospital. These calculations are summarized in the second column of this table. "Feeling that I am part of a patient care team" has the equivalent value of a $244,800 increase in pay. Figures such as this one are more meaningful than an abstract number from an attitude scale.

Nurses' perceived need for additional training appears in Table 1 [25-1]. To plan for in-service training it was necessary to estimate the demand for various training programs. Respondents' first choices are reported in Table 5 [25-5]. It will be noted that the demand for training differs according to whether the nurse has a diploma, an associate degree or a bachelor's degree. (Variations in demand across segments are common in marketing.) These data will make it possible to make an estimate of the number of nurses who would take each training opportunity if it were offered.

Some nurses wanted courses for which they could receive college credit. The demand for these courses also varied according to the basic training that the nurse received. These data were also collected so that arrangements could be made with nearby universities.

How Was the Research Used?

Six months and then several years after the research report was submitted the author conducted follow-up interviews to see if the findings had been applied. The feedback was heartening. A team approach was being used to staff the services. In-service training was decentralized to the level of specific nursing services. The monetized utility data had been used to support budget requests. Turnover had been reduced. While marketing research cannot take all of the credit, it did provide important information for the decisions that produced the results.

Table 25-4 Perceived Benefits by Client Nurses*

Benefit	Client Hospital Nurses ($)	Annualized Perceived Value** ($)
Feeling that I am part of a patient care team	68	244,800
Working the shift of my choice	54	194,400
Assignments consistent with my training	54	194,400
Availability of nurse preceptors at the clinical unit level	44	158,400
Knowing my work schedule a month in advance	41	147,600
Improved cleanliness	37	133,200
Better equipment	34	122,400
Better parking facilities	29	104,400
Better supervision of my work	23	82,800
A minibus that picks me up at home and returns me after work	3	10,800
Day-care services for my children at no cost to me	3	10,800
Better social life	0	0

*Number of respondents = 90. Dollars are equivalent monthly pay increases.

**The annualized perceived value of a benefit for client nurses is computed by multiplying the monthly pay equivalent shown in Table 4 [25-4] times 12 to yield an annual rate per nurse. This figure is then multiplied by the average number of client nurses.

Source: G. David Hughes, "Can Marketing Help Recruit and Retain Nurses?" *Health Care Management Review* 4, no. 3, Aspen Systems Corporation, Germantown, Md., (Summer 1979): 65. Reprinted by permission.

Table 25-5 Estimated Demand for Various Training Programs

First Choice Training/ Experience	Nurse Training Program (%)			
	Diploma	Associate Degree of Nursing	Bachelor's Degree	Total
Practice/Experience				
Anesthesia	0.0	0.0	2.7	1.2
Emergency room	7.7	28.6	2.7	7.2
Inhalation therapy	7.7	0.0	2.7	4.8
ICU/CCU	2.6	0.0	5.4	3.6
Nurse clinics	0.0	14.3	0.0	1.2
Ob/Gyn	0.0	0.0	5.4	2.4
Operating room	5.1	14.3	0.0	3.6
Pediatrics	0.0	0.0	2.7	1.2
Pediatric ICU	0.0	0.0	2.7	1.2
Psychiatry	2.6	14.3	0.0	2.4
Public health	2.6	0.0	2.7	2.4
Other	0.0	0.0	10.8	4.8
Practitioners				
Family nurse practitioner	7.7	0.0	5.4	6.0
Midwife	2.6	0.0	0.0	1.2
Pediatric nurse	0.0	0.0	8.1	3.6
Other	0.0	0.0	5.4	2.4
Further education				
MS	0.0	0.0	8.1	3.6
Other	5.1	14.3	2.7	4.8
Training				
Cardiac	15.4	14.3	10.8	13.3
Leadership	12.8	0.0	2.7	7.2
Management	2.6	0.0	2.7	2.4
Pharmacy	0.0	0.0	2.7	1.2
Physical assessment	5.1	0.0	2.7	3.6
Renal	2.6	0.0	0.0	1.2
Other	15.4	0.0	5.4	9.6
Miscellaneous				
Other	2.6	0.0	5.4	3.6
Sample size	39	7	37	83
Percent in each program	47.0	8.4	44.6	100.0

Source: G. David Hughes, "Can Marketing Help Recruit and Retain Nurses?" *Health Care Management Review* 4, no. 3, Aspen Systems Corporation, Germantown, Md., (Summer 1979): 66. Reprinted by permission.

In conclusion, the success of this application of marketing research techniques was in seeing the parallels between the critical questions in marketing and those in the recruiting and retention of nurses. These parallels made it possible to apply or adapt research techniques with known properties. Using known techniques lowers the costs and increases the probability that research will improve decision making.[5]

Hughes's conclusions all point to one vital fact: a nurse who stays with your institution is a satisfied nurse. Let us therefore proceed on the assumption that the first step in retention is job satisfaction.

According to a three-part job satisfaction study conducted by *Nursing 78* magazine:

A satisfied nurse is one who:

- works in a setting with adequate staffing
- spends a lot of her time on direct patient care
- has interesting, challenging work
- has the authority to do the work the way it should be done
- rates team spirit among her co-workers as high
- has a supervisor she trusts
- gets recognition and feedback on her work
- enjoys a supportive nursing administration
- gets a response to her suggestions and complaints

- has a hospital administration she respects
- has a feeling of accomplishment at the end of the day.

The study surveyed some 17,000 nurses and asked:

What would be the most important consideration if *you* were looking for a new job? Would it be more money? An opportunity to choose your working hours? A nursing administration that stands behind its nurses? A nurse/patient staffing ratio that allows quality care? Or would it be the chance to spend more time with patients and less paperwork?

The answer turned out to be *opportunity for professional growth.*

The answer isn't surprising when you think about it, the study points out:

Over 30 years ago, social scientist Abraham Maslow suggested that human needs are hierarchical. Once the physiological, security, and companionship needs are at least partially met, self-esteem and the esteem of others become important. Then, even when a person is well respected, there's still something more he wants: Maslow calls it self-actualization, the need to realize one's potential to the fullest. Or, in this case, the opportunity for professional growth.[6]

ASSURING JOB SATISFACTION

If job satisfaction at your institution is at less than optimum level, you are defeating yourself. We hope you will consider putting some of the following suggestions into work.

Committees to Review Problems

Establish committees with members representing all levels of the nursing staff. These committees should be directed to address such topics as staffing and scheduling, including the amount of rotation an individual does in a week or a month as well as the number of weekends a nurse must work within a given period. You might wish to put your hands on a study conducted by the Stanford Research Institute in Menlo Park, California, for the National Institute for Occupational Safety and Health, an agency of the Department of Health, Education, and Welfare. It determined that:

rotation between the shifts may harm the health and well-being of the shift worker. Compared to nurses on fixed shifts, the nurses on rotating shifts

tend to have more serious ailments, more industrial accidents, more clinic visits, more digestive problems, more trouble sleeping, more fatigue, more menstrual problems, higher use of alcohol, poorer sex lives, and less satisfaction in their personal lives.[7]

Next, the committee might look at nursing practice policies with a view toward improving direct patient care. You might want to investigate the nurse mentor system currently in use at Children's Hospital of San Francisco. It has helped to solve that hospital's problems of a chronic regional shortage of registered nurses, regularly rising costs, lack of recognition for individual interpersonal and clinical expertise, and lack of an ongoing staff development program. The system involves a primary team nursing function with a nurse mentor as the role model and leader. The mentor, aided by two or three assistants, is responsible for total patient care for a specific group of patients for each eight-hour shift. Since the establishment of the nurse mentor system, there has been a marked decrease in employee tardiness, absenteeism, and turnover, and a decided improvement in the quality of patient care.[8]

Don't forget a committee that gives staff members an opportunity to voice their opinions about such personnel policies as uniform dress guidelines and the method by which employees are evaluated for job performance. Look at your own policies before they start to become insurmountable problems. Here are some problems we've heard about in various hospitals.

One RN, who works the 7 A.M. to 3:30 P.M. shift in a busy operating room, said that there have been so many emergency cases at night that she and three other RNs have been working on call one or two nights a week, plus every fourth weekend. They get paid for on-call time and overtime, but they don't get any guaranteed time off after being on call. Curiously, a weekend on call is considered time off, no matter how many hours they work. Morale in the department is very low (understandably). The nurses sent a grievance letter to administration requesting time off after being on call. Their request was denied, for financial reasons. The director of nursing only compounded the problem by telling the four RNs, "It was your choice to work in the OR." The four RNs are tired of getting the runaround, and they're just plain tired. It would not surprise us if they are reading the help-wanted ads.

An RN has worked part-time in a hospital for nine years. She received a letter stating that her workdays were being cut from three days a week to every other weekend. All part-time nurses were getting the same cut. Such a step seems an unfeeling and less than intelligent way to reward someone for nine years of faithful service. At the least, a supervisor should have sat down with the part-time nurse and discussed the reasons for the cut. You never know when you are going to need her loyalty again!

There is a full-time RN on the 3-to-11 shift who seldom gets a break during the eight hours. Because of staffing problems, she can't even leave the unit to eat. And she can't order a dinner tray because the food service is closed by the time she has helped the patients with their trays. Although there is no law that says a break is required on an eight-hour shift, how about the moral obligation to this employee? Isn't there some way she can be relieved so that she can sit down and eat a sandwich and return to her patients with a better attitude?

A former secretary fulfilled a lifelong ambition and graduated from an associate degree program. Her first nursing job provided two days of orientation, after which she was told that the other nurses would answer her questions. But when she did ask questions, she was reported to the head nurse. She took another job, again with two days of orientation. Again, the other nurses were too busy to answer questions. At this point she became very frustrated, and, despite high grades in school and excellent evaluations from instructors, she is thinking she is not cut out for nursing. We think, instead, that nursing let her down and owes her a longer, more comprehensive orientation.

In all of these instances, a committee where grievances could be voiced and policies discussed might prevent resignations and decrease turnover.

Above all, establish a joint practice committee that involves physicians. Discuss new, congruent roles for the nurse and the physician that may lead to a better working relationship between the two staffs. An excellent resource for stimulating interaction between nurses and physicians and producing documents and guidelines for their interaction has been the National Joint Practice Commission (NJPC). A recent issue of *Hospitals* magazine cited a report on the NJPC's Third National Conference on Joint Practice, held in Dallas. According to findings released at the conference, "If physicians and nurses can continue to discuss their differences without getting bogged down in semantics, there's hope for progress."[9] There are several examples of hospitals where interaction is successfully at work.

Guidelines for Pulling

"Floating" or "being pulled" on a regular basis has always been a major complaint of staff nurses. Often the nurse is looked upon as a body that can simply be moved from one area to another to help out, rather than as an individual who has special skills that may not be applicable from one area to another. In many institutions, particularly those with high turnovers, pulling is a fact of life. Too many institutions have learned the hard way the costs of forcing nurses into the float pool. They've ended up with nurses who are frustrated by their unfamiliarity with procedures in special areas, and they've jeopardized their patients through a loss of continuity of qualified care. But if the problems caused by pulling are addressed in an honest, adult, professional manner, it is very possible that the frustration level of nurses will be reduced.

First of all, be sure to tell applicants at the time of the first interview that pulling may occur. Second, when nursing administration has no choice and must resort to floating and pulling, to irregular rotation patterns, and to time-off patterns that do not make for a happy nursing staff, offer the staff nurses a chance to discuss these decisions. Be sure they understand the reasons for them. Ask for their suggestions. If you are making every effort to be fair to all employees, show them proof of your efforts. Nurses who understand what is going on and are involved in decision making accept decisions more easily.

Finally, provide the supervisors who are involved with staffing with some concrete guidelines for pulling and make these guidelines known to the nursing staff. Try to limit pulling within basic job areas. For example, a medical/surgical nurse can be moved only to another medical/surgical unit, or an ob/gyn nurse to another ob/gyn area. Avoid asking a nurse from pediatrics to work in coronary care. It is also best to avoid pulling charge nurses. Be sure that nurses who are pulled work under the direct supervision of an experienced staff member. Try not to pull the same nurses all the time, and also avoid pulling a new graduate whose lack of experience limits flexibility. Be sure the pulled nurse does not end up with the "worst" patient in terms of physical care. Generally it is this patient who should get the attention of regular staff members, as they are most familiar with that patient's problems; it should not be the newcomer to the unit.

Inform the charge nurse of these guidelines so that the nurses pulled to a new area will at least be able to work in an atmosphere of minimal frustration. Also, advise everyone in the area receiving pulled nurses to spend a few minutes orienting them to the area, offering help, and thanking them for the job they are doing.

Adequate Staffing

In practically every survey and study, adequate staffing is listed as one of the most important factors in creating job satisfaction. If you are engaged in a formal recruitment program, your hospital is already demonstrating an activity to secure additional nurses. But what do you do until you have hired all of the nurses you need?

First, plan a realistic method for delivery of patient care based on the number and kinds of staff currently available. Don't try to do primary nursing when you have personnel only for a team or functional approach. Set guidelines for the system you have chosen, and carry them out as efficiently as possible on a 24-hour basis. A single system is less frustrating to employees than a fragmented system that changes with each shift. Inform your staff of your system; ask for opinions and suggestions; and describe your plans to change the system as more nurses are hired.

Salaries and Benefits

Compare the salary and benefit program you offer with that of your major competitors. And look at the level of RN salaries as compared to other professionals and nonprofessionals within your organization. Often, where nonnursing employees have been unionized, the bargaining unit employees are paid on a higher ratio to the work done than are nurses. Benefit packages may also be more attractive under the union. Such inequality can lead to decreased job satisfaction among employees who feel they are being treated unfairly, and to some grave internal problems.

Open-Door Policy

Be sure that the door to nursing and hospital administration is open to staff nurses. Create an atmosphere that encourages nurses to voice complaints and offer suggestions. Prove that you are listening to these suggestions and opinions by always trying to provide answers—if not immediately, then at some specified later date. Whether these answers are positive or negative, an answer is generally what the employee is after. An open-door policy will help the nurse establish an identity as a contributing member of the total health care team.

Here are three instances where an open-door policy might make the difference in retaining a nurse.

An RN has worked at her hospital for two years. She enjoys nursing, but is thinking of giving it up and looking for another job. She's very discouraged because her supervisor has given her a poor job evaluation, and one that she feels is very unfair. She needs to talk to somebody, but feels that nursing administration doesn't really care about her as an individual.

Another RN was a head nurse on a medical/surgical unit for two years. He was demoted to staff nurse because of a patient complaint. He is not satisfied with the recommendation of the grievance committee that he work as an assistant head nurse for a three-month probation period and he has started to look for another job.

A nurse earned her BSN ten years ago and has worked as a staff nurse ever since. Recently, she was diagnosed as having multiple sclerosis. The condition does not seriously interfere with her work, except when she is fatigued. To ease the fatigue, she has cut back her schedule to three days a week and has been transferred to a smaller unit. This nurse was a straight A student and is taking courses at the local university, and doing well. She knows she has limitations, but she dearly loves nursing and wants to continue in the profession. There should be a place for her. Perhaps if she felt comfortable about sitting down with nursing administration, there could be a resolution to this problem that would satisfy the staffing needs of her employer and help a dedicated nurse retain her self-esteem.

Other Suggestions

The above suggestions relate to five areas that, if improved, can increase job satisfaction among nurses and, in turn, help to increase your rate of retention. There are, in addition, other steps you can take with the same goal. We suggest that you concentrate on the following ten areas:

1. Think of the initial interview as the first step in retention. Be very honest; tell the applicant what you have to offer as well as what you don't have. Avoid creating disappointments and an employee who may resign shortly after orientation.

2. Look at your orientation program as a part of your retention plan. Are you providing the new employee with adequate guidance and direction to function in the manner your institution expects? Provide a comprehensive program for the new graduate that includes intensive management skills instruction and/or review. It will help to make a smoother transition from student to confident practitioner.

3. Reinterview new employees at various times after employment. Such interviews may uncover areas of concern or dissatisfaction that you will be able to deal with at once, and so prevent the individual from leaving your hospital frustrated and needlessly upset.

4. Of course, the exit interview has been traditionally considered the time for learning of employee problems. Be sure that the results of these interviews are directed in a constructive manner to the proper individuals for evaluation and possible action or correction.

5. Ongoing communication with all levels of the nursing staff, from the director or chief administrator to the ward secretary and nursing assistant, must also be considered as a very important part of your retention program. Good communication can be achieved through regular meetings, newsletters, unit-level meetings (aside from the traditional staff-level meetings) with the director of nursing and the director's staff, and the involvement of all levels of the nursing staff on various patient care committees as well as policy and procedure committees for the nursing department. Make the employees realize that you need their input in matters that involve their work situations.

6. Staff nurses look for ongoing educational opportunities. Be sure that you offer the chance for the nursing staff on all shifts to participate in in-house programs and in programs outside the institution.

7. Be sure your staff members are aware that nursing administration always offers them promotional opportunities before looking outside of the hospital to fill positions. Utilize a well-planned procedure for posting job openings, one that is fair to all employees.

8. Opportunities for horizontal mobility are as important to nurses as traditional vertical mobility. Consider programs that offer the nurse who does not want a leadership position recognition for her clinical excellence.

9. Your mobility plan should also include a well-defined and strictly observed transfer policy that is fair to each employee and allows for mobility within the institution for the purpose of professional growth and development.

10. Last, but certainly not least, be very sure that your salary and benefits plan is competitive for your geographic area of the country.

Salaries

If you're not up to date on this final but very important aspect of your retention program, the October 1979 issue of *Nursing 79* magazine is a good source of information on the specifics that affect an individual nurse's paycheck. Some points made in an article by Marjorie A. Godfrey are:

Differentials for Shift Work

Virtually all hospitals pay a premium for evening and night work. The average additional amount paid to RN's for the 3-to-11 shift is 37¢ an hour.

The nurse on the 11-to-7 shift averages an extra 42¢ an hour. But the nurse who rotates shifts may find the extra 42¢ hardly compensates for the resulting stress and strain of a constantly changing schedule.

Education

Despite the increasing emphasis on education, seven out of ten hospitals pay no differential at all for increased education.

The survey turned up an added benefit of exactly 8¢ an hour in the average starting salary for the nurse with a bachelor's degree, by comparison with the earning rate of the nurse *without* a bachelor's degree. The nurse with her bachelor's degree begins at $5.55 an hour; the diploma and AD graduate at $5.47.

Specialty Areas Pay Dividends

Two years ago, only 20% of the hospitals responding paid higher salaries to operating room (OR) or intensive care unit (ICU) nurses, and only 10% boosted salaries for delivery room nurses. This time, 35% pay extra to ICU-CCU nurses; 31%, to OR nurses; and 20%, to delivery room nurses.

Bigger Is Better

Three other factors influence salaries: the size of the hospital, the type of hospital, and the existence of a collective bargaining agreement.

Nurses can earn more money by working in a large hospital. In a small hospital (under 50 beds), a staff nurse starts out at an average salary of $5.29; in a medium hospital (51 to 199 beds), at $5.43; in a large hospital (200 beds and over), at $5.70.[10]

The suggestions we've given in this article are meant only to get you started on your retention planning. Undoubtedly you can add suggestions of your own, and it's worth the effort to do so. Then, act on them. Remember, a nurse retained is a nurse recruited. Providing an employment setting that allows for psychological rewards as well as intellectual stimulation and recognition for a job well done will not only help you retain the nurses you already have, but will be an added attraction for those you hope to recruit.

NOTES

1. Aaron Levenstein, J. D., "The Art & Science of Supervision," *Supervisor Nurse*, February 1977, p. 74.

2. Ibid., p. 74.

3. Daniel Yankelovich, "The New Psychological Contracts at Work," *Psychology Today*, May 1978, p. 47.

4. Todd W. Baumgardt, "Symposium on Issues and Trends in Nurse Recruitment," *National Association of Nurse Recruiters Newsletter* 3, no. 6 (January 1979).

5. G. David Hughes, "Can Marketing Help Recruit and Retain Nurses?" *Health Care Management Review* 4, no. 3 (Summer 1979): 61–66.

6. Marjorie A. Godfrey and *Nursing 78*, "Job Satisfaction," *Nursing 78*, June 1978, pp. 81, 82.

7. *Health Consequences of Shift Work*, HEW Publication No. 78-154.

8. Jo Hohman, "Nurse Mentor System Cuts Costs, Boosts Quality of Patient Care," *Hospitals, JAHA*, January 1, 1979, p. 93.

9. "HOSPITALS Headlines," *Hospitals, JAHA*, December 16, 1978, p. 17.

10. Marjorie A. Godfrey and *Nursing 79*, "The Dollars and Sense of Nurses' Salaries," *Nursing 79*, October 1979, pp. 98–99. Reprinted with permission.

26. Employee Opinion Surveys—Sometimes Painful, Always Helpful

LAWRENCE C. BASSETT

Periodic physical examinations are vital to ensure good personal health. While odds are high for a clean bill of health, sometimes unexpected problems are diagnosed and proper treatment can be started.

Just as preventive medicine has proved its worth, employee opinion surveys can protect the good health of an organization. But for the same reasons that an individual may shy away from preventive action, so do many health care organizations.

SECTION I: SHOULD AN OPINION SURVEY BE UNDERTAKEN?

Typically, four barriers lead managers to put off assessments of employee attitudes.

1. The 'Lack of Obvious Symptoms' Barrier

Many individuals and managements discover too late problems that existed for a long time, albeit out of sight or disguised. Organizational insulation frequently prevents employee dissatisfaction from reaching the proper ears and eyes. Furthermore, self-deceiving managers fail to realize the significance of messages that are communicated in more subtle and indirect ways. Such values vary among groups. What an employee considers important a busy administrator may view as a minor matter.

For instance, an executive may consider the problem of poor lighting in the employees' parking lot trivial as compared to other budgetary demands. Employees, however, may have little patience with an administration that is more concerned with dollars than personnel safety.

Some feel that surveys "only stir up trouble" and "put things in people's minds." This argument is without merit, for if trouble is "stirred" it's a good indication that trouble exists—and the survey bringing it to light is warranted.

Attitude assessments in various forms should be part of a regular program of preventative management. Crisis management is expensive and frequently unsuccessful, but early knowledge of potential problems permits action that is constructive, rather than remedial. Effective managers cast aside the old and erroneous adage: Don't go looking for trouble . . . trouble will find you.

Another argument that there is no time for a study is counterproductive, particularly for the manager who then becomes occupied with a problem that could have been avoided if it had been detected early. Even in organizations that believe they have good internal monitoring, it is prudent to suspect certain information will be suppressed consciously or overlooked unconsciously by managers who feel threatened by that information.

2. The 'I Don't Want To Hear Bad News' Barrier

The unknown stimulates fear, so switches are turned off to avoid hearing bad news. Less secure administrations fear that problems may be traced to a dislike of or a lack of confidence in management itself. For managers to learn that what they have been doing is neither appreciated nor respected can be demoralizing and threatening, particularly if the information is to be reviewed by higher levels and ultimately by a board of trustees.

Whether it's personal health or organizational well-being, playing the ostrich can be irreparably harmful when problems finally explode and demand action. The act of facing reality is a sign of a mature management. Anxiety over the unknown often proves unwarranted since many studies indicate that, in general, things are going well. Positive findings give confidence to administration and in fact may reinforce its position when seeking approval for new policies or changes from a recalcitrant board.

When making any sort of self-examination, individuals hope for the best. No one likes failure. But failure is less blameworthy if a reasonable course of action is followed to learn all relevant facts in advance. Coping with disappointments and surprises is the hallmark of a flexible management that can make the most out of adverse events. Indeed, many managements have been able to design strategies around negative results that can be used to plan for change and thus parlayed into strengths.

3. The Expense Barrier: 'How Can I Justify the Cost?''

Of course, management must consider cost-effectiveness and financial priorities. There will be times when an examination or a survey is inappropriate; however, the expense argument frequently is more an excuse than a justified decision.

When a skeptical board, medical staff, or employee group is pressuring for more personnel or equipment, some kind of study must be made to determine the balance between cost and estimated gain. Methods to conduct the study with attention to both elements should be analyzed and decided after a decision is made regarding the desirability of a study, not before it.

Unless the hospital has a poor history of acting on results of similar studies, employees usually are very receptive to a survey of their ideas, attitudes, and opinions. Employees feel good communication is worth a

price and the cost of a study usually is a tiny fraction of the hospital's total budget. Moreover, even skeptical employees, when included in a study, have positive attitudes toward the process since it recognizes their importance and affords a way for them to present management with ideas that otherwise might go unheard. Frequently, a study is perceived by persons in professional categories as an effective way of communicating more sophisticated ideas that they feel will improve patient care.

As pressures mount on health care institutions, a team effort is vital. A properly conducted opinion study provides an excellent vehicle for promoting this concept when its results are given to employee task forces to analyze or to plan action.

When considering costs, it also is important to note that health care institutions that have properly implemented employee attitude and opinion studies have saved money. It's a rare study that doesn't produce suggestions, ideas, or recommendations or improve the bottom line. Even when employees are pleased with the organization, management saves money by changing its priorities based upon survey findings. For example, the redesign of an insurance package and the postponement of the implementation of a benefit have resulted from information gathered from employees. Management was able to determine that that particular improvement or increased benefit would not have brought about more positive employee relations value at that time.

Surveys do uncover needs that may increase costs, but some rises in expenditures frequently are preordained long before a study takes place. Avoiding surveys in order to avoid spending money on employee programs is unrealistic. A survey will help management decide where best to spend the available dollars.

The cost of a study actually is low when put into perspective. For example, an institution with 1,000 employees could conduct a full study for a cost of about 1/100 of 1% of payroll—less, if some of the considerations discussed later are used. The cost for smaller organizations might be a bit higher since the overhead for a survey would not go down proportionately, but the cost for a larger institution would not increase in direct proportion to number of employees. Further saving is possible if a group of institutions conducts a group survey.

4. The 'Unwillingness-to-Deal-with-Survey-Findings' Barrier

The value of an opinion study depends on two factors: (1) speedy return of information to employees and (2) timely action on its findings and recommendations. For example, employees will appreciate the delivery of a long-sought vending machine if it arrives one month after a study, rather than after a year's deliberations. Employees see quick attention as a sign that administration is listening; it also evidences management's credibility, responsiveness, and respect. Plans that percolate for months merely raise levels of expectations, so the possibilities for disappointment increase when and if they finally are implemented. Major programs often lose impact because of longtime anticipation. Organizations with suggestion systems can attest to the fact that the speed with which ideas are implemented can be more important than the size of the reward.

Implementation of survey results can be made difficult and time-consuming if the decision-making process in the organization is allowed to stall. Yet this frequently happens if it deals with possible changes in personnel. Another example: while a survey never should be designed to reveal confidences or to put the finger on any supervisor, there may be times when personnel changes are appropriate. More frequently than not, survey results confirm, rather than contradict, administration's prior feelings. The reluctance to reprimand or dismiss an ineffective supervisor, especially one with long-term service, not only delays the inevitable but also hurts administration's reputation and image.

Delays in analyzing and implementing study findings can be minimized by preparation and presurvey planning. It is advisable to designate in advance members of administration or of the management staff as a team to handle suggestions or recommendations.

Feedback sessions with employees can be scheduled even before the survey begins, based on projections of when the findings will be available. Such an action usually raises the level of participation and lets employees know that results will be shared with them. This can be an important factor in ensuring a greater level of participation. Some administrations hesitate to provide feedback to employees on the assumption that the results might be construed as a commitment to actions the health care institution cannot or will not take; this may appear to be valid, but experience has shown otherwise.

Employees, more than any administrator, can anticipate a survey's results since they supply the information and have ideas as to how to remedy the situation. The hospital grapevine may be more effective than official channels. Publicizing the findings to employees lets them know administration has received the message. The manner in which feedback is given, including round-the-clock meetings by administration

and the surveyors, also can enhance positive employee attitudes. Even negative information can be presented in a constructive way. Avoiding discussion on matters about which employees have been thinking and seeking solutions does not minimize those thoughts or hopes. But an administration that responds to the employees' message and promptly reveals its position—for instance, the rationale for declining to act on a given suggestion—reduces skepticism and increases credibility. Employees want respect. Providing answers as to why something will not happen will be accepted far more readily with full disclosure than no answer and no action. Employees do not expect to score 100 percent.

The most important preparation is psychological. Administration and the board need to be prepared to accept the findings and be committed to action. Prior commitment to accept the survey results and to react to them appropriately reduces decision-making time in terms of reviews and deliberations.

SECTION II: IMPLEMENTING AN OPINION STUDY

Who Should Do It?

Administration must determine the depth and nature of the study before deciding the "by whom" and "how." The objectives of the survey must be delineated prior to determining the efficacy of an in-house study. When the depth and nature of the study have been decided, the surveyors should be selected after considering several criteria: surveyor credibility, survey methods, presentation of results, and whether any surveyors should help implement the recommendations.

First, the surveyors must have credibility with employees. There must be complete confidence in the survey team or answers will be distorted. Any suspicion that information might not be kept confidential will lead to unsatisfactory results. Ironically, employees tend to accept strangers more easily and readily than people they know. Thus, in-house surveys rarely are as successful as those done by outsiders. Employees generally feel that outsiders are acceptable, indeed preferred, if they are specialists in conducting such programs. The surveyors usually have optimum credibility even though they are selected by management. There are times, however, when the employee relations department or certain members of administration have the positive reputation that enables them to coordinate or carry out at least some form of survey.

The second important question pertains to the survey methods. Surveys can be limited to certain groups, carried out through interviews, use of questionnaires only, or, still better, a combination of these approaches. A series of interviews with a sample of 5 percent to 10 percent adds a qualitative element to the tabulations and promotes lively, realistic interpretations. The interviews enable the surveyors to gain an insight into the personality of the organization and the relative weight employees put on different matters.

A survey conducted strictly through interviews has some deficiencies. In unstructured face-to-face interviews, employees tend to express negatives—the things that bother them. A surveyor can get the feeling that little is going right when actually many positive features, which do indeed exist, just haven't been mentioned. A written questionnaire evokes answers over the whole range and reminds employees to discuss the more positive aspects of the organization that might be neglected during an interview.

Questionnaires should be easy to complete and analyze. Computers can tabulate answers quickly, making it possible to obtain cross-correlations and patterns. In addition, the questionnaire should offer open-ended questions to which employees can introduce new thoughts not included in the survey or to give further thought to a given area.

The third question relates to how the results will be presented. Even the best information, when not properly analyzed and summarized, can make an otherwise successful process counterproductive. With the use of computers, it's possible to have enormous quantities of statistical printouts. However, unless there are preplanned questions around which the data are compiled, interpretation of the information becomes subjective or confusing. A well-programmed survey can easily compare and correlate answers from different age groups, sections of the organization, and other combinations to determine whether patterns exist that reveal information not apparent at first glance.

A report should include the rationale behind the surveyors' interpretation of answers and the patterns of response. Such clarification gives meaning to what otherwise might be confusing statistics. As noted, personal interviews provide the needed insights.

While a few managements can transform raw data into decisive action, most are helped by reports that include recommendations. If the surveyors are experienced, they will be able both to interpret the findings and to make specific recommendations.

The last question pertains to whether the surveyors are capable of assisting in implementing the recommendations. There are advantages to retaining surveyors who have the capability of helping implement

the recommendations. This can be construed as self-serving for the surveyors, but in actuality employees see this as an important part of follow-through by management that indicates "they mean business."

The question of whether or not the survey should be done by the organization's own staff depends on its feasibility and how much detail is sought. In-house studies are less expensive, but much may be lost in the process. The feasibility of using an organization's own staff rests upon how sure management is of the surveyors' credibility.

Conducting the Study

Using Outside Surveyors

While most professional surveyors have a modus operandi, the organization should be sure certain criteria are observed.

Employees must feel convenienced and at ease. If questionnaires are to be completed, arrangements must be made for this to be done during the employee's shift in a comfortable setting with sufficient privacy. Each employee must feel unpressured and be confident the answers are unobserved. The most successful location to administer the questionnaires is in the employee's own work area; familiar surroundings tend to reduce inhibitions.

Since a good sampling of interviews is important, some surveyors seek interviews with small groups of employees in addition to individual sessions. Depending upon the institution's normal internal relationships, employees who are accustomed to talking openly with each other (head nurses, technologists, and other groups) not only speak more freely with their peers but can remind each other of points that may have been overlooked. Group interviews should not displace all individual interviews, but they are effective in getting participation by larger numbers of employees and verifying much of the information supplied by individuals.

Surveys Done In-House

When a health care organization conducts the survey by itself, neutral, objective interviewing may not be feasible, acceptable, or credible; this may mandate the use of a questionnaire as the sole survey instrument. No one on the management staff should administer the questionnaire, even if that individual appears to possess an unequivocal position of respect. Questionnaires should be placed into closed containers and employees should be notified that results will be tabulated by persons hired from the outside. It is rare that employees will accept having questionnaires reviewed directly by the institution's staff. It also is inadvisable.

Questionnaires administered in-house also have a drawback in that certain details in questions may have to be eliminated if it appears that confidentiality might be compromised.

Cooperative Studies

There may be times when it makes sense for two or more health care institutions to conduct a joint study. This can minimize overhead costs of questionnaire design and administration, computer time, and other factors while the results can be nearly as comprehensive as if each institution conducted its own study. Surveys sponsored and coordinated by associations or groups of hospitals have an additional benefit in that they allow valid comparisons on key points and permit the accurate tracking of changes. Confidentiality can be maintained for each participating institution, although the preparation stage might be more extensive since the needs of all participants would have to be accommodated in the program's design.

Other Considerations

When feasible, any study should include all members of the organization's staff, including those from the medical and dental staff, volunteers, and students attending schools sponsored or operated by the institution. The added cost of including these groups usually is minimal but the results can be meaningful in comparing how they perceive the organization. Any outcome that might lead to facilitating their contribution to overall patient care justifies the cost.

A survey should not be a one-time effort. When properly administered and conducted periodically, a series of surveys can measure and evaluate progress by comparing employee attitudes, opinions, and feelings at different times. If properly planned, follow-up surveys need not be as extensive or as expensive. By proper planning of the original questionnaire, it is possible to conduct brief surveys every two or three years to review key points.

Although normally undesirable, the focus of surveys at times may have to be narrowed intentionally to include only supervisory and management staff. A survey of the entire organization may be inappropriate, for instance during union organizing, although management might seek the information to assess its internal strength. Most supervisors represent at least an insight into the values and sentiments of their employees. They can shed light on the environment in the institution, although there is the danger that some facts will be concealed and weaker supervisors may present distorted pictures of their departments. More often than not, sufficient information can be gathered to obtain conclusions and to develop a proper perspective, but the limitations of this approach must be considered.

Designing a Questionnaire

Questionnaires should permit easy tabulation. Key punching is the usual method and no special electronic readers are required. With computer capabilities expanding, however, it is now possible to use a mark-sensor that enables a machine to read the answers directly and save time and cost. However, key punching of information may be preferred.

In designing the survey, questions should be included that verify previously acquired information, since to ensure the validity of results a correlation should be made of points raised in different forms.

ONE FINAL WORD

Peoples' views differ, sometimes sharply, about the use and value of employee opinion and attitude surveys. These feelings usually relate to the individual's personal experience with other studies. With any tool, how it is used and by whom it is used makes the difference. If administration is to be responsive and efficient, it must have all the facts. An enlightened management recognizes that an employee opinion study is the best way to obtain objective and complete data. Management realizes that a well-conducted employee study is invaluable.

Surveys are not to be feared, and the cost makes them an excellent value. A flexible, forward-looking management that seeks ways to ensure the health care organization can cope with change, meet new challenges, and maintain forward momentum should welcome the opportunities a survey provides. Removing the barriers that stand in the way is not a formidable task; attempting to cope with crises brought on unnecessarily is indeed formidable. Periodic health examinations accompanied by proper diagnosis and treatment have produced sound health for the persons involved. Periodic employee opinion and attitude studies accompanied by proper diagnosis and "treatment" can provide sound organizational health for the concerned institution.

27. How to Reduce the Turnover of Hospital Nurses[*]

JAMES L. PRICE and CHARLES W. MUELLER

The high turnover rate of hospital nurses is well known. A 1962 study of 428 nonfederal hospitals, for example, found a crude turnover rate of 58 percent among nurses.[1] The high level of this rate is apparent when it is compared to the turnover of teachers and social workers, who have educational requirements and sex distributions similar to hospital nurses. A national sample of 2,179 school districts in fifty states and the District of Columbia from the fall of 1959 to the fall of 1960[2] found a crude turnover rate of 13 percent for elementary and secondary teachers. A 1964 study of 171 state and local welfare organizations[3] reported a 30 percent crude turnover rate among social workers. The turnover rate of nurses, therefore, is more than four times that of the teachers and almost twice that of social workers.[4]

High nursing turnover seriously complicates the health care institution's goal of providing quality care for its patients. Nurses are especially important to the hospital because they are the most highly trained professionals whose presence is continuous. Physicians, the highest trained of all, spend very little time in the hospital visiting their patients; licensed practical nurses, who spend the most time with patients, have limited professional training. Since nurses are such a critically important group, and since job performance generally improves with experience, it is desirable to have a large core of experienced nurses in each unit for the day, evening, and night shifts. With a crude turnover rate of approximately 60 percent, such a staffing pattern is impossible to achieve. The experienced nurses must be spread very thinly among the units, thereby complicating the task of providing quality patient care. Nursing turnover, in short, threatens hospital effectiveness.[5, 6]

Not only is the provision of quality patient care threatened, but the care that is available becomes very expensive to maintain. One careful study[7] of turnover among nurses in a large metropolitan general hospital estimates that the institution incurred a minimum cost of about $420 to replace each nurse who left. Since these figures pertain to 1965, contemporary costs of course are significantly higher. If hospitals could reduce their nursing turnover significantly while maintaining existing standards of patient care, productivity would be increased noticeably—output would remain the same (existing standards of patient care) while one input (costs of nursing turnover) would decrease.[8, 9] Productivity often is referred to as efficiency.

*We would like to thank the Division of Nursing, Bureau of Health Manpower (RO2-NU-00593), and the American Nurses' Foundation for funds to perform this research. Dr. Myrtle K. Aydelotte (Executive Director, American Nurses' Association, and Professor, College of Nursing, University of Iowa) greatly encouraged us when we were most in need of support. The cooperation of the employees in the seven hospitals we studied was truly extraordinary; we extend our heartfelt thanks to them and hope that our research will be of some assistance in the performance of their work. And, last but not least, we would like to thank our many colleagues—too many to list in this brief space—who have read and criticized various drafts of this paper.

All nursing turnover obviously is not detrimental to hospital effectiveness. High turnover, for instance, probably makes it easier for hospitals to introduce change because traditional procedures are weakened by the movement of employees in and out; in an environment of rapidly evolving health care technology such as exists today, the quality of patient care is likely to be improved by many of these changes. Nor is all nursing turnover necessarily destructive to productivity. When relatively incompetent nurses leave, for example, costs are likely to be reduced and patient care improved. The main body of the literature, nevertheless, has focused on the negative impact of turnover on effectiveness and productivity, thereby ignoring possible benefits for the organization.[10, 11] However, the authors' belief, which we cannot support empirically in a rigorous fashion, is that when nursing turnover approximates 60 percent, its net impact on effectiveness and productivity probably is negative.

The authors have conducted an empirical study of the determinants of hospital nurse turnover and, based on its findings, make recommendations to reduce this turnover. Before the recommendations are discussed, the empirical study is described and its findings summarized.

THE EMPIRICAL STUDY

The focus of the study[12] was on voluntary leaving (quits). The study excluded layoffs, dismissals, retirements, deaths, and resignations due to serious illness because they are types of involuntary leaving. Transfers and promotions, since they take place within hospitals, also were excluded. (To simplify this presentation, turnover is used as a substitute for voluntary leaving.)

The turnover literature suggests that the following 11 determinants produce variations in turnover: opportunity, routinization, participation, instrumental communication, integration, pay, distributive justice, promotional opportunity, professionalism, general training, and kinship responsibility. The literature suggests two additional variables, job satisfaction and intent to stay, which the authors hypothesize to intervene between the determinants and turnover. Intent to stay is viewed as a component of commitment.[13] Definitions of these determinants and intervening variables are presented in Exhibit 27-1.

The relationships among the variables (causal model) are depicted in Figure 27-1. As is apparent from this diagram, alternative jobs outside the hospital serve to increase directly the amount of turnover.

Seven determinants have an indirect impact on turnover through job satisfaction. One, repetitive work, decreases job satisfaction; the six others—participating in job-related decisions, being informed about job-related issues, having close friends employed by the same organization, receiving good pay, being fairly compensated, having an opportunity to obtain a better job in the organization—all increase job satisfaction. As that satisfaction increases, individuals evidence greater intent to stay with the organization. Three determinants have an indirect impact on turnover through intent to stay. Increased dedication to occupational standards of performance and general occupational socialization serve to decrease intent to stay, whereas obligations to local kin serve to increase intent to stay. Finally, the model indicates that intent to stay has a direct negative impact on turnover.

None of the variables defined in Exhibit 27-1 refers to "correlates," such as age, length of service, existence of a union, vested pension funds, and so forth. Correlates (sometimes termed demographic variables) are not included in the model because they do not indicate the means whereby they produce variations in turnover. Age illustrates this. Some literature[14] supports a negative relationship between age and turnover: younger members usually have higher rates of turnover than older members. Age, however, does not indicate *how* the younger age produces higher rates of turnover. An answer to the "how" question must be sought among the variables defined in the exhibit. Younger members, for instance, have higher rates of turnover than older members because the younger nurses usually have the most routine jobs, participate little in decision making, lack knowledge about their work, have fewer close friends, receive less pay, and have few local obligations to kin. In short, it is not age per se that produces variations in turnover, but routinization, participation, instrumental communication, integration, pay, and kinship responsibility, all of which are correlated with age.

The correlates of turnover are not totally ignored, however. The correlates are used to check the adequacy of the causal model and to specify the conditions under which the model operates.[15] One of the correlates, age, also is used as the basis for one of the recommendations.

The site of the study was seven voluntary, short-term, general hospitals. Six were of medium size, between 100 and 500 beds; the seventh had 620 beds, so it was not substantially different from the others. Five of the hospitals were in Iowa and two in Illinois. The communities in which they were located were between 50,000 and 250,000. All of the hospitals were church

Exhibit 27-1 Determinants and Intervening Variables: Definitions and Measures

Variable	Definition	No. of Questions	Sample Questions Addressed to Nurses*
Opportunity	The availability of alternative jobs in the organization's environment	4	How easy would it be for *you* to find a nursing job with another employer? How would you describe the number of *available nursing jobs,* with all types of employers, for a nurse with your qualifications?
Routinization	The degree to which a job is repetitive	4	To what extent are the activities that make up your job *routine?* How much *repetitiveness* is there in the activities that make up your job?
Participation	The degree of power that an individual exercises concerning the job	4	For each of the following decisions, please indicate *how much say you actually have* in making these decisions: (a) How you do your job; (b) Sequence of your job activities; (c) Speed at which you work; (d) Changing how you do your job.
Instrumental Communication	The degree to which information about the job is transmitted by an organization to its members	7	How well *informed* are you about each of the following aspects of *your job* in the hospital: Priority of work to be done? Technical knowledge? Nature of equipment used?
Integration	The degree to which an individual has close friends among organizational members	4	*While you are actually working,* how often do you see your close friends among hospital employees? How often do you see your close friends among hospital employees *during breaks,* such as for coffee and lunch?
Pay	The amount of money, or equivalents, distributed in return for service	1	Total yearly income from nursing before taxes and other deductions.
Distributive Justice	The degree to which rewards and punishments are related to the amount of input into the organization	3	*Compared to the effort that you put into your job,* how do you feel about the pay you receive in the hospital? (a) Compared with the effort, my pay is very poor, (b) Poor, (c) About right, (d) Good, (e) Very good.

*A complete description of the items used is available upon request from the authors.

Exhibit 27-1 continued

Variable	Definition	No. of Questions	Sample Questions Addressed to Nurses
Promotional Opportunity	The amount of potential movement from lower to higher strata within an organization	8	How much do you agree or disagree with each of the following statements about *promotional opportunities* for a person with your qualifications somewhere in the hospital?: There is little chance to get ahead. There is a very good opportunity for advancement.
Professionalism	The degree of dedication to occupational standards of performance	3	How many *memberships* do you have in *professional associations,* such as American Nurses' Association, Association of Operating Room Nurses, Critical Care Nurse Association, and so forth? How often do you generally *attend meetings* (district, state, and national) of a professional association?
General Training	The degree to which the occupational socialization of an individual results in the ability to increase the productivity of different organizations	1	How much *professional schooling in nursing* have you had? (a) Associate, (b) Diploma, (c) Baccalaureate, (d) Graduate degree(s).
Kinship Responsibility	The degree of an individual's obligations to relatives in the community an employer is located	3	Index based on marital status, presence of children, and importance given to being a parent.
Job Satisfaction	The degree to which individuals like their jobs	7	How much do you *agree* or *disagree* with each of the following statements about your job? I find real enjoyment in my job; I am fairly well satisfied with my job; I definitely dislike my job.
Intent to Stay	The estimated likelihood of continued membership in an organization	2	Which of the following statements most clearly reflects your feelings about your *future in the hospital?* (a) Definitely will not leave, (b) Probably will not leave, (c) Uncertain, (d) Probably will leave, (e) Definitely will leave.

Figure 27-1 The Causal Model of Turnover

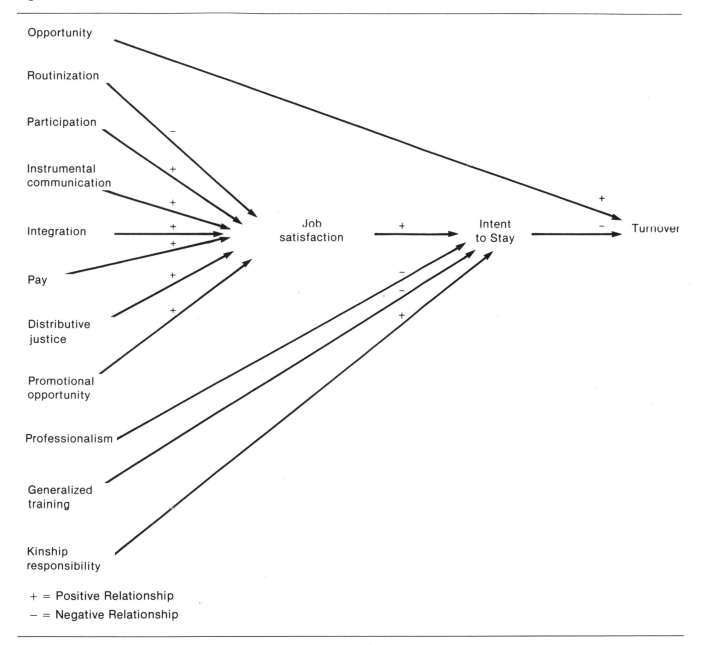

+ = Positive Relationship

− = Negative Relationship

operated—four were Protestant and three were Roman Catholic.

The researchers distributed questionnaires, mostly by mail, to the homes of 1,383 nurses in August 1976. The nurses were requested to return the completed questionnaires to the researchers at the University of Iowa. The response rate was 80 percent since 1,101 questionnaires were returned.

The final sample consisted of 1,091 nonsupervisory registered nurses. Nurses with three types of training were employed by the hospitals: associate (N = 140),

diploma (N = 770), and baccalaureate-graduate (N = 174).[16] Both full-time (N = 674) and part-time (N = 415) nurses were included in the sample.[17]

In September 1977 each hospital (usually the nursing director and/or personnel officer) received a list of its nurses who had returned the questionnaires to the researchers. The hospital was requested to indicate the names of the nurses no longer employed there as of October 1, 1977.[18] It also was asked to indicate nurses who had died, retired, or had been dismissed.[19] One of the researchers visited each hospital in October 1977 to collect and cross-check these data.

Between August 1976 and October 1977, 221 nurses (20 percent) had left the hospitals. Since this study was concerned only with voluntary leaving, ten nurses (of the 221) who left involuntarily were dropped from the analysis. This results in an N of 1,091, for which the rate of voluntary leaving is 19 percent.[20, 21]

Two units were used to analyze the data: the individual and the immediate work group. When the individual is the unit, turnover is a dichotomous variable (each individual is either a leaver or a stayer) and the determinants are measured for each nurse. When the immediate work group (the nursing unit) is used to analyze the data, turnover is a rate for each unit and the pooled scores of the nurses who are members of the units are used to measure the determinants. When the individual is the unit of analysis, the causal model is estimated five times—once for the entire sample of nurses and once each for four categories of nurses: full time under 30, full time 30 and over, part time under 30, and part time 30 and over.[22]

The data were analyzed by multiple regression and path analytic techniques.[23, 24] These techniques allow an ordering of the determinants in terms of their net influence on turnover and an estimation of how important, overall, they are in explaining why some nurses stay and others decide to leave.[25] Although the causal model represented by Figure 27-1 constitutes a synthesis of material from diverse sources concerning what is known about the causes of turnover, the analysis was designed to determine if all of the determinants in the model are important and which of those are the most important.

MAJOR FINDINGS OF THE EMPIRICAL STUDY

The findings are presented separately from the two units of analysis (the individual and the nursing units). Since the similarities outweigh the differences, and because it is easier to make general recommendations based on similarities among the nurses, the differences found among the four categories of nurses are not discussed here. As previously indicated, the individual also is the unit of analysis when the four categories of nurses are used to analyze the data.

The Entire Sample

Only five determinants from the causal model were especially important when the individual was used as the unit of analysis: intent to stay, opportunity, general training, job satisfaction, and kinship responsibility.[26] The determinants whose increase resulted in reduc-

tions in turnover were intent to stay (which was viewed as a component of commitment), job satisfaction, and the existence of local kin. The determinants whose increase produced greater turnover were many available jobs outside the hospitals and training that prepared the nurses to operate in diverse settings. It was assumed that the training of baccalaureate nurses was the most general and diploma nurses the most specific, with the associate nurses located between these two extremes.

The Four Categories of Nurses

The separate analysis of the four categories of nurses defined by age and amount of time worked indicated that six determinants were important for at least three categories of nurses: intent to stay and job satisfaction, as in the total sample, as well as routinization, participation, instrumental communication, and promotional opportunity. The five determinants whose increase produced less turnover were intent to stay, job satisfaction, participation in making job-related decisions, the receipt of work-related information, and the chance to get ahead occupationally in the hospitals. Increased repetitiveness of work resulted indirectly in greater turnover.

The Nursing Units

Four determinants, all of which were significant when the individual was the unit of analysis, also were important when the immediate work group was used as the unit of analysis: intent to stay, job satisfaction, kinship responsibility, and general training.[27] When nursing units are composed of nurses with high average levels of intent to stay, job satisfaction, and the existence of local kin, these units as a consequence are likely to have low rates of turnover. Nursing units with high percentages of baccalaureate nurses, however, are likely to have high turnover.

The explained variance, that is, the explanatory completeness of the model, for the different units of analysis and categories of nurses is as follows: the entire sample, 17 percent; full time under 30, 15 percent; full time 30 and over, 18 percent; part time under 30, 26 percent; part time 30 and over, 12 percent; and the nursing units, 26 percent.[28] These explained variances compare favorably with other research on the determinants of turnover.[29] The practical significance of these explained variances is indicated in the concluding section of this article.

The empirical study yielded nine determinants that influence turnover and thus can be used as a basis for recommendations to reduce hospital nurses' turnover: opportunity, intent to stay, job satisfaction, general training, kinship responsibility, routinization, participation, instrumental communication, and promotional opportunity. However, three of these—opportunity, intent to stay, and job satisfaction—are not directly manipulable and thus are of little practical assistance in making recommendations. Although the availability of more outside jobs directly increases turnover, hospitals have little or no capacity to influence the job market for nurses. Thus recommendations about opportunity are of little practical importance. Although increased intent to stay (which suggests increased commitment) directly produces less turnover, hospitals must be informed as to how this factor can be increased. Thus recommendations specifically about intent to stay also are not too helpful. Finally, although greater job satisfaction indirectly decreases turnover by its positive impact on intent to stay, hospitals require information as to how job satisfaction can be increased—thus recommendations specifically about this subject also are not very informative. Exclusion of recommendations directly involving opportunity, intent to stay, and job satisfaction leaves six determinants that can serve as the basis for recommendations.

As indicated, correlates such as age and length of service were not part of the causal model. Correlates, however, can serve as the basis of the recommendations that appear in the next section. The findings about the relationship between age and turnover are relevant.[30] Turnover rates decreased sharply for older nurses: part time under 30, 30 percent turnover; full time under 30, 24 percent; part time 30 and over, 11 percent; and full time 30 and over, 8 percent. As may be recalled, the rate of turnover for all the nurses was 19 percent.

The primary purpose is to make recommendations based on the findings of the empirical research. However, one recommendation (Number 8) is not based on the research but was suggested by the 1976 work of the noted turnover researchers from the Republic of South Africa, Roux Van der Merwe and Sylvia Miller.[31] Their recommendation on the necessity of obtaining more data on turnover is so basic that its inclusion seemed essential.

RECOMMENDATIONS TO REDUCE TURNOVER

Eight recommendations, or sets of recommendations in most instances, are presented. However, four preliminary comments are pertinent:

1. Suggestions about how to implement the recommendations will be mostly ignored because these proposals differ greatly in the ease of their implementation. Some can be carried out easily, whereas others—for legal, financial, or administrative reasons—can be implemented only with considerable difficulty, if at all. Legal considerations are very important; the law must be obeyed scrupulously in implementing the recommendations.
2. A cost-benefit perspective is essential because all of the recommendations involve both costs and benefits. It is assumed that the benefits will be substantially greater than the costs, especially over a period of several years.
3. It should be emphasized that quality patient care, not the reduction of turnover, is the goal of the hospitals studied. Turnover, as was indicated in the introductory comments, does result in improvements in patient care in some instances. However, it is assumed that excessive turnover is harmful to the patients and costly for the hospital, and it is excessive turnover that should be reduced.
4. Finally, the recommendations are not arranged in order of importance. The first recommendation, for instance, will not necessarily result in greater reduction in turnover than any of the others.

1. Allow Voluntary Transfers between Nursing Units

(This recommendation is based on the findings concerning routinization.)

Because of the staffing needs of the hospital when they are hired, nurses with specialized training often are assigned to units where they have little or no opportunity to make use of their special skills and knowledge. Still other nurses develop special interests, expanded by extra education of various types, that are underutilized by the hospitals. Transfers between nursing units would permit better use of these special skills and knowledge and both nurses and patients should benefit. Some of the complaints about repetitive work seem to be the result of insufficient use of special skills and knowledge.

Such transfers must be voluntary, of course. If the nurses are not willing to transfer, such movement constitutes a punishment and decreases job satisfaction and commitment. It is necessary only to note the hostility to "pulling" among nurses—involuntary transfers for one shift—to appreciate the necessity of keeping the moves voluntary.

A policy of allowing transfers requires that vacancies throughout the nursing department be posted officially in some manner. Many nurses will learn about forthcoming vacancies informally. Such channels, however, are not too reliable and often are unfair. Information transmitted informally is not always accurate and often is kept among a few close friends. Organizations therefore should depend primarily upon formal means to transmit information about vacancies.

The mechanics of such transfers are not difficult to manage. A nurse in a specialized unit (such as cardiac intensive care) resigns, the vacancy is posted officially throughout the nursing department, the resigning nurse is replaced by one already employed (in a general medical unit, for instance), and, finally, a new nurse is hired to fill the vacancy created by the transfer out.

It is important to emphasize that to allow voluntary transfers between units is not to institute a system of "musical chairs" among the nurses. Too frequent transfers would be just as harmful as allowing no transfers.

2. Hold Regular and Brief Meetings of the Nursing Units during Working Hours

(The findings concerning participation and instrumental communication are the basis of this recommendation.)

"Regular" means scheduled at a specific time. The frequency of the meetings naturally will vary for the different units, but once a week seems to be sufficient. The scheduling of the meetings should be arranged so that the maximum number of part-time nurses can attend, because these are the individuals for whom the sessions are especially important. Brief meetings are essential because of the needs of the patients and the cost of staff time. Seldom should a session last longer than about 45 minutes.

"Unit meetings" refers to assembling all, or substantially all, of the members of a unit at a specific place. Individual meetings between the unit supervisor and a staff nurse, for instance, are important but are not an adequate substitute for unit meetings. Since there are three shifts of nurses, there will have to be three meetings of each unit. This will require two extra visits to the hospital by the unit supervisor, but it is more fitting to inconvenience the supervisor than the staff nurses since the conduct of meetings is a responsibility of the supervisor.

These sessions constitute a pressure to communicate work-related information and to allow partici-

pation in making work-related decisions. For example, a supervisor who meets regularly with the members of the unit will be constrained by the pressure of the group to share information and to allow greater participation in its operation. The meetings also provide an opportunity for supervisors to receive information from the staff nurses and for the latter to communicate among themselves. Upward and horizontal communication are as important as downward communication.

All organizations must plan for the regular transmission of work-related information. However, this is particularly difficult to bring about adequately in hospitals because of the constant pressure to care for sick patients, their regular arrivals and departures, the necessity of three different work shifts, and the mixture of full-time and part-time workers. Hospitals thus must make a special effort to do what is much easier for other organizations.

The mere existence of unit meetings, of course, does not guarantee better communication or greater participation in decision making. A minimum of information may be communicated and the meetings may allow for no sharing of power. The quality of the meetings is all-important; without a genuine sharing of information and power, the sessions may be too costly to be a regular feature of hospital operations. Unit supervisors must know how to conduct meetings so that information and power are shared.

3. Promote Primarily from within the Nursing Department

(The findings regarding promotional opportunity are the basis for this recommendation.)

This type of promotional policy allows maximum use of existing opportunities for promotion. The present career structure allows for relatively few promotional opportunities for nurses; these limited openings should be reserved primarily for the current staff members. Implementation of such a policy naturally will require an official posting of vacancies for existing staff before outsiders are notified.

Hospitals cannot, of course, promote entirely from within. Situations sometimes arise when the existing staff does not possess the needed qualifications or when an outsider clearly has superior competence. However, these situations are relatively rare. When higher positions, mostly nursing unit supervisors, are available within the department, the burden of proof should be on the person who wishes to hire an outsider.

4. Create an Alternate Career Structure for Staff Nurses

(This recommendation is based on findings regarding participation and promotional opportunity.)

A career is a succession of related and ranked occupations through which persons move in a predictable sequence.[32] The occupations in a career are ranked in terms of money, prestige, power, rights, and responsibilities. The career commonly available to most hospital nurses consists of the following sequence: staff nurse, unit supervisor, assistant nursing director, and nursing director. Most notable is the fact that this career mostly consists of administrative positions; only the lowest, that of staff nurse, is primarily professional.

For instance, there might be four steps in an alternate career for staff nurses: staff nurse $_1$ through staff nurse $_4$. Each step should result in a significant increase in money, prestige, rights, and responsibilities. Without these increases, a genuine alternate career does not exist. Administrative rights and responsibilities probably will increase somewhat as a nurse progresses through the sequence of occupations. What is essential, however, is that each occupation in the sequence consists primarily of professional rights and responsibilities. What is proposed here is a professional career structure for hospital nurses.

Pay and number of persons supervised will not always be correlated if an alternate career structure is established. Some of the experienced staff nurse $_4$s, will make more money than the unit supervisors. An alternate career structure thus departs in some instances from a civil service type of organizational structure in which pay always is related to the number of persons supervised.

Advanced training, such as possession of a master's degree, should not be a prerequisite for movement to the position of staff nurse $_4$; nor should any specific type of education, such as a baccalaureate degree, be preferred. What is absolutely basic is competence. There should be a steady progression of increased competence *as a nurse* as the individual moves from staff nurse $_1$ to staff nurse $_4$. For a hospital to have a genuine alternate career structure, there also should be a sizeable distribution of nurses throughout the sequence. One or two staff nurses in a large hospital, for instance, hardly constitute a genuine alternate career structure.

An alternate career for staff nurses would create more opportunity for in-house promotion. Although this system would be especially attractive to full-time nurses who are under 30, the system also would be attractive to the three other categories of nurses. An alternative career would mean that a staff nurse need not become an administrator to receive significant increases in money, prestige, power, rights, and responsibilities, but could enjoy such benefits by remaining a staff nurse. Implementation of this recommendation would be especially important in view of the greater proportion of women who work full time for longer periods of their life. The recommendation thus is consistent with what seems to be a major change in the role of women in American society. Since an alternate career structure would mean more power for the top of the career structure—the staff nurse $_3$ and the staff nurse $_4$—the result should be less dissatisfaction about the making of job-related decisions. Nurses who are strongly motivated to participate in making job-related decisions probably will be staff nurse $_3$s and staff nurse $_4$s. They now are relatively powerless staff nurses.

5. Recruit More Diploma Nurses

(The responses on the general training issue are the basis for this recommendation.)

Nurses with baccalaureate and/or graduate degrees naturally will continue to be hired. Their links with universities provide a source of new ideas and an emphasis on professionalism that hospitals can ill afford to lose. The recommendation means simply that, if turnover is to be reduced, relatively more of the nursing staff should be diploma nurses.

This recommendation is contrary to the current emphasis on baccalaureate training as the preferred route. Reduced turnover, of course, is not the main goal of hospitals. It may be that patient care is improved in the long run by greater emphasis on baccalaureate training. The authors believe this to be the case. They also believe that adjustments are required by both hospitals and baccalaureate nurses if the quality of patient care is to be improved. This study, however, focuses only on turnover and the results indicate that nurses with baccalaureate training have higher rates of turnover than those without such training. One cost of the current emphasis on baccalaureate training probably will be more turnover. This cost, to emphasize a point made previously, must be weighed against the many long-term benefits for the patients that are likely to result from an increased emphasis on baccalaureate training.

6. Hire More Local Nurses Who Are Married and Who Have Children

(The findings about kinship responsibility are the basis for this recommendation.)

A local nurse is one who has been born and reared in the community in which the hospital is located. Local nurses are likely to have parents and siblings living in the area who constitute a constraint not to leave the hospital. Marriage and children create relatives that further constrain turnover. In addition to this kinship responsibility, local nurses are likely to have close friends working in the hospital. These generally will be the result of long residence in the community and may constrain turnover slightly.[33]

Aggressive recruiting will be necessary to locate local nurses who are married and who have children. Many of these nurses will have left the labor force and will not respond to the typical newspaper advertisement. The existing staff generally will be aware of many of these nurses in the community and can serve as valuable aids in recruiting.

Since many local nurses will have left the labor force, they usually will require special training before they can start working again. Public schools in the area, such as community colleges, should provide regular nurse refresher courses since the benefits of such training will accrue to no single work organization. Hospitals cannot be expected to provide costly training that can benefit other organizations that might employ the nurses who have taken the refresher courses. Even with refresher courses at community colleges, these nurses will require extra training by hospitals. The hospitals may have to provide extra flexibility in working hours to accommodate these nurses. There is nothing sacred, for example, about three eight-hour shifts. This extra training and flexible scheduling will be costly for the hospitals, but will be less than the considerable benefits received by the lower turnover of these nurses.

Competence must not be compromised by this recommendation. When competence levels are approximately equal, preference should be given to local nurses who are married and who have children. None of the recommendations in this section, it should be emphasized, are intended to suggest violation of merit criteria in the recruitment, promotion, and retention of nurses. Weakening of merit criteria threatens the provision of quality care for patients, and such weakening is unacceptable.

7. Hire More Nurses Who Are 30 and Over

(This recommendation is based on the survey's findings about age.)

Previous comments about local nurses who are married and who have children also are applicable to the nurses 30 and older. Aggressive recruitment will be needed to locate and hire these nurses and, once hired, extra training will be necessary since many of them will have been out of the labor force for some time. The extra costs, however, should be less than the benefits because of reduced turnover among these nurses.

Nurses under 30 will continue to be hired. The recommendation means that, if other things are approximately equal, especially competence, then preference should be given to the older nurses.

It should be noted that it is likely that a single individual will possess several qualities emphasized by these recommendations. A local nurse who is married and who has children, for instance, also is likely to be a diploma trained nurse who is 30 or over. Such a nurse thus satisfies three of the recommendations. Each recommendation, however, should contribute separately toward reducing turnover.

8. Obtain Better Data about Turnover

Most hospitals calculate crude turnover rates for their nursing departments. The number of leavers during a period, usually a year, is divided by the average number of nurses employed during that time. A common way of obtaining the average number employed is to add the number employed at the beginning and end of the period and divide by two. Crude turnover rates also are calculated for nursing units within the nursing department. This rate also is used for the hospital as a unit of analysis.

The crude turnover rate is a helpful measure because it indicates the volume of turnover, and the greater the volume, the greater the cost. Hospitals also should calculate the median length of service for all nurses who leave.[34, 35] The median is better than the arithmetic mean because the distribution of leavers is highly skewed. Most of the leavers, for instance, consist of short-service nurses. With the median length of service for leavers, the hospital will know where nursing turnover is occurring in terms of length of service. It makes a big difference, for example, whether or not turnover is occurring among the long-service nurses or the short-service nurses. Costs are greater and the quality of patient care is more threatened when there is turnover of long-service nurses. The median length of service of the leavers thus is an excellent complement to the commonly used crude turnover rate.

Care should be exercised in calculating these rates for small nursing units. The turnover of a single nurse in a small unit will make a major difference in either of these statistics. If the size of the unit is smaller than 20, this fact should be noted and the rates should be viewed with caution.[36]

SUMMARY AND CONCLUSION

Eight steps that hospitals can take to reduce the turnover of their nurses have been suggested. Hospitals can allow voluntary transfers between nursing units, hold regular and brief meetings of the units during working hours, promote primarily from within the nursing department, create an alternate career structure for staff nurses, recruit more diploma nurses, hire more local nurses who are married and who have children, hire more nurses who are 30 and older, and obtain better data about turnover by calculating the median length of service for all nurses who leave as a supplement to the commonly used crude turnover rate.

Three cautions are in order. First, based on the data in this survey, it must be pointed out that the recommendations, if implemented, will not result in a drastic reduction in the turnover of hospital nurses. The highest explained variance was 26 percent. This means that, where the study was most successful, 74 percent of the variation in turnover could not be explained. This fact alone should inject a sobering note into the discussion. Even more sobering, however, is the fact that the authors could make no specific recommendations based on three very important determinants—opportunity, intent to stay, and job satisfaction.

The total effects on turnover of these three determinants far exceed the total impact of the six determinants on which the recommendations are based—general training, kinship responsibility, routinization, participation, instrumental communication, and promotional opportunity.[37] Opportunity and intent to stay have larger total effects because they primarily operate directly to influence turnover, whereas the six determinants on which the recommendations are based indirectly influence turnover.[38]

However, the authors believe, and here we go beyond the data, that the causal model is better than the empirical findings indicate.[39] The comments at this point thus are conservative. Even if the model is better than the findings indicate, and it will require further research to check this possibility, it is best not to expect too much from any set of recommendations.

Second, the authors recognize that even though implementation of the recommendations should reduce turnover, some could have unanticipated costs that will nullify the intended benefits. In addition, the manner of implementing the recommendations is all-important. Sound recommendations, based on the very best research, can have basically harmful effects on a hospital if they are implemented clumsily.

Third, other recommendations probably can be derived from the findings of this research. The authors have not exhausted the universe of recommendations consistent with the findings.

The virtue of these recommendations is that they indicate an empirically-based course of action that should reduce the turnover of hospital nurses. Although implementation of the recommendations probably will not result in a drastic reduction in nursing turnover, and other recommendations may be equally consistent with these findings, the proposals do provide a guide to cope with the difficult problem of excessive turnover of hospital nurses. Movement toward a solution of this problem should result in better patient care at reduced cost.

NOTES

1. American Nurses' Association, *Spot Check of Current Hospital Employment Conditions* (Kansas City, Mo.: American Nurses' Association, Research and Statistics Unit, 1962). The 52.8 percent in this spot check seems to refer only to the first 11 months of 1962. Based on that span, the yearly estimate is 57.6 percent, rounded to 58 percent.

2. Frank Lindenfield, *Teacher Turnover in Public Elementary and Secondary Schools, 1959–1960* (Washington, D.C.: U.S. Government Printing Office, 1963).

3. U.S. Children's Bureau, *Child Welfare Statistics, 1964* (U.S. Department of Health, Education, and Welfare, Statistical Series 82, 1965).

4. Jerome P. Lysaught, *An Abstract for Action* (New York: McGraw-Hill Book Co., 1970), pp. 132, 146. The present situation, of course, could be different from the historical periods described in the three studies cited above. Lysaught presents more recent data that suggest the situation has not changed basically, at least with respect to nurses.

5. James L. Price, "The Study of Organizational Effectiveness," *Sociological Quarterly* 13 (1972): 3–15.

6. —————, *Organizational Effectiveness* (Homewood, Ill.: Irwin, 1968).

7. Murray Melbin and Doris L. Taub, "The High Cost of Replacing a Nurse," *Hospitals, JAHA* 40 (1966): 112–122.

8. Solomon Fabricant, *A Primer on Productivity* (New York: Random House, Inc., 1969).

9. John W. Kendrick, *Understanding Productivity* (Baltimore: Johns Hopkins Press, 1977).

10. James L. Price, *The Study of Turnover* (Ames, Iowa: The Iowa State University Press, 1977): 110–119. This includes an extended discussion of the impact of turnovers on organizational effectiveness.

11. Dan R. Dalton and William D. Tudor, "Turnover Turned Over: An Expanded and Positive Perspective," *The Academy of Management Review* 4 (1979): 225–235.

12. James L. Price and Charles W. Mueller, *Professional Turnover: The Case of Nurses* (Jamaica, N.Y.: SP Medical and Scientific Books, 1980).

13. Richard T. Mowday, Richard M. Steers, and Lyman W. Porter, "The Measurement of Organizational Commitment," *Journal of Vocational Behavior* 14 (1979): 224–247. Our view of the commitment is the same as the one advanced by Porter and his colleagues as described in this article.

14. Price, *The Study of Turnover*, pp. 28–29.

15. Price and Mueller, *Professional Turnover,* Chapters 5–7. This work offers more detail about the use of the correlates.

16. The total N does not add up to 1,091 because in seven cases data concerning type of training were missing.

17. Two nurses did not indicate whether they worked full time or part time.

18. Nurses who submitted letters of resignation effective by October 1, 1977, also were considered as leavers.

19. Nurses who resigned because of very serious illness also were considered to be involuntary leavers.

20. This 19 percent refers to the instability rate and not the crude turnover rate. Use of the latter, as in our introductory comments, would yield a considerably higher statistic.

21. Price, *The Study of Turnovers,* pp. 11–23, includes a discussion of different measures of turnover.

22. Age and amount of time worked (whether full time or part time) are used to obtain these four categories of nurses. This is use of the correlates of turnover to specify our causal model.

23. Fred N. Kerlinger and Elazar J. Pedhazur, *Multiple Regression in Behavioral Research* (New York: Holt, Rinehart, and Winston, 1973).

24. Otis D. Duncan, "Path Analysis: Sociological Examples," *American Journal of Sociology* 72 (1966): 1–16.

25. Net influence refers to a determinant's impact, with the influence of other determinants controlled statistically.

26. The reference here is to the total effects for these determinants. Total effects are calculated by means of the techniques used in path analysis.

27. As was the case when the individual was the unit of analysis, the reference is to total effects.

28. We refer here to the adjusted explained variance. Adjustments are made for the number of variables in the causal model and the size of the sample.

29. Price and Mueller, *Professional Turnover,* Chapter 5.

30. No recommendations are based on length of service and amount of time worked. Although the rate of turnover is higher for the short-service nurse, we do not see how a practical recommendation can be based on this finding. No recommendation is based on amount of time worked because, contrary to what we had been led to expect by hospital administrators, there was no relationship between turnover and amount of time worked. Full-time nurses had a turnover rate of 20 percent, part-time nurses a rate of 19 percent.

31. Roux Van der Merwe and Sylvia Miller, *Measuring Absence and Labor Turnover* (Johannesburg, Republic of South Africa: McGraw-Hill Book Co., 1976).

32. Magali Sarfatti Larson, *The Rise of Professionalism* (Berkeley, Calif.: University of California Press, 1977), p. 70.

33. The "slightly" should be emphasized since integration—that is, close friends in the hospital—did not turn out to be a very important determinant of turnover in our research.

34. Van der Merwe and Miller, *Measuring Absence,* pp. 32–64.

35. Price, *The Study of Turnover,* pp. 11–23. Both this work and the one by Van der Merwe and Miller contain material about the median length of service for leavers.

36. Van der Merwe and Miller, *Measuring Absence,* p. 57.

37. Price and Mueller, *Professional Turnover,* Chapter 5. This provides more information about total effects.

38. Job satisfaction also has an indirect impact on turnover through intent to stay. (As previously indicated, all of these causal relationships are depicted in Figure 27-1.) No recommendations, however, are based on job satisfaction, so the nature of its impact on turnover is not material at this point.

39. We think our causal model is better than our findings indicate because of theoretical and methodological improvements that could be made in our research. These points are discussed in Price and Mueller, *Professional Turnover,* Chapter 8. It should be emphasized that our theory and methodology are basically sound. All research can be improved, and our study is no exception.

28. The Vanishing Operating Room Nurses

HAROLD LAUFMAN

The operating room is getting only a negligible trickle of recruits from the 12,000 nurses graduating from nursing schools each year. For those who are aware that the operating room nurse is vanishing, there seems to be little to do but look for substitute personnel to fill the gap. Medical and nursing administrators, educators, and surgeons concerned with this problem admit defeat in their efforts to get nursing schools to recognize the needs and train undergraduate nurses in operating room work.

ORIGINS OF THE PROBLEM

The two watchdog associations that control the educational programs and certification of nurses in the United States, the American Nurses' Association (ANA) and the National League for Nursing (NLN), have held steadfast in their refusal to make operating room nursing a required part of the undergraduate curriculum. Officially, these associations do not object to individual nursing schools' giving courses in operating room nursing, but that training is not a requirement for certification. Nor do they object to a graduate R.N.'s taking postgraduate training in operating room nursing. But a career in the operating room certainly is not encouraged.

Curiously, almost nowhere in the pamphlet literature of the NLN are the words "surgery" or "operat-

ing room" to be found. Virtually every other specialty of nursing is listed or described, such as obstetrics, social service, psychiatry, pediatrics, and so on—but not surgery.

Ironically, the cover of a fund-raising brochure of the NLN portrays an operating room scene with nurses merrily assisting the surgical team, giving the false impression that the operating room nurse is a product of the NLN's educational philosophy.

Interviews that this writer has had with the leaders who set educational policy for nurses reveal that in their opinion, operating room duty isn't nursing.

Nurse educators believe that the nurse in the operating room is not a nurse, but is an instrument passer, a cleanup maid, or an insensitive technician who doesn't mind taking guff from hot-tempered surgeons. These are actual words used by distinguished nurse educators to support their stand against educating undergraduates for a career in operating room nursing.

The Association of Operating Room Nurses (AORN), a group of 29,000 nurses who are operating room specialists, has no voice whatsoever in undergraduate nursing training. The AORN was formed in 1957 by a few hundred nurses making a career of the operating room who wanted to share their daily problems. By 1970 the AORN had 5,000 members. As a testament to the intensity of interest in such an organization, and to the chagrin of the ANA, the AORN has grown to its present size which, despite its growth by leaps and bounds, represents only 40 to 50 percent of

393

all nurses working in operating rooms in the United States. But many more are needed.

One operating room supervisor commented that at their early meetings, members of the AORN used to discuss operating room techniques, materials handling, and operating room management methods, and cry on each others' shoulders about the fate of their dying race. Their small band did, indeed, have a lot to cry about.

In 1969, the AORN published a "white paper"[1] that started out with a list of legitimate grievances about the plight of the operating room nurse but ended up with a kind of pledge of allegiance to the parent ANA, thereby blowing a big chance of airing the entire problem and its issues.

According to Jerry Peers, executive director of the AORN and architect of its growth to its present strength, the ANA finally is becoming a bit more receptive to undergraduate operating room training. Today, most nursing schools have some kind of operating room observation sessions ranging in length from a few hours to a few days. In some diploma schools, the undergraduate follows a patient through the surgical unit, whereas in associate program schools there is no exposure at all to the operating room. Baccalaureate programs in large university centers, on the other hand, have reinstated undergraduate operating room training on their own, despite educational guidelines of the ANA or NLN.

OPERATING ROOM TECHNICIANS

Out of desperation for operating room nursing personnel, a shortage that has been mounting exponentially since the end of World War II, medical personnel groups agreed that armed forces operating room technicians would be employed to take the place of nurses in civilian hospitals. This seemed feasible because of the satisfactory experiences during the war with enlisted personnel who were trained to be operating room technicians in the armed services. However, the supply of such persons, so plentiful in the wake of World War II and the Korean War, dropped off greatly with the relatively small yield of veterans of the Vietnam War who were willing to take civilian jobs as operating room technicians.

The Office of Economic Opportunity (OEO) then was prevailed upon to offer career training grants to hospitals and medical universities to train the employable unemployed to become operating room technicians. To carry out this program, however, it was necessary for already overworked operating room nurse personnel to be assigned to teaching. In many large

inner-city hospitals, these weary nurses took on the additional burden of training their replacements while they carried a full schedule of operating room duties. The budgets of most hospitals had no room for a full-time inservice training nurse. Usually such a person worked part time at operating room duties and part time as inservice instructor. Most government-funded programs have been discontinued for lack of funding.

To compound this inequity, the hospital workers' union regulations required that technicians be paid for overtime, where in the 1950s and 1960s the nurses had no union to make demands for them. Operating room nurses who had to assist in the middle-of-the-night emergency operations or in those that extended well past their regular working day never were compensated on an overtime basis in the past. It was considered part of their dedication to duty. So here was the paradoxical situation of the nurse working overtime for nothing, side by side with pupils who collected overtime pay for overtime duty. In time, this disparity was corrected by individual hospitals only under threat of a walkout by the operating room nurses, but as far as the author knows, it still is only an on-paper policy.

It is well known that among all the nurses in the various specialties, no group is more mobile than those who work in operating rooms. If they are experienced, they know they can get a good job in operating room nursing anywhere they go. Operating room staffing patterns, accordingly, suffer further.

But the turnover of techs also is very high. In a survey conducted by the AORN, there is a trend to fill tech positions with nurses in hospitals where they can be recruited. For many years, the AORN has taken the position that techs may serve as scrubbed assistants at the instrument table but should not serve as circulating nurses. Only a nurse should serve in the more responsible circulation or ambulatory role. The survey showed that circulating personnel in operating rooms throughout the country were mostly nurses, and only very seldom were techs.

On the other hand, regulations of the Department of Health, Education, and Welfare (now the Department of Health and Human Services) permit techs to circulate in the operating room. The AORN is waging a legal battle to have these regulations rescinded.

Not only have surgeons felt the pinch of losing surgical nurses but their work has been hampered further by the loss of surgical assistants because of a reduction in surgical residencies. As a result, surgeons have had to turn to professional assistants (P.A.s—Physicians Assistants) and technicians trained in operating techniques for surgical staff. Aside from the genuine grief most surgeons feel about the loss of the "good ole"

OR nurse,[2] a look into the uncertain future raises the question of where to find the PAs and technicians. Surgeons now are performing some 20 million operations each year.

Moreover, the complexity of the procedures places greater demands upon surgical assistance. As the situation now stands, the nation is faced with a paradoxical situation in which the need for operating room nurses and technicians is becoming greater while the supply of nurses of all kinds is becoming smaller and the pool of surgical PAs and technicians is not growing fast enough. Unless this problem is solved, it is obvious that its effects will be felt in the availability to the public of surgical services in general. It is not uncommon even now for the daily schedule of elective surgical operations to be curtailed in large urban hospitals for lack of nursing or support personnel.

THE ADVENT OF SURGICAL PAs

If surgically trained physician assistants had not become available in the past decade, they would have had to be invented by surgeons to fulfill a need created by two paradoxical situations: (1) the paradox of too many surgical residents being trained vs. the dire need for surgical assistants and house surgeons in hospitals; and (2) the paradox of the paucity of trained surgical nurses vs. the discouragement of surgical nursing as a career for nurses.[3]

Until the 1960s, a large proportion of surgical residency positions for young M.D.s were filled by foreign-schooled residents. The prime reason for this situation was that there were more residency positions than American medical school graduates could fill. The reason so many positions were available in the 1950s and the 60s was the direct outgrowth of a combination of factors, including the acceptance by the specialty surgical boards of a nationwide network of Veterans Administration hospitals as well as the rapid increase in the amount of operative surgery being performed in all hospitals in the wake of burgeoning numbers of new hospital beds. A study carried out jointly by the American Surgical Association and the American College of Surgeons in 1973 showed that more surgeons were being trained than could possibly find staff appointments after certification. Surgeons must have staff appointments in a hospital in order to practice their specialty. So the recommendation was to reduce the number of available surgical residents.

How, then, could all the surgical house staff work get done in a training hospital if there were fewer surgical residents? One answer was supplied by the advent of surgical P.A.s.

Physician assistants, many of whom are former members of the military medical corps, military nurses, or medical technicians were conceived as a new health profession in the 1960s. About 60 training programs now are recognized by the various federal health education agencies and the medical associations. Upon certification, P.A.s go into various medical specialties for which they get additional training. Most of the country's 10,000 registered P.A.s work in physicians' offices or clinics. About a third of them are in hospitals, where they are assigned to various medical specialty services such as surgery, pathology, medicine, neurology, and so on. More and more hospitals, especially those with more than 400 beds, are hiring P.A.s to perform many of the necessary tasks previously done by medical or surgical residents.

P.A.s on surgical services not only assist at surgical operations but carry out routine patient-oriented tasks such as history taking, physical examinations, and prescribing certain forms of treatment under a physician's guidance. This has led to some friction between the nursing staff and the P.A.s, reaching a peak when nurses are asked to carry out orders or prescriptions for a patient written by someone who is not a physician. Surgical nurses bridle when a P.A. is allowed to suture a surgical wound or do other quasi-surgical tasks that they never were permitted to do. In other instances, the duties of the P.A. and those of the surgical nurse overlap, but in such cases both the P.A. and the nurse will have been taught by a physician to do the task, whereas the strictly nursing duties will have been taught by a nurse.

The paucity of surgically trained nurses also has been a factor in opening the door to surgical P.A.s. A distinction is made between the role of the surgical nurse in the operating room and that of the P.A. The nurse's role traditionally is that of supervisor, circulating nurse, or scrub nurse, while the role of the P.A. is that of a second or third surgical assistant. The P.A. goes on patient rounds while, lamentably, the operating room nurse usually does not. The duties of operating room nurses have been taken over, in their absence, mostly by operating room technicians, while the P.A.s have assumed a role somewhere between the surgical assistant's function and the resident's floor duties. Yet the presence of P.A.s has lightened the blow of the missing operating room nurse by their assumption of some advanced nurse duties when technicians do not perform them.

According to Ms. Peers, more and more nurses are trying to get appointments as first surgical assistant, thus vying with P.A.s who have assumed this role at the bidding of surgeons. This trend distresses the

AORN. While the association is trying to clarify nurses' rightful place in the operating room, their competitive attitude toward P.A.s seems to be a dominant constraint. Surgical nurses are reluctant to take orders from P.A.s. They feel that if they are to work in the operating room, and they are just as qualified as P.A.s to do P.A. work, they want to get the salary of a P.A. This is an understandable position, but was overlooked by the surgeons who hailed the advent of P.A.s. To the P.A., surgical assisting is a job. To the nurse, it is a matter of prestige.

JOB DESCRIPTION OF THE SURGICAL NURSE

Great concern over the problem of the disappearing operating room nurse has been expressed for years. The American College of Surgeons, the surgical societies, and the American Medical Association, as well as government agencies, all have been looking for solutions. However, the board of regents of the American College of Surgeons has not supplied an answer to the AORN's request for a job description of the nonsurgeon first assistant. The House of Delegates of the AORN adopted a resolution stating that in the absence of other surgical assistance, a nurse may assume the role as first surgical assistant. Although, in truth, this has been done tacitly for many years, the AORN would like to get a clear statement of approval from the American College of Surgeons.

A perusal of the minutes of some of the meetings of concerned surgeons stretching over many years, as well as interviews with nursing educators who are responsible for setting educational policy, have turned up two curiously interdependent facts, aside from the absence of undergraduate surgical training for nurses:

1. The job definition or description of a nurse is not, and never has been, clear. That is, different people have different ideas of what a nurse's job definition is.
2. The nursing profession has further confounded the issue by taking on the mantle of an independent health care profession, more in competition with the medical profession than in collaboration with it.

Nursing traditionally has been looked upon by the general public as a profession of people with mercy (angels of mercy), compassion for the sick and disabled, and altruism that went beyond mere job description. However, in today's changing world with its inflation and cost-of-living demands, the nation sees the development of unions, strikes, and the threat of walkouts by hospital workers, licensed practical nurses (L.P.N.s), nurses' aides, and even some R.N.s, just as is the case with police and fire forces, school teachers, and other public servants. With this changing picture, it might be useful to review briefly the history of nursing[4] with an eye toward the changing concepts of the nurse's job description through the ages, especially surgical nursing. If history is prologue, perhaps something can be learned of present and future trends.

CHANGING CONCEPT OF NURSING THROUGH HISTORY

Ever since the first nurses were appointed by the bishops of the early Christian church as laywomen who would visit the sick in their homes, the definition of a nurse has been sought. As with most other professions, the role of the nurse in society has changed with the times. Oddly enough, these changes have not always followed scientific advances in medicine. In fact, the history of nursing follows the history of religion, war, social reform, suffrage, women's liberation, and socioeconomic conditions at least as much as it does the history of medicine.

The Early Christian Era

There is no record of nursing, and there may not have been any nursing as we know it, in the first large hospitals such as the huge one founded by Emperor Constantine in AD 330, and the one built about the same time in Caesarea (now part of Israel) by the Greeks.

During the Middle Ages, when the only medicine being practiced was what was left of the Roman traditions and the ecclesiastical medicine of the monasteries, three nursing orders—of men—became prominent. These were the Knights of St. John, the Teutonic Knights, and the Knights of St. Lazarus. These were the knights who went into battle with the crusaders and then retired to attend the sick and wounded. They dressed wounds and offered comforting words. When the Crusaders learned from the Arabs how to establish a hospital, the knights devoted themselves to tending personal and psychological needs. Here, then, were two great influences shaping nursing practice in the Middle Ages—the religious and the military. The care of the sick was considered more a religious than a medical duty. Three orders for women who tended only female patients in special hospitals were designated to correspond with the three male orders of knight hospitalers and were named after the male orders. Regular religious orders thus began to staff the hospitals.

When the Hôtel Dieu in Paris opened its doors in AD 650, it was staffed by a small group of volunteers who looked after the sick. They remained a self-governing religious nursing order called the Augustinian Sisters for 600 years until Pope Innocent IV in 1250 caused them to be cloistered under the rigid rules of St. Augustine. To the present day, in European countries and in England, a nurse is referred to as a "sister" whether or not she belongs to a religious order. Parallel developments took place in other European countries, such as Italy, Germany, and elsewhere. In Italy, it was St. Catherine of Sienna who organized a form of nursing within a religious order; in Germany it was St. Hildegarde, a Benedictine abbess who trained young noblewomen in the care of the sick in her abbey.

In the Middle Ages the human body was considered inferior to the soul and unclean, and therefore it was considered improper for the nurses to perform certain procedures such as enemas or vaginal douches. At the Hôtel Dieu, as at other hospitals, an important duty of the sisters was to minister to the spiritual needs of patients, and religious considerations dominated every activity.

Although a number of notable lay groups of nursing were organized in the Middle Ages, only a few, such as the Beguines of Flanders, flourished as independents for any length of time. Others were managed by religious orders and were cloistered, such as the Order of the Visitation of St. Mary's.

Nursing in Social Reform

Since historians look upon nursing as a social function, nursing was said to have reached its own "dark age" after the Reformation, and they trace today's status of nursing largely to the subsequent developments of social reform.

In the Americas, the early Spanish explorers and the French were emigrants from the split of European nations into Catholic and Protestant states. Their missionaries—Dominicans, Franciscans, and Jesuits—gave rise to corresponding nursing orders. The clergy was largely responsible for care of the sick and wounded. The first American hospital was established by Cortez in 1524 in Mexico City, but the nature of the nursing there is an unknown quantity today. In 1638 the Ursuline Sisters, accompanied by Augustinian nuns, staffed the new Hôtel Dieu in Quebec for teaching nursing as well as caring for the sick.

In the nineteenth and early twentieth centuries, nursing became part of the advancing science and art of medical care, but it was primarily a community ser-

vice. Changes in nursing care of this period reflected the emancipation of women. This movement, in turn, owed much of its impetus to the Industrial Revolution. It has been said that without the various fights for human rights first expressed in the eighteenth century and later as one of the principles of the French Revolution, nursing might have developed as a craft and not as a profession.

The Nightingale Concept of Nursing

Although the training and organization of Protestant nurses had begun before Florence Nightingale, it is generally agreed that she was the one most important influence in the development of nursing as a profession and career as it is known today. However, only part of her life efforts were devoted to the advancement of care of the sick. Her contributions to reforms in the military, the public health service, and public health in Great Britain fall more within the realm of social welfare and public health than they do that of hospital nursing or nursing education.

Her only formal training as a nurse was a three-month stint at the Fliedners' institution at Kaiserworth in Germany, when at the age of 31 in 1851 she accompanied her mother and sister on a trip to "take the cure" at Carlsbad and stayed to work at the hospital. As a young debutante, her interest in hospital reform was so keen that she became something of an authority on the subject before she had even this meager training. In fact, after Miss Nightingale's brief visit to Kaiserworth, she published a 32-page pamphlet with the ponderous title, "The Institution of Kaiserworth on the Rhine for the Practical Training of Deaconesses Under the Direction of the Rev. Paster Fliedner, Embracing the Support and Care of a Hospital, Infant and Industrial Schools and a Female Penitentiary."

When she was appointed superintendent of a nursing home for governesses in London, she soon reorganized the institution. But she quickly became restless, wanting to visit other hospitals and collect facts for nursing reforms. She apparently realized, perhaps because of her own lack of organized training, that before reform could be launched some type of school for the training of reliable and qualified nurses must be organized. She became a consultant to hospitals and to doctors who were beginning to recognize the need for trained nurses.

A fact about Miss Nightingale that present-day nurse educators might well ponder is her realization of the importance of nurses in surgery. In fact, when a Dr. Bowman, a well-known surgeon of the day, was to perform a difficult operation on a patient under chloroform, the new anesthetic, Miss Nightingale agreed to assist as his operating room nurse. Here, certainly, was Florence Nightingale's recognition of the importance of the nurse in the operating room, the very role deemphasized by present-day nursing educators.

Miss Nightingale's definition of what constitutes a good nurse may be reread with profit:

A woman who takes a sentimental view of nursing [which she calls "ministering"] is of course, worse than useless. A woman possessed with the idea that she is making a sacrifice will never do; and a woman who thinks that any kind of nursing work is "beneath a nurse" will simply be in the way.

For us who nurse, our nursing is a thing, which, unless in it we are making progress every year, every month, every week, take my word for it we are going back. The more experience we gain, the more progress we can make. The progress you make in your year's training with us is as nothing to what you must make each year after your training is over. A woman who thinks of herself "Now I am a full nurse, a skillful nurse. I have learnt all there is to be learnt" take my word for it, she does not know what a nurse is, and she will never know: she has gone back already. Conceit and nursing cannot exist in the same person.[5]

Nursing in America

American nursing developed not only on the precepts of Florence Nightingale but also on independent experiences gained in the Revolutionary War, the Civil War, and the Spanish-American War. Two kinds of nursing developed out of the Civil War: a regular Army Nursing Service and an organization sponsored by private citizens out of which grew the Sanitary Commission. The health and welfare of troops were their central interests, and here again the line between nursing and social service becomes all but unrecognizable.

By the turn of the twentieth century, it became obvious that alumnae associations of the many nursing schools that had been springing up were not a cohesive enough group to carry on a nationwide professional organization. The Nurses' Alumnae Association of the United States and Canada, originally formed in 1897, became the American Nurses' Association in 1911. Its original purposes were "(1) to establish and to maintain a code of ethics, (2) to elevate standards of nursing education, and (3) to promote the usefulness and honor, the financial and other interests of the nursing profession."

Sections of the ANA that have developed include: government nursing section, private duty section, general staff or institutional section, men's nursing section, administrators of nursing section, and industrial nursing section. In 1948, the ANA adopted a platform emphasizing "the expanding role of the American nurse in world affairs, increasing participation of the nurse in national affairs, and expansion of the nursing service to meet the health care needs of the American people."

Another kind of nurses' society, the National League for Nursing, grew out of an exhibit at the 1893 World's Fair in Chicago at which nurses from anywhere could meet and get acquainted. The NLN controls reforms in nursing education and maintains a service that prints, distributes, and grades state board examinations. In 1950, at a convention in Atlantic City, nurses voted to have two national organizations, the American Nurses' Association and the National League for Nursing, and listed the joint and independent activities of the two groups. The AORN was not organized until 1957.

HOW TO DEFINE NURSING?

How, then, in the light of this brief history, can today's nurse be defined? Perhaps it is not too simplistic to say that a nurse is a health care professional who tends the sick in collaboration with other professionals. But such a definition implies cooperation, not competition, involving all health care professionals from technician through medical specialist.

It would include all specialty categories from social medicine through surgery, and would be operational within the framework of changes of the times. Moreover, this definition would allow for individual judgment and action in matters within the capabilities of the nurse, but would recognize the interdependency between nurses and doctors, including surgeons, on the one hand, and between nurses and technical or support personnel, on the other.

The definition does not interfere with any of the declared precepts of the ANA, NLN, nor those of any specialty nursing, medical, or other group, and, equally important, does not restrict an individual's education or field of interest.

WHY WAS OR NURSING DELETED FROM CURRICULA?

As far as the author is able to determine, the decision to omit operating room experience as a required part of undergraduate nursing education grew from two main stems:

1. an effort to make the undergraduate period more attractive to the recruit than an apprenticeship in any environment the student might not like
2. a conviction on the part of nurse educators that operating room duty falls more properly in the realm of technicians than nurses because of its relative absence of personal patient contact and its technical nature.

The reasons behind these beliefs were expressed to the authors by middle-aged nurse educators influential in formulating undergraduate curricula, who remember with a great deal of unpleasantness their own nursing student days of operating room duty. They tell of having to scrub floors, walls, and sinks; clean instruments; pass instruments to surgeons during operations; and do menial, unprofessional tasks, only to be rewarded by rudeness (and even cruelty) from surgeons and operating room supervisors. They recall several student nurses' dropping out of training during or after their period of operating room experience.

The unhappy memories of these distinguished educators undoubtedly are accurate, the effect of their experiences upon their psyches is understandable, and their efforts to correct the situation certainly are commendable. But when they were asked how recently they had revisited an operating room, none had done so for several years. None was aware of the fact that operating room nurses today no longer scrub floors; that instrument passing during operations is largely being done by technicians or by nurses who are considered to be part of the surgical team, and that for almost every rude, heartless surgeon, there is a kind thoughtful one.

These nurse educators are the ones who believe that operating room training should be withheld until the graduate period—that is, after the RN or baccalaureate. In the author's opinion, this concept might be reasonable provided there was at least enough exposure to the operating room during the undergraduate period to have whetted the appetite of the students. If the individuals never are exposed to it, how can they know whether or not they would like it? After all, some of the former classmates of today's antioperating-room educators were attracted to it even in the old days, and today are operating room supervisors, teachers, and leaders in OR nurse training.

Moreover, if nurses are truly coprofessionals with physicians, they should understand that in medical school many courses are required and offered, some of which will appeal to students more than others. A med-

ical school education without exposure to courses in surgery, surgical physiology, and surgical pathology can hardly be called a good medical education, no matter what specialty is pursued later. Not all medical students become surgeons, but unless some practical exposure to the subject is experienced, how can the student know? Sometimes a student is influenced positively or negatively by a teacher, by a fellow student, or by an incident. But without the exposure, the education is incomplete.

In response to this opinion, nurse educators contend there are "too many specialties" filling the nurse undergraduate's time to allow for surgery in the curriculum. A moment's reflection on this comment reveals a selectivity borne of obvious prejudice. The fact is that surgical care is a major segment of all patient care and is among the fastest growing of medical specialties. Until three decades ago, no more than 30 percent of the hospitalized patients in civilian life were admitted for surgical operations. A decade ago, this figure reached 50 percent. Today, it is close to 60 percent in many hospitals. Here, then, is an undeniable trend that will require more and more nurses, in the writer's estimation, not only in the operating room but in surgical intensive care units, in surgical clinics, and in other surgical patient care areas.

The close interdependence between surgery and surgical intensive care nursing was exemplified a few years ago by a threat of surgeons and surgical nurses to strike or quit a hospital in New York because the administrator, in an ill-fated effort to economize, announced that he was closing the surgical intensive care unit after the day shift and on weekends. The surgeons argued that they could not possibly take care of the surgical load without the ICU and its nursing care. After a public clamor and newspaper publicity, the surgeons won out, and the unit stayed open.

A thought to think upon: would nurse-educators change their minds in favor of undergraduate operating room nurse education if they themselves had to undergo a surgical operation? How would they react to being greeted in the holding area of the surgical suite not by a nurse, but by technicians and other nonnurse personnel? How would they react to being attended to in the recovery room or surgical intensive care unit by strictly nonnurse attendants? Such a situation is happening today in some hospitals.

HIGH TURNOVER RATE OF OR NURSES

The National Commission for the Study of Nursing and Nursing Education recognizes that high withdrawal rates of nurses from the profession, high turnover, and frustration symptoms still plague nursing today. In the light of such an analysis, perhaps nurse educators should reexamine their stand on surgical education. The situation has existed for 20 years. Removal of surgical training from the undergraduate curriculum did not prevent dropouts or high turnover, but did create a drastic shortage of surgical nurses in the face of an increase in nurse practitioners, and may be largely responsible for today's dilemma.

Despite the efforts of nurse-educators to make nursing a more attractive career, the ranks of R.N.s of all types are being depleted at a rapid pace. Graduate nurses are quitting the profession and going into other pursuits. The reasons given for this exodus are comparatively low wages for hard work, too rigorous a routine for young nurses, and the loss of the facade of glamor from the profession. It has been estimated that the present population of 1,500,000 R.N.s in the United States will shrink by 400,000 by 1985 at the present rate of depletion. This prediction alone could further deplete the ranks of operating room nurses by one-third if they leave the fold at the same rate as others. However, nurses who chose an operating room career tend to remain in that field despite their tendency to flit from one OR job to another, so their ranks may not diminish as much as those of others. Nonetheless, the shortage of OR nurses is a hard fact.

In other words, it would appear that nursing education has painted itself into a corner by deemphasizing appropriate education in specific areas of needs, such as surgery, and overemphasizing ego-satisfying but not necessarily crucially needed careers in nursing.

NURSING AS AN INDEPENDENT HEALTH CARE PROFESSION

The ANA appears to be trying to alter the job definition of nursing by endorsing the development of nurse practitioners. It can only be assumed that this is the result of an effort to upgrade the lot of the nurse and perhaps persuade more nurses to remain in the profession and not leave the fold. Nurses now are being encouraged to consider themselves a separate wing of the patient care scene, independent of the doctor, practicing diagnostic and therapeutic medicine on their own. No matter how lightly one wishes to view this scene, the now-accepted term of nurse practitioner translates into nurse-doctor. Nurse practitioners may hang out a shingle, act as primary physicians, and refer patients to specialist-physicians much the way a general practitioner M.D. refers patients to specialist M.D.s. The big difference is that the R.N. practitioner, at least at this writing, needs no special qualifications other than the R.N. certification in order to be a nurse-practitioner and to assume the responsibilities of a primary care physician.

An operating room nurse by definition is one who helps, supports, or assists the surgeon rather than one who performs the operation. If the next step is the emergence of the nurse-surgeon, then it is to be hoped that proper qualifications would be demanded by those in charge of certifying and qualifying surgeons, rather than a lack of reaction so far shown by organized medicine to the emergence of the nurse practitioner.

Reflecting on this probability, it can be wondered whether today's movement to make nursing an independent health care profession might have had its origin either in a "get-even" complex or in an effort to make the nursing profession more attractive than the nurse-educators find it.

Interestingly, the medical profession, including surgical specialists, do not generally consider themselves as an independent health care profession. Conversations the author has had with many fellow surgeons reveal the genuine feeling surgeons have about the *inter*dependence of the three legs of any medical care effort—medicine, nursing, and administration, not necessarily in that order. One leg cannot hold its own without the two others in today's world of sophisticated medical care.

In settings such as day-to-day patient care and contact, either inside or outside the hospital, the nurse certainly is the dominant health care person. In other settings such as institutional medicine and the efficient management of hospitals, administration assumes an especially dominant role. In still other settings, such as diagnostic and therapeutic medicine in all its specialties, the physician, either generalist or specialist, is the dominant provider of direct patient care. But in all settings, all three play the same role; the only difference is one of degree.

The illogic of attempting to make nursing an independent health care profession for whatever reason is equalled only by the illogic of assuming that medicine can be made an independent profession without the need for nursing and administration. The "separate-but-equal" philosophy professed by the ANA policysetters cannot work in all situations for the very reason of the nature of medical care itself. Some situations require dominance of nurses, others dominance of physicians, and still others dominance of administrators.

In the operating room, the surgeon of necessity must assume the dominant role most of the time. The surgeon relinquishes this role to the anesthesiologist for the physiological support of the patient under anesthesia. The surgeon also may relinquish the dominant role by designating an assistant to perform a maneuver during an operation or to close an incision. The assistant may be a resident or intern M.D., or it may be a P.A., or a nurse. In any case, a surgeon who designates someone else to do a part of the operation remains the legally responsible party in the event of a mishap. Knowing this, the surgeon must have full confidence in the designee's capabilities.

BENEFITS OF OR EDUCATION

Naomi Nisenson, R.N., the late operating room supervisor of Montefiore Hospital, New York, always maintained that the undergraduate nurse would gain immeasurably in education, in maturity, and in stature by receiving up-to-date exposure to the role of the nurse in the operating room. She outlined the following points:

1. *Direct patient care.* Nurses in the operating room are charged with the responsibility of establishing and maintaining aseptic techniques and an aseptic environment.

   Nurses are responsible for the patient's physical and psychological comfort during the preoperative holding period, in the operating room up to the moment of unconsciousness, as well as in the waking period during the crucial period in recovery room or intensive care unit.

   The postanesthesia recovery period places on the nurse a direct patient care responsibility unmatched in any other area of nursing except that in other intensive care environments.

2. *The OR as an educational laboratory.* No better laboratory can be provided for the student nurse to observe, learn and participate in:

   a. teamwork
   b. participation in patient safety and comfort
   c. aseptic techniques
   d. preoperative maneuvers, medications, and psychological management
   e. direct visualization of normal and abnormal anatomy, physiologic responses and actual pathology as encountered in the patient. Such direct exposure cannot be matched by any amount of viewing of slides or motion pictures.

3. *Preparation for all other fields of specialization.* How many nurses have actually seen a heart valve and watched it being inserted; ob-

served the heart sewed up, and then resume its own beat after the extracorporeal pump is disconnected from the patient? How many have actually watched a coronary artery shunt, a blood vessel graft, or a kidney graft? How many have helped during an operation to replace an entire hip joint with a metal-and-plastic prosthesis? A nurse's direct benefits from being present during any of these or other surgical operations include clearer understanding of postoperative limitations in activity, alimentation, physiological changes, and dependency on good nursing management.

Even the nurse who is a primary care practitioner can be a better one if she has had OR experience in her educational period. She is better able to recognize the problems of the surgical patient, or the one who may need surgery. She will have acquired a keener insight into the needs of all patients, nonsurgical as well as surgical. She is cognizant of what the patient had to experience, or will have to experience, while in the hospital, and is in a position to understand the finer nuances of contraindications to surgery and post-operative rehabilitation. In short, no matter what specialty a nurse ends up practicing, whether it be public health, primary care or psychiatry, an educational experience in the OR forms an essential part of her professional capability.

A patient should not cease to exist with respect to nursing once that patient goes through the OR doors.[6]

SUPPRESSION WITHOUT REPRESENTATION

In the world of industry, when decisions are made for the distribution and assignment of personnel, management science requires specific job descriptions, definitions of staffing requirements, and an orderly process of analysis of needs and capabilities. Such analyses usually are carried out by industrial engineers or systems engineers.

The history of nursing reveals that the job description of nurses parallels closely the socioeconomic as much as it does the technological history of the world. Hence, it should not be surprising that the current uncertain job description for nurses reflects an amalgam of today's confused world. As throughout history, today's socioeconomic conditions have led to demands for higher wages, formation of unions, equal rights requirements and the development of social care nursing, while technological and scientific advances are responsible for the development of specialist nurse education in such fields as intensive care nursing, nuclear medicine nursing, and special procedure nursing. But strangely, the operating room, where some of the greatest leaps in technology have been made, has eluded, or more accurately has been bypassed, by those to whom nurse education is entrusted.

To the best of the author's knowledge, no management science study preceded the decision of the NLN to exclude operating room nursing from the undergraduate curriculum. Yet this decision was made and has resulted in depriving operating rooms of nurses. It also has resulted in almost depriving surgical nurses of their identity.

But not quite. There still are enough dedicated operating room nurses to demand representation on decision-making committees of the ANA and NLN, or to work outside these structures, to restore the operating room nurse to a rightful place in the sun.

NOTES

1. "Definition and Objective for Clinical Practice of Professional Operating Room Nursing," *AORN Journal* 10 (1967): 4–47.
2. Harold Laufman, "What's Happened to the Good Ole OR Nurse?" *AORN Journal* 17 (1973): 61–70.
3. *Nurse Clinician and Physician's Assistant: The Relationship Between Two Emerging Practitioner Concepts*. The National Commission for the Study of Nursing and Nursing Education, February 12, 1971.
4. A. E. Pavey, *The Story of the Growth of Nursing* (London: Faber and Faber, Ltd., 1938), p. 296.
5. Florence Nightingale, The Institution of Kaiserworth on the Rhine for the Practical Training of Deaconesses. Privately published, London, 1853.
6. Naomi Nisenson, "Comments on What's Happened to the Good Ole OR Nurse?" by Harold Laufman in *AORN Journal* 17 (1973): 61–70.

29. Medical Center Activities Program

INEZ GREENSTADT

Many companies and medical centers offer extra benefits to employees, volunteers, and students through various types of activities programs. The type of program offered depends on many factors, the most important of which is the philosophy of the institution. The philosophy is reflected in funding for the program, which is the second major factor. The third factor is where the institution is located in conjunction with the types of facilities and opportunities available for use in an activities program.

Before an organization can consider an activities program, a number of key questions must be addressed:

1. What is our philosophy concerning employees, volunteers, and students?
2. What are our objectives?
3. How will the program be organized and administered?
4. How much will it cost?
5. How will the costs be met?
6. What facilities are available?
7. What kinds of programs are needed?
8. What about liability?

Each institution will have to seek out answers to these questions, which of course will vary with each group.

SUGGESTED ACTIVITIES PROGRAM OBJECTIVES

Companies or health care institutions thinking about developing or expanding an activities program can consider these general objectives:

1. Providing opportunities to participate in various activities.
2. Providing and developing opportunities to express needs and interests.
3. Developing channels of communication between members and management.
4. Acting as a positive force in maintaining the morale of members.
5. Providing discounts and various types of consumer information.
6. Strengthening and improving relationships among students, volunteers, employees, and management.
7. Giving opportunities to develop leadership qualities.
8. Improving and maintaining the physical and mental health of employees and students.
9. Reducing employee-student apathy, absenteeism, and turnover.
10. Fostering good community relations through employee-student-volunteer involvement and contributions.

11. Promoting continuing personal and professional educational opportunities.

12. Providing an activities-consumer program that assists in the recruitment of students, staff, and volunteers.

13. Assisting in preparing employees for retirement and providing recreational services to retirees.

14. Assisting employees, students, and their families in planning vacation and leisure activities.

15. Offering assistance to employees and students. (The type of assistance offered will depend on the qualifications of the person(s) working in the program.)

16. Assisting patients, their families, and friends during the hospital experience by offering recreational-consumer information.

These objectives are the ones used to develop the activities-consumer program in The Mount Sinai Medical Center in New York City. This case history also presents general information that might be helpful in establishing similar programs.

CASE HISTORY OF AN ACTIVITIES PROGRAM

The Mount Sinai Medical Center probably has one of the most comprehensive activities programs for employees, volunteers, and students in the country. The program reflects the attitudes and values of the center's board of directors and administration. Mount Sinai has some 7,000 employees, including 800 residents and interns, as well as 1,000 students from many schools. The major student body consists of about 600 medical and graduate students. The Medical Center also has a medical faculty of about 1,200, plus 300 volunteers. The center fortunately is located adjacent to one of New York's greatest recreational areas— Central Park. The center also has many facilities for recreational activities; i.e., two gymnasiums, several auditoriums, and many meeting rooms. The varied recreational opportunities available in New York City make it possible to provide comprehensive programs for students and staff.

The activities program grew out of one provided for nursing students in the center. The school of nursing provided funds for the creation of a program for students involving socials, special interest groups, and theater, concert, and opera tickets. The program administrator was asked to expand it and make it available to the entire medical center when the nursing school closed in 1970.

At present, the recreational-consumer program is divided into four parts: the ticket program, the activities program, the consumer program, and the general counseling and recreational program. To have an effective program, it is necessary to have at least one person responsible for it. The assistants can be either volunteers or employees whose assignments are considered part of their work time.

The Mount Sinai program is run by volunteers, student interns, and paid personnel. The director is aided by a recreational assistant who is responsible for student activities and an administrative assistant in charge of office procedures. The salary for the recreational director is paid out of the personnel department's budget. The recreational assistant is paid by a federal grant plus personnel department funds. The personnel department provides $3,000 annually for program expenses. The funds are used for office supplies, professional memberships, travel and meetings, books and periodicals, refreshments for committee meetings, and parties for those who donate their services to the program.

The Ticket Program

In view of the fact that the medical center is located in an area that is the center for all kinds of events— from track meets to concerts—the ticket program probably is the most popular activity. In the course of a year, 40,000 tickets are distributed to students, patients, volunteers, and staff. Some of the tickets are donated to the institution but the majority are obtained at a substantial discount. In the case of a top hit, tickets are bought at full price. If an event is offered, employees and students may request at least two tickets, and if the supply is substantial they may obtain tickets for families and friends.

At Mount Sinai, those who wish to participate in the ticket program obtain membership cards for a $5 fee (employees and volunteers) or $2.50 (students). Members' cards are marked according to the number of tickets obtained. Each card is valid for ten tickets. The cards bear no expiration date, and members may obtain as many as they wish. If members leave the institution without completing their cards, they can request a refund. The monies accumulated from these fees are given to the medical center.

It should be feasible for almost any institution to offer a ticket program. If an institution is not convenient to the entertainment center, buses or other transportation can be used to convey people to the events. Should transportation be required, it usually is advisable to combine the tickets with some sort of dinner arrangement; discount dinner arrangements can be made if a group is involved. At Mount Sinai, dinners are not too popular so they rarely are included.

To offer a complete ticket program, a cooperative effort with other groups can be considered. Mount Sinai Hospital cooperates with four other groups in its program, often making joint purchases of tickets or exchanging them for different events. To obtain a discount on tickets, (or even to buy tickets to popular shows) a minimum order—usually 20 to 25 tickets—must be placed. By pooling resources, tickets to all kinds of events can be ordered, providing a complete program.

For an institution interested in starting a ticket program, the following suggestions are offered:

1. Place one person in complete charge of the program. That person can have assistants, but one person must be responsible.
2. Arrange for some kind of service charge. The membership card can be used as a receipt, and the fees can be used to offset salaries and other expenses.
3. Limit the hours when tickets may be obtained. At Mount Sinai, tickets are distributed from 9 to 9:30 a.m. and from 12:30 p.m. to 5:30 p.m. The hours may be determined by the number of tickets available and the population of the institution.
4. Work out a system to take care of night personnel so that no one is deprived of the service.
5. Try to obtain tickets for events that would interest all types of people.
6. Make sure the person responsible for the program is knowledgeable with regard to the events or has material available to explain them to the group.
7. Develop an effective method of informing people about the available events. Mount Sinai uses a taped message announcing all events, bulletin boards, and the weekly newsletter that is distributed to all major departments.
8. Take no reservations without payment. This is most crucial in formulating a good program. To assure fair service for all, develop a program that facilitates payments by employees and students. The only difficulty encountered at Mount Sinai occurs when there is a deviation from procedures.
9. Establish a policy that once someone has purchased a ticket, it is theirs. If they wish to resell it, Mount Sinai will list it again, but will not return the service charge nor their money. Any-

one who buys the ticket pays the owner of the ticket, not the medical center.
10. Consider the possibility of having a theater club checking account.
11. Ask the volunteer department to assign people to work with the ticket program. Mount Sinai has had seven volunteers helping. In addition, employees assist during lunch periods.
12. Feel that the ticket program is worthwhile. It is a wonderful way to help employees, volunteers, and students enjoy their leisure time and get them out of the often depressing, all-consuming hospital atmosphere.

The Activities Program

The second important program is the Employee-Student Activities Association. This association was started three years ago by the recreational director, assisted by student interns studying recreation. At the time, there were a few activities (symphony orchestra, bowling teams, basketball and softball teams, and a few special classes). The recreational director decided to try to develop a more comprehensive program, and used the interns to help organize it. The recreational director selected about 20 persons from all walks of life to be on the planning committee. The people selected were those who seemed to be creative and interested in a wide variety of things. The committee members had a series of meetings at lunch time, developed preliminary questionnaires and took them back to their departments for distribution. The committee submitted its findings to administration for suggestions and approval. After several conferences, the following guidelines were developed for all activities:

1. The activity must be consistent with the general philosophy of The Medical Center.
2. The activity must meet all safety standards and must be covered legally.
3. All special interest groups must be self-sustaining. The Medical Center provides space for meetings and prints notices about activities. All other expenses must be borne by members of the group.
4. All leaders must be volunteers. The volunteers can lead groups only during their off-duty hours. Volunteers also could be outsiders who would register with the volunteer department.
5. All groups must hold their sessions during employee and student off-duty hours. If an event is scheduled during the lunch period, lunch may be eaten during the meeting.

6. The director of recreational activities coordinates all group activities until the Employee-Student Activities Committee is firmly established with officers, committees, and written rules and regulations.
7. The director of recreational activities acts as the adviser to the group and as the liaison with administration.
8. Any activity must be cancelled if the space is needed for official Medical Center business.
9. Employee volunteers who take leadership positions that may involve telephone calls at work, or some other time commitment during the workday, must obtain permission from their supervisors before assuming the responsibility.
10. All committee chairpersons, officers, and group leaders must follow established Medical Center procedures in making room reservations, use of bulletin boards, writing publicity materials, care and use of space reserved, etc. The director of recreational activities advises the groups concerning correct procedures.

In 1977, the committee recruited a number of volunteer leaders, found space, and sent a memo to all students and employees outlining the program. The committee encouraged suggestions from everyone in The Medical Center. In the beginning, the following activities were offered:

indoor gardening
sketching and drawing
macrame
backgammon
exercise classes
volleyball
beginners tennis
beginners Spanish
beginners French
conversational French
chess
special programs on:
  jogging
  bicycling
  sailing

The bowling league, softball and basketball teams, and symphony orchestra were encouraged to keep the members informed about their activities, and representatives from these continuing groups were asked to join the general committee.

During the first year, the recreational director and the student interns assumed all responsibility for the program. As leaders emerged, they were encouraged

to be a part of the planning committee to develop bylaws for the association. Monthly lunch-hour meetings were held with departmental representatives and all others interested. Gradually, the group decided on an internal structure and completed its bylaws. The group concluded that the executive committee should be composed of a president, vice-president, secretary, treasurer, and director of publicity. The following standing committees were established: sports and physical fitness, educational and cultural, games and creative activities, social and special events, and consumer and civic action. It was hoped that all the activities would fit into one of these categories and that the head of each standing committee would be in close touch with the leaders of all groups under their jurisdiction. The executive committee and the chairperson of the standing committee compose the steering committee. The adviser is the director of recreational activities, whose function was defined as follows:

1. Act as management's adviser to the executive committee.
2. Be responsible for reporting to the executive and steering committees any relevant administration policies; provide as much information or insight as needed on administration procedures.
3. Be responsible for working with the committees to obtain administrative approval for all major new proposals.
4. Assist in the development of programs appropriate to fulfilling the goals of the association.
5. Solicit and supervise field work students and any other persons to work with the Employee-Student Activities Association.

The volunteer leader idea has proved to be a very positive force. These volunteers' resourcefulness, creativity, talent, and genuine interest in people were impressive. The following list of activities sponsored by The Medical Center in the last three years does not include social events, holiday parties, and religious observances sponsored by various departments. For example, the medical and graduate students sponsor many events each year, independent of the Employee-Student Activities Association. The recreational office offers assistance to the schools and other departments in planning their own events.

ACTIVITIES IN THE MOUNT SINAI MEDICAL CENTER—1977–1980

All activities were led by volunteers unless marked *. The activities using outside facilities are marked #.

Languages

Intermediate French
Beginners French
Conversational French
Beginners Spanish
Conversational Spanish
Beginners Hebrew
Conversational Hebrew
Beginners Italian
Conversational Italian
Beginners Arabic
Conversational Hungarian

Special Interest Groups

Knitting and Crocheting
Bible Study
Photography Class
Overeaters Anonymous
  (two groups)
Lose Weight Discussion Groups
Home Computer Group
Gourmet Cooking Classes
Crewel and Quilting
Juggling
New Games
Macrame
Indoor Gardening
Music—Drama—Art
Guitar (Beginners)
Guitar (Intermediate)
Choral Group*
Mount Sinai Symphony Orchestra*
Performing Dance Group
Disco Dancing
Hustle Dancing
Hebrew Dancing
Sketching and Drawing

Table Games

Beginners and Advanced Bridge
Beginners and Advanced Chess
Beginners and Advanced Backgammon

Physical Programs

Basketball Teams
Softball Teams
Bowling League #
Soccer Teams
Karate Classes
Yoga Classes
Exercise Classes

---

*Leader was paid from funds in special grants.

Horseback Riding* #
Beginners Tennis
Intermediate Tennis #
Volleyball
Squash Club #

Special Events Sponsored in the Last Two Years

Yearly Arts Festival
  (for one week)
Makeup Workshops
Nutrition Workshops and participation in special
  programs
Stop Smoking Clinics with American Cancer
  Society
Meditation Seminar
Fix It Workshops with Handivan (plumbing and
  electric wiring)
Fashion Show
Disco Parties
Wine and Cheese Parties
Interior Decorating Workshops
Tips on Bicycling
Tips on Jogging
Tips on Sailing
Tips on Skiing
Day Trips
Weekend Trips
Workshops on Consumer Buying
Workshops in Banking
Ounce of Prevention (see details later in this
  article)

Ideas Being Considered

Disco Roller Skating
Outdoor Roller Skating
Evening of Wine with Live Classical Music
Literary Journal
More Trips
Retirement Seminar
Kite Workshop
Estate Planning
Travel Workshops
Share Your Hobby Meetings
The Great Clearance Sale (giving everyone a
  chance to recycle anything they wish)

Other Activities

Swimming and other gym activities are available
  in the nearby YMHA, where discount
  memberships have been arranged. Discounts
  also are available with other health clubs. A
  listing of free pools is available.

Perhaps the most prestigious program was the one in which heads of medical departments talked about their specialties. A committee was established that worked with the Employee Health Service in scheduling the events. The programs were not offered to the community, but future programs were to be publicized and anyone in the community invited to attend. The idea that a Medical Center is willing to educate the public in what is going on in medicine is appealing. Too often, citizens/employees feel they are not allowed to participate or even to comprehend what is happening in medicine. Developing public forums on medicine should be very helpful to everyone. Mount Sinai cast itself as a pioneer in letting the public meet its top doctors to hear what they have to say.

This is the schedule for the Ounce of Prevention Program:

January 8:   THE POST-HOLIDAY BLUES . . . The Blahs, Depression, and Other Sorrows.
February 5: THE AIR AROUND US: What You Should Know About Environmental Pollution.
March 5:   KEEP SMILING: Dental Care from Milk Teeth to Maturity.
April 2:   WHAT ABOUT WEIGHT: Calories and Carbohydrates.
May 7:   SHAPE UP FOR SUMMER: Exercise for Everyone.

The activities program has been one of the most exciting offered in The Medical Center and has only scratched the surface. Additional programs were to be started when a more effective means of communication with employees, volunteers, and students could be developed. Any medical center or hospital has many experts available. They range from experts in child care, nutrition, home repairs, air conditioning, basic health information, and psychiatric information to employees and students with special interests who are willing (and often eager) to share their knowledge with others.

If it should be decided that leaders would be hired for some special groups, they would be asked to accept a payment lower than it would be outside and the group would be very careful in its selection of such leaders. Any paid leader would have to be approved by the steering committee. The group doubted that it would go in the direction of paying leaders but believed it soon would start asking all members to make a small contribution when they joined an activity. The money would be used for special events for the group

and for a present for the leader at the end of the course.

The Consumer Program

The third major sequence is the consumer program. It often is possible to obtain discounts from many different sources, simply by asking. Often, local merchants are willing to give employees and students a discount if they show their I.D. cards. To develop a program, a form should be prepared requesting the group contacted to fill in all of the necessary information. This should include discount rates, the items covered, method of identification, length of time the discount will be allowed, and hours and location of the agency. Many companies are located in areas that have established buying services. If the area has buying services, investigate the potential of one in the organization. Many times there is a fee involved for membership, but it usually is waived if the group joining is sufficiently large.

At Mount Sinai, discounts are available for health clubs, restaurants, eyeglasses, luggage, records, furniture, major appliances, hotels, car rentals, magazines, clothing, shoes, Disneyland and Disney World as well as other tourist attractions, cars, florists, etc. The group belongs to four buying services, and employees and students are encouraged to check with all four when they anticipate making large purchases. Catalogues also are available for discount buying.

The office has a number of books listing various discount stores in the area. Copies of consumer reports and yearly buyers' guide are available. Material regarding funeral societies is made available, as well as data on dental groups that charge low fees, and lists of other places where employees and students can obtain services at a discount. Directories are available listing varied goods and services at discounts and regular prices.

The recreational director is knowledgeable about travel, and assistance is given to employees and students planning vacations. Many companies sponsor group travel activities, but this has not been developed at Mount Sinai. Several attempts were made to sponsor group travel opportunities, but it was found that interest could not be generated despite the apparent savings. However, an institution probably could achieve a considerable saving if all travel could be booked through the same agent, and if group rates could be used in sending people to conferences and conventions. A travel agent also could help professionals to combine seminars and meetings with their vacation plans. Several agencies specialize in this type of package and are eager to cooperate in establishing tax deductible vacations. The program also has its own directory of favorite restaurants.

Mount Sinai presents employees and students with opportunities to advertise goods and/or services they wish to make available to others. This is done by established bulletin boards, listings in the weekly intrainstitutional newspaper, and a directory of services in the recreational-consumer office. Notices are posted to help personnel form car pools, locate apartments, roommates, or to lease their apartments or sell their homes. This program has been well received.

The General Counseling and Recreation Program

The fourth part of the recreational-consumer program is the general counseling and recreation program. The recreational director is knowledgeable about schools, religious organizations, social clubs, and many other opportunities available in the area. This person spends time with new personnel and students, giving them an orientation to the New York City area, answering questions about special interests, and is ready to aid them in finding answers to their questions and/or needs. In addition, the Employee Health Service sponsors a special employee assistance program that offers personal counseling.

The counseling in the recreational office is geared toward assisting people to make social contacts and to obtain information that might enhance the quality of their lives. For example, the recreational director may encourage individuals to join a social club where special opportunities could be offered to develop their interests. Or, the director might give them a listing of adult education courses they might enjoy. If they have guests from out of town, the director will plan an entire week of activities for the visitors and furnish them with city maps and directories. The director assists in planning weddings and special events and helps in many diverse areas. Any employee or student can make an appointment to discuss special interests and needs.

In the general recreational program, the recreational office works with many groups in The Medical Center that ask for assistance. The office helps medical and graduate students in their orientation and general activity programs. Training is given to student leaders, and students are encouraged to initiate different types of programs. They also are given assistance in their fund-raising endeavors. Student memberships for museums and the YMHA are distributed from the recreational office. Office personnel schedule rooms for socials and also are responsible for the gymnasium schedule. The office compiled a student directory, including information about New York City. This will supplement the student handbook, which contains official information needed by all students. The office recently became responsible for the annual Medical Center Art Festival, which had been sponsored by the public relations department.

The recreational director is one of the managers in the personnel department, attends all managers' meetings, helps develop recruitment programs, gives orientations to all new employees, and participates in general Medical Center programs.

The Recreational director worked with other groups in planning a program in retirement counseling as well as a more comprehensive program for Medical Center retirees. Retirees are invited to an annual cocktail party and a few participate in the ticket program. One volunteered to work with the recreational director in planning activities for retirees. Retirees can obtain books on retirement, lists of discounts, listings of agencies and organizations that can offer assistance and information to senior citizens, etc.

The tentative outline for the retirement counseling program is as follows:

1. *Social Security:* Ask someone from Social Security to talk to employees about all of the ins and outs of the program. Request that the speaker include information about Medicare and Medicaid.
2. *Benefits:* Schedule meetings with all employees to discuss the benefits the institution offers. It may be necessary to schedule different meetings if the benefit plan varies for the different in-house groups. Include information on medical plans for retirees, retirement benefits, optional plans for annuity programs, insurance programs, etc.
3. *Finance:* Arrange for an authority to talk to the general group about making financial plans for retirement. This individual should discuss the development of realistic plans concerning budgeting, income, and expenses. Information should be available about retirement communities, ways to invest money to help plan for retirement, and general information.
4. *Legal:* Arrange for a lawyer to inform the group about wills, taxes, and contracts. Often, the intrainstitutional legal department can provide this service. Income taxes should be discussed to provide information on deductions that might be available.
5. *Physical and Mental Health:* Members of the medical staff should be asked to present a program discussing potential problems and how to

deal with them. This can be a positive program about nutrition, exercise, etc.

6. *Second Careers, Leisure, and Use of Time:* This program can be organized to give information about possible second careers, supplemented with ways individuals can develop interests to help them use leisure time.

If a program on retirement is offered, all members of the recreation staff should attend since planning for retirement should begin well in advance. Therefore, publicity should be geared to include all employees, also with the hope that many younger employees will elect to participate. If there are any costs involved in establishing the program, a fee could be established for participants. Or, even if no cost is incurred, it might be advantageous to have a small registration fee. This fee will help in determining how large an audience will be present. Presentations can be made either at lunch time or after work; after-work sessions probably are more effective.

STARTING A RECREATIONAL-CONSUMER PROGRAM

For those interested in starting a recreational-consumer program some recommendations are offered. Initially, answer the questions listed in the first part of this article. On the basis of those answers, do not be afraid to start in a minor way. At the outset, it may be possible to offer only a few discounts and directories. The most important decision is the selection of the person or persons who will be responsible for the program. Appoint an individual who is energetic, creative, and sincerely interested in people. If possible, create an advisory committee. Almost any medical center has an area, whether it is in personnel, health services, benefits, etc., where many people come for various types of services. Ask someone who has contact with all types of individuals to help organize a planning committee, or ask department heads to select representatives for the committee. Be sure that the people responsible for the program know how much time they can spend on it and that they have some kind of budget. As stated previously, goals and general rules should be established as soon as possible. Most important of all, obtain support and approval of management.

In addition to the advisory committee, the institution should try to cooperate with others in the area. It may be worthwhile to trade some of each other's spaces. For example, Agency A may let Agency B use its gym if Agency B will include Agency A's employees in its ticket program, or some other exchange. There may be enough interest to establish some sort of competitive sports teams from different institutions.

Become a member of a local chapter of the National Industrial Recreation Association and join the national association. A listing of some of the services offered by this association is on the last page of this article. If the institution does not wish to join IRDA, some other group may be available; "outside" ideas can be very helpful.

If the hospital does have a program, encourage those responsible to participate in conferences, workshops, and other programs that might be helpful. Contact local schools to ascertain whether recreational interns or other students are available to assist in programming. Also, the hospital's volunteer department should be requested to assist.

As mentioned, Mount Sinai's recreational director originally was responsible for a program for 325 nursing students. The success of this program paved the way for the current one. In some institutions, there is no such central position; the program is run by a committee of students and employees who are recognized by management.

Management usually indicates the amount of time each individual can spend on the program during the work week. Often, this type of program works as long as someone in administration supervises it. Any sort of program is better than none, and every medical center or hospital should try to provide opportunities for recreation in some form, supplemented by discounts for its group.

Those interested in obtaining copies of the lists of discounts available to Mount Sinai employees and students, copies of the bylaws covering its Employee-Student Activities Club, or copies of articles written about the program, may contact the author and the information will be furnished.

Those thinking of starting a program may find that funding is a major obstacle. If personnel already on staff are used, funds for the program can be raised by charging a service fee for tickets, a registration fee for courses, and/or asking vendors who are desirous of offering discounts in the institution to reimburse the hospital with a portion of those discounts. Many institutions use the profits from their vending machines to totally support their recreational program. If vending or other machines can be installed, they might produce sufficient funds to employ a full-time recreational director. If management recognizes that the program can help retain employees, it may channel funds from recruitment or from the general budget into the operation. For example, it costs $2,000 in The Mount Sinai Medical Center to recruit one nurse. If this program is instrumental in retaining 20 nurses a year, it more than pays for itself. When the program is measured in dollars, it has been found that it costs less than $5 per person to support it for one year. Members of the theater club save at least that amount every time they obtain a ticket.

In New York, the Women's Auxiliary of St. Luke's-Roosevelt Hospital decided to support a recreational program for its personnel, financed by a ticket donation fee of $1 per ticket and by special fundraising activities. The president of the auxiliary visited Mount Sinai and hired one of its volunteers to administer and create the program. The two hospitals now are working closely and Mount Sinai has found that the new program has helped expand its own program.

Other medical centers in New York have recreational programs, each one funded in a different way.

In summarizing the complete recreational-consumer program in The Mount Sinai Medical Center, there is no question that it saves money for all participants, broadens horizons, and enriches lives. The program is used to recruit and retain students, staff, and volunteers. Thus far, it has not been able to determine whether it is effective in reducing absenteeism or in increasing productivity. However, the program does help the group think more positively about experiences in The Medical Center. It is helpful in developing leadership qualities. Its members like the program—they like the way they see people interacting from all walks of life. The members think they are a positive force in supporting preventive medicine, and hope they also are a creative force in people's lives.

30. Hospital Merger: The Human Resources Impact (The St. Francis-St. George Experience)

WILLIAM M. COPELAND

The purpose of this article is to share the experience of merging the administrative structures of two separate hospitals into one corporate entity. The objective was to have the merger complete, with a smoothly functioning corporate staff ready to move into a new building constructed to replace both existing physical plants. These two existing hospitals were sponsored by different orders of religious sisters; the new corporation is sponsored by both of these orders and by the local archdiocese. Compounding the difficulty of merging two staffs and moving into a new building is that the new hospital will have approximately 46 fewer beds than the two organizations had previously. Needing fewer employees, management had to plan carefully to avoid the potentially explosive morale problem that would result if the employees became unsure of their futures with the organization.

In addition to staff feelings of insecurity, there were two sets of management groups that were, with the normal infighting and jealousy to be expected in this situation, competing for the same jobs. Not only did the inevitable reductions unsettle staff and administration, but physicians who customarily admitted patients to the two hospitals faced a reduction in the number of beds available. These two medical staffs understandably were loyal to their respective institutions. In addition, management had to consider the allegiance of each institution's own area community and a health planning environment that was less than conducive to the entire process. Despite management's recognition

that these problems would exist, both institutions acknowledged that only by combining their resources into a single facility would more efficient health care delivery result.

The type of merger discussed here, where two hospitals join assets, allows a sharing of management expertise and fiscal resources, which leads to more efficient utilization of the assets at the new institution's disposal. Joint purchasing arrangements and cooperative laundry activities between hospitals have demonstrated that shared activities save money, but merger into one overall management structure brings this efficiency to all operations of the new institution. This increased efficiency is why the federal government has pushed the shared systems development and why, during the last 15 years, there has been increased emphasis on developing the kind of shared systems that mergers can produce.

The impetus for this new trend toward merger came from the planning legislation originally enacted in 1972, (P.L. 92-603).[1] While its overall goal was to stem the rapidly increasing cost of hospital care, the legislation's major thrust was to generate increased efficiency in the utilization of the health resources available.

Concurrent with ever-increasing government pressure, substantial changes were occurring within the hospital industry itself. Hospitals were becoming big business. It was becoming increasingly apparent that this new, emerging industry would have to adopt more efficient management practices if it was to survive. Hospital administrations have begun to use systems support such as management engineering and data processing. These help management to improve the efficiency of hospital operations. In addition, the prerequisite for employment at the top levels of hospital management is increasingly becoming at least a master of hospital and health administration (MHA) or a related master's degree. In fact, the MHA is almost a necessity for admission to the American College of Hospital Administrators, the industry's most prestigious professional association. In short, professional management has come on the scene.

One of the manners by which the hospital industry has manifested this turn to modern management practice is the trend toward sharing services involving two or more organizations, or actually merging those organizations into a multihospital system or single organization. It is this latter situation that is addressed in this article—the merger of St. Francis and St. George Hospitals into St. Francis-St. George Hospital, Inc.

THE BACKGROUND

St. Francis Hospital is located in the western section of Cincinnati. It was founded by the Franciscan Sisters of the Poor, headquartered in Brooklyn, New York. The order sponsors 14 hospitals throughout the eastern United States. Construction of St. Francis Hospital began in 1886 and the first patients were admitted January 2, 1889. The purpose of the hospital at first was primarily to care for aged, infirm, and incurable patients. With the addition of east and west wings in 1900, the first acute care patients were admitted. St. Francis now is certified to operate 247 acute care beds, 204 of which are being used for short-term acute care and 43 for alcoholism treatment.

Early in the 1970s, St. Francis officials embarked on a program to correct serious long-range problems resulting not only from the fact that the hospital was situated in an old neighborhood but also from its antiquated building. The hospital was rapidly becoming uneconomical to operate. Remodeling projects were required to meet fire and safety regulations. The building had been expanded and renovated so frequently that various departments were experiencing difficulties in functional integration. A market evaluation indicated that the population of the area in the immediate vicinity of St. Francis was declining, and that future occupancy levels would decrease as patients began patronizing other hospitals with more modern facilities. St. Francis recognized that replacement of its physical facilities was mandatory but also was aware that new

construction would require a new site. The current site was 10.34 acres on an almost 45-degree hillside. It was at this point that management initiated discussions with St. George Hospital.

St. George Hospital is in the suburban Western Hills part of the city and serves not only that section but also the southwestern portion of Hamilton County. Both of these areas in recent years have experienced considerable growth in population and residential development. In 1944, the hospital purchased a building to provide extended care treatment. In 1968, a new building with 75 acute care beds was constructed to replace the original. Subsequent alterations have resulted in an 84-bed complement. The hospital was founded by the Dominican Sisters of St. Mary of the Springs, whose headquarters are located in Columbus, Ohio. The Dominican Sisters is a Roman Catholic order with a membership of 545. The order operates 44 schools, St. George being its only hospital.

St. George Hospital was overcrowded almost from its opening. Census figures of the hospital in recent years consistently were above 90 percent, which, combined with an extremely heavy emergency room/ outpatient load, strained the institution's limited facilities. Expansion was an absolute necessity, but its limited land area, 12.16 acres, and residential location inhibited additional building there. Even while plans were being developed to expand the building to accommodate 300 beds, management decided against this method in favor of combining with St. Francis to construct a new hospital at a new site.

The New Organization Begins

In 1975, an organization called St. Francis-St. George Hospital, Inc., came into being. It should be noted that this new corporate entity did not replace either the St. Francis or the St. George Corporations. Both of these organizations and their boards of trustees remained intact and continued to manage their respective institutions. The newly established corporation was commissioned to plan for the new institution and to acquire a site for the new building.

Having three organizations with separate operational and planning responsibilities created a significant interface problem: there was no one centralized authority directing the activities of this consortium. It became apparent to everyone that a new corporation, responsible for both operational and planning activities, was mandatory.

To answer this need, the St. Francis and St. George corporations were merged into one corporate entity in March 1977 and a new board of trustees appointed.

Two very significant actions were taken at this time: (1) a project director was contracted to facilitate the development of the new hospital and (2) the board selected a management and operations committee to oversee the dual continuing hospital operations. The two hospital administrators reported directly to this committee because a chief executive officer had not been selected for the new corporation at this point.

An executive staff subcommittee (a subcommittee of the board's planning committee) was formed to coordinate the merger activities and to work with the project director so that the transition from two hospitals to one could occur in an orderly fashion. Unfortunately, committee management did not appear to be the answer, and it was becoming increasingly clear that a chief executive officer, who would be responsible for all the activities of the corporation, was needed to provide essential leadership. Early in 1978, a search committee was formed and subsequently hired a CEO.

The Corporate Organization Develops

With this appointment, a new corporate organization was developed, with all of its functions reporting to the president. The new organization included an executive vice-president and four vice-presidents, who supervised the line operations of patient services, therapeutic and diagnostic services, general services, and finance. In addition, the following staff offices were created: medical staff services, program planning, development, personnel, and religious programs. These agencies were headed by corporate directors with executive level status. The president, executive vice-president, and all vice-presidents were made officers of the corporation, with the president serving as a member of the board of trustees.

The management and operations committee, which previously had assumed the functions of the CEO, was discontinued. The executive staff subcommittee became the executive staff, acting in an advisory capacity to the president. This high-level advisory body was composed of the president as chairman, the executive vice-president, the vice-presidents, and the corporate directors. This influential body proved to be the foundation of the system developed to make the merger work. It was candid and open and provided a forum to discuss problems and develop workable solutions. It also proved to be a valuable tool in dealing with a rather unusual corporate structure.

Usually an organization composed of two or more units has separate managers appointed to direct the operations of each. Unlike this traditional structure, St. Francis-St. George granted all vice-presidents and corporate directors the authority over their respective divisions and agencies in both hospitals. For instance, the vice-president for patient services held the director of nursing accountable for all nursing activities. The rationale was to create an organizational structure equally adaptable to a single unit or to multiple units. The reorganized administrative structure would be ready to transfer to the new facility upon completion of the building. This ambitious scheme for reorganization was developed at this point only on paper. The much more difficult task of implementation was still to come.

To initiate the process, each vice-president and corporate director produced a Gantt Chart that delineated goals and projected target dates. The first major goal had been achieved by the end of 1979—the majority of departments were merged and joint department managers had been selected. Achievement of this goal was a rather long process that, in some instances, required the replacement of both existing department heads and the appointment of an entirely new manager. In most cases, however, one of the current department managers was appointed, the other either remaining in a supervisory position in one of the hospitals, choosing another position within the hospital, or terminating employment completely.

Sometimes, particularly where the structure of the department in each of the two hospitals was not compatible with the reorganization scheme, three to five previously existing departments were merged into one. A notable example was the admitting and outpatient registration function. At one of the facilities these were distinct departments; at the other there was a department of patient registration. The operations of both hospitals were combined to form a department of patient registration. Two of the managers sought employment elsewhere and the head of the previous department assumed responsibility for the entire operation.

FEARS AND THEIR PROBLEMS

With the merging of departments progressing at such a rapid pace, a staffing plan was developed for the new hospital. Since the new facility was to have 46 fewer beds than the existing hospitals, the plan called for approximately 100 fewer employees. Understandably, employees feared that all 100 full-time equivalent employees to be let go would come from their institution. Management's attempts to allay these fears didn't have equal impact on employee morale as did the rumor mill. As if to underscore the difficulty in getting accurate information to employees, two other problems affected morale. There was much concern in each hospital that the management of the other would take over and impose its management concepts. Coupled with this was concern that the unique caring attitude characterized in the Christian Catholic philosophy would be lost in the process of relocating to the new institution. Because so many changes were taking place simultaneously, radical changes in the lines of communication between management and employees were imperative.

The Attitude Survey

The first step was to request Don Rowe Associates, the consulting firm that had worked very closely with management throughout the entire process, to conduct an attitude survey. The results were revealing. Although problems were identified, the survey indicated that the morale of St. Francis-St. George employees was better than the national average for all hospitals previously surveyed by the firm. It is interesting to note that the hospitals upon which the average was based supposedly were stable and were not experiencing the kinds of unsettling changes that St. Francis-St. George was witnessing. Management was both surprised and pleased with the positiveness of the overall results, but realized that its communications problems demanded immediate attention.

Communication between management and staff was complicated further by the fact that the corporation had two hospitals located in separate facilities five miles apart, but the executive offices, the project office, and the purchasing department all were situated elsewhere. Mechanisms had to be developed that could bridge the geographical isolation and bring the employees together as one group. The birthday breakfast seemed to be a step in the right direction.

A breakfast for all employees during the month of their birthdays had been a program at St. George Hospital for a year and a half. It allowed the St. George administrator to meet and break bread with employees whose birthdays were celebrated in a given month. The purpose of this program was twofold: it permitted the chief executive officer to recognize and breakfast with every employee at least once a year and it provided a forum for open and candid discussion of employees' concerns. An additional, though unexpected, benefit was that other employees who wanted questions answered would relay them to breakfast attendees. The program, therefore, reached a larger group than those targeted specifically. Moreover, the questions and their answers were published in the employee newsletter.

The breakfast was a successful tool whose structure necessarily was altered somewhat so that it could be adapted to a two-hospital operation. Two months were combined, allowing for a monthly gathering at each hospital on alternate months. The birthday breakfast was used by management as a forum to discuss corporate policy, personnel policy, or environmental factors that would have an impact on employees, their future, or the future of the hospital organization.

Publications and Other Efforts

Another method that helped with communications was the issuance of four new publications, each specifically designed to reach a different audience: a twice-monthly publication for employees, a monthly publication for managers, a monthly publication for physicians, and a quarterly publication designed to reach members of the community. The public relations staff was expanded so that the quality of communications to these audiences was improved.

Several other steps were taken. An automatic telephone or recorded answering device, called The Action Line, was installed. This instrument proved indispensable in identifying concerns and responding to questions that otherwise would not have been recognized or answered simply because they would not have been asked openly of management. A speakers' bureau was organized in which all members of the executive staff participated. The members repeated the St. Francis-St. George story at luncheon meetings, dinner engagements, wherever they were invited, in an effort to keep the community informed.

All of these activities had an effect; nevertheless, more assistance was needed. Management had to utilize whatever forum was available—the newspapers, television, radio, public meetings—with candid and open discussion of the concerns of the employees and the community. The lesson to be learned from the experience is that in the dynamic atmosphere of a merger, communications never can keep pace with the rapid change. Management should recognize that there will be a never-ending problem, requiring unrestricted and lively discussion of the issues in a straightforward manner.

Anticipating the problems far enough in advance to identify and correct them was difficult. The most critical needs were to convey accurate and up-to-date information and to deal with the morale problem generated by the necessity to reduce the staff by 100. To deal with this employee fear, several personnel programs were developed.

A Skills Inventory Backfires

A skills inventory was taken in which every employee in the organization completed a questionnaire designed to identify academic, practical, and experience capabilities. The intent was to use the skills inventory as a tool in the placement, either within the organization or externally, of employees who would be displaced. Unfortunately, the device was perceived as a vehicle by which all selections of employees for positions in the new hospital would be made. Consequently, the accuracy of the resulting information was questionable, and rather than providing management information to assist employees, it further deflated morale. Again, communications failed.

Other measures taken to reassure employees about the reduction in staff included a reanalysis of the staffing plan by the staff committee and the development of a placement service. The staff committee involved the vice-presidents functioning as a subcommittee of the board-level planning committee. This group verified the accuracy of the preliminary staffing projections; with that accomplished, the transition committee could proceed with confidence. The placement service helped find jobs for displaced employees and identified departments that would suffer the most. With this information in hand, plans were developed to ease the transition in the affected areas.

The transition committee was organized as a working group charged to produce a systematic plan for the move into the new facility, including not only equipment and patients but also the transition of the work force. The director of program planning was appointed chairman, and representatives from the various functions, as members of the committee, were assigned the responsibility for accomplishing the move. Each of these members was delegated the responsibility for developing one portion of the move plan. Once developed, each plan was coordinated through the committee and became a subsystem of the entire program. It was essential that these subsystems interface with each other so the move could be systematic and unnecessary problems could be avoided.

Last, and vitally important in this planning process, was the Operation Witness program. Designed by the director of religious programs, the program sought to alleviate employee concern that the caring attitude, which was such a vital part of health care delivery at both St. Francis and St. George, not disappear in the transition. The primary purpose of the Witness program was to ensure that the Christian spirit of caring and providing health care on a holistic basis (spiritually as well as physically) would not be lost.

PROBLEMS IN ORGANIZATIONAL STRUCTURE

With a year of experience behind the new corporation, it became evident that there were inherent problems in the organizational structure. Not only was there some degree of fragmentation in the line operating departments (as a result of their division between the president and executive vice-president), but some of the staff services (such as internal auditing and management engineering) were not being allocated their fair share of supervision. In addition, there was considerable detachment among the corporate level committees that made recommendations to the executive staff. Little coordination existed among those committees and, in many cases, responsibilities and lines of authority were not defined clearly.

In an effort to rectify the situation, a revised organizational structure was developed in which the president assumed responsibility for all line functions. All staff activities, with the exception of three, were transferred to the executive vice-president. This officer also assumed the chairmanship of the majority of corporate level committees and initiated a process of reviewing and streamlining them. Their authority and responsibilities were delineated specifically in a new corporate policy. Some committees were eliminated and their responsibilities transferred either to the line or staff division having that function.

The staff departments that continued to report directly to the president were planning, development, and medical staff services. Program planning was responsible for the transition committee. This staff function also was assigned to develop two to three new projects for submission to the local health systems agency for approval during the year. The president felt that it was crucial to maintain direct responsibility for this activity.

The development office was in the process of conducting an $8 million fund-raising campaign. While more than $6 million of this goal already had been realized, the remaining three years of the campaign were the most critical and the balance of this goal would be the most difficult portion to achieve. Therefore, the president believed that the compelling nature of this activity made it imperative that he keep immediate supervision over it.

Medical Staff Transition

Medical staff services was experiencing a transition of its own with the merging of the two staffs. The president retained the responsibility for this activity also because of the dynamic characteristics of the new joint medical staff. This merger became effective January 1, 1980, and faced an inordinate number of problems in its first year.

The two medical staffs worked closely with each other in developing this joint staff, an accomplishment that did not occur easily but ultimately succeeded as the result of tremendous effort and cooperation. Most of the credit for achieving this merger must be extended to the staff leadership. Management, on the other hand, remained in a supportive role while taking steps that greatly assisted the leaders. The first and most important of these steps was the development of a department called medical staff services.

Medical staff services is not, in itself, a unique term. A majority of hospitals have a department with that name or something similar. The difference at St. Francis-St. George, however, is the conceptual nature by which this department was organized.

There has been a trend in the last decade, to implement a concept called the medical director.[2, 3, 4]. The management of St. Francis-St. George Hospital, while finding the medical director concept valid from a theoretical aspect, had practical problems with implementation. Most notable among these was the medical staff's open opposition to the idea. The primary factor was the staff members' reluctance to subject themselves organizationally to the control of the chief executive officer.[5] The medical director theory does exactly that: it installs a physician, who is a director of the medical staff and who reports directly to the chief executive officer.[6] The management of St. Francis-St. George sought to avoid such a confrontation.

The Medical Director

The primary advantage of having a medical director is that it relieves the part-time medical staff president, who has a practice of his own, from the administrative burdens of managing the medical staff and places these duties instead with the medical director, who is a full-time physician/employee of the hospital. The management of St. Francis-St. George Hospital thought this was a laudable result. But the administration realized that this result could be achieved, at least in substantial part, by creating a staff level person with the academic training and experience to have a level of competence to carry out the administrative activities of the medical staff. This person would do so under the direction of the president of the medical staff and the chief executive officer of the hospital. This method had the advantage of leaving medical judgments/decisions with the physician, who is selected by the

medical staff. Such a function was created at St. Francis-St. George and proved very successful.

While a detailed discussion of the nonphysician director of the medical staff services is beyond the scope of this article, it is necessary at this point to explain how this position operates. It was established in answer to a need for coordination, cooperation, and more direct integration of the medical staff activities into the mainstream of a dynamic hospital organization. Here, it was necessary to combine two community hospitals whose physicians had a vested interest in the survival of the fledgling organization as a whole, yet these two groups held dearly to the self-government concept of their respective medical staffs. Management did not want to usurp authority; rather, it needed a vehicle by which the hospital could provide the physician group with a person who could coordinate the activities of the medical staff with the operational aspects of the institution.

As Williams points out,[7] since the board of trustees is responsible for the quality of medicine practiced in the hospital, and it is the chief executive officer who is charged with the accountability for monitoring that care to ensure its adequacy, the conclusion could be drawn that the medical staff director, a physician, should report to the chief executive officer.

The management of St. Francis-St. George was not convinced that the hospital had to have a paid physician/medical director reporting to the CEO to make certain that this quality assurance feature was carried out. Rather, it felt that if the elected senior medical staff officer was given the support of administration and was relieved of administrative duties that it was not necessary to perform personally, the job of quality assurance supervision could be handled efficiently by this elected staff official. Such proved to be the case and, remarkably, the elected officials of the staff even found time to develop a joint medical staff organization and compose a set of bylaws by which the joint staff could be governed. It is significant to note that the nonphysician director of medical staff services provided the staff support in the form of research, education, and advice and greatly assisted in the development of the joint structure.

Achieving the Merger

Turning away now from how the medical staff services organization assisted the medical staff in its merger activities, a look at the manner by which those merger activities were accomplished is in order.

First, a committee including key representatives from each of the two staffs was established to develop bylaws for the merged staff. The new bylaws were scrutinized item by item, approved by the two executive committees, by the general staff, and by the board of trustees. Problems were encountered making the organization consistent with the standards of the Joint Committee on Accreditation of Hospitals, but minor revisions of one section of the bylaws after discussion with representatives from the Joint Commission resolved the situation. Otherwise, few significant problems were encountered. The ease of this merger can be attributed, in large measure, to the advice and counsel of the director of medical staff services. The differences of opinion that did exist fell in three distinct categories: (1) organizational structure of the medical staff, (2) medical staff committee structure, and (3) the composition of the combined medical executive committee. These issues were resolved through compromise and the resulting medical staff organization was one that could be accepted by all.

The combined medical staff bylaws included a provision that should be embraced by all medical staffs contemplating consolidation: physician appointments were made to staff categories with prerogatives, privileges, and responsibilities equivalent to those held by these doctors at their hospitals before the merger. The board of trustees approved these provisions and they became effective immediately upon consolidation.

While the bylaws were being developed, the two medical staffs were attempting to combine many of their committees. First to be organized were the ad hoc chart committee and the credentials committee. Since different chart systems existed at each hospital, the respective executive committees of the medical staffs appointed members to an ad hoc chart committee. This panel was charged with developing a common chart system that would be received willingly by both staffs. Through the efforts of participating physicians, nurses, and paramedical personnel, this process resulted in the production of a new chart system. A byproduct was that a closer working relationship was fostered between physician and hospital. Similarly, the combined credentials committee developed a single application format and procedure.

Because the separate staffs were to be dissolved, a method of transition to the new structure was devised. First, the president of the combined staff was chosen during a run-off election of the presidents-elect of the two hospitals staffs. The physician receiving the greatest number of votes assumed the presidency for a one-year term beginning in or during 1980, while the runner-up held the title president-elect during 1980 and assumed the presidency in January 1981. Second, the two executive committees acted as the nominating committees to draft separate slates for the remaining elected officers. In addition, the past presidents of both hospitals served on the medical executive committee for calendar 1980.

The role of the chief executive officer in the merger of the medical staffs was basically that of adviser. This role was mandated in order to ensure that the resulting combined medical staff bylaws met the requirements of such third parties as the JCAH. The CEO also had to make certain that the new organization would be as compatible as possible with the new hospital structure, and that an avenue existed for a free exchange of ideas between administration and the changing medical staffs.

IMPLICATIONS AND CONCLUSIONS

Several conclusions can be drawn from the experience of the St. Francis-St. George Hospital's merger activities. Chief among these is that regardless of what management attempts to do there will be a significant communications problem. Rumors will run rampant. It is absolutely essential that the chief executive officer answer all questions in as candid a manner as possible. When a question cannot be answered because the information is confidential or because a staff person is involved, the CEO should say just that. Never, under any circumstance, should the CEO avoid relaying information to employees; to the contrary, the executive always should keep them aware of any development.

The second major conclusion is that a formal planning program is critical. There should be a formal committee organized to coordinate the overall planning activities. All planning functions must be routed through this central source so that fragmentation, redundancy, and, most importantly, the uncontrolled "doing one's own thing," does not exist.

The planning should be accomplished by all the people involved in the move themselves. They should have representatives on the planning and transition committees. But just as important as making the people responsible for the planning themselves, there must be central coordination. It must function in a systematic manner. If it does not, disorganization will occur, with a very high probability that the entire process will fail and chaos will result.

NOTES

1. P.L. 92-603, 1972.
2. Kenneth Williams, "Practical Applications of the Medical Audit," *Hospital Progress,* January 1965, pp. 109–111.

3. —————— , "The Role of the Medical Director," *Hospital Progress*, June 1978, pp. 50–57.

4. P. Rogatz, "The Case for the Medical Director," *Trustee*, June 1979, pp. 21–25.

5. William M. Copeland, "Hospital Responsibility for Basic Care Provided by Medical Staff Members: 'Am I My Brother's Keeper?'" 5 *Northern Kentucky Law Review*, 1978, pp. 28–33.

6. K. Williams, "The Role of the Medical Director," *Hospital Progress*, June 1978, pp. 50–57.

7. Ibid.

31. A Key Resource for Personnel Executives: The Hospital Management Engineer

LARRY E. SHEAR

Today's hospital personnel executive is confronted with a myriad of issues ranging from legislative and federal guidelines through to the day-to-day management of salary programs, labor relations, recruitment/ retention, budgeting, and employee morale. Seen as a vital support to the administration, to middle management, and to the employees, the personnel executive has evolved into an essential component of the hospital's top-level decision-making team, as well as being a key resource to deal directly with virtually any topic related to people and the work environment. This excludes few situations not calling for consultation with the personnel executive. Short of meeting these expectations to seemingly be a "master of all trades," the personnel executive more frequently is calling upon the talents of the hospital management engineer for support.

SHARING A COMMON PURPOSE

Without reviewing the history of management engineering from its purported origination in the late 1800s to its evolution into hospitals in the last 20 years, it is only necessary to point out the wide acceptance and use of the specialty today. The vast majority of larger hospitals and medical centers now have full-time management engineers on staff or have access to similar services through state associations or proprietary consulting firms. Many of these hospitals increasingly

show organizational linkages between the personnel executive and the management engineer. In quite a few, the functions report to the same individual, while in others they participate on similar committees and task forces. Regardless of reporting relationships, however, both positions are viewed as necessary resources to the executive administrator, sharing a common purpose in creating a climate for change for the betterment of the organization and its employees.

MANAGEMENT ENGINEERING OBJECTIVES

The primary objectives of the management engineering functions focus on the application of technical and managerial skills to:

- design organizational and operational systems to advance the institution to greater levels of effectiveness;
- establish the environment necessary to accept and implement new concepts and designs that will affect the overall level of performance of the organization;
- assist the organization in the management processes of planning, researching, analyzing, solving, implementing, and measuring the results of specific undertakings.

Figure 31-1 Organizational Relationships

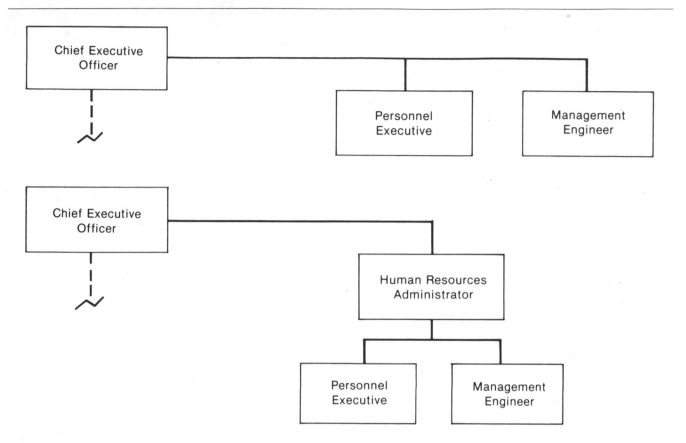

Note: The crooked dark lines indicate that the organizational structure is extended beyond the functions that appear to include the remaining hospital departments.

In this context, the roles and responsibilities of the personnel executive parallel those of the management engineer and offer a forum for dynamic joint collaboration on key issues of operation and organization.

The levels of sensitivity each discipline brings to the task necessitate a recognition of human values and expectations that can help provide an improved working environment. This recognition extends directly to the employee as an individual, the functional job, the working climate, training, the organization, and the management information network that contribute to the overall advancement of the organization as a whole.

SUPPORTING THE PERSONNEL EXECUTIVE

1. *The employee:* Vital in any organization as a means of acknowledgment and reward, employee recognition plays a highly impressionable role in health care, principally because of the various and varying levels of specialized talents and unique training backgrounds found in hospitals. The development of specific job tasks, their relationship to the total effort, and the contributory and necessary part they play is defined via management engineering job description development and procedural integration, preceded by systems design. Management engineering efforts form the structure for employee recognition via desk audits as well as by incentive plans through the establishment of productivity criteria, work station design, work simplification, and environmental assessment—all directed at providing an increased level of work life for the individual.

2. *The job:* The management engineer may be instrumental in establishing the objectives of a particular job or position. Quantifiable performance standards may be set, recruitment criteria determined, educational/experience levels recognized,

and federal/state licensure guidelines incorporated. Through needs determination of a given job function, the management engineer is most helpful in aiding the personnel function in defining the job correctly and accurately to allow not only for placement but also for appropriate classification.

3. *The work environment:* Work area design, workflow, work distribution, and equipment selection all fall within the realm of expertise of the management engineer. Making an employee's working conditions as satisfying as possible leads to higher levels of output. Recognition of health and safety factors, regulations, and human factors (ergonomics) provides an increased insight into improving the overall working environment.

4. *Functional management:* The management engineer can be instrumental in assisting first-line management with problem solving and in creating an atmosphere conducive to resolving issues. Through participation in task forces, committees, and departmental meetings, an objective perspective is applied to ensure that fundamental human resource management techniques are in operation and that total efforts are contributing to the hospital's own goals and objectives.

5. *Training for the job:* Through participation in the training process, the management engineer can present the technical aspects of a job function in a manner that blends the task into the total hospital process. The combining of the technical and humanistic orientation forms a firm level of job understanding and contribution for the new or retrained employee.

6. *The organization:* The personnel executive is involved actively in any number of organizational systems that could be facilitated best with the assistance of a management engineer:

- position control
- budget development
- labor standards
- labor performance control systems
- career ladder development programming
- benefits package analysis (cost/benefit)
- MBO program coordination
- data analysis/union negotiation

7. *Management information:* The statistical and analytical background of a management engineer lends itself quite directly to the support of the personnel department in the provision of integrated personnel management systems, automated data base networks, turnover reporting analysis and protocols, forms design, and statistical analysis. Possible areas of support also include survey criteria, questionnaire development, sampling plans, and data analysis—all of which are helpful in assessing benefits reviews, attitude surveys, and so forth.

In toto, the resources offered by the management engineer serve as a valuable component of the overall personnel function in almost every area of involvement. The analytic tool brought to the task, as well as the ability to apply objective perspective—taking into account human values as well as organizational needs—makes the management engineer vital to the survival of a hospital in today's health care market.

Exhibit 31-1 Mission/Purpose of the Management Engineering Function

The management engineering function exists to serve and assist its management with the ultimate purpose of achieving and maintaining the highest degree of patient care at the lowest reasonable cost, through the effective application of resources—human, equipment, facility, and fiscal. Toward this goal, management engineering strives to provide those services which are responsive to organizational and employee needs; to a continually changing health care environment; and to dynamically technological and humanistic health care settings. It actively recognizes its role as both a manager of resources and a systems analyst in dealing with managerial/administrative needs and organizational systems required to pursue institutional aims and objectives. Management engineering further recognizes its role as a facilitator and coordinator in directing multidisciplinary approaches to the hospital environment, through planned integration of service disciplines inclusive of those expertises such as are related to organizational development, health planning personnel management, quality assurance, operations research, and other such functions which traditionally interface through staff support efforts.

Source: Larry E. Shear, editor, reprinted with permission of Pacific Health Resources, Los Angeles, California, © 1980.

Exhibit 31-2 Integrating the Personnel Function and the Management Engineer

Personnel/Human Resource Activity	The Management Engineer's Role
Goal setting and management by objectives	needs identification, coordination, performance standards, costs
Management and organizational effectiveness	operational audits, identification of management deficiencies
Employee and management opinion surveys	questionnaire development, sampling plan, statistical validity of results
Employee communication programs	needs identification, coordination
Supervisory assessment	trained assessment, recognition, and identification
Supervisory principles training	participation in hospital operations
Evaluation reviews of personnel administrative systems	criteria analysis, review, sampling, policy, procedure development
Establishment of performance appraisal and evaluation processes	financial impact analysis, desk audits, needs determination
Installation of job evaluation and wage administration programs	budgeting
Benefits plan analysis and construction	cost/benefit analysis
Safety and security surveys and programming	audit, operations, compliance with code/standards review

A CASE STUDY

The Lutheran Hospital Society of Southern California and its multihospital cooperative system has been using the concept of departmental or service integration for a number of years. Its management engineering department and personnel department function jointly on efforts through the system's human resources committee.

This committee, which also includes participants from hospital administration and the training department, has focused efforts on initiating a number of highly successful undertakings. The joint activities of the two functions have resulted in establishing the needs requirements for a totally automated personnel administration information system, including the ultimate method of implementation and evaluation. Further efforts have involved the creation of a position control system for the network's seven hospitals that includes policies, procedures, protocols, and budgetary control mechanisms. Working with the personnel directors in each of the hospitals permitted the mutual

development of labor performance standards in personnel departments on a predetermined time standard program.

Collaboration on the development of performance standards allowed for the setting of guidelines that ultimately were adopted by the entire organization to measure accomplishments. This, coupled with an analytical process to monitor objective-setting programs, provided for evaluation of the organization's progress toward formalized goals and formed the basis for performance reviews. In the area of training, management engineering's organizational review and operations audit process provided a needs assessment highlighting points that were identified as requiring skills development. The process also solicited employee perspectives and opinions insofar as the overall hospital was perceived. Management engineering surveys assisted in relieving recruitment problems in key areas where regional shortages existed. By realigning nursing functions and altering skill mixes, surveys defined needs more specifically, resulting in a real sense of personnel needs and considerable dollar savings.

A number of these collaborative efforts by the Lutheran Hospital Society are explored now in greater detail to provide a higher level of understanding for these new and successful programs.

The Society's CARE Program

Faced with the need for advanced management information and human resource data, the Lutheran Hospital Society embarked on a program development project utilizing its human resources committee under the task force direction of the management engineering component. This effort yielded a program, active since 1977, called CARE, an acronym for *Control Assurance and Resource Effectiveness.*

CARE is designed to be a result-oriented program related directly to the hospital system's goals and objective-setting process. The integration of the budgetary and objectives processes, combined with industry-tested work measurement techniques, provides the basis for the program. This integrated management information system permits labor performance to be reviewed on the timely basis necessary to react effectively. Unlike some management programming activities, CARE is based upon a continuity of effort. It is not designed to be a one-shot panacea to be implemented on a short-term basis. Rather, it is a continuing process, viewed as a continuing task of fundamental managing. Because the CARE philosophy recognizes that each institution functions somewhat differently, that hospital's own objectives and expectations are built into the program. In this way, CARE becomes a process that relates so closely to the organization that it is responsive to the conditions and circumstances prevailing in the surrounding systems.

The implementation of the CARE program has resulted in a program that:

- monitors labor performance MBO results
- forecasts personnel needs by providing standard guidelines
- provides a training aid to resource utilization and monitoring
- allows for the projection and impact of wage and salary plans and budget implications

Previous systems used or reviewed by the society had faced a number of problems. In developing the CARE format, an attempt was made to address these problems jointly with the operational managers of participating hospitals in concert with the human resources committee. These problems, briefly, included:

- *Untimeliness:* Receiving a report two months after the situation has occurred is of little value. It already is after the fact and too late to react.
- *Data Inaccuracies:* Converting weekly or biweekly payroll information into monthly formats gives close approximations, but can be quite misleading, especially during periods that contain a holiday.
- *Inclusion of Extraneous Information and Details:* Many reports are so cumbersome it is difficult to pick out critical criteria.
- *Inability to Delineate Problems Properly:* Past data or trends can be analyzed only by digging out old reports. Hence, it is not known readily whether the numbers of a current report represent an improvement or a decline.
- *Standards of Measurement:* Systems using standards that are outdated, complex, or unrealistic provide little integrity to the program.
- *Inflexibility:* Many systems provide for reporting only on a monthly basis, which meets many hospital requests, but many institutions have needs beyond the monthly capabilities.

The product of this joint effort involving management engineers and human resource committee components resulted in what has now evolved into a meaningful and important segment of the overall multihospital information network of the Lutheran Hospital Society. This product is summarized in Exhibit 31-4, with Table 31-1 illustrating one of the output formats.

Quality Assurance Programs

To assist the society in dealing with risk management, approval by the Joint Committee on Accreditation of Hospitals, and safety, the management engineering function also collaborated on the development of a quality assurance program. The principal objective was to provide administration with a tool for management control and a system for evaluating the quality of care given. Within this framework, the quality assurance program:

- assists the personnel department in identifying specific quality deficiencies and training/ recruitment needs;
- provides a measure indicating the relative level of quality of care given and service provided;
- enables administration to monitor quality in a systematic fashion and on a continuous basis;
- provides continuous return of information in order to permit necessary corrective action in matters of JCAH compliance, and safety factors;

Exhibit 31-3 The CARE Components

The CARE program is made up of three inter-related elements:

- *The Vital Signs Report:* This is the continuous reporting mechanism through which departmental profiles are generated. It is the name given to the reports issued in synchronization with payroll runs to display key indicators, including financial data, payroll information, and performance indexes.
- *The Comparative Report:* This is a periodic (bimonthly) publication that reviews the operational characteristics of specific departments via a side-by-side profile of similar institutions. Specifically, it views organizational structures as well as staffing philosophies, policy variations, equipment resources, maintenance requirements, operational procedures, and financial indicators.
- *Budget Simulation:* All data and CARE reporting results are retained in the computer data bank. With the accumulation of this information, projections may be made on personnel needs, which then may be used in budgeting, in variable planning schemes, and in satisfying various statistical needs in quantifying future requirements.

Source: Reprinted from "C.A.R.E.—A Control Assurance and Resource Effectiveness Program for the Health Care Manager," with permission of Pacific Health Resources, Los Angeles, California, © 1979.

- provides a means of establishing staffing patterns based upon optimum personnel utilization and assured quality of care.

Through this mechanism, the hospital administration and personnel executive could identify deficiencies in qualitative aspects, personnel needs, training and education, and specific areas of development through the MBO program.

Through the quality assurance program, the management engineering function provides:

- full and complete documentation of the program, including forms, processes, program description, and update material as it becomes available;
- an orientation to the program for administration, nursing supervision, and head nurses in collaboration with the training function;

- assistance as needed in the selection of a quality assurance coordinator to maintain the program in-house in collaboration with the personnel department;
- training of the individual selected to maintain the quality assurance program;
- forms, policies, procedures, and job description designed for the hospital's particular needs;
- statistically developed sampling plans to ensure data reliability;
- implementation plans to introduce the program throughout the hospital.

LHS's Position Control Network

The position control system, developed by the management engineering and personnel staffs, serves as an additional management tool. In conjunction with the labor distribution and CARE reports, the position control network provides information on the use of the work force. It also serves as a communication mechanism among department heads, the personnel department, and the hospital administration regarding departmental staffing needs.

The system provides the means for establishment and review of personnel budgets by department, and for monitoring of these budgets (profiles) on a continuing basis. It controls hiring and promotions through the use of personnel requisition. While department heads continue to assume responsibility for budget recommendations and implementation, the review and approval process provides administration with up-to-date information on the staffing status and needs of each department.

The establishment of department personnel profiles requires the manager to think of staffing needs not only in terms of numbers but also of classifications, and to consider the personnel structure needed to provide service and manage resources efficiently and effectively. Since the position control system is an integral part of the budgeting operation, the manager is expected to plan the personnel needs of the department in advance. Once the profiles are approved, changes may be made only with the administrator's approval.

Management engineering expertise also assisted with the development of the policies and procedures associated with the position control network, inclusive of audit trails, as suggested by the following excerpt from the LHS policy guide:

So that the position control system will serve as a management tool, reports regarding the status of the personnel budget will be generated monthly.

Table 31-1 CARE Vital Signs Reporting System*

```
7T4 FLOOR                          HOSPITAL
PAGE 009   AS/OF 10-11-80

DEPARTMENT NUMBER  6082
UNIT BED CAPACITY  49
```

C.A.R.E.
VITAL SIGNS REPORT

PACIFIC HEALTH RESOURCES
Management Sciences Division
1423 SOUTH GRAND AVENUE, LOS ANGELES, CALIFORNIA 90015
C.A.R.E. LINE: (213) 742-6436

```
UNIT OF MEASUREMENT   PATIENT DAYS
REPORT STATUS         INTERIM STANDARD
C.A.R.E. FORMULA      5.70 HRS/PAT DAY

PERFORMANCE OBJECTIVE (5.95 HRS/PT DAY)   96
REGISTRY HOURLY RATE  $11.25
```

PERIOD ENDING	SERVICE UNITS	HOURS DISTRIBUTION						TOTAL COSTS	COST/ U.O.S.	PAYROLL DISTRIBUTION			INDICATORS		
		PAID F.T.E.	WORKED P.E.	DIFF. FTE-PE	O/T HOURS	CONTR. HOURS	AV/HR RATE			REQUIRED P.E. COST	WORKED P.E. COST	DIFF. WORK-REQ	REQ. HRS/ U. OF S.	WORKED HRS/ U. OF S.	PERF INDX
10-13-79	1,280	111.13	95.94	15.19	247.8	1469.0	7.38	55,589	51.24	53,844	56,542	2,798	5.700	5.996	95%
10-27-79	635	56.18	49.39	6.79	153.0	752.0	7.48	33,642	52.98	27,074	29,554	2,480	5.700	6.222	91%
11-10-79	629	54.41	49.79	4.62	121.0	784.0	7.52	32,746	52.14	25,919	29,955	3,036	5.700	6.343	89%
11-24-79	631	59.58	49.80	8.73	344.1	880.0	7.59	35,036	57.11	27,659	30,539	2,980	5.700	6.314	90%
12-08-79	629	59.58	51.39	7.19	157.7	1032.0	7.46	34,946	55.65	26,704	30,567	3,953	5.700	6.546	87%
12-22-79	583	53.52	46.85	6.66	147.5	760.0	7.72	33,047	56.68	25,654	28,943	3,289	5.700	6.431	88%
01-05-80	516	49.37	41.74	7.13	455.3	712.0	7.94	30,662	59.42	23,059	26,179	3,120	5.700	6.471	88%
01-19-80	626	57.20	43.95	8.35	872.0	712.0	7.49	34,259	54.73	26,726	29,272	2,546	5.700	6.243	91%
02-02-80	634	56.85	43.85	8.82	159.0	872.0	7.51	34,594	54.56	26,501	30,456	2,955	5.700	6.312	90%
02-16-80	613	56.35	50.03	6.82	146.5	1135.0	7.56	33,513	54.67	27,356	31,016	2,955	5.700	6.693	85%
03-01-80	634	57.31	51.29	4.15	135.7	1056.0	7.57	34,989	55.19	27,016	31,425	4,069	5.700	6.548	87%
03-15-80	590	57.81	51.89	5.92	120.2	1152.0	7.55	35,745	60.58	27,425	31,929	6,202	5.700	6.693	80%
03-29-80	593	54.15	52.17	6.25	200.2	992.0	7.65	33,273	55.55	25,727	30,924	4,224	5.700	7.074	86%
04-12-80	590	52.36	48.05	3.72	146.3	784.0	7.92	33,771	57.24	27,106	30,983	3,877	5.700	6.515	67%
04-26-80	600	52.29	48.97	4.31	59.5	758.0	8.06	35,375	58.95	28,933	33,142	4,209	5.700	6.529	67%
05-10-80	602	52.53	49.74	3.32	87.9	904.0	8.46	36,344	60.37	27,356	33,507	4,615	5.700	6.610	67%
05-24-80	569	51.02	47.97	4.24	95.5	1008.0	8.42	34,640	60.88	27,535	32,583	5,047	5.700	6.745	84%
06-07-80	572	47.97	50.58	3.05	91.5	1016.0	8.49	34,892	60.37	29,083	35,449	6,366	5.700	6.948	82%
06-21-80	596	55.23	50.58	5.63	286.5	1232.0	8.92	39,444	68.96	29,083	30,315	2,298	5.700	6.165	92%
07-05-80	619	50.13	45.73	4.20	76.5	800.0	8.25	33,106	55.55	28,027	34,597	4,606	5.700	6.575	86%
07-19-80	612	50.00	50.88	9.12	290.0	1152.0	8.50	39,804	65.92	29,991	31,204	2,983	5.700	6.302	90%
08-02-80	603	57.51	43.21	9.30	132.2	736.0	8.09	37,230	60.83	29,221	31,204	1,809	5.700	6.057	94%
08-16-80	598	52.13	45.73	6.40	53.0	648.0	8.17	34,063	56.50	28,081	29,890	3,586	5.700	6.501	87%
08-30-80	543	50.41	44.13	6.28	105.5	576.0	8.55	33,217	61.17	25,504	29,090	3,561	5.700	6.397	89%
09-13-80	598	57.24	47.92	9.42	158.1	784.0	8.55	39,168	55.50	29,144	32,705	1,972	5.700	6.088	93%
09-27-80	601	57.46	44.84	10.59	196.4	992.0	8.71	39,910	55.70	29,735	32,528	2,793	5.700	6.235	91%
10-11-80	595	51.65	44.38	10.62	105.0	904.0	8.88	36,704	61.69	30,117	31,881	1,764	5.700	6.034	94%
** ALL	16,881	56.91	50.07	6.84	4549.9	24816.	8.01	985,191	58.35	770,735	866,257	95,521	5.700	6.406	89%
** STR 1	595	51.55	44.39	6.77	105.0	904.0	8.86	36,704	61.69	30,117	31,881	1,764	5.700	6.034	94%
** YTL	595	51.55	44.38	6.77	105.0	904.0	8.88	35,704	61.69	30,117	31,881	1,764	5.700	6.034	94%

*The cumulative report is synchronized with payroll to display a hospital department's profile.

Source: Reprinted from "C.A.R.E.—A Control Assurance and Resource Effectiveness Program for the Health Care Manager," with permission of Pacific Health Resources, Los Angeles, California. © 1979.

These reports are the Monthly Position Control Report and the Monthly Change of Status Report. The Monthly Position Control Report shows, for each budget unit or department, the current number of budgeted FTE's and explains any variance between the two numbers. For example, if, in the laboratory, 12.5 FTE's are budgeted and 11.5 FTE's are filled, the "Variances" column will show "1 Laboratory Assistant vacant." The Change of Status Report shows the names and positions of all incoming and outgoing employees, as well as those undergoing a change of status such as a promotion or an interdepartmental transfer. These two reports verify the transactions approved through the personnel requisitions. They are completed by the personnel supervisor and forwarded to the hospital administrator at the end of each month.

Collaborating on Training Programs

With a fundamental and inherent commitment to education and the development process, the Lutheran Hospital Society provides a considerable number of structured opportunities for professional growth. One program offers experiences in viewing the hospital as a total system, as opposed to individual departmental modules. With such a systems approach, individuals can gain the exposure and experience of dealing with organizational goals and the composite contribution each lends to the achievement of those objectives.

Introduced through training professionals, the Continuing Operational Review and Evaluation (CORE) program is supplemented by workshop sessions on implementation techniques conducted by management engineering personnel and a unique blend of organizational theory with health care systems reality. The tools and techniques presented include:

- staffing and scheduling
- work simplification
- budgeting
- organizational charting
- information analysis
- problem solving
- work sampling
- work distribution

Staffing Standards for Personnel Departments

Determining the size of staff required in a personnel department is a constantly perplexing issue. Given new requirements imposed by government, added

program services, and expanding hospital staff, the staffing of a personnel office always is changing. The management engineering staff of LHS worked very closely with the Council of Personnel Executives—COPE (a component of the human resources committee) in defining the role of the personnel department and then in quantifying labor needs.

This role was defined in the form of a listing of activities that could be measured, and included:

1. Benefit Enrollment Meetings
   Preretirement counselling
   ERISA (Employee Retirement Income Security Act)
   Workers compensation
   Appeals hearings
   Leave of absence benefits
   Insurance
2. Performance Evaluations
   Personnel requests
   Job evaluations
   Turnover reporting
   Annual surveys
   Payroll
3. Recruitment
   Servicing
   Selection
   Processing
   Orientation
   Work volume
4. Employee relations
   Policy interpretation
   Career counselling
   Employee activities
5. Administrative

Each activity was defined through the group, represented by the seven hospitals; data were gathered as to how much time was expended, how frequently the activity occurred, and how many persons and at which skill levels would be required.

THE ORGANIZATIONAL REVIEW PROCESS

The organizational review process is a mechanism adapted to review a hospital organization and operation in a manner very similar to an accountant's annual audit. Its purpose is to highlight strengths and weaknesses in a hospital while identifying methods of potential improvement. Typically, the personnel executive and the management engineer collaborate on such efforts in a team approach that focuses upon:

Exhibit 31-4 Standards Development for Personnel Departments

SAMPLE FORMAT

The following questionnaire deals with the *BENEFITS* section of our project to develop standards for your departments. The data obtained from these questions will help us to focus in on the major differences brought out on the previous, overall questionnaire. Please complete all portions of the questionnaire, indicating "N/A" if a question is not applicable to your hospital. Feel free to add any supplemental data on a separate sheet of paper. Please return the completed questionnaire to the November meeting of C.O.P.E. or within a few days of that meeting to Management Engineering. An analysis of your responses will then be presented at the December C.O.P.E. meeting. Thank you very much for your cooperation. (C.O.P.E.—Council of Personnel Executives)

H O S P I T A L _____

1. How often are enrollment meetings held for new employees? _____
   Are the meetings with individuals or with a group? _____ If with a group, are they hospital-wide or by department? _____ Who conducts these meetings? _____ How long does the meeting last? _____ What method is used to follow up enrollment? (memo, phone call, etc.) __ _____

2. Do you provide pre-retirement counselling for your employees? _____
   If yes, how many do you counsel each week? _____ How much time is spent each week counselling? _____ Who does the counselling? _____

3. In one week, how much time is spent on ERISA compliance? _____

4. Who processes Workers Compensation claims? _____ How many claims do you currently have pending? _____ How much time does this involve each week? _____
   _____

5. Who represents the hospital at Unemployment Appeals Hearings? _____
   How many cases do you currently have pending? _____ How much time each week on this process? _____

6. Do you collect money for L.O.A. benefits? _____ If yes, how many employees are you currently collecting from? What is your procedure in processing the money and how much time is involved?

Source: Reprinted from "Standards Development for Personnel Departments," with permission of Pacific Health Resources, Los Angeles, California, © 1980.

- policies and goals
- organization
- planning and budgeting
- controlling
- communications
- management information
- personnel
- materials management
- operations

The end result materializes into an operational strategic plan identifying educational needs, management development potentials, compliance issues, employee attitude/opinion results, and work improvement situations. Recommendations are offered, supported by specific findings, with quantifiable potential benefits noted, thus providing a hospital with a sense of what is at issue in setting priorities.

SUMMARY

It is only through a mutual level of participation that the problems facing today's health care environment can be addressed from all perspectives, resulting in optimized and long-lasting solutions. The partnership of the personnel executive and the management engineer offers a positive step toward resolving the people problems of the future created by advancing technology, shortages in staff, and the generally increasing complexity of health care issues.

Exhibit 31-5 Sample Organizational Review Output

Recommendation	Supportive Findings	Potential Benefits
Issues of accountability should be addressed and clarified at all levels of the organization. Responsibility, authority, and accountability should be consistent.	The overruns in the annual budget indicated several problems. Investigation revealed that one of the prime problems was that department managers perceived minimal accountability for their budget. They generally expressed confusion over accountability for performance measures as well. Inconsistencies existed among the various administrative personnel regarding the accountability and responsibility placed at the department manager level. In some cases, this level is responsible for revenue and expenses; in other cases, revenue alone. Revenue-over-expense ratio in some cases is used. With regard to CARE standards, the view was generally held that if they could not be met, they should be changed. This attitude arose from the fact that minimal accountability was expected for these as well. Rather, an explanation would suffice. These problems were most severe in the nursing department; many head nurses and supervisors did not know what they were responsible for, fiscally or managerially. While a step was taken in involving the head nurses in budget development, it is not enough. It must be followed up by vigorous enforcement and understanding of accountability.	Strengthening accountability will improve budget performance significantly. In the case of the previous budget, savings could have amounted to $1,750,000; similar results could be expected this fiscal year. Controlling of personnel expense, through use of the CARE report, will account for most of the dollar savings, and improve productivity and morale.

PART II

EMPLOYEE BENEFITS

INTRODUCTION

Employee fringe benefits now constitute nearly one third of payroll costs, amounting to an average of $5,560 per worker annually, as reported in a U.S. Chamber of Commerce survey issued at the end of 1980. According to the survey American workers received some $390 billion in benefits during 1979, representing 31.8 percent of total wages and salaries paid that year; for hospitals the comparable cost was 28.2 percent. It is significant to note that the percentage of payroll costs constituting benefits in hospitals rose appreciably between 1977 and 1979. These benefits included Social Security taxes, insurance premiums, and pension premiums, as well as vacation, holiday, and sick pay. One of the authors in this section points out that this growth may be accounted for, in part, by several trends:

- sophistication of employee expectation
- the realization of the purchasing power of group benefits programs
- tax advantages to employees when benefits are prepaid
- increased competition for recruitment and retention of workers in the marketplace

There is a major shift in the primary responsibility for supplying retirement income from individuals and their families to the employer. Employees look at the total benefit plan as a means of reducing or offsetting entirely the financial loss that they can incur due to death, disability, medical expense, and retirement. But as another of the authors comments, the employer also gains since plans in the area of employee benefits are a means of:

- attracting or retaining competent employees
- increasing and/or maintaining employee morale and productivity
- increasing the employee's income through the tax shelter of the employer-paid benefits

Hospitals are paying the greater share of the costs of employee benefits. The scope of benefits continues to widen. The choice offered to employees is more varied and is directed toward providing them a greater tax advantage. The nation is witnessing ever-increasing governmental pressure toward changes in vesting requirements, improvements, early retirement payout, and heightened interest in portability.

The human resources manager must become more knowledgeable and sophisticated in the greater health protection necessary to attract and to retain employees. Dental, drug, psychiatric, and optical plans are being developed at a faster pace than ever before. Employee benefits management is an integral part of human resources management. The administration of employee benefits mandates intensive planning, close supervision, and integrated direction by the human resources manager.

1. Benefits Plan Design Issues Today and through the 1980s

ANNA M. RAPPAPORT

Reprinted with permission from *Topics in Health Care Financing, Employee Benefits*, Vol. 6, No. 3, Spring 1980, Alex W. Steinforth, Issue Editor. Aspen Systems Corporation, Germantown, Md., © 1980.

Our society is very security minded; people feel they have a right to security; both government and employers spend large sums on security. A U.S. Chamber of Commerce survey states that in 1977 total employee benefits cost 36.7 percent of pay; for hospitals the comparable cost was 25.7 percent of pay.[1] Benefits in the Chamber of Commerce survey include legally required benefits, pensions and welfare benefits, time not worked and miscellaneous benefits. The 1980 fiscal year budget of the U.S. government shows that 39 percent of U.S. federal expenditures are for direct benefit payments to individuals.[2]

Trend data in the Chamber of Commerce study show steady increases in employer expenditures for benefits as a percentage of payroll. Trend data in the federal budget show steady increases in expenditures for security. Employers should therefore be increasingly concerned about benefits today, since they represent a significant and growing operating expense and play a major role in employee satisfaction. In addition, the environment in which an employer must provide benefits is constantly changing as new laws and regulations create additional obligations, and as the family patterns, demographics and expectations of the work force evolve.

GENERAL CONSIDERATIONS

Employer Goals in the Establishment of a Benefit Program

An employer has a number of goals which its benefit program should meet. Often benefit programs have evolved over a period of years, and these goals have become "generally understood," and then forgotten. The programs should provide for a reasonable and adequate level of employee financial security. Financial security is the employee's ability to maintain a reasonable living standard even when the employee's paycheck has stopped. Employee benefits fill this gap, provide for the payment of medical care costs, and aid employees in establishing capital accumulation and savings programs. They should aid the employer in attracting and retaining the type of work force needed.

More specifically, an ideal retirement program, including Social Security benefits, should permit the career employee to retire at normal retirement age and maintain a standard of living equal to the preretirement standard of living. A 1979 Harris Poll stated that 81 percent of employees, 84 percent of retirees and 82 percent of business leaders felt that this was an appropriate goal for a retirement plan.[3] Life and health insurance benefits, Social Security and a reasonable amount of individual coverage should permit dependents to maintain their standard of living after the premature death of the breadwinner. Benefits are needed for dependent children until they reach adulthood and have completed their education. Benefits are needed for dependent spouses during periods when they are required for child care, to help make possible an adjustment to a new self-sufficient status and to provide income after retirement age. In addition, death benefits are needed to take care of final expenses and, in some cases, estate taxes. Disability benefits should permit a disabled employee to maintain a somewhat lower standard of living during the period of disability.

The level of disability benefits should be such as to provide an incentive to return to work upon recovery.

Medical care reimbursement programs should protect the employee from unusual and catastrophic health care costs. Many programs also pay for a substantial portion of normal health care expenses.

The adequacy of programs which replace lost income is often measured in terms of replacement ratios. A replacement ratio is the ratio of the benefit after payments begin to the regular earnings of the employee just prior to commencement of benefit payments. Replacement ratios can be calculated on the basis of before- or after-tax earnings or income. In considering benefit adequacy, taxes before and after regular income stops need to be taken into account, as do work-related expenses and a reasonable level of savings. An employer may wish to look at pension benefits on a basis that includes postretirement spouse's benefits and cost-of-living increases after retirement.

Benefits should be designed and communicated so that employees can understand and appreciate them. A benefit which is not understood will not aid in attracting and keeping good employees, or in promoting good labor relations.

Design Considerations

Employee benefit plan design is a continuous process. Virtually all employers have programs, and they are continually updating them to reflect changing conditions. Benefit adequacy and the satisfaction of employee needs are usually of primary concern. Cost is also a consideration, and the employer is constantly balancing desired benefits and available funds to determine the mix that best meets employee needs within available resources.

An employer must consider the needs of different groups of employees in selecting desired benefits and in setting priorities. The hospital work force consists of a mixture of full-time and part-time employees. Long-term workers may change their work schedules from time to time. The staff will include a wide variety of skill levels ranging from highly paid professionals to low-paid unskilled workers. Some of the workers will be planning a career in health care, and others will be temporary with high rates of termination.

A hospital's employees will be members of different types of families. The U.S. work force consists of workers living in four basic family patterns or households: two-income husband-wife families, one-worker husband-wife families, single-adult households with dependents and single-adult households without dependents. It is possible that in 1980 the work force will be composed as follows:

Husband or wife in two-income family	45%
Earning spouse in one-income family	20%
Single worker with dependents	10%
Single worker without dependents	25%

The needs of different employees vary, and the needs of a particular employee may change over time. Dependents' benefits are extremely important to some employees and worthless to others. Medical care benefits may not be important to someone who is already covered as a spouse in a plan which provides equivalent benefits. Life-insurance needs differ by individual. Priorities change at different times in the life cycle, and for individuals with fluctuating family patterns. A benefit program should be able to accommodate workers in different circumstances and at different times in their life cycles.

The traditional approach to benefit design has been to develop a single pattern of benefits, with some completely paid for by the employer, some cost-shared and some paid for solely by the employee. The working husband, dependent wife and minor children model has served as the family prototype around which this pattern was built. The employee's only choice has been whether to participate in contributory coverages. This benefit pattern was chosen to represent a compromise which would best meet the needs of a majority of the work force.

Table 1-1 shows different family types and their need for benefits. There are very large differences in the need for medical care and death benefit protection. The table does not show differences in willingness of individuals to assume risks and differences in priorities. These factors would determine which employee might choose more vacation compared to another benefit, and which employee might be willing to increase deductibles, if given the option to do so.

The factors which will determine the pattern of benefits that best fits a particular employee are:

- family situation;
- availability of other sources of benefits;
- willingness to assume risks;
- priorities of the individuals; and
- general financial situation.

A new approach to benefit plan design is currently developing in the United States. This approach provides for flexible benefits and permits individual em-

Table 1-1 Household Types and Benefits Needed

| | Does Household Have Income and Benefits Source Other Than Worker | Medical Benefits Needed for | | | Death Benefits Needed for | | | Disability Benefits Needed | Retirement Benefits Needed |
| | | | | | Final Expenses | Support of Dependents | | | |
		Worker	Spouse	Children		Spouse	Children		
Two-worker couple— no dependent children	Yes	Yes*	*	No	Yes	No†	No	Yes	Yes
Two-worker couple— with dependent children	Yes	Yes*	*	Yes*	Yes	No†	Yes	Yes	Yes
One-worker couple— no dependent children	No	Yes	Yes	No	Yes	Yes	No	Yes	Yes
One-worker couple— with dependent children	No	Yes	Yes	Yes	Yes	Yes	Yes	Yes	Yes
Single—no dependent children	No	Yes	No	No	Yes	No	No	Yes	Yes
Single—with dependent children	No	Yes	No	Yes	Yes	No	Yes	Yes	Yes

*Coverage needed only once. Both can be covered under one spouse's plan, or each can be covered as worker. If both have coverage, there is overlapping coverage and duplication so that couple could be better off if one spouse could choose other coverage.

†Either or both spouses may wish to provide some income to survivor in order to supplement the survivor's earnings. Living expenses for one person are more than 50% of the living expenses of two. Needs vary depending on the income mix of the spouses.

Note: "Spouse" is used here to refer to either partner in a couple maintaining a household involving a sharing of income and expenses.

ployees to tailor a benefit package that best fits individual needs. This new approach is in the experimental stage, and as of July 1979 three employers, TRW, American Can and the Educational Testing Service, were experimenting with flexible benefits. Each of these programs involves a core of benefits provided by the employer for all employees, together with numerical credits which allow employees to select additional benefits beyond the core. Whether this method will work out well over the long term remains to be seen. However, it seems inevitable that over the next ten years employers will increasingly recognize the need to respond to differences in employee needs, and so will provide choices to employees.

Benefit design should be reviewed to see how a particular benefit pattern will position an employer relative to the labor market in which it is operating. While competitive considerations are secondary to sound design, they should not be totally ignored. This is more important at times when, or in areas where, the labor market is tight. Although in most situations, levels of current pay are considerably more important than benefits in employment decisions, the employer may wish to determine to what extent benefits are a factor.

Tax considerations also play a major role in the design of benefit programs. Employer funds can be used to purchase benefits for the employee which are not immediately taxable to the employee, even though they are tax deductible to the tax-paying employer. The tax-favored status of these programs, however, depends on their being designed to meet federal regulatory requirements.

Table 1-2 summarizes the tax aspects of income replacement and other fringe-benefit programs. An employer who desires a total benefit program that is partly contributory should consider the taxation of various benefits in order to decide which of these should be contributory. For example, disability income benefits become tax free if provided solely by employee contributions. In contrast, there is no change in the taxation of medical-reimbursement benefits if the employee pays for them. However, as shown in Table 1-2, an employee can deduct part of his or her contributions toward medical care insurance as an itemized deduction in computing federal income taxes. Hence channeling employee contributions to a disability income or medical program rather than to a program where there are no tax benefits is beneficial to employees. The effect of allocating such contributions between disability and medical programs varies depending on the circumstances of the employee.

The rules cited here are general principles. Any application of these principles in a specific situation should be checked with the hospital's attorney to make sure that it applies after considering all of the facts and circumstances.

Table 1-2 Taxation of Benefits

	Part I—Income Replacement Programs*	
	Employee Contributions	Taxation of Income
Qualified pension or other retirement plan	Not tax deductible	Employer-provided benefit fully taxable
Disability income		Employer-provided benefit taxable†
Survivor benefits payable after death‡	Not tax deductible	Lump sum value of income included in employee's estate—interest part of periodic payments is taxable income
Social Security	Not tax deductible	Tax exempt

	Part II—Other Programs	
	Employee Contributions	Taxation of Benefits
Life insurance‡	Not tax deductible	Benefits included in employee estate
Medical reimbursement	See Note	Benefits do not create taxable income
Tax-sheltered annuities	Employee contributions from before-tax income	Benefits fully taxable as ordinary income
Thrift programs	Not tax deductible	Investment income tax deferred / Benefits based on employer contribution taxed as ordinary income

*Employer contributions to these programs are tax deductible.

†Up to $100/week of income paid in lieu of wages may be excluded from gross earnings in some circumstances. This exclusion is phased out for taxpayers earning over $15,000 per year.

‡If the value of benefits exceeds $50,000, then employee is taxed annually on the employer contribution excess over $50,000.

Note: Employee contribution—½ of expenses for medical care insurance up to $150 are itemized deductions, balance of expenses are medical expenses; medical expenses in excess of 3% of adjusted gross income are deductible as itemized deductions. No deduction is available unless employee itemizes deductions.

Sample Hospital Benefit Program

Table 1-3 shows a sample of the type of benefit program that might be provided by a hospital. The program provides coverage for a variety of risks, and is complex and expensive.

Nearly all larger employers provide some protection to cover loss of income at death, disability and retirement, and for payment of medical expenses. However, there is considerable variation in the level and design of the benefits and in the split between employer versus employee contributions. Some employers pay for all benefits whereas others expect their employees to make a significant contribution.

RETIREMENT AND PENSION PLAN DESIGN ISSUES

Pension Plan Income Needed

Under current law, except with respect to certain highly paid employees, an employer cannot require an employee to retire prior to age 70. Therefore the level of pension benefits will probably be a major factor in individual retirement decisions prior to age 70. Retirement is unlikely until the total of pension benefit plus Social Security, together with other sources of income, are viewed as adequate. For most people this will mean the ability to maintain a living standard generally comparable, but perhaps somewhat lower, than the standard of living prior to retirement.

The employer should consider whether employees are to be encouraged to remain until 70, to retire at normal retirement age or to retire early. Employee groups subject to liberal early-retirement benefits have high early-retirement rates. Benefit plans and other personnel practices should be designed to support the employer's policy with respect to retirement.

Benefits projected to retirement are usually evaluated by means of replacement ratios. A replacement ratio expresses various types of retirement benefits—i.e., Social Security benefits, private plan benefits, or a combination of the two—as a percentage of the compensation earned in the year before retirement. Social Security benefits under the current law are

Table 1-3 Sample Benefit Program

Risk	Primary Protection	Other Protection Paid for by Employer Dollars	How Dependents Are Covered
Death in active service	Group life insurance—one times salary plus survivor benefit targeted to produce total income of 20%–60% of predeath salary depending on circumstances	Social Security survivor benefit Social Security lump-sum benefit Pension plan pre-retirement death benefits Accidental death and dismemberment Tax sheltered annuity account balance	As beneficiaries Survivor income paid to stated dependents
Disability	*Short-Term* 75% of pay up to 90 days 60% of pay between 90 and 180 days *Long-Term* 60% of pay to age 65 offset by benefits from Social Security and Worker's Compensation	Social Security disability benefits Worker's Compensation Waiver of premium in group life Continued medical care coverage during disability Continued pension plan accrual (State short-term disability program in certain states)	Indirectly—disabled worker shares income
Medical care	Medical expenses paid subject to deductible, coinsurance and certain inside limits	Dental Vision care	Directly—via dependent coverage
Retirement	Pension payable at 65—annual accrual is 1½% of pay to taxable wage base plus 2½% of excess	Tax sheltered annuity program (nonprofit hospitals only) Postretirement life insurance of $2,000/year Postretirement Medicare supplement	Indirectly—via income shared with dependents
Other benefits	Educational assistance Thrift or savings plan Prepaid legal coverage		

designed to replace a decreasing percentage of pay as income levels rise.

The approximate level of benefits at retirement age 65 provided by the current law is as follows:

1980 Pay	*Initial Primary Social Security Benefit As a Percentage of Pay before Retirement*
$ 7,500	46%
10,000	42%
15,000	37%
25,000	27%
50,000	14%

These replacement ratios are based on the assumptions that the employee will work for all of adult life, that 1980 salaries for the individual will increase over the working life span at the same rate as average salaries for all persons covered under the system. The benefit formula in the law provides approximately level replacement ratios regardless of retirement year, provided that earnings increase at the same rate as average earnings of all covered workers.

The private plan should be designed to provide a total benefit, including Social Security, which will meet the employer's goals. These goals should be set for the career employee taking into account both the amount of income needed to maintain preretirement living standards and the employer's philosophy as to whether living standards should be fully or partly maintained after recognizing taxes and expenses related to working.

Table 1-4 illustrates the amount of income needed to maintain full living standards for a single employee. The total benefit needed ranges from 72 percent of pay for an employee earning $10,000 per year to 51 percent for an employee earning $50,000. For a married employee with a nonworking spouse, the comparable range is from 75 to 55 percent. The procedure set forth in Table 1-4 should be modified for state taxes and should reflect local conditions as to work-related expenses. Savings assumptions can be developed after discussion with the plan sponsor.

Table 1-5 shows how needs change for a married employee with a dependent spouse.

Type of Pension Benefit Formula

The most fundamental design decision is the choice of the basic type of formula. Most hospital plans con-

Table 1-4 Retirement Income Needed to Replace 100% of Preretirement After-Tax Spendable Income for a Single Employee

	$10,000	$15,000	$25,000	$50,000
(1) 1979 salary at age 64				
(2) Net spendable income after taxes, savings and work-related expenses				
(a) Social Security taxes	600	900	1,400	1,400
(b) Federal income taxes	1,400	2,600	6,000	18,100
(c) Savings percentage	0	4%	6%	10%
(d) Savings	0	600	1,500	5,000
(e) Work-related expenses (assume 7.5% of gross pay)	800	1,100	1,900	3,800
Net spendable income before retirement = (1) − (2a) − (2b) (2d) − (2e)	7,200	9,800	14,200	21,700
(3) Income needed after retirement for 100% replacement of net spendable income at 65				
(a) Estimated Social Security benefit	4,900	6,300	6,600	6,600
(b) Income needed from other sources after tax: 2(f) − 3(a)	2,300	3,500	7,600	15,100
(c) Additional income needed to pay tax on 3(b)*	0	200	1,100	3,800
(d) Income at 65 needed to replace 100% of net spendable income: 3(b) + 3(c)	2,300	3,700	8,700	18,900
(4) Replacement ratios as % of gross income for 100% of replacement of spendable income:				
(a) Social Security 3(a) ÷ (1)	49%	42%	26%	13%
(b) Other sources 3(d) ÷ (1)	23%	25%	35%	38%
(c) Total 4(a) + 4(b)	72%	67%	61%	51%

*Based on assumption that standard deduction applies.

Table 1-5 Retirement Income Needed to Replace 100% of Preretirement After-Tax Spendable Income for a Married Employee with a Dependent Spouse

	$10,000	$15,000	$25,000	$50,000
(1) 1979 salary at age 64				
(2) Net spendable income after taxes, savings and work-related expenses				
(a) Social Security taxes	600	900	1,400	1,400
(b) Federal income taxes	1,100	2,100	4,600	15,000
(c) Savings percentage	0	4%	6%	10%
(d) Savings	0	600	1,500	5,000
(e) Work-related expenses (assume 7.5% of gross pay)	800	1,100	1,900	3,800
(f) Net spendable income before retirement = (1) − (2a) − (2b) (2d) − (2e)	7,500	10,300	15,600	24,800
(3) Income needed after retirement for 100% replacement of net spendable income at 65				
(a) Estimated Social Security benefit—employee	4,900	6,300	6,600	6,600
(b) Estimated Social Security benefit—spouse	2,500	3,200	3,300	3,300
(c) Income needed from other sources after tax: 2(f) − 3(a) − 3(b)	100	800	5,700	14,900
(d) Additional income needed to pay tax on 3(c)*	0	0	400	2,600
(e) Income at 65 needed to replace 100% of net spendable income: 3(c) + 3(d)	100	800	6,100	17,500
(4) Replacement ratios as % of gross income for 100% of replacement of spendable income:				
(a) Employee Social Security 3(a) ÷ (1)	49%	42%	26%	13%
(b) Spouse's Social Security	25%	21%	13%	7%
(c) Other sources 3(e) ÷ (1)	1%	5%	24%	35%
(d) Total 4(a) + 4(b) + 4(c)	75%	68%	63%	55%

*Based on assumption that standard deduction applies.

tain either a career-average salary or final-average pay type of formula.

Under career-average salary plans, the benefit earned each year is related to the compensation paid in that year. Under a typical final-average pay plan, the level benefit earned for each year of service is determined by applying a formula to the average pay during the last five years of work. Career-average salary plans are well suited to situations where the work force includes many employees who periodically change their work schedules or many employees who have a mix of actual hours of work and hours when they are on call and available for work, because benefits are related to actual earnings in each year. Under final-average pay plans, the benefit will not accurately reflect such an irregular work history.

Inflation seems to be a persistent part of our current economic environment. Benefits paid under career-average salary plans are not self-adjusting for inflation prior to retirement. Instead the plan sponsor periodically has the option of updating accrued benefits in order to reflect inflation since they were earned. Final-average pay plans are automatically self-adjusting for inflation prior to retirement in that the entire benefit is related to earnings during the period shortly before retirement.

The question as to which type of formula is better is often asked. Both have advantages and disadvantages. The career-average salary plan requires periodic amendments to keep the plan up to date. This allows the employer discretion as to when and to what extent the plan will be updated, thus allowing the employer to

evaluate the financial considerations when making the choice. The employer also gets credit from its employees for making a plan improvement. A final-average pay plan offers better protection to employees, but the employer has less control over future costs and usually incurs a higher initial cost.

It is interesting to note that many union-negotiated plans are flat dollar plans, a form of career-average plan under which the benefit earned is a level amount for each year of service. The union traditionally bargains for increases in the benefit to be earned either in future years only or in both future and past years. The use of this type of plan enables the union to "win" benefit increases for its members on a periodic basis.

A comparison of the two types of plans appears in Table 1-6.

Integration

An analysis of Social Security benefits shows that they are significantly higher as a percentage of income for lower paid employees than for higher paid employees. The Social Security system is designed to achieve this result because social adequacy is one of its major goals. However, an employer probably will want to provide a more consistent benefit to all employees as a percentage of pay. Therefore, the private plan benefit needed to maintain the preretirement living standard will be higher as a percentage of pay for higher-paid employees than for lower paid employees.

The Internal Revenue Code does not allow plans to discriminate in favor of higher paid employees. How-

Table 1-6 Comparison of Career Average and Final Pay Plans

	Career Average	*Final Average*
Benefit formula	Specified accrual in each plan year; total benefit is sum of individual yearly accruals	Benefit based on final average earnings and total credited service
Handling of inflation before retirement	No automatic adjustment. Employer may periodically update benefits	Benefit adjusts automatically
Employee relations	Employer can improve plan periodically via update—good for employee relations	No plan improvement needed and hence no "credit" for employer
Financial risks	Employer has discretion over plan improvements—financing of updates by level payments over 10–30 year period	Benefit increases due to salary increases prefunded to extent provided by salary scale—excess of pay increases over salary scale leads to actuarial loss
Timing of updates	Completely at discretion of employer (unless subject to union negotiation)	N/A
Method of accommodating erratic work history	Each year's accrual reflects actual earnings so accruals track the history	No provision: however partial year's credit may be given
Accrued benefit	Sum of prior accruals	Based on application of formula

ever, in measuring discrimination, the employer is allowed to recognize Social Security benefits in the plan formula because a portion (historically 50 percent) of the Social Security tax is paid by the employer. The process by which Social Security benefits are recognized in the plan formula is called "integration," and several different methods of integration are permitted. Detailed regulations give rules and limits for integration.[4]

Plan sponsors should periodically review the replacement ratios resulting from all employer-provided benefit plans plus Social Security. If the pattern between higher and lower paid employees is not satisfactory, the integration method and level should be reviewed to see if a better result can be achieved. Many plans were designed some time ago and are integrated based on the prior Social Security law. Since major revisions were made to the Social Security law in both 1972 and 1977, a review may be especially appropriate at this time.

Design Issues of the 1980s

The Employee Retirement Income Security Act (ERISA) of 1974, signed into law on Labor Day in 1974, vastly expanded regulation of benefit plans and brought with it major changes in the legal requirements for most pension plans in the United States. The ERISA introduced a number of minimum requirements for pension plan provisions in areas such as eligibility, vesting, joint and survivor annuities, preretirement death benefits, and treatment of employee contributions.

The outlook for the 1980s is that further required changes in benefit plans seem very likely, and that these changes will be in response to a number of issues including:

- pressure on current and future retirees resulting from inflation;
- pressure on employers resulting from inflation, and cost pressure on health care facilities resulting from public pressure and possible legislation designed to contain and limit the increase in health care costs;
- age discrimination legislation and regulations;
- sex discrimination legislation and regulations;
- concern about equity between persons covered by qualified pension plans who terminate employment on a nonvested basis, and persons not covered and therefore eligible for individual retirement accounts.

The most difficult and controversial design issue of the 1980s is likely to be response to inflation, primarily in the form of cost-of-living increases after retirement. This issue will also arise in the form of pressure for final-average pay pension plans, or for past service updates in existing career-average pay plans. At present, employers quite commonly provide pension benefits updated for inflation up to the time of retirement, utilizing one of the methods previously described, but most private employers do not provide for automatic cost-of-living increases after retirement. A 1979 Harris Poll indicated that cost-of-living increases are the design issue of most concern to both retirees and active employees.[5] Retirees participating in that study state that they are badly hurt by inflation. A 1978 study by the Conference Board, a national business research organization, showed that inflation was a major concern of retired executives.[6]

Social Security benefits are indexed by the Consumer Price Index. Other public plans include full or partial indexing. The effect of this indexing is anomalous. It serves to add great credence to the arguments of those who demand indexing in the private sector, while at the same time it greatly increases the cost of the public plan benefits. Demographic trends, interacting with inflation and pay-as-you-go funding, will make many public plans and Social Security far more expensive than they appear to be today, and quite possibly too expensive for the American public. The real cost of these plans is slowly being recognized.

Postretirement indexing will be a bargaining issue for the most powerful unions in the next few years, and it will increasingly get the attention of legislators. The issue will be studied in Washington. The cost of such indexing is high and open ended. Groups representing older Americans can be expected to place higher priority on this issue.

The other side of the inflation picture will be increased pressure on health care facilities, as employers, to keep costs under control, and possible regulation of benefits as part of general wage price control programs or health care cost containment. Employers will increasingly search for trade-offs (ways to reduce costs in one area) while at the same time introducing other improvements or responding to an increase in the cost of another benefit.

In the long run, an increase in the normal retirement age seems the most likely way to reduce employer pension costs, and also Social Security costs. This would seem unlikely to occur in the next five or ten years, but very likely will take place before the turn of the century as the age distribution of the population shifts upward.

Another method of increasing retirement income without increasing employer costs is to have the employees pay for the increase in benefits themselves. A nonprofit hospital can use a tax-sheltered annuity program to supplement a noncontributory pension plan and permit employees to use before-tax dollars to help pay for their retirements. The 1979 Harris Poll indicates that much of the public is willing to help pay for their own retirement.[7] Use of a supplemental tax-sheltered annuity permits a structure whereby all employees can participate in the basic plan whether they choose to contribute to the supplemental plan or not. The tax-sheltered annuity may also be useful for providing additional benefits for higher-paid personnel without changing the basic structure of the pension plan. The hospital can pay for these benefits on a discriminatory basis by granting pay increases which are to be used for the tax-sheltered annuity contribution.

Employee contributions to pay for benefits are likely to get increased attention during the next decade. Four bills before Congress in 1979 would either permit tax deductibility of employee contributions or permit all employees to establish Individual Retirement Accounts, whether or not they are currently covered by pension plans. At present, employees can establish Individual Retirement Accounts only if they are not covered by qualified pension plans. This has led to concern about equity between employees not so covered, and those who are covered but never receive any benefits because they leave employment on a nonvested basis. The potential legislative areas to watch for during the next decade are:

- expansion of Individual Retirement Accounts and liberalization of the rules governing their establishment;
- tax deductibility of employee contributions to pension plans up to a stated maximum level;
- requirements that employers accept voluntary employee contributions in all qualified pension plans, together with restrictions on mandatory employee contributions.

During 1978 and 1979 the federal government expanded age discrimination regulation, with the passage of the Age Discrimination in Employment Act of 1978 (ADEA), and the promulgation in May 1979 of an Interpretative Bulletin setting forth requirements with respect to benefit plans. The 1978 legislation prohibits mandatory retirement before age 70 except for highly paid executives. It requires significant changes in many welfare plans, but will have little effect on defined benefit pension plans. Under this legislation, pension benefits may be frozen at normal retirement age, usually age 65. Legislation to ban all age-based mandatory retirement has already been introduced in Congress and passed in several states. We can also expect pressure for mandated pension plan accruals beyond normal retirement age, and this too will probably be a legislative issue in the next decade.

Another area which will give rise to pension plan design issues is problems arising from sex discrimination and the relative treatment of men and women. On an immediate basis, proposed regulations under the Equal Pay Act would require that benefits payable to men and women under all optional forms of payment be equal. This may require the use of the same mortality tables for men and women (commonly referred to as unisex tables) for determination of optional methods of payment in pension plans. Ian Lanoff, Administrator, Pension and Welfare Benefit Programs Division of the Department of Labor, is looking into the effect of pension benefits on women. Current studies of this issue are focusing on differences in the life patterns of men and women, and whether women are disadvantaged as a result of these differences.[8] During the 1980s we can expect a number of questions to be asked, with the result that minimum design specifications may become more stringent.

The interaction of vesting and eligibility with work patterns is currently under study. Today there is confusion as to the rights of spouses to pension benefits in divorce cases. This area will be clarified by court decisions, and probably eventually by legislation. We can also expect requirements for earlier preretirement death benefits.

Capital Accumulation Programs

Defined benefit pension plans are designed to provide stipulated benefits payable as regular income, and income is the key reason for establishing these plans. Defined contribution plans are designed around capital accumulation, whereby the accumulation may or may not be converted to income.

Various forms of defined contribution programs can be used in conjunction with defined benefit pension plans to provide a means of capital accumulation on an advantageous basis. The funds accumulated may be used either for additional periodic retirement income, for other retirement needs or, in the case of thrift plans, for needs before retirement. An employer may offer a capital accumulation facility to its employees without participating directly, or may offer to match a portion of the employee's contribution. The most popular forms of capital accumulation programs are tax-sheltered annuities, where available, and thrift plans. These programs offer the employee the chance for automatic savings through payroll deduction. Many of these plans offer investment vehicles more attractive than available elsewhere, particularly when the taxation of the programs is considered. A program may offer a choice of investment in one or more equity funds, and in a fixed income fund with interest guaranteed at a rate as high as 9 percent. Many insurance carriers offer special contracts designed for investment of the funds generated by these programs, and tailored to the needs of these programs. Nonprofit hospitals operating under Section 501(c)(3) of the Internal Revenue Code can sponsor tax-sheltered annuity programs. Under these programs, the employee can generally contribute up to 16 2/3 percent of income on a before-tax basis into the tax-sheltered annuity. The money accumulates on a tax-free basis until the annuity income is received. At that point the employee pays tax on both the amount put into the annuity and the investment income. A special use of this type of program is to provide supplemental retirement income for higher paid employees.

These programs, since the benefits are immediately vested, offer a benefit with immediate value to the younger employee for whom retirement is remote. Even though the benefit may not be payable for many years, the employee can see the dollar amount of an accumulation account. An employer contribution to a capital accumulation program is often an alternative to an improvement in a pension plan.

DISABILITY AND MEDICAL REIMBURSEMENT ISSUES

Recent changes in disability experience, family patterns and the legal environment are affecting disability plans. The legal environment in which employers provide disability coverage, a major employee need, has changed dramatically in the last few years. The 1977 Social Security Amendments reduced the level of disability benefits, particularly for employees who become disabled at early ages. The Interpretative Bulletin setting forth requirements with respect to the ADEA requires an extension of disability coverage beyond age 65, the traditional age at which employers have cut off disability protection. The 1978 pregnancy disability legislation requires that, for benefit purposes, disability resulting from pregnancy be treated the same as any other disability for benefit purposes. The disability claim costs experienced by the Social Security system have generally increased while legal requirements have forced employers to expand coverage.

The existence of a second income in the two-income family has added a new element to the financial picture which determines employee needs and which will determine employee motivation to return to work. Furthermore, public attitudes indicate a decline in the work ethic and an increasing interest in getting something for nothing.

All of these factors mean that employers will need to manage disability programs well in the 1980s, and that both benefit design and claims management will be important.

As with regular retirement benefits, Social Security benefits provide the first layer of disability coverage. Social Security benefits are not available until the employee has been disabled five months, and may not be payable to every disabled employee. The combined benefit level should be low enough such that there is an incentive to return to work. If benefits are fully paid for by employee contributions, disability income is tax free, so that there is an advantage in allocating employee contributions first to disability programs. Limited amounts of benefits paid for by employer dollars are also tax free. Claim costs can be expected to increase as the ratio of disability benefit to earnings increases.

In many situations, an older disabled employee may have a choice between a disability benefit and a retirement benefit. This problem will become more acute as employers modify their plans to comply with ADEA requirements. The Interpretative Bulletin relating to ADEA offers several alternatives with respect to disability coverage after age 65:

- continue disability coverage to age 70;
- provide five years of disability income for persons disabled after age 60, but in no case pay disability income after age 70;
- using a graded schedule of benefit periods, shorten the benefit period at each age in order to equalize cost at the higher ages;
- use a decreasing schedule of benefits at the higher ages in order to cost equalize with the next younger age before the decrease starts;
- use a "package approach" to equalize costs of more than one benefit.

Over the long term it will be essential that disability and retirement programs be designed to work together. Otherwise, employers may find disability programs being used for retirement, with resulting high claim costs.

Short-term disability may be covered by either a formal or informal sick leave program. In the current environment, informal programs should be formalized and claim procedures reviewed. Outside claims administration may be preferable even though claims were once handled inside. Some of the areas to watch for in short-term programs are:

- use of employer-paid physicians for review of medical status of claimants;
- benefit levels that encourage return to work;
- review of claims procedures to see that appropriate and complete information is developed for each type of disability.

The legal requirement to cover pregnancy-related disability for the first time in 1979 has provided many employers an incentive to review and update their handling of short-term disability claims.

Disability benefits are also included in Social Security and other employer-provided benefit plans. Many pension plans continue accruals during disability, particularly if the employer provides a long-term disability program. Others make provision for payment of a disability pension on a basis more favorable than the regular early retirement provision. Life insurance premiums are usually waived during periods of disability, up to a specified maximum age.

Medical care plan issues over the next decade will depend greatly on how much, if any, national health insurance Congress chooses to legislate. The comments here assume no national health insurance. The major emphasis is likely to be on containing employer costs. There are three directions which can be pursued in order to achieve this end:

1. increase the portion of the medical expenses paid by the individual through the use of higher deductibles or more coinsurance;
2. decrease the employer's share of the cost through a higher employee contribution;
3. design the benefit structure so as to create a favorable climate for change in the patterns of care.

The trend in the recent past has been to reduce the amount the employee has to pay, but this may reverse over the next few years as cost pressures grow. The greatest opportunity lies in the area of encouraging changes in the pattern of care. Second-opinion programs can reduce surgery and are beneficial for all concerned. However, employees may be reluctant to seek second opinions, and public education will be needed before this becomes accepted practice. Benefit schedules can be designed to encourage maximum use of outpatient facilities whenever medically sound. In the past, benefit structures often had the reverse effect. Hospitals, as medical care experts, are in a position to play a leadership role in promoting benefit design which encourages efficient use of health care facilities.

The work force in a hospital provides some difficult questions as to who should reasonably be eligible for benefits and how benefit levels should be structured. Traditionally, benefit programs have covered only full-time workers. Under ERISA, employees who work at least 1,000 hours in a year must be included in pension plans. Part-time work is common, and many part-timers work on a regular basis. Hospital part-time workers may include professionals. The general social climate points to pressure, and possible regulation, which would require coverage of more employees.

DEATH BENEFIT ISSUES

Death benefits have been and remain an important part of an employer-sponsored fringe-benefit program. The challenge of the 1980s will be to keep benefit design simple, need related, logical and understandable to the employee.

Survivor income, for the lifetime of the spouse, until the children reach adulthood or for a temporary readjustment period, is the most fundamental need to be covered. In addition, there is a need to have funds for final expenses.

Employer-sponsored life insurance can also be used for estate building and conservation and to provide funds to pay estate taxes.

Employer philosophies as to the purposes and goals of employer-sponsored death benefits vary and should be identified.

The factors to be considered in death benefit design are the multiple sources of benefits, different tax treatment of benefits provided in different ways and differing needs of the various segments of the work force. The fact that Social Security provides survivor benefits and a small lump sum death benefit may also influence benefit design.

An analysis of death benefits currently provided in employer plans indicates that in some cases the amounts provided are high relative to employee needs. There is also likely to be an abrupt increase in death benefit protection when an employee reaches eligibility for pension plan death benefits. There may be other discontinuities as well.

The ADEA requirements call for continuation of death benefit coverage to age 70 while in active employment, but permit benefit reductions for cost equalization. Employers with large lump-sum benefits may wish to reduce these benefits and shift to a program with a heavier emphasis on survivor income. A coordinated survivor-income program would provide a benefit at a predetermined level but with offsets for benefits provided from other employer-paid benefit sources. This is one method of simplifying the structure.

Death benefits before and after retirement and the method of reduction are likely to get increased attention in the 1980s. A large benefit drop at date of retirement is likely to encourage sick employees to continue in active employment, or to remain on disability, since often disabled employees get the same life insurance coverage as active employees, whereas retired employees do not. A method of handling this problem is to gradually reduce benefits with advancing age, instead of abruptly at retirement. Under the cost-equalization provisions of ADEA, benefits for active employees can be reduced either on an age-by-age basis, or on a five-year average-age-grouping basis. The five-year age grouping allows benefits at ages 60 to 64 to be reduced between 30 percent and 35 percent at age 65, if they are then held level from ages 65 to 69, based on commonly used tables. Single year-by-year reductions of about 8 percent per year will equalize costs.

Death benefits are much more important to some employee groups than to others. If an employer offers an optional benefit program, some employees may choose to exchange part of their death benefits for other types of benefits.

THE 1980s—YEARS OF CHALLENGE

The basic principles underlying benefit design in the 1980s will be the same as they have been in the 1970s and in past decades. Employer goals, employee needs and employer resources will be cornerstones on which benefit design rests. The specific problems employers must face, however, may be somewhat different. The 1970s brought a vast expansion of regulation of benefit patterns and huge increases in Social Security benefits and taxes.

The 1970s also were a time of expansion of the definition of employee rights and of issues relating to discrimination, and these concepts formed the basis of expanded regulation. The 1970s were difficult economically, with wage increases and price increases at higher levels than in previous decades, which slowed the rise in living standards.

It is not possible to predict how things will change in the 1980s, but we know that change is inevitable. Sound design today requires flexibility and planning, with the expectation that changes will inevitably be required. It calls for study of the present and tracking of emerging trends so that tomorrow's problems will be identified as early as possible. It requires an understanding of the needs and value systems of our society, because law and regulation respond to these values.

As we enter the 1980s, benefits managers will have to respond to growing demands of employees, growing economic pressures and new regulation. The 1980s will be years of challenge.

NOTES

1. Chamber of Commerce of the United States of America, *Employee Benefits, 1977* (Washington, D.C.: The Chamber of Commerce, 1978).
2. U.S. Executive Office of the President, Office of Management and Budget, *The United States Budget in Brief, Fiscal Year 1980* (1979).
3. Louis Harris, et al., *1979 Study of American Attitudes Toward Pensions and Retirement* (New York: Johnson & Higgins, 1979): iv.
4. U.S. Internal Revenue Service, Revenue Ruling 71-446 (1971).
5. Harris, *1979 Study of American Attitudes,* p. 64.
6. *The Productive Retirement Years of Former Managers,* Report No. 747 (New York: The Conference Board, Inc., 1978): 6.
7. Harris, *1979 Study of American Attitudes,* p. 31.
8. U.S. Department of Justice, Task Force on Sex Discrimination, Civil Rights Division, *The Pension Game: American Pension System from the Viewpoint of the Average Woman* (Washington, D.C.: U.S. Government Printing Office, 1979).

2. Some Fundamentals of Employee Benefits Administration

FRANK J. MALOUFF

Following World War II, employee benefits accounted for virtually no percentage of the total compensation paid to workers. As business enters the 1980s, benefits account for a third or more of the total compensation paid. This growth may be accounted for in part by several trends:

- sophistication of employee expectations
- the realization of the purchasing power of group benefits programs
- tax advantages to employees when benefits are prepaid
- increased competition for recruitment and retention of workers in the marketplace

As the growth of the benefits sector continues, the need arises for a more systematized approach to administration of employee benefits. This article looks at some of the fundamentals of employee benefits programs and identifies suggestions and trends that impact on current activities. These are derived from the author's experience administering a major benefits program. Critical philosophical issues of benefits administration, including communication of benefits and the "cafeteria" approach, are considered at the end of the article.

EMPLOYEE HEALTH BENEFITS

Abraham Maslow[1] suggests that following primal concerns with salary compensation on a job, an employee turns quickly to security, including concerns for individual and family health. Given the rapid increase in the costs of health care, virtually no benefits program today excludes at least some health insurance provisions.

Major Medical Health Insurance

There are four major characteristics of major medical health insurance programs: (1) blanket coverage, (2) an insurance deductible, (3) percentage participation by insured employees, and (4) maximum amount of coverage. These plans usually define blanket coverage to include inpatient hospitalization expenses and limited outpatient benefits for medical situations that are nonroutine in nature.[2] More routine situations such as annual physical examinations and well-baby care may not be included in some plans.

Like automobile insurance, major medical plans require the insured to exceed a deductible amount of expenses before the provisions become operable. These deductibles may be in the ballpark of $100 annually for the employee or a total of $200 annually for the employee and dependents. Deductibles reduce claim administration expense by limiting the number of small claims that the insured probably can manage anyway. This allows more benefit dollars to go for serious and large losses. When employees have bills in excess of the deductible, they may file for the entire sum for reimbursement.

The percentage participation characteristic of major medical plans often is called coinsurance. After satisfying the deductible, employees may share in a small amount of their medical expenses on part or all of the coverage. The employees may retain responsibility for 20 percent to 25 percent of the expense, with the plan assuming the remainder.

Many coinsurance plans exclude expenditures over a certain limit. This protects the employee from major catastrophic losses and is a low-cost addition to the plan. For example, a plan might feature a $200 family deductible and 80 percent-20 percent coinsurance on the first $5,000 coverage, with 100 percent of expenses above $5,000 paid. Given this type of plan, employees can determine their maximum liability to be $1,200 annually—$200 for the deductible and $1,000 for 20 percent of the next $5,000.

The final characteristic of major medical plans is the maximum amount. Some plans may limit benefits paid to an amount such as $500,000 in a lifetime. More and more plans are eliminating the maximum in favor of unlimited coverage. Curiously, some employees react more favorably to an absurdly high arbitrary maximum (i.e., $100 million lifetime maximum), than a simple "unlimited lifetime maximum."

Major medical plans are more desirable to younger groups of employees or where workers pay a majority of the premium costs. Major medical plans are among the most reasonable from the premium cost standpoint.

Comprehensive Health Insurance Plans

Comprehensive plans often specify limits to be paid for specific health care services such as hospitalization, inpatient drugs, or surgery. These plans usually carry more expensive premium schedules since deductibles and coinsurance may be eliminated. These plans are more common when the company pays the majority or all of the premium.

With the growth of health care in the gross national product and as a percentage of personal expenses, there is a definite trend toward this type of plan. This is especially true among companies with union-negotiated benefits packages and in areas of high competition for skilled workers.

Such plans usually emphasize the nature of their benefits with descriptive names such as "first dollar" plans to indicate that expenses are paid from the first dollar of expense. To provide coverages over the contractual amounts and to cover catastrophic illness, many comprehensive plans also contain major medical clauses. With the majority of medical expenses being covered in the comprehensive portion of the plan, the catastrophic major medical is available at extremely low cost.

Health Maintenance Organizations (HMOs)

Perhaps the fastest growing sector in the health insurance industry is the band of health maintenance organizations (HMOs) across the country. These organizations represent an innovation in health delivery systems designed to provide comprehensive health services with cost controls. Cost control is achieved by organizational recognition of the physician as the primary consumer as well as provider of health services. Incentives to physicians are built into the plan through extensive peer review and standards of care. Use of physician extenders and incentives for patient use of preventive services also contribute to the cost savings of HMOs.

HMO care is provided on a capitation basis. Therefore, no matter what level of services the patient uses, the cost remains virtually constant. HMOs are popular among families with small children because of the services available for routine care and normal childhood illnesses. HMOs often offer the most comprehensive services of any health insurance plan, including: physician services, inpatient hospitalization, outpatient care, emergency services, diagnostic laboratory and radiology, preventive health services, and routine care.

Much of the growth of HMOs can be attributed to the federal Health Maintenance Organizations Act of 1973. This legislation requires employers to offer HMO plans to employees if the company:

- has 25 or more employees
- pays minimum wages
- has employees in the service area of a qualified HMO
- is approached by the HMO[3]

Medicare Supplements

Some employers provide benefits for eligible employees and retirees that fill the gap between regular Medicare provisions and the company's regular health plan. These plans appear under a variety of names (i.e., Medigap) and usually are relatively low cost.

Many such plans will not cover items under Part B of Medicare, whether or not the person has enrolled for such coverage. Therefore, the employer should take steps in these cases to ensure that eligible employees do in fact enroll for Medicare Part B.

Pregnancy Benefits

The biggest furor of the last few years in health insurance benefits has been that caused by the Pregnancy Discrimination Act of 1978, which applied to health benefits plans as of April 29, 1979. That law mandates that pregnancy benefits be provided on the same basis as nonpregnancy disabilities. Employers of 15 or more employees must comply with this act.

While not all requirements are clear, it appears that health benefit plans must:

- provide eligibility for maternity benefits on the same basis as other benefits, not on the "conception basis"* that prevailed in the 1970s
- provide maternity benefits without requiring female employees to elect dependent coverage to be eligible
- make appropriate changes if maternity benefits are treated differently in any aspect of plan design (i.e., deductibles, coinsurance, extension of benefits)

One major issue on requirements for maternity coverage of dependent wives and dependent children remains unclear.[4,5,6]

Self-Insurance Plans

Some large employers are finding it attractive to develop self-insurance plans as cost-saving devices. These plans do not necessarily have to be developed around an employer hospital. The author has worked with a plan for house staff in Denver that allows members to obtain care at any hospital.

Many self-insured plans are modeled after the La Habra Plan from that city in California. La Habra self-funded its employees for $720 each annually. Employee claims were paid from this amount. Any medical deduction qualifying under Internal Revenue regulations was eligible for reimbursement under the plan.

Employees could draw on this $720. However, if the employee filed no claims, the individual received a bonus of $720 at year's end. When claims exceeded $720, the employee paid 100 percent of the expenses up to $1,000, when an umbrella major medical clause paid 100 percent of costs over that.[7]

The plan for house staff associated with the University of Colorado Health Sciences Center is a more tra-

ditional combination of comprehensive benefit limits and major medical coverage. The plan covers 800 house officers to a specified aggregate stop-loss each year. An umbrella policy covers claims in excess of the stop-loss and individual claims in excess of $40,000. Since its inception, the plan has been successful in increasing benefits and maintaining premiums at virtually a constant level.

Some Medical Insurance Trends

As benefits packages are improved, certain low-cost additions are being added to health insurance plans. These often include vision care, breakage of glasses, home health coverage, alcoholism treatment plans, and hearing care. These improvements often are made on a coinsurance basis or as part of major medical insurance provisions.

One extremely popular and cost-saving improvement is coverage for a second opinion in prospective surgery cases. Potential cost savings, especially for rated plans, appear to be far in excess of any additional premium or contribution costs.

LIFE INSURANCE BENEFITS

The American Council of Life Insurance reports that the growth of group life insurance in the period 1956–1977 was almost tenfold. Protection of $12.4 billion was purchased in 1957, $118 billion in 1977.[8]

Group life insurance, accidental death and dismemberment, and disability insurance remain a relatively inexpensive benefit. It is especially attractive to the younger work force, which usually does not seek large amounts of individual life coverage.

Term Life Insurance

Benefit life insurance most commonly involves either term insurance plans with one face amount for all ages, or decreasing term insurance plans with lesser face amounts for older employees.

Group rated plans with single premiums usually pay higher premium amounts. This can mean that premiums are very high for employees under a certain age (around 40) and very low for others. Large employee groups may find that administration of the plan is simpler under these structures. Smaller plans may find it advantageous to provide data on the ages of employees and rate the plan on that basis. Under these plans, the premium for older employees is higher.

Decreasing term insurance plans usually provide one premium rate, with the face amount determined by

---

*The manner in which the "conception basis" had been applied was that the insurance company which covered this benefit at the time of conception was the company which paid the maternity benefits. This is no longer true.

age. This is difficult to structure if the face amount is low initially.

Even nondecreasing plans usually limit the amount of insurance a retiree may carry in a benefits package. It is common in these cases to substantially reduce the amount available to the retiree to perhaps 20 percent to 25 percent of the preretirement amount. At some point these retiree coverages become virtually certain claims for the carrier.

Internal Revenue Service regulations limit to $50,000 the amount of life insurance that may be prepaid for an employee. On an employee pay basis, these amounts may go higher. Usually they are based on some multiple of the annual salary. In other words, the employer may pay for an employee's coverage up to $500,000. However, an employee can opt for more coverage at his or her own expense.

Some companies offer a small option for prepaid life insurance, with a higher option available for employee purchase. A common practice is to differentiate life insurance benefits between executive and nonexecutive groups. The issue of any differentiation is one an institution must consider in light of its own philosophies and objectives.

Accidental Death and Dismemberment (AD&D)

AD&D coverage often is combined with employee group term life. It is very inexpensive, running about 5¢ to 7¢ per month per $1,000 coverage. Eligibility usually is the same as for life coverage. AD&D plans stop at retirement; however, past practices of also terminating coverage at age 65 have been dropped since the Age Discrimination Act amendments of 1979.[9]

AD&D benefits most often are tied to group life coverage. Many pay equal to total group life (basic and any supplemental coverage). Premium payment may be either contributory or noncontributory for basic coverage. Supplemental virtually always is contributory on the part of the employee.

Short-Term Disability

Some institutions fund their own short-term disability plans through accrued sick leave policies. Others may provide a certain number of days for hospitalization, but maintain purchased short-term salary reimbursement insurance. The advantage to the latter may be to decrease the overall cost of lost time by reducing the number of questionable sick days—or "mental health" days.

Some plans reimburse after a minimum period of three to seven days. Reimbursement then may be retroactive. However, employees may then be sure to remain off the job until the minimum period passes, even if the illness no longer persists.

In some instances, employers who provide accrued sick leave are reassessing their policies to tie in time off bonuses for employees who do not use their benefits. Few employers of any size have subjective policies for determination of paid or nonpaid time on an individual basis. The problems of consistency in these plans are enormous.

The issues raised in health benefits plans by the Pregnancy Discrimination Act of 1978 are applicable here also. The act may be responsible for either a substantial rise in the cost of such programs, or their reduction in scope over time—or both. However, institutions must research any reductions in plans carefully before making changes if they are to maintain compliance with the law.

Long-Term Disability

Despite the requirement by most states for employers to purchase Workers' Compensation Insurance for employees injured as a result of the job, many employers provide long-term disability (LTD) plans on either a prepaid or subscription basis.

Workers' Compensation plans vary, but often provide a percentage of salary for employees whose injuries qualify. These may have weekly limits. Compensation for lost benefits usually is not made. Social Security benefits also may come into play for long-term disabled employees. However, those receiving benefits from separate disability plans may not be eligible to receive payments from Social Security.

There is a trend among some employers to assist employees in appealing denied Social Security benefits. In many cases, these appeals may save LTD plans substantial payouts. There also may be corresponding savings in health insurance benefits for the disabled.

The following are suggested features in the design of LTD plans:

- initiation at around 26 weeks
- some maximum benefit level to discourage abuse
- limits on LTD and pension benefits paid to the same person
- coordination of benefits with other plans to eliminate duplicated coverages
- benefit levels set at less than full take-home pay
- payment for rehabilitative services to reduce long-term claims[10]

Travel Insurance

Another inexpensive group insurance coverage may be obtained for travel. Some medical facilities cover faculty and executives for business travel. This coverage may be obtained for larger groups based on average number of days in travel status a year. Premiums are surprisingly low.

Some plans also offer voluntary travel insurance coverage. However, the premiums may multiply several times for such voluntary coverage. Blanket annual coverage for groups seems to be the best bargain.

DENTAL INSURANCE BENEFITS

Dental insurance is perhaps the hottest benefit item of the late 1970s and early 1980s. Much hard data exist to indicate the value of preventive dental care in reducing later expenses, so most dental programs cover at least part of the cost of preventive care.

Protecting against adverse selection is an extremely important factor in dental insurance plan design. Few plans will be written without at least 75 percent of the group's members participating. Mandatory coverage also is very prevalent. Employer contributions seem to be an important incentive in boosting participation. Many plans contribute the entire cost of the employee's premium and some even contribute to the premium for dependents.

Dental plan benefits often are on a coinsurance basis. Some do pay 100 percent for scheduled preventive care. The most restrictive benefits in many plans are for orthodontia. Indeed, such benefits are omitted entirely from some plans.

RETIREMENT BENEFITS

Interest in employee retirement benefits has increased in the last few years, mainly because of inflation and of public concern over the stability of the Social Security program. Changes in the mandatory retirement age notwithstanding, interest is shifting to early retirement benefits and supplemental retirement and annuity plans.

Social Security (FICA)

There are two major parts to the Social Security (FICA) retirement plan: Old Age Survivors and Disability Insurance (OASDI) and Medicare benefits. Unless workers are included in a qualified alternative retirement plan, they must be covered by Social Security.

Employer and employee each pay half of the deductions for Social Security. There has been a trend in recent years to the employer's paying the entire premium. The major complication of this concept is the taxability of the added employer contribution.

Faced with a work force of growing age and the ever-present problem of inflation, Social Security contributions have increased rapidly. Most workers will be paying Social Security on virtually every dollar of their earnings by 1983.

It is virtually impossible for most employees to trace the mechanism for determining Social Security benefits. Benefits are paid based on a primary insurance amount (PIA), which itself comes from computation of average monthly earnings (AME). The AME formula involves calculation of seven different segments.

The formula is weighted to favor lower income brackets. In the AME formula, early marginal dollars of AME produce more PIA than do late marginal dollars of AME. As a package, Social Security benefits are estimated to be equal to about 75 percent of the yearly salary subject to Social Security taxes.[11]

Supplemental and Private Retirement Plans

There is much interest, therefore, in supplementing Social Security benefits with other plans. Integration or nonintegration with Social Security are concerns of importance for employers seeking additional coverage. Plans in which the amount of money contributed varies, but the eventual benefit is determined in advance, are called defined benefit plans. If the contributions to the fund are fixed, but actual benefits are not known, the plan is a defined contribution plan.[12]

Vesting of benefits is an important variable in evaluating retirement plans. Vesting defines the level of benefits that an employee cannot lose, even if the individual terminates before retirement. Some plans are vested immediately, while others use a percentage based on the number of years of service.

The Employee Retirement Income Security Act of 1974 (ERISA) defines three alternative vesting schedules. Plans may adopt one of these or a schedule that vests earlier than the minimums defined. ERISA's alternative vesting schedules are:

Cliff Vesting:	Full vesting after ten years' service, with no vesting before then.
Graded Vesting:	25 percent vesting after five years of service, with 5 per-

cent additional vesting each year up to ten years, plus an additional 10 percent for each year thereafter. This formula vests 100 percent after 15 years.

Rule-of-45 Vesting: 50 percent vesting for an employee with at least five years' service when age and service add up to 45, plus 10 percent additional vesting each year for five years.

Integration of plans with Social Security usually is accomplished in one of three ways: (1) the offset mechanism provides for private plan benefits to be reduced by Social Security payments; (2) excess only plans include only earnings in excess of the integration level; (3) step rate plans provide for one benefit rate for covered earnings and a higher rate for excess earnings. The step rate approach is extremely popular.

Annuities

Much attention has been paid to annuity plans in the last few years, particularly because of the extremely high interest rates. More than 500 companies sell annuity plans. These may be contributory by the employer or voluntary.

The IRS regulations provide for annuity options for qualified educational institutions. A major feature of annuity programs is the exclusion of contributions from immediate taxation. Annuity contributions are made by reduction of taxable income, rather than deduction from taxable income.

Contributions to annuity programs as governed by the IRS are defined as maximum exclusion calculations. These calculations examine the amount of service, salary level, other retirement contributions, and past salary excluded in determining maximum participation in an annuity.

Participants may elect to credit contributions to fixed or variable portions of the annuity plan. Fixed plans guarantee a level of return. These funds usually are invested in government bonds or other similar securities. Earning levels often are banded to rates defined each fiscal quarter. For example, many companies will apply interest for each quarter. Therefore, if the rate of interest for the first quarter is 12 percent, that is the rate they will apply to first quarter payments as long as that money is in the annuity. If the interest rate for the second quarter increases to 13 percent, that is the rate the companies will apply to that portion of the money as long as it is in the annuity. This is what is known as earning levels being *banded to rates*.

Variable plans base eventual earnings on the performance of stocks, corporate bonds, or similar securities. Most plans allow participants to split between fixed and variable contributions. Variable plans may offer options between different types of investment portfolios. For example, variable options may be available separately for stocks and for bonds.

Annuities often charge administrative fees for transactions or "load fees" off the top for contributions. Many "no load" plans are available, but virtually all plans have some mechanism for recovering administrative charges.

TIME OFF BENEFITS

Social psychologists indicate that time off is an increasingly important concern of workers—from television host Johnny Carson to professional and nonprofessional employees of health institutions.

The early 1970s witnessed a trend to expanded types of time off. Some employers developed separate categories of leave to cover holidays, vacation, sick time, on-the-job injuries, funerals, jury duty, maternity, active military service, military reserve summer camp, educational opportunities, and others. The trend now may be reversing itself as employees seek to maximize time under their own control, rather than time off for which they may or may not qualify. Employers, too, may find the reversal of the trend appealing as a way to reduce administrative bureaucracy in the control of the various types of time off.

For purposes of this discussion, the major categories of time off are examined separately; others are considered only briefly.

Holidays

Standard practices vary greatly in the number of paid holidays a year granted employees, from a minimum of five or six to 12 or more. Among the holidays employers may grant are:

New Years Day
Washington's Birthday
Lincoln's Birthday
Memorial Day
Independence Day
Labor Day
Columbus Day
Veterans' Day
Election Day

Thanksgiving Day
Christmas Day
Employee's birthday
Floating holidays

Some trends are very evident. Washington and Lincoln's Birthdays may be combined into one President's Day. Columbus Day and Veterans' Day may be omitted. They also may be combined into extra days at Thanksgiving or Christmas. Some traditional holidays may be replaced by employee-selected floating holidays.

Vacation and Personal Leave

The federal government is the traditional leader in vacation, with some agencies granting what amounts to one month per year paid leave to all levels of employees. This is known as annual leave or personal leave. In industry, the traditional standard has been two weeks per year. However, that figure is increasing. Often more senior employees earn more leave in all job categories.

In institutions that condense the various types of leave into fewer categories, the titles annual or personal leave are popular. Employees may be granted a few more days' leave than just those planned for vacation purposes. However, they are expected to use these extra days to cover funerals and similar commitments.

Many institutions regulate the use of personal leave, especially when such leave may be accrued. Maximum accruals are common. Practices vary, but normally some payment may be made at retirement or termination for earned but unused personal leave.

It is common to see earning schedules based on the month, rather than on an entire year. This simplifies some practices in administering personal leave benefits, but may be slightly more costly as benefits for part-years are provided.

Sick and Health Leave

Some of the most interesting changes in time off benefits have come in sick and health leave practices. Major changes occurred as a result of the Pregnancy Discrimination Act of 1978. The cost of sick leave has brought about others.

In previous years, one common practice was to grant special maternity leave to female employees who were pregnant. The Pregnancy Discrimination Act (P.L. 95-555) now prohibits treating maternity different from other medical conditions. The law states that "women affected by pregnancy, childbirth and related conditions shall be treated the same for all employment-related purposes, including receipt of benefits under fringe benefits plans, as other persons not so affected, but similar in the ability or inability to work."

Employers must consider maternity like any other disability condition. This may force them to reconsider the amount of disability coverage for any condition. Reductions in the number of weeks given are a distinct possibility in redesigned benefits programs. The growth of new disability plans also is in doubt.

Employers also are beginning to limit sick leave to offset increased utilization of one-day incidents. This trend has not met with much resistance where sick leave reductions are negotiated in favor of more flexible time off policies. Conversion mechanisms of unused sick leave to annual leave are becoming popular. These mechanisms seek to give employees incentives for not using sick leave unless it is absolutely necessary.

Educational Leave

After money issues, perhaps the most important concern of health professionals is for continuing education. In some states continuing education is mandatory for relicensure. Many health institutions are beginning to budget for educational leave with pay for professional employees.

Other educational leave mechanisms may provide for paid or nonpaid time for employees to pursue credit courses at local colleges and universities. These benefits are separate from educational assistance programs (discussed later in this article). Educational assistance provides funding for course work for individual employees.

Other Types of Paid Leave

Some institutions do provide for specific leave mechanisms for situations such as family funerals, military service, and jury duty. Funeral leave also may be allowable under sick leave provisions in isolated cases. State of Colorado employees may use up to five days' funeral leave with pay for the funeral of each immediate family member, including most close relatives except cousins.[13] This is a very liberal example of this type of leave, however.

The Department of Defense has been signing contracts with employers since the Vietnam conflict to allow reservists and National Guard members time off for summer camp responsibilities. The intent of these agreements is to provide the soldier/employee time to meet this commitment without being penalized personal vacation time. Often these agreements include provisions for the employer either to make up any money difference from military pay or to allow the employee to keep both military and institutional pay.

Similar provisions may be found for jury and witness duty. Since jury duty is the responsibility of every citizen and since courts make only token compensation for this service, many employers provide for employees to complete this duty without loss of pay or benefits.

Leave without Pay

Many employers provide for leave without pay, although this is used infrequently in most cases. However, with changes that may result from the Pregnancy Discrimination Act and sociocultural changes, employees may increase the number of requests for this type of leave. Employers may want to assess their policies on leave without pay in light of potential increases in utilization and their institutional employment philosophies.

OTHER BENEFITS

A lot of benefit mileage can be gotten from some relatively simple programs that impact an employee's life style. These include educational assistance, industrial discounts, free banking, employee credit unions, legal insurance, automobile insurance, and in-house benefits. These can be extremely visible while requiring a minimum of administrative resources.

Educational Assistance

Advanced educational opportunity is becoming more and more an expectation of every American. Employers find educational assistance programs very popular in their work force, especially so in health institutions. For example, the changes in the structure of nursing education place more and more emphasis on the degreed Registered Nurse. Diploma program graduates are seeking academic credit to complete their degrees in increasing numbers.

Other employees are working for college degrees and advanced degrees on a part-time basis. Some of the educational assistance programs in health institutions reimburse employees for job-related course work. Others place no restrictions on the type of courses. Such programs may be perceived as big differences between institutions in a competitive employment community.

Health institutions that do not have such programs may find rich opportunities to establish tuition assistance plans by negotiation with local colleges. Academic institutions may be responsive to bartering assistance for the use of space or instructional resources. Affiliation agreements for colleges may include provisions for assistance for employees of the health institution.

Industrial Discount Programs

Many businesses are responsive to establishing discount programs for groups of employees.[14] In fact, many seek to initiate these programs as marketing devices. Institutional discount arrangements commonly are available from car rental companies, motel and hotel chains, dinner clubs, major and minor league sports franchises, and chain discount stores. These arrangements are not limited to business use, but are available for personal use of employees.

Most arrangements can be made simply for the asking. The motivation of commercial firms in granting these discounts is to establish patronage patterns for their product or service. A car rental discount may bring in not only the business of frequent users, but also contacts from an employee who may rent only once every several years.

Health institutions that develop these programs may want to establish some of the following policies:

- The institution may supply information about a discount program, but this does not mean it endorses the product or service.
- The institution cannot intercede for either the employee or the vendor in the commercial relationship.
- The institution cannot provide "front money" for discounts. (Vendors may desire this, but it is often discarded quickly, given this policy.)

Free Banking

Virtually every employee maintains a business relationship with a bank. Health institutions may easily negotiate accounts providing for no service charge and/or no minimum balance checking for their employees. Other services such as free traveler's checks, discounts on safe deposit boxes, free notary service (to name a few) also are available.

Banks are most responsive to these discounts in return for automatic deposit arrangements for the institution's payroll. The bank and the health institution also benefit in most cases. The health institution may find savings in payroll costs by reducing or completely eliminating the expense of producing checks. Advantages to the bank include increased cash flow by handling the payroll and increased business in other areas as a result of the relationship with the employees.

Health institutions may find it advantageous to include free employee banking in specifications to banks for placing institutional operating and development accounts.

In some cases health institutions may only transfer payroll funds through a private bank. Employees then may choose either a full-service checking account without charge or a limited service account. In a limited service arrangement, the employee writes a single check for the amount of salary due each payday. This allows the employee to obtain cash or transfer funds to another banking institution.

Credit Unions

Single health institutions or groups of health institutions may sponsor employee credit unions. The services provided by a credit union are well known. Additional value may be gained through credit unions that can seek out and administer discount programs for members. Some credit unions also provide checking account services, traveler's checks, credit card services, group automobile or legal insurance, and the like.

Legal Insurance and Automobile Insurance

Group plans may be available in competitive markets for legal or automobile insurance. For little or no premium consideration, group legal clinics may provide coverage for one consultation (often 30 minutes) without charge and group rates for other services.

Application of the group insurance concept to automobile insurance may or may not be practical. Institutions may be able to obtain employee discounts in the placement of larger liability or malpractice insurance accounts in the community. It is clear that leverage is available to health institutions that pursue linkages between their large purchases and employee discounts.

In-House Benefits

Health institutions traditionally have provided services or discounts internally to employees. These should be emphasized when communicating benefits

to workers. House benefits may include cafeteria discounts, hospitalization discounts, parking, and others.

Unemployment Insurance

Most employees do not consider unemployment insurance in their benefits packages. Few understand the funding of this program. When claims are made, the employee no longer is a part of the institution. Larger employers are charged directly for their unemployment experience; others may be in pooled groups.

Maximum weekly payments exist in most states, ranging from $70 to $172 weekly. Claimants may be granted full or partial awards for up to 26 weeks.[15]

Workers' Compensation

Most states also require employers to purchase Workers' Compensation insurance against the possibility that their employees will be injured or become ill as a result of the job. Workers' Compensation pools provide for partial salary losses and rehabilitative services in most cases. Again, few employees are aware that the institution is purchasing this benefit for them.

NEW TRENDS IN BENEFITS PHILOSOPHY

Two new trends are appearing more frequently in the design of benefits programs: (1) an increased emphasis on communicating information on the programs to employees, (2) a cafeteria approach to specific benefits.

One valid generalization that can be made about benefits is that employees know little about their specific programs. Health institutions are finding that it is more important than ever to communicate details of their programs to their employees. This trend may be due in part to increased unionization and the desire of administrations to counter this movement.

Employee benefits reports may be produced internally or bought under contract with a specialized firm. These generally cost a few dollars per year per employee. It makes sense to spend a minimal amount of money to explain the thousands of dollars in benefits given employees each year.

In contracting for benefits reports, there is a privacy issue to be considered. Employee financial information for the most part is private. Some release on an individual basis may be necessary under the laws of particular states.

As for the cafeteria approach to specific items, this concept provides for a certain amount of dollars to be spent on core benefits. Employees then may elect to use flexible credit dollars toward certain plans or coverages for inclusion in their benefits programs. They may elect dependent coverage in health insurance, for example, or additional coverages or plans. About the only restriction to the cafeteria approach is group term life, which is subject to IRS regulations.

The primary consideration in this approach seems to be, again, one of communication of benefits. Unless employees are knowledgeable about the programs offered, they may be at a disadvantage in making choices.[16]

Both of these concepts highlight the need for planned communication of benefits to employees. Whatever programs an institution may choose, communication to employees is an imperative that should be built into administration of the plans at the outset.

SOME FINAL REMARKS

Health institutions may find it difficult to cope with fiduciary management, other regulations such as ERISA, and trends in employee benefits administration.[17] Many institutions simply are not large enough to justify expenditures for a large benefits staff. For these reasons health institutions may find it especially attractive to contract with benefits consultants. Both national and local firms are available in most cities.

Services provided include researching benefits plans and design of comprehensive programs for individual employers. The value of a consultant's contacts in the industry alone is worthy of note. Consultants may provide a highly acceptable alternative to supplement benefits administration for both small and large institutions.

Consultants often are reimbursed either by retainer or by a percentage of premiums paid. In larger accounts, especially, this percentage may come from the carrier or may be built into the premium structure.

NOTES

1. A. H. Maslow, "A Theory of Human Motivation," *Psychological Review,* Vol. 50, pp. 370-396 (1943).
2. Albert H. Mowbray, Ralph H. Blanchard, and C. Arthur Williams, Jr., *Insurance,* 6th ed. (New York: McGraw-Hill Book Co., 1969), passim.
3. _____ , "Typical HMO Contract," *Employee Benefits Developments,* May 1978, p. 4.
4. 42 USC §2000e-2(a)(1)(1970).
5. Patricia M. Lines, "Update: New Rights For Pregnant Employees," *Personnel Journal* 58, no. 1 (January 1979): 33-36.
6. Paul S. Greenlaw and Diana L. Foderaro, "Some Further Implications of the Pregnancy Discrimination Act," *Personnel Journal* 59, no. 1 (January 1980): 36-43.
7. Samuel C. Walker, "Improving Cost and Motivational Expectation of Employee Benefits Plans," *Personnel Journal* 56, no. 10 (November 1977): 570-572.
8. _____ , "Group Life Has Staggering Growth," *Employee Benefits Developments,* July 1978, p. 3.
9. _____ , "AD&D Coverage," *Employee Benefits Developments,* March 1980, pp. 1-4.
10. _____ ," Long Term Disability Plan Design: Rehabilitation Is Important Factor," *Employee Benefits Developments,* May 1979, pp. 1-4.
11. Paul E. Burke, "Methods of Integrating Social Security With Private Pension Plans," *Personnel Journal* 56, no. 10 (November 1977): 566-569.
12. U.S. Department of Labor, "Know Your Pension Plan" (pamphlet) (Washington, D.C.: U.S. Government Printing Office, 1979), passim.
13. "Rules & Regulations of the Colorado State Personnel System" 6-3-2, April 1980, p. 84.
14. Hoyt W. Doyel and John D. McMillan, "Low Cost Benefits Suggestions," *Personnel Administrator* 25, no. 5 (May 1980).
15. U.S. Department of Labor, "Unemployment Insurance: How It Works" (pamphlet) (Washington, D.C.: U.S. Government Printing Office, 1979), passim.
16. Robert Krogman, "What Employees Need To Know About Benefits Plans," *Personnel Administrator,* 25, no. 5 (May 1980).
17. William I. Rupert, III, "ERISA: Compliance May Be Easier Than You Expect and Pay Unexpected Dividends," *Personnel Journal* 55, no. 4 (April 1976): 179-184.

GENERAL REFERENCES

Changing Times magazine.
Joseph J. Famularo, ed., *Handbook of Modern Personnel Administration* (New York: McGraw-Hill Book Co., 1972).
Hospitals, Journal of the American Hospital Association.

3. Employee Benefits Administration

GERALD R. GURALNIK and JOSEPH K. SAPORA

Perhaps no issues in twentieth century American social/economic events offer more insights into the changing nature of social philosophy and responsibility than those dealing with retirement and health care "rights." This article deals with pension changes.

Since the turn of this century, the nation has witnessed a major shift of the primary responsibility for supplying retirement income from the individual and the family to the employer, based upon tax policy.

Part of this pressure may be traced to the fact that because of science and improved living conditions, increasingly large numbers of persons are surviving their working years into retirement. Current demographic studies demonstrate a significant upward shift in the ratio of retired to active working lives, which suggest the increasing cost of these plans in the near future.

The post-1960s inflation trends, which many believe will continue at least just below double digit levels for the next two decades, have had a serious cost impact on retirement plans and Social Security. The deterioration of pension purchasing power has raised the serious problem of postretirement inflation adjustments, which could add tremendously to current expense.

Pension costs (defined benefits, tax sheltered annuities, special deferred compensation agreements) when combined with Social Security expenses (employer cost only) already are typically 12 percent to 15 percent of covered payroll—and rising.

The retirement arena has become the focal point of a number of other social changes, including issues of sex discrimination, age discrimination, and the right to work beyond age 65, as well as the right to a continuation of basic living standards. In one way or another, these are a part of the dialogue, open or subtle, within each institution.

When these social and personnel matters are coupled with the growing fiscal pressures on the operating budgets and reimbursement rates of institutions, these matters become an important part of corporate fiscal planning—for health care institutions or any others.

RETIREMENT SYSTEMS IN THE U.S.

The development of the American retirement system, which is very much different from those of Europe or Asia, may form a useful setting in which to understand current events and focus on future institutional policy.

The earliest efforts to formalize the retirement income process for employees in America came during the last half of the nineteenth century. New York City established a fund for retired policemen. The emerging railroad industry, in an effort to assure personnel performance to safeguard passengers and equipment through mandated retirement of older workers, offered benefits that covered 50 percent of those employees by 1910. In both cases, the pension issue arose in what is recognized as a "hazardous" industry, where age is presumed to have a direct correlation with risk and reduced physical efficiency.

By 1910, about 100 pension plans were in existence. Within the next ten years, the total increased to about 250 and included such industries as public utilities, iron and steel, oil, banking and some manufacturing. The American Federation of Labor (AFL) began its pressure for retirement benefits for its members as part of the collective bargaining effort.

Generally, the retirement plans of this period were discretionary, typically paid for by the employer, awarding benefits under a series of specified conditions, but containing no legal obligation to do so.

The Revenue Act of 1921 provided income tax exemption for stock bonus and profit-sharing trusts. By 1926, taking the form of a floor amendment to the Revenue Act of that year, this status was extended to pension plans. This change—using tax incentives as a means of encouraging the start of private plans—was a reflection of two influences. The first was that since 1909 corporate income tax had become a new fact of business life. The second was the desire on the part of companies that had plans to take tax deductions for the expenses of the plan, to improve cash flow and to reduce costs. By the middle of that decade, the number of private plans exceeded 300, covered about 3 million employees, and paid benefits to 42,000 retirees.

During the 1920s, state and municipal governments began to adopt retirement plans. In 1921, the Civil Service Retirement Act provided coverage for most federal employees. Benefits were paid to current retirees as contributions were being made, not generally prefunded.

By 1930, 15 percent of all privately employed, non-farm workers were covered by pension programs.

Four other major events—after granting tax exempt status—helped shape the future of the development of these plans:

1. the passage of the Social Security Act of 1935
2. the emergence of the Congress of Industrial Organizations
3. the wage freeze during World War II
4. the Supreme Court decision in the Inland Steel case in 1949

Social Security contributions became effective in 1937 and benefits started in 1940. The Roosevelt effort clearly was implemented to permit the retirement of the aged to open up jobs for the younger unemployed and to create purchasing demand by revenue transfer through payment of retirement benefits. Private plans began to see themselves in relation to the Social Security program.

By 1940, more than 4 million employees were covered by retirement programs, with annual benefits totalling $140 million and annual employee/employer contributions more than $300 million. The decade of the 1930s witnessed a tripling of assets to $2.4 billion.

A major change in the philosophy of the use of the tax deduction incentive to affect plan design occurred when the Internal Revenue Code of 1942 for the first time stated that the deduction would be afforded a "tax qualified" plan only if it could meet the test of not discriminating in favor of highly paid managerial or supervisory personnel with respect to benefits, coverage, and the financing of the program.

During World War II, the economic stabilization (freeze) mandate did not include contributions to private plans. As a result, in the five-year period to 1945, some 2.25 million workers were added to the pension system, since unions could not negotiate wage increases and had to turn to fringe benefits.

Prior to the Inland Steel vs. United Steel Workers of America case in 1949, unions, although increasingly sensitive to the pension need, were reluctant to press the issue too hard. These benefits, while tax deductible, still were at the option of the company. Unions were concerned that so long as pensions were gratuitous and not a subject for collective bargaining, they could represent a political/economic threat to worker organizing actions. The decision in the Inland Steel case that year held that pension plans no longer were purely voluntary for the employer, but instead were subject to collective bargaining rights under the National Labor Relations Act. The Congress of Industrial Organizations (CIO), of which the Steelworkers were members, stepped up its pension negotiation efforts in steel, auto, and other mass production industries.

By 1950, almost 10 million persons were covered by plans, including almost 25 percent of those in private industry. Pension fund assets grew to $12 billion and benefit payments to $370 million. Total annual contributions were some $2.0 billion, with the employers' contribution growing to 80 percent of that total contribution from about 60 percent just ten years earlier.

The next event that further enhanced the growth of coverage in the private pension system was the Welfare and Pension Disclosure Act of 1958 and its extension in 1962 to include the self-employed. Over the two decades ending in 1970 the total covered tripled again. The number of retirees increased by 1,000 percent and their benefits 20 times. Some 30 million persons became participants—almost 50 percent of the industrial labor force. The pensioner rolls swelled to 4.7 million with annual benefits of almost $7.5 billion. Fund assets continued their growth to $137 billion.

The hospital industry, in large part, did not need income tax deductions since it operated principally as voluntary, not-for-profit, or government institutions. There was a key personnel problem, particularly regarding health care institutions' ability to retain physicians on staff in competition with the very substantial and growing economic lure of private practice. In an effort to reduce this problem and give the institutions a bargaining point, Congress created the Technical Amendments Act of 1958 that permitted, for those that qualified as §501(c)(3) organizations under Internal Revenue regulations, the use of tax sheltered annuities (TSAs). Since then, the TSA method has grown. It permits selectivity without dealing with the antidiscrimination rules required of private qualified plans. In addition, many institutions have extended this coverage to broader employee groups either as a primary plan or, more often, as a supplement to a basic plan. It is noteworthy that unions in the health care field never have seriously addressed this as a benefit, preferring to concentrate on developing the traditional defined benefit plan.

The Employee Retirement Income Security Act of 1974 (ERISA) continued the theme of nondiscriminatory practices. It added many significant requirements for participation, vesting, and funding. Perhaps its most radical and fundamental additions to legislated pension history, however, were (1) the establishment of a contingent employer liability beyond the contributions made and the plan's assets, and (2) new rules governing collective and individual fiduciary responsibility. Under the first new rule, in the event of plan termination, a plan sponsor is required to assure payment of the value of the vested benefit even beyond the contributions made and beyond the assets in the fund. The Pension Benefit Guarantee Corporation (PBGC) was created to federally guarantee at least the basic amount of vested benefit for the plan's participants and beneficiaries. Under the second new rule, the plan's fiduciary was jointly and personally liable to conduct the fund in the sole interest of the participant. (This important legislation is discussed in detail later.)

As a fitting close to this section of benefits history, it should be noted that major social issues such as minimum benefits; full, immediate vesting and portability; inflation protection for retirees; sex and age discrimination, and the rights of participants to control the economic power represented by investable pension assets became the subjects of study by the President's Commission on Pension Policy. This commission was to report its study findings and recommendations to Congress in 1981. The scope of its research reached to the fiber of the American pension system. Its delibera-

tions and comments may have far-reaching implications for every institution or corporation.

MAJOR TYPES OF PLANS AND HOW THEY WORK

There is a variety of private pension plans. For comparative purposes and for general understanding, they may be classified into two broad categories: defined benefit plans and defined contribution plans.

Defined Benefit Plans

These are so named because the amount of pension benefit for each individual is defined by a formula and must be definitely determinable. The annual contribution requirement to finance this benefit is then a function of the size of that ultimate pension expectancy.

Within this category, there are two types of formulas, those defined as a percentage of pay and those expressed as a fixed, or flat, dollar amount. In both cases, it is typical for a plan to multiply the function by years of service with the institution, thus rewarding those with longer term service by affording them greater benefits at retirement. The flat dollar type generally is seen in union-negotiated plans or those covering hourly workers.

The percentage of pay formula method, which usually covers salaried personnel, may be expressed in career average pay (CAP) or final average pay (FAP) terms.

The *career average pay plan* generally bases its benefits on the earnings either during each year of service, or on an average of the total salary earned during a career. This approach tends to produce a lesser, albeit less expensive, benefit in an inflationary economy. Organizations that employ the career average method tend to review the program for important benefit improvement every three to five years to hedge continuous inflation pressures. Thus, these costs usually start lower and increase periodically as this plan tends to be improved over time to relate to the more liberal FAP plan.

The *final average pay plan* bases benefits on the earnings of the participant, generally during the last five years of service. Government-sponsored plans generally have moved this up to the last three years of service (or the three highest-paid years). The theory of this method is the desire to make the ultimate benefit payable at retirement automatically inflation proof by relating it to the average salary just before retirement. This method assumes that pay moves up with inflation. This is preretirement only. As a function of pension expense, this automatic inflation-proofing feature is costlier than the other type—the career average plan—assuming no changes in the pension formula over the years.

Defined Contribution Plans

In these plans, the employer establishes the amount of contribution the institution desires to make on behalf of each participant. There is no definition of a definitely determinable benefit. The amounts set aside each year accumulate, along with the investment earnings, in separate participant accounts—almost like a bank passbook. The contributions may be defined as a percentage of pay or a flat annual amount per salary range.

The amount of the benefit is determined by the value of the account balance at retirement. It may be paid out of the trust fund, using a preset annuity purchase table, or the fund may ask for competitive bids from insurers, on behalf of the participant, to provide a retirement annuity. As an alternative, the balance may be "rolled over" into an individual retirement account (IRA). There are three types of such plans in the health care industry:

1. money purchase pension plan
2. profit sharing, thrift plan in proprietary institutions
3. tax sheltered annuity for institutions that qualify under §501(c)(3) of the Internal Revenue Code.

The principal defined contribution vehicle used in the hospital and health care homes industry is the tax sheltered annuity. Under this program, employees may arrange with the employer to divert a portion of their current or future salary, before taxes, to be accumulated to purchase retirement annuity benefits in accordance with the tax deferral provisions in §§403(b) and 415 of the IRS Code.

If this program is fully employer-paid, it may set aside an annual amount equal to 25 percent of the employee's compensation for the year, but not exceeding $25,000 (adjusted for cost of living). If the employer purchases less than the maximum allowance, an employee may buy the remainder, as a salary reduction, so long as it falls within the individual's own exclusion allowances under IRS regulations.

Benefits for past years of service with the institution during which no plan was in existence may be funded via a separate agreement to be added to the ultimate benefit under the TSA.

An employer who is providing a basic defined benefit plan may want to use this individual selective method as a supplemental program. A special calculation has to be made to determine the total allowable excess contribution since the participant already is covered by a tax-qualified plan. In any event, the tax sheltered annuity program is fully vested from inception.

The annuity investment vehicles cover the spectrum from fixed guaranteed types to fully variable types. Participants, if permitted, often select a mix of each.

Social Security

This is another of the building blocks that make up total retirement income. It is federally mandated and cocontributory between employer and employee. It is a defined benefit structure of the career average type. A number of other nonpension federal benefits (survivor insurance, disability insurance, Medicare, black lung benefits, Supplemental Security Income, etc.) are not covered in this article but provide valuable information to employees and employers.

Legislation in 1950 and subsequently provided for voluntary inclusion of state and local governments and nonprofit organizations in Social Security, under certain conditions. Currently, about 90 percent of the 4 million employees of nonprofit organizations have elected coverage under Social Security. About 90 percent of all jobs in the United States are now covered by Social Security.

Old Age, Survivor, and Disability Insurance (OASDI)

This federal program provides:

- monthly benefits for employees who retire after attaining age 62, plus a benefit for their eligible spouse and dependents
- monthly benefits for disabled employees and their spouse and dependents
- monthly benefits for eligible survivorship of a deceased employee and a lump sum death benefit

The amount of monthly benefits relates to the average earnings on which Social Security taxes were paid through the larger portion of the employee's lifetime. Benefits for the lower wage earner are higher as a percentage of pay and contributions. Benefits are not paid on income in excess of the Social Security earnings maximum. The earnings are indexed to relate to the changing patterns of nationwide income in an inflationary economy.

Because of inflation, retirees receive increases each July if the Consumer Price Index grows by more than 3 percent in the preceding 12 months.

Social Security benefits are not subject to income tax.

Medicare benefits are provided for both hospital and medical care for citizens age 65 and older. The hospital portion is automatic, the medical portion elective.

The retirement benefits are funded exclusively at this point by a payroll tax paid equally by employee and employer. In 1981, that tax rose to 6.65 percent of the maximum taxable earnings—or a combined total of 13.3 percent. By 1990, this rate is scheduled to go to 7.15 percent, or a total of 15.3 percent. Even modest estimates expect this to exceed 8.0 percent each by the year 2000 and 12 percent each by 2025 (given the assumed demographic changes).

The contribution rate is multiplied by the maximum taxable earnings—and that, too, is rising. In 1981, that level reached $29,700 and was to continue its rise each year thereafter based upon the rate of increase of the average earnings of all employees nationwide.

Social Security is not prefunded like a private plan. It is a "pay-as-you-go" method in which the current working generation's tax revenue goes to pay for the benefits of the current retirees (intergenerational transfer payments). Since it is not prefunded, changing demographics, even though anticipated in the legislated contribution rate, have a sharpened effect on future benefits as well as on the contribution levels. In fact, pressures for change from a separately defined tax to the general tax funding method stemmed from the realization that the actuarial bases upon which the funding percentages were established were deemed too liberal. As a result, future funding will require rates to rise again. This tax, for many young and lower wage people, is now larger than their net income tax burden and represents a political as well as an economic problem. It also may require either benefit reductions or later retirement ages as alternatives to increased contributions.

EMPLOYEE RETIREMENT INCOME SECURITY ACT OF 1974 (ERISA)

Prior to the advent of the Employee Retirement Income Security Act (ERISA) in 1974, the typical hospital or home (other than proprietary) was not required to "qualify" its pension plan with the IRS. Many did not since the issue of obtaining a tax deduction for contributions was not a motivating influence in not-

for-profit or government-sponsored institutions. In fact, a number of institutions maintained unfunded plans and elected to add to their budget each year only the anticipated pension expense for the current year's retirees. By not seeking tax qualification, institutions found themselves not subject to the typical IRS requirements for minimum participation and nondiscriminatory benefits nor to the more formal rules of advanced funding of the liability. For many organizations this permitted certain flexibilities for a while. By the 1960s, and more so currently, the patterns changed for external and internal actuarial, financial, and accounting reasons.

To meet the rapidly increasing pension liabilities, the institutions developed more level, prefunded costs, and entered them into both their budgets and reimbursement rate requests. To the extent that union organization of employees was successful, pensions became a bargaining issue and new, joint-managed pension funds arose. Even though it was not important to gain a current tax deduction on contributions, tax qualification became the standard approach for providing a basic set of written rules governing the plan's design, requiring that the assets be held in a separate trust and that there be an assured minimum level of funding.

Then ERISA came, established in late 1974 but effective in most cases as of January, 1976. Its new requirements were based upon the deferred wage theory of pensions and substantially voided the reward-for-long-service concept. What it did not do was to mandate that each employer must implement a plan for its employees. Nor did ERISA mandate a minimum benefit level. The act regulates plans already in existence and requires all, other than certain government and church employee-benefit programs, to comply with its requirements. This includes institutions in the health care industry. The major burden of ERISA compliance clearly falls on the defined benefit pension plans, although defined contribution plans and others also are affected (particularly in the fiduciary standards and disclosure areas).

The following is a thumbnail sketch of ERISA's major provisions regarding pension plans. It is designed to introduce the key issues but is not meant to be complete or in depth. When detailed interpretations are required, the health care institution's legal counsel should be consulted.

A. Eligibility and Participation

All full-time employees over 25 years of age with more than one year of service, hired earlier than five years before the plan's normal retirement age (usually

65), must be included. If the plan has a mandatory employee contribution, the worker may elect not to join even if the individual meets these criteria, unless joining is a condition of employment.

A year of service is achieved by working 1,000 hours in a year. If a participant leaves employment before being vested, a break in service occurs. The participant must not lose credit for that past employment, after one year of work from the date of returning to the job, if the length of the total absence is less than the service earned before leaving. An employee vested at termination must be assured those years of credited service represented by the accrued benefit in the form of a deferred retirement benefit. Being a participant does not confer automatic employment rights.

B. Vesting

There are three general vesting (ownership of benefits) rules that may be used by a plan:

1. 100 percent vesting after completing 10 years of service; or
2. a schedule of increased vesting starting with 25 percent at the end of five years' service, an additional 5 percent for each of the next five years, and 10 percent for each of the final five years of service, becoming 100 percent vested after 15 years of service; or
3. the "Rule of 45," which vests 50 percent when the participant's age and service total 45 (e.g., age 35 and 10 years of service) and an added 10 percent for each additional year of service thereafter to 100 percent. A minimum of five years of service is required.

C. Maximum Benefits Permitted

For defined benefits plans, the employer may not provide more than the lesser of 100 percent of the average of the last three years' salary, or $75,000. This $75,000 ceiling is adjusted annually for cost-of-living increases. In 1980, the figure was over $109,000.

For defined contribution plans, the yearly contributions to a participant's account may not exceed the lesser of 25 percent of annual compensation or $25,000 (which also is subject to cost-of-living adjustments). In 1980, it was about $37,000.

Where two such qualified plans are afforded (dual plan maximum), a combined formula provides a "1.4" rule. The employer is not automatically permitted to enjoy both maximums as two separate plans unless the formulas jointly meet this test.

D. Automatic Death Benefits

The defined benefit plan (and the defined contribution plan, if it provides an annuity benefit option at retirement) must provide the participant an opportunity to protect the spouse in the event of early death after retirement. To do this, the subscriber must be provided with an automatic option of a joint and 50 percent survivor annuity on an actuarial equivalent basis (unless a benefit option of equal financial value is selected).

ERISA requires that a plan that offers an early retirement benefit be required to provide a preretirement death benefit option, also in the form of an actuarial equivalent, joint and 50 percent survivor annuity.

E. Funding Requirements

In general, the current year's annual costs, as they accrue, plus an amortization payment toward past benefit costs, must be paid in order to satisfy the minimum funding standards.

For single-employer plans, the amortization period for the past service liability (for pre-ERISA past service benefits) may be no longer than 40 years. For new benefits improvements, no more than 30 years must be used. As few as 10 years may be used to increase the funding level, if desired.

The actuarial assumptions recommended by the enrolled actuary (EA) must be reasonable in the aggregate. Gains, or losses, relative to actual experience vs. those assumptions generally must be amortized over 15 years. A full actuarial evaluation must be performed not less frequently than every three years. The EA must certify to the IRS and the Labor Department as to the reasonability of the actuarial assumptions, the valuation cost methods, and the minimum funding compliance each year (on Schedule B of Form 5500).

Each plan must continue to satisfy the minimum funding standard account to comply. If it does not, a series of remedies is prescribed to bring it back into compliance: greater contribution requirements over a short period of time (usually five years) at interest, the freezing of all benefit improvements during the repayment period, a penalty tax for failure to follow the program. Meeting these assumptions and obligations above generally should avoid a deficit.

Multiemployer plans (jointly managed union-negotiated plans) are permitted to amortize their past service costs over 40 years and their gains and losses against actuarial assumptions over 20 years.

F. Benefits Guarantee Insurance

Prior to ERISA's passage, the participant's total benefits claim was limited to the proportion of the benefit that was considered funded by the assets of the Fund. The employer, or institution, had no further liability.

A new ERISA agency, the Pension Benefit Guarantee Corporation (PBGC), was created to deal with the benefits obligations of the plan (benefits) and the plan sponsor in the event of a plan termination. ERISA stated that participants who are at least vested have a right to receive their fully accrued benefits, deferred to normal retirement date, whether or not the plan's assets are sufficient. The original benefit guarantee originally extended up to a maximum of $750 per month, but is adjusted each year by the increased cost of living. (Since defined contribution plans have no past service liability, they are not an issue for the PBGC.)

These ERISA provisions originally covered single employer plans only. It wasn't until passage of the Multiemployer Pension Plan Amendments Act of 1980 that multiemployer plans also became covered.

In the event that the employer terminates the plan and there is not enough money in the trust to pay for the insured, vested benefits, the PBGC is authorized to place a lien of up to 30 percent of the employer's net worth. Coverage of newer plan benefits is phased in at the rate of 20 percent of their values each year for five years. Multiemployer plans are subject to a different payoff requirement for such benefits, namely, over not longer than 20 years.

To help finance this guarantee, the PBGC is authorized to charge every covered plan annual premiums. Originally, these were set at one dollar per participant for single employer plans and fifty cents per participant for multiemployer plans. As of 1981, the rates had grown to $2.60 for single employer plans and to $1.40 for multiemployer plans, phasing up to $2.60 by 1989.

G. Fiduciary Responsibility

Before ERISA, the issue of the individual's or plan sponsor's responsibility to this type of trust was bounded by old court guidelines established out of the personal trust experience. ERISA tried to cope with needed changes.

The current guiding principle is that anyone agreeing to undertake responsibility for managing a plan or investing trust assets must be aware that all actions must be conducted in the sole interest of the participants and beneficiaries. Further, anyone accepting that responsibility must have knowledge of the requirements, since lack of expertise is not a permissible excuse for failure to serve well.

Failure to adhere to that principle can subject each party to legal action (individually as well as collectively), including both fines and jail sentences.

For investment purposes, the act redefined the "prudent man" rule as guide for action. This includes such requirements as diversification of investments, general limitations on investment percentages in any one company, seeking a reasonable rate of competitive return, protecting principle, and providing for the emerging pension payments.

Defined contribution plans tend to be more vulnerable to fiduciary liability risk in the investment area. In the defined benefit plans, the employer can and must (by the ERISA funding rules) make up for deficiencies in the investment program in order to continue funding the plan soundly. However, in this type plan, there is no makeup for losses since the contribution is established and there are no ERISA funding rules. ERISA requires the naming of a plan administrator as the primary fiduciary. The act requires the bonding of all persons who handle funds or property. It empowers the fiduciary (often the Board of the Institution) to delegate responsibility for day-to-day administration or for the investment of assets. But that body must retain ultimate policy control. If investment responsibility is delegated to an investment manager, such an agreement and the legal obligations must be enunciated carefully.

The Plan Administrator must retain an Enrolled Actuary for a Defined Benefit Plan who will be required to perform an actuarial valuation not less frequently than every three years—annually if deemed necessary by the actuary because of the course of events.

The trust for either type of plan also must retain an independent account to review the books, records, and transactions of the Fund annually. Both the actuary and the auditor have responsibilities placed upon them by ERISA to certify the compliance of the plan and trust in each of their separate disciplines. Their advice, if followed reasonably, offers the fiduciary important information for policymaking and affords comfort in terms of liability exposure.

H. Report, Disclosure, and Recordkeeping Requirements

When the board names an administrator for the daily activities of the plan, that person must undertake to do the following, among other required tasks:

1. Maintain the records of the plan and fund in enough detail to permit accurate and timely compliance with ERISA requirements on behalf of the participants. These must be held for at least six years after the date the material was in effect or due to be reported.
2. Provide annual statements to any participant who requests it showing accrued and vested benefits.
3. Notify eligible participants of their rights to preretirement death benefit information necessary to make an informed choice.
4. Advise terminating participants who are vested, in writing, of their vested accrued benefits (or account balances, if it is a defined contribution plan). Copies of the deferred, vested notices are required to be sent to the Social Security Administration annually. For those who are nonvested at termination, they must be advised of their break-in-service rights.
5. Provide a summary plan description (SPD), every tenth year (or fifth year if there are major plan changes) that is "written in a manner calculated to be understood by the average plan participant" and that is "sufficiently accurate and comprehensive to reasonably apprise such participants and beneficiaries of their rights and obligations under the plan."
6. Issue a summary annual report (SAR) detailing the required financial and transaction information reflecting the conduct of the business of the trust.
7. Make available at the principal office of the administrator and other places, the:

   - plan description
   - latest annual report
   - documents under which the plan was started or is operated (plan document, trust agreement, collective bargaining agreement)

Critical dates are associated with compliance in each area of responsibility. The premailed government forms describe those dates in the instructions. Other internal forms should be scheduled and parties made accountable for each responsibility.

DESIGNING A RETIREMENT BENEFITS PROGRAM

Whichever pension technique is used to accomplish the task, each institution generally addresses four main questions in plan design:

1. What are the component parts that go into providing that level of replacement income?
2. What do we believe are the amounts and types of benefits this institution should expect its retiring employees to enjoy?
3. What benefits are being provided by our competitors for our labor supply?
4. What will our institution's budget currently permit, in an effort to fund that ultimately desired program?

It is useful to point out that no program should be static and unchanging. These are dynamic considerations, affected by both external and internal pressures. This fact becomes one of the basic design principles affecting judgments. For example, it may be both unwise and uneconomical to focus on implementing the ultimate program immediately since the institution's view of what is ultimate may undergo radical change over time at least in part because of changing legislation, economics, and community, and competitive pressures for personnel.

Within each of those broader questions, there are underlying issues that the institution must deal with to arrive at an effective program.

Component Parts

The private sector in general has come to agree that a soundly designed program should consider a building block approach when trying to arrive at a level of benefits to replace working life income. These blocks include:

- Social Security benefit values
- private pension plan benefits
- personal savings

For many institutions and companies, this multitiered program idea suggests the wisdom of designing a pension formula that integrates with the Social Security program. A typical pension formula would establish the overall benefit level objective for both these programs combined. (Either career average or final average pay plans may be so coordinated.) In doing so, the law permits the institution to take credit, in the plan formula, for the fact that Social Security benefits have been provided by the employer for earnings up to the taxable wage base but not for earnings over that amount.

One way this formula technique may be accomplished is by subtracting a portion of Social Security from the pension plan benefit (offset type). Alternatively, the formula may provide a higher percentage for salary in excess of the maximum taxable wage base, upon which Social Security taxes are paid, and a lower amount on the earnings below that level. Both approaches are governed by IRS regulations.

The advantages of this method are to avoid duplication of costs, prevent total retirement benefits from exceeding net take-home working pay, and consciously establish an appropriate replacement ratio relative to salary or wages earned before retirement, to be funded by the institution.

Both defined benefit and defined contribution plans may use the Social Security integration method. Tax sheltered annuity plans do not generally use this planning tool.

Amounts and Types of Benefits

This subject reflects the current dialogue that extends the concept of guaranteed annual wages (income floors) during the working lifetime to the postretirement period. These questions are being asked:

- What is a reasonable level of retirement income?
- Should this program provide a minimum retirement income that, when compared to preretirement after-tax income, will provide a standard of living of equal relative value?
- What percentage should it be? 60 percent? 70 percent? 80 percent? including Social Security?
- Should the institution peg its formulas to the assumption that the employee with 25, 30, or more years of service with the hospital is the one whose standard of living the plan is aimed at showing? It could be argued that a much shorter work history with the institution suggests that that person served more than one employer during a working lifetime and will receive multiple benefits.

Inflation impact is a significant influence. Earlier, formulas using Final Average Pay or Career Average methods were discussed. The FAP clearly was designed to provide automatically a postretirement benefit that most nearly reflects the economic conditions just prior to retirement. The Career Average formula can keep pace with inflation only to the extent that it is increased periodically.

Many companies and institutions have new pressures growing from their current retirees and the soon-to-retire for post-retirement inflation adjustments to otherwise fixed benefits (at the time of retirement). Social Security has provided for benefits changes automatically on an annual basis. An institution's plan is likely to be pressured to consider these possibilities and its priority vis-à-vis other considered program improvements. The cost of the various ways of implementing some inflation relief is high, specifically if implemented on an automatic (vs. an ad hoc) basis.

OTHER BENEFITS DESIGN CONSIDERATIONS

When defining the desired replacement ratio, care must be taken to define the salary or wages upon which that ratio is based. It could be restricted to base pay, base pay with shift differential, include overtime pay, or even other allowances. The broadest definition usually used by a Plan is the employee's W-2 reported pay, or W-2 pay including TSA contributions. This important decision affects not only the benefits levels but also the costs of the plan.

When establishing or improving the defined benefit plan, it is worthwhile to define the program in terms of the needs of the various groups of employees. Sometimes it is useful to design the benefits formula differently as between past and future service. One may be lesser than the other (usually the past service formula) based upon the needed emphasis, given the target budget. This is a method of designing formulas that assist in controlling costs according to economic conditions. (This approach also generally is applicable to tax sheltered annuity type programs or to profit-sharing plans at proprietary institutions.) Although previously earned benefits may not be reduced, designing a past-service formula lower than that of future-service formula, or raising only the existing future service formula, (in the event of benefit improvement requirements) not only can control costs but also can direct contributions toward the most effective use, and can limit employer liability.

The Early Retirement Factor

Early retirement considerations do play an important role in pension plan design and in the human resource policy at institutions. The early retirement opportunity usually is based upon a combination of age and service. The immediate payout provided by the plan is usually the amount accrued to that time, reduced actuarially to reflect the participant's receiving benefits for a longer period. The benefit also may be deferred, in full, to normal retirement age. If the institution includes the early retirement feature, ERISA requires that it offer a preretirement death benefit.

Early retirement may be subsidized by the plan rather than providing an actuarial equivalent reduction in benefits. This will produce a larger immediate benefit and tend to encourage early retirement on a voluntary basis. Plans also organize the benefit payment in early retirement in such a fashion as to produce a level amount of total retirement income including Social Security. It does this by granting a larger amount before Social Security eligibility and an actuarially reduced lesser amount when Social Security does begin its payments. This produces a level total retirement income.

Recent amendments to the Age Discrimination in Employment Act (ADEA) prohibit a plan, with limited exceptions, from invoking mandatory retirement before the participant reaches age 70. Late retirement benefits may be calculated for those who choose to continue to work beyond normal retirement age (usually age 65) on a frozen basis, which means no service accruals or salary increases need be recognized. The plan also is not required to increase the benefits accrued to age 65 on an actuarial equivalent basis to actual deferred retirement date even though no benefits were paid for that period. The plan may choose to continue accruals or even pay the actuarial equivalent as a matter of institutional policy.

As a result of ERISA's imposing certain statutory benefit maximums on both defined benefit and defined contribution plans, some organizations, in order to provide full benefit programs to their most senior executives affected by these maxims, have turned to providing supplementary programs. These usually are provided on a selective basis and often on a nonqualified (with the IRS) basis.

For institutions that qualify for, and have implemented, tax sheltered annuity plans, the recent Manhart vs. City of Los Angeles case and the subsequent conforming regulations of the Equal Employment Opportunity Commission on the issue of sex discrimination have caused important plan revisions to be made equalizing contributions and benefits for males and females. Mortality tables had to be revised to effect these benefits purchases.

Previously, given the use of generally accepted group mortality tables, the rule was that a plan recognizing the mortality differences in the aggregate could provide either equal benefits or equal contributions. The issue of equality now may not be based upon aggregate mortality tables but is required to deal with each individual's life experience separately. To do this, many plans are turning to one or another form of "unisex tables" in which general cost compromises or averages are calculated between male and female mortality group experience.

Where early retirement benefits are provided, these sex discrimination considerations have direct implications on the amount of benefit afforded the spouse of an employee under the preretirement death benefit joint-life annuity option. Similar adjustments must be made for participants selecting the joint annuity postretirement option.

Should the Plan Require Employee Contributions?

One reason for requiring a contribution from the employee is the possibility of providing a better plan than might otherwise be the case, given the institution's budget. Another reason is that by requiring a contribution, the employee feels a part of the plan and takes a greater interest in its development. The savings, or thrift, feature of the employee contribution frequently is useful. Although the employee's monies are paid with after-tax dollars, the earnings on the savings are tax free until the benefit or proceeds are received. For many, this could be better than bank savings and the contributions are always owned (fully-vested) by the participant.

A drawback is that lower-paid employees sometimes feel the added deduction from the paycheck, when combined with Social Security taxes, is too severe a burden on their current living needs. This can have a significant impact on the number of employees who elect to participate in the plan, if it is optional.

The maximum mandatory contribution permitted by law to defined benefit and standard defined contribution plans is 6 percent of salary. Voluntary contributions are permitted up to an additional 10 percent of pay. The employee contribution allowance for tax sheltered annuities is the same as though it were noncontributory.

ACTUARIAL ASSUMPTIONS AND COST METHODS

The cost of a defined benefit plan is the value of the benefits paid out plus the expense of administering the plan, minus the investment yield achieved in the course of prefunding the program. (The cost of a defined contribution plan is the defined percent of pay that the institution decides it wishes to contribute.)

Actuarial assumptions are the estimates made by the defined benefit plan's actuary of the probability of personnel and investment experience the program is expected to develop in the future. These are not precise elements fixed for all time but estimates based upon recognition of the past history of the organization, recent history of economic affairs, and projections as to what the future course of events is likely to demonstrate. These actuarial assumptions are applied mathematically to the plan's benefit promise, the results of which calculation establish the institution's current and projected liabilities.

This pension liability (mortgage) becomes the basis for establishing the funding program for the plan over the years of its existence. Since experiences change, so will cost requirements to fund the plan. Recognizing this, most organizations elect to value their plan actuarially each year to determine current costs. Further confirming the estimated nature of the actuarial assumptions, ERISA requires that the assumptions and results be reviewed at least each three years but certified as being valid in the aggregate by the enrolled actuary not less frequently than every year on Schedule B of Form 5500. ERISA's concern is to protect the financial soundness of the plan for the participant and assure the reasonability of the contribution. It must be remembered, however, that the actuary only recommends these assumptions. It is the fiduciary (board) that adopts them and has the power to reject them in whole or in part if it feels it justified and necessary. If it does so reject or modify, the board would either debate the selection of assumptions with the current actuary or hire another. If the actuary is changed, the reason must be noted on the next Schedule B.

Actuarial Assumptions Defined

A. *Interest Assumption*—the first great variable—is the rate of return the fund reasonably expects to earn, over the long term, on its current assets and future contributions. ERISA requires that the various invested assets must be valued at market to determine the rate of return.

The hired investment manager(s) proposes to earn amounts equal to or in excess of the assumption without undue exposure to risk. If this is done (depending upon the size of the excess), the excess may be used to offset other assumption losses, reduce plan expenses if there are no other losses, or improve benefits without additional cost to the institution.

Notwithstanding current investment opportunities, the interest rate assumption, being a long-term consideration, tends to be more conservative than rates of return available currently on prime, fixed income obligations, especially if a substantial percentage of the assets is invested in common stock.

B. *Salary Assumption*—the second great variable—refers to the estimate of future salary and wage increases for personnel. In an era of significant inflation, the size of salary changes has been generating large actuarial losses. Few organizations are prepared to anticipate the real effect by raising this scale to as much as 7 percent or 8 percent—which would have a significant impact, but would be more realistic. The general view has been to use a 4 percent to 6 percent salary scale that produces actuarial "losses" each year that the institution hopes will be offset by "gains" from investment yields in excess of that assumption.

Historically, the belief has been that the yield on assets would exceed the interest assumption by as much as the salary increases would exceed the salary assumption, the offset allowing for relatively level costs. Unfortunately, recent history has not demonstrated that, and major actuarial losses have occurred on both counts, raising pension costs precipitously.

For some time, the general view has been that the interest assumption should never exceed the salary assumption by more than 1½ percent (e.g., 6 percent–4½ percent). The current trend is to narrow that to 1 percent or an equal percentage in order to achieve a more realistic view of the costs of the plan.

C. *Mortality Assumption* is the table the plan uses to define, by age and sex, the probability of survival of current and future participants and retirees. The actuary usually recommends the table believed most reasonably to reflect the group being covered.

These tables are developed from the experience of populations much larger than most groups included in a plan. There are likely to be some gains or losses each year because the experiences of a smaller group will vary from the table.

D. *Turnover Assumption* is the table that attempts to assess the number of participants who will continue covered employment to retirement. It presumes the rate of voluntary or involuntary termination of employment. The higher the expected turnover, the lower the current costs of the pension plan since fewer are expected to actually retire. These factors also relate to the vesting provision. The earlier the vesting, the less likely that the affect of turnover will be important as a cost factor. (Under tax sheltered annuity plans, the contributions are vested immediately so employee turnover has no cost effect and turnover assumptions are not used.)

The IRS sometimes looks at actual turnover experience as evidence of the validity and reasonability of the vesting schedule as it relates to possible de facto discrimination. If the IRS sees that too many participants, especially the lower paid vs. higher paid, tend to lose benefits because of termination, it probably would require that the vesting schedule be lowered (increased cost) to provide some benefits for those many who seem to leave before they become vested.

E. *Age at Retirement* is the assumption that predicts when employees are expected to retire. This has not been a major issue until the last few years when a trendline has developed toward earlier retirement along with the increased rate of entry of women into employment, changes in Social Security opportunities, and the new rules (ADEA) on age discrimination dealing with mandatory retirement for defined benefit and defined contribution plans.

F. *Other assumptions* of lesser importance are those to assess the impact of the administrative cost of the plan, or the rate of disability, if such benefits are afforded.

Actuarial Cost Methods

Deciding upon and understanding the issues involving the proper use of actuarial cost methods for defined benefit plans is a bit more complicated.

The actuary's recommendation of a cost method is based upon the type of plan and represents the expert's assessment of the most realistic way the program will be able both to maintain its cash flow requirements and to pay off the liability created by the pension promise.

When the typical defined benefit plan is established, it generally recognizes two parts to its benefit formula—the past service benefit and the future service benefit. The former is based on the years of service employees worked for the institution before the plan came into being. This generates an initial liability that will be funded over 30 or 40 years, at interest, like a mortgage. The size of that liability is determined by such factors as the benefit formula, the salary to which that formula will be applied (final average pay, or career average pay, or the salary the year before the plan started, etc.), and the funding method and actuarial assumptions adopted by the plan.

The future service benefit is based on each year of service between when the plan started and normal retirement date. For each of those future years, the actuary, to determine the costs for the current year, applies the retirement formula to the age, sex, salary based upon the actuarial funding method, and assumptions.

For final average pay plans, there generally are four funding methods that actuaries recommend to establish current and future costs: the entry age normal, frozen initial liability, attained age normal, and aggregate methods. Each of these is an acceptable method under ERISA.

The principal difference between these techniques is their treatment of the funding of the past service liabil-

ity. The aggregate method, for example, does not recognize the past service liability separately over, for example, 30 or 40 years but funds it as part of the current service cost each year. It tends to be the highest cost method. But if the institution has a newer plan, a mature population, and a formula that permits very early normal retirement with high benefits levels, it may need this method to provide proper funding for cash flow.

The typical procedure used by FAP plans is the Frozen Initial Liability method. Here the past service liability is established as frozen at the commencement of the plan, and is amortized over 30 or 40 years. In addition, a current cost (normal cost) is determined to fund the future service benefits. The two funding pieces make up the annual contribution requirement. The key advantage of this method, over others such as the Aggregate method for a single employer plan, is the contribution flexibility allowed in funding past service liability from a maximum dollar amount over a 10-year period to a minimum amount over 40 years.

If an institution provides a Career Average plan of benefits, the actuary typically will employ the Unit Credit method. This technique values the benefits as they are earned (accrued) each year. This technique tends to result in an increased cost each year, all things being equal on the actuarial assumptions. For a hospital with a Career Average plan, this could become both a serious budgeting problem and one of establishing costs for reimbursement rate purposes. This has become especially difficult during these years of high inflation and larger salary increases as the costs under this method have tended to increase at an even faster rate. To anticipate this occurrence, and smooth out these increases, actuaries have begun to recommend various methods based on projected payroll. The impact of this leveling technique would be to pay more currently than under prior techniques but to avoid very precipitous rises in pension expense.

The dual issues of realistic actuarial assumptions and proper cost methods are important to the entire human resources planning effort. Benefit improvements, anticipating institutional benefits cost patterns, and the ability to absorb costs occasioned by legislated changes are part of this consciousness.

FUNDING VEHICLES FOR CONTRIBUTIONS AND ASSETS

The issues of how and where to invest employer contributions to optimize return, assure safety of principal, or in the case of defined benefit plans to try to keep plan costs in balance, are the hard questions of the day. This is partly true as well for the TSA plan, where fine investment rates of return can produce higher levels of potential benefits and the satisfaction that makes the program more worthwhile to the participant and the institution.

To comply with ERISA, the plan assets must be set aside in a separate trust (or similar vehicle) so that they are fully separated from the general assets of the institution. Even though the plan administrator has control over the trust, these monies generally are for the exclusive benefit of the participants on whose behalf they have been contributed.

Typical investment vehicles available to an institution's plan are:

For Tax Sheltered Annuities for qualifying (education-based) institutions: Insurance companies that offer individual or group annuity programs. They usually provide optional vehicles into which participants may elect to place their annual contributions. They range from fixed income guarantees to variable investment trusts (such as a common stock mutual fund), or a combination of both.

Some such TSA investment opportunities are available at banks and in certain bond purchases as well, but the insurance route is the most universally adopted method for tax sheltered annuity plans.

For Other Defined Benefit and Contribution Plans: It is the responsibility of the plan sponsor to develop the investment policy and method aided by advice from the actuary and accountant. Care in the development of the trust agreement should provide the plan sponsor the opportunity to delegate much of the investment responsibility to the investment manager.

Whoever is selected for that position, it remains the obligation of the plan sponsor to regularly monitor the manager's absolute and comparative performance and to retain both the power and responsibility to make changes if the results are subpar.

Under ERISA, the "prudent man" definition suggests that unless the plan sponsor is an expert in the field of investment, or is willing to bear the risk personally, that individual ought to seek professional advice as to how best to invest the assets of the fund. Paying a fee for this general advice, including help in monitoring performance, may be a wise decision.

The investment vehicles available to qualified defined benefit plans are the same as for profit-sharing, thrift, savings, or money purchase programs.

The plan sponsors may develop a trust agreement for a bank's trust department to act as investment manager as well as custodian. The bank, depending upon the size of the fund and its flow of contributions, may operate the trust as a separate entity or it may pool all or a portion of the assets with other funds of

similarly qualified plans. Usually, banks have several pooled trusts—real estate, common stock, money market, short-term cash, etc., into which the board or committee may direct portions of the assets.

On the other hand, a fund may contract to be served by an independent investment manager (e.g., a stock brokerage firm). In this approach the manager directs the investments of the fund while a bank acts as custodian for the trust.

It is not unusual for a plan to retain an investment adviser on a fee basis, separate from a bank or investment brokerage firm, to give investment advice where the expert has no vested interest in the sales or purchases of securities. This presumes a level of investment objectivity on behalf of the fund.

If the fund's assets and its annual contributions are sufficiently large, some plan sponsors choose to divide the operation among different managers for balance, diversification of expertise, and competitive performance. (Care must be taken to consider the administrative cost of doing so, since the manager's fee schedules usually start at a high rate and descend as asset volume grows.)

Another major resource is the insurance company, which over the many years of retirement plan history has played a historic part. Its traditional role of assuming a risk for a premium was the basis for the original individual and group annuity purchases made by some of the earliest defined benefit plans in the United States. Insurers now offer a wide range of investment products geared to the various sizes and needs of plans. They range from traditional individual policy insured vehicles to group investment contracts that, in most respects, duplicate the functions performed by banks and investment brokers.

Insurers do offer products structured to cover each individual through one or another form of whole life insurance policies, individual annuities, or single life policies with a separate investment trust (side fund). Few employers in the health care industry are likely to use these products, which are geared to plans covering fewer than 100 lives.

Generally, institutions with several hundred or more participants that wish to use an insurer will turn to their group products ranging from deposit administration (DA) contracts, to guaranteed investment contracts (GIC), to the "Investment Only" management fee agreement. Each of these are insurance company answers to the other investment organizations' entry into the pension trust investment field.

The DA typically is a fixed income investment plan without a guaranteed rate (payable as earned). It is generally targeted for smaller groups. The monies are held in the general assets of the insurer until a participant retires, at which point an annuity is purchased. The GIC program is fully guaranteed with a fixed rate of return. In addition, it will credit added interest based upon the new money rates earned by the insurer each year in the investment of its general assets. These dollars also are held in the insurer's general account. The Immediate Participation Guarantee (IPG) is a plan that usually invests in common stock equities and other such programs. The actual yield and actual expenses are credited to the fund as they occur each year. The investment only program is similar to the IPG but is stripped of all expense loadings of the insurer other than the costs of investing. It performs much like the activity of the bank trust department.

It is important when considering these investment arrangements to have the contractual provisions carefully reviewed for such items as withdrawal rights, annuity purchase methods and rates, investment return, expense charges, etc. They often are negotiable.

To provide these programs competitively, the insurers have built up investment research and administrative staffs mirroring the banking and Wall Street firms' capabilities. The critical change that permitted insurers to compete at these levels was the acceptance by the Securities and Exchange Commission (SEC) some years ago of their right to engage in these investment practices in separate SEC-approved funds without violating their State Insurance Department regulations regarding the insurers' other publicly held assets.

Even today, one of the most attractive investment opportunities afforded by the insurance industry is the fixed income fund. Insurers lend money long term; banks generally lend money for a short time (under five years). As a result, insurers can and do make available unique longer term rates of return, many of them in the private placement market. (This market refers to large loans made directly with institutions or even nations.) Pension funds find fertile field in an insurer's guaranteed offerings for some portion of the trust's assets.

Insurers' performance in the common stock equity market generally has rivalled that of the other investing agencies. However, their experience in the real estate field has led them to develop certain pooled trusts that have performed very successfully. Ordinarily their rules limit the percentage (usually 10 percent) or the total assets that may be invested in this or other specialty pooled funds.

COLLECTIVELY BARGAINED PLANS

In general, labor unions that represent health care industry employers have not concentrated their retirement focus on the use of tax sheltered annuities since these are available only to the limited number of institutions that qualify under §501(c)(3) of the IRS code. Except for some defined contribution (target-type) plans in the proprietary hospital sector, the typical union-negotiated program is of the defined benefit type.

Unionized employees are covered in retirement plans in several different ways. One is a program sponsored by the employer but organized separately from the plan covering nonunion employees. This plan may be managed by the employer alone or jointly with the union. In either event, for ERISA purposes it is treated as a single employer plan (unless the union arrangement covered many other employers as well). The benefits may be the same or different for the union and nonunion groups, depending upon the negotiated agreement. Even though the plans are separate but are administered and invested in common, ERISA provides that the benefits no longer need to be comparable so long as all the benefits issues were on the bargaining table.

In some cases all employees participate in one plan for the entire institution. Since union negotiations usually occur every two or three years, institutions tend to focus on that period of collective bargaining to arrange for changes in the plan. The negotiated changes are likely to become applicable to all employees in the institution. Ordinarily, the institution will not alter benefits during the interim period unless it consults with the union for approval as regards its own membership. Not to do so might establish the basis for a union grievance and an unfair labor practice charge. ERISA designates this method as a single employer plan.

Where the union participates in the company plan, it usually negotiates benefits, not contributions. As in a typical corporate defined benefit plan, the company essentially underwrites the plan's pension cost. Since the benefit is defined, the required employer contributions will vary based upon actuarial experience. Favorable experience reduces costs and unfavorable experience increases them since the employer must make up the funding difference.

Over the last 25 years, many more unionized employees have become participants in an area, or regional, jointly managed retirement plan and trust. ERISA designates these as multiemployer plans. They have certain compliance requirements that tend to be more liberal than those of the single employer plans. These constitute groups of employers that, through collective bargaining, have agreed to make stipulated and equal contributions to a common pooled trust with common benefits, rules, and regulations for all contributing institutions. A distinguishing feature of multiemployer plans is that employees have portability of service credits when they move from one institution to another. This is the portability of service principle ERISA cited in permitting multiemployer plans to have more liberalized rules for compliance than do single employer plans.

Jointly managed, multiemployer plans were created in 1947 by the Taft-Hartley Act. The law required that employers and union maintain equal representation in the management of the plan's affairs, from benefits decisions to contribution adequacy, to the investment of the assets, and to the general administration of the plan. This was done to separate the plan from union-only management and required contributing employers to share equally in the responsibility.

In a typical multiemployer union fund, the process is reversed. Here the contributions are established first; then the benefits are decided upon with the help of the actuary (target plan). Those established benefits then are reported to the employees much as though they were a defined benefit plan. In this case, with the contributions fixed, actuarial gains do not reduce costs but can be used to fund new benefits in the next negotiations. Actuarial losses usually are made up by the employer if the union wins on such a contract demand in the collective bargaining agreement. Funding deficiencies rarely are made up by reducing benefits in these types of plans.

Social Investing and Prudence

Unions have long held the belief that pension contributions were an extension of wages and that their members, through the collective bargaining process, had agreed to forego current compensation in favor of deferred benefits. The pension contributions were part of the settlement package. In their mind, therefore, the unions reserved the ultimate right to the say in what happened to the program and how it should be administered.

Recently a new theory has been developing that proposes that the union and its members have the right to direct the investment of the plan's assets into socially useful channels—including prohibiting purchases of equity in corporations that are perceived to be antiunion, or are "runaway shops," or are perceived to be flagrant violators of regulations of the EEOC or of the Occupational Safety and Health Administration.

Given the increasing union sensitivity to the economic and political power inherent in directing the investment of pension fund assets, it is unimportant whether a Fund is jointly managed or is the single-employer type that includes union members. The pressure is likely to grow in either case for the right to direct the use of the assets. The Labor Department and others have been offering alternative definitions on the possible acceptability of, or conflicts inherent in, such a course that now is referred to as social investing. The liability of the fiduciaries is unclear at this writing.

ERISA has required that the funds be invested "solely in the interest of the participants and beneficiaries" as a matter of fiduciary obligation. Unions argue that these social investment activities—if still producing a reasonable (not necessarily maximum) rate of return on investment—are solely in their participants' interests. This type of investment activity, they say, also represents job protection (the key to getting benefits at all) as well as reduction of injury and death, and maintains the principle of equal treatment for both sexes.

Potential for Conflicts of Interest

A major problem for plan sponsors, be they single-employer or multiemployer programs, is how to perform prudently solely on behalf of the participants, given the fact that each side wears at least two hats—one as trustee of a pension fund and the other as a party to the process of collective bargaining. It often is difficult to separate the influences during the decision process. For example, an employer might want contributions to fund the plan to be as low as acceptable. A union might share that view but for different reasons. It might feel that additional contributions could be used to purchase greater benefits rather than to fund the plan more fully. On the one hand, the participants would appreciate a more securely funded plan, especially in private industry where their institution, or plant, could go out of business. On the other hand, they also would want improved benefits, especially if they were nearing retirement age.

In the health care industry, the most vulnerable area of exposure, to which the trustees of a jointly managed fund should be highly sensitive in their decision processes, is in the management of a welfare plan. When the plan provides hospital and medical care benefits, the trustees, as in a jointly administered program, not only represent the participants but also both sides at the collective bargaining table. However, in this case, institutional employers are both users (i.e., employees go to the hospital for care) and providers of some of the services—the vendors.

Items that could pose conflicts of interest are the price of services, the hospital's (home's) policy on admission, length of stay, ancillary service charges, and so forth, each of which has an impact on the fund's costs. By implication, these concerns for objectivity also could be a factor in the benefits and funding decision process for a single-employer fund in this industry covering all participants, both union and nonunion.

While multiemployer plans have employee service portability built into them, this same pooling also presumes a joint employer benefit liability as well. If one contributing employer goes into bankruptcy, then the issue of the outstanding liability for its participants becomes a financial concern of the remaining employers. This issue was a key provision of the Multiemployer Pension Plan Amendments Act of 1980. This act requires that employers who become bankrupt or otherwise withdraw from a multiemployer plan must be held responsible for their share of the plan's unfunded vested liability. The important ramification here is that employers cannot arbitrarily discontinue participation, leaving remaining employers to fund vested benefits.

The health care industry, formerly believed to be invulnerable to bankruptcy, experienced these economic problems in the 1970s, and they are likely to continue through the 1980s. Such considerations have become a real concern where they are in multiemployer plans. The portability feature tends to increase the number of participants who become vested, thus increasing the potential financial exposure in the event of hospital failure.

MAKING THE PROGRAM UNDERSTANDABLE

For many years, participants' understanding of their pension benefits was dealt with at three levels:

1. The Plan Sponsor usually published a booklet describing the program and its benefits.
2. The Plan Sponsor may have published a brief individual annual statement of accrued or projected benefits, perhaps containing a reiteration of the highlights of the plan.
3. The Plan Sponsor, when a participant was approaching retirement age, would work through the personnel department (or the fund administrative office, if a multiemployer plan) to provide help in describing benefit entitlements, estimated Social Security benefit, and other information. This usually would be done on request.

ERISA not only has defined more of the information that must be transmitted to participants and beneficiaries, and its frequency, but also has mandated that these communications be drafted in a prompt

enough manner and clear enough language so that the participants will understand them.

Even before the advent of ERISA, but further encouraged by the agency, many companies and funds began to install better organized programs of communications with employees and better preretirement counseling systems. The general perception is that not only do the covered employees deserve clear information and assistance in planning their futures but also that such activity is a good investment, reaping rewards of job satisfaction, feelings of long-term security, reduced turnover, and a sense of the dignity of retirement under the company's program.

Although the systems discussed here may not be practical for every institution, they can be used for both active and preretirement counseling purposes.

For Employees

Clear and accurate pension booklets should be published with as many worksheets (with examples) as will allow employees to work out their own scenarios. Some find it useful, as a Part 2 of this booklet, to publish the entire text of the plan (with amendments) as reference.

Prominence should be given to the "don'ts" of the plan, with explanations as to why they are included. ERISA requires much of this in the form of a summary plan description (SPD).

Interesting and informative annual statements should be distributed describing each of the critical benefit values the employee has gained since the previous year as well as projected pension and Social Security benefits at normal retirement age. These statements also might describe the other benefits and fringes available and/or used during the year as reminder of the breadth of the overall employee benefit program and the percentage of pay contribution being allocated by the employer for these purposes.

Prompt, clearly readable "Terminated Vested" notices and "Break-in-Service" notices should be issued. The other employees will appreciate the attitude expressed by these publications for their fairness and completeness. They also are required by ERISA.

An easily readable annual financial statement, or Summary Annual Report, with simple explanations, should be provided. Many participants are not familiar with financial presentations. It would be helpful to have the principal points summarized in an introductory page, calling attention to key items and comparisons. This presentation represents the security feeling confirmation in the plan's promise.

A procedure should be developed through which employees may ask questions, seek information, and receive answers in an organized way from the personnel/benefits department. Some employers establish personnel counseling hours. Some plans suggest written questions and provide written answers. Some use the institution's newsletter to publish a column on benefits in general—even printing employees' questions and answers (with their permission).

Institutions and funds could consider conducting new participant classes explaining the benefits program in some detail.

For Those Near Retirement

If the plan affords early retirement benefits, the employer can offer a preretirement death benefit option. Under this option, if an active employee dies after becoming eligible for early retirement, an annuity is payable to his or her spouse as though the deceased had retired and elected a joint life annuity with at least 50 percent payable to a surviving beneficiary.

Aside from being an ERISA requirement, this provides an opportunity to be helpful to the long-term employee who qualifies for such a benefit. A useful instrument is a well-drafted worksheet showing, step by step, how the benefits evolve, both before and after retirement, if the option is selected. It should include explanations, with examples, of the reasons for the actuarial equivalent values. The importance and complexity of this choice requires at least one employee counseling session with a knowledgeable person from the human resources benefits department.

As participants draw within one year of actual retirement, the institution would do well to establish a personal retirement counseling service. Employees should be afforded opportunities to discuss their anticipated retirement problems and concerns with staff people qualified to help them work out solutions. These reviews may help the employee decide either to retire or to stay at work beyond normal retirement age.

The subjects with which counselors find themselves dealing are:

1. a detailed estimate of the retirement benefits expected and the values under each of the retirement options made available by the plan;
2. a full explanation of the Social Security retirement program, including how it relates to the institution's benefits plan;
3. a review of Medicare benefits and the continuous supplemental benefits provided by the institution; this would include the cost of Part B and the life insurance that will continue into retirement;

4. a series of educational sessions, using lecturers from government agencies and social agencies, dealing with:

   - general health and nutrition
   - shopping habits
   - financial planning
   - postretirement taxation
   - housing arrangements
   - leisure time activities and resources
   - legal issues
   - life style adjustments (psychological)
   - resource organizations available to help with all sorts of concerns and needs

To the extent that the institution wishes, it may continue contacts into retirement by, among other things, interviews in its house newspaper, keeping retirees notified about company activities by sending information along with the retirement check, or inviting them to social and retirement celebrations.

Interchanges of information between retirees and the institution can enhance morale throughout the hospital and reaffirm the value of the program.

SUMMARY OF OPEN ISSUES

It is useful to conclude by delineating a number of upcoming issues in the retirement field. Institutions that follow these issues (some legislative) carefully can find them helpful in planning, in avoiding duplications, and in balancing benefits and costs. These points involve:

1. various forms of postretirement inflation adjustment (perhaps automatic cost-of-living adjustments, with maximums) that may become a mandatory subject of collective bargaining;
2. earlier vesting rules, probably similar to the government's 4-40 type (40 percent after four years of service, scaled up to 100 percent after ten years);
3. minimum benefit requirements for any participant who achieves retirement age;
4. required continued benefit accruals and wage increases after age 65 if the employee elects to continue to work;
5. preretirement death benefit option choices, to be made available when an employee becomes vested rather than upon reaching early retirement time;

6. liberalization of part-time and seasonal employment definitions to require more of those workers to be covered;

7. possible tax deductibility of employees' mandatory contributions in the same fashion as the IRA program but with a lower maximum;

8. reverse discrimination court cases developing as the EEOC presses to implement unisex tables that might reduce benefits to males proportionally;

9. elimination of excess pay only formulas that provide benefits only to employees whose pay exceeds the Social Security wage maximums;

10. new integration rules for plans that choose to define their benefits in combination with Social Security;

11. increases in the per-participant cost of premiums to the Pension Benefit Guaranty Corp. (PBGC) as the multiemployer plans become covered and if an economic recession occurs;

12. Medicare removed from Social Security tax payments and shifted onto the general tax role, but without a change in the dual contribution rates (6.65 percent each for 1981) to protect Social Security's needs through 2000;

13. possible requirements that employees who have become vested and who terminate employment will have the option to elect to roll over their accrued benefits into an IRA or to the plan of their next employer;

14. action by many more, if not most, plans to integrate their retirement programs with Social Security benefits to avoid duplication;

15. liberalization of early retirement benefits by many plans to encourage more participants to retire earlier;

16. federal legislation regarding benefit plans for public employees, i.e., a PERISA (Public Employee Retirement Security Act) analogous to ERISA. PERISA probably would be limited in scope, initially, however, to disclosure and fiduciary requirements.

Many other issues will arise, especially subsequent to the report of the President's Commission on Pension Policy.

4. Employee Benefit Communications

JAMES D. HAWTHORNE

Reprinted with permission from *Topics in Health Care Financing, Employee Benefits,* Vol. 6, No. 3,
Spring/1980, Issue Editor: Alex W. Steinforth, Aspen Systems Corporation,
Germantown, Md. © 1980.

The basic communication process that all individuals take for granted involves the development of a message for a specific audience, the transmission of that message to that specific audience and the analysis of feedback resulting from the impact of the message on that receiver. The communication of employee benefits involves this same information flow.

The continuous use of various media is essential to a meaningful flow of benefit information. One medium is not enough to help an organization reach its goals and achieve understanding and effective use of employee benefits.

MAJOR ROLE

While the role of employee benefit communications has been given increased recognition by hospital administrators over the past few years, there are still many hospitals that have limited such communications to the first series of orientation meetings, one or two employee benefit plan booklets or an initial audiovisual presentation about the hospital, which includes information about benefits.

To give minimum attention to budgeting and staffing for adequate communication seems inconsistent with the need to solve or reduce the severe human resource problems that face hospitals. Such problems include competition for qualified people, insufficient professional knowledge, high turnover, excessive absenteeism, waste and negative attitudes. In view of these and other such overlapping problems, the role of employee benefit communications serves a number of interrelated goals.

The major role of benefit communications is to reinforce the benefit program objectives established by the institution. These objectives often include attracting good employees, boosting employee morale, minimizing or reducing turnover, increasing job satisfaction, motivating employees, enhancing the organization's image among employees and in the community, putting compensation dollars to better use, keeping the union out or reducing its influence and enhancing emotional security.

Because the benefit *communication* objectives are meant to reinforce the benefit *program* objectives, they are often one and the same. Benefit *communication* objectives that can be added to the aforementioned list are orienting new employees, building loyalty to employer, creating job pride, encouraging career employment, increasing awareness of benefits, increasing understanding and appreciation of benefits, promoting effective use of benefits, conveying the value of benefits, reducing absenteeism and showing evidence of legal compliance.

TRENDS

Growing Sophistication

While there remains much room for growth, the role of benefit communications over the past ten years has become more important to employers, especially with the impetus provided by the Employee Retirement Income Security Act of 1974 (ERISA). With this increased importance, the media or "products" used to transmit benefit information have become more "sophisticated;" many are produced by communications specialists.

The most common media are employee handbooks, annual benefit statements and audiovisual aids. Other media occasionally used to communicate employee benefits are surveys, questionnaires, posters for high-traffic areas, benefit newsletters, direct mail pieces, brochures, claim kits, displays, house organ articles, live presentations or conferences and special events emphasizing benefits and benefit values.

While the production and use of these products have increased, many employers still produce employee communication tools on an infrequent and sporadic basis, thus making them less effective in reaching the goals described. More time, money and energy should be allocated to developing ongoing communication programs that help maximize the return on multimillion dollar investments in direct and indirect compensation.

Top Management Awareness

Recent surveys indicate that top management is becoming more aware of the role that benefit communications play in protecting the investment an organization has made in its benefit program. Therefore, management is willing to spend more money for programs to help employees understand, appreciate and use their benefits. To achieve this goal, more professional communicators will be employed, and a greater variety of products or media will be used to reinforce benefit messages and compete successfully with other media for employees' attention.

Benefit Identity Programs

Another trend is toward greater use of "benefit identity programs." A benefit identity program utilizes a logo or theme (developed especially for the subject of benefits) applied to all media used in an employer's benefit communications program. A well-designed logo or theme can serve, through repetitive use, to bind different media together by creating a relationship from one medium to another and providing graphic consistency from piece to piece.

Because employers are producing a greater number and variety of media and are recognizing the value of identity programs that can unify the media efforts, a "campaign" approach to communicating benefits is emerging. This approach is much like an advertising campaign, in which the message development, media mix, media timing and general budget are planned at least a year in advance to meet previously established objectives for specific audiences.

IMPLICATIONS FOR HEALTH CARE INDUSTRY

Employee Satisfaction

What does this mean to hospitals in particular? Hospitals need to attract and retain qualified personnel. In view of the continued shortage of qualified medical personnel in many areas of the country, it is important that hospital administrators intensify their efforts to recruit and retain qualified people. Well-executed benefit communication pieces can help administrators achieve this objective. For example, a well-written and graphically appealing comprehensive description of a hospital's entire benefits package can impress prospective candidates and help them judge the importance placed on the financial security and well-being of each employee.

The greater the shortage, the greater the competition among hospitals for qualified medical personnel and the higher the level of mobility of people seeking to improve their situations. In this type of competitive environment, it is especially true that a particular benefits program and the success of efforts to communicate it could provide the competitive edge needed by the hospital. If a given hospital already has a high turnover, the personnel shortage is likely to be worse. Also intensifying the personnel shortage is the rapid expansion of medical technology, which has further increased the need for knowledgeable individuals.

New employees are usually enthusiastic about their new positions and excited about the potential the future holds for them. These highly desirable attitudes must be nourished through proper communication and orientation. Proper handling of the benefit communications program can reassure new employees, keep them motivated and reinforce their fresh outlooks and positive attitudes. Good communications will contribute to their peace of mind and will foster these positive attitudes, as well as encourage productivity and quality work.

Hospitals need positively motivated personnel in light of increased public scrutiny. Employees who are happy about their situations and secure about their financial futures and their physical well-being are more apt to support the profession and the institution that employs them. If employees know the hospital administration is concerned about their attitudes and well-being, they are apt to show concern for the well-being of the hospital—to say nothing of the well-being of the patients.

Because of the shortage of qualified medical personnel, hospital administration often looks to part-time employees to help meet human resource requirements. Benefits that are offered to this group are often especially appreciated, because part-time people are frequently not offered benefits. Therefore, benefits can become quite effective in attracting and retaining qualified part-time personnel.

Cost Reductions

Benefit communications can often reduce the cost and misuse of benefits if employees feel positive about their employer and appreciate benefits that are, in fact, paid for *by the hospital* (through the premiums on experience-rated plans) and not by the insurance company. Also, employees who are more knowledgeable about claims procedure, and do what they are supposed to do, reduce administrative costs through more efficient claim handling.

For a hospital that is actively implementing cost-containment techniques, it is vital that those techniques and the use of them be communicated. For example, consider a second-opinion program. If employees do not know that a plan will pay for second opinions, few second opinions will be requested. The same principle applies to elective outpatient surgery. If a plan will pay for certain procedures to be performed on an outpatient basis at a higher rate than on an inpatient basis, employees will take advantage of it—if they know about it.

Improved Coordination

Benefit communications can and should be a vital part of other employee communications that address issues of employee attitudes, morale, job satisfaction, pride, employee goals and career service. It is natural to coordinate benefit communications with these work environment issues. Communication can and should be based on the premise that the more employees know, the more supportive they will be.

Examples of good coordination of benefit communications with other general employee communications are emerging employment philosophies, policies and procedures with benefit plan explanations, utilizing benefits as recruiting instruments, designing new employee orientation that stresses benefits as well as acquainting new employees with career opportunities throughout the hospital, circulating attitude surveys on benefits and other compensation and stressing safety and benefits.

Benefit communications, though just one part of employee communications, touch all parts of general employee communications.

STEPS TO GOOD COMMUNICATIONS

In view of the many positive reasons for budgeting and producing benefit communications, it appears desirable to create and maintain an ongoing communications plan that uses media that present an organized, unified and consistent identity. The steps to such an end are few.

Identify Needs

First, identify or confirm the communication needs at the hospital. On what subjects? To whom? When? What are the management needs, employee needs or employer/employee needs? What are the priorities? The hospital administrator might know these needs through everyday experience or may want to research such needs through a professional study and analysis.

Analyze the Audience

Second, analyze the audience. Find out what the audience knows about the benefits, what they think they know and why they think the way they do. A formal survey is very helpful in determining these audience characteristics. In the absence of such a survey, the following questions can help determine audience characteristics.

1. Are there employee groups that require special information or a special communications program?
2. What kind of information should be given to new employees?
3. What might be the thoughts or expectations of an audience before and after information is received?
4. What are the anticipated reactions to certain messages?
5. What is the size of the intended audience for each message?
6. Are there any physical limitations that may restrict the size of the audience?

Develop the Message

Third, develop the message. This is the process of identifying the content. To do so, the following questions are important:

1. What is the subject?
2. What should the audience do (or not do) or think (or not think) as a result of the communication?
3. What needs clarification, emphasis or reinforcement?
   - Important plan features or provisions?
   - Important plan changes?
   - Plan objectives?
   - Other?

4. What benefits or plan provisions does management feel employees are

   - most aware of?
   - least aware of?
   - most appreciative of?
   - least appreciative of?

5. What are the most frequent employee questions or comments?
6. What might be included in expectation of upcoming events or changes?

Other considerations in the development of content are whether there should be photographs, line artwork, graphs, tables, charts, the feelings expressed by photographs, the feelings that need to be conveyed, the tone of the writing to be used, the style of the writing to be used and the format of the messages.

Writing style can be formal or informal, technical or nontechnical, light or serious, dialogue or narrative. It is important that the client and writer mutually establish the style, especially if outside writers or consultants are utilized. The client must also provide unannotated, accurate and up-to-date source documents, and must be willing to specify what the writer is expected to do. This will avoid later inconsistencies, errors, incongruities and inaccuracies. The writer will provide a first draft. The first draft is not meant to be perfect; it is made to be modified and for the incorporation of material that the writer has inadvertently (or on occasion, purposefully) omitted. Time spent with the writer, in the beginning, can minimize areas that might later be considered deficient.

Select the Medium

Fourth, select the medium. Once the overall message or messages are audience-defined, it is necessary to select the medium or media best-suited to transmit the message(s). The media selected might make some minor adjustments necessary. For example, if it was decided that a set of booklets would be more effective than one all-inclusive, it would require some modification of the writing.

Selection of and production considerations for choosing the method or media are as follows:

1. What methods or media are being used *now* to communicate benefits to employees?
2. What are the strengths and weaknesses of these methods?
3. What medium or channel of communications best

   - meets communications objectives?
   - accommodates the scope of content to be conveyed?
   - reaches the total intended audience in such a manner as to impress, inform or cause action?
   - suits physical limitations of facilities?
   - fits sequence or timing required?

4. What equipment is readily available?
5. What methods of distribution (mailing list, bulletin boards, etc.) are immediately available?
6. How much can be spent?
7. What is a realistic date and the proper time to communicate?

Media or "methods of transmission" are the tools for maintaining and controlling the process of communications. A seemingly endless variety is available to the benefits communicator for transmitting benefit messages (information) and feedback; imagination, budget and time are the only limitations.

Establish the Schedule

Fifth, establish the schedule. Employee handbooks can take about six months to write and produce, assuming all approvals are given at a reasonable pace. Employee benefit statements usually take from 14 to 18 weeks, depending on how elaborate the statements are and the availability of unannotated data. Audiovisual aids can take two to three months. Other printed materials take a like amount of time, assuming source material is all in place. Schedules should be developed after consideration of the date the information is needed. However, to expect to produce a communication effort on an unrealistic schedule only jeopardizes the quality and the effectiveness of the project. Therefore, ample time should be allowed for all parties to fulfill their responsibilities to the best of their abilities. For most productions, schedules should be thought of in terms of a target date. There are many components in the construction of a communications project, and a delay in any one of them can delay the development of the others. The worst way to approach production of a project is to assign an arbitrary date and have everyone rush to meet it *when it is not necessary*.

Establish a Budget

Sixth, establish a budget. The cost of a communication project depends on the scale of the program and type of media. Cost is a measure of time and energy expended. The usual project estimate will include time and expense charges for research and review of source material, the writing of drafts, word processing or typing, editing and proofreading, design and layout, finished art, and printing or duplicating. And the cost of any containers or special equipment that may be necessary to deliver the finished product is an additional consideration.

In every project circumstances arise that may increase or decrease costs. For planning purposes, the following rough cost estimates are offered. For a coordinated set of booklets distributed among 1,000 employees, the cost may range from $15,000 to $25,000. An employee benefit statement for 1,000 employees may range from $8,500 to $15,000. Audiovisual aids that are 12 to 15 minutes and consist of 100 slides and a professional recording may range from $10,000 to more than $18,000.

The value of any medium of communications is best realized when the project has been planned and derived from well-developed project objectives. To relate cost to objectives, the following questions should be answered.

1. How much is being spent on employee benefits?
2. Is the hospital receiving a good rate of return on its employee benefit ''investment''?
3. How much *is* being spent to explain the hospital's benefit ''investment'' to employees?
4. How much *should* the hospital be spending?

   - A percent of benefit costs?
   - A per-employee amount?
   - A dollar amount level?
   - A project or program fee?

5. How *important* is meeting the hospital's objective(s)?

Evaluate the Program

The seventh and last step, which is very often overlooked, is program evaluation. Many employers fail to evaluate the message/media effectiveness with either formal or informal techniques. Proper evaluation can define the results of the project and improve future efforts.

The following are some considerations that may be helpful in establishing an evaluation or feedback program.

1. Is a response system in place

   - for channeling and answering questions, complaints, and comments correctly and positively?
   - for obtaining feedback on specific communication efforts and materials?

2. If not, can and should one be established?
3. What will indicate that the hospital's efforts are successfully meeting its goals?
4. What changes does the hospital expect in the employees' actions or attitudes as a result of its efforts to communicate?
5. What actions will indicate these changes? What will be the evidence of a successful effort or campaign?
6. When should a meeting be held to review projects and, if necessary, implement additional strategies to attain the hospital's goals?
7. When will it be appropriate for implementation of the next benefit communication effort?

Employee communications and benefit communications must be frequent if the effort is to prosper and succeed. It is vital that new information be pumped through the system regularly, continually and with a purpose.

5. ERISA and Benefit Funds

NOEL ARNOLD LEVIN

This article is based on parts of a book, *Fiduciary Responsibility* (International Foundation of Employee Benefit Plans, Bluemound, Wis., © 1980). The author and publisher acknowledge with appreciation the permission of the foundation for use of this material, and of the Practicing Law Institute, New York, for use of material by this author published by the institute in books titled *Labor-Management Benefit Plans* (1971) and *ERISA and Labor-Management Benefit Plans* (1975).

INTRODUCTION

The principles of fiduciary responsibility as we know them today date back for centuries in English common law. In general, individuals are entrusted with fiduciary responsibility, or act in a fiduciary capacity, when they have a duty, created by their undertaking, to act primarily for another's benefit in matters connected with that enterprise.

The concept of trusteeship, which is one principle of fiduciary responsibility, also had its origins hundreds of years ago in English common law. Essentially, a trustee is one who has the legal title to property in which another person or persons have the equitable interests. The beneficiaries have the right to the principal or the income of the trust, or both. The job of the trustee is to safeguard and manage the property being held for the benefit of the beneficiary and ultimately to pay all or part of it to the beneficiary or apply it for the beneficiary's use.

Several kinds of trusts now exist.

EMPLOYEE BENEFIT TRUSTS

The major category of trust analyzed here is the form arising out of the employment relationship. In this category are trusts set up to provide pensions; hospital, medical, or life insurance; or certain other benefits, for the employees of certain employers. Frequently, but not always, these trusts are set up as a result of collective bargaining between union and management. In many instances, however, the trust may be instituted unilaterally by the management of a health care institution; in such cases, the union that represents the workers may not participate in the actual establishment or operation of the trust. However, union consent is required. Indeed, many institutions that have no union have established trusts for profit sharing, pensions, and/or welfare purposes.

For those engaged in the health care industries, these trusts have a double significance. First, as with other employees, unionized workers often bargain for and obtain the trust vehicle for benefits. Health care personnel executives therefore must be concerned with both the bargaining about and administration of these trusts. These areas require careful scrutiny and expert management. Second, many of the payments for services to health care facilities are made either by the trust fund directly or by the insurers for these funds. For this reason, even institutions without funds for their own employees should be concerned with the operation of benefit funds since these may be large payers to the facility.

The trust vehicle is more advantageous than simply having the employer pay the employees and letting them obtain benefits individually and directly for these reasons:

1. There are substantial economies of volume. Group health or life insurance or pensions cover-

ing thousands of persons obviously are cheaper to purchase than a policy for each individual. The costs of administration generally decline as the size of the group increases. Economies of scale are achieved whether the benefits are provided by an insurer or are self-insured.

2. There are tax benefits to both employer and employee, the latter getting particular advantage. When an employer pays money into a qualified trust, the money is deductible as an expense of the business. However, in the case of a trust, the dollar value of the benefits accruing to or purchased for the worker is not taxed to that individual as value received in lieu of wages at the time of payment. Thus, the pension or hospital benefits are bought with pretax dollars instead of aftertax dollars, usually giving additional purchasing power of 20 percent or more, depending on the individual's bracket. The value received in health or hospitalization coverage paid for by employers seldom is taxed. (In particular circumstances uninsured benefits paid by an employer may be taxed.) The dollars ultimately received from pension or deferred profit-sharing plans generally are taxed to the individual only after the person is retired and therefore in a lower bracket. Consequently, the tax would be less than when the employee is under 65 and has a higher income.

3. With only minor qualifications, the income received by a trust fund from dividends and interest, as well as from capital gains, is free of all taxation. As a result, trust funds can grow at approximately double the rate of a corporation or an individual in the 50 percent bracket.

4. Trust funds cannot be dissipated. They block the spendthrift and create a form of compulsory insurance. The individual generally has no option to pass up or overlook health or other insurance protection or pension security and, in effect, such necessary coverage is provided without the employee's having the opportunity to otherwise spend the dollars that pay for this.

ADMINISTRATION

When trusts are established pursuant to labor-management contracts, they may be administered in any of six ways.

First, the trust may be managed unilaterally by the employer alone. In these cases, the employer is solely responsible for the selection of a trustee or trustees, and for the administration of the trust. Neither the union itself nor its officials participate in the formal management of the trust, although in some cases they may act in advisory capacities or as observers. Despite the broad scope of management power in this kind of arrangement, the health care institution nevertheless must either (a) make contributions to the trust in a set amount determined by the collective bargaining agreement or (b) make payments that when coupled with the rate of return on investment and other factors are sufficient to provide certain benefits called for in the union agreement. When such trusts are set up by institutions that do not have unions, management generally has total and unilateral control not only over the trust but also over contributions and/or benefits.

Second, trust funds may be run by the union or its officials alone. The only funds so constituted today are those in existence prior to January 1, 1946. The passage of the Labor Management Relations Act of 1947, commonly referred to as the Taft-Hartley Act, banned the establishment of funds managed by a union alone but permitted those already in existence to continue in operation. There are only a small number of such negotiated plans. Obviously, this type of trust is not growing as fast as others, since these funds can develop only by virtue of higher contributions and broader membership, not as a result of collective bargaining.

Third, neither employer nor employees' representatives administer the trust, although the employer is the contributor. Instead, an independent third party (usually a bank or insurance company) is trustee. These trusts are relatively few. If they existed before there was a union, they frequently are converted to joint fund management when a union enters the picture and requests participation in administration.

Fourth, employee benefit funds set up by municipalities, states, and other government agencies at first were dominated by senior government officials who often were popularly elected representatives. These funds are not necessarily covered by the requirements of Taft-Hartley and the Employment Retirement Income Security Act of 1974 (ERISA) but do have to comply with other laws or regulations, particularly Internal Revenue Service requirements. These are becoming similar to Taft-Hartley type funds since union representatives are gaining greater participation.

Fifth, pension trusts for self-employed persons, either individuals or partnerships, may be set up for their benefit and that of their employees. These are often called H.R. 10 or Keogh plans after the bill's numerical designation and sponsoring congressman. The individual entrepreneur or partners as a rule can be covered only if all of the employees with three or more years of service are covered. There are various legal requirements that must be adhered to, including the ages that the monies can be withdrawn, etc. ERISA provides for Individual Retirement Accounts (IRAs). These are for persons not covered by any other plan. With very little formality or red tape, these individuals may pay into their IRAs $1,500 a year or 15 percent of their income, whichever is less. In the case of a nonworking spouse, an additional contribution of up to $250 a year may be made provided that the aggregate contribution does not exceed 15 percent of the income of the wage earner and in no event more than $1,750.

TAFT-HARTLEY FUNDS

The sixth type, joint labor-management trust, also is known as the Taft-Hartley fund because it must be set up and operated in accordance with that law. Such a trust must meet certain well-defined standards. It operates in the private employee sector. The Taft-Hartley Act outlawed employer payments to unions or union representatives except for a few specific purposes listed in the law. One of these exceptions is a trust fund established for the sole and exclusive benefit of the employees and their families and dependents.

Failure to comply with the Taft-Hartley law makes the parties liable to criminal sanctions and the trust itself illegal. If the trust is not in compliance with Taft-Hartley, payments by the employer violate the law. These legal requirements are clear and generally easy to comply with. The conditions in § 302(c)(5) of the Taft-Hartley Act are:

1. The payments must be held in trust for the sole and exclusive benefit of eligible employees and their families and dependents.
2. A joint board of trustees on which management and labor are equally represented and have equal power must administer the fund.
3. An audit by an independent accountant must be made at least annually.
4. An impartial arbitrator must be provided to break a deadlock in case the trustees do not agree and become stalemated.
5. The basis upon which the payments are made must be set forth in a written agreement.
6. The purposes of the trust are limited to certain specific functions. They can pay for health, hospital, and disability or life insurance. They can pay for pensions or annuities. They may provide for apprenticeship training, vacation or holiday funds, day care centers, scholarships, and group legal services.

MULTIEMPLOYER FUNDS

Under ERISA § 3 (37), as amended by the Multiemployer Pension Plan Amendments Act of 1980, a multiemployer plan generally is defined as one to which more than one employer is required to contribute and that is maintained under one or more collective bargaining agreements with an employee organization. A plan that does not meet these criteria will not be considered a multiemployer program. Thus, if a group of employers agree among themselves to establish a common pension and/or welfare plan for their respective employees, the result would not be a multiemployer program because it was not maintained under an agreement with a union.

The distinctions between multiemployer and multiple employer plans are more than definitional. Certain sections of ERISA treat multiemployer plans differently from all others, including multiple employer plans. The two areas where this different treatment is most evident are the pension plan funding and termination sections of the act.

ERISA established basic, minimum standards for funding pension plans. Generally, the act requires strict adherence to a schedule for amortization of past service costs (the expense of retirement benefits based on an employee's years of service with an employer before the inception of the plan). These costs must be amortized over a period not to exceed 30 years. If they are increased or decreased because of subsequent plan amendments, these changes are to be amortized separately over no more than a 30-year period. (Plans that existed prior to January 1, 1974, may be amortized over 40 years.)

Multiemployer programs generally are subject to the same funding requirements as other plans, except that pursuant to the Multiemployer Pension Plan Amendments Act of 1980 future increases in past service liabilities can be amortized over 30 years (rather than 40 years) and future experience losses over 15 years (rather than 20 years).

Because it was known that many pension plans would incur substantial, and in some cases devastating, costs in complying with these funding standards, ERISA allows amendments to be made on a retroactive basis, with certain restrictions to decrease program liabilities.

In the pension plan termination sections of ERISA, multiemployer programs are treated differently from others. When a covered single-employer defined benefit plan is terminated, the Pension Benefit Guaranty Corporation (PBGC) will determine whether the program's assets are sufficient to pay benefits that the PBGC by law guarantees. If the assets are sufficient, the PBGC will allow the plan to be terminated by its own trustees. On the other hand, if the assets are not sufficient, the PBGC will take it over and administer its assets as trustee. If there is a deficiency in the assets, the PBGC must depend on its reserves, made up of premium contributions from other plans, to assure that participants will receive their guaranteed benefits. Further, the employer who sponsored the terminated plan would be liable to the PBGC for the deficiency in an amount up to 30 percent of its net worth. If the sponsoring employer has substantial net worth, the PBGC may recover the total deficiency and not have to tap its own insurance reserves. However, the more likely situation would find the sponsoring employer with no, or a negative, net worth, resulting in no recovery by the PBGC.

PLAN TERMINATION AMENDMENTS

Mandatory coverage of single employer plans has been effective since ERISA's date of enactment, September 2, 1974. However, coverage by the PBGC of a terminating multiemployer pension plan did not become mandatory until August 1, 1980. While the act does give the PBGC the discretionary authority to cover multiemployer plans before that date, the PBGC has exercised this discretion in extremely limited circumstances. (There were only a handful by 1980.)

Congress in 1980 enacted the Multiemployer Pension Plan Amendments Act of 1980—legislation proposed by the PBGC to amend the multiemployer plan termination insurance provisions of ERISA. The PBGC recognized that when coverage of such terminations became mandatory, there was an immediate potential for large claims on its insurance system. Many of the multiemployer plans covered by the PBGC tend to be concentrated in declining industries or in those characterized by irregular employment, small employers, and little or no net worth among the contributing companies. For many of these plans, the costs of continuing the plan may be much greater than the employer obligations, and terminations may be inevitable. Employers with some, or even substantial, net worth may withdraw to limit their own liability. Such withdrawals, though, actually could accelerate plan terminations. The net result, in the opinion of the PBGC, would be a substantial drain on the insurance system and would yield little hope of recovering deficiencies from employers.

The PBGC reported to Congress that in the instances where it had exercised its discretion and covered terminated multiemployer plans, it found that the employer liability generally covered only 20 percent of the deficiencies, with the remainder being paid by the agency.

The legislation drastically revised the ERISA pension plan termination program for multiemployer funds. It provided for liability for an employer that stopped contributing to a multiemployer pension plan. The liability would be a fractional share of the unfunded vested benefits more or less equal to the employer's proportional share. This liability would be paid off until the withdrawal liability is amortized, but subject to a 20-year "cap." The payment rate would be determined by multiplying the highest contribution rate of the employer over the ten years preceding withdrawal times the highest three-year average contribution base. There are specific exemptions to the obligation such as those relating to the construction industry, certain very small employers, etc. Partial withdrawal was provided for and annual multiemployer premiums to PBGC were set to rise to $2.60 per participant.

The PBGC's insurance liability was modified to guarantee less than the fully vested amount, and funds that did not meet precise funding requirements could have lower guarantees. An insurable event under ERISA is insolvency of the plan, not termination, as had been the case. For a plan in financial difficulty, accelerating funding and other protective measures will result. Contributions erroneously made may be returned to employers under certain circumstances.

REGULATION OF BENEFIT FUNDS

Employee benefit plans were subject to only sporadic regulation until 1962. Some states had specific laws pertaining to these plans; other states regulated them only indirectly under general trust law and then usually after a problem occurred. Regulation, as a rule, came as the result of misconduct and in the form of investigation and sometimes punishment for delinquencies. There was no systematic method of avoiding such problems in advance.

There were, of course, Internal Revenue Code requirements with which pension and welfare funds had to comply, and there was some monitoring of Taft-Hartley trusts by the IRS, but it was done on a limited basis at best.

Congress recognized the need for some regulation of funds but, unwilling to revamp the entire system, amended the Welfare and Pension Plans Disclosure Act (WPPDA) in 1962. Originally enacted in 1958 as a result of information elicited during the course of the Senate's McClellan Committee investigation into labor-management practices, the act was designed primarily to require reporting and disclosure of operational data of private pension funds.

The act applied to health, welfare, and pension plans with 26 or more participants that were established or maintained by employers engaged in commerce, by an employee organization representing workers engaged in commerce, or by both. "Participants" included employees or former employees covered by the plan. This act applied to all benefit funds, including Taft-Hartley plans.

Bonding regulations in the act required trustees to purchase a fidelity bond and maintain it in force. The bond was to be updated at the start of each reporting year in an amount equal to 10 percent of the total of plan funds handled during the previous reporting year. The minimum bond was $1,000, the maximum $500,000. The bond had to be purchased from an acceptable surety company. There were other legal requirements. The bonding requirements under ERISA are basically the same as under the WPPDA, which was repealed by ERISA.

Despite passage of the Welfare and Pension Plan Disclosure Act, many still were concerned about the employee benefit field in general and pension trusts in particular. This had been called the largest pool of unregulated money in the United States. Private sector pension plans are estimated to aggregate about $250 billion in assets. Before the end of the century, private and public plans are expected to have assets exceeding a trillion dollars. Concern increased because of the tremendous impact of these funds on the securities market. Consternation was generated by horror stories—many of them true—of people who had worked a lifetime and were deprived of pension benefits when they were ready to retire. This loss occurred either because the pension fund or sponsoring company was bankrupt or because of highly restrictive technical requirements, some of which were considered unfair by many people.

Concern grew when Studebaker was unable to pay 100 cents on the dollar for pensions. This tragedy was repeated in many smaller situations, causing hardship for thousands of workers and their families. Unions became alarmed, particularly since these defaults occurred in the relatively good economic climate of the 1960s. Responsible corporate executives also were disturbed, and fair-minded, socially conscious people all over the country were upset.

A piecemeal state-by-state approach did not make sense because many funds crossed state lines and the problem was national. After a long period of gestation, beginning in the late 1960s, several bills crystallized.

The House bill was less controlling than the Senate one. For example, the House was willing to let estab-lished practices stand unless they were specifically found to be harmful. The Senate, on the other hand, set forth in detail what transactions were prohibited. A tremendous amount of work took place before an acceptable compromise bill was enacted. That bill was ERISA.

ERISA

The Employee Retirement Income Security Act of 1974 (ERISA) was signed by President Ford September 2, 1974. It was considered by the president, the law's sponsors, and many others to be the most significant piece of social legislation since the enactment of Social Security nearly 40 years earlier.

The intent of ERISA is to protect the well-being and security of millions of workers and their dependents affected by the operation of employee benefit plans. This intent is carried out through various means. First, ERISA requires the administrators of employee benefit plans to make numerous reports to the three government agencies with jurisdiction over compliance—the Department of Labor, the Internal Revenue Service, and the Pension Benefit Guaranty Corporation. ERISA also requires the administrators to disclose certain information to plan participants and beneficiaries and to provide specific detailed information to these individuals upon request. Second, ERISA sets minimum standards for participation, vesting, funding, and benefit accrual. Third, ERISA establishes the PBGC to insure pensions in the event a covered pension plan terminates without sufficient funds to meet its vested obligations. Finally, ERISA establishes federal standards for weighing fiduciary conduct and procedures for their enforcement.

FIDUCIARY STANDARDS

Any examination of the federal standards governing the conduct of fiduciaries must necessarily begin with the definition of a "fiduciary" under ERISA. Section 3(21)(A) provides that a person is a fiduciary with respect to a plan to the extent that the individual:

1. exercises any discretionary authority or control over the management or disposition of its assets;
2. provides investment advice for a fee or other compensation, direct or indirect, with respect to any monies or other property of the plan, or has any authority or responsibility to do so;
3. has any discretionary authority or discretionary responsibility in the administration of a plan;

4. has been designated by a "named fiduciary" to carry out fiduciary responsibilities (other than trustee responsibilities) under the plan.

There is little question that under this broad definition, named fiduciaries, fund trustees, administrators (more often called fund managers), and investment managers all are fiduciaries. There still is a question whether other individuals having dealings with employee benefit funds, such as professional advisers, are subject to the standards. Interpretive Bulletins from the Department of Labor appear to exempt actuaries, attorneys, accountants, and investment aides without discretionary authority.

The important point to note, though, is that the true test of fiduciary status is not an individual's title nor what the trust indenture defines as the person's responsibility, but what the individual actually does.

THE 'PRUDENT MAN' RULE

ERISA establishes federal standards for fiduciary conduct and specifically preempts state law. It provides that, in general, the preemption provision should not be construed to exempt or relieve any person from any state law regulating insurance, banking, or securities, or prohibit the use of any generally applicable state criminal law.

The fiduciary standard, on the surface, seems to be the "prudent man" rule, but a careful reading indicates that it is more detailed, refined, comprehensive, and stringent. The act provides that a fiduciary must discharge the duties of the role "with the care, skill, prudence, and diligence under the circumstances then prevailing that a prudent man acting in a like capacity and familiar with such matters would use in the conduct of an enterprise of a like character and with like aims." The standard further provides that a fiduciary must discharge these duties solely in the interest of participants and beneficiaries and for the exclusive purpose of providing benefits to participants and their beneficiaries and defraying reasonable expenses of administering the plan. The standard adds a new dimension to previous law by specifically requiring that a fiduciary must diversify the investment of the assets of a plan so as to minimize the risk of large losses, unless it clearly is prudent not to do so.

Compliance with the act's "prudent man" rule is determined by analysis of all the facts and circumstances at the time of any alleged impropriety. It must be emphasized that the act adds a new dimension to the established common law "prudent man" rule by requiring a fiduciary to conform functional conduct with that of a prudent man who is "familiar with such matters." Given this new criterion, some commentators state that a presumption of expertise is imposed on the conduct of fiduciaries. While this may be too strong a reading of the "familiar with such matters" standard, clearly trustees and other fiduciaries must have a meaningful degree of familiarity with the issues with which they deal.

COFIDUCIARY RESPONSIBILITY

The act contains separate provisions that set out the circumstances in which a fiduciary is liable for a breach of duty by a cofiduciary. Liability for a cofiduciary's breach of duty arises if the fiduciary:

1. has participated knowingly in or knowingly has undertaken to conceal an act or omission of the other fiduciary, knowing that such an act or omission is a breach;
2. has enabled the other fiduciaries to commit a breach by failing to comply with the general fiduciary duty (i.e., the "prudent man" rule) in administration of the specific responsibilities that give rise to the fiduciary status; or
3. has knowledge of a breach by such other fiduciary, unless the individual makes reasonable efforts under the circumstances to remedy the breach.

In the first instance, a fiduciary must have knowledge of the misconduct of another fiduciary and also must participate in the impropriety or undertake to conceal the other's actions. This kind of liability is premised on action and not on lack of it.

In the second case, liability occurs when a fiduciary, through failure to adhere to the general "prudent man" rule, allows a breach of duty by a fellow fiduciary. The Congressional Conference Report on the act cites an example of two cotrustees jointly managing the plan assets. Trustee A improperly allows trustee B to have custody of all the assets and makes no inquiry as to Trustee B's conduct. If B thereby is enabled to sell the property and embezzle the proceeds, A is liable for a breach of fiduciary duty.

The potential for liability under this provision is considerable. Trustees and other fiduciaries must recognize that they not only must be prudent with respect to the conduct of their own affairs, but also must be vigilant as to the conduct of other fiduciaries.

Liability in the third case arises when a fiduciary has knowledge of a breach of duty by a fellow fiduciary and fails to take reasonable efforts to remedy that breach. The critical element is what is "reasonable." It is difficult to give precise guidance because the "necessary" steps will hinge on the circumstances of the particular case. However, the Conference Report does give some indication of the conduct expected.

It states that a trustee may be required to cure a cofiduciary's impropriety, assuming that the trustee has the proper authority. As an alternative, a trustee might be required "to notify the plan's sponsor of the breach, or to proceed to an appropriate federal court for instructions, or bring the matter to the attention of the Secretary of Labor." The Conference Report adds that the proper remedy will turn on the facts and circumstances in each case and "may be affected by the relationship of the fiduciary to the plan and to the cofiduciary, the duties and responsibilities of the fiduciary in question, and the nature of the breach."

These comments seem to imply that affirmative action is required. A mere negative vote against the improper action or a resignation by the trustee who believes misconduct is occurring probably will be deemed too passive and therefore an insufficient response. The political consequences for the "virtuous" trustee may be unpleasant, of course, but appear inevitable. A trustee's or other fiduciary's potential liability for breach of duty by a cofiduciary is the same as that for a breach of the "prudent man" rule or any of the other duties.

PROHIBITED TRANSACTIONS

The act prohibits a fiduciary from causing a plan to engage in certain prohibited transactions with a party in interest. The term "party in interest" is defined broadly as including anyone who directly or indirectly is associated with the plan.

The act prohibits a rather broad list of transactions between the plan and a "party in interest:" the sale, exchange, or leasing of any property; the lending of money or other extension or credit (except under special circumstances); the furnishing of goods, services, or facilities; and the transfer of assets of the plan to, use by, or for the benefit of, a party in interest. Basically, the prohibited transaction section is designed to codify what long has been considered improper for fiduciaries—a conflict of interest. The ERISA provision, however, is more precise in that it spells out in detail what is banned and is broader since it includes parties in interest as well as fiduciaries. Moreover, under the prohibited transaction rules, even if the dealings benefitted both the party in interest and the fund and were not unconscionable, a breach of ERISA still would occur.

The act prohibits transactions involving self-dealing or breach of the duty of loyalty by the fiduciary. Specifically, the act bans a fiduciary from dealing with the assets of a plan in the individual's own interest or account, acting on behalf of any party whose interests are adverse to the interest of the plan or plan participants or beneficiaries, or receiving any consideration for a personal account from any party dealing with the plan in connection with the transaction involving its assets.

The act excludes a number of specific transactions from the broad list of prohibited dealings and provides for a procedure whereby a proposed transaction may be granted an exemption from the prohibited provisions. Exceptions to the general January 1, 1975, effective date provide for transition periods of several years for phasing out "party in interest transactions" involving loans, leases, sales, and the provision of services between a plan and a party in interest.

In this writer's opinion, overly strict interpretations of the law will prove to be counterproductive. Many practices that funds could engage in that are for the benefit of both parties to the transaction, or even to the fund only, are prohibited. For example, Corporation Q, a contributing employer to a pension fund, wishes to sell a building that the fund could use as a headquarters. Q needs cash, which the fund has. The price Q is seeking is below the value set by three impartial appraisers. Nevertheless, the purchase technically would be a prohibited transaction. While it is all very well to point out that exemptions may be obtained, Corporation Q needs cash now and is not willing to wait a long while for legal opinions, Department of Labor advice, exemptions, or hearings. Thus an ideal building investment may be lost to the fund.

Another example: Welfare Fund X pays benefits for all its members for maternity care and delivery. Welfare Fund X covers painters in eight counties in the Southwest. In one county there is only one large medical center with facilities for deliveries known as County General Hospital. County General employs six painters full time. They are covered by a collective bargaining agreement with the local painters' union and contributions are made on their behalf to Welfare Fund X. The wife of a painter suddenly suffers labor pains. Obviously, her husband is not going to drive 100 miles across the desert to a noncontributing employer when he and his family live ten blocks from County General Hospital. He takes his wife—now in labor—to County General where she is delivered of a fine set of twins. He applies subsequently to Welfare Fund X to pay the hospital bill pursuant to the trust plan. Will the payment from the fund to a contributing employer (a party in interest) be a prohibited transaction? Is it within the "services" statutory exemption? This is a problem not yet fully clarified but it would appear to fall within the exemption. It is essential that it be so construed, since this is not an isolated type of transaction that can be considered unique but one that could occur many times over.

DELEGATION OF FIDUCIARY DUTY

Trustees' delegation and allocation of fiduciary duties, and their rights to limit their liability, are indeed intricate aspects of the act's fiduciary part. The act requires that any allocation or delegation of any trustee or fiduciary duty or duties take place pursuant to a written procedure embodied in the plan or trust agreement. To the extent that any of the trustees contemplate allocating or delegating any of their fiduciary duties, they must make absolutely certain that such a delegation or allocation is under written authority in the trust agreement.

It appears, at this point, that informal allocations will not satisfy the intent of the act. Moreover, this writer believes it would not suffice to have allocation spelled out in detail—no matter how clear and legalistic—if the practice is contrary to normal. Thus, if a trustee interferes in the activities of another trustee's committee or function, this behavior on a consistent basis may be deemed to vitiate the written clause and the relief it provides.

CONCLUSION

The challenges to trustees are many. However, pension and welfare funds are very significant parts of the total compensation package. An abdication by management of a health care institution of the exercise of its responsibilities will lead to greater control either by the federal government, unions, or both. Unless management wants these alternatives, it must participate actively in the direction of joint funds, select effective and educated trustees, and support them.

6. Self-Insuring Workers' Compensation: Does It Really Save?

KARL R. BIRKY

This article was prepared jointly with R. E. Harrington, Inc., Columbus, Ohio, a national unemployment and workers' compensation cost control consulting company. Reprinted with permission from *Topics in Health Care Financing,* Cost Containment Part II, Vol. 3, No. 4, Summer/1977, Issue Editor, William O. Cleverley, Ph.D., by Aspen Systems Corporation, Germantown, Md. © 1977.

Workers' compensation is the single largest commercial line of insurance in existence with 1974 premiums approaching the $5.5 billion level. This has been the result of yearly increases in the medical care industry and in benefit levels.

INSURING WORKERS' COMPENSATION

Currently every state, except Louisiana, requires employers to insure their workers' compensation or to demonstrate their ability to self-insure these obligations. Workers' compensation liability can be covered through a private insurance carrier or state insurance program, or an employer can establish a self-insurance program. Each state regulates the types of programs which an employer may use.

Private Insurance Carrier

Described in Table 6-1 are the types of programs employers may use for insuring their workers' compensation losses in various states. Forty-four states permit private insurers to insure an employer's workers' compensation liability. Private insurers, which paid 52 percent of all the workers' compensation claims in 1975,[1] can generally be divided into two categories: (1) Proprietary (or stock) and (2) Mutual insurance companies. Proprietary insurers are owned by profit-seeking stockholders and have similar rights

and responsibilities to stockholders in profit corporations not engaged in insurance. Mutual insurance companies are very similar to proprietary insurance companies except that the stockholders are the policyholders and any dividends paid are paid to the policyholders.

State Administered Programs

State administered workers' compensation programs are found in 18 states and paid 35 percent of all workers' compensation losses in the United States in 1975.[2] These funds, which enjoy a tax-free status, operate much the same as private funds, collecting premiums based on experience ratings, reserving funds for future losses, making actuarial studies and servicing claims. Employers in 12 of these states find their state fund competing with private insurers for a share of the workers' compensation insurance market. Some state funds have been very competitive and insure a major segment of the market, while others predominantly insure poor risk employers unable to obtain insurance privately.

In addition to these 12 competitive state funds, there are six exclusive (or monopolistic) state funds. Private insurers in exclusive fund states are not permitted to insure workers' compensation claims, although two exclusive fund states, as well as *all* competitive fund states, permit employers to self-insure their losses and

Table 6-1 Methods Available to Employers in Various States for Insuring Workers' Compensation Losses

	States Permitting Self-Insurance		State Not Permitting Self-Insurance	Total
States permitting Private Insurance:				
1. With no State Fund	31 remaining states		Texas	32
2. With a competitive State Fund	Arizona	Montana	none	12
	California	New York		
	Colorado	Oklahoma		
	Idaho	Oregon		
	Maryland	Pennsylvania		
	Michigan	Utah		
States not permitting Private Insurance:				
Exclusive State Fund	Ohio		Nevada	6
	West Virginia		North Dakota	
			Washington	
			Wyoming	
Total		45	5	50

Source: C. A. Williams, Jr., *Insurance Arrangements Under Workmen's Compensation,* U.S. Department of Labor Bulletin No. 317 (Washington, D.C.: Government Printing Office, 1969), pp. 27–28.

to purchase specific excess insurance from private insurers. One distinct advantage of an exclusive state fund is the ability to increase premiums without fear of losing customers since they have a captive market.

Self-Insurance

Even though numerically only one percent of all employers self-insure their workers' compensation claims, self-insurers in the 46 states that permit self-insurance paid 12 percent of all losses in 1975.[3] This does not result from self-insurers having higher claims per employee, but from the fact that self-insurers are generally larger employers, often with an insurance or risk management department. In recent years the self-insurance approach has gained substantial recognition. Through the implementation of a self-insurance program, many hospitals have fulfilled their insurance needs, minimized their risks, and generated a substantial cash flow savings. Although not all employers can qualify for self-insurance, a hospital paying in excess of $70,000 in premiums a year should explore this alternative. It is important to note that no matter which one of the three alternatives a hospital currently uses or is considering, the hospital will always pay the total cost of a valid workers' compensation claim.

BACKGROUND

Before considering the potential benefits or disadvantages of self-insuring a hospital's workers' compensation liability, it is important to first understand how the typical workers' compensation self-insurance program operates. In most cases, self-insurance provides for the administration and payment of workers' compensation claims directly from hospital funds rather than through an insurance carrier. Typically, self-insured employers will retain only a specified amount of risk per incident, imposing a retention limit of, for instance, $100,000 per incident. Employers will then purchase "specific excess" insurance from a carrier to protect against the infrequent, yet possible, catastrophic loss in excess of $100,000. In addition, some employers may also purchase "aggregate excess" insurance which provides a stop loss for the total cost of all accidents during a specific period of time. Self-insurance, then, is really a policy of hospital-assumed risk combined with coverage of catastrophic losses by an insurance carrier.

When viewing self-insurance as an alternative, a hospital should consider not only the potential benefits of a successful self-insurance program, but also the disadvantages that may result if an improper decision to self-insure is made, or an improperly administered program is instituted. Fortunately, the predictability of workers' compensation losses, in comparison to other exposures, provides the controller or risk manager a methodology whereby he can forecast his future liability with some degree of accuracy. At the same time, however, a detailed understanding of the not-so-obvious costs—sometimes referred to as the hidden costs of self-insurance, must be developed.

Of course, only in those hospitals where the advantages of self-insurance significantly outweigh the disadvantages should self-insurance be considered. It is important, therefore, to first determine what the advantages and disadvantages may be for an individual hospital.

As indicated earlier, a hospital is going to pay for the cost of a claim regardless of whether it does so through an insurance carrier, a state fund system, or from hospital funds by way of a self-insured program. However, there can be considerable advantages to the self-insured method, particularly in cash retention (cash flow).

An insurance carrier, and to a similar extent a state fund system, calculates and collects premiums on the basis of incurred loss (current year paid losses and anticipated future costs), overhead and administrative costs plus profit. This calculation covers a short period of time—the rating period—even though the entire cost of the claim may not be totally paid for many years in the future. This is necessary because the carrier or state fund generally retains liability for claims even after the company may have cancelled the policy. Thus most hospitals must immediately pay premiums that have been adjusted to include the anticipated cost of the claim that may take years to pay out.

ADVANTAGES OF SELF-INSURANCE

1. In contrast to the insurance carrier and state fund methodology, one benefit of self-insurance is that a hospital will pay claims liability only when it becomes due. The current year premium expense that normally would have been spent with an insurance carrier for future claims payment is now free for other hospital uses.

In fact, by comparing and averaging the annual reports of leading private insurers of workers' compensation, it was found that private insurers pay 30 percent of the total losses in the year of injury. The 70 percent of the total losses not paid out are invested by the insurer or used internally if the hospital self-insures. Subsequent payouts were 30 percent in the first year after injury, and 18, 12 and 10 percent in subsequent years. (See Table 6-2.) This cash flow principle is one of the most significant advantages of a self-insurance program.

2. Another potential benefit that may result from a self-insurance program is the ability to retain a significant portion of the insurance premium dollar that was going to insurance carrier sales and advertising costs, administration and profit. Utilizing insurance industry standards, this could amount to 30 percent or more of the premium.[4]

3. Once self-insured, many employers believe they now have a more effective claims handling program than was available to them under conventional coverage. This occurs, first of all, because under self-insurance an employer may be able to pay legitimate claims with greater promptness, thereby improving employee relations. In addition, fraudulent claims can be handled more effectively since the employer is directly involved with the claims and their processing.

4. Still another advantage is that under a self-insured program an employer will not be penalized for the poor loss experience of other employers in the same industry. Also, an employer will not be penalized for his own previous poor experience years as may

Table 6-2 Payout Schedule of Incurred Liability

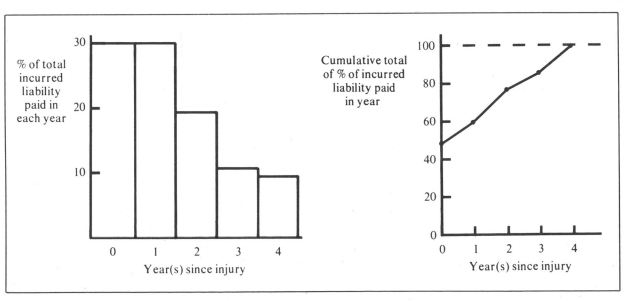

occur under the modification provisions of an insurance carrier's plan.

5. Finally, each workers' compensation loss is predictable within a fairly narrow range because the size of the loss is limited by a rigidly prescribed formula. Hospital management often believes that insuring any type of predictable loss is an expensive luxury. They state that predictable losses should be planned for, not insured. Under self-insurance, the only insurance that needs to be purchased is excess insurance, which will insure the hospital against the infrequent, yet possible, catastrophic loss. In other cases, aggregate excess insurance may be purchased to ensure against total loss in any one particular year. The cost of excess insurance to provide coverage for liability beyond a maximum limit is modest in comparison to public liability or other insurance claims which are subject to litigation.

DISADVANTAGES

As with any approach to a business problem, there are always disadvantages that deserve very careful consideration. Let's discuss the more predominant ones.

1. Loss control, or the prevention and control of occupational accidents, is an extremely important function that a self-insured hospital must emphasize. If the hospital is not confident that an effective program of loss control will accompany the move to self-insurance, very serious doubts should be raised about whether self-insurance is appropriate.

Loss control is the first line of defense against claims. Its prime function is to continually seek out and correct any unsafe working conditions that may contribute to accidents. To be most effective, loss control personnel must be completely familiar with management's philosophy relative to performance standards. They must continually review existing job descriptions and evaluate new job responsibilities as they relate to established safety standards. While loss control effectiveness is extremely important under an insurance carrier program, it may have increased significance for the potential self-insured.

2. It goes without saying that only hospitals with sufficient financial stability to be comfortable assuming a fair amount of risk over the years should consider self-insurance. This, by the way, will not be only the hospital's concern. Each state's regulatory commission will be very interested in this area when an employer files an application to qualify as a self-insured employer.

3. Finally, self-insurance may not be appropriate unless the hospital's management is interested in it not only as a means to improve the overall cost of workers' compensation, but also as a method to demonstrate management's direct involvement, understanding and concern for work-related accidents. The decision to self-insure must be made conscious of the fact that self-insuring is a long-term commitment. Losses incurred while self-insuring must continue to be paid by the employer even if the employer begins insuring with an insurance carrier.

When initially considering self-insurance, a hospital must look at its size, loss experience, financial stability, future claims administration plans as a self-insurer, and whether it will be able to fairly, promptly, and over a long period of time, meet the overall obligations of self-insuring. Before approving a hospital to initiate a self-insurance program, the state regulatory commission will examine each of these areas.

CASE STUDY OF SELF-INSURING HOSPITALS

Seventeen Ohio hospitals that self-insure their workers' compensation were examined to determine whether significant benefits were being realized in the programs. Benefits accruing to the hospitals potentially would arise from two areas: differences in the amount of payment and in the timing of payments. If self-insuring hospitals could pay only valid claims and return employees to work more quickly than the state fund, or if payments could be deferred by retaining in the hospital those funds normally paid in premiums and benefit payments made from these funds over an extended period of time, savings would be realized.

Of course, since Ohio is an exclusive fund state, which permits employers to self-insure their workers' compensation, all hospitals not self-insuring their claims were insured with the state fund. It is worth noting that the Ohio state fund had the largest total benefits payments of any state fund in the country in 1975.[5] Aggregate data was obtained for benefit payments made by the state fund for all hospitals it insured for comparison with a sample of the 46 self-insuring hospitals in Ohio.

Self-Insured vs. State Fund Results

This self-selected sample of 17 hospitals, having an average bed size of 391 beds, and an average 1976 payroll of $10.5 million, had been self-insuring an average of 43 months. The self-insurance programs had been in place in 11 hospitals for more than 36 months.

Consequently the experiences of thcsc 11 hospitals were analyzed in more detail and compared to the state fund's experience for the hospitals it insured. Interestingly enough, these 11 hospitals averaged payments of 13.1 cents per $100 of payroll for 1974 injuries from the time of injury until December 31, 1975. A similar examination of claims payments actually made by the state fund shows that the state fund paid 23.2 cents/$100 of payroll in the same period for all state-insured hospital employees.

These comparisons were only between actual losses paid and do not include administrative costs, reserves, or interest income on reserves. The Ohio Bureau of Workmen's Compensation increased its administrative fees from 6 cents/$100 of payroll to 9.5 cents/$100 of payroll in January 1977.[6] Fccs charged by sclf-insurance service agencies for administering a self-insurance program are very comparable, averaging four cents to six cents/$100 of payroll. The Ohio state fund realized a 6.68 percent return on its invested funds in 1975.[7]

Another significant difference in the amounts paid was found when the average self-insured hospital's losses actually paid through December 31, 1976 for injuries in 1974 and 1975 were compared to the losses the state fund paid for all the hospital employees it insured the previous year: 1973 and 1974 injuries paid through December 31, 1975. Information of state fund payments was available only through December 31, 1975 for the years 1971, 1972, 1973, and 1974. Information for the self-insuring hospitals, on the other hand, was available only for years 1974, 1975 and 1976 through December 31, 1976. Therefore, except for the preceding comparison, dissimilar periods were compared. The assumption was made that costs of workers' compensation claims were increasing; this assumption is reinforced by the steadily increasing premiums.

State payments through December 31, 1975 for injuries that occurred in 1973 and 1974 were 27.0 cents/$100 of payroll. Self-insuring hospitals paid 16.4 cents/$100 through December 31, 1976 for injuries that occurred in 1974 and 1975. The assumption has been made that the medical costs as well as benefit levels increased from 1973 to 1974 and 1974 to 1975. Even if one assumes no increase, the 10.6 cents difference in loss payouts is interesting and significant.

Other similar comparisons were made and in every case the self-insuring hospitals paid significantly less on the average for their workers' compensation losses than the state paid for all the hospital employees it insured.

Clearly the self-insuring Ohio hospitals in the sample paid less than the state fund paid for similar injuries.

Additionally, when one considers that self-insuring hospitals had paid 13.1 cents/$100 of payroll in the years 1974 and 1975 for 1974 injuries, and that the 1974 average premium, including a six cents administrative fee, was 84 cents/$100 of payroll, the cash flow advantages become apparent. Rather than paying the 84 cents/$100 of payroll into the state fund in 1974, these premiums were retained and as of the end of 1975 only 13.1 cents/$100 of payroll had been paid out for claims in addition to self-insurance administrative fees, state fund fees and excess coverage insurance.

In fact, C. Arthur Williams, Jr., in a study done for the U.S. Department of Labor in 1969, concluded that ". . . self-insurers probably have the lowest costs, followed by employers insured, respectively, by exclusive state funds, competitive state funds, and private insurers."[8] He also found that exclusive state funds paid out 95 cents in benefits for every premium dollar.[9]

Deferred Payment Benefits

In Table 6-3 we examine the benefits of deferring payments (timing differences) through a self-insurance program by making assumptions for a hypothetical insurer and completing a future value analysis.

The example illustrated in Table 6-3 is very theoretical, assuming as it does $1000 premiums and $1000 losses each year. A hospital with premiums of $100,000 could *increase* its cash flow in seven years by $206,800. The example has not included the administrative costs of self-insuring or of an insurance carrier. Administrative costs in the state funds and self-insurance are, as discussed earlier, very comparable in most respects and do not significantly affect the analysis at the theoretical level. Commercial insurers on the average had a much lower benefit-to-premium ratio than state funds,[10] and the inclusion of administrative fees in a comparison with self-insurers would favor self-insurers.

An estimate of the payout schedule for the Ohio state fund was developed from the 1972, 1973 and 1974 annual reports of the Industrial Commission of Ohio and Ohio Bureau of Workmen's Compensation and indicates a payout of benefits for the state fund as shown in Table 6-4.[11]

If this payout schedule is used in the preceding example and premiums and losses remain $1000, the net future value of self-insuring, at 14 years without consideration for other expenses, is $7,995 at a four percent discount rate, $11,512 at eight percent and $16,544 at 12 percent.

Hospitals considering self-insurance will want to consider a similar analysis, done either internally or by

Table 6-3 Seven-Year Self-Insured Evaluation

Assumptions:
1. Premiums less administrative fees are $1000 per year.
2. Incurred liability (total eventual losses) are $1000 per year.
3. Claims are paid according to the following payout schedule. Derived from private insurance data for workers' compensation.

Year after injury	0	1	2	3	4
% of incurred liability paid	30	30	18	12	10

	Year of Payment						
	1977	1978	1979	1980	1981	1982	1983
Insurance Premium Cost:	1000	1000	1000	1000	1000	1000	1000
Self-Insured Cost:							
1977 injuries	300	300	180	120	100	0	0
1978 injuries		300	300	180	120	100	0
1979 injuries			300	300	180	120	100
1980 injuries				300	300	180	120
1981 injuries					300	300	180
1982 injuries						300	300
1983 injuries							300
Total losses in year	300	600	780	900	1000	1000	1000
Retention (Premium less losses):	700	400	220	100	0	0	0
Interest Earnings on Retention: @ 8%							
Current year's retention @ 4%							
(½ year @ 8%):	28	16	9	4	0	0	0
Cumulative retention:		56	88	106	114	114	114
Total Interest Earnings:	28	72	97	110	114	114	114
Total Retention:	728	472	317	210	114	114	114
Total Cumulative Retention:	728	1200	1517	1726	1840	1954	2068

a self-insurance specialist, which includes all actual costs of self-insuring, the actual loss experience of the hospital and actual premiums currently being paid.

THE THIRD PARTY REIMBURSEMENT DILEMMA

Hospitals, dealing as they do with third party payers—in particular, cost payers—will want to know the regulations concerning self-insurance programs and the effects of these regulations on the benefits. Before discussing the regulations it is important to re-emphasize the importance of establishing reserves for losses in any self-insurance program. Self-insurance is a planned risk retention program; improper planning and reserving can have serious consequences for a hospital. Hospitals can reserve funds through various mechanisms the most common being (1) trusteed reserve funds, and (2) non-trusteed reserve funds.

The *Provider Reimbursement Manual* does not specifically deal with workers' compensation or with self-insurance programs for insuring workers' compensation claims. However, the regulations for unemploy-ment compensation are assumed to apply for workers' compensation programs and deal with self-insurance programs for insuring unemployment compensation. Section 2122.5 paragraph C of Revision 165 of the manual indicates that costs of premiums and other fees for workers' compensation insurance are allowable costs if insurance is obtained from a state fund, commercial insurer or a joint insurance fund. Funds deposited in a reserve account are not allowable costs, which is consistent with generally acceptable accounting principles to date. Moreover, any income earned from investment of the funds of the reserve account must be used to offset a provider's allowable interest expense under the Medicare program.[12]

In a February 3, 1977 Administrative Bulletin No. 1117 from Blue Cross Medicare Administration (Chicago) to Directors of Federal Programs and Reimbursement Managers, The Bureau of Health Insurance responded to questions posed by the Blue Cross Association clarifying Section 2122.5C of the PRM.

Question #1

Section 2122.5C states: ". . . any income earned from investment of the funds of the reserve account

Table 6-4 Estimated Payout Schedule for Ohio State Fund

Year after injury	0	1	2	3	4	5	6	7	8	9	10	11	12	13
% of incurred liability paid	13	10	9	8	7	7	7	6	5	5	5	4	4	10

must be used to offset a provider's allowable interest expense under the Medicare Program.''

Since the Medicare Program did not participate in the establishment of the fund, as contributions to the reserve account are not allowable costs, why should interest income on these funds be offset against interest expense? . . .

Answer #1

". . . A reserve fund for unemployment compensation costs is clearly an investment of a provider's general funds. . . . Such funds could come from Medicare or other patient revenues or from borrowed funds or from intermingled general funds used for all types of operating expenses.''

Question #2

. . . If a provider were to establish an unrelated trustee, having sole control over the unemployment compensation reserve, would the provider be able to claim the payments as cost (provided the contributions were based on an actuarial determination and did not exceed the payments that would have been made to a state)? . . .

Answer #2

"Where a provider establishes an unrelated trustee having sole control over the unemployment compensation reserve, this procedure essentially consists of a single provider establishing its own reserve account to meet unemployment compensation costs. Accordingly, under current Medicare policies, such a plan would be considered a self-insurance program and the costs of payments to such a reserve would not be allowable. Moreover, we believe the joint unemployment insurance programs provide an adequate remedy in such situations."[13]

It would appear that self-insuring hospitals wanting to establish separate reserve funds must do so through some type of joint insurance program. As illustrated in Table 6-5, an examination of the effects of these regulations on the hypothetical insurer is dramatic and insightful. The same assumptions have been made and additionally it is assumed that 60 percent of the hospitals' revenues are cost based. Total cumulative retention from the self-insurance program is decreased from $2068 to $672 in the seven year period. Obviously hospitals looking for cost-saving mechanisms become frustrated when the majority of the savings from a self-insurance reserve fund is passed on to the cost paying reimbursers. Hospitals in states that do not permit joint insurance programs must lose much of the reserve interest income, find an alternative method of reserving, or not reserve at all. Certainly none of the alternatives is attractive and perhaps a concerted effort should be made to permit retention of interest income and/or the expensing of contributions to an actuarily sound reserve fund. Potential savings do exist for the hospital and ultimately the consumer, in spite of these restrictions. Many hospitals will want to examine closely the self-insuring of their workers' compensation liability as a cost-saving alternative.

The primary goal a hospital considering self-insurance should set is "to make a proper decision" whether or not to self-insure. This objective can be reached if the correct study methodology is exercised in a truly analytical manner. But self-insurance is not a "try it and see" alternative. It is a critical decision that deserves the highest level of management attention. If properly made and executed, however, a workers' compensation self-insurance program can achieve dramatic results for a hospital.

Table 6-5   Seven-Year Self-Insured Evaluation with Cost Payer Adjustments

Assumptions:
1. Premiums less administrative fees are $1000 per year.
2. Incurred liability (total eventual losses) are $1000 per year.
3. Claims are paid according to the following payout schedule derived from private Insurance Data for Workers' Compensation.

Year after injury	0	1	2	3	4
% of incurred liability	30	30	18	12	10

4. Revenues are 60% cost based.

	1977	1978	1979	1980	1981	1982	1983
	1000	1000	1000	1000	1000	1000	1000
Self-Insured Cost:							
1977 injuries	300	300	180	120	100	0	0
1978 injuries		300	300	180	120	100	0
1979 injuries			300	300	180	120	100
1980 injuries				300	300	180	120
1981 injuries					300	300	180
1982 injuries						300	300
1983 injuries							300
Total losses in year:	300	600	780	900	1000	1000	1000
Retention (Premium less losses):	700	400	220	100	0	0	0
Retention after cost payer adjustments:	280	160	88	40	0	0	0
Interest Earnings on Retention @ 8%:							
Current year's retention @ 4% (½ year @ 8%):	11.2	6.4	3.5	1.6	0	0	0
Cumulative Retention:		22.4	35.2	42.2	45.4	45.4	45.4
Total Interest Earnings:	11.2	28.8	38.7	43.8	45.4	45.4	45.4
Interest Earnings after cost payer adjustments:	4.5	11.5	15.5	17.5	18.2	18.2	18.2
Total Retention after cost payer adjustments:	284.5	171.5	103.5	57.5	18.2	18.2	18.2
Total Cumulative Retention after cost payer adjustments:	284.5	456.0	559.5	617.0	635.2	653.4	671.6

NOTES

1. D. N. Price, "Workers' Compensation: Coverage, Payments, and Costs, 1975," *Social Security Bulletin* 40, no. 1 (January 1977): 35.
2. Idem.
3. Idem.
4. C. A. Williams, Jr., *Insurance Arrangements Under Workmen's Compensation.* U.S. Department of Labor Bulletin No. 317 (Washington, D.C.: Government Printing Office, 1969): 200.
5. Price, p. 35.
6. "Compensation System to Get $20 Million Boost from Rates," *The Columbus Dispatch* (Columbus, Ohio, January 7, 1977).
7. Industrial Commission of Ohio and Ohio Bureau of Workmen's Compensation, *1975 Annual Report* (Columbus, Ohio, 1976), p. 7.
8. Williams, p. 200.
9. Idem.
10. Idem.
11. Industrial Commission of Ohio and Ohio Bureau of Workmen's Compensation, *1972 Annual Report;* the *1973 Annual Report;* the *1974 Annual Report* (Columbus, Ohio 1973, 1974, 1975) p. 15 (1972), p. 13 (1973) and p. 10 (1974).
12. U.S. Department of Health, Education and Welfare, *Provider Reimbursement Manual* Section 2122.5C (September 1976).
13. Letter from Medicare and CHAMPUS Administration, Blue Cross Association, Chicago, to Directors of Federal Programs and Reimbursement Managers, Administrative Bulletin No. 1117 (February 3, 1977).

7. Preretirement Planning Programs

ROBERT H. WILCOX

Reprinted with permission from *Topics in Health Care Financing, Employee Benefits*, Vol. 6, No. 3, Spring/1980, Issue Editor: Alex W. Steinforth, Aspen Systems Corporation, Germantown, Md. © 1980.

Retirement, like schooling and career, is a phase of life that offers many alternatives, and many pitfalls. The more one can prepare for the eventuality of retirement, the more likely one will find those years rich and fulfilling. Clearly, the opportunity that most Americans have to prepare for retirement is excellent because they have ample time to consider the options, and they can base their decisions on the multitude of life's experiences that has gone before. Yet employees in a wide range of occupations give little prior thought to their retirement, and as a result often end up confronting seemingly insurmountable psychological hurdles. For this reason alone, a preretirement planning program, thoughtfully designed and maintained, can become one of the most valuable employee benefits that an employer can offer.

The advantages of a preretirement planning program to both employee and employer are numerous and compelling. Such a program facilitates the entire process of retirement, instilling the positive concept of opening up the life rather than shutting it down. It can also be regarded as a gesture of loyalty to employees, repaying the loyalty they have shown throughout their working years. A positive effect on general morale is likely to result, from which the employer should benefit through improved employee performance on the job. Furthermore, to the extent that a preretirement program is publicized beyond the institution's walls, the employer's public relations image is enhanced, and ties with the community are strengthened.

MISCONCEPTIONS ABOUT AGING AND RETIREMENT

Any attempt at preretirement counseling of employees must be understood in the context of widely prevalent misconceptions in U.S. society concerning aging and retirement. Dr. Robert Butler, author of *Why Survive? Being Old in America*, calls these attitudes "the genuine tragedy of old age in America," and goes on to paint a picture of U.S. society as one that is "extremely harsh to live in when one is old . . . the (aging) process has been made unnecessarily and at times excruciatingly painful, humiliating, debilitating, and isolating through insensitivity, ignorance and poverty . . . for the most part, the elderly struggle to exist in an inhospitable world."[1] Despite the efforts of many, both in and out of our government, such attitudes persist and are slow to change.[2,3]

The basic misconception about aging is that a direct relationship exists between advancing numerical age and declining competence and ability. This concept has evolved in a number of forms, which Jack Ossofsky, executive director of the National Council on the Aging, has collectively termed "the myths of aging."[4] Such myths characterize elderly people as poor, sick, depressed, isolated, nonfunctional and much alike in their misery. They ignore statistical realities that clearly disprove each point, such as the facts that older employees as a group show less absenteeism than younger ones, and that an overwhelming majority of men and women over age 65 are self-sufficient. The real danger of these misconceptions is that older people themselves may tend to believe them. It is a common observation about human behavior that when people are regarded in a certain way, they tend to follow that role model; if they are treated with respect, however, they will usually respond in kind. Old age, it must be remembered, is a status that everyone can expect to enter, and its "arithmetic of life," as developmental psychologist Gail Sheehy calls it, inexorably computes its numbers for everyone eventually.[5]

Misconceptions concerning retirement are no less persistent, although they are of more recent origin. The institution of retirement, it is interesting to note, is a product of the industrial revolution and is scarcely 100 years old. The first national old age Social Security and pension system, in fact, was established by Bismarck in Germany in 1889. The United States did not follow suit until the Social Security Act of 1935, and the choice of age 65 as the retirement age was based on very little scientific evidence.[6] From that point forward, the magic age of 65 became a very real though arbitrary crossroads in working life, regarded by countless workers, with varying degrees of anticipation and fear, as that moment when usefulness on the job ends and life style must change abruptly. With the passage of the Age Discrimination in Employment Act of 1978, it is evident that U.S. society is moving toward a less rigid concept of retirement. However, the consequence of this legislation is not so much a postponement of retirement decisions as it is an increase in the options and hence the uncertainties of many prospective retirees. As with the concept of aging, the institution of retirement and attitudes toward it are influenced only slowly by such legislation, and the role of preretirement planning remains crucial in counteracting existing misconceptions.

TYPES OF PRERETIREMENT PROGRAMS

The concept of formalized preretirement planning originated in the early 1950s on the campuses of the Universities of Michigan and Chicago. Today the types of programs that can be developed to communicate retirement information and options to employees are many and varied. They range from simple individualized counseling by a personnel or benefits representative, to elaborate life- and career-planning seminars conducted by a staff of experts with the most sophisticated audiovisual methods available.[7] The choice of which approach to take within this scope of possibilities depends on the philosophy and objectives of the company or institution. Such factors as the degree of commitment to the personal well-being of the employee, the importance of establishment of ties with the community, and the willingness to invest administrative time and money will determine the complexity of the program selected. Pilot programs at optimal locations with small groups of the eligible employee population provide an excellent means of experimenting with the concept. The most important consideration is that the end result be a preretirement program ideally suited to the unique needs of the particular employer and employees.

The establishment of preretirement programs as integral parts of a total benefits picture is a growing trend among employers. In a comprehensive survey of 269 business organizations, conducted in 1976 by Prentice-Hall and the American Society for Personnel Administration, it was found that 75 percent of the respondents offered some form of preretirement communication. Of the hospitals reporting, four out of every five were conducting individual preretirement counseling, and one of every three was offering group planning sessions. Furthermore, exactly half of the respondents in the health care area indicated that they had intentions of either initiating or modifying preretirement planning programs "in the near future."[8] More recently the Dartnell Institute of Business Research reported, based on their 1978 survey of comparable scope, that 40 percent of their respondents offer some form of preretirement counseling, and that nearly three-quarters of these had taken this step within the last five years.[9] From these data, it is clear that employers are recognizing the need for preretirement planning for their employees and are acting upon that realization, both in business in general and in the health care field in particular.

Individual Counseling

At minimum, individuals approaching retirement should be counseled at least once by a knowledgeable representative of the institution's personnel or benefits unit or department. A call-up system keyed to employee age is necessary to identify eligible individuals and determine their dates of retirement, although both early and postponed retirement would have to be taken into account. Meetings held with eligible employees should focus on the organization's retirement benefits, and the preparation of individualized retirement benefits statements covering such items as retirement annuities, life insurance, hospitalization and medical care, stock or savings plan, etc., gives structure and direction to the discussion. To cover additional topics effectively, the counselor may wish to supplement the conversation with booklets and handouts. Local sources of such literature might be public health and welfare departments, district offices of the Social Security Administration, the mayor's office in larger cities, and state departments of human resources, and much of this information is likely to be available at little or no cost. Reference can also be made to the growing numbers of books and publications that provide a thorough inventory of retirement issues and options.[10-12] In addition, bulletins on retirement, produced by the employer and sent to the homes of the eligible employees, are an inexpensive but efficient way of relaying information in the institution's style. It can be seen from these methods that the individual approach to retirement counseling need not be confining, and its success is a direct function of the ability and resourcefulness of the counselor.

Group Seminars

Although much can be accomplished in individual meetings, and indeed such meetings should never be eliminated entirely, the term *preretirement planning program* usually refers to some kind of group concept. Much of the information that is necessary and helpful in preretirement planning is similar for all employees, and the most efficient way of reaching people with a common message is through a group context. In a hospital setting, where demands on employee time are ongoing and largely unpredictable, the time available for such sessions may be limited, and attention must be given to covering the most essential material. Packages of various kinds, featuring prerecorded information and supplementary literature, address the problem of tight scheduling but may sacrifice the personal touch. The most effective method of communicating retirement issues is usually the group seminar, in which employees can relate the material to their own experiences and allay some fears by sharing the experiences with peers. Such programs can be run by educational institutions or consulting firms with varying degrees of participation by representatives of the employer, and the inclusion of guest presentations on particular topics lends added credibility to the sessions. In short, a group approach to preretirement planning is a highly visible indication that the employer is committed to transmitting retirement information to employees in the most complete and accurate manner possible.

PROGRAM CONTENT

Once the decision is made to establish a preretirement counseling effort using group seminar sessions, the subject matter must be determined and evaluated. Clearly, greatest attention should be focused on subjects that are most important to prospective retirees. In conversations with older people—both employees who are nearing retirement and former employees who have already retired—three themes seem to reappear with greatest frequency. One is uncertainty about the financial aspects of retirement, including what the organization's benefit programs have to offer. Another is concern about the physical process of aging, and how good health can be maintained into old age. And a third is a general feeling, which some find difficult to express, concerning the necessity of adjusting emotionally or psychologically to the very different world of retirement. If it becomes necessary to deal with the gamut of retirement planning in the space of two or three hours, these three topics of finances, health and psychological adjustment would require coverage above all else.

Most experts are in agreement about the additional topics to be identified in an expanded preretirement program. Such subjects include relocation and housing, legal services, employment, education, leisure and travel, and volunteer and community services. Several of these might be grouped together as one session, depending on the time intervals available. The specific topics to be chosen ultimately depend on the particular needs and preferences identified by the employer and its employees.

Psychological Adjustment to Retirement

The impact of psychological adjustment issues on prospective retirees is of great interest, if for no other reason than that it illustrates how the intangible aspects of retired life are perceived to be every bit as important as the material ones—and, in some cases, even more important. In many ways, psychological adjustment represents the foundation for dealing with all the other ramifications of retirement, and therefore constitutes the ideal first session in a preretirement planning program. It is vital that such a session be conducted with patience and sensitivity, as it serves to set the tone for all that follows. The counselor must empathize with the individual who will suddenly face a morning without a job to do and a routine to follow. An excellent way to achieve this effect is to involve previous retirees on a panel or at the podium, to provide such a perspective directly. Then, brief self-evaluation questionnaires can be advanced to enable employees to better anticipate their own strengths and weaknesses in adjusting to retirement. The main point to be emphasized during this session is that retirement is merely another phase in the normal life process, and that success in this phase simply draws on the successes of all previous phases of life. Each employee who retires today is, after all, fundamentally the same individual who was on the job yesterday and will be faced with defining successful retirement in his or her own unique way.

Specific psychological watchwords and pitfalls can be identified and discussed. Philip Harsham, senior editor of *Medical Economics,* outlines four symptoms that are common to health care professionals approaching retirement: reluctance to shed the professional image, inability to create structured tasks, disinclination to remain mentally and physically active, and failure to assay emotional needs.[13] To counteract these tendencies, one could advance several guidelines for a successful adjustment to retirement at any level, including the maintenance of a positive attitude, the insistence on goal orientation, the retention of an up-to-date outlook on life, and a reminder to count one's blessings. Speaking such phrases is simple, and provides no automatic assurance that everyone's adjustment will necessarily occur more smoothly, but the counselor should realize that such messages, effectively presented, may well have a lasting impact on a number of the participants.

Benefits and Financial Aspects

An organization can provide an outstanding benefits program for its retirees, and yet go largely unappreciated due to its lack of communication and understanding. The preretirement planning seminar affords an excellent vehicle for a thorough discussion of retirement benefits, placed in the context of financial considerations in retirement. Indeed, one of the most severe adjustments for the employee approaching retirement is a financial one, and a reduced standard of living is inevitable in many cases. But a reduction in expenses will also accompany retirement. A systematic balance sheet to estimate and anticipate income and expenses is essential in determining the feasibility of a variety of retirement activities, and many employees will have had very little experience with some of the concepts involved. In the health care literature, studies appear from time to time that are very helpful in the area of preretirement financial planning, especially at the professional level.[14,15] In the seminar itself, it is quite possible that the hospital administrator is sufficiently versed in these issues to offer assistance, or even to preside over the session. In addition to retirement benefits, items that might be covered include Social Security, stocks and bonds, mortgages, medical care costs, consumer tips and senior citizen discounts.

Health Considerations

Aging is a process that begins at birth, and the mere passage of time does not cause diseases of old age. The number of years that a person has lived has little general scientific significance in predicting that individual's health pattern.[16] Nevertheless, a person's susceptibility to physical problems usually does increase with age, as does one's concern about them. At any age, individuals often tend to take their health for granted; as they near retirement age, the penalties for this tendency loom larger. There is no greater tragedy than the worker who has looked forward to retirement for years, only to be unable to enjoy it when it finally arrives due to ill health. For this reason alone, the topic of health considerations requires a position of prominence in preretirement planning, and administrators of such a program for employees in the health care industry should encounter little difficulty in identifying a qualified speaker close at hand. Possible points for discussion in such a session are the importance of preventive care and checkups, the value of exercise and diet, the systems of the body and their diseases, sensory systems, longevity, sexuality, and insurance and Medicare.

Additional Topics

The flexibility to include topics beyond the three just discussed adds a richer dimension to the preretirement planning program. The subject of relocation and housing, for example, breaks down to the questions of whether to move at all, and where to move. The topic of legal services can be used to explore the details of estate planning, wills, laws, trusts and contracts. Employment encompasses the possibility of extending the current career, the opportunity to develop a second career, and other options such as part-time work, temporary assignments, jobsharing and flexible careers. Education relates to the multitude of day and evening courses often available in the community, as well as correspondence courses, seminars and conventions. A session on leisure and travel should stress the concept of leisure as an active process, requiring careful planning to avoid the squandering of the precious commodity known as *free time.* Finally, volunteer and community services deserve particular emphasis if the organization wishes to encourage a link between the employee and the community—especially in the health care industry, where a large number of retirees are inclined to return to the hospital or clinic in a volunteer capacity.

A program that systematically includes each of the foregoing topics may well require a final session to tie it all together. During such a session, the participants could be guided in how to construct a balance sheet of retirement pros and cons, so that they can arrive at realistic retirement plans on their own. And if the topics that have been described sound like a cross section of life itself, that is exactly as intended, because activities during the retirement phase reflect a scope and diversity that is similar to and evolves from all of life's previous phases.

LOGISTICAL QUESTIONS

The practical side of the preretirement counseling effort is one of logistics. The preretirement planning program must itself be planned carefully before it becomes reality, which means certain logistical questions must be asked and answered.[17] Several of the most important of these questions are presented here. It should be remembered that there is no right answer in each case, but rather one that would ultimately be determined by the employee's own needs and preferences.

Initiating a Program

Successful preretirement planning programs originate from a variety of sources. The initial idea may have been mentioned at the highest levels of the organization, or may have evolved from comments made by the employees themselves. Such a program is often conceived and developed within the personnel or human resources department. Regardless of the moving force during the initial stages, however, the structure of the project must be consistent with and reflective of the philosophy of the employer, or it will be unlikely to succeed. Furthermore, the wholehearted support of top management must be received and retained throughout the venture. If the program is to be at all ambitious, a planning committee consisting of representatives from various segments of the organization would probably be necessary to ensure that it is formulated sensibly and that it runs smoothly.

Identifying the Coordinator(s)

Regardless of the quality of the material to be presented, much depends on how it is communicated by the coordinator. This person will provide the continuity for the entire program and will represent the focal point for all of the participants. For this reason, it is essential that one individual, with strong communi-

cation skills and a sensitive manner, be chosen to occupy this position. If possible, such a person should be selected from inside the organization. All else being equal, credibility is probably greater if an older person occupies this role, although personality usually proves to be more important than age in this regard. Nevertheless, the younger coordinator may prefer to have a more experienced representative of the organization share the spotlight for certain segments of the program. During the specialized sessions, guest speakers can be utilized to supplement the coordinator, such as a physician, an attorney, a psychologist or a social worker in the community. In addition, previous retirees should be included to provide firsthand insights on what to expect in retirement.

Deciding on Time, Place and Format

Some employers have found that preretirement planning can be accomplished effectively during an intensive all-day format, where the participants constitute a captive audience directing full attention to the presentations. Such a program becomes almost mandatory when attendees are brought in from outlying locations. However, in the health care industry, where it is exceptionally difficult for employees to be removed from their jobs for long periods, this arrangement is probably not advisable. Instead, a more traditional educational format should be adopted: the establishment of weekly sessions, perhaps five to eight in number, each approximately two hours. Such an approach provides enough time for each self-contained retirement topic to be discussed in some detail and allows for a question period at the end. In addition, the spacing of the sessions gives the participants an opportunity to digest the preceding subject and prepare for the next. Participation is usually better if the sessions occur during working time, although the individual commitment is greater if employee time is used. This distinction may break down in hospital environments, however, where prospective attendees are drawn from several shifts, and some ingenuity of scheduling may be necessary to maximize participation. Another consideration is the inclusion of the spouse, which acknowledges that retirement decisions necessarily involve the total family unit; if spouses are invited, a late afternoon or early evening time period is preferable.

Selecting and Notifying the Participants

Determining who will attend the preretirement planning program will depend on the age range selected, and the size of the eligible employee pool within the range. It should be remembered that the needs of these employees will differ: the 50-year-old individual may be intrigued by the topics of education and second careers, while the 64-year-old is likely to be more concerned with specific details of such programs as Social Security and Medicare.

Although a thorough approach to preretirement planning is generally more effective with employees who are not on the brink of retirement, it is the imminent retirees who must be reached first at the onset of a new program. Therefore, it is recommended that the individuals closest to retirement be the initial participants. Contact with these people should be made individually, with care and tact, so that follow-up memoranda announcing the program do not embarrass or affront. In meetings with these employees, it should be stressed that personal aspects of their retirement plans are none of the institution's business, and that their preferences concerning what is or is not to be shared with the group will be honored without question. Of course, those employees who decide not to participate should not be compelled to do so.

Ensuring Feedback and Follow-Up

As with any course or seminar, the preretirement planning program will lose much of its impact if feedback and follow-up techniques are not built in. The best method of obtaining feedback is to prepare, well in advance, short evaluation sheets to be completed by each participant at the conclusion of the final session. Such devices often provide valuable input that may not be readily apparent from the administrator's perspective. Once the program has ended, the most important follow-up is to ensure that those individuals very close to retirement receive proper individual benefits counseling. Although the group coordinator may not be involved in this counseling, he or she will at least be able to help identify such individuals. If it is decided that former participants will be allowed to reattend individual sessions for purposes of "brushing up," these employees should be kept informed as to when the program will be repeated. After retirement, former employees should be contacted periodically to ensure that they are receiving their checks and organization literature on time, and that there are no major problems of adjustment. Further gestures designed to maintain contact with retired employees include subscriptions to retirement magazines, invitations to events sponsored by the institution, establishment of a retirees' club or a "homecoming" day, and reimbursement for annual physical examinations. In addition, formal counseling sessions with groups of retirees may be advisable, especially to keep them abreast of legis-

lation and procedural changes that may directly affect them. With such a detailed attitude and approach to follow-up, the organization conveys the message that retirees have not been severed from their domain but have merely changed status within it.

THE FUTURE OF PRERETIREMENT PLANNING

The future of preretirement planning in the United States can be best understood in light of demographic trends and projections. In an address before the American Academy of Political and Social Science on April 8, 1978, former Secretary of HEW Joseph A. Califano outlined four such trends.[18] First, life expectancies are increasing steadily, so that people who reach age 65 today can look forward to living 16 more years, on the average—approximately 14 years for men, but 18 years for women. Second, the postwar "baby boom" will reappear as a "senior boom" early in the twenty-first century, so that 18 percent of the population can be expected to be age 65 or over by the year 2030. Third, the option of early retirement is becoming steadily more popular, with 41 percent of workers aged 45 to 54 indicating they intend to retire before 65. Fourth, as a consequence of the foregoing trends, the ratio of active to retired workers is expected to drop from six to one today to three to one by 2030. Added to these trends are such factors as the liberalization of mandatory retirement laws, the greater availability of flexible work arrangements and the increasing difficulty of funding both pension plans and the Social Security system.[19] If a scenario of the future can be deciphered from these varied indicators, it is that older workers will become more plentiful, encounter more options, endure more uncertainties about traditional retirement possibilities and most certainly require more frequent and effective counseling to deal with these new realities.

In the field of health care, which is characterized by high public visibility and a well-educated, dedicated, but mobile work force, a concise but attractive preretirement planning program represents a very persuasive employee benefit. The major precautionary note in this projection is the issue of cost containment, which screams out today from the pages of almost every health care periodical.[20,21] A precise cost-benefit analysis of preretirement counseling is not available even from experts in the field, owing to its newness, so employee feedback on existing programs becomes an essential evaluation tool within a given organization, and long-term concepts of investment and payoff become necessary. In this regard, perhaps the most significant trend in the health care industry is the movement toward multihospital systems, which enjoyed a 10 percent growth rate in 1978, and are projected to expand at least as much in 1979.[22, 23] As more and more health care institutions opt for the multihospital approach, short-term cost stresses can be withstood through a philosophy and structure more akin to that of industrial corporations, and such projects as preretirement planning programs can be assimilated more economically into the health care environment.

Adjustment to retirement, after all, is just another aspect of adjustment to life, and to the extent that an organization can utilize its power to provide a measure of guidance, both employee and employer will profit.

NOTES

1. R. N. Butler, *Why Survive? Being Old in America* (New York: Harper & Row, Inc., 1975).

2. C. H. Percy, *Growing Old in the Country of the Young* (New York: McGraw-Hill Book Co., 1974).

3. R. Gross, B. Gross, and S. Seidman, eds. *The New Old: Struggling for Decent Aging* (Garden City, N.Y.: Anchor Press/Doubleday, 1978).

4. National Council on the Aging, Inc., *Facts and Myths About Aging* (Washington, D.C.: The Council, 1976).

5. G. Sheehy, *Passages: Predictable Crises of Adult Life* (New York: E. P. Dutton & Co., 1976).

6. G. C. Pati, and R. C. Jacobs, "Mandatory Retirement at 70: Separating Substance from Politics." *The Personnel Administrator* 24, no. 2 (February 1979): 19–24.

7. C. E. Kozoll, *Pre-retirement Planning for Employees* (Chicago: The Dartnell Corp., 1979).

8. *P-H/ASPA Survey: New Directions in Employee Pre-retirement Planning Programs* (Englewood Cliffs, N.J.: Prentice-Hall, Inc., 1976).

9. Dartnell Institute of Business Research. *Target Survey: Pre-retirement Counseling Taking Hold* (Chicago: The Dartnell Corp., 1978).

10. J. Adler, *The Retirement Book* (New York: Morrow, 1975).

11. J. C. Buckley, *The Retirement Handbook* (New York: Harper & Row, Inc., 1977).

12. HEW. *Planning for the Later Years*, DHEW Pub. No. P-3000 (Washington, D.C.: Government Printing Office, 1967).

13. P. Harsham, "Four Reasons Why Retirement Goes Sour," *Medical Economics* (March 6, 1978), pp. 182–193.

14. L. Farber, "Are You Shortchanging Your Retirement Plan?" *Medical Economics* (March 20, 1978), pp. 197–208.

15. Litton Industries, Inc., "Retirement: Do It On Your Own Terms" in "1979 Financial Planning Guide," *Medical Economics* (November 6, 1978), pp. 181–210.

16. T. Anderson, "The Aging Process," *Profit Sharing* (February 1979), pp. 11–16.

17. R. G. Martorana, "Preparing the Employee for Retirement," *Profit Sharing* (February 1979), pp. 17–21.

18. J. Califano, "*The Aging of America: Questions for the Four Generation Society*" (Washington, D.C.: Government Printing Office, April 8, 1978).

19. S. H. Rhine, *Older Workers and Retirement*, Conference Board Report No. 738 (New York: The Conference Board, 1978).

20. D. E. L. Johnson, "Basic Assumptions Are Being Reviewed," *Modern Healthcare* 8, no. 1 (January 1978): 54–55.

21. J. T. Foster, "Cost Containment: Are Hospitals Taking a Bum Rap?" *Hospitals*, JAHA, 53, no. 7 (April 1, 1979): 70–73.

22. V. DiPaolo, "Chains Grow with Unbundled Services," *Modern Healthcare* 9, no. 1 (January 1979): 54–55.

23. D. E. L. Johnson, "87 Multihospital Systems Grew 10%, Predict 9% Expansion in 1979," *Modern Healthcare*, 9, no. 4 (April 1979): 46–51.

PART III

LABOR RELATIONS

INTRODUCTION

With the passage of the 1974 Health Care Amendments to the National Labor Relations (Taft-Hartley) Act (P.L. 93-360), labor relations in health care facilities now are subject to a complex body of statutory, administrative, and case law. Human resources administrators have a critical need for a fundamental knowledge of labor relations and labor law if the industry is to increase productivity in the provision of patient care services. Health care administrators, faced simultaneously with demands for more and higher quality services and with closer examination of medical costs by consumers and government, have become particularly concerned about the threat of union organization and collective bargaining.

The growth of unions in the health care industry is paralleling the spread of industrial unions in the 30s and 40s. Human resources administrators must understand what sparks the union organizing campaign at a health care facility. The health care professional, who has the responsibility for dealing with unions either during organizational campaigns or in formal relationships after a certification from the National Labor Relations Board, has an awesome requirement to become familiar with the laws involving that relationship. From the organizing campaign through dealings with the NLRB, with mediators and arbitrators, and with boards of inquiry, there is a pressing need to keep current. What are employer unfair labor practices? Union unfair labor practices? Election procedures?

Negotiating techniques? Notice requirements? Grievance and arbitration procedures?

One of the most important interpersonal relationships within the hospital is between employee and supervisor. The organization reflects its style through the supervisor's attitudes toward employee grievances. Taking disciplinary action against an employee places the burden of proof upon the supervisor. The final step in most grievance procedures is arbitration. The human resources manager must become an expert in that field. More than one-quarter of all cases submitted to arbitration dealt with discipline.

One of the distinctive differences between collective bargaining in private business enterprises on the one hand and voluntary hospitals and nursing homes on the other hand is the absence of market restraints in the health care industry. That industry does not face the competitive product and market forces to the same extent as does private business and depends on public and private insurance companies for most of its operating revenue.

Therefore, labor-management decisions that affect the cost of delivery of health care services strongly affect consumers. The challenge for the hospital industry is to develop an approach to collective bargaining that is highly sensitive to the possibility of strikes, but that is not permeated, undermined, and diluted by fear of such actions. Such an approach, as well as a reduction of the possibility of strikes over terms and conditions of employment, can be achieved by the retention of experienced and knowledgeable labor relations executives and counsel.

1. Hospital Labor Unions: Description and Analysis

ROGER FELDMAN, RICHARD HOFFBECK,
and LUNG-FEI LEE

This project was supported by Grant Number HS 03649 from the National Center for Health Services Research, Office of the Assistant Secretary for Health.

INTRODUCTION

Widespread interest in labor relations in the health services industry can be dated to the publication in 1972 of a classic book by Norman Metzger and Dennis D. Pointer.[1] The book, *Labor-Management Relations in the Health Services Industry: Theory and Practice,* traced the development of collective bargaining in the health services industry's 7,000 hospitals.

Metzger and Pointer noted that there had been a dramatic increase in collective employee activity—for example, the number of hospitals receiving formal requests for recognition from employee organizations increased 102 percent from 1967 to 1970 (from 5.7 to 10.5 percent of all hospitals registered by the American Hospital Association (AHA).[2] However, in 1967, the latest year for which data were available for that study, only 7.7 percent of hospitals had a negotiated contract.[3]

By 1970, an AHA survey[4] indicated that one out of every seven hospitals (14.7 percent) had a collective bargaining contract. Clearly, hospital unionism was on the rise.

On August 25, 1974, an event occurred that may have "marked the end of one era and the beginning of another."[5] This was the day that the Taft-Hartley amendments (P.L. 93-360) took effect, bringing voluntary not-for-profit hospitals under the coverage of the National Labor Relations Act (NLRA). The National Labor Relations Board (NLRB) was empowered to conduct secret elections and order nonprofit hospitals to bargain with the unions chosen by a majority of the employees voting in such elections. Unions often had cited unavailability of these election procedures as a major roadblock to organizing efforts. Speaking for hospital management at a 1975 symposium sponsored by the AHA, Irvin G. Wilmot, executive vice-president of the New York University Medical Center, said that unionization had spurted since passage of the amendments.[6] He noted that, according to some union leaders' forecasts, 50 percent of all hospitals and 70 percent of urban hospitals were likely to have some form of union organization by 1980.

The NLRA amendments have now (in mid-1980) been in effect for six years. Data are available for at least some of those years that permit a redrawing of the picture of hospital unionism in the postamendment world. The focus here is on both the extent of unionism and its distribution across different types of hospitals. Were the predictions by labor leaders regarding the extent of unionism accurate? Can trends be forecast? Have the characteristics of hospitals favorable to unionism, such as federal ownership and large size, changed significantly since the Metzger-Pointer study? These are some of the questions addressed in this article.

The evidence on the spread of hospital unionization after 1974 is required and an estimate of an equation provided that can be used to forecast the extent of unionization and the effect of the amendments. To summarize the findings in advance: the authors expect unionization to spread rapidly during the 1980s, reaching perhaps 65 percent of all hospitals by the end of the decade. The 1974 amendments had a positive effect on the spread of unionization, but the estimates suggest that it is not as large as popularly believed: about 3 percent of all hospitals will be unionized as a direct consequence of the 1974 amendments. The rest of the spread of unionization results from factors that were present already in 1974.

The second objective is to describe the distribution of unionization across different types of hospitals in 1977 and depict them in tables that can be compared to the Metzger and Pointer study earlier.

Data for the analysis are taken from a survey conducted at the University of North Carolina in spring and summer of 1977.[7] A major advantage of this dataset over the surveys analyzed by Metzger and Pointer is it looks at four hospital occupations: registered nurses, licensed practical nurses and technical employees, office clerical staff, and service and maintenance workers. The characteristics of unionization in each occupation are analyzed separately. Another novel feature of this survey is a profile of the major unions currently organizing hospital employees—which unions are active and where, how many collective bargaining agreements are in effect, and how many employees are covered. This analysis, which is separate for the four occupations mentioned, should be of interest to labor relations experts.

The third section of the article is a statistical analysis of occupation-specific data on unionization and hospital wage determination. The answers to two questions are sought: by how much do unions raise wages, and how important are potential wage gains as a determinant of unionization? Many studies of the first question indicate that unions raise wages, although the union effect differs between industries and points in time.[8] The findings suggest that hospital unions raise wages from 3.40 percent for R.N.s to 7.85 percent for service and maintenance employees; the gains for L.P.N.s and office clerical workers are 5.61 and 7.43 percent, respectively.

It has been asserted[9] that health care facilities that do not pay competitive wages are most vulnerable to union organization. The findings here support this assertion: for all four occupations studied, the probability of a collective bargaining contract increases significantly as the potential wage gain from unionization grows.

The fourth section answers the questions raised here with a mixture of tabular description and statistical analysis. For readers not trained in research disciplines such as economics or industrial relations, the

statistical analysis may appear unnecessarily difficult; wherever possible, an attempt is made to explain results in pragmatic terms, emphasizing their practical significance.

THE SPREAD OF HOSPITAL UNIONIZATION AFTER 1974

Hospital unionization already was on the rise before the 1974 amendments—the percent of those with at least one collective bargaining agreement had increased from 7.7 in 1967 to 14.7 in 1970. However, the majority of these were either government-owned or investor-owned hospitals already covered by either the National Labor Relations Act, the Executive Order on Collective Bargaining for Federal Employees (1962), or state labor laws.[10]

The 1974 amendments appear to have increased health industry union activity, with much of it in nonprofit hospitals. The number of representation ("R") petitions from the health industry to the NLRB increased from 461 during fiscal year 1974 to 1,659 in fiscal year 1975.[11] The health industry includes hospitals, nursing homes, and other related health care facilities such as ambulatory clinics. From August 1974 through mid-May 1975, 140 contested hospital elections were held and not-for-profit institutions were involved in 90.4 percent of them, according to Joseph Rosmann of the AHA.[12] Elections had been completed in 82 cases, and employees had selected unions in 40.

To determine the impact of the 1974 amendments on the health care industry, the Federal Mediation and Conciliation Service (FMCS) in 1979 conducted a study[13] for the U.S. Department of Labor. This study covered the period from August 25, 1974, through December 31, 1976. During these two and a half years, FMCS reported that 2,585 collective bargaining contracts were negotiated in the health care industry, involving 414,000 workers in bargaining units, or one-quarter of the 1.7 million persons employed by those establishments.[14,15] It estimated that 70 percent of these contracts involved hospitals, 25 percent were in nursing homes, and 5 percent were in other health facilities.[16] The Service Employees International Union (SEIU) was the largest health industry union, with 839 contracts and 156,099 covered employees.[17]

Of the total number of contracts, 745 or close to 30 percent involved initial agreements.[18] An increased pace of collective bargaining activity is revealed by trends in the ratio of initial to total contracts: it rose from 24 percent in the first three months after the amendments took effect to 33 percent during the rest of the study period.[19]

Although the FMCS report is a valuable guide, it has two weaknesses: first, hospital data are not presented separately from other health care institutions; and, second, since the report covers only the period after the 1974 amendments, it does not have a control group for a "before-and-after" statistical test.

The data analyzed here are from a survey at the University of North Carolina in 1977 (henceforth referred to as the Hospital Survey) that addressed both of these problems. A sample of all U.S. hospitals was surveyed.[20] From responses to the question, "Did you have a union representation election or elections in the last 12 months?" the level of union organizing activity was projected.[21] Table 1-1 shows that 676 hospitals (about 10 percent) had a union election. Broken down by bed size, most elections occurred in hospitals with 100 to 200 beds but, proportionately, elections were most common in larger hospitals with 400 or more beds.

Ten years earlier Metzger and Pointer also had looked at the distribution of union representation requests by hospital size. They found[22] that large hospitals were much more likely to receive a representation request than small hospitals. Similar results were found by the AHA in 1970.[23] The authors' data, therefore, represent the continuation of a trend in which union activity concentrates in large hospitals.[24] But an attenuation of the trend was discovered. When the sample was split into approximately equal parts, it was found that those with more than 100 beds accounted for 52 percent of all hospitals and 70 percent of all institutions experiencing a union election. The same size group in 1967 accounted for 45.5 percent of all hospitals and 85.6 percent of all representation requests. Therefore, elections are less concentrated than

they used to be—an indication (explored in the next section) that unionization is seeping down from the largest hospitals to the smallest.

Breakdown of the Four Occupations

As noted, the survey broke the elections down by four occupations: registered nurses, licensed practical nurses and technical workers, office clerical staff, and service and maintenance employees. These four groups were chosen to reflect definitions of appropriate bargaining units currently favored by the NLRB.[25,26]

The number of elections by occupation ranges from 300 to almost 400, indicating that unionization efforts are active in all four groups. A total of 1,406 occupation-specific elections were held. If this is expressed in terms of elections per hospital, it can be seen that they "come in two's:" approximately 2.1 elections were held in each hospital in which a vote took place. In other words, occupations tend to organize together. This may be due to mutual problems, such as poor working conditions perceived by all occupations, or it may indicate that a single union is organizing several occupations.[27]

When "win rates" were computed for each occupation, registered nurses' unions won 45 percent of elections where the outcome was not contested (only 29 contested elections were found, but 25 of those involved R.N.s). L.P.N.s won 43 percent of their elections. Office clerical workers were least successful (38 percent), and service and maintenance employees most successful (51 percent). Overall, the union win rate was 44 percent. This is considerably lower than

Table 1-1 Distribution of Union Elections[1] by Hospital Size

Total Beds, 1975	Number and (%) of Hospitals		Number and (%) of Elections		No. and (%) of Elections by Occupation			
					R.N.	L.P.N.	Clerical	Service
0–25	287	(4)	27	(4)	18	24	20	16
25–50	1,482	(21)	50	(7)	15	36	42	25
50–100	1,614	(23)	127	(19)	93	62	45	45
100–200	1,522	(22)	161	(24)	47	75	68	124
200–300	820	(12)	64	(9)	30	37	44	42
300–400	407	(6)	54	(8)	19	27	5	24
400–500	316	(5)	82	(12)	11	61	34	41
500–	558	(8)	111	(16)	70	71	75	77
Totals	7,006[2]	(101)[3]	676	(99)[3]	303	393	333	394

[1]Based on answers to the question, "Did you have a union representation election or elections in the last 12 months?"

[2]The total number of hospitals in the universe is 7,129. The number in each table will be different, and less than 7,129, because of the exclusion of cases with missing values.

[3]Percentages may not add to 100 due to rounding.

the 62.5 percent win rate found by Rosmann[28] during the first year of the Taft-Hartley amendments. But Rosmann noted that "this win rate may decline, because historical studies have shown that unions have been more successful in organizing new fields."[29] The data in this article were collected during the third year of the amendments. Perhaps the decline forecast by Rosmann had set in by that time. In any case, the overall win rate found was below the average (50 percent) for all industries in the U.S.[30]

The union elections also were broken down by hospital ownership (see Table 1-2). The industry is dominated numerically by nonprofit institutions, which account for about half of all U.S. hospitals and also half of union elections. These ratios have not changed since 1967, when Metzger and Pointer[31] found that nonprofit hospitals accounted for 51.5 percent of all hospitals and 52.1 percent of all requests for union recognition. Thus, the 1974 amendments do not seem to have increased the pace of unionization in nonprofit hospitals in relation to other groups.

For-profit hospitals had less than their proportionate share of union elections, and federal hospitals had more. These results also are similar to Metzger and Pointer's finding.

On the Hospital Survey, every hospital with a signed collective bargaining agreement was asked to indicate how many years the agreement had been in effect. A cumulative count of unionized hospitals, shown in column 3 of Table 1-3, indicates that hospital labor organizing originated around 1940. This estimate accords fairly well with Metzger and Pointer's historical account,[32] which reported that the first successful hospital organizing drive occurred in 1936 when the American Federation of Labor organized engine room, laundry and dietary employees, and nurses' aides and orderlies in San Francisco. Hospital unions were fairly inactive during World War II and had contracts in less than 1 percent of all hospitals until about 1952. But since then, the percentage of unionized hospitals has grown rapidly, reaching 6.1 percent in 1967, 9.4 percent in 1970, and 18.4 percent in 1975.[33]

Analysis of the Trend

Tables 1-4 and 1-5 present the results of a statistical analysis of the trend in hospital unionization. A "logistic" equation is used. This is commonly employed[34,35] to explain data where the dependent variable is a proportion, e.g., the proportion of hospitals that are unionized. Obviously, this proportion must fall between zero and one; the logistic equation, which looks like an elongated "S" curve with the lower tail approaching 0 percent unionized and the upper tail approaching 100 percent unionized, fits this theoretical specification.[36]

The estimates of the coefficients of the logistic equation are reported in Table 1-4. Model 1 uses a dummy variable called 1974 Law that takes the value of zero for all years before the 1974 amendments and one for years afterward (1975 and 1976). Model 1 implies that the amendments caused a one-time jump in the pace of hospital unionization. Model 2, on the other hand, represents the amendments with Post-Law Trend, a variable that equals zero before 1975 and equals the value of the Time Trend in 1975 and 1976 (Time Trend is scaled so that 1975 equals 75). Model 2 implies that the amendments caused a permanent speed-up in the pace of hospital unionization.

The data are found to be consistent with both models. In both cases there is a positive time trend in unionization and, depending on which model is used, a statistically significant ($\alpha < .01$ in a one-tailed t-test) effect of the 1974 amendments. Model 2 gives a marginally better fit to the data.

The estimated coefficients from Table 1-4 are used to predict the percent of hospitals unionized in selected past and future years in Table 1-5.[37] Both models underestimate the proportion of unionized hospitals in 1970 but are quite accurate in 1976. The predictions for 1976 and future years are made both with and without the 1974 amendments. A comparison of the two values provides an idea of the contribution of the amendments to the spread of hospital unionism. By 1990, the authors predict that about 65 percent of

Table 1-2   Union Elections by Hospital Ownership

Ownership	No. and (%) of Hospitals		No. and (%) of Elections		No. and (%) of Elections by Occupation			
					R.N.	L.P.N.	Clerical	Service
Nonprofit	3,587	(51)	346	(51)	95	165	113	171
For-profit	690	(10)	45	(7)	14	29	13	29
State and local	2,361	(34)	207	(31)	158	144	149	139
Federal	367	(5)	77	(11)	36	36	59	56
Totals	7,005	(100)	675	(100)	303	374	334	395

Table 1-3 Hospitals and Unionized Hospitals, by Year

Year	All Hospitals[1]	Unionized Hospitals[2]	Column 3 ÷ Column 2
1976	7,082	1,424	.201
1975	7,156	1,319	.184
1974	7,174	1,112	.115
1973	7,123	912	.128
1972	7,061	817	.116
1971	7,097	734	.103
1970	7,123	668	.094
1969	7,144	572	.080
1968	7,137	501	.070
1967	7,172	434	.061
1966	7,160	328	.046
1965	7,123	272	.038
1964	7,127	229	.032
1963	7,138	222	.031
1962	7,028	207	.029
1961	6,923	152	.022
1960	6,876	141	.021
1959	6,845	114	.017
1958	6,786	106	.016
1957	6,818	105	.015
1956	6,966	79	.011
1955	6,956	78	.011
1954	6,970	73	.010
1953	6,978	73	.010
1952	6,903	73	.011
1951	6,832	41	.006
1950	6,788	36	.005
1949	6,277	36	.006
1948	6,160	30	.005
1947	6,173	25	.004
1946	6,125	20	.003
1945	6,511	20	.003
1944	6,611	20	.003
1943	6,655	19	.003
1942	6,345	19	.003
1941	6,358	5	.001
1940	6,291	5	.001
1939	6,226	0	.000

[1]*Sources: 1972–1976, American Hospital Association Guide to the Health Care Field* (Chicago: The American Hospital Association, 1977), p. 3; *1960–1971, Hospital Statistics* (Chicago: The American Hospital Association, 1971), p. 12; *1946–1959, Hospitals, JAHA,* 39 part 2 (August 1, 1965): 48; *1940–1945, Hospitals, JAHA* 29, part 2 (August 1955): 6. Data from 1940–1945 reflect all U.S. hospitals This statistical discrepancy is unimportant; since so few hospitals were organized during this period, the unionized/all hospitals ratio is not affected by the choice of a denominator. The number of registered hospitals in a given year is tabulated by the AHA on March 31 of the following year. Thus, there were 7,082 AHA-registered hospitals on March 31, 1977.

[2]Hospital Survey, weighted to the population of all AHA-registered hospitals.

all hospitals will have one or more union contracts. Without the amendments, about 62 percent would have been unionized. Therefore, the anticipated contribution of the amendments will be about 3 percentage points in 1990. Most of the increase in unionization would have occurred anyway. These predictions should be interpreted with caution since they are based solely on extrapolation of past trends. Some of the variables that may be causing the secular increase in unionization are discussed after a look at the cross-sectional causes of unionization in the final section of this article.

THE DISTRIBUTION OF HOSPITAL UNIONIZATION IN 1977

In 1967, Metzger and Pointer[38] examined the distribution of union contracts across different types of hospitals. They found the following associations:

Table 1-4 Logistic Equations for the Time Trend of Hospital Unionism

Independent Variable	Model 1 Coefficient (t-value)		Model 2 Coefficient (t-value)	
Constant	−12.321	(67.779)	−12.319	(67.761)
Time Trend	.143	(52.312)	.143	(52.293)
1974 Law	.112	(2.828)	---	---
Postlaw Trend	---	---	.00149	(2.836)
Mean Square Error	2.151		2.149	

- Hospital ownership and control patterns appear to influence significantly the probability of having a contract, with federal hospitals having far more negotiated agreements than would be expected based on numbers alone, and proprietary hospitals far fewer.[39]
- "The extent of collective bargaining organization and facility size (as measured by adult bed capacity) are perfectly and positively correlated."[40]
- Hospital unions are found most frequently in the Pacific and Middle Atlantic states, the least frequently in the South (South Atlantic and East and West South Central states).[41,42]

They also noted that the penetration of unions, as measured by the proportion of employees organized, was greater in government hospitals (federal, state, and local) than in nongovernment hospitals, and was greater in larger facilities.[43]

Ten years later, data from the Hospital Survey confirm that unionism still is related to hospital ownership, size, and location. Table 1-6 shows that federal hospitals account for 5 percent of all such institutions but 19 percent of those with unions. For-profit hospitals are 10 percent of the total and 5 percent of the unionized group. If anything, these associations have become more pronounced since 1967, when federal hospitals had about 2.9 times their proportionate share

of union contracts and for-profit hospitals had .63 of their share.[44]

A similar pattern of disproportionate representation is shown for each occupation in Table 1-6. In addition, it appears that clerical employees are especially likely to organize in government hospitals.

Table 1-7 shows that large hospitals are more likely to have a union than small hospitals.[45] This relation has been stable or increasing for 10 years. Hospitals with more than 300 beds accounted for 17 percent of all such institutions and 35.6 percent of all union contracts in 1967;[46] this same group represented 18 percent of all hospitals and 39 percent of unionized ones in 1977. By occupation, no distinctive departures from this pattern are noticeable.

By region of the country, union contracts are proportionately most common in Pacific states, which have 12 percent of all hospitals and 22 percent of unionized ones (Table 1-8). East North Central, Middle Atlantic and New England states also account for more than their proportionate share of unionism, while the South and Mountain states are underrepresented. Nurses (R.N.s and L.P.N.s) appear to be relatively more organized in Pacific states than other occupations but less organized in East North Central states.

Metzger and Pointer noted that union penetration was greater in government hospitals and large hospitals. While this may have been superficially true, it

Table 1-5 Actual and Predicted Percent of Hospitals Unionized

Year	Actual Percent of Hospitals Unionized	Predicted Percent of Hospitals Unionized with (and without) 1974 Amendments			
		Model 1		Model 2	
1970	9.4	---	(8.7)	---	(8.8)
1976	20.1	20.1	(18.4)	20.2	(18.4)
1980	---	30.8	(28.5)	31.0	(28.5)
1985	---	47.6	(44.8)	48.0	(44.9)
1990	---	65.0	(62.3)	65.5	(62.4)

Table 1-6 Unions by Hospital Ownership

Ownership	Number and (Percent) of Hospitals		Number and (%) of Hospitals with Union		No. and (%) of Unionized Hospitals by Occupation							
					R.N.		L.P.N.		Clerical		Service	
Nonprofit	3,605	(51)	679	(42)	374	(36)	414	(33)	231	(23)	573	(39)
For-profit	692	(10)	80	(5)	44	(4)	62	(5)	35	(3)	62	(4)
State and local	2,399	(34)	568	(35)	451	(43)	498	(39)	444	(44)	531	(37)
Federal	371	(5)	309	(19)	178	(17)	291	(23)	300	(30)	286	(20)
Totals	7,067	(100)	1,636	(101)	1,047	(100)	1,265	(100)	1,010	(100)	1,452	(100)

should not be inferred that it is true for workers in individual bargaining units. When a particular group of employees, e.g., R.N.s, is covered by a union contract in a hospital, the authors' data show that 100 percent of the R.N.s in that hospital are organized.[47] The only exceptions occur in so-called ''right-to-work'' states, where employees in the bargaining unit do not have to belong to the union.[48] The percentage of employees organized in union hospitals is less than 100 percent in right-to-work states. Table 1-9 shows that union organization in such states is roughly 80 to 90 percent. Organization also appears to be greater in Northern than in Southern right-to-work states (although this observation is based on a small sample of hospitals in Iowa, Kansas, Nebraska, and South Dakota).

Greater union penetration in government hospitals and large hospitals is not due to different levels of organization within a bargaining unit but to the number of occupations covered in these institutions. Table 1-10 shows that the number of occupations covered by contracts is an increasing function of both bed size and government ownership.

The Hospital Survey requested the name of the union representing each covered group of employees. The answers are shown in Tables 1-11 through 1-14. The survey finds 1,073 contracts covering 132,105 reg-istered nurses, with more contracts (309) in the Pacific region than in any other. It can be seen in Table 1-11 that, with the exception of unions representing government employees, registered nurses most often are organized by state nurses' associations. As might be expected, the associations with most contracts are found in California and populous Northern states such as New York, Pennsylvania, Massachusetts, and Michigan.

Licensed practical nurses and technical employees are covered by 1,245 contracts, most frequently (317 times) in Pacific states. The American Federation of State, County, and Municipal Employees (AFSCME) has more contracts than any other union representing L.P.N.s, but the data indicate that the California Medical Laboratory Technicians represent more L.P.N.s and technical employees than any other union.[49]

Several unions appear on the list for all non-R.N. occupations. These include AFSCME, the American Federation of Government Employees, and the Service Employees International Union, among others.[50] Several industrial unions, such as the Steelworkers, Teamsters, Operating Engineers, and Communication Workers also are organizing hospital employees but, with the exception of service and maintenance employees, do not have a significant foothold.

Table 1-7 Unions by Hospital Size

Total Beds 1975	Number and (Percent) of Hospitals		Number and (%) of Hospitals with Union		No. and (%) of Unionized Hospitals by Occupation							
					R.N.		L.P.N.		Clerical		Service	
0–25	287	(4)	23	(1)	18	(2)	23	(2)	23	(2)	16	(1)
25–50	1,510	(21)	191	(12)	114	(11)	103	(8)	95	(9)	148	(10)
50–100	1,616	(23)	199	(12)	122	(12)	147	(12)	104	(10)	128	(9)
100–200	1,544	(22)	361	(22)	228	(22)	301	(24)	196	(19)	321	(22)
200–300	831	(12)	220	(13)	120	(11)	162	(13)	146	(14)	202	(14)
300–400	406	(6)	140	(9)	83	(8)	83	(7)	61	(6)	130	(9)
400–500	316	(4)	113	(7)	58	(6)	82	(6)	48	(5)	112	(8)
500–	558	(8)	389	(23)	304	(29)	364	(29)	338	(33)	396	(27)
Totals	7,068	(100)	1,636	(99)	1,047	(101)	1,265	(101)	1,011	(98)	1,453	(100)

Table 1-8   Hospital Unions by Region of Country

| Region | No. and (Percent) of Hospitals | | No. and (%) of Hospitals with Union | | No. and (Percent) of Unionized Hospitals by Occupation | | | | | | | |
					R.N.		L.P.N.		Clerical		Service	
New England	364	(5)	103	(6)	74	(7)	85	(7)	80	(8)	97	(7)
Middle Atlantic	962	(14)	418	(26)	253	(24)	301	(24)	251	(25)	378	(26)
South Atlantic	637	(9)	96	(6)	50	(5)	75	(6)	70	(7)	94	(6)
East North Central	1,657	(23)	407	(25)	220	(21)	280	(22)	242	(24)	379	(26)
East South Central	497	(7)	46	(3)	32	(3)	44	(3)	45	(4)	46	(3)
West North Central	468	(7)	120	(7)	62	(6)	88	(7)	49	(5)	108	(7)
West South Central	1,081	(15)	47	(3)	34	(3)	44	(3)	46	(5)	44	(3)
Mountain	524	(7)	40	(2)	14	(1)	29	(2)	38	(4)	43	(3)
Pacific	878	(12)	361	(22)	307	(29)	322	(25)	193	(19)	268	(18)
Totals	7,068	(99)	1,638	(100)	1,046	(99)	1,268	(99)	1,014	(101)	1,457	(99)

In estimating the national coverage by all unions of hospital employees in four occupations, it was found that about 29 percent of all R.N.s in hospitals were represented by collective bargaining agreements in 1977. The rate in each of the three other occupations was 33 percent.[51] Altogether these four groups account for 2,250,000 workers, 700,000 of whom are represented by labor unions.

STATISTICAL ANALYSIS OF UNIONIZATION AND WAGE DETERMINATION

In the previous section, it was found that hospital unions were concentrated in federal hospitals, large hospitals, and certain regions of the country. Those findings were based on comparisons of unionization rates with one independent variable (hospital ownership, size, or region) at a time. Such two-way comparisons can be misleading if other variables excluded from the evaluation are correlated with the included variable. For example, federal hospitals tend to be large (Table 1-11), so the association of federal ownership and unionization may mask a more fundamental size-unionization relation.

In addition, the descriptive comparisons overlooked the association of wages and unionization, despite the assertion by Pointer and Metzger[52] that "Unions will select the health care facilities that are the most vulnerable: those who do not pay competitive wages. . . ." Low earnings clearly are a key issue to potential union members.[53] Comparisons of nonunion and union hospitals that do not consider wages would be incomplete.

These remarks suggest that unionization should be examined with a multivariate model that includes wages. However, the effect of pay is confounded by a relation that runs the other way—from unionization to wages. In other words, the unionization-wages question is a simultaneous one.

Table 1-9   Right-to-Work vs. Percent of Employees Organized in Union Hospitals

| Occupation | % Organized in Union Hospitals in Right-to-Work States | NORTH | | SOUTH | |
		No. of Hospitals in RTW States	% Organized in Union Hospitals	No. of Hospitals in RTW States	% Organized in Union Hospitals
R.N.	.79	10	.88	87	.78
L.P.N.	.80	16	100	101	.77
Clerical	.84	16	.88	102	.84
Service	.88	15	.97	119	.87

Table 1-10 Number of Contracts Per Unionized Hospital, by Hospital Size and Ownership

Hospital Ownership	Hospital Size*		Weighted Row Averages**
	Small	Large	
Nonprofit	2.34	2.44	2.39
For-profit	2.44	2.68	2.56
State and local	3.045	3.71	3.38
Federal	3.36	3.57	3.47
Weighted Column Averages	2.80	3.10	2.95 Overall Average

*Hospital size is defined in relation to the median size in each ownership category. "Small" nonprofit hospitals have fewer than 200 beds. The corresponding cutoff points are 100 beds in for-profit hospitals, 300 in state and local hospitals, and 400 in federal hospitals.

**Weights for column averages are the proportions of hospitals in each ownership class; row weights are the proportions in each size class.

This section reviews the evidence on the causes of unionization and the union effect on wages. A simultaneous model of hospital unionization and wage determination is postulated and its coefficients estimated by statistical techniques. Variables in the model are chosen with reference to economic theory. Thus, the authors view these results as tests of the theory, and interpret statistically significant positive coefficients as evidence that particular variables cause unionization, in the sense that higher values of these variables increase the probability that a hospital will be unionized.

Causes of Unionization

The reasons why hospital unions form are discussed often. Unfortunately, little quantitative evidence is available. Union leaders stress the economic and humanitarian benefits.[54] Hospital workers respond to a number of concerns:

- low wages and slow advancement
- inadequate benefits
- lack of job status or a feeling of dignity
- lack of recognition by or communication with management

Table 1-11 Major Unions Organizing R.N.s

Union	No. of Contracts	No. of Covered Employees	Location of Most Contracts (State or Region)
California Nurse Association	86	37,623	California (86)
Washington Nurses	77	3,752	Washington (77)
New York Nurses	75	18,477	New York (75)
American Federation of Government Employees	68	3,895	South Atlantic (19)
Pennsylvania Nurses Association	67	8,197	Pennsylvania (67)
Massachusetts Nurses Association	59	6,630	Massachusetts (59)
Michigan Nurses Association	53	3,633	Michigan (53)
Civil Service Employees Association	52	6,267	Middle Atlantic (52)
National Federation of Federal Employees	36	2,046	West South Central (14)
American Federation of State, County, Municipal Employees (AFSCME)	35	938	East North Central (26)
Oregon Nurses Association	28	2,746	Oregon (28)
Illinois Nurses Association	26	1,907	Illinois (26)
Ohio Civil Service Employees Association	26	407	Ohio (26)
Other State Nurses Assns.	45	6,503	Hawaii (19)
Other/Not Identified[1]	340	29,084	Pacific (83)
Totals	1,073	132,105	Pacific (309)

[1]Includes Hospital and Institution Workers, Communications Workers of America, Hospital Employee Labor Programs, Service Employees International Union, Steelworkers, Teamsters, United Nurses-California, New Jersey Civil Service, Oregon State Employee Association, and District 1199 of the Retail-Wholesale-Department Store Union.

Table 1-12   Major Unions Organizing L.P.N.s and Technical Employees

Union	No. of Contracts	No. of Covered Employees	Location of Most Contracts (State or Region)
AFSCME	187	21,305	East North Central (108)
American Federation of Government Employees	184	23,704	South Atlantic (34)
Service Employees International Union	71	11,788	East North Central (40)
Licensed Practical Nurses—Minnesota	53	1,740	Minnesota (53)
Civil Service Employees Association	52	18,157	Middle Atlantic (52)
Licensed Practical Nurses—Washington	47	3,499	Washington (47)
National Federation of Federal Employees	45	3,865	West South Central (14)
Hospital and Institution Workers	30	2,707	Pacific (29)
Licensed Practical Nurses—New York	27	3,205	New York (27)
California Medical Laboratory Technicians	24	38,189	California (24)
Steelworkers	22	1,998	East North Central (10)
Hospital Employee Labor Programs	21	268	Pacific (19)
Other State L.P.N. Associations	45	2,348	Pennsylvania (19)
Other/Not Identified[1]	437	59,478	Middle Atlantic (107)
Totals	1,245	192,251	Pacific (317)

[1]Includes Pottery and Allied Workers, Communication Workers of America, Firemen and Oilers, Office and Professional Employees International Union, Public Service Employees Union, Teamsters, Radiation Technologists-Santa Clara, unnamed professional associations, Oregon Nurse Association, Oregon Society of Radiological Technologists, Ohio Civil Service Employees Association, Oregon State Employee Association, and District 1199 of the Retail-Wholesale-Department Store Union.

- poor job security
- desire for increased voice in decision making
- poor work schedule
- lack of a grievance procedure
- inadequate staffing
- supervisory favoritism or arbitrary behavior
- work outside of job description[55]

Federal mediators note that wages are the top issue in health care bargaining but account for only 18 percent of the demands.[56] Other issues are duration of the contract, union security problems, and working conditions. In a pilot study[57] undertaken by three researchers, names of nonprofit hospitals were obtained from the NLRB election reports and 78 hospital and union representatives were mailed questionnaires containing ten issues to which the respondents were asked to assign priorities. Wages were rated as a high priority item, with less emphasis on fringe benefits.

Supply and Demand Roles

Economists[58,59] view union membership as an asset that is expected to yield returns to those who join, in return for which they are obliged to pay certain costs. This view places the unionization decision into the economists' familiar model of supply and demand; in this case, the union supplies services and workers demand them.

The model is quite general in that it can be applied to traditional labor unions and also nontraditional organizations such as professional nurses' associations or the American Medical Association. Most of the work on the supply of union services has been done on these nontraditional organizations.

In a seminal study, Stigler[60] proposed that "every industry that has enough political power to utilize the state will seek to control entry." Occupational licensure is one way to control entry. Stigler gathered state-level data on the year of licensure for 11 occupations. Explanatory variables were the urban concentration of each occupation and the ratio of each job's aggregate size to that of the state's labor force. These variables were designed to measure the costs to an occupation of using the state's political power to obtain licensing. According to the empirical results, urbanization is the stronger influence on regulatory success—the higher the degree of occupational urbanization, the earlier in time the group achieved licensure. Larger occupations also achieved licensure earlier.

Begun and Feldman[61] in 1979 applied Stigler's theory to the optometric profession. They measured the content of regulatory policy by a sum of dummy variables representing the presence or absence of certain regulatory goals, e.g., bans on price advertising by optometrists. Independent variables included characteristics of both the interest groups concerned with the

Table 1-13 Major Unions Organizing Clerical Workers

Union	No. of Contracts	No. of Covered Employees	Location of Most Contracts (State or Region)
American Federation of Government Employees	190	16,417	South Atlantic (34)
AFSCME	167	12,652	East North Central (71)
Civil Service Employees Association	57	3,698	Middle Atlantic (57)
Service Employees International Union	48	7,976	East North Central (65) and Pacific (15)
National Federation of Federal Employees	47	3,249	West South Central (14)
Office and Professional Employees International	37	1,627	Pacific (30)
Hospital Employee Labor Programs	27	538	Pacific (19)
Steelworkers	27	1,704	East North Central (10)
Hospital and Institution Workers	26	56,886	Pacific (26)
Ohio Civil Service	26	224	Ohio (26)
Other/Not Identified[1]	347	31,833	Middle Atlantic (78)
Totals	999	136,804	Middle Atlantic (249)

[1]Includes Carpenters and Joiners, Communication Workers of America, Firemen and Oilers, Retail Clerks International Union, Public Service Employees Union, Teamsters, Oregon State Employees Association, and District 1199 of the Retail-Wholesale-Department Store Union.

regulations and of the state political system. Begun and Feldman contended that these variables more accurately measured the costs to optometrists of using the state political system than did Stigler's proxy variables. Their findings supported the argument that more regulations are acquired when the costs to the profession are low, for example, when competing interest groups are few and poorly organized.

In the hospital industry, it already has been noted that large hospitals, federal institutions, and those in certain regions (mainly outside the South) are unionized more often. These findings may be explained by low costs of supplying unionization associated with each predisposing characteristic. Hospital size could be associated positively with unionization if there are certain fixed costs to the union of conducting an organizing campaign.[62] Fixed costs are spread over more workers in large hospitals.

The costs to a union of organizing in federal hospitals are low because of historically favorable treatment given to federal employees' associations.[63,64] Executive Order 10988, issued by President Kennedy on January 17, 1962, gave all federal employees the right to join or not to join organizations of their own choosing that would represent them regarding the terms of their employment. A supplementary order, in May 1963, spelled out unfair labor practices similar to those contained in Sections 8(a) and 8(b) of the Taft-Hartley Act.[65] The same collective bargaining rights were not extended to private nonprofit hospitals until the 1974 Taft-Hartley amendments.

The reasons why Southern hospitals and, for that matter, Southern workers generally, are poorly organized are complex. Right-to-work laws may raise the costs of organizing a union. Right-to-work laws create the "free rider" problem in which nonunion employees receive the benefits of a contract without contributing to the support of the union. Since the South is a right-to-work section,[66] this may explain why so few workers there are unionized.

However, unionization in the South also may lag because its workers do not want to be unionized. Since workers' feelings toward unions belong on the demand side of the model, attention now turns toward demand variables.

Quality of Employment Factors

In 1977, the Survey Research Center at the University of Michigan conducted the Quality of Employment Survey. Attitudes and experiences of a representative sample of the labor force were surveyed on a variety of questions related to their working lives. The researchers found that, when other variables were controlled, nonunion workers were less likely to support unionization if they held a "negative" image of unions.[67] Negative image was defined by workers' agreement with a series of statements that unions exert undue influence over the private lives of union members as well as public elections, legislation, and the process of government. Southerners were more likely to agree with these negative images than were non-Southern workers. So it appears that workers' at-

Table 1-14 Major Unions Organizing Service and Maintenance Workers

Union	No. of Contracts	No. of Covered Employees	Location of Most Contracts (State or Region)
AFSCME	220	41,418	East North Central (128)
American Federation of Government Employees	173	19,595	South Atlantic (38)
Operating Engineers	144	15,949	Pacific (55)
Service Employees International Union	97	13,968	Pacific (38)
Teamsters	50	7,867	East North Central (23)
Civil Service Employees Association	40	15,514	Middle Atlantic (40)
National Federation of Federal Employees	39	2,817	West South Central (14)
Hospital Employee Labor Programs	34	5,133	Pacific (19)
Communication Workers of America	30	7,136	Middle Atlantic (19)
Hospital and Institution Workers	28	28,535	Pacific (26)
Steelworkers	26	2,465	East North Central (10)
Other/Not Identified[1]	560	77,350	East North Central (127)
Totals	1,441	237,747	Middle Atlantic (381)

[1]Includes Pottery and Allied Workers, Carpenters and Joiners, Firemen and Oilers, Hotel and Restaurant Employees and Bartenders International Union, Laborers International Union, Machinists and Aerospace, Office and Professional Employees International Union, Retail Clerks International Union, Plant Guard Workers, Public Service Employees Union, Ohio Civil Service Employees Association, Oregon State Employee Association, and District 1199.

titudes in the South have a negative effect on their support for unions.

The size-and-unionization association mentioned earlier also may have some demand-side characteristics in the model of supply and demand for unionization. Conventional wisdom holds that workers in small establishments have more satisfactory interpersonal relations with their supervisors than do those in large establishments.[68] Actually, the Quality of Life Survey found that employees in both the smallest (fewer than 10 workers) and largest (1,000 or more) establishments were least willing to join unions. This may indicate that medium-size establishments are big enough to be impersonal, yet too small to use sophisticated or enlightened personnel management techniques.

Low Wages As a Unionizing Factor

Low earnings clearly are a key issue to potential union members. There really are two issues here: (1) to what extent do unions raise wages; and (2) what is the quantitative significance of potential wage gains on the decision to unionize?

To date, the most comprehensive study of union wage effects has been the 1963 analysis by Prof. H. Gregg Lewis.[69] He concludes that unions universally raise members' wages. This result is strong in some industries (15 to 25 percent in skilled building trades and mining) and weak in others (0 to 5 percent in footwear, cotton textiles, and common building labor).

Several studies have investigated the impact of unions on the wages of hospital employees. Sloan and Elnicki (1978) estimate a wage equation for R.N.s only.[70] They include a dummy variable that equals 1 if a given hospital has a collective bargaining unit covering R.N.s. They conclude that these bargaining units have a small effect on the starting monthly salary of an R.N. The only coefficient significant at the 5 percent level (out of 5 estimated equations) implied that unions raised the starting salary by 3.9 percent.[71]

C. R. Link and J. H. Landon (1975)[72] reached slightly different conclusions. Their analysis also examined the union impact on R.N. starting salaries. They differentiated their analysis by including measures of the proportion of nurses in a hospital who were unionized. When at least 75 percent of R.N.s in a hospital were unionized, annual starting salaries of B.S. degree and diploma nurses rose by $500 to $800. This is about 5 to 10 percent of starting salaries.

M. D. Fottler (1977) was concerned with how unionization altered wage rates for nonprofessional hospital employees.[73] He regressed a weighted average of weekly wages for six nonprofessional occupations on the percent of nonprofessional hospital employees in each city covered by a collective bargaining agreement. One interesting aspect of Fottler's study was his disaggregation of data into private and public hospitals. This allowed him to determine which category was affected most by unions. He concluded that unions raised weekly wages by 4.5 to 8.2 percent, with private hospitals feeling the greater impact. Since wages of nonprofessional employees are approximately 25 percent of total hospital costs, the union impact on total costs was 1 to 2 percent.

R. W. Hurd took a different approach.[74] He found that nurses' wages were depressed in cities where the eight largest hospitals accounted for a larger percentage of employment. Concentration of employment in a few hospitals implies market power that enables hospitals to hold wages down, according to Hurd.

Davis estimated the effect of the threat of unionization on the average wage rate in given hospitals.[75] In a 1973 report, she used two different measures of the union threat effect. The threat effect[76] occurs when nonunion employers raise wages to forestall the organization of their work force. It usually is assumed that the threat effect is greater as organization in the market area increases. The percent of nonagricultural workers who belong to a union in the area around the hospital usually was found to have a negative and statistically insignificant effect on wages. A dummy variable was used that took the value 1 if a particular state had a law requiring nongovernmental nonprofit hospitals to recognize a collective bargaining unit when the majority of employees of the unit requested it. The coefficient of this variable was always positive and sometimes significant at the $\alpha = 5$ percent level. Davis admits that the effect of unions on wage rates cannot be determined conclusively in this study because she did not measure the extent of unionization within the hospital.

Brian E. Becker (1977) studied the impact of unions on wages and fringe benefits in a three-state area—Illinois, Wisconsin, and Minnesota. He found that unions raised occupational rates for nonprofessional hospital employees by approximately 5 percent.[77]

Roger Feldman and Richard Scheffler (1979) analyzed data from the Hospital Survey used for this article.[78] They found that unionization appeared to be more important for less hospital-specific labor such as secretaries and housekeepers than for nurses. The overall effect of unions on R.N. and L.P.N. wages averaged about 8 percent, as compared to roughly 11 to 12 percent for secretaries and housekeepers in hospitals.

Some of these studies are flawed by data problems. For example, the principal data source used by Sloan and Elnicki was a mailed questionnaire of 982 hospitals conducted in 1973. Slightly more than 500 usable responses were received. Only 12 percent of the respondents had collective bargaining agreements covering professional nurses. By the time of this article's survey, 23 percent of all U.S. hospitals had at least one collective bargaining agreement (see Table 1-6).

The Becker study was conducted more recently, but it is doubtful that his three-state results can be generalized to the whole country. Both Wisconsin and Minnesota have a large number of union contracts, and Minnesota required the resolution of disputes by compulsory arbitration.[79] In addition, only 144 of the 563 hospitals he surveyed (26 percent) responded to the questionnaire. Predictions concerning union-nonunion wage differences were based on only 36 unionized hospitals.

From Earnings to Unionization

All of these studies also are flawed by the potential confounding of the effect of unionization on earnings by the relation that runs the other way, from earnings to unionization. This relation has not escaped the attention of other labor economists, however. Schmidt and Strauss[80] postulated a model where earnings and union membership are related. Heckman[81] made the probability of being in a union depend not on actual earnings but rather on the level of earnings in the absence of a union. The underlying choice is assumed to depend on the potential gains from union membership. Schmidt reexamined the question with a model that explicitly includes the union-nonunion wage differential.[82] His data were based on 912 individuals from the 1967 Survey of Economic Opportunity. He found that unions raise wages but, surprisingly, large potential wage gains do not significantly increase the probability of individual union membership.

Lung-Fei Lee[83] in 1978 published the most rigorous theoretical and empirical study of the simultaneous relation between unionism and wage rates. The sample used in the estimation consisted of observations on 3,720 operative (blue-collar) workers, 1,925 of whom belonged to a union and 1,795 did not. His empirical results show that the most powerful factor determining unionism is the union/nonunion wage differential. Lee criticizes the Schmidt-Strauss contrary result as having no basis in rational choice behavior. Lee also finds that the union/nonunion wage differential for the whole sample is 17 percent. Unionism has the strongest effects on wage increments in mining and construction industries and, in all cases, the differential markedly increases with the extent of union organization in an industry.

In summary of the two issues pertaining to unions and wage gains: unions in the hospital industry appear to raise wages by small but usually significant amounts, although this conclusion is based on studies that have problems of data and/or methodology; and the union/nonunion wage differential is the most powerful factor determining unionism, according to Lee's study. This result was based on a survey of blue-collar workers, so it may not be applicable to the hospital industry.

Estimation of a Model

This section estimates a version of Lee's model for the hospital industry. Lee predicts that workers will join a union if the percentage wage differential from joining exceeds their "reservation wage." The reservation wage, which summarizes their receptivity to the union, depends on the characteristics of the person and the costs of becoming a union member.

Lee's model describes the individual worker's choice behavior, whereas the data on which this article is based pertain to bargaining units. Can it be assumed that individual choices can be aggregated, i.e., added up in some way, so the relations that hold for the individual still hold for the bargaining unit? Conceptually, the cost-of-unionization variables do not present an aggregation problem. This is because the union is selling its services to workers and, as a first approximation, the price charged to each worker may be equal. Aggregation of the benefits of unionism is more troublesome. Benefits may be perceived differently by different workers and, in some cases, one group may get higher wages from unionization while another group does not gain. This could happen if workers with very dissimilar interests were thrown together into the same bargaining unit. In this case, the average wage gain across the whole bargaining group is not a good predictor of whether its members will vote to unionize. That decision depends on the numbers of workers in the winning and losing camps, the strength of their interests at stake, and their ability to organize and articulate these interests.[84]

While the authors do not have a definitive answer to the aggregation problem, they believe the design of their study, which focuses on four separate occupations, is superior to the analysis of the whole hospital labor force. The NLRB chose these occupations as bargaining units because employees in them have common interests distinct from other occupations. With the possible exception of linking L.P.N.s and technical employees, the NLRB unit decisions appear not to have had a major impact on the collective bargaining process in hospitals.[85]

Variables in the Model

Variables in the model of wages and unionism are described in Table 1-15. Estimation of the model proceeds in two steps. First, regression analysis is used to obtain predicted wage rates for nonunion and union occupations. Variables in the wages equations were chosen largely from the Feldman and Scheffler[86] analysis of occupation-specific wage setting in individual hospitals. Estimates of the coefficients of the wages equations for nonunion and union workers are presented in Tables 1-16 and 1-17.

Second, the predicted percentage wage gain from unionization is used, along with other variables related to the workers' reservation wage, in a probit analysis (Table 1-18) of union status. Probit analysis is a technique specially suited to "either/or" choices such as to join or not to join a union.[87]

The first variable examined is fringe benefits. These are included in the wages equations to standardize pay for other forms of compensation.[88] The hypothesis being investigated is that wages are lower in hospitals with more generous fringe benefits. This would occur if hospitals and employees bargain (formally or informally) for total compensation and make trade-offs within the overall package between wages and fringe benefits. An alternative possibility is that wages and fringe benefits are related directly because of the personal income tax exemption that increases the attractiveness of fringe benefits to high-income employees. The data support this explanation since, for all occupations in both union and nonunion samples, wages are related positively to fringe benefits.

The union sample includes two variables, *union time* (the number of years before 1977 that this occupation has been unionized) and *job action* (a strike or slowdown in this occupation in 1977) that do not appear in the nonunion wage equations. The exclusion of union time is obvious. Job action was left out because, in the sample, job actions occurred almost entirely in union hospitals.[89] The number of years organized was found to have a positive effect on wages in union occupations. This gain is largest for service and maintenance employees (about one-half of one percent per year) and smallest for R.N.s. Job action also has a positive coefficient, except in the case of R.N.s, indicating that strikes usually are associated with higher wages in the union sample.

Hosbarg is the percent of hospitals in the state with collective bargaining agreements in 1975. A positive coefficient on this variable in the nonunion sample might indicate that nonunion hospitals raise wages to forestall the threat of union organization. In the union sample, it might be argued that unions have more bargaining power if more hospitals in the area are organized. But neither effect is indicated by the data: the coefficient of Hosbarg is negative in all equations and it sometimes is statistically significant.

Table 1-15 Variables in the Models of Wages and Unionism

Variable	Definition
ℓn R.N. wage	Natural log of average annual salary for full-time registered staff nurse with 3-year diploma, 1976–77.
ℓn L.P.N. wage	Natural log of average annual salary for full-time licensed practical nurse with two years' experience at this hospital, 1976–77.
ℓn Secretary wage	Natural log of average hourly wage for full-time general secretary, 1977.
ℓn Housekeeper wage	Natural log of hourly wage for full-time housekeeping employees, 1977.
R.N. union[1]	The hospital has a signed collective bargaining agreement or memorandum of understanding with a union or employee association representing R.N.s, 1977.
L.P.N. union[1]	L.P.N.s represented by collective bargaining, 1977.
Secretary union[1]	Secretaries represented by collective bargaining, 1977.
Housekeeper union[1]	Housekeepers represented by collective bargaining, 1977.
Union time	Number of years prior to 1977 this occupation has been unionized (nonunion occupation = 0).
Fringe benefits	Average annual cost per employee of all fringe benefits ($1,000s), 1977.
Job action[1]	A strike or slowdown in this occupation, 1977.
Hosbarg	Percent of hospitals in state with a collective bargaining agreement, 1975.
Sandl[1,2]	State or local government hospital ownership.
NFP[1,2]	Not-for-profit hospital.
Profit[1,2]	Proprietary hospital.
Concentration	County four-hospital bed concentration ratio in 1975.
Beds	Total number of beds in this hospital, 1975.
Hospitals	Total number of hospitals in the county, 1973.
Income	County per capita income ($1,000s), 1972.
Urban	County urbanization index in 1972.
Section[1]	Hospital is located in Northeast, Middle Atlantic, West North Central, or Pacific state.
Right-to-work[1]	State right-to-work law, 1977.
M.D. office wage	County average annual wage of employees in offices of physicians and surgeons ($1,000s), 1973.
Retail wage	County average annual wage of employees in wholesale and retail trade ($1,000s), 1973.
Service wage	County average annual wage of employees in service industries ($1,000s), 1973.
AFDC	Average monthly state aid for dependent children per recipient family ($100s), 1977.
Selectivity	Selectivity variable for this occupation.

[1]Indicates dummy variable equal one for positive responses.
[2]Omitted ownership category is federal hospitals.
Sources: ℓn R.N. wage through Job action, from the Hospital Survey conducted by Feldman and Scheffler;[78] Hosbarg through Hospitals, *1975 Annual Survey of Hospitals* (Chicago: American Hospital Association, 1975); Income and Urban, *Medicare/Medicaid Reimbursement Study* (Washington, D.C.: The Institute of Medicine, 1975); Right-to-work, data supplied by the National Right to Work Committee, Fairfax, Va.; M.D. office wage through service wage, *County Business Patterns* (Washington, D.C.: U.S. Bureau of the Census, 1974); AFDC, *Public Assistance Statistics, February 1977* (Washington, D.C.: National Center for Social Statistics, USDHEW Publ. No. (SRS) 77-03100, June, 1977). All money variables have been divided by a 1977 state cost-of-living index from W. McMahon and Carroll Melton, "Measuring Cost of Living Variation," *Industrial Relations,* 17, no. 3 (October, 1978): 324–332.

Three variables—*Sandl* (state of local government hospital ownership), *NFP* (not-for-profit), and *profit* (propriety)—present the effect of hospital ownership (relative to federal hospitals) on wages. They show a consistent pattern that nonunion federal hospitals pay higher wages than other nonunion hospitals, but the wage gap either diminishes or reverses in union hospitals. In other words, labor unions close the wage gap between federal and nonfederal hospitals. Within the samples, it appears that nonunion/nonfederal L.P.N.s are at a smaller wage disadvantage than other nonunion/nonfederal employees, and in the union sample, nonfederal L.P.N.s get the largest wage premiums.

Table 1-16   Estimates of the Nonunion Wages Equations[1]

VARIABLE	ℓn R.N. WAGE EQUATION Coefficient (t-value)	ℓn L.P.N. WAGE EQUATION Coefficient (t-value)	ℓn SECRETARY WAGE EQUATION Coefficient (t-value)	ℓn HOUSEKEEPER WAGE EQUATION Coefficient (t-value)
Fringe benefits	.0218 (1.860)	.0303 (2.377)	.0640 (4.466)	.00146 (.0823)
Hosbarg	−.383 (4.206)	−.168 (1.911)	−.0307 (.349)	−.01812 (.631)
Sandl	−.147 (4.790)	−.0435 (1.083)	−.263 (5.396)	−.401 (4.109)
NFP	−.129 (4.981)	−.0410 (1.086)	−.244 (5.258)	−.424 (4.485)
Profit	−.0941 (2.797)	−.00102 (.025)	−.229 (4.456)	−.512 (5.309)
Concentration	−.240 (5.806)	−.163 (4.331)	−.142 (2.450)	−.243 (4.149)
Beds	.0000292 (.553)	.0000472 (.864)	.000128 (1.759)	.0000785 (.769)
Income	−.0554 (2.642)	.0372 (1.740)	.143 (6.827)	−.0157 (.529)
Section	−.00607 (.175)	−.0461 (1.218)	−.0305 (.870)	.0580 (1.074)
M.D. office wage	.245 (6.803)	.0277 (.779)	--- ---	--- ---
Retail wage	--- ---	--- ---	−.269 (1.600)	--- ---
Service wage	--- ---	--- ---	--- ---	.825 (7.174)
AFDC	−.000403 (1.448)	−.000486 (1.801)	−.00115 (4.052)	−.000393 (.914)
Right-to-work	.0164 (.401)	−.0789 (1.731)	−.0507 (1.177)	−.146 (2.303)
Constant	9.563 (34.916)	8.982 (33.588)	1.401 (5.069)	1.476 (2.993)
Number of observations	224	169	232	108
$\overline{R}^2$	31.6	24.2	42.2	51.4

[1]For technical reasons, the wages equations include squared terms for each continuous independent variable. Coefficients and t-statistics in Tables 1-16 and 1-17 are evaluated at the mean values of the independent variables.

Hospital *concentration* (county four-hospital bed concentration in 1975) basically is a measure of fewness of buyers of labor. A common finding of studies reviewed is that fewness of buyers depresses the wages of sellers of labor.[90] This is one case of the general economic theory that fewness of competitors enhances the market power of a firm. The results show that concentration has a negative and statistically significant effect on wages in all nonunion occupations. In the union sample, concentration has two sign reversals from negative to positive. This lends support to Galbraith's well-known claim that

market power of unions is a countervailing force to the market power of hospitals.[91]

Hospital bed size (*beds*) is a control variable used as a proxy for the skills of the labor force. It is well known that large hospitals have more complex facilities and services, such as cobalt therapy, open-heart surgery, and renal dialysis,[92] than small hospitals. Skilled employees who operate these complex facilities can be expected to receive premium wages. Results for both samples indicate that workers in large hospitals receive premium wages, although the premium usually is not statistically significant.

Table 1-17   Estimates of the Union Wage Equations

VARIABLE	ℓn R.N. WAGE EQUATION Coefficient (t-value)	ℓn L.P.N. WAGE EQUATION Coefficient (t-value)	ℓn SECRETARY WAGE EQUATION Coefficient (t-value)	ℓn HOUSEKEEPER WAGE EQUATION Coefficient (t-value)
Union time	.00280 (.928)	.00298 (1.580)	.00315 (1.210)	.00441 (1.901)
Job action	−.0165 (.172)	.0979 (2.596)	.126 (2.126)	.0647 (1.476)
Fringe benefits	.0496 (3.519)	.0345 (3.669)	.0463 (3.334)	.0400 (3.307)
Hosbarg	−.406 (−3.955)	−.482 (6.608)	−.300 (2.792)	−.0783 (.854)
Sandl	−.0658 (1.933)	.0699 (3.037)	−.170 (6.210)	−.319 (11.001)
NFP	−.0372 (1.072)	.109 (4.263)	−.120 (3.199)	−.318 (9.851)
Profit	.00316 (.063)	.178 (4.664)	.0558 (.813)	−.252 (5.230)
Concentration	.0184 (.278)	−.164 (3.585)	.0490 (.766)	−.223 (4.480)
Beds	−.36 × 10⁻⁶ (.0084)	.0000474 (1.647)	.0000421 (1.183)	.0000411 (1.152)
Income	.0655 (2.257)	.0624 (3.331)	.0941 (3.767)	.0466 (2.150)
Section	−.0914 (1.610)	−.00287 (.087)	−.00980 (.241)	.0572 (1.261)
M.D. office wage	.0151 (.305)	−.0705 (2.040)	--- ---	--- ---
Retail wage	--- ---	--- ---	.662 (3.214)	--- ---
Service wage	--- ---	--- ---	--- ---	.502 (5.556)
AFDC	.00144 (3.465)	−.000599 (2.224)	−.000450 (1.328)	−.000617 (1.705)
Right-to-work	−.00437 (.064)	−.0228 (.587)	−.00708 (.162)	−.106 (1.973)
Constant	8.868 (22.073)	9.034 (32.434)	.874 (2.168)	1.278 (3.734)
Number of observations	135	175	144	169
$\overline{R}^2$	24.3	39.9	36.5	57.7

Demand variables will have a positive impact on wages if hospital labor markets are noncompetitive.[93] Although many factors affect the demand for hospital care, including insurance, income, out-of-pocket costs, and illness, the analysis was able to account for only per capita real income (*income*)—(county per capita income in $1,000s in 1972). Because of an omitted variables problem, the authors do not place any confidence in the magnitude of the income coefficients, although they all have the expected positive sign in the union wages equations and are statistically significant.[94]

Section is a dummy variable that indicates that the hospital is located in states in one of four areas of the country—the Northeast, Middle Atlantic, West North Central, or Pacific states. These regions have proportionately more unionized hospitals than the rest of the country (see Table 1-8). However, no consistent relation between real wages, i.e., wages adjusted for the cost of living, and section is found. Housekeepers

Table 1-18 Structural Estimates of the Union Status Equations

VARIABLE	R.N. UNION EQUATION Coefficient (t-value)	L.P.N. UNION EQUATION Coefficient (t-value)	SECRETARY UNION EQUATION Coefficient (t-value)	HOUSEKEEPER UNION EQUATION Coefficient (t-value)
Predicted Wage difference	6.010 (2.531)	9.967 (2.263)	9.966 (2.313)	8.698 (3.157)
Fringe benefits	−.0240 (.196)	.111 (.703)	.188 (.00693)	−.156 (.00597)
Hosbarg	2.193 (2.685)	2.661 (2.614)	2.357 (1.750)	.367 (.300)
Sandl	−.467 (1.201)	−2.429 (3.426)	−2.298 (3.132)	−2.253 (2.175)
NFP	−1.057 (2.749)	−3.345 (4.094)	−3.305 (4.024)	−3.456 (3.223)
Profit	−.993 (2.034)	−3.517 (3.693)	−5.130 (3.345)	−4.959 (3.661)
Concentration	−.798 (1.241)	.170 (.235)	−1.599 (1.721)	−.768 (.800)
Beds	.00125 (2.841)	.00151 (2.736)	.00161 (2.410)	.00161 (2.271)
Income	−.0107 (.0423)	.749 (2.172)	.666 (1.468)	.324 (.900)
Urban	−.0513 (.647)	−.0912 (.972)	−.0382 (.451)	.267 (1.761)
Section	.291 (.705)	−1.069 (1.919)	−.483 (.927)	−1.324 (1.985)
Right-to-work	.956 (2.089)	−1.439 (1.958)	−.448 (.719)	−1.115 (1.499)
Constant	−.487 (.401)	−.859 (.608)	−.605 (.348)	.675 (.328)
X^2 (df=12)	75.501	141.859	187.677	142.009

are the only occupation with higher wages in these sections (this relation applies to both union and nonunion groups). While it may be risky to make too much out of this result, it is consistent with the fact that the rate of return to schooling is higher in the South.[95] The control states for section are mainly Southern, and housekeepers are relatively unskilled, so it is not surprising that relatively lower wages for unskilled labor are found in the South.

Job Opportunities outside Hospitals

The next four variables control for employment opportunities outside of hospitals. The hypothesis is that hospital wages will be higher where alternative opportunities, as measured by alternative wage levels, are better. Alternative employments may be different for each occupation. The list selected was one that could be defined by county. For hospital R.N.s and L.P.N.s, the alternative employment is in offices of physicians and surgeons; wholesale and retail trade is postulated to be the alternative employment for secretaries, and service industry for service and maintenance workers. Average monthly state aid to families with dependent children (AFDC) per recipient family is included. In states where AFDC payments are generous, hospital wages may have to be higher in order to attract people into the work force.

In general hospital wages are found to be higher where alternative employment opportunities are better. Six out of eight estimated coefficients are positive, although the alternative wage effects for nonunion secretaries and unionized L.P.N.s are negative. The effect of AFDC payments on hospital wages is ambiguous and typically opposite to expectations. It is positive only for nonunion R.N.s.

This may indicate a weak attachment to the labor force among nonunion R.N.s.

The final variable in the wage analysis is a dummy variable to indicate the presence of a state *right-to-work* law. Evidence is found that, except for nonunion R.N.s, right-to-work legislation is associated with lower wage rates.

Union Status Equations

Table 1-18 presents estimates of the union status equations. The key result is that hospital employees unionize to obtain higher wages: the predicted wage difference from unionization has a positive and statistically significant impact on organizing in all occupations. To assess the quantitative significance of this coefficient, it is necessary first to measure the predicted wage difference and, second, to multiply this value by its coefficient and evaluate the resulting change in the probability of unionization.[96] Predicted wage differences are obtained by using the union wage equation to estimate what the average nonunion worker would gain by unionization. The results indicate that unionization would increase R.N.s' wages by 3.40 percent and L.P.N.s' by 5.61 percent. The gains for nonprofessional occupations would be larger: 7.43 percent for office clerical employees and 7.85 percent for service and maintenance workers.

The survey finds that these potential wage gains have a large quantitative impact on the probability of unionization. Without the possibility of potential wage gains, the probability that R.N.s would unionize, given the sample mean values of other variables, would fall from .375 to .30, L.P.N.s .49 to .30, clerical workers .38 to .15, and service workers, .61 to .34. The percentage decrease is smallest for R.N.s (20 percent) and largest for clerical workers (61 percent) but in all cases the extent of unionization would drop significantly.

The results pertaining to potential wage gains from unionism and the magnitude of the *predicted wage difference* coefficient are interesting in their own right. In particular, why do unions raise wages less for R.N.s and L.P.N.s than for nonprofessional employees? And why does the predicted wage gain have a smaller impact on union status for R.N.s than for the other occupations? There are several suggestions, but no definitive answers, to these questions.

Reasons for Lack of Impact

One reason why unions do not have much impact on nurses' wages is that R.N.s and L.P.N.s may be close substitutes in production. Sloan[97] has noted that there is a substantial amount of interstate variation in R.N.-to-population ratios. But if L.P.N.s and aides-orderlies are added to R.N.s, interstate variations almost disappear in the resulting ratios. He says,[98] "Clearly, employers of nursing personnel substitute less skilled personnel for professional nurses in geographic areas in which professional nurses are relatively scarce." Sloan's evidence suggests that an attempt by a union of R.N.s and L.P.N.s to raise wages will cause hospitals to substitute against the expensive labor, thus confronting the union with a painful trade-off between employment and wages and, presumably, causing it to moderate its wage demands. If this suggestion is correct, it follows that NLRB bargaining unit decisions might well consider the community of interests between R.N.s and L.P.N.s.

A second reason for low union wage effects is that nurses' unions are not, in some sense, as "tough" as those representing nonprofessional employees. Registered nurses have been ambivalent about taking job actions to support their bargaining demands. From 1950 to 1958 the American Nurses' Association (ANA) endorsed a no-strike policy, and for two more years took a neutral stand in disputes that did not involve nurses.[99,100] It was not until 1970 that the ANA House of Delegates recommended that state associations work with other employer organizations to further mutual concerns. During the 18-year tenure of the no-strike policy, nurses generally bargained with their employers from a position of extreme weakness,[101] typically having recourse only to mass resignations to back up their bargaining positions. Contrast this to more aggressive nonprofessional unions such as District 1199, which has used the strike weapon even in situations where it has specifically been illegal to do so,[102] and the relatively poor performance of nurses' unions in the bargaining arena may be understood.

A third explanation for the effects of low union wages is that R.N.s are more concerned with nonwage benefits than are the other occupations. A survey[103] of nurses (including those who did not favor unions) found that the answer given most often as to why they were organizing was "to make management listen." This surpassed the importance of wages and fringe benefits. What do nurses want management to listen to? For one thing, 59 percent of the nurses responding wanted more say in the quality of patient care. Other demands are that they have a voice in nursing assignments and that they be enabled to participate more fully in continuing education.[104] To the extent that nurses are willing to trade off between wages and nonwage benefits in contract negotiations, this will be reflected in lower union wages effects. Under this interpretation, low union wage effects do not represent bargaining weakness or ineptitude but rather imply that nurses are concentrating on other goals.

This interpretation is supported by the size of the coefficient of predicted wage difference in Table 1-18. A given percentage wage difference will have only about two-thirds the effect in the R.N. union status equation as in the other equations. The finding here supports the subjective survey data mentioned earlier—apparently, wage gains are not as important to nurses who are considering unionizing as they are to other occupations.

The Importance of Fringe Benefits

In contrast to predicted wage gains, the level of fringe benefits does not affect union status for any occupation.

Hospital ownership and size affect unionization for all occupations. Large hospitals and federal hospitals are more likely to be unionized than others. Thus, the multivariate analysis affirms the results of the two-way comparisons (Tables 1-6 and 1-7) presented earlier.

On the other hand, section of the country becomes insignificant or negative when control is injected for other geographic factors such as right-to-work and Hosbarg (the number of hospitals in the state with collective bargaining agreements in 1975). Hosbarg has a positive effect on unionization and right-to-work has a negative effect, except for R.N.s. The positive association of right-to-work and R.N. unions is further evidence that these nurses perceive different costs and benefits of unionization than do other occupations. In a similar vein, high per capita income increases the probability of union representation for all occupations except R.N.s.

Urbanization does not affect unionization. This finding contrasts with Stigler's study and suggests that urbanization is not an appropriate general proxy for the costs of unionization.[105]

Hospital concentration has a negative effect on unionization in three occupations and is statistically significant (at $\alpha = .05$ in a one-tailed t-test) for secretaries. It already has been demonstrated (Table 1-16) that concentration reduces wages for nonunion workers, so the present finding implies that concentration has an additional indirect effect by reducing the probability of unionization and thereby reducing wages.

Reconciling the Cross-Section and Time Series Results

The previous section showed that unionism, at a point in time—1977—depends powerfully on predicted wage gains, hospital ownership, and bed size. But the earlier analysis of time series data from 1940 to 1976 used only the passage of time and a variable for the 1974 Taft-Hartley amendments to explain the proportion of hospitals with collective bargaining agreements. In these concluding comments, the two sections should be reconciled and some trends to watch for in hospital unionization suggested.

The time series analysis of unionization was essentially "atheoretical," or lacking any basis in economic theory, for the obvious reason that the passage of time by itself can explain little. However, time can be correlated with changes in the average value of theoretically relevant variables, such as hospital bed size. Between 1968 and 1978, the average number of beds in community hospitals increased from 138 to 167.[106] But this trend cannot explain much of the increase in unionization over the time period.

Another possibility is that the whole cross-section relation is shifting upward over time, i.e., for given values of predisposing variables, the probability of unionization is higher now than it was 10 years ago. This possibility is likely and, in fact, the use of the dummy variable for the 1974 amendments was an attempt to introduce structural shift into the equation. However, the predicted path of unionism is raised only about three percentage points by the amendments. What accounts for the rest of the increase?

Unfortunately, few of the possible structural shifts can be tied to a specific event such as the 1974 amendments. This means that they cannot easily be analyzed statistically, although they have influenced the course of hospital unionization and, in all probability, will continue to do so in the future. Two qualitative structural shifts merit discussion: (1) increased receptivity by workers for unionization and (2) increased willingness of unions to organize hospital workers.

Hospital employees, especially professionals, have long been ambivalent about collective bargaining. It appears to conflict with their professed ideology of service to clients and the public. Thus nurses took a stand in favor of collective bargaining, but for 18 years refused to endorse strikes. However, these attitudes have been changing, as shown by the ANA's action in rescinding its no-strike doctrine. Several reasons may explain the new trend.

First, nurses can observe that other white-collar employees are becoming increasingly unionized.[107] Second, nurses can observe probargaining sentiments among physicians; for example, more than half of the doctors in one survey indicated that they were willing to join a physicians' union. Nearly two-thirds affirmed physicians' right to strike and 56 percent said they would treat only emergency cases in the event of a strike.[108] It will be very difficult for nurses to accept a passive role if physicians become more militant. Finally, special forms of collective bargaining will evolve to deal with the unionism-professionalism conflict. Nurses may tend toward modified collective bargaining that stresses the following:

- shared governance
- different levels of nursing practice
- developing nurse competence, e.g., professional leaves and continuing education
- quality of care[109]

CONCLUSION

The authors suggest that collective bargaining will become increasingly attractive to professional hospital employees and that their bargaining demands will extend beyond wages and working conditions to include a role in the governance of the institution.

Hospital labor organizing has lagged behind the unionization of the industrial work force, in part because the labor movement shunned such workers. Two union representatives attributed labor's failure to venture into this field to a number of factors, including:

- Hospital employees were among the lowest paid workers in the country. Their organization could hardly swell union treasuries.
- Hospitals were widely dispersed in thousands of communities and the work force was further divided into numerous departments within each institution, making organization more difficult.
- A large number of the workers were blacks, Spanish-speaking, and members of other minority groups.[110]

The last point is important because it has been alleged that unions discriminate against minorities and women.[111]

Recent changes in the health industry wage structure have negated the influence of the first point. The pay differential between hospital service workers and others decreased rapidly in the late 1960s and had disappeared entirely by the early 1970s.[112] Earnings for allied health personnel (wage and salary workers with less than 18 years of schooling), standardized for color, age, sex, and schooling, rose from 86 percent of the all-industry norm in 1959 to 95 percent in 1969.[113] The increases for health workers in hospitals exceeded those in other settings and were particularly rapid for R.N.s and L.P.N.s.[114] The reasons for this

catch-up are complex (the authors attribute it to increased demand for hospital services because of better insurance coverage) but in any case, hospital workers no longer are relatively underpaid. Thus, unions have a reason to take a second look at these workers.[115]

A more important reason is that unions' traditional base in manufacturing industries is shrinking. The level of union membership increased by 4.3 million or 25 percent during the period 1953–1970, but as a percent of the nonagricultural labor force declined from 34.1 to 30.1.[116] This trend was examined by Moore and Newman, whose statistical analysis supported the "saturationist" position that "significant changes have occurred in the structure and composition of the American labor force which have caused the past determinants to union growth to be inoperable in the future."[117]

If this contention is correct, then the hospital industry, with its rapidly expanding work force,[118] may be one of the last frontiers for union organizing. It remains to be seen how unions will meet this challenge, and how hospitals will respond.

NOTES

1. Norman Metzger and Dennis D. Pointer, *Labor-Management Relations in the Health Services Industry: Theory and Practice* (Washington, D.C.: Science and Health Publications, Inc., 1972).

2. Ibid., p. 81.

3. Id.

4. "AHA Research Capsules—No. 6," *Hospitals, JAHA* 46 (April 1, 1972): 216–218.

5. *Taft-Hartley Amendments: Implications for the Health Care Field* (Chicago: American Hospital Association, 1976), p. 1.

6. Ibid., p. 2.

7. Richard Waddell, "UNC Project on Hospital Labor Markets," Final Report on Project 2544-1416, Research Triangle Institute, July 15, 1977.

8. C. J. Parsley, "Labor Union Effects on Wage Gains: A Survey of Recent Literature," *Journal of Economic Literature* 18, no. 1 (March 1980): 1–31.

9. Dennis D. Pointer and Norman Metzger, *The National Labor Relations Act* (New York: Spectrum Publications, Inc., 1975), pp. 181–182.

10. Joseph Rosmann, "One Year Under Taft-Hartley," *Hospitals, JAHA* 49 (December 16, 1975): 64–68.

11. Ibid.

12. Ibid.

13. Lucretia Dewey Tanner, Harriet Goldberg Weinstein, and Alice Lynn Ahmuty, *Impact of the 1974 Health Care Amendments to the NLRA on Collective Bargaining in the Health Care Industry* (Washington, D.C.: Federal Mediation and Conciliation Service, U.S. Government Printing Office, 1979).

14. Ibid., p. 126.

15. The number of contracts *negotiated* during any period does not equal the number of collective bargaining agreements *in effect* during that span since some may be negotiated two or more times and others may be in effect throughout the period without being re-

negotiated. However, most health sector contracts are of two years' duration. FMCS estimates that only 185 contracts were renegotiated during the two and a half years of the study period. An unknown number of three-year contracts were negotiated just before the effective date of the 1974 amendments. Despite these data limitations, FMCS contends that contract negotiations closely approximate private sector bargaining in health care facilities.

16. Tanner et al., p. 126.

17. Ibid., p. 66.

18. Ibid., p. 127.

19. Ibid., p. 128.

20. Unionization data were collected by using a stratified national probability sample of 1,200 hospitals drawn from the 7,129 institutions responding to the AHA's 1975 Annual Survey. The sample was stratified into four geographical regions, four types of hospital ownership, and the presence or absence of a collective bargaining agreement in 1975. Two mailings of a questionnaire and a telephone follow-up yielded a response of 942 cases, or 78.5 percent of the sample. A test for nonresponse bias showed that the sample was representative of all union and nonunion hospitals. The data generated by the survey included the number and types of personnel employed in the hospital, costs of fringe benefits to the institution, presence or absence of collective bargaining agreements, types and numbers of employees covered by union contracts, the length of time the agreement had been in effect, and histories of collective bargaining, including job actions and strikes. Annual salary or hourly wage rates were collected for R.N. staff nurses with a three-year diploma, L.P.N.s with two years' experience at this hospital, general secretaries, and housekeeping employees.

21. Union representation elections exclude contract renegotiations. Thus, the picture presented here is of union organizing activity, or "new" unionization attempts.

22. Metzger and Pointer, *Labor-Management Relations.*

23. "AHA Research Capsules."

24. The reader is cautioned that two-way comparisons, such as Table 1-1, which relate union elections and hospital size, do not control for other variables that affect voting. Uncontrolled variables may have shifted between 1967 and 1977. In addition, the authors examined union elections while Metzger and Pointer looked at requests for recognition. Some requests may be withdrawn before the election and others may be pending at any time. The last factor, at least, is unimportant—only 50 hospitals had elections pending at the time of this survey.

25. Rosmann, "One Year."

26. W. H. Pyle, "Organizing in the Health Care Industry: NLRB Unit Decisions Under the 1974 Amendments and Organizational Activity on the Employer's Premises," paper presented at Retail Clerks Attorneys Conference, Monterey, Calif., September 12–15, 1976.

27. See Tables 1-11 through 1-14.

28. Rosmann.

29. Ibid., p. 64.

30. Ibid.

31. Metzger and Pointer, Table V-1.

32. Ibid., p. 23.

33. The unionization estimates from the authors' Hospital Survey and an AHA survey were fairly close for 1967 (6.1 percent vs. the AHA's 7.7 percent) but differ widely in 1970 (9.4 percent vs. 14.7 percent). A resurvey by the AHA in 1975 found that 1,407 (22.7 percent) of 5,574 responding hospitals had a union (very few of the 955 nonrespondents probably had one). This again is fairly close to our 1975 estimate of 18.4 percent unionized hospitals. We cannot explain the discrepancy in 1970, but tend to trust our survey because the AHA data would indicate that unionization doubled between

1967 and 1970 and then grew only about 54 percent in the next five years. Our data, on the other hand, indicate a smoother pattern of growth without an anomalous jump between 1967 and 1970.

34. Duane E. Leigh, *An Analysis of the Interrelation Between Unions, Race, and Wage and Nonwage Competition,* Final report prepared for the Employment and Training Administration, U.S. Department of Labor, under Research and Development Grant 91-53-77-06, April 1978, p. 27.

35. Richard Dusansky, "The Market for Non-physician Hospital Personnel," Mimeographed. State University of New York at Stony Brook, Economic Research Bureau, 1980.

36. Formally, the logistic equation is $\ln\frac{P}{1-P} = \beta X$ where P is the probability of unionization, X represents a column vector of explanatory variables, and β is a row vector of coefficients to be estimated. This equation was estimated by ordinary least squares, using the proportion of unionized hospitals as an empirical measure of the probability of unionization. Since this approximation introduces heteroscedosticity, each variable in the equation is multiplied by $\sqrt{n_t p_t(1-p)_t}$, where n_t is the number of hospitals in year t and p_t is the proportion of unionized hospitals in year t. (See H. Theil, *Principles of Econometrics* (New York: John Wiley & Sons, Inc., 1971), p. 635.

37. An estimate for $\hat{P}$ is obtained by solving the equation, $\hat{P} = e^{\hat{\beta}X}/(1 + e^{\hat{\beta}X})$, where $\hat{\beta}$ are the estimated logistic coefficients.

38. Metzger and Pointer.

39. Ibid., pp. 86–88.

40. Ibid., p. 89.

41. Ibid., p. 91.

42. Regional definitions used in this article are:

New England (NE): Connecticut, Maine, Massachusetts, New Hampshire, Rhode Island, Vermont.

Middle Atlantic (MA): New Jersey, New York, Pennsylvania.

South Atlantic (SA): Delaware, District of Columbia, Florida, Georgia, Maryland, North Carolina, South Carolina, Virginia, West Virginia.

East North Central (ENC): Illinois, Indiana, Michigan, Ohio, Wisconsin.

East South Central (ESC): Alabama, Kentucky, Mississippi, Tennessee.

West North Central (WNC): Iowa, Kansas, Minnesota, Missouri, Nebraska, North Dakota, South Dakota.

West South Central (WSC): Arkansas, Louisiana, Oklahoma, Texas.

Mountain (M): Arizona, Colorado, Idaho, Montana, Nevada, New Mexico, Utah, Wyoming.

Pacific: Alaska, California, Hawaii, Oregon, Washington.

43. This interpretation of Table V-6 (in Metzger and Pointer, p. 90), is questionable. Unions had more penetration in the largest hospitals (500+ beds) than the smallest (up to 25 beds), but the relation was not monotonic for intermediate bed sizes.

44. Metzger and Pointer, Table V-3.

45. The rank ordering of size and the percent of hospitals with a union contract is increasing monotonically except for a very slight reversal between hospitals with 25 to 50 beds and those with 50 to 100 beds.

46. Metzger and Pointer, Table V-5.

47. This finding is tentative because of possible measurement error in the union penetration ratio, which was computed as the number of organized employees in an occupation divided by the total number of organized employees in that occupation. To be exact, the denominator should include part-time employees and should exclude

those who are not part of the bargaining unit. For example, 100 percent of R.N.s rarely are covered since supervisory nurses are exempt under NLRB decisions.

48. Edwin F. Beal, Edward D. Wickersham, and Philip Kienast, *The Practice of Collective Bargaining*, 4th ed. (Homewood, Ill.: Richard D. Irwin, Inc.), p. 308.

49. The California Medical Laboratory Technicians recently joined with the Marine Engineers Beneficial Association to organize technical employees in hospitals in that state.

50. Tables 1-11 through 1-14 are organized so the major unions in each occupation, as measured by the number of contracts, are listed separately. After this, minor unions and answers that could not be coded (e.g., AFL-CIO) are listed together in a single "Other/Not Identified" group. One unfortunate exception occurred because of a coding error that places District 1199 of the Retail-Wholesale-Department Store Union in the "not identified" category. District 1199 membership therefore must be estimated from other sources. In 1976, District 1199 had 80,000 members, 62,000 of whom were located in New York, New Jersey, and Connecticut (Tanner et al., p. 81). Districts 1199-E in Baltimore and 1199-C in Philadelphia represented an additional 7,500 and 6,000 members, respectively. It is estimated that about 65,000 members worked in hospitals (personal communication from Norman Metzger to the first author). District 1199 represented few R.N.s but actively organized L.P.N.s, clerical, and especially service employees. Therefore, District 1199 must be considered as a major union organizing these occupations, in addition to those indicated in Tables 1-12, 1-13, and 1-14.

51. The denominators for our coverage rates are: R.N.s, 461,456; L.P.N.s, 626,977; clerical, 420,816; and service and maintenance, 717,563.

52. Pointer and Metzger, p. 181.

53. *Taft-Hartley Amendments* (AHA), p. 2.

54. Leon J. Davis and Moe Foner, "Organization and Unionization of Health Workers in the United States: The Trade Union Perspective," *International Journal of Health Services* 5, no. 1 (1975): 19–26.

55. "AHA Research Capsules."

56. Tanner et al., p. 132.

57. Ken DeMarko, James W. Robinson, and Ernest C. Houck, "A Pilot Study of the Initial Bargaining Demands by Newly-Organized Employees of Health Care Institutions," *Labor Law Journal* 29, No. 5 (May 1978): 275–291.

58. John H. Pencavel, "The Demand for Union Services: An Exercise," *Industrial and Labor Relations Review* 24, no. 2 (January 1971): 180–190.

59. Orley Ashenfelter and George F. Johnson, "Unionism, Relative Wages and Labor Quality in U.S. Manufacturing Industries," *International Economic Review* 13, no. 3 (October 1972): 488–508.

60. George J. Stigler, "The Theory of Economic Regulation," *Bell Journal of Economics and Management Science* 2 (Spring 1972): 3–21.

61. James W. Begun and Roger D. Feldman, *A Social and Economic Analysis of Professional Regulations in Optometry*, Final report prepared for the National Center for Health Services Research, Office of the Assistant Secretary for Health (OASH), under Grant No. 1-RO1-HS-03085-01, August 31, 1979.

62. As one union executive put the issue of fixed costs, "Some of our best organizers really work for a period of weeks or months to build an organizing committee, and that means that not a single person has yet signed a card or has made any commitment in terms of paper or material . . ." (Metzger and Pointer, p. 261).

63. Metzger and Pointer, p. 57.

64. Pointer and Metzger, pp. 21–22.

65. Section 8(a) spells out unfair labor practices for employers, who are forbidden to interfere with employees' rights to organize;

Section 8(b) enumerates unfair labor practices by unions. (Labor Management Relations Act, 1947, as Amended by Pub. L. 86-257, 1959).

66. All states in the South except Delaware, the District of Columbia, Maryland, West Virginia, Oklahoma, and Kentucky have right-to-work laws.

67. Thomas A. Kochan, "How American Workers View Labor Unions," *Monthly Labor Review*, U.S. Department of Labor 102, no. 4 (April 1979): 23–31.

68. Ibid.

69. H. G. Lewis, *Unionism and Relative Wages in the United States: An Empirical Inquiry* (Chicago: University of Chicago Press, 1963).

70. Frank A. Sloan and Richard A. Elnicki, "Professional Nurse Wage-Setting in Hospitals," Ch. 3 in Frank A. Sloan, ed., *Equalizing Access to Nursing Services: The Geographical Dimension*, DHEW Publication No. HRA 78-51 (Washington, D.C.: U.S. Government Printing Office, March 1978), pp. 57–86.

71. When nonwage benefits were included in the wage equation, the union wage effect was 2.7 percent, but was statistically insignificant (t = 1.5).

72. C. R. Link and J. H. Landon, "Monopsony and Union Power in the Market for Nurses," *Southern Economic Journal* 41, no. 4 (April 1975): 649–659.

73. M. D. Fottler, "The Union Impact on Hospital Wages," *Industrial and Labor Relations Review* 30, no. 3 (April 1977): 342–355.

74. R. W. Hurd, "Equilibrium Vacancies in a Labor Market Dominated by Non-Profit Firms: The 'Shortage' of Nurses," *Review of Economics and Statistics* 55, no. 2 (May 1973): 234–240.

75. K. Davis, "Theories of Hospital Inflation: Some Empirical Evidence," *Journal of Human Resources* 8, no. 2 (Spring 1973): 181–201.

76. Sherwin Rosen, "Trade Union Power, Threat Effects, and the Extent of Organization," *Review of Economic Studies*, April 1969, pp. 185–196.

77. Brian E. Becker, "Union Impact on Wages and Fringe Benefits of Hospital Nonprofessionals," *Quarterly Review of Economics and Business* 19, No. 4 (Winter 1979): 27–44.

78. Roger Feldman and Richard Scheffler, "Unionization and Hospital Compensation," forthcoming in *Industrial and Labor Review*, 1981.

79. Tanner et al., p. 34.

80. Peter Schmidt and Robert P. Strauss, "A Multiple Logit Analysis of Industrial Employment Patterns," *International Economic Review* 17, no. 1 (February 1976): 204–212.

81. J. Heckman, "Simultaneous Equations Models With Both Continuous and Discrete Endogenous Variables With and Without Structural Shift in the Equation," in S. Goldfeld and R. E. Quandt, eds., *Studies in Nonlinear Estimation* (Cambridge, Mass.: Ballinger Publishing Co., 1976).

82. Peter Schmidt, "Estimation of a Simultaneous Equations Model With Jointly Dependent Continuous and Qualitative Variables: The Union-Earnings Question Revisited," *International Economic Review* 19, no. 2 (June 1978): 453–465.

83. Lung-Fei Lee, "Unionism and Wage Rates: A Simultaneous Equations Model With Qualitative and Limited Dependent Variables," *International Economic Review* 19, no. 2 (June 1978): 415–433.

84. A classic example occurred in 1980 in Minnesota when the state legislature created by fiat a single faculty unit for the Twin Cities (Minneapolis and St. Paul) campus of the University of Minnesota, negating previously established separate bargaining units for the law school and health sciences faculty. (Memorandum from James C. O'Neill of Kelley, Torrison, and O'Neill, attorneys, to University of Minnesota health sciences instructional employees,

April 28, 1980.) The health sciences faculty sought to reestablish a separate bargaining unit via a technical provision in the new law. Should this fail, the faculty undoubtedly would oppose collective bargaining because of the fear that this would lower its members' relative income status within the entire faculty.

85. For a more thorough discussion of unit determination, see Tanner et al., pp. 394–406.

86. Feldman and Scheffler.

87. If $I^* > 0$ worker, i ,is in the union, otherwise not, where $I^* = \delta_0 + \delta_1 ((W_{ui} - W_{ni})/W_{ni}) + \delta_2 X + \epsilon$. W_{ni} is the worker's nonunion wage, W_{ui} is the individual's union wage, X is a vector of other variables (costs of unionization and personal characteristics) that influence the reservation wage, and ϵ is a random error term.

88. Ideally, separate equations should have been estimated for occupation-specific fringe benefits. A pretest of the Hospital Survey revealed, however, that respondents could not calculate separate levels for each occupation.

89. Because of the small numbers involved, it is advisable not to generalize this association of strikes and unions to all U.S. hospitals. The FMCS surveyed all 129 strikes in the health care industry between August 25, 1974, and December 13, 1976. Strikes typically (two out of every five times) involved disputes over first contracts. (See Tanner et al., pp. 320, 322.)

90. See Sloan and Elnicki[70] for a summary of the evidence on market concentration and wages. Sloan and Elnicki[70], and Hurd[74], expect that concentration should reduce R.N.s' wages most. In comparison to L.P.N.s and nonprofessional employees, R.N.s have the fewest employment opportunities outside the hospital.

91. John Kenneth Galbraith, *American Capitalism: The Concept of Countervailing Power* (Boston: Houghton-Mifflin Co., 1952), pp. 122–148.

92. Louise B. Russell, *Technology in Hospitals* (Washington, D.C.: The Brookings Institution, 1979), pp. 99–131.

93. Sloan and Elnicki, pp. 57–86.

94. Feldman and Scheffler[78] also found significant positive coefficients for nominal per capita income in nominal wages equations that controlled for a separate cost-of-living variable.

95. Barry R. Chiswick, *Income Equality: Regional Analyses Within a Human Capital Framework* (New York: Columbia University Press, 1974), p. 23.

96. If $\hat{I}^*$ is denoted as the estimated probit equation, then the probability that an occupation is unionized is $\dfrac{1}{\sqrt{2\pi}} \int_{-\infty}^{\hat{I}^*} e^{-\frac{1}{2}z} \, dz$. The probability that the occupation is not unionized is one minus this expression.

97. Sloan and Elnicki, pp. 57–86.

98. Ibid., p. 51.

99. Tanner et al., pp. 92–94.

100. Joseph A. Alutto, "The Professional Association and Collective Bargaining: The Case of the American Nurses' Association," in M. F. Arnold, et al., eds., *Administering Health Systems: Issues and Perspectives* (Chicago: Aldine-Atherton, 1971), pp. 103–126.

101. Michael H. Miller, "Nurses' Right to Strike," *Journal of Nursing Administration,* February 1975, pp. 35–39.

102. Robert K. Match, Arnold H. Goldstein, and Harold L. Light, "Unionization, Strikes, Threatened Strikes, and Hospitals—the View From Hospital Management," *International Journal of Health Services* 5, no. 1 (1975): 27–36.

103. Marjorie Godfrey, "Someone Should Represent Nurses," *Nursing 76,* June 1976, pp. 73–85.

104. Thomas P. Herzog, "The National Labor Relations Act and the ANA: A Dilemma of Professionalism," *Journal of Nursing Administration,* October 1976, pp. 33–35.

105. Begun and Feldman[61] (p. 100) included urbanization in their study of professional regulation in optometry because nonurban optometry is characterized by the classic "professional" approach to occupational development. Competition and commercialism are downplayed in this setting. They found that urbanization lessens the chance of optometry's attaining its professional goals. Three different results on the urbanization variable (Stigler[60]—positive, Begun and Feldman[61]—negative, and the present study—nil) suggest that the importance of this factor depends on the specific occupation being studied.

106. *Hospital Statistics, 1979 Edition* (Chicago: American Hospital Association, 1979), p. vii.

107. Ronald G. Ehrenberg, *The Demand of State and Local Government Employees: An Economic Analysis* (Lexington, Mass.: D.C. Heath and Co., 1972), p. 4.

108. "Labor Relations Update," *Hospitals, JAHA* 50 (February 1, 1976): 44.

109. Virginia S. Cleland, "Shared Governance in a Professional Model of Collective Bargaining," *Journal of Nursing Administration,* May 1978, pp. 39–43.

110. Davis and Foner, "Organization and Unionization," pp. 20–21.

111. See Orley Ashenfelter, "Discrimination and Trade Unions," in O. Ashenfelter and A. Rees, *Discrimination in Labor Markets, 1973* (pp. 88–112) for a discussion of discrimination and trade unions. This issue may not be important in the health care industry because the union movement and civil rights have been closely allied in hospitals (Davis and Foner; see also, Jonathan Rivin, "The Impacts of Unionization on Unskilled Hospital Workers and the Hospital Industry." Unpublished B.A. thesis. Cambridge, Mass.: Harvard College, 1977, p. 49).

112. Rivin, p. 14.

113. Victor R. Fuchs, "The Earnings of Allied Health Personnel—Are Health Workers Underpaid?" *Explorations in Economic Research* 3, no. 3 (Summer 1976): 408–432.

114. Ibid.

115. Ibid.

116. William J. Moore and Robert J. Newman, "On the Prospects for American Trade Union Growth: A Cross-Section Analysis," *Review of Economics and Statistics* 54, no. 4 (January 1975): 435–445.

117. Ibid.

118. Rivin, Table 1-2.

2. Labor Agreements in the Hospital Industry: A Study of Trends in Collective Bargaining Output from 1974 through 1981

HERVEY A. JURIS and GAIL ANN BENTIVEGNA

When researchers talk of the output of the collective bargaining process, they mean the web of rules, both formal and informal, that the parties have mutually agreed will govern their work relationship over a certain period of time. Many of these rules find their way into the labor agreement. This then becomes a basis by which parties compare one relationship to another. Although this is an imperfect measure of bargaining outcomes, in the sense that informal agreements are not part of the labor contract, contractual language is a step forward from sole reliance on wage data in making such comparisons. This is true because of the trade-offs between wages and other terms and conditions of employment that are made in the bargaining process.

Because of a desire to create such a data base, as well as to tap the rich vein of hospital bargaining experience that predated the 1974 amendments to the National Labor Relations Act, the senior author in that year entered into an agreement with the American Hospital Association (AHA) to collect and analyze as many contracts as it could obtain. In all, 817 contracts were collected during 1974 and 75 and a summary prepared that concentrated on the elements that distinguish hospital contracts from those in all industry generally. This summary was reported in *Labor Law Journal,* August 1977. That analysis predicted that as bargaining matured, contracts in the hospital industry would become indistinguishable from those in all other industries, including steel, autos, meat packing, police, fire, etc. Contracts continued to be collected through 1980.

This article reports the results of a summary analysis of 613 hospital collective bargaining agreements from 393 hospitals in 1978 and 79. By comparing current patterns with those established through 1977 and reported in the previous article, trends can be identified, earlier predictions tested, and new predictions generated.

THE POPULATION AND THE SAMPLE

To set the trend analysis in perspective, the reader is referred to Tables 2-1 and 2-2. Table 2-1 reports the results of a special topic survey sent to 7,012 hospitals by the AHA in October 1979 (5,663 responded) and Table 2-2 a survey sent to 7,165 hospitals in September, 1975 (6,199 replied). Of the hospitals answering the 1979 current survey, 24 percent (1,371) reported that they had at least one union contract in force. This number has remained relatively constant during the previous four years—between 23 percent and 24 percent. Unionized hospitals, in contrast to all responding institutions, still are more likely to be in Standard Metropolitan Statistical Areas (SMSAs) of more than 1 million, to represent disproportionately larger bed size categories, to be publicly owned, and to be more heavily concentrated in the West and North Central regions of the United States. The AHA requested the 1,371 unionized hospitals in the 1979 survey to send it all of their contracts. The 613 contracts

Table 2-1 Extent and Nature of Unionization of U.S. Hospitals (1979)

Hospital Characteristics	Percentage of Hospitals Reporting			
	All U.S. Hospitals (N=7,012)	Responding Hospitals (N=5,663)	Unionized Hospitals (N=1,371)	Contract Sample (N=393 Hospitals)
SMSA Size				
Non-SMSA	45.6	44.9	28.2	29.0
Fewer than 250,000	9.5	10.0	12.0	9.9
250,000–1 million	17.7	18.3	19.2	18.3
More than 1 million	27.2	26.8	40.7	42.7
Bed size category				
0–99	46.5	43.9	23.3	20.1
100–199	22.7	22.6	22.5	25.4
200–399	18.0	19.6	26.4	30.3
400+	12.8	13.9	27.8	24.2
Control				
Government, nonfederal	31.8	31.3	31.7	23.4
Government, federal	5.2	5.8	19.5	—
Church	10.5	11.4	6.6	12.5
Voluntary	39.7	41.5	38.2	61.3
Proprietary	12.6	10.0	4.0	2.8
Region				
West (Pacific)	12.5	11.5	19.9	24.2
North East (New England & Mid Atlantic)	17.0	17.7	32.1	30.1
North Central	28.0	29.9	29.9	39.4
Other	42.4	40.9	18.1	6.4

Source: Reprinted with permission from *Special Survey on Selected Hospital Topics,* American Hospital Association, Hospital Data Center, October 1979.

submitted were negotiated in 1977, 1978, and 1979, and are expiring in the 1972–82 period.

The profile of the 393 hospitals that supplied the 613 contracts showed them to be representative of the 1979 population of unionized hospitals with respect to SMSA size, bed size category, and region. The only significant sample variation from the population is type of ownership: this sample is weighted slightly toward not-for-profit hospitals. (Federal hospitals were dropped from the data base because many of the conditions of employment for their employees are the result of a legislative process rather than of the collective bargaining relationship.) On the basis of this analysis, the authors feel comfortable drawing inferences from the sample regarding practices and trends in the unionized sector of the hospital industry.

SOME FINDINGS FROM THIS STUDY

In general, the scope of provisions in hospital contracts continues to be quite broad, covering most issues conventionally found in mature labor-management relationships in industry. This is consistent with the 1977 prediction that as hospital bargaining matured, output would imitate the patterns of other unionized industries.[1] Because of space limitations, this discussion focuses on areas in which there was divergence in 1977 and convergence today.

Contract Duration

Hospital contract duration periods (Table 2-3) were substantially shorter than all-industry contracts from 1974 through 1977, when almost one-quarter ran for one year or less. By 1979 only 2 percent of all hospital contracts were for one year or less—a pattern identical to the current all-industry situation. The proportion of hospital and all-industry contracts of four years or longer also is identical, 3 percent. By 1979, almost all hospital contract periods were for two (42 percent) or three (53 percent) years, a trend to be expected as bargaining relationships mature.

The slightly smaller proportion of three-year contracts in hospitals relative to those in the private sector appears related to the high proportion of local and state government institutions with annual or biannual

Table 2-2   Extent and Nature of Unionization of U.S. Hospitals (1975)

Hospital Characteristics	Percentage of Hospitals Reporting			
	All U.S. Hospitals (N=7,165)	Responding Hospitals (N=6,199)	Unionized Hospitals (N=1,418)	Contract Sample (N=576 Hospitals)
SMSA Size				
Non-SMSA	46	46	26	27
Fewer than 250,000	9	9	10	8
250,000–1 million	17	18	18	14
More than 1 million	28	28	46	51
Bed size category				
0–99	49	46	23	21
100–199	22	22	22	24
200–399	17	18	26	28
400+	13	14	29	28
Control				
Government, nonfederal	32	32	31	35
Government, federal	5	6	20	1
Church	11	12	7	11
Voluntary	39	39	36	49
Proprietary	13	11	6	4
Region				
West	13	12	22	28
North East	18	18	34	31
North Central	28	30	28	31
Other	41	40	16	10

Source: Reprinted with permission from *Special Survey on Selected Hospital Topics,* American Hospital Association, Hospital Data Center, September 1975.

budgets, the high rates of inflation in effect when many hospital contracts were negotiated, and the relative absence of cost-of-living allowance (COLA) clauses in those agreements. Subsample analysis of duration provisions for 1974 through 1977 shows that professional contracts were somewhat shorter and nonprofessional contracts somewhat longer.[2] These patterns have remained stable through 1980. It was predicted that over time as bargaining matured, contract duration would lengthen, reliance on reopeners decrease, and the inclusion of COLAs increase. Table 2-3 illustrates that all these trends have occurred.

Union Security

Union security was another area of significant difference. In 1977, union shop provisions were found in 63 percent of the all-industry sample, but in only 30 percent of the contracts in the authors' hospital sample; by 1980, union shop provisions were 62 percent of the all-industry sample and 38 percent of the hospital group. However, there is significant intraindustry variance among hospitals disaggregated by control, city size, and bargaining unit.

In the 1974–77 survey, 46 percent of the private hospitals had union shops as compared to 6 percent of the public hospitals; the current figures are approximately half of the private hospitals and 7 percent for public ones. The major trend in union security is a sharp drop in open shop from 57 percent in the 1977 survey to 16 percent in the current one for public hospitals, and from 19 percent in 1977 to 3 percent in 1980 for private hospitals. In 1974 through 1977, agency shops and maintenance of membership provisions showed a slightly higher incidence in the public sector, while modified union shop was twice as prevalent in private hospitals as in public institutions. By 1980, the proportion of modified union shop clauses in private institutions was two-and-a-half times greater than in public hospitals.

Professional and technical units are more likely to have open shop clauses; nonprofessional and combination units are more likely to have union shops. About half of the union security clauses in cities with more than 1 million population are union shop, as opposed to 66 percent in 1977. In 1974 through 1977, contracts negotiated in cities below 250,000 were much less likely to contain union shop provisions than were large

Table 2-3   Duration of Contract, COLA, and Reopeners

Contract Clause	Percentage of Contracts Reporting			
	Hospital Contracts 1974–1977 (N = 817)	All-Industry 1975 (N = 400)	Hospital Contracts 1978–1981 (N = 613)	All-Industry 1979 (N = 400)
Length of contract				
1 year or less	23	5	2	2
2 years	50	21	42	22
3 years	25	70	53	73
4 years or more	—	—	3	3
Deferred increases	65	88	86	95
Wage reopeners	29	8	9	8
Cost of living allowances	7	36	15	49

urban areas. By 1980, contracts negotiated in cities of 100,000 to 250,000 showed a union shop increase— approximately one-third, as compared with half of those in larger cities.

Other elements of union security in hospitals are comparable to all-industry patterns. Dues checkoff currently appears in 88 percent of the hospital contracts and in 86 percent of the BNA sample, compared to 79 percent and 86 percent in 1977. As might be expected in the absence of strong union security provisions, clauses prohibiting employer discrimination for union membership currently appear in 57 percent of the hospital contracts as opposed to 49 percent of the BNA sample contracts, compared to 59 percent and 43 percent in 1977. The pattern of increased emphasis on union security in health care, particularly in the private sector, is approaching the all-industry pattern.

In the area of individual and job security, several provisions are noteworthy. Seniority today seems to be used in promotion and in transfer roughly to the same extent that it is in all-industry. Seventy percent of the hospital contracts and 67 percent of the BNA sample use seniority in some degree for promotion, compared to 66 percent and 69 percent in 1977; 36 percent of the hospitals and 44 percent of the BNA sample use seniority in transfers, as opposed to 44 percent and 48 percent in 1977.

A distinction emerges, however, when seniority is the sole or deciding factor. Because of the nature of licensure and occupational restrictions in the hospital industry, it would be expected that seniority would be less likely to be such a factor in promotions. This is in fact the case. Seniority is listed in 31 percent of the hospital contracts as the sole or deciding factor in promotions, a 14 percent increase over the 17 percent in 1977; this is compared with 42 percent of the industry sample now and 38 percent in 1977. Seniority is mentioned as a secondary factor in an additional 22 percent of the industry agreements and 37 percent of the hospital cases; in 1977, these factors were 25 percent and 40 percent.

Transfers, Layoffs, Recalls, etc.

With respect to transfer, for which occupational and licensure limitations are less important, 36 percent of the hospital contracts call for seniority to be the sole or determining factor as opposed to 30 percent of the industry sample. This is a significant change from 1974–77 when 65 percent of the hospital contracts and 31 percent in the industry sample named seniority as the sole factor in transfers. Seniority is mentioned in the current survey as a secondary factor in approximately 12 percent of the industry agreements in addition to the value reported earlier, down from 15 percent in 1977.

Provisions for seniority in layoff now occur in 86 percent of the hospital contracts as opposed to 83 percent of those in industry, and for seniority in recall in 80 percent of the hospital contracts and 78 percent in industry. In 1974–77, use of seniority in layoff was 75 percent in the hospital contracts and 85 percent in industry; in recall, it was 66 percent as opposed to 75 percent. Severance pay appears in only 6 percent of the hospital contracts as against 37 percent of the industry sample, decreases from the earlier survey's figures of 9 percent and 39 percent. Limits on subcontracting occur in 19 percent of the hospital contracts (up from 10 percent since 1977) vs. 44 percent in industry (40 percent in 1977), and limitations on crew size in 3 percent of the hospital contracts (5 percent in 1977); the authors have no comparable data for the all-industry sample.

Each of the last five items (layoff, recall, severance, subcontracting, and crew size) may reflect the fact that until very recently with cost passthrough, significant economic constraints did not exist in the hospital industry. As hospitals continue to face economic difficulties because of prospective rate review and any Federal restrictions on rising costs, these types of protective provisions can be expected to increase in importance to a level comparable to the private sector, where the demand for labor has been more price elastic over time.

Discipline, Due Process, and Grievances

In the area of discipline and due process, there currently seems to be very little difference between the two sectors. Ninety percent of contracts in hospitals and 96 percent in industry provide for discipline and discharge; in 1977, these sectors were more divergent—82 percent and 97 percent. Cause or just cause are specified in 87 percent of hospital contracts and 80 percent of industry; in the earlier survey, these figures were 76 percent and 79 percent. Discharge for specific offenses is provided in 65 percent of the industry contracts but in only 36 percent of those in hospitals. However, these figures show greater convergence than in 1974–77, when 66 percent of the industry contracts provided for discharge for certain offenses and only 8 percent of the hospital agreements did. Many hospital and industry contracts contain both general clauses and a specific list of offenses leading to automatic discharge.

Ninety-nine percent of both hospital and industry contracts have grievance procedures, which does not reflect much change from the 97 percent and 98 percent in 1977. However, whereas 83 percent of the industry contracts put limitations on what constitutes a grievance, only 39 percent of the hospital contracts appear to, although this is up significantly from the 1977 figures of 68 percent and 22 percent. Arbitration is the final step in 96 percent of the industry sample and in 92 percent of the hospitals; the industry percentage was the same in 1977, when hospitals were at 88 percent.

Wage-Related Provisions

Although no data were collected on wages per se, a great deal were assembled on wage-related provisions. With respect to hours and overtime, the frequency of premiums for the sixth and seventh day is reasonably the same for both groups—usually less than a quarter of all contracts. However, the number of hospital contracts providing premium pay for Saturday as a regularly scheduled day (16 percent) or for Sunday as a regularly scheduled day (18 percent) is significantly smaller than in the BNA sample, which reports that 50 percent of the contracts pay a premium for Saturday work per se and 64 percent for Sunday. These figures show a slight change from 1977, when the figures for hospitals were 11 percent and 14 percent, respectively, and the BNA reported 52 percent and 68 percent. Currently, shift differentials are found in 92 percent of the hospital contracts and 79 percent of the BNA sample, a significant change from the earlier poll in which 58 percent of the hospital agreements provided shift differentials and the all-industry sample 82 percent. The incidence of shift differentials decreases slightly with increases in SMSA size.

Report pay and unscheduled callback pay are significantly lower in the hospital sample than in the BNA report, while scheduled standby pay for persons on call is significantly higher in the hospital contracts, as would be expected—58 percent vs. 3 percent, up from the 1977 figures of 46 percent and 3 percent.

Time Off, Leaves, Holidays, Overtime

In the benefit area, major differences involve holidays and paid sick leave. Table 2-4 shows that the hospital industry is behind the all-industry sample in number of holidays and in the rate of pay for holiday hours worked. However, the most striking difference is in paid sick leave, which is included in 95 percent of the hospital contracts and in just one quarter of the BNA sample.

This difference was even more dramatic in the 1974–77 survey, with paid sick leave in 94 percent of the hospital contracts and in only 3 percent of the BNA group. To investigate the possibility that the deficit in holidays was compensated for by paid sick leave, a frequency distribution of total paid days off (holidays plus personal days plus paid sick leave but exclusive of vacations) was computed.

These data are presented in Table 2-5, then disaggregated (Table 2-6) by bargaining unit, control (ownership), SMSA size, bed size, region, and single hospital vs. multiple hospital system status.

While comparable data on the range of total paid days off is not available for the BNA sample, it does appear that the hospital industry is generous in time off; the mode is 20 days—more than half the contracts provide 20 to 22 paid days off. With vacations included, the industry is well on the way to a four-day work week. The most generous provisions for paid

Table 2-4 Holiday and Holiday Pay Provisions

Contract Clause	Percentage of Contracts Reporting			
	Hospital Contracts 1974–1977 (N = 817)	All-Industry 1975 (N = 400)	Hospital Contracts 1978–1981 (N = 613)	All-Industry 1979 (N = 400)
Provision for paid holidays	95	97	97	99
Number of paid holidays				
6 or less	10	6	10	3
7	23	10	20	8
8	23	12	33	11
9	11	29	14	17
10	23	42	12	27
11	—	—	4	15
12 and more	—	—	7	17
Compensation for holiday work*				
Equal time off	53	NA	15	NA
1½ times regular pay	0	2	4	1
2 times regular pay	8	16	19	17
2¼ or 2½ times regular pay	17	43	42	45
3 or more times regular pay	2	32	2	33

*Effective rate of pay—i.e., 8 hours holiday pay plus rate for hours worked; 2 times equals 8 hours for the holiday plus straight time for hours worked.

time off occur in the Northeast, in relatively large hospitals, or in urban areas with more than 250,000 in population.

Professional Contracts

Finally professional contracts were examined to see whether they differed in scope from other hospital con-

Table 2-5 Total Paid Days Off (Exclusive of Vacation)

Number of Days Off (Holidays and personal days and paid sick days)*	Hospital Contracts (%)	
	1974–77	1978–81
1–9	7	3
10–18	14	9
19	16	6
20	17	21
21	10	17
22	10	20
23–25	16	19
26 or more	10	5

*Seven percent of the 817 contracts for 1974–1977 contained language on paid holidays, personal days, or paid sick leave too vague for inclusion in the table. The frequencies presented here are for N=759. For 1978–81, 11 percent of the 613 contracts had language on paid holidays, personal days, or paid sick leave too vague for inclusion here. The frequencies presented here are for N=542.

tracts. Based on the literature on nonhealth professionals (teachers, engineers, professors, police), professional contracts in hospitals were expected to contain the same full range of traditional clauses as all other contracts as well as provision for some kind of professional issues decision-making apparatus. This turned out to be true: 46 percent of the current hospital contracts provide for joint study committees, over 42 percent in 1977.

Professional associations that represent R.N.s particularly negotiate for the establishment of labor-management committees. These committees, composed of administrators and unionized R.N.s, address topics such as patient care, peer review, and communication with management. They generally exclude traditional collective bargaining issues such as determination of salaries and benefits and procedures for settling grievances. Because these committees usually are advisory bodies, management is not obligated to implement their suggestions.

Much of the decision-making authority that traditionally has been reserved for the director of nursing and other managers now appears on the agendas of the labor-management committees. Although directors of nursing may not be particularly committed to the concept of a professional association functioning like a union or to a union/management committee debating professional issues, R.N.s and L.P.N.s continue to use this kind of collective bargaining as a means to resolve both professional and economic issues.

Table 2-6 Total Paid Days Off (Exclusive of Vacation)—Disaggregated

	NUMBER OF PAID DAYS OFF					
	(Percent of Hospital Contracts)					
	Less Than 20 Days*		20 Days		More Than 20 Days	
	1974–77	1978–81	1974–77	1978–81	1974–77	1978–81
By Bargaining Unit						
Professional	38	17	21	20	41	63
Technical	35	13	22	33	43	54
Nonprofessional	41	21	19	23	40	56
Combination	35	17	11	14	54	69
By Control (Ownership)						
Government	30	14	17	17	53	69
Church-related	52	25	29	34	18	41
Other nonprofit	40	17	15	20	45	63
Proprietary	36	25	14	19	50	56
By SMSA Size (Population)						
Less than 50,000	46	21	27	35	27	44
50,000–250,000	44	33	23	21	33	46
250,000–1,000,000	38	17	16	7	46	76
More than 1,000,000	32	11	11	17	58	72
By Bed Size						
0–99 beds	43	25	24	26	33	49
100–199 beds	38	16	25	35	37	49
200–399 beds	36	12	17	12	47	75
400–plus beds	43	19	8	12	49	69
By Single v. Multiple Hospital System						
Single	39	17	19	21	42	62
Multiple	29	11	9	23	62	66
By Region						
Northeast	24	4	4	3	72	93
North Central	58	28	16	28	26	44
West	29	13	26	32	44	55

*In 1974–77, 38 percent of professional contracts provided less than 20 days, 21 percent 20 days, and 41 percent more than 20 days. For 1978–81, 17 percent provided less than 20 days, 20 percent 20 days, and 63 percent more than 20 days.

In related areas because of the nature of occupational licensing in the industry and because of legislative pressures for continuing education and professional upgrading, 55 percent of the contracts provide for educational leave, up from the 47 percent that did in 1977. The highest incidence of educational leave occurs in contracts negotiated by professional and technical employees. BNA does not report comparable data on either joint study committees or educational leave for the private sector.

SUMMARY

The purpose of this article has been to explore the relationship between hospital industry contracts and those from an all-industry sample, as well as to look at change over time. In general, the scope of bargaining in each set seems quite similar, with distinct differences in depth of coverage on certain issues. These differences result, in part, from the high proportion of unionized professionals and of publicly owned hospitals. Despite these differences, as early as 1978 hospital collective bargaining covered most of the issues that occur in mature industrial bargaining. The 1977 prediction in the earlier article that major differences would narrow is illustrated here, particularly in the areas of duration, union security, individual security, discipline, and due process. Main differences involve paid time off, education, and committee structures, the last two associated primarily with professional employees.

The contracts in this industry are developing in a way indistinguishable from steel, autos, meat packing, police, or fire. To the authors, at least, this is additional evidence to support the thesis that it is the nature of the employment relationship that leads to unionization, that the grievances of workers with respect to that environment appear to be generic, and that they become manifest in similar contractual provisions and language.

On the basis of these findings, it is likely that in the future hospital managers may feel safe monitoring general trends in health care by following published reports of all-industry developments such as those in BNA's *Basic Patterns in Union Contracts* or the Bureau of Labor Statistics' *Current Wage Developments*. For the resolution of local issues in bargaining, however, managers still will require a detailed analysis of contract provisions in their particular markets.

NOTES

1. *Basic Patterns in Union Contracts,* 8th and 9th eds. (Washington, D.C.: Bureau of National Affairs, 1975 and 1976). These analyses are derived from 400 labor contracts from 5,000 in all industries. The all-industry frequency figures used here are based on those contracts. BNA cautions that this sample may not approximate patterns in the private unionized sector. (The 1974 hospital data are from tables in a paper presented by the senior author at the 1977 Annual Spring meeting of the Industrial Relations Research Association and reprinted in the *Labor Law Journal* (published by the Commerce Clearing House), August 1977, pp. 504–511.)

2. *Professional contracts* are defined as those covering units that include some or all of the following: registered nurses, physicians, house staff, social workers, dieticians, and allied professionals. *Nonprofessionals* refer to service, maintenance, and clerical occupations. *Technical* unit personnel include x-ray and laboratory technicians, licensed practical nurses, and similar occupations. *Combined* means a unit with two or more of the first three classifications—for example, a unit of L.P.N.s and service employees. *Control* and *Region* are defined in Tables 2-1 and 2-2.

3. Health Care Industry under the National Labor Relations Act

SAMUEL M. KAYNARD

*The comments in this article are the personal opinions of the author and are not to be construed as any official statements of the National Labor Relations Board or the General Counsel of the NLRB.

INTRODUCTION

On August 25, 1974, a Sunday, the health care institution amendments to the National Labor Relations Act (referred to as the NLRA or the act) took effect and extended its coverage to some 1.4 million employees. These amendments repealed the exemption incorporated into the act in 1947 and brought health care institutions under its umbrella. The amended act now embraces employers, labor organizations, and employees in the health care industry in the private sector, excluding municipal, state, and federal institutions.

The interpretation and implementation of these amendments by the National Labor Relations Board (NLRB) has generated much controversy, in part because of the nature of the development of collective bargaining in the health care industry, particularly in nonprofit hospitals by virtue of their exemption from the act since 1947 and their coverage under state labor relations laws and other legislation applicable to them.

These factors involved inclusion of supervisors and guards in units; proliferation of units; the development of the law relating to for-profit and proprietary hospitals and nursing homes and charitable institutions under the act; the particular nature of the institutions themselves and the nature of their personnel, such as M.D.s, Registered Nurses (R.N.s), Licensed Practical Nurses (L.P.N.s), professionals, etc. Most interestingly, the controversy has been heightened by the hopes and aspirations, perhaps now somewhat deflated, of those who sought the amendments that the act would provide a cure for the problems and difficulties that confronted them in collective bargaining outside its coverage or "protection."

Some of the issues that have generated controversy are:

- Which health care institutions are subject to the jurisdiction of the act under the amendments?
- What is the impact of public funds?
- What is the impact of the First Amendment and freedom of religion?
- What are the appropriate units for collective bargaining in the industry—"wall to wall" overall units?
- What breakdown among the different categories of employees is fair and effective from the viewpoint of the workers and the health care institution and are such units consistent with the intent of the amendments?
- Are registered nurses sufficiently separate to warrant a unit apart from other professionals?
- Can the nurses' associations, which historically have included supervisors in their higher echelons, represent such nurses?
- Are interns and residents "employees" and therefore covered by the act or "students" and not within its purview?

537

- Should the board carve out certain maintenance "craft" groups of employees and separate them from other service and maintenance personnel?
- Perhaps, most important of all, what limits are to be imposed upon the unions in striking and/or picketing health care institutions?[1]

In the years that the health care amendments have been in existence, the NLRB and the courts have addressed these and other issues; some have been resolved, some remain subject to final resolution, most still are the subject of philosophical, practical, and legal differences.

JURISDICTION AND COVERAGE

Threshold issues confronting the NLRB were the questions of which organizations were covered by the term "health care institution" and what monetary jurisdictional requirement, if any, must such institutions satisfy.

Health Care Institution

The amendments introduced a new term—health care institution. In 1935, when the NLRA (the Wagner Act) was passed, there was no exemption from its coverage relating to hospitals or health care institutions.[2] In 1947, when the Wagner Act was amended by the Labor Management Relations Act (Taft-Hartley), the definition of the term "employer" (Section 2(2)) was changed to exclude "any corporation or association operating a hospital, if no part of the net earnings inures to the benefit of any private shareholder or individual. . . ." This removed nonprofit hospitals from the statutory jurisdiction of the act; however, proprietary institutions remained covered. The NLRB, using its discretion, for the most part did not exercise such jurisdiction until 1967 when it concluded that it would effectuate the purposes of the act to do so.[3]

In 1974, although the thrust of the legislation was to bring back under the act the not-for-profit, voluntary hospitals, the amendments actually encompassed the "health care institution," which was defined (Section 2(14)) to include "any hospital, convalescent hospital, health clinic, nursing home, extended care facility, or other institution devoted to the care of sick, infirm or aged persons."

In determining which facilities come under health care institution, the board has asserted jurisdiction not only over hospitals and nursing homes but also over other facilities it had declined to encompass on the ground that they were not health care institutions or

because their activities were purely local in nature. Thus, the board now has asserted jurisdiction over outpatient clinics engaged in providing abortion and gynecological care services,[4] a for-profit community hemodialysis unit,[5] day care facilities,[6] half-way houses,[7] homes for retarded persons,[8] dental facilities,[9] practice of medicine by doctors,[10] treatment facilities for adolescents involved in drug or alcohol abuse,[11] facilities for rehabilitation of drug abusers,[12] and homes for neglected and/or disturbed children.[13]

The board has refused to cover under health care institutions organizations that are vocational rather than medical in nature[14] but has asserted jurisdiction over a facility whose purpose is rehabilitation rather than institutionalization.[15] Nor, according to the legislative history, is the term "health care institution" intended to cover "purely administrative health connected facilities" such as insurance companies specializing in medical coverage; Blue Cross; Blue Shield; commercially operated health spas, diet clinics, or muscle building organizations; medical laboratories testing human medical specimens;[16] diagnostic medical laboratories conducting tests for hospitals, nursing homes, clinics, doctors;[17] or blood banks.[18]

JURISDICTIONAL STANDARDS

The board established, in *East Oakland Community Health Alliance, Inc.*,[19] the discretionary standards for assertion of jurisdiction over health care institutions: gross annual revenue of $100,000 for nursing homes, visiting nurse associations, and related facilities, and $250,000 for hospitals and all other types of health institutions.[20]

In determining whether to assert jurisdiction over a health care facility, the board has been called upon to assess various factors, including the impact of the infusion of public funds into the institution, and whether the relationship and close ties of the government to the institution require nonassertion of jurisdiction as an exempt public employer under the act.[21] In the past, the board was guided by whether there was an "intimate connection" between the institution and the government, in determining whether the employing entity shared the immunity of the related exempt institution.[22] The board since has abandoned the "intimate connection test" and has substituted the twofold test: "whether the employer itself meets the definition of 'employer' in Section 2(2) of the Act, and, if so, determine whether the employer has *sufficient control over the employment conditions of its employees to enable it to bargain with a labor organization as their representative*"[23] (emphasis supplied).

The board has applied the new *National Transportation* test to assert jurisdiction over health care institutions despite the "close ties to an exempt government entity"[23a] or the fiscal control by and accountability to the State,[23b] where the facts disclose that the health care has "autonomy in determining its employer-employee relations policies"[23c] and "retains sufficient control over the employment conditions of its employees to enable it to bargain with a labor organization as the representative of its employees,"[23d] e.g., "can negotiate and has contracted concerning a large range of non-cost items,"[23e] the governmental limitations "do not prohibit the (institution) from granting increased wages and benefits."[23f]

Similarly, the board has been confronted with the impact of the First Amendment of the Constitution on the issue of the assertion of jurisdiction over a hospital which was operated by a religious order. Thus, in *St. Elizabeth Community Hospital*,[24] the Board rejected the contention "that the Board lacked jurisdiction over (the Hospital) because the application of the Act to (the Hospital's) operations violates both the free exercise and establishment clauses of the first amendment of the Constitution." That decision was prior to the Supreme Court's decision in *The Catholic Bishop of Chicago v. NLRB*,[25] which presented a similar issue in the context of a university.

In *The Catholic Bishop of Chicago*, the Supreme Court rejected the board's assertion of jurisdiction over church-operated schools "in the absence of a clear expression of Congress' intent to bring teachers in church-operated schools within the jurisdiction of the Board." The Court declined "to construe the Act in a manner that could in turn call upon the Court to resolve difficult and sensitive questions arising out of the guarantees of the First Amendment religious clauses."

Following the Court decision in *Catholic Bishop of Chicago*, the board has restated its conclusion that the legislative history of the act "manifests a clearly expressed affirmative intention that the Board assert jurisdiction" over a health care institution that is owned by and functions as an arm of a church (here, the Seventh Day Adventist Church) and "such an intention was expressed in the legislative history" of the 1974 amendments.[26]

NO-SOLICITATION/NO-DISTRIBUTION RULES

One of the fundamental issues presented by the act, from its very inception, has been the clash between the right of private property and the rights of an employee

under Section 7 to "self-organization, to form, join or assist labor organizations . . . and to engage in other concerted activities . . . and the right to refrain from any or all of such activities . . ." on the property of the employer during working hours.

Is the common law action of trespass superseded by the right to organize and the concomitant rights arising under the First Amendment? Can the employer tell employees: "This is my property. While you are working for me, while you are on my property, you cannot engage in union activities"? Can the employer tell the union and its organizers: "This is my property. Get off it. Don't come on my property. If you trespass, I will have you arrested"? Can the employee reply: "I have rights also. I have a right to engage in union activities. I will do so on my time, even on your property"? Can unions assert: "We have a right to come on your property and solicit your employees. That's the only way we can reach them"?

The accommodation between these two obviously divergent rights has been made in broad terms by both the board and the courts.[27] As a result, the employer's right to use and restrict private property has been recognized but the absolute right to that private property has been tempered somewhat to give effect to the right of the employee and the union to engage in union and other concerted activities. In simple terms, which is always dangerous and rarely simple, the accommodation may be stated as follows:

"Employees: work time is for work; nonwork time (lunch time, coffee breaks, etc.) is employees' time. You can talk 'union' during your nonwork time. You can distribute your union literature on nonwork time but only in nonworking areas."

"Union: private property is private property, but under special circumstances, if you demonstrate that you truly cannot reach the employees, you may come on my property under limited conditions. But don't abuse the privilege."

"Employer: be careful, you cannot 'post' your property completely during working hours against union activity by employees or unions. The threat to arrest cannot be made loosely."

Tranquility and Employee/Union Rights

Needless to say, as indicated, the simply stated rules become subject to various refinements by the board and the courts, e.g., a distinction between oral solicitation and distribution of materials, working hours vs. working time, work areas vs. nonwork areas, rules promulgated or applied discriminatorily, special rules for special enterprises (retail establishments), rules governing areas open to the public, activities by employees and by nonemployees or off-duty employees, etc.

It is not surprising, therefore, that one of the prime concerns of health care institutions was the extent to which they could promulgate no-solicitation, no-distribution rules and thus limit, inter alia, union activity on their premises. The institutions argued that the nature of their operations—providing patient care—mandated broad no-solicitation, no-distribution rules so as to limit and severely restrict union activities on the premises. Asserting their prime concern for patient care, the hospitals wanted to be "sanitized" and "antiseptic," free from union activities on their premises. The hospitals sought generally the right to ban such activities by employees and union organizers to ensure patient care free from outside distractions, pressures, and disturbances, which they felt was a natural concomitant of such activity.

The board recognized that "the primary function of a hospital is patient care and that a tranquil atmosphere is necessary to carrying out that function."[28] But it also recognized that not all hospital and health care personnel were involved directly in patient care, that for every person "above ground" who is involved in patient care there are others involved in indirect services "below ground" not in direct contact with patients; while certain areas of the hospital are involved directly in patient care and should be free from such possible intervention, there are other areas where such activity would not affect patients adversely.

The board undertook to accommodate the need for a "tranquil atmosphere" and the right of employees to engage in concerted or union activities, distinguishing between patient care areas and other areas in the hospital. Thus, "a hospital may be warranted in prohibiting solicitation even on nonworking time in *strictly patient care areas,* such as the patients' rooms, operating rooms, and in places where patients receive treatment, such as x-ray and therapy areas. Solicitation at any time in those areas might be unsettling to the patients—particularly those who are seriously ill and thus need quiet and peace of mind. Consequently, banning solicitation on nonworking time in such areas as described above would seem justified in hospitals. . . ." (Emphasis supplied.)

As to other nonpatient care areas where visitors and patients have access, the board concluded that "the possibility of any disruption in patient care resulting from solicitation or distribution of literature is remote. As to the restrictions in *patient access areas* such as cafeterias, lounges, and the like, we do not perceive how patients would be affected adversely by such activities. On balance, the interests of patients well enough to frequent such areas do not outweigh those

of the employees to discuss or solicit union representation." (Emphasis supplied.) The board thus concluded that hospitals may be justified in imposing somewhat more stringent prohibitions on solicitations than are generally prohibited. However, the board indicated that these were presumptions and that a hospital may be able to impose more stringent rules if it can establish the need for them, i.e., showing a disruption to patients.

The Supreme Court's Decisions

Beth Israel Hospital

The Supreme Court generally upheld the board's no-solicitation and no-distribution rules and presumptions as applied to health care institutions, with some caveats. In the *Beth Israel* case,[29] the hospital had promulgated a rule that permitted employees to solicit and distribute literature on nonworking time in "employee locker rooms and certain adjacent rest rooms. Elsewhere within the Hospital, including patient-care and all other work areas, and areas open to the public such as lobbies, cafeteria and coffee shop, corridors, elevators, gift shop, etc., there is to be no solicitation nor distribution of literature."[30] The board held that while a hospital could prohibit solicitation and distribution in "immediate patient care areas," it could not limit such activity in lounges and cafeterias, absent a showing of disruption to patients. The NLRB required, inter alia, that the hospital "rescind its written rule prohibiting distribution of union literature and union solicitation in its cafeteria and coffee shop." The narrow question presented to the Court was the propriety of the board's order requiring the hospital to rescind the rules as applied to the cafeteria and coffee shop.

A five-member majority of the Court concluded that the board had properly found that a ban on solicitation in the cafeteria, a "natural gathering area for employees," was unlawful. However, although upholding the board, the Court issued a caveat: that the interest of providing health care to patients may require the board to use "a more finely calibrated scale" in applying its rules. Thus, the Court noted that "the availability of one part of a health care facility for organizational activity might be regarded as a factor required to be considered in evaluating the permissibility of restrictions in other areas of the same facility." Accordingly, inasmuch as *Beth Israel* involved only the cafeteria and coffee areas of the hospital, the Supreme Court did not discuss the *St. John's* general rules and presumptions and the scope of "immediate patient care areas." The Court spoke to those issues in *Baptist Hospital*.

Baptist Hospital

In the *Baptist Hospital* case, the hospital had barred solicitation in all areas open to patients or visitors. The board concluded that the rule was overly broad and that the hospital had not overcome the presumption that such a rule was invalid insofar as it applied to solicitation outside "immediate patient care areas." The Court of Appeals for the Sixth Circuit[31] denied enforcement of the board's order. That court found that the hospital had presented sufficient evidence of ill effects on patient care to justify its broad no-solicitation rule in all areas.

The Supreme Court,[32] by an 8-1 majority, agreed in part with the hospital and the Sixth Circuit and in part with the board. Thus, the Court generally approved the board's rules and presumptions regarding no-solicitation, no-distribution rules. It agreed with the board that, with regard to the cafeteria, gift shop, and ground lobbies, the hospital had failed to supply sufficient evidence to establish that activity in those areas was harmful to patient care. But the Court agreed with the hospital and the Sixth Circuit that, with respect to corridors and sitting rooms adjoining or accessible to patient rooms, there was substantial evidence to support the hospital's ban on solicitation, finding that the evidence indicated that those areas were involved in patient care and therapy. The Court further specifically noted "the availability of . . . alternative locations for solicitation" on nonwork time in other areas even under the hospital's no-solicitation rule. Though not dispositive, the Court pointed out, this lends support to the validity of the hospital's ban on such activities in other areas.

More important than the specific conclusions in *Baptist Hospital* is the approach the Supreme Court took in reviewing the NLRB conclusions. There were four separate concurring opinions and, although they agreed as to the result, they disagreed as to the weight to be given to the NLRB's "expertise" in the area.

The Court suggested that the board review "the scope and application of its presumption" and instructed the board to undertake a "continuous review of the usefulness of its presumption." Some of the justices stated that the "evidence of record in this case and other similar cases . . . cast serious doubt on a presumption as to hospitals so sweeping that it embraces solicitation in the corridors and sitting rooms on floors occupied by patients." To overcome the board's presumption, the Court pointed out that the hospital need only show that solicitation was likely either to

disrupt patient care or disturb patients. The Court declared: "Solicitation may disrupt patient care if it interferes with the health-care activities of doctors, nurses, and staff even though not conducted in the presence of patients. And solicitation that does not impede the efforts of those charged with the responsibility of caring for patients nonetheless may disturb patients exposed to it."

The Supreme Court cast serious doubt on the board's approach to the issue in hospitals, pointing out that "the experience to date raises serious doubts as to whether the Board's interpretation of its present presumption adequately takes into account the medical practices and methods of treatment incident to the delivery of patient care services in a modern hospital."

General Counsel's Guidelines

Since the *Baptist Hospital* decision, the NLRB has remanded for further hearing various cases involving no-solicitation, no-distribution rules to review evidence consistent with the Court's ruling. Similarly, all other cases involving similar issues must consider the questions raised by *Baptist Hospital*. Thus, the general counsel of the NLRB has suggested that "some of the factors that should be considered include the nature of the services rendered in each area; problems caused by the movement of patients or emergency equipment; physical separation of the area in question from patient-oriented areas; and whether an area of predominantly public or employee use also has an important patient-care function."[33]

Also to be used is a refinement and amplification of the extent and scope of "immediate patient care areas" to determine whether the term goes beyond areas mentioned in *St. John's,* namely, "patients' rooms, operating rooms, and places where patients receive treatment, such as x-ray and therapy areas;" and whether patient care areas include "such places as corridors adjacent to patients' rooms, operating rooms and treatment 'areas,' sitting rooms on patient floors accessible to or used by patients; and elevators or stairways used substantially to transport patients." Similarly, "special attention should be given to the availability of alternative channels of communications."

As indicated, there is a distinction between solicitation and distribution. As for solicitation, a rule is presumptively unlawful insofar as it prohibits such activity by employees during their nonworking time on the employer's premises other than in "immediate patient care areas" as modified by the Supreme Court in both *Beth Israel* and *Baptist Hospital*. A ban on employees' distribution of literature during working hours is presumptively lawful in all working areas as well as in immediate patient care areas.

Restraints on Nonemployees

Further, in assessing the propriety of no-solicitation, no-distribution rules in health care institutions, the rules have been viewed primarily from the viewpoint of employee activity in the hospital. However, as in other private sector institutions, the breadth of restrictions of such activities by nonemployees on the facility's premises or property likewise is of paramount concern. Generally, the board and the courts have applied more stringent rules to the activities of nonemployee organizers on private property. Thus, generally, an employer may prohibit nonemployee union organizers from distributing literature and soliciting on hospital property if the employees can be reached reasonably in any other manner.[34]

In *Babcock & Wilcox,* the Supreme Court held that "an employer may validly post his property against nonemployee distribution of union literature if reasonable efforts by the union through other available channels of communication will enable it to reach the employees with its message and if the employer's notice or order does not discriminate against the union by allowing other distribution."[35]

Other Distributions and Cafeteria

Query: What if a hospital has permitted community health-related solicitation or distribution on its premises and denied similar access to nonemployee union organizations?[36] Does that "discriminate against the union by allowing other distribution?"

In *Rochester General Hospital,*[37] the board held that "work-related activities that assisted the hospital in carrying out its community health care functions and responsibilities" did not constitute "disparate application of a valid no-solicitation, no-distribution rule as to require the [hospital] to waive its rule and permit access to its employees by nonemployee union organizers." This included such activities as Red Cross postering and blood collection in the hospital for the blood bank, postering of sales by a volunteer group that donates all the proceeds to the hospital, displaying of pharmaceutical products that doctors might prescribe and the hospital pharmacy therefore might purchase, and displaying of medical books of interest to the doctors.

Another question: If a hospital has a public coffee shop that is available to the public, can it exclude a nonemployee union organizer from that cafeteria?

Some guidance can be found in the board's decision involving a public restaurant in a retail establishment. In *Marshall Field & Company,*[38] the board disagreed with the employer's contention that prohibition of all solicitation in the store's public restaurant was lawful. The board found no violation in the circumstances there, however, because in practice the employer did permit nonemployee organizers to meet with its workers in the restaurant "by appointment" as long as the organizers did not circulate from table to table. The board ruled that, as distinguished from a blanket proscription, such restricted use of the restaurants would ensure that "solicitation is carried on in the public restaurant as an incident to the normal use of such facilities."

Applying this principle to hospitals, it may be argued that the hospital may preclude general union activity by a nonemployee in the public cafeteria, e.g., "table hopping," but may not preclude the union organizer from "meeting by appointment" there with employees. However, even in the "by appointment only" situation, the hospital may be able to exclude the organizer where the circumstances are such as to create a reasonable apprehension that the nonemployee would not comply with the "appointment only" rule, e.g., the organizer would violate the rule in other respects by soliciting employees in their work areas during their working time.

REPRESENTATION ELECTION PROCEEDINGS

Every industry regards itself to be sui generis and thus seeks to impress upon the board that special rules should be applied to it. The health care industry similarily has sought to impress the board with its distinctiveness. As discussed previously, hospitals made such an argument in connection with the propriety of their broad no-solicitation and no-distribution rules.

In the representation election area of the board's processes, the industry similarly has sought to distinguish itself from other commercial enterprises and to have special rules for itself. One of the major issues involves unit determinations in health care institutions. Needless to say, the determination of the appropriate collective bargaining unit is of uppermost importance in connection with organizational activities in health care institutions, and very often is the determining factor in the ultimate success of the union campaign. Hospitals have sought broad units, encompassing all or major segments of their personnel and have argued vociferously against proliferation of units.

In its efforts for special consideration, the health care industry has had some assists from the legislative history and some courts, as well as from the NLRB, but apparently not enough, according to some critics of the board.

"Due consideration should be given by the Board to preventing proliferation of bargaining units in the health care industry."[39] Thus did the House and Senate reports direct the board to act in the establishment of appropriate collective bargaining units in the health care industry.

In 1975, less than a year after the passage of health care amendments, the board issued a series of bargaining unit cases[40] and acknowledged the congressional directive. Thus, the board stated, "our consideration of all issues concerning the composition of appropriate units in the health care industry must necessarily take place against this background of avoidance of undue proliferation."[41]

The board established, generally, units of (1) professional employees, (2) registered nurses, (3) technical employees, (4) service and maintenance employees, (5) business office clericals, and (6) guards. Subsequently, the board, although adhering basically to those unit determinations, engrafted some modifications.

The NLRB's adherence to its unit pronouncements and subsequent modifications at times have provoked strong reactions by the courts, as well as from health care institutions.

Registered Nurses and Professional Employees

When the NLRB established guidelines in 1975 for unit determinations at health care institutions, it concluded that a unit of registered nurses (R.N.s) was appropriate "if they are so sought and so desire" in view of the fact that they have a singular history of representation and a unique separateness or community of interest not shared with other professional employees.[42]

The board expressly left open the question whether, in the absence of a separate petition seeking R.N.s, it would direct an election only in an overall professional unit, including registered nurses, or whether, if sought, it would find appropriate and direct an election in a unit of all professional employees, excluding R.N.s.[43]

The St. Francis Hospital Benchmark

In *St. Francis Hospital of Lynwood*,[44] the board reiterated its position that a unit of registered nurses was an appropriate entity. The facts and the nature of the proceedings are interesting and of importance, in view of the subsequent court action. St. Francis Hospital is a nonprofit institution that has 1,440 employees, including 220 registered nurses. The United Nurses Association filed a representation petition for a unit of R.N.s. At the representation hearing, the hospital argued that the unit should include all professional employees rather than only registered nurses and it sought to present evidence in support of that position.

The hearing officer refused to allow such evidence, relying upon the *Mercy Hospital* and *Methodist Hospital* cases (*supra,* n. 42) as establishing the propriety of separate units of registered nurses. The regional director sustained the exclusionary ruling of the hearing officer but permitted the hospital to make an offer of proof. The hospital did so but argued that it was necessarily limited. The regional director held that a unit of registered nurses was appropriate and again rejected the hospital's claim that the hearing officer had committed prejudicial error in refusing to admit evidence relating to the propriety of an overall professional unit. The board denied the hospital's request for review of the regional director's decision.

In the subsequent board-conducted election, the union won and was certified as to the exclusive bargaining representative of a unit of registered nurses. St. Francis refused to bargain with the union. The union filed an unfair labor practice charge and complaint was issued against the hospital. The hospital admitted its refusal to bargain but challenged the propriety of the unit and reiterated its previous arguments. The NLRB granted a motion for summary judgment and reaffirmed the refusal to admit evidence relating to the propriety of an all professional bargaining unit. The board ordered the hospital to bargain with the union on a unit of R.N.s.

The Court of Appeals for the Ninth Circuit[45] refused to enforce the board's order. The court was critical of the board's per se approach—that a bargaining unit of registered nurses was irrebuttably appropriate when sought in a nonprofit hospital—as being inconsistent with the congressional directive to prevent an undue proliferation of bargaining units in the health care industry. "This is not to say," the court stated, "that a determination of a bargaining unit composed exclusively of registered nurses can never be valid. Rather, the problem lies in a rule that such a unit is always valid and its concomitant procedural quirk which excludes any consideration of evidence to the contrary." Accordingly, the court remanded the case to the board for action, consistent with its opinion, to determine the appropriate unit, based upon a full independent evaluation of all the factors and evidence. The board has accepted the remand of the case, and the hearing has been reopened to take additional testimony on the issue of the propriety of a unit of registered nurses at that hospital.

It must be emphasized that the court did not conclude that the board could not find a unit of registered nurses appropriate. While rejecting the board's policy of approving units limited to R.N.s, the court's criticism was directed primarily at the fact that the hospital was not permitted to introduce evidence to demonstrate that an R.N. unit was inappropriate there. Despite its differences with the board on the basis for unit determinations in the health care industry,[46] the court did state that the NLRB could find a bargaining unit of R.N.s appropriate if one were sought "so long as it is clear in each case that a proper determination had been made" and that the board could use presumptions "so long as the interested parties are given the opportunity to effectively present evidence to rebut the presumption."

Thus, the basic difference between the board and the court appears to be not on the appropriateness of a unit of registered nurses but rather on the elucidation of the basis for such findings in the particular health care institution under consideration and a rejection of a blanket per se unit determination. It would appear, then, that if on remand the board evaluates the evidence presented by the hospital and concludes that it does not demonstrate that a unit of R.N.s is inappropriate, the court still may enforce the board's order. But there is a caveat: the court did indicate some of the factors it regarded as important or unimportant and particularly took the board to task for relying on the "community of interest" in determining that a unit of R.N.s was appropriate.[47]

In considering this issue, it is necessary to be mindful of the Supreme Court's admonition to the NLRB in the *Beth Israel* and *Baptist Hospital* cases that the board's presumptions as to hospital no-solicitation, no-distribution rules must be considered against the background of evidence introduced by the institution relating to its particular circumstances, and the court's comment that the presumptions may be rebutted effectively on a case-by-case, location-by-location basis.

Newton-Wellesley Hospital

On July 31, 1980, the board apparently gave its answer to the Ninth Circuit on the registered nurses unit issue in *Newton-Wellesley Hospital*.[48] The board found a unit of R.N.s appropriate notwithstanding the hospital's contention that only a unit of all professional employees was appropriate. The board acceded in part to the Ninth Circuit's criticism in *St. Francis Hospital*, and concluded that "so much of the Board's *St. Francis* decision as may be read to establish an irrebuttable

presumption of the appropriateness of registered nurse units in all cases, without regard to particular circumstances, should be disavowed and that (s)uch a *per se* approach to unit determinations is inconsistent with the Board's Section 9(b) responsibility to decide 'in each case' whether the requested unit is appropriate." However, to the court's rejection of the NLRB's application of the traditional "community-of-interest" test in the health care industry, the board noted that "the court's disagreement with our approach may be largely semantic."

The board stated: "Our inquiry—though perhaps not articulated in every case—necessarily proceeds to a further determination whether the interests of the group sought are sufficiently distinct from those of other employees to warrant the establishment of a separate unit. We respectfully suggest that, at least to that extent, the test of disparateness described by the court is, in practice, already encompassed logically within the community-of-interest test as we historically have applied it, and, accordingly, we interpret the court's direction to the Board to be one of emphasis or degree, and not embracing a distinction of kind."

Noting that "at the time the 1974 amendments were passed, the Board had utilized the community-of-interest test for 39 years," the NLRB concluded that the amendments did not require it to forego consideration of that standard in such health care cases; however, it did recognize that any "community-of-interest" evaluation must accommodate the congressional admonition to avoid proliferation of bargaining units in that field.

The board has continued to follow the policy enunciated in *Newton-Wellesley* and assessed the appropriateness of a separate unit of registered nurses in light of the facts of each case. Thus in *Mount Airy Foundation d/b/a Mount Airy Psychiatric Center*,[48a] the board concludes that, under the facts of that case, the separate unit of registered nurses sought by the petitioner therein was inappropriate and the unit must include the non-nurse team leaders who hold master's degrees and charge nurses who are not registered nurses but hold master's degrees.

Registered Nurses As Supervisors

A collateral issue that has been presented by the organizing efforts of registered nurses is their status as supervisors under the act and the impact of that status on the entities seeking to be certified as their bargaining representatives.

In a health care institution, registered nurses often are classified as supervisory nurses, charge nurses, or head nurses and in the performance of their duties may direct their attention and actions not only vis-à-vis patients or other nurses, but also upon other hospital personnel, e.g., licensed practical nurses, aides, therapists, etc. Thus, the question may be presented whether particular nurses are supervisors within the meaning of the act and so generally not covered as employees. In reaching such a determination, the board has applied its traditional tests, namely, whether the nurse exercises any of the traditional indicia of supervisory authority vis-à-vis nurses under Section 2(11), e.g., authority to make effective recommendations as to hiring, firing, assignment, transfer, discipline, or directing nurses that are not routine in nature but require exercising independent judgment, etc.

However, in so assessing the supervising status of nurses, the board has distinguished the performance of supervisory activities from the duties and functions that are the "exercise of professional judgment" incidental to their proper and efficient treatment of patients; in the latter event the nurses are not supervisors under the act.[49] Similarly, as indicated, the duties of R.N.s extend beyond their relationship to other nurses in the unit, impact upon other hospital personnel, and may reflect the exercise of "supervisory authority" over such nonnurse personnel. In determining whether such exercise of supervisory authority vis-à-vis nonunit personnel (e.g., L.P.N.s, aides, orderlies, clericals) is sufficient to classify such nurses as supervisors under the act, the board has applied the *Adelphi* rule,[50] namely, individuals who do not spend 50 percent of their time in supervising duties of nonunit individuals are not supervisors in their unit.

Qualification for Certification

The supervisory status of nurses and their organization into associations for the purpose of bargaining has raised the question of the qualification of such entities for certification under the NLRA in view of the fact that such groups may have supervisory R.N.s as members and officers. Can an organization that admits supervisors to membership and has them among its officers be certified as a collective bargaining representative for nonsupervisory personnel?

Preliminarily, some basic observations are in order. The board has recognized that units and contracts that include supervisors are not unlawful per se. Similarly, the inclusion of supervisors as members of a labor organization does not, in and of itself, render that union unlawful or disqualify it as such within the meaning of the act.[51] The conclusions may vary depending in part upon the numerical ratio of supervisors, the nature of the participation, and the duties and functions they

seek to perform in the collective bargaining relationship.[52]

The board has considered under what circumstances such labor organizations could qualify or be disqualified, for certification.[53] The issue surfaced again when nurses' groups affiliated with the American Nurses' Association, Inc. (ANA) sought an election and certification as the collective bargaining representative of a unit of R.N.s. The history and development of the doctrine by the board and the courts are interesting.

In *Anne Arundel I*,[54] the Maryland Nurses' Association, Inc. (MNA) and the ANA filed a petition for certification of a unit of registered nurses at Anne Arundel General Hospital. The hospital contended that the MNA was not a bona fide labor organization within the meaning of the act because it was influenced, dominated, and controlled by supervisors, inasmuch as its officers and directors included supervisors.

The board concluded that MNA was a bona fide labor organization "inasmuch as the Petitioner, through its Anne Arundel Professional Chapter, has delegated its collective-bargaining authority respecting the Employer's employees to its Anne Arundel Hospital Professional Chapter, independent of ANA or other MNA influences, and as that chapter admits no supervisors to its membership, and has no employer supervisors as its officers or directors," the board concluded that MNA "in its collective-bargaining process is not subject to the influence, domination, or control of supervisors as defined in the Act."[55]

Subsequently, the board certified the MNA and directed the hospital to bargain with it.[56] The U.S. Court of Appeals for the Fourth Circuit, on August 31, 1977, denied enforcement of the board's order.[57] The court majority found that "delegation of the bargaining function to [the local Anne Arundel Professional Chapter] was *sine qua non* to certification of MNA;" by issuing such "conditional certification," the board was seeking to avoid "the difficult problem of whether an employer can be forced to bargain with a labor organization which allows the employer's supervisors to be members." The court concluded that the act required that the "certified labor organization be willing and able to bargain" and prohibited the NLRB "from certifying MNA to bargain on condition that it not bargain." It found that the board in effect had certified a "different labor organization than that petitioning." The court concluded that the board had exceeded its authority inasmuch as "under the Act the Board may not certify a bargaining agent on condition that it not bargain."

The dissent by Judge Hall, adopting the unpublished panel opinion of the late Judge Craven (*supra*, n. 57), argued that the employer was attempting "to turn the statutory offense of 'employer domination' into an excuse for refusing to bargain;'' that a holding that the presence of other employers' supervisors "somehow flaws the integrity of the bargaining representative" could be based only upon some conflict of interest, and that the employer failed to show that a real or potential conflict of interest existed.

While the *Anne Arundel* case was going through its board and court processes, the NLRB had before it a petition filed by the California Nurses' Association (CNA), a/w ANA, involving a unit of registered nurses at Sierra Vista Hospital, Inc. In *Sierra Vista I*,[58] the board on August 31, 1976, had reaffirmed its certification of CNA, finding in accord with *Anne Arundel* that the CNA had "effectively delegated its collective bargaining authority, which it had acquired by virtue of the Board's certification here, to an autonomous local unit of non-supervisory registered nurses, and that said local is properly exercising this authority on its behalf." Subsequently, the board in *Sierra Vista II*[59] directed the hospital to bargain with CNA.

'Present Danger' or *'Conflict of Interest' Principle*

When the Fourth Circuit issued its decision in *Anne Arundel* rejecting the board's "conditional certification" principle, the NLRB reconsidered the principle in *Sierra Vista* and issued a supplemental decision, referred to as *Sierra Vista III*.[60] The board abandoned the *Anne Arundel* doctrine and concluded that it "will not condition certification of nurses' associations on the delegation of their bargaining authority to autonomous chapters of locals." In its place, the NLRB established a "present danger" or "conflict-of-interest" test, with the burden on the employer to establish that the presence of supervisors in the labor organization seeking certification created such "danger" or "conflict," a concept found in Judge Hall's dissent in *Anne Arundel*.

On the one hand, the NLRB held that a nurses' association is a labor organization under the act as long as it exists for the purpose of bargaining and admitting employees to membership although it accepts supervisors, even in substantial numbers.

On the other hand, the board recognized that such a labor union may be disqualified from NLRB certification and bargaining rights because of a potential conflict of interest resulting from the admission of supervisors and the role they play in the organization. This potential for disqualification steme from the statutory right "employees have to be represented in collective bargaining negotiations by individuals who have a single-minded loyalty to their interests" and the possi-

ble conflict created when "supervisors admitted to membership in a labor organization can, in certain circumstances, compromise that statutory interest."

In considering the possible "danger" or "conflict," a distinction is to be made between a nurses' association that (1) has supervisors of the employer involved in the NLRB certification proceeding and (2) has supervisors of an employer otter than the employer involved in the proceedings.

Thus, in the first situation, "active participation in the affairs of a labor organization by supervisors employed by the employer with whom that labor organization seeks to bargain can give rise to questions about the labor organization's ability to deal with the employer at arm's length."[61]

In the second situation, "the active, internal union participation of supervisors of a third-party employer (i.e., an employer other than the one with whom the labor organization seeks to bargain) does not present the danger that an employer may be 'bargaining with itself.' But it may operate, nonetheless, to disqualify a labor organization from acting as a bargaining representative for particular employees. Although, in such cases, the legitimate interest of an employer in the loyalty of its supervisors is not in issue (the active supervisors are not its own), the presence of supervisors of third-party employers may impinge upon the employees' right to a bargaining representative whose undivided concern is for their interests. Not because, . . . there is an inherent conflict between all supervisors and all employees, but because of the possible relations between the employer with whom bargaining is sought and the employer or employers of the supervisor participating in the bargaining process."[62]

Accordingly, in view of the membership and participation of supervisors in the nurses' association, the board established, in place of the "conditional certification" doctrine, the "conflict-of-interest" test. The disqualification of the association as representing a unit of nurses "would depend on a demonstrated connection between the employer of those unit employees and the employer or employers of those supervisors and, with respect to this possibility, we stress that the participation of supervisors (of third-party employers), even if constituting a majority of a nurses' association's board of directors, would not in and of itself necessarily require disqualification, absent some other demonstrated conflict of interest, for we do not assume an 'inherent' conflict between supervisors and employees in the bargaining process." The burden is to establish such a conflict of interest; absent meeting such burden, the association would not be disqualified for certification, notwithstanding the presence of supervisors in that organization and among its officers.

Finally, there is the procedural issue whether such supervisory participation in the affairs of the labor organization can be litigated in the representation hearing. The board[63] concluded that it was a proper forum, even though such issues may involve unfair labor practice matters such as employer domination or interference with or assistance to labor organizations in violation of Section 8(a)(2). The NLRB, in the representation case, will consider evidence to determine whether there is a "clear and present danger" of conflict of interest that compromises the association's bargaining integrity.

The board has applied the *Sierra Vista* "conflict of interest" test in subsequent cases involving various nurses" associations and similar organizations. Thus, in the *Sierra Vista* case itself, in order to provide the parties with an opportunity to fully litigate the conflict of interest issue, the Board rescinded its denial of the hospital's earlier motion to revoke California Nurses' Association's (CNA) certification and its decision granting the General Counsel's Motion for Summary Judgment and remanded the case to the Regional Director for a hearing to determine issues raised by the hospital's motion to revoke CNA's certification, namely, whether or not the presence of supervisors as officers in, on the board of directors of, or in other positions to speak for or bargain on behalf of CNA disqualifies that association as the collective bargaining representative of the hospital's nonsupervisory nurses.

Pursuant to the board's remand order, a hearing was conducted, but the hospital declined to produce any evidence, taking the position that the board's decision to remand the case for further hearing "constituted an attempt by the Board to improve its chances of prevailing in the court of appeals in the related unfair labor practice case against the (hospital). The (hospital) further objected to being called into a hearing controlled by what it characterized as its 'adversary.'" The hearing closed with taking of evidence.

Thereafter, the board concluded that, inasmuch as it is the employer's burden to prove that there is a clear and present danger of conflict of interest, Sierra Vista Hospital had failed to meet the burden of proving a conflict of interest sufficient to prevent CNA from representing the registered nurses at Sierra Vista Hospital and, accordingly, the board denied the motion to revoke the certification previously issued to CNA.[63a]

In other cases, the board has similarly evaluated the conflict of interest issue on the particular facts in each case and has concluded that a particular labor organization is or is not qualified to act as the collective bargaining representative. Thus, e.g., the labor organization was found not to be disqualified in *Baptist Hospitals, Inc. d/b/a Western Baptist Hospital* (Kentucky Nurses' Association), 246 NLRB No. 25 (1979); *Lancaster Osteopathic Hospital Association, Inc.* (Pennsylvania Nurses Association), 246 NLRB No. 96 (1979); *The Arlington Hospital Association, Inc., t/a Arlington Hospital* (District of Columbia Nurses Association a/w American Nurses Association), 246 NLRB No. 159 (1979); *The Sidney Farber Cancer Institute* (Massachusetts Nurses Association), 247 NLRB No. 1 (1980); *Healdsburg General Hospital* (California Nurses Association), 247 NLRB No. 30 (1980); *Lodi Memorial Hospital Association, Inc.* (California Nurses Association), 249 NLRB No. 121 (1980); *French Hospital Medical Center* (California Union of Health Care Professionals, Service Employees International Union, AFL-CIO, Local 723), 254 NLRB No. 83 (1981).

But, in *Exeter Hospital* (Exeter Hospital Nurse Subcommittee), 248 NLRB 377 (1980), the board found that the labor organization was not qualified to represent the employees for collective bargaining purposes. The board concluded that "the involvement of supervisors in the . . . organization presents a clear and present danger of a conflict of interest which would interfere with the collective bargaining process. By occupying the important office of chairperson and by serving as shift representatives, supervisors are clearly in a position to play a crucial role in the Petitioner's internal affairs. Consequently, permitting representation by the Petitioner would jeopardize the employees' right to a bargaining representative which is exclusively concerned with their interests, and the Employer's right to loyalty from its own supervisors."[63b]

A different kind of conflict of interest issue, wherein a health care institution sought to disqualify a nurses' association as the collective bargaining representative, was presented to the board in *Visiting Nurses Association, Inc., Serving Alameda County* (California Nurses Association a/w The American Nurses Association).[63c] In that case, the employer contended that there was a conflict of interest between the petitioner, California Nurses Association (CNA), and the employer, because the CNA was engaged in competition with the employer through the Nurses Professional Registry, Inc. (Registry) of the Alameda County Nurses Association (ACNA), which is one of the 10 regional associations comprising the CNA.

The Employer is a licensed home health care agency engaged, *inter alia*, in providing part-time registered nurses and home health care aides to homes in Alameda County and sends registered nurses to hospitals to engage in discharge planning for the patients. The Registry was established by the ACNA and directly employs health care practitioners who it places as temporary employees in hospitals, and it also acts as a placement agency for private duty care practitioners who work in patients' homes. The board concluded that, in accordance with its longstanding policy that "a union which is also a business rival of an employer is precluded from acting as the collective bargaining representative of the employer's employees,"[63d] the CNA was precluded from representing the employer's employees, inasmuch as the Registry, which is a creature of the ACNA, which in turn is a regional arm of the CNA, is in substantial competition with the employer in providing home nursing services.[63e]

Interns and Residents—'Employee' Status

One of the initial issues to confront the board under the amendments was whether certain house staff members of a hospital—interns, residents, and fellows—were employees under the act.[64] In its first decision on this matter, *Cedars-Sinai Medical Center*,[65] the board majority concluded that although interns, residents, and clinical fellows comprising a hospital house staff possessed "certain employee characteristics," they were "primarily engaged in graduate training" and "their status is therefore that of students rather than employees" as defined in the act."[66] The majority found "they participate in these programs not for the purpose of earning a living; instead they are there to pursue the graduate medical education that is a requirement for the practice of medicine."

The board dismissed the petition filed by the House Staff Association for an election in the unit of interns, residents, and fellows. In his dissent, Member Fanning argued that these persons were employees since they performed medical services, received payment for their services with federal and state monies, received fringe benefits, and received no grades or examinations. He stated, "Certainly, there is a didactic component to the work of any initiate, but simply because an individual is 'learning' while performing this service cannot possibly be said to mark that individual as 'primarily a student' and, therefore, not an 'employee' for purposes of our statute." The board continued to follow this precedent.[67]

Whereupon Physicians' National House Staff Association filed a petition asking the District Court for the District of Columbia to (1) vacate the NLRB's dismissal of various election certification petitions; (2) declare that house staff associations are labor organizations and their members employees under the act; and (3) order the board to assume jurisdiction. The NLRB moved to dismiss the suit on the ground that the federal district court did not have jurisdiction because the act provides for judicial review only of unfair labor practice orders of the board, as distinguished from orders relating to petitions for elections and certifications under the act. The district court granted the NLRB's motion to dismiss[68] for lack of jurisdiction, under the doctrine of *Leedom* v. *Kyne*,[69] which holds that that court does not have jurisdiction to review NLRB actions in representation election proceedings except in a very narrow area and that judicial review is limited to unfair labor practice orders.

The House Staff Association appealed to the U.S. Court of Appeals for the District of Columbia, asserting that the narrow exception of *Leedom* v. *Kyne* was applicable. Initially, a panel of the Court of Appeals reversed the lower court and concluded that the court did have jurisdiction under that exception. The panel concluded that in light of the legislative history of the health care amendments, house staff were employees and, accordingly, "as employees under the NLRA, house staff may not be deprived of rights 'assured to them by Congress' . . . . We reach this conclusion not on the basis of factual characteristics of the hospital industry or the work performed by house staff, but on the terms of the statute itself and its legislative history." However, in May 1979, upon application by the NLRB for reconsideration by the full court en banc, the Court of Appeals granted the motion for reconsideration and withdrew its opinion.

On July 11, 1980, the Court of Appeals by a five-to-four decision reversed the finding of its own three-member panel[70] and concluded that the NLRB had not exceeded its delegated powers when it ruled that hospital interns and residents were students and not employees subject to the NLRA; that the court was not empowered to review the board's decision, absent a showing that the board had acted without statutory authority; that Congress had not intended to classify house staff as employees when it enacted the 1974 amendments; and the defeat of H.R. 2222 in the House of Representatives in November 1979 that would specifically have overruled the board's decision in *Cedars-Sinai* demonstrated that Congress was satisfied with the board's decision.

The court declared, "The 1974 amendments gave the Board jurisdiction over private, non-profit hospitals. The National Labor Relations Act does not expressly command the Board to find that members of house staffs are employees. The decision is not reviewable in District Court."

The court acknowledged that the board's decision may never be reviewed. The dissenting judges argued that Congress had approved the amendments with the "clear assumption" that house staff doctors were employees; they also raised the propriety of the court-majority in improperly taking into account the action of the House in 1979 in determining the intention of the whole Congress in 1974. Physicians National House Staff Association v. Murphy (Fanning).[70a]

In view of the fact that the NLRA preempts state laws, plus the decision that interns and residents are not "employees" under the act but that hospitals are covered, interns and residents currently do not enjoy any rights or have any obligations under the NLRA or any state statutes. In the area of labor relations, it may be said that they are in a "no person" land.[71]

In considering the composition of a unit of professionals in the health care industry, thought must be given to the impact of the Supreme Court's decision in *Yeshiva*.[72] In this case, the board had certified a unit of faculty members of a large private university. The Court reversed, concluding that in view of the role played by the faculty members of that university on such matters as appointments, curriculum, degree requirements, and the like, they were managerial employees under the act and thus not subject to it. Thus, in hospitals where units may include doctors who are members of the teaching faculty and units of doctors who are members of the different departments and disciplines, it can be anticipated that some arguments may be advanced concerning their status as employees in light of the Supreme Court pronouncement in *Yeshiva*.

Service and Maintenance Employees

The board majority has established as appropriate a unit of service and maintenance employees.[73] In so concluding, it rejected the contention that the appropriate unit should be expanded to include technical employees (as argued by the employer and urged by the dissent). Similarly, in its initial determinations the board rejected overtures to establish, as appropriate, smaller units carved out of the service and maintenance unit. Thus, the board majority[74] found inappropriate a unit of stationary engineers, concluding that these engineers did not possess a community of interest sufficiently separate and distinct to remove them from a broader unit, particularly in view of the legislative history of the health care amendments. The dissents argued that the stationary engineers possessed an apparent singular homogeneous community of interest in and among themselves and enough apart from other employees to warrant a separate unit.

Subsequently, however, the majority concluded that such limited units may in fact be found appropriate, much to the dismay of the hospitals and some courts of appeals. The continuing dispute between the board, on the one hand, and the health care industry and the courts of appeals on the other hand, and the differences among board members on the issue of carrying out smaller "craft" type units from the overall service and maintenance groups, is reminiscent of the dispute in the 1940s in the American Federation of Labor between the industrial horizontal unions and the craft vertical unions that led ultimately to the establishment of and the split off of what became the Congress of Industrial Organizations. Whereas there, the dispute was within the unions, with the resultant rift between labor organizations, the differences here are between members of the board and between the board and the courts and health care institutions.

In *Allegheny I*,[75] a three-member panel of the board issued a decision on July 19, 1977, finding that it was proper to extend comity to the certification of the union in a unit of maintenance department employees, issued by the Pennsylvania Labor Relations Board (PLRB) prior to the official date of the NLRA health care amendments on August 25, 1974,[76] and that the hospital had unlawfully refused to bargain with the union. In so concluding, the board was called upon to consider the propriety of the unit determination of the PLRB under the NLRA inasmuch as the hospital contended, inter alia, that the PLRB-certified unit was inappropriate. The board concluded that such a limited unit of maintenance employees was consistent with its prior determinations in the health care industry.

The Boiler Operators Case

In a somewhat similar earlier case, the NLRB had found appropriate a unit of boiler operators and had directed St. Vincent's Hospital to bargain with the certified union. The board did so "on the basis of its traditional standards which have long recognized that units of licensed boiler room employees may constitute a separate appropriate unit."[77] St. Vincent's Hospital refused to bargain with the union and appealed the board's order to the Court of Appeals for the Third Circuit. On December 15, 1977, that Court denied enforcement of the board's order.[78] The court concluded that the NLRB's finding that the hospital's boiler operators were an appropriate collective bargaining group constituted an unwarranted proliferation of such units in this industry contrary to the intent of Congress, chided the board for its "inconsistent" decisions in determining such units and disagreed with the board's application of "traditional" standards to the health care industry.

In view of these comments,[79] the board reconsidered its *Allegheny* decision and subsequently issued a supplemental finding, *Allegheny II,*[80] in which it addressed itself in great detail in the court's criticisms. The board, "[a]fter carefully reconsidering the legislative history of the 1974 amendments . . . concluded that, with all due respect to the Court, Congress did not intend to prohibit such units" and did not "preclude the Board from relying on its traditional community of interest criteria in making unit determinations in the health care industry." The board reaffirmed its prior determination of a unit of maintenance department employees.

As expected, Allegheny General Hospital refused to abide by the board's directive to bargain and appealed to the Third Circuit. The court again rejected the board's order,[81] declaring that "the NLRB must respect the applicable decisions of the Court." In reaffirming its prior conclusion that the board unit determination was improper, the court pointed out that its decision was buttressed by the fact that the "United States Courts of Appeals for the Second and Seventh Circuits have recently refused to enforce Board orders that were based on the use of traditional bargaining unit standards to determine hospital bargaining units," citing *NLRB v. Mercy Hospital*[82] and *NLRB v. W. Suburban Hospital.*[83]

The Maintenance Employees Case

As indicated by the *Allegheny* decision, the third case worthy of note in this unit determination situation involved *Mercy Hospital* in the Second Circuit.[84] Here, too, the NLRB had certified a limited unit consisting of maintenance employees of the hospital. The Second Circuit denied enforcement of the board's order and remanded the case, pointing out that "[i]n its decision certifying the bargaining unit the Board did not discuss the weight—if any—which it gave to the Congressional admonition against the proliferation of bargaining units in the health care field. We therefore remand to the Board for consideration of the propriety of a standard affording appropriate deference to the mandate of Congress."

The court stated that, in the 1974 amendments, "Congress was expressing concern not only that health care institutions be spared the egregious unit proliferation of the construction trades but that less extreme unit fragmentation arising from application of usual industrial unit criteria could also impede effective delivery of health care services." Further, it said, "when the Board makes a unit determination for health care institution employees, traditional community of interest factors must be put in balance against the public interest in preventing fragmentation in the health care field." This requires an evaluation of the

factors in each particular hospital, and the board's "decision must specify 'the manner in which its unit determination . . . implement[s] or reflect[s]'" the congressional admonition against undue proliferation of units.

On April 14, 1980, the Supreme Court denied the board's petition for certiorari and the NLRB reconsidered *Mercy Hospital,* which was expected to be a vehicle for a further explication of its determination of units in the health care industry as the board made the "independent evaluation" required by the Second Circuit.[85]

In this connection it is important to note what the court did and did not do in *Mercy Hospital.* It rejected the board's position, articulated in *Allegheny II* (*supra,* n. 80), that Congress approved of the use of the traditional community-of-interest test in determining the appropriateness of bargaining units in health care institutions, and that the congressional admonition against undue proliferation of units was not directed against the use of the test but against the practice of allowing employees to be grouped according to craft skills and job functions. The Second Circuit did not hold that the board could find a separate maintenance unit. Rather, it said that such a determination could not be based solely on traditional community-of-interest considerations. In remanding the case, the court did not spell out what considerations it expected the board to weigh in order to overcome the injunction against undue proliferation or state the circumstances in which community of interest could override concern about undue proliferation.

Limited Maintenance or 'Craft' Units

What the board would do on this issue of limited maintenance or "craft" units in the health care industry in the face of rejections of its position by courts of appeals for three circuits[86] and perhaps even by the Supreme Court, was an interesting question.

Ordinarily, the Supreme Court's denial of certiorari does not mean that it agrees with the circuit court on the merits. However, in view of the fact that three circuits had disagreed with the NLRB on the legal issue and the board had sought certiorari to clarify an important point, it could be argued that the Supreme Court, in its refusal to hear the case, was agreeing with the circuit courts that the board had misinterpreted congressional intent concerning the admonition against proliferation of bargaining units in health care institutions and, perhaps, also indicating disagreement with the board's reliance on traditional "community-of-interest" principles in determining hospital units. It may be argued that the court did not mandate abandonment of the board's determination of limited maintenance units but rather required the NLRB to make such decisions on grounds other than the traditional "community of interest," on a case-by-case basis.

The board may have responded already to the criticisms of the circuit courts on the issue of undue proliferation, the per se argument, and the use of the "community of interest" in establishing units in the health care field.

Thus, on July 3, 1980, several months after the Supreme Court denied certiorari in the *Mercy Hospital* case (*supra,* n. 84), the board issued its decision in *Newton-Wellesley,*[87] involving a unit of nurses. In response to the Ninth Circuit on the issue of registered nurses (*St. Francis Hospital of Lynwood, supra* n. 44, 45), the NLRB reaffirmed the separate unit and commented that its difference with the court may be one of "semantics;" disavowed any per se rule in its unit determinations; and on the "community-of-interest" test, asserted that the 1974 amendments "clearly [do] not require the Board to forego consideration of the community of interest among employees within the health care industry" in making unit determinations. The board concluded with the observation, "we recognize that any community of interests evaluation must accommodate the admonition to avoid proliferation of bargaining units in the health care field. The Board's efforts to effect such an accommodation should be manifest . . . from the number of situations in which the Board has refused to approve units that, in any other context, would amount to appropriate units."[88]

Similarly, in fashioning appropriate collective bargaining units in nursing homes, as distinguished from hospitals, the board has not limited itself to the five, six, or seven units described above. Thus, it has found appropriate a unit of all nonprofessional employees in accordance with the agreement of the parties,[89] and a unit of R.N.s and L.P.N.s, as sought by the petitioner, although contested by the nursing home.[90]

In a 1980 case decided by the board prior to the denial of certiorari by the Supreme Court in *Mercy Hospital,* the NLRB majority, in finding appropriate a unit of the plant operations department in a hospital, commented that the "court's decisions in *Memorial Hospital, St. Vincent's,* and *Allegheny General* did not announce a *per se* rule prescribing certification of such a unit, but rather have reminded the Board that when exercising its discretion in determining bargaining units in the health care industry it has the added responsibility of balancing the employees' interest in adequate representation against the special consideration of avoiding disruption in that industry. Because of this extra consideration, we find that the nature of the

work performed and job responsibilities of all the plant operations employees . . . mandates their inclusion in the unit."[91] The board's decision was expected to go before the same Third Circuit Court on appeal.

Finally, the NLRB, either in an effort to stem the tide of adverse court decisions, to extend an olive branch to the health care industry, or to allay any fears that the board might proliferate units in the industry, in 1980 reiterated its commitment to the congressional admonition against proliferation of units.

It noted that "in the approximately six years since the passage of the health care amendments and the Board's initial entry into the determination of appropriate units in the industry, we have had frequent occasions to apply and reevaluate our original unit decisions in a variety of factual settings, and in the light of the arguments and briefs filed by a wide range of employers, unions and other interested parties. From them we have gained a better perspective on both the realities of employment in the health care industry and the impact of our unit determinations on that industry. Although individual Board members may differ about whether the maximum number of units that conceivably may be appropriate in the industry is four, five, six, or seven, we emphasize that . . . we cannot foresee any circumstances or combination of factors that would cause us to conclude that any additional units are appropriate in the industry.[92] Perhaps this will lay the matter to rest—possible but not probable.

Technical Employees

In *Barnert Memorial Hospital Center,*[93] the board majority found appropriate a unit of technical employees separate from service and maintenance workers; the dissenting members argued that the congressional mandate against proliferation of units required a broad unit encompassing technical employees along with the service and maintenance employees.

In *St. Catherine's Hospital of Dominican Sisters of Kenosha, Wisconsin, Inc.,*[94] the majority, cognizant of the warning against undue proliferation of units, found that licensed practical nurses should be included in the unit of technical employees. However, in *Bay Medical Center,*[95] on the basis of bargaining history by which the parties had voluntarily established a separate unit for practical nurses, the board majority made an exception and excluded the L.P.N.s from the technical unit found appropriate there, emphasizing that this was an exception restricted to the facts in the case.

Business Office Clericals

The NLRB decided that "in the health care field, as in the industrial sphere, there is some distinction between business office clericals, who perform mainly business type functions, and other types of clerical employees whose work is more closely related to the function performed by personnel in the service and maintenance unit.[96] Accordingly, the board found, as separately appropriate, units that consisted of business office clericals.[97] These units included switchboard operators; those involved in admitting, patient billing, and the credit department; accounts payable clerks, business office cashiers, and electronic data processing coordinators. The board excluded medical records employees and ward clerks, finding that they did not share a community of interest with the business office clericals but rather with a broader unit of service and maintenance employees.[98]

Unit Clarification

When hospitals and other health care institutions were not subject to the jurisdiction of the NLRA, either by virtue of the statutory exclusion or the board's self-imposed withholding of its authority, they were subject to various state laws and agencies governing their labor relations that had regulations different from those under the act, particularly for supervisors and guards. As a result, many of the collective bargaining agreements between hospitals and labor organizations included supervisors and guards in their units and coverage. When the 1974 amendments brought hospitals and health care institutions under the act, supervisors, guards, managerial persons, and independent contractors were excluded as employees under the NLRA.[99]

The act circumscribes the board's powers and authority with respect to guards: "the Board shall not . . . decide that any unit is appropriate for such purposes if it includes, together with other employees, any individual employed as a guard to enforce against employees and other persons rules to protect property of the employer or to protect the safety of persons on the employer's premises; but no labor organization shall be certified as the representative of employees in a bargaining unit of guards if such organization admits to membership, or is affiliated directly or indirectly with an organization which admits to membership, employees other than guards."[100] Indeed, one of the reasons that prompted hospitals to seek coverage under the NLRA was these differences and their desire to exclude such individuals from the bargaining agreements that covered their other personnel.

So, suppose after the effective date of the health care amendments (August 25, 1974) a hospital has a collective bargaining agreement covering its personnel that includes supervisors, managerial persons, guards,

and independent contractors. How can these individuals be excluded from the coverage of the contract? Of course, one method is to have the parties modify the contract to exclude them, a solution not always feasible. The problem is further complicated if the parties disagree as to whether these persons are, in fact, supervisors, guards, etc. A procedure available under the board's rules is the unit clarification (UC) proceeding.

Under the unit clarification procedure, a petition may be filed by the employer and/or labor organization in a collective bargaining relationship to exclude from the unit individuals who are not employees under the act, e.g., supervisors, managerial persons, independent contractors, or others who should not be included, i.e., guards. In this proceeding, the board is asked to determine the status of the contested individuals and, if required, to exclude them from the unit. The unit clarification proceeding cannot be used as a substitute for a representation petition; its function is to clarify the status of particular individuals or groups and, if necessary, "clarify" them in or out of the unit. A unit clarification petition should be filed toward the end of the contract period; the 60–90-day or 90–120-day rule governing the filing of representation petitions does not apply to unit clarification petitions.[101] Although no precise time frame is established for filing such petitions, they would be inappropriate when filed in the early or middle stages of a contract term when they would be disruptive of voluntarily continued bargaining relationships.[102] "Ordinarily such petitions are appropriately filed shortly before the expiration of the collective bargaining agreement. At that time, when the parties are preparing for negotiations on a new contract, unit clarification may spare them an unnecessary labor dispute."[103] Health care institutions have availed themselves of the unit clarification procedures developed by the board.[104]

TIMELINESS OF REPRESENTATION PETITION

The NLRB over the years has established basic rules for the timely filing of a representation petition for an election where there is a lawful collective bargaining agreement in effect covering the employees involved. The board has held that such a contract may be a bar to a petition for the duration of the contract, but at most for a three-year period.[105] Further, for a petition to be timely filed, it must be submitted more than 60 but not more than 90 days prior to the expiration of the contract covering the unit involved, subject to the three-year contract bar rule.[106] Thus, the present rules as to the timely filing of representation petitions permit a 30-day "open period" between the 90th and 60th days before expiration of the agreement, followed by a 60-day "insulated period" during which no petition can be timely filed. This insulated period coincides with the obligations under Section 8(d) of the act regarding the 60 days required for notices to the other parties of contract termination or modification and the 30 days required for notices to the mediation services. These requirements were designed to "prevent the threat of overhanging rivalry and uncertainty during the bargaining period."[107]

The 1974 amendments changed Section 8(d) specifically to provide that in collective bargaining contracts involving health care institutions, any party desiring to open the agreement must give at least 90 days' notice to the other party and 60 days' notice to the Federal Mediation and Conciliation Service before contract expiration.[108] In view of these requirements, "designed to encourage and facilitate bargaining between the parties during the 90 days prior to contract expiration and to promote the stability of on-going bargaining relationships," the board in *Trinity Lutheran Hospital*[109] modified the length of the insulated period for contracts in health care institutions to 90 days to coincide with the 90 days' notice provision. Accordingly, in any contract involving a health care institution, to be timely a petition must be filed more than 90 days but not over 120 days before the terminal date, subject, of course, to the three-year contract bar rule.

Union Security Provision

The act permits the parties to a collective bargaining agreement to negotiate and include in the contract a limited form of union security. Simply stated, the act permits a union security provision that requires an employee to become a member of the union that is the lawful collective bargaining representative after 30 days (seven days in the construction industry) and to maintain membership as a condition of employment.[110]

The union security provision may take the form of the 30-day union shop provision described above,[111] the agency shop provision,[112] or the maintenance of membership provision.[113] The obligation of membership under a union security provision can be complied with by the payment of dues and initiation fees.[114] As the Supreme Court stated in *NLRB v. General Motors Corp.*, "It is permissible to condition employment upon membership, but membership, insofar as it has significance to employment rights, may in turn be conditioned only upon payment of fees and dues. 'Membership' as a condition of employment is whittled down to its financial core."

In 1974, the amendments, apparently in consideration of "the problem of potential conflict between an employee's religious beliefs and collective bargaining responsibilities"[115] provided that workers' obligations under a union security provision in a health care institution under certain circumstances can be satisfied by payments to specified charitable organizations rather than as dues and initiation fees to the union. Thus Section 19 of the act states:

> Any employee of a health care institution who is a member of and adheres to established and traditional tenets or teachings of a bona fide religion, body, or sect which has historically held conscientious objections to joining or financially supporting labor organizations shall not be required to join or financially support any labor organization as a condition of employment; except that such employee may be required, in lieu of periodic dues and initiation fees, to pay sums equal to such dues and initiation fees to a nonreligious charitable fund exempt from taxation under section 501(c)(3) of the Internal Revenue Code, chosen by such employee from a list of at least three such funds, designated in a contract between such institution and a labor organization, or if the contract fails to designate such funds, then to any such fund chosen by the employee.

STRIKES AND/OR PICKETING

One of the prime concerns of Congress in considering legislation governing health care institutions was the effect of strikes and/or picketing upon their patients. To meet this problem and to minimize to some extent any possible adverse impact on patient care, Congress added Section 8(g) to the act and modified Section 8(d) insofar as it applies to health care institutions.

In enacting the 1974 amendments, Congress was concerned with two interests. On the one hand, it sought to give recognition to the right of employees of health care institutions, particularly nonprofit hospitals, to organize and bargain collectively as was granted to employees in other industries; on the other hand, it sought to recognize the need and grant protection to these institutions in order to assure continuity of patient care. In an effort to balance these interests, Congress extended and guaranteed bargaining rights to these employees and, at the same time, added Section

8(g) requiring a labor organization to give ten days' written notice before striking or picketing at a health care institution;[116] in addition, it modified Section 8(d) to extend the loss of employee status to workers who engage in a strike proscribed by Section 8(g),[117] and modified Section 8(d) notice requirements where such institutions are involved.[118]

The intent of Section 8(g) in requiring a labor organization to give at least 10 days' written notice to the institution and to the Federal Mediation and Conciliation Service before engaging in any strike, picketing or other concerted refusal to work was to give the health care institution time to prepare itself and its patients against the effects of such activities.

Several answered and unanswered questions have been raised as to the meaning and application of Section 8(g).

Threat to Strike or Picket

In his initial interpretation of Section 8(g), the general counsel of the NLRB argued that a threat to strike or picket came within the notice provisions of Section 8(g). The board disagreed in *Greater Pennsylvania Avenue Nursing Center, Inc.*[119] The facts are interesting. The labor organization involved was the collective bargaining representative of the service and maintenance employees of the proprietary nursing home. The collective bargaining contract provided that the union should have reasonable opportunity to visit the premises and confer with the employees. In February 1976, during an influenza epidemic, the nursing home decided to bar visitors from the home. When the ban was applied to a representative of the union, the union and the home discussed the situation. When the home persisted in its position in view of the epidemic, the union official announced he would strike the facility at 6 o'clock the next morning.

As a result of this threat, the home undertook intensive preparations to ensure continued operations in the event of a strike and to minimize the effects upon the patients. When the home asked union officials during the day whether there would be a strike, the answer was "maybe yes, maybe no." The union had not given prior written notification to the home or the Mediation Service of an intention to strike. In fact, no strike occurred.

The general counsel argued that the intent, purpose, and legislative history of Section 8(g) supported the conclusion that a threat came within the notice requirements of the section. The administrative law judge concluded to the contrary that neither the language nor the legislative history supported such a find-

ing but rather mandated for the opposite conclusion. The board adopted the administrative law judge's conclusion. Accordingly, a union's threat to engage in a strike or other economic action against a health care institution without complying with the ten-day notice provisions of Section 8(g) does not constitute a violation if the threat was not carried out.

However, it should be noted that while such a threat may not constitute a violation of Section 8(g), when made in conjunction with an organizing campaign or a demand for recognition, it may be relevant to establish a violation of Section 8(b)(7)(C) or to trigger an expedited election under certain circumstances.[120]

Strike/Picketing without Authorization

Section 8(g) appears, on its face, to apply only to striking or picketing by a labor organization. Query: Does the section's notice requirement apply to a work stoppage where no labor organization is involved and does such activity by workers result in a loss of employee status under Section 8(d) or subject them to discharge or other discipline?

In *Walker Methodist Residence & Health Care Center,*[121] the board was confronted with those issues and concluded that Section 8(g) applied only to strikes and picketing by a labor organization, that employees who engaged in such activity independently of their union did not lose their status as employees and, further, since they were engaged in protected concerted activity they could not be discharged for doing so.

In *Walker Methodist,* several nurses of the facility of approximately 500 patients became dissatisfied with understaffing of their evening shift and lack of supplies—matters that had been the subject of several discussions with the administration. On this day, four nurses' aides sought to discuss this grievance with the shift supervisor; she could not speak with them because she was "counting narcotics." The aides decided to leave the floor until the supervisor was ready to see them; they removed their name tags and went to the break room. Shortly thereafter, the supervisor discussed the grievance for about 10 or 15 minutes and they all returned to the floor and completed their shift. Two days later, two aides were discharged for "unauthorized absence from the floor."

The NLRB concluded that the language and legislative history of the amendments led to the conclusion that Section 8(g) applied only to striking or picketing by a labor organization and did not embrace any work stoppage by employees. "Congress was concerned that sudden, massive strikes [by labor organizations] could endanger the lives and health of patients in health care institutions. . . . A brief work stoppage by a few unorganized employees simply was not the type of disruption with which Congress was concerned.''

''The legislative history stresses that the purpose of the notice provision is to allow a health care institution to make arrangements for the continuity of patient care in the event of a strike or picketing by a labor organization,'' the board said, ''Placing the duties of advance warning on labor organization is warranted because a strike involving a labor organization is likely to last longer and involve a greater number of employees than a work stoppage by unorganized employees. Further, a strike by a labor organization is of greater concern because the presence of a picket line has the potential for interfering with receipt of supplies and making both replacements and non-striking employees unwilling to work.''[122]

The board declared that the loss of employee status referred to in Section 8(d)—that workers who participate in a strike or picketing of a labor organization in violation of 8(g) lose their status as employees under the act—does not apply where there is no Section 8(g) violation because the activity was not labor organization activity. ''A holding that Section 8(d) applies in the instant case would lead to the incongruous result that employees who are under no obligation to give a 10-day written notice prior to striking are nonetheless deprived of their protection under the Act if they engage in a strike without giving such notice.'' Accordingly, the nurses' aides did not lose their status as employees under the act.

Finally, the board concluded that since the work stoppage by the nurses' aides was for the purpose of presenting a grievance, a protected Section 7 activity, it was protected concerted activity unless it was unlawful, violent, in breach of contract, or indefensible, stating: ''The Board has not held work stoppages against health care institutions to be outside the protection of the Act.'' Accordingly, the discharge or discipline of the nurses' aides for engaging in such work stoppage was held to be in violation of the act.

The significance and importance of the board's conclusion that, in assessing the propriety of concerted activities of employees of health care institutions, ''it will apply the same standards of conduct to health care institutions as to other enterprises''[123] are highlighted by its decision in *Montefiore Hospital and Medical Center*.[124] Montefiore Hospital operated an outpatient clinic servicing a low income population. Its primary service was the availability of physicians to examine these clients and to provide health maintenance and preventive care on a continuing basis. The majority of the hospital's staff were represented by a union that

engaged in a lawful strike after giving proper notice under Section 8(g).

Two doctors employed by the hospital at the clinic, who were not represented by any labor organization, joined the strike in a sympathy gesture and participated in the picketing. While on the picket line, the two doctors approached prospective patients who were attempting to enter the clinic and, after identifying themselves as clinic physicians, informed these individuals that there was a strike involving most clinic workers, that normal facilities were not available, that the clinic was not then a full-service facility, and that the individuals would receive better medical care at a full-service nonstruck facility. After the strike, the two doctors were discharged on the grounds that they had abandoned their duties without notice, had obstructed persons seeking medical care, and had disparaged the medical services available at the clinic. Subsequently, the hospital reinstated the two doctors and converted their discharges to suspensions without pay on their assurances that they would not repeat such conduct in the future. The legality of the discharges and suspensions without pay were put in issue by a complaint issued by the NLRB general counsel.

The administrative law judge concluded that the hospital had violated the act by discharging the two doctors who had engaged in a sympathy strike that was protected concerted activity. However, the law judge found that insofar as the discharges were based on the doctors' attempts to persuade patients not to enter the struck clinic, they were not for unlawful reasons and that back pay was not warranted. He held that such activity constituted picket line misconduct sufficient to remove the doctors from the act's protection because they not only had improperly rendered ''medical advice'' but also had used their professional status in their attempt to prevent prospective patients from seeking medical care at the clinic. The law judge concluded that physicians could engage in such conduct on a protected basis only if they ascertained the condition for which the individuals sought treatment and either provided adequate medical care or saw that the patients received such care elsewhere.

The board agreed with the administrative law judge that the hospital had violated the act by discharging the two doctors whose sympathy strike was protected concerted activity, but disagreed with the judge that they had lost the protection of the act because of their alleged picket line misconduct. The board concluded that the doctors' activities were not improper because their statements did not constitute ''medical advice'' because they did no more than reflect the fact of the strike and picketing and the apparent impact on the clinic's operations, namely, a strike-depleted staff unable to provide full and adequate medical service. In the context of the prospective patients' seeking services of a nonemergency nature, the board held that there was no reason to require the picketing doctors to make even a tentative diagnosis of the individuals' medical condition before urging them to seek care elsewhere. As long as such appeals and attempts to discourage patronage were not accompanied by, nor made in the form of, threats of violence or the like, and did not disparage the product or service, the board ruled, they were privileged and their authors were entitled to the protection of the act. The board perceived "no basis for drawing . . . a distinction between physicians and non-physicians who choose to picket." Accordingly, the board directed that the doctors who had been reinstated be made whole for any loss of pay. In so concluding, the board made special note that "[t]here is no contention . . . that [the doctors] sought to turn away any cases which would be described as emergencies . . . . If the situation does arise we will deal with it in the context in which it occurs."

The Court of Appeals for the Second Circuit agreed, in part, and disagreed, in part, with the board's conclusions.[124a] Preliminarily, the Court agreed with the board that there was no obligation on the part of the two part-time doctors, who were engaging in a sympathy strike, to give a 10-day notice under Section 8(g) of the Act of their intention to strike, because Section 8(g) applied only to the above organizations. The Court then further agreed with the board that the two doctors were "engaged in protected activity when they went on strike in sympathy with the union employees."

But, the Court disagreed with the board in evaluating the propriety of the conduct of the doctors during their strike and picket activity. The Court concluded that the two doctors "lost their protection when they discouraged patients from entering the clinic by telling them, in reckless disregard of the truth or falsity of their statements that they could not be taken care of there; . . . the Board was in error in granting back pay . . . for the period during which the doctors were discharged for their activity;" and the "Board was also in error when it ordered immediate action on the doctors' applications for permanent admitting privileges, since the delay was in response to unprotected activity," i.e., the doctors' action on the picket line.

However, the Court agreed with the board in concluding that "the Hospital acted unlawfully by denying (the doctors) full-time positions because they had filed unfair labor practice charges with the Board," and the Court adopted the board order that the doctors be offered full-time positions and be made whole for any wages they lost due to the improper delay.

NOTICE REQUIREMENTS UNDER SECTION 8(g)

As previously indicated, the essence of Section 8(g) is that a labor organization is required to give written notice to a health institution and the Mediation Service at least ten days "before engaging in any strike, picketing or other concerted refusal to work at any health care institution."

Section 8(g) expressly provides that the notice "shall state the date and time" of the start of the intended strike or picketing. However, questions arise:

1. To whom at the institution must the union send the notice?
2. How should it be sent?
3. When does the ten-day period begin, upon transmittal or receipt?
4. Should there be separate notices and times specified for striking and picketing?
5. Should the notice specify the unit(s) involved?

One further question, of grave and great importance: What happens when a notice is given under Section 8(g) but the picketing or strike does not take place on the stated date?

In the general counsel's view, "for a labor organization to comply with Section 8(g), (a) the 8(g) notice should be served on someone who has been designated to receive the notice or through whom the institution will actually be notified; (b) the notice should be personally delivered or sent by mail or by telegram; (c) the ten-day period begins upon receipt of the notice by the employer and FMCS; (d) the notice should specify the dates and times of both strike and picket conduct, if both are contemplated; and (e) the notice should also indicate which unit(s) will be involved in the planned action."[125]

However, the board has been somewhat more lenient and flexible. It discussed some of these issues in *Bio-Medical Applications of New Orleans.*[126] In that case the union was certified as the bargaining representative of the employer's hemodialysis technicians on December 31, 1975. On March 8, 1976, after the parties were unsuccessful in reaching a collective bargaining agreement, the union sent by certified mail a notice of initial dispute to the employer and to Federal Mediation and Conciliation Service, stating that unless agreement was reached by April 6, the union would consider a strike. On July 20 the union, located in New Orleans, sent by certified mail to the Mediation Service office in Atlanta and to the employer in New Orleans a notice of intent to strike at 7 a.m. on August 2.

The FMCS received the strike notice on July 23, but the employer did not until September 2; apparently there was insufficient postage and it finally was delivered after twice going between the post office and the employer. On July 23, FMCS advised the employer that it had received the ten-day notice and, pursuant to the Mediation Service request, the parties met on July 29 but made no progress; no mention was made of the impending strike at this meeting. On the afternoon of August 2, the day the strike was scheduled to begin, the employer received a telegram from the union stating that the strike would commence the next day, August 3. On the morning of August 3, the union set up a picket line at the facility and the strike began.

Because the parties were unable to resolve their differences, the employer made preparations for the impending strike. On the afternoon of the day the strike was scheduled to begin, the employer received a telegram from the union stating that the walkout would begin the next day. A week after the strike began, the union telegraphed the employer that the strikers were unconditionally offering to return to work and, on the same day, ten striking employees unsuccessfully sought reinstatement. The administrative law judge dismissed the union complaint against the employer alleging unlawful discharge and refusal to reinstate the strikers. The law judge found that the workers had lost their status as employees under Section 8(d) of the act because the union had failed to satisfy the notice requirements of Section 8(g).

The administrative law judge stated some basic Board law:

Where a statute "requires notice to be given or served without prescribing the manner in which it should be done, actual notice is required and the notice is ineffective until received by the person to be served." This requirement has been relaxed in exceptional circumstances where the party required to give notice has failed despite a conscientious effort to comply. The law judge concluded that the union was less than conscientious about compliance because it mailed the notice with insufficient postage, should have inquired of the Postal Service concerning the "fate" of its strike notice, and failed to mention the impending strike at the bargaining session.

The board reversed the administrative law judge and, although conceding that the union did not comply with the literal terms of Section 8(g), concluded that it had taken reasonable steps to comply with the regulation and therefore "it would be inequitable to hold the union responsible for the untimely service of the notice when no reason for the delay can be attributed to it." The board noted that the employer made no mention of not having received the notice at the negotiation meet-

ing with the union of FMCS, that the Postal Service should have followed its policy of delivering the certified letter to the recipient and collecting the postage due or returning it to the sender, and that the employer actually had ten days' notice from the FMCS and had the opportunity to make, and in fact made, arrangements to ensure patient care.

The board issued a caveat: "In reaching the result herein, however, we wish to make it clear that we by no means are condoning a union's disregard for the provisions of Section 8(g). Thus, we stress that in the instant case the union made reasonable efforts to give the employer a ten-day written notice of its intent to strike and the employer had actual ten days' notice of such intent, the employer had the opportunity and in fact did make arrangements to insure continuity of patient care during the strike . . ."

Where a union has given proper notice under Section 8(g) of its intention to strike or picket on a fixed time and date, but does not do so, what are its options if it wishes to strike thereafter? The answers are found in part in Section 8(g), in the legislative history, and in board cases.

Thus, Section 8(g) itself permits the parties to agree to a new time where such mutual agreements are in writing. It is suggested that the FMCS also should be advised of such agreements. Further, of course, the union may give a new Section 8(g) ten-day notice. However, the legislative history of Section 8(g) indicates that repeated serving of ten-day notices upon a health care facility may be construed as constituting evidence of the union's refusal to bargain in good faith. Similarly, repeated intermittent striking or picketing, even where notices are given, might constitute evidence of a union's refusal to bargain in good faith.[127]

With certain limitations, the union may unilaterally extend the time of the start of picketing or striking as set in the initial ten-day notice. Congress laid down the limitations in the legislative deliberations.

The 10-day notice is intended to give health care institutions sufficient advance notice of a strike or picketing to permit them to make arrangements for the continuity of patient care. It is not the intention of the Committee that a labor organization shall be required to commence a strike or picketing at the precise time specified in the notice; on the other hand, it would be inconsistent with the Committee's intent if a labor organization failed to act within a reasonable time after the time specified in the notice. Thus, it would be unreasonable, in the Committee's judgment, if a strike or picketing commenced more than 72 hours after the time specified in the notice. In addition, since the purpose of the notice is to give a health care institution advance notice of the actual commencement of a strike or picketing, if a labor organization does not strike at the time specified in the notice, at least 12 hours notice should be given of the actual time for commencement of the action.

The board adopted those instructions. Thus, in *Bio-Medical Applications*,[128] the board stated, "it is clear that Congress . . . not only contemplated, but specifically approved a labor organization's extension of the time set forth in the initial 10-day notice for the commencement of a strike by unilateral notification to the employer, at least in circumstances in which the postponement of the strike is between twelve and seventy-two hours of the time set forth in the initial notice and where there is at least 12 hours advance notice given to the employer of the postponement." Similarly, as the board stated in *Federal Hill Nursing Center*,[129] "Congress also made it clear that it did not intend such unilateral extensions to be open-ended, but, rather, indicated that in its opinion any unilateral extension beyond a period of 72 hours would be unreasonable, with the further *caveat* that, even within the 72-hour period, a union should give the health care facility at least 12 hours' notice of the actual time that the strike or picketing will commence." In *Federal Hill*, the board found that the union had violated Section 8(g) when, without giving any notice of the delay in the start of picketing and in the absence of any agreement between the parties, began actual picketing 80½ hours after the time stated in its initial notice.

An open question is the form and delivery of the 12-hour notice. The general counsel said that "since the institution has already been put on formal notice of the threatened activity, oral notice should be sufficient, as long as it is given to one capable of receiving that original 8(g) notice . . . and because the legislation contemplates an important role by FMCS in settling disputes in the health care industry . . . FMCS should similarly be given a 12-hour notice."[130]

In one case, the general counsel of the NLRB considered the legality of picketing under Section 8(g) where the union began picketing on the tenth day after the institution had received notice of an intent to picket, instead of picketing on the eleventh day, after ten full days had elapsed.[131] The general counsel was prepared to argue that such picketing on the tenth day was in violation of Section 8(g) and that Congress intended that labor organizations give health care institutions ten full days after notice in which to make preparations for patient care.[132]

Sympathy Picketing

Suppose a union, after giving proper and timely notices under Section 8(g), pickets a health care institution; then another union starts sympathy picketing at the facility without giving the 10 days' notice of its intention to do so. Does that "sympathetic" union violate Section 8(g)?

The board answered the question in *First Health Care Corp.*[133] In that case, a union gave timely 8(g) notices, went out on strike, and picketed a health care institution. Approximately two weeks into the strike, four officers of another union that did not represent any employees at the facility joined the picket line in sympathy and picketed for an hour and a half without giving 8(g) notices.

A board majority concluded that the sympathy picketing by the second union violated Section 8(g) because the latter union failed to give its own notices and could not rely upon the prior notices of the first union. The majority reasoned that "It may well be that suppliers, non-striking employees, and strike replacements who may be willing to cross one union's picket line, will refuse to do so if another labor organization begins picketing."

Indeed, in assessing the impact of threatened picketing and the steps it may take to avoid its impact and provide continuity of patient care, a health care institution may well consider the nature of the union, the type of service involved, the nature of the unit involved, etc., and the sudden injection of another union may change all its calculations and plans. Therefore, the majority said, it is essential that any labor organization give notice under Section 8(g) that it intends to picket. Note that whereas in the *First Health Care* case, the second union did not represent any employees at the institution, the same rule would be applicable to a second union that does represent workers at the facility.

The dissenters in *First Health Care* relied on the fact that "the brief presence of [the other union's] pickets did not basically change the character of the picketing, did not broaden its objectives, and did not generate any new or economic pressures on [the employer]."

The Court of Appeals for the Second Circuit, announcing its decision from the bench after oral argument, denied enforcement of the board's order on the ground that the violation found was de minimis. Apparently, the court did not reject the legal principle that underlies the board's decision, i.e., that the 8(g) notice requirements apply to sympathy picketing. It merely held that the union's conduct in failing to give notice before its four officers joined the picket line for an hour and a half was de minimis.

Informational Picketing

Is all picketing at a health care institution within the ambit of Section 8(g)? In *United Hospitals of Newark*[134] the union was certified and opened negotiations. In the midst of this process, the union advised FMCS that a dispute existed that was subject to mediation. About four weeks later, the union, without giving notice to either the employer or FMCS, staged a demonstration, with 25 employees carrying placards in front of the employer's main entrance to demonstrate support for the negotiating committee. Only employees who were off duty participated in the picketing, access to the main entrance was not blocked physically, and no one was requested not to enter the facility. A majority of the board concluded that the 8(g) notice requirement referred to *any* picketing activities even if they were informational and unrelated to a work stoppage and that the picketing fell within the proscription of the section since the union had failed to provide the requisite notice. The majority noted the "potential disruption inherent in any act of picketing . . . irrespective of the picketers' intent or self regulation . . . ," thereby creating a risk of interrupting the flow of health care services. The dissent argued that the union's informational picketing was tantamount to handbilling and therefore outside the proscription of Section 8(g).[135] The dissent would read the section as referring to picketing that was related to some form of work stoppage and therefore did not embrace this form of informational picketing.

Excused Noncompliance with Section 8(g)

Are there special circumstances where a union can engage in a strike or picketing without complying with the notice requirements of Section 8(g)? The answer is in the affirmative, it would appear, but under what special circumstances?

In *CHC Corp.*,[136] the board gave an example of one set of special circumstances. The union was the recognized representative of the service and maintenance employees of the nursing home. Under the collective bargaining agreement, the union and the employer were required to hold periodic meetings to discuss and resolve grievances. The "strike" for 5 to 15 minutes occurred after postponement and cancellation of a scheduled grievance session and evidence that the employer was avoiding meeting with the union, engaging in subterfuge and unreasonable conduct.[137] The board concluded that the unannounced 15-minute walkout did not violate the 8(g) notice provision because the union's members were "goaded beyond endurance"

by the actions of the employer. The board commented that "there is a high duty of care owed to the patients in health care institutions but an employer also owes some duties to his employees and their representative. Certainly, Section 8(g) was not intended to license deliberate and blatant frustration of the bargaining process. . . . Section 8(g) of the Act was intended to guarantee continuity of services to patients, but not at the cost of abridging the traditional rights of employees under the Act. In this case, the [employer] flouted the rights of the employees and spurned its collective bargaining obligation under the Act."[138]

Similarly, where an employer has committed "serious" or "flagrant" unfair labor practices,[139] a union could protest by striking or picketing without complying with the notice requirements of Section 8(g).[140]

Likewise, a labor organization may be released "from its obligation not to engage in [a strike or picketing or other] economic action during the course of the ten-day notice period" where the health care institution has abused the waiting period. Thus, according to the Senate Committee Report, it was contemplated that after a union has given proper 10-day notices, the institution "should remain free to take whatever action is necessary to maintain health care, but not to use the ten-day period to undermine the bargaining relationship that would otherwise exist. For example, the employer would not be free to bring in large numbers of supervisory help, nurses, staff and other personnel from other facilities for replacement purposes. It would clearly be free to receive supplies, but it would not be free to take extraordinary steps to stock up on ordinary supplies for an unduly extended period. While not necessarily a violation of the Act, violation of these principles would serve to release the labor organization from its obligation not to engage in economic action during the course of the ten-day notice period."[141] However, this leaves open and unanswered the question of precisely what activities during the ten-day period "undermine the bargaining relationship," what actions the institution may take to provide continuity of care for its patients, and what steps it may take to withstand the strike or the picketing.

It has been argued that where an employer's action might destroy the union's representative status (e.g., hiring permanent replacements for all union members during the ten days), such action may justify a union's immediate action without full compliance with the ten-day waiting period. Undoubtedly, the answer lies in an evaluation of the total circumstances and the institution's actions during the ten-day period, e.g., "the permanency of the replacements, the number and type of supplies being ordered, the nature of the patients' illnesses, and the willingness of the union to permit the passage of supplies and personnel through its patient lines.''[142]

It should be noted, however, whatever limitations are thus imposed upon institutions during the ten-day waiting period, these limitations do not stay the employer's actions after the picketing has commenced, if those activities are otherwise lawful.

INTERROGATION OF EMPLOYEES ON INTENT TO STRIKE

Another collateral issue presented by Section 8(g) and its admitted purpose to afford the health care institution an opportunity to prepare for threatened strike or picketing is what action the facility may take to determine whether its employees will honor a strike or picketing. In *Preterm, Inc.,*[143] the union, which had been certified and engaged in collective bargaining negotiations for a first contract, sent the institution a ten-day notice of intention to strike as required by Section 8(g). Thereafter, the employer, through its supervisor, for scheduling purposes questioned 11 employees as to whether they intended to report for work on the strike's first day, telling those who declined to respond that it would be assumed that they were not coming to work and therefore were putting their jobs in jeopardy.

Subsequently, the employer circulated to its employees a questionnaire on the same subject that stated that its purpose was to facilitate the scheduling of incoming patients and the availability of employees to take care of them. It assured them that no reprisals would be taken against them whatever their decision might be. The board concluded that a health care institution that had received a 10-day strike notice could properly attempt to determine the need for replacements by asking employees if they intend to strike since, in enacting Section 8(g), Congress was concerned about ensuring the continuity of patient health care. The board deemed the questionnaire lawful because it contained the safeguards outlined in *Johnnie's Poultry Co.* and *John Bishop Poultry Co.*[144] and *Strucksnes Construction Co. Inc.,*[145] which regulate the manner in which such interrogation is conducted. To lessen the inherently coercive effect of the polling on its employees, the employer had an obligation to explain fully the purpose of the questioning, to assure the workers that no reprisals would be taken against them as a result of their response, and to refrain from otherwise creating a coercive atmosphere. The hospital had fulfilled these obligations with respect to the questionnaire and therefore that conduct was lawful,

but it had not fulfilled the requirements on the supervisors' questioning of employees when the supervisor stated that if workers failed to respond it would be assumed they would not report for work and thus put their jobs in jeopardy. The board concluded that such statements could be construed as a threat to discharge the strikers and thus exceeded the bounds of permissible inquiry and violated Section 8(a)(1) of the act.

Picketing and 'Common Situs'

The issue presented is whether a labor organization violated Section 8(g) by picketing at the premises of a health care facility in connection with a dispute involving an employer other than the institution performing work at that common situs without first giving ten days' written notice of its intent to do so to the institution and to the FMCS. Initially, the board had concluded that such picketing generally would violate Section 8(g). This doctrine came to be referred to as *Lein-Steenberg*.[146] The *Lein-Steenberg* doctrine was rejected by two courts of appeals[147] and subsequently, in view of those reversals and a change in the composition of the NLRB, *Lein-Steenberg* was reversed in principle and replaced by *Henry C. Beck Company*[148] and *St. Mary's Hospital of Roswell, Inc.*[149]

In *Lein-Steenberg,* the union had a dispute with a subcontractor working on alterations at a hospital. A reserved gate was established, reserved solely for the subcontractor's use. The union engaged in area standards picketing at the reserved gate and its picket signs indicated that the dispute was only with the subcontractor. Although some employees of the general contractor and other subcontractors honored the picket line, no hospital employees did so, and hospital service was not disrupted. In *Mercy Hospital of Laredo,* the union engaged in recognitional picketing of the general contractor that was working on a project to expand the laundry facilities of the hospital. The picketing took place at the contractor's reserved gate adjacent to the hospital's emergency rooms. There was no allegation that any hospital employees ceased work or that the union's picketing had any adverse impact on the facility. In both cases, the unions failed to notify either the hospitals or the FMCS of their intent to picket.

The issue presented was whether such picketing violated Section 8(g). A majority of the board (then-Chairman Murphy and Members Penello and Kennedy) held that the unions had violated the section. The board concluded that in the plain language of the section, the intent was to apply the notice provisions to any picketing on the premises of a health care institution rather than only to picketing directed against a facility. It argued that a strike on hospital premises might interrupt patient care and that the 8(g) requirement of notice was not an imposition on the union. Members Fanning and Jenkins dissented. In their view, the majority's interpretation of 8(g) was supported neither by the literal language nor the legislative history of that provision. They maintained that the notice requirement was not intended to encompass disputes between nonhealth care parties.

The Court of Appeals for the District of Columbia denied enforcement of the board's orders in both *Lein Steenberg* and *Mercy Hospital*.[150] The court concluded that Section 8(g) applied only to unions representing health care institution employees.[151] The court disagreed with the board that "the statutory language is unambiguous." Turning to the legislative history, the court was "struck by" the absence of any reference to the labor activity of nonhealth care employees, commenting that "the legislative silence is most eloquent." The court concluded that Congress had not intended the 8(g) notice provisions to apply to unions representing nonhealth care employees. Moreover, it found its reading of the section consonant with its relationship to Section 8(d). The court noted that Section 8(d), which is referred to specifically in Section 8(g), authorizes the FMCS to assist in resolving disputes involving "employees of a health care institution." Since Congress gave the FMCS no power over the activities of nonhealth care employees, the court stated that there was no reason why these employees should be required to notify FMCS of their intent to picket.

In December 1979, the board majority (now consisting of Chairman Fanning and Members Jenkins who had been the dissenters in *Lein Steenberg* augmented by subsequently appointed Member Truesdale and with the concurrence of Member Murphy) issued its decision in *Henry C. Beck Company*,[152] reversed *Lein-Steenberg* and decided that "Section 8(g) does not require a labor union . . . to give notice of its intention to engage in concerted activity against an employer which is not a health care institution, simply because the activity is to take place at the premises of a neutral health care institution. . . ." Instead, "Section 8(g) becomes operational only when the concerted activity is directed against the health care institution. . . . Congress did not intend for Section 8(g) to apply to . . . concerted activity simply because it occurred on the premises of a health care institution." In this case, Beck was constructing a new five-story hospital that subsequently would be connected by a breezeway with an existing outpatient center. The union had a dispute with one of the subcontractors and picketed adjacent to the health care institution at reserved gates. The board concluded that the picketing

was not directed at the institution, the union was not required to give notice of its intent to picket, and the picketing was lawful.

In *St. Mary's Hospital of Roswell, Inc.*,[153] the board extended the rule of *Henry C. Beck* and concluded that a union had no statutory obligation to notify the institution or FMCS of its intention to picket at the facility where the union, which had a dispute with the general contractor constructing a nursing home on the hospital's premises, engaged in picketing at the entrance with signs directed against the contractor. The hospital had not established a reserved gate for the contractor and the board found that the union had carefully sought to comply with the traditional standards for common situs picketing[154] and that there was no evidence that it had tried unlawfully to enmesh the hospital in its dispute with the construction contractor.

However, there are some caveats. In reversing *Lein-Steenberg*, the board, in *Henry C. Beck*, made it clear that "with all due respect to the two courts of appeals, we do not agree, nor do we hold, that Congress intended that Section 8(g) should apply only where the union engaged in the concerted activity represents or seeks to represent health care employees." Thus, in *St. Joseph Hospital*,[155] the board found that Section 8(g) applied to picketing by the Painters Union, even assuming that the picketing was not intended to forward any representational purpose. The board made it clear that in its view "such activity is to be regulated by Section 8(g) whether or not it is related to bargaining, and, moreover, even in instances where it would constitute 'stranger picketing'."[156]

Similarly, it must be emphasized that both the board and the courts, in reversing *Lein-Steenberg*, did not pass upon the question "whether employees engaged in work activities necessary to the present operation of a health care institution, but not employed directly by the institution, should be deemed health care employees,"[157] or so related as to impose upon a union that has a dispute concerning such workers the notice requirements of Section 8(g). For example, a hospital has a contractual relationship with a security service company to furnish uniformed guards; the guards are paid, supervised, and controlled by the security company and not by the hospital; a union has a recognitional dispute with the security company; the union pickets the entrances to the hospital where the guards are working with signs stating that its dispute is with the guard security company; the picketing occurs without the union's giving the requisite ten-day notice; during the picketing, there is no interruption of deliveries or adverse impact upon the hospital's health-related activities. Query: Does such picketing activity aimed at employees not employed directly by the hospital at its premises fall within Section 8(g)? It is submitted that the answer lies in an evaluation of the board decision and rationale in *St. Joseph's Hospital*,[158] the board's reversal of *Lein-Steenberg*[159] in *Henry C. Beck Company*,[160] the court opinions in *Lein-Steenberg* and *Mercy Hospital of Laredo*[161] and *Hoffman Co.*,[162] and the questions unanswered in those cases by the board and the courts as noted *supra* and *St. Mary's Hospital at Roswell, Inc.*[163] explicating *Henry C. Beck*. It is clear that the board and the courts have not decided the issue.

CONCLUSION

Congress in its wisdom turned over to the NLRB the health care area on August 25, 1974, more than half a decade ago. How has the board handled its sensitive responsibilities in this field that touches directly a million and a half employees and every one of us indirectly?

It has provided a set of workable rules and basic precedents that have made it possible for both management and employees through their representatives to negotiate their way around quicksand and land mine traps and deal with issues of professionalisms and units ranging from doctors to boiler operators, from nurses to cleaning persons. It has balanced free speech and ''hospital area'' safety and solicitation rights as against the protection of patient privacy. It has carried out the congressional mandate as to the control of strikes and picketing.

Each individual will have to decide and evaluate the scorecard of NLRB performance, but the author would suggest that for efforts, performance, independence of thought, and commitment to the aims and goals of the health care amendments, the National Labor Relations Board is entitled to high marks.

NOTES

1. In addition to repealing the previous exemption for nonprofit hospitals in Section 2(2) of the act and defining the term ''health care institution'' in Section 2(14), the amendments included a new subsection (g) to Section 8, dealing with notice requirements by labor organizations ''before engaging in any strike, picketing or other concerted refusal to work at any health care institution;'' and amended Section 8(d) relating to duty to bargain, with particular reference to health care institutions.

2. *See Central Dispensary and Emergency Hosp.*, 44 NLRB 533 (1942), *affd.* 145 F.2d 852 (D.C. Cir. 1944), *cert. denied*, 324 U.S. 847 (1945).

3. *Flatbush Gen. Hosp.*, 126 NLRB 144 (1960); *Butte Medical Properties*, 168 NLRB 266 (1967); *University Nursing Home*, 168 NLRB 263 (1967). *See also Drexel Home, Inc.*, 182 NLRB 1045 (1970).

4. *Charles Circle Clinic*, 215 NLRB 382 (1974); *Planned Parenthood Ass'n of Miami*, 217 NLRB 1098 (1975).

5. *Bio Medical Applications of San Diego*, 216 NLRB 631 (1975).

6. *Lutheran Welfare Servs. of Illinois*, 216 NLRB 518 (1975); *Young World*, 216 NLRB 520 (1975).

7. *Baker Places, Inc.*, 219 NLRB 86 (1975).

8. *Lutheran Ass'n for Retarded Children, d/b/a Home of Guiding Hands*, 218 NLRB 1278 (1975); *Beverly Farm Foundation*, 218 NLRB 1275 (1975); *Resident Home for the Mentally Retarded of Hamilton County*, 239 NLRB No. 2 (1978).

9. *Jack L. Williams, D.D.S.*, 219 NLRB 1045 (1975), *enforced* 538 F.2d 337 (9th Cir. 1976).

10. *Family Doctor Medical Group*, 226 NLRB 118 (1976).

11. *Pius XII Schools, Inc.*, 218 NLRB 711 (1975).

12. *Sodat, Inc.*, 218 NLRB 1327 (1975).

13. *St. Peter's School*, 220 NLRB 480 (1975). A side effect of the health care amendments has been their impact on the assertion of jurisdiction over noncommercial activities of other nonprofit charitable organizations. In the past, the board has refused to assert jurisdiction over a facility that had provided education and treatment for emotionally disturbed children, *Ming Quong Children's Center*, 210 NLRB 899 (1974). However, with the passage of the amendments and the deletion of the nonprofit hospital exemption from Section 2(2), the board overruled Ming Quong and asserted jurisdiction over such a facility. *The Rhode Island Catholic Orphan Asylum a/k/a St. Aloysius Home*, 224 NLRB 1344 (1976). The board concluded that the deletion of the nonprofit exemption foreclosed the NLRB from refusing to assert jurisdiction over a nonprofit organization because of its charitable purposes.

14. *Abilities and Goodwill*, 226 NLRB 1224 (1976).

15. *Chicago School & Workshop for the Retarded*, 225 NLRB 1207 (1976).

16. *Boston Medical Laboratory, Inc.*, 235 NLRB 1271 (1978); *Center for Laboratory Medicine, Inc.*, 234 NLRB 387 (1978).

17. *Damon Medical Laboratory, Inc.*, 234 NLRB 333 (1978).

18. *San Diego Blood Bank*, 219 NLRB 116 (1975); *Sacramento Foundation Blood Bank*, 220 NLRB 904 (1975).

19. 218 NLRB 1270 (1975) (Chairman Murphy and Members Jenkins and Penello; Member Fanning concurring in part and dissenting in part.)

20. The majority extended the $250,000 standard previously applied to proprietary hospitals to nonprofit hospitals and to other types of health care institutions and limited the $100,000 standard as previously enunciated for nursing homes. Member Fanning concurred with the $100,000 standard for nursing homes and related facilities but dissented from the $250,000 standard for other institutions on the ground that Congress had made no distinction among the various components of the industry.

21. Section 2(2) excludes from the definition of employer ''the United States or any wholly owned government corporation, or any Federal Reserve Bank, or any State or political subdivisional thereof. . . .''

22. *See Bishop Randal Hosp.*, 217 NLRB 1129 (1975); *Camden-Clark Memorial Hosp.*, 221 NLRB 945 (1975); *Morristown-Hamblen Hosp. Ass'n*, 226 NLRB 76 (1976); *Grey Nuns of the Sacred Heart*, 221 NLRB 1215 (1975); *Toledo Dist. Nurse Ass'n*, 216 NLRB 743 (1975).

23. *National Transportation Serv., Inc.*, 240 NLRB No. 99 (1979), 100 LRRM 1263. *See Catholic Bishop of Chicago, A Corporation Sole, Dept. of Federated Programs*, 235 NLRB 776 (1978); *Mon Valley United Health Services, Inc.*, 238 NLRB No. 129 (1978); *Lutheran Hosps. and Homes Society of America*, 233 NLRB No. 81 (1977), *enf. denied* _____ F.2d _____ (10th Cir. 1980).

23a. *Loma Prieta Regional Center, Inc.*, 241 NLRB No. 165 (1979).

23b. *Ibid.*

23c. *Ibid.*

23d. *D.T. Watson Home for Crippled Children*, 242 NLRB No. 187 (1979).

23e. *Loma Prieta Regional Center, Inc., supra.*

23f. *D.T. Watson Home for Crippled Children, supra.*

24. 237 NLRB 849 (1978). *See also Motherhouse of the Sisters of Charity of Cincinnati, Ohio*, 232 NLRB 318 (1977). It should be noted that, although the board asserted jurisdiction in this case, it concluded that inasmuch as the nursing home involved was "essentially maintained for the purpose of enabling infirm members of the order to continue the practice of their religion and their existence as part of the religious community" it would not effectuate the policies of the act to direct an election in the petitioned-for unit.

25. 440 U.S. 490 (1979).

26. *Mid American Health Services, Inc.*, 247 NLRB No. 109 (1979).

27. *See,* e.g., *Republic Aviation Corp.* v. *NLRB*, 324 U.S. 793 (1945); *Peyton Packing Co.*, 49 NLRB 828 (1943), enf'd 142 F.2d 1009 (5th Cir. 1944); *Essex Int'l, Inc.*, 211 NLRB No. 112 (1974); *Stoddard-Quirk Mfg. Co.*, 138 NLRB 615 (1962); *NLRB* v. *Babcock & Wilcox Co.*, 351 U.S. 105 (1956); *Hudgens* v. *NLRB*, 424 U.S. 507 (1975), 230 NLRB No. 73 (1977); *Sears Roebuck & Co.* v. *San Diego County Dist. Council of Carpenters*, 436 U.S. 180 (1978); *Giant Food Markets*, 241 NLRB No. 105 (1979); *May's Department Stores*, 59 NLRB 976 (1944), enf'd. 154 F.2d 533 (8th Cir. 1946); *GTE Lenkurt* 204 NLRB 921 (1973); *East Bay Newspapers, Inc.*, 225 NLRB 1148 (1976).

28. *St. John's Hosp. and School of Nursing, Inc.*, 222 NLRB 1150 (1976), enf. denied 557 F.2d 1368 (10th Cir. 1977).

29. *Beth Israel Hosp.* v. *NLRB*, 437 U.S. 483 (1978).

30. The rule in *Beth Israel Hospital* provided:

> There is to be no soliciting of the general public (patients, visitors) on Hospital property. Soliciting and the distribution of literature to B.I. employees may be done by other B.I. employees, when neither individual is on his or her working time, in employee-only areas, employee locker rooms and certain adjacent rest rooms. Elsewhere within the Hospital, including patient-care and all other work areas, and areas open to the public such as lobbies, cafeteria and coffee shop, corridors, elevators, gift shop, etc., there is to be no solicitation nor distribution of literature.
> Solicitation or distribution of literature on Hospital property by non-employees is expressly prohibited at all times.
> Consistent with our long-standing practices, the annual appeal campaigns of the United Fund and of the Combined Jewish Philanthropies for voluntary charitable gifts will continue to be carried out by the hospital.

31. 576 F.2d 107 (1978).

32. 442 U.S. 773 (1979); 101 LRRM 2556.

33. "Guidelines for Handling No-Solicitation, No-Distribution Rules in Health Care Facilities," issued by the General Counsel of the NLRB, October 5, 1979.

34. *NLRB* v. *Babcock & Wilcox Co.*, 351 U.S. 105 (1956); *see also, Sears, Roebuck & Co.* v. *San Diego County Dist. Council of Carpenters*, 436 U.S. 180 (1978); *Hudgens* v. *NLRB*, 424 U.S. 507 (1975); *Central Hardware Co.* v. *NLRB*, 407 U.S. 539 (1972).

35. *In Central Hardware Co.*, v. *NLRB, supra*, n. 34, the Supreme Court applied the same nonemployee distribution rule to a case involving the nonemployee no-solicitation rule.

36. Note the rule promulgated by *Beth Israel, supra*, n. 29.

37. 234 NLRB 253 (1978).

38. 98 NLRB 88 (1952), modified on other grounds and *enforced* 200 F.2d 375 (7th Cir. 1952).

39. S. Conf. Rep. No. 988, 93rd Cong., 2nd Sess.; S. Rep. No. 766, 93rd Cong., 2nd Sess. 5 (1974); H. Rep. No. 1051, 93rd Cong., 2nd Sess. 7 (1974).

40. *Mercy Hosps. of Sacramento, Inc.*, 217 NLRB 765 (1975); *Nathan and Miriam Barnert Memorial Hosp., Ass'n*, 217 NLRB 775 (1975); *St. Catherine's Hosp. of Dominican Sisters, Inc.*, 217 NLRB 787 (1975); *Newington Children's Hosp.*, 217 NLRB 793 (1975); *Duke Univ.*, 217 NLRB 799 (1975); *Mt. Airy Foundation*, 217 NLRB 802 (1975); *Shriners Hosps. for Crippled Children*, 217 NLRB 806 (1975).

41. *Mercy Hosps. of Sacramento*, 217 NLRB 765, 766 (1975). The NLRB's concern with the Congressional mandate against proliferation of units in the health care industry and the importance of establishing appropriate collective bargaining units is further reflected in the board's refusal to accept units stipulated by the parties for an election where such stipulations "contravene the provision or purposes of the Act or well settled Board policy." *Otis Hosp., Inc.*, 219 NLRB 164 (1975). Although in *Otis Hosp.*, the board accepted the unit limited to L.P.N.s agreed upon by the parties notwithstanding its conclusion that generally L.P.N.s should be included in the unit of technical employees, in *Barnert Memorial Hosp., supra*, n. 40, the board rejected the stipulated unit of technical employees that had excluded the L.P.N.s.

42. *Mercy Hosp. of Sacramento*, 217 NLRB 765 (1975). *See* also, *Methodist Hosp. of Sacramento, Inc.*, 223 NLRB 1509 (1976).

43. In *Dominican Santa Cruz Hosp.*, 218 NLRB No. 182 (1975), the board found an appropriate unit of professionals excluding registered nurses, even where no labor organization was seeking to represent them, but it observed that an all-professional unit including R.N.s might also be appropriate.

44. 232 NLRB 32 (1977).

45. 601 F.2d 404 (9th Cir. 1979); 101 LRRM 2943.

46. Thus, the court stated that the community of interest test was not dispositive; rather, in the health care industry the board must emphasize a disparity of interests between R.N.s and other professionals as a means of balancing hospital employees' right to representation with the Congressional directive to avoid undue proliferation. Moreover, the court indicated that the factors relied upon in *Mercy* (*supra*, n. 42)—such as the fact that R.N.s must be on duty around the clock, that their duties are nondelegable, and that they have certain license and educational requirements—did not establish a sufficient disparity of interests from other professionals, particularly in view of the hospital's proffered evidence concerning similar attributes of other professionals. The court also questioned the appropriateness of relying upon requirements imposed by state law or other regulatory bodies to establish either a community or disparity of interest because such reliance could impede the development of uniform national labor policy. Finally, the court indicated that the board's decisions in the area did not sufficiently set out the history of collective bargaining by R.N.s, and suggested that the hospital's proffered statistics concerning such units called into question the board's conclusion in *Mercy* that R.N.s had a singular and impressive history of collective bargaining in separate units.

47. *See supra*, n. 46.

48. 250 NLRB No. 86 (1980).

48a. 253 NLRB No. 139 (1981).

49. *Trustees of Noble Hosp.*, 218 NLRB No. 221 (1975); *Wing Memorial Hosp. Ass'n*, 217 NLRB No. 172 (1975); *Western Medical Enterprises d/b/a Driftwood Convalescent Hosp.*, 217 NLRB No. 183 (1975); *Gnaden Huetten Memorial Hosp.*, 219 NLRB 235 (1975); *Mount Airy Foundation d/b/a Mount Airy Psychiatric Center*, 253 NLRB No. 139 (1981).

50. *Adelphi Univ.*, 195 NLRB 639 (1972). *See also Texas Inst. for Rehabilitation*, 228 NLRB 578 (1977).

51. *See Graham Transportation Co.*, 124 NLRB 960 (1959). *See also Chicago Calumet Stevedoring*, 146 NLRB 116 (1964); *Marine & Marketing Corp.*

52. *See Sakrete of Northern California v. NLRB* 332 F.2d 902, 908 (9th Cir. 1964), *cert. denied* 379 U.S. 961; *Int'l. Organization of Masters, Mates & Pilots of America, Inc., AFL-CIO (Chicago Calumet Stevedoring Co., Inc.,)* 144 NLRB 1172 (1963), 146 NLRB 116 (1964), 351 F.2 771 C.A. D.C. (1965); *Nassau and Suffolk Contractors Ass'n*, 118 NLRB 174 (1957).

53. *New York City Omnibus Corp.*, 104 NLRB 579 (1953); *Brunswick Pulp & Paper Co.*, 152 NLRB 973 (1965); *Buckeye Village Market, Inc.*, 175 NLRB 271 (1969); *International Paper Co.*, 172 NLRB No. 933 (1968).

54. 217 NLRB 848 (1975).

55. The board found:

> no supervisors hired by the Employer are included as its officers and directors. Furthermore, none of the Employer's supervisors serve on the Council of Professional Employment Activities, inasmuch as the policy of the Anne Arundel Professional Chapter, which is represented on the Council, excludes supervisors. . . .
>
> The Anne Arundel Hospital Professional Chapter has a negotiating committee which is elected by the general membership of the Employer's employees. The members take part in the bargaining process by selecting the bargaining items and collaborating with the negotiating committee, and, according to uncontroverted testimony, an agreement, if reached, would be ratified by the membership. Should the Petitioner be certified, the membership of the Professional Chapter, working with the negotiating committee, would determine the bargaining goals and issues.

56. 221 NLRB 305 (1975).

57. *NLRB v. Annapolis Emergency Hospital Ass'n, Inc., (Anne Arundel)*, 561 F.2d 524 (4th Cir. 1977). It is interesting to note that the case was argued initially before a panel of the Fourth Circuit consisting of Judge Craven, Judge Hall, and Judge Winter; a decision was prepared by Judge Craven in which Judge Hall concurred enforcing the board's order, with Judge Winter dissenting. Before the panel decisions were filed, a motion was made within the court to rehear the case en banc and the motion carried. Before reargument en banc, Judge Craven died. After reargument en banc, the full court, with the exception of Judge Hall, voted to deny enforcement of the board's order and adopted the panel opinion of Judge Winter that previously had been the dissent. Judge Hall dissented and adopted the panel opinion of Judge Craven that previously had been the majority.

58. 225 NLRB 1086 (1976).

59. 229 NLRB 232 (1977).

60. 241 NLRB No. 107 (1979). (Chairman Fanning, Members Jenkins, Pennello, and Murphy; Member Truesdale dissenting in part).

61. To guard against such possibility, the board has held "that an employer has a duty to refuse to bargain where the presence of that employer's supervisors on the opposite side of the bargaining table poses a conflict between those interests."

62. In view of that potential conflict of interest, the board has held that an employer "may lawfully refuse to bargain with a bargaining representative which itself was in a competing business; that an employer may refuse to bargain where the union's bargaining team included an agent of a union representing employees of a principal competitor; since trade secrets might be revealed, that agent's pres-

ence as a negotiator raised a clear and present danger to meaningful bargaining."

63. Member Truesdale, although agreeing with the abandonment of the *Arundel* rule, would not litigate what he regards as an unfair labor practice matter in a representation proceeding.

63a. *Sierra Vista Hospital*, 249 NLRB No. 66 (1980). *See also Sierra Vista Hospital, Inc.*, 249 NLRB No. 66 (1980).

63b. *See also Sav-On Drugs, Inc.* (Guild for Professional Pharmacists) 243 NLRB No. 149 (1979). The "conflict of interest" issue was also explored in a proceeding involving a unit of registered nurses at North Shore University Hospital located in Manhasset, New York, and the New York Nurses' Association. The matter is still pending before the Administrative Law Judge.

63c. 254 NLRB No. 5 (1981).

63d. *See Bausch & Lomb Optical Company*, 108 NLRB 1555 (1954).

63e. *See Lodi Memorial Hospital Association, supra, Healdsburg General Hospital, supra, Sierra Vista Hospital, Inc., supra*, where the board found that the CNA was not disqualified by reason of any alleged supervisory conflict of interest.

64. Section 2(3) defines the term "employee" under the act. It makes no specific reference to health care institutions.

65. 223 NLRB 251 (1976) (Chairman Murphy and Members Jenkins, Pennello, and Walthers; Member Fanning dissenting).

66. The majority also found that the petitioner, Cedars-Sinai House Staff Association, was not a labor organization since it was composed solely of interns, residents, and clinical fellows.

67. *St. Christopher's Hosp.*, 223 NLRB 166 (1976); *Univ. of Chicago*, 223 NLRB 2032 (1976); *St. Clare's Hosp.*, 223 NLRB 1022 (1976); *Kansas City Gen. Hosp.*, 225 NLRB 108 (1976); *Wayne State Univ.*, 226 NLRB 1062 (1976).

68. 443 F.Supp. 806 (D.C.D.C. 1978) 97 LRRM 2444.

69. 358 U.S. 184 (1958).

70. Note the similarity of the en banc action in the *Arundel* case that reversed a panel of the court.

70a. F.2d (C.A.D.C. 1980). On December 8, 1980, Physicians National House Staff Association filed a petition for a unit of certiorari in the U.S. Supreme Court. The NLRB has filed an opposition to the granting of such unit.

71. It should be noted that although the intern-resident employee issue was involved indirectly in *NLRB v. Committee of Interns and Residents*, 566 F.2d 810 (2nd Cir. 1977) *cert. denied*, 435 U.S. 904 (1978), the issue was not passed upon. In that case, the NLRB successfully argued to the Second Circuit that even though the board will not assert jurisdiction over the interns, residents, and fellows of a hospital subject to its jurisdiction, national labor policy preempts any state jurisdiction over house staff. In agreeing with the board on the preemption issue, the Second Circuit expressly withheld judgment on the nonemployee status of house staff as found by the board. *See also Kansas City Gen. Hosp.*, 225 NLRB 108 (1976).

72. *NLRB v. Yeshiva Univ.*, 444 U.S. 672 (1980).

73. In *Barnert Memorial Hosp. Center*, 217 NLRB 765 (1975) the board majority directed an election in a separate service and maintenance unit, excluding technical employees. A similar unit was found appropriate in *St. Catherine's Hosp. of Dominican Sisters of Kenosha, Wisconsin, Inc.*, 217 NLRB 787 (1975); included in the service and maintenance unit were all employees who were not technicians, professionals, or office clericals. In *Newington Children's Hosp.*, 217 NLRB 793 (1975) the board majority directed an election in a service and maintenance unit, including hospital clericals but excluding technical employees.

74. *Shriners Hosps. for Crippled Children*, 217 NLRB 806 (1975).

75. 230 NLRB 954 (1977).

76. The union petitioned the PLRB for a unit of engineering and maintenance department employees of the hospital on April 6, 1971.

After hearings, the PLRB ordered an election, which was held on June 15, 1972, with the union winning 44 to 12. The PLRB certified the results on July 12, 1972. On November 6, 1972, the PLRB issued its final order dismissing the hospital's exceptions and certifying the union.

The hospital then petitioned the Court of Common Pleas of Allegheny County, Pa., to set aside the PLRB order. That court dismissed the hospital's appeal on July 20, 1973. On July 23, 1974, the Commonwealth Court of Pennsylvania affirmed the decision of the Court of Common Pleas and in November 1974, the Pennsylvania Supreme Court denied the hospital's petition.

In the meantime, on August 25, 1974, the health care amendments to the act became effective. On December 30, 1974, the hospital asked the PLRB to vacate its order on the ground that the health care amendments preempted state jurisdiction. The PLRB returned the hospital's motion, noting that the Pennsylvania Supreme Court had closed all proceedings by denying the hospital's petition in November 1974, and that the PLRB's jurisdiction had been preempted by the health care amendments.

On March 13, 1975, the NLRB issued an advisory opinion (216 NLRB 1001) indicating it would assert jurisdiction over the hospital with respect to unfair labor practices.

On April 7, 1975, a complaint was issued against the hospital alleging, inter alia, that the PLRB-certified unit was appropriate and that the hospital had violated the act by refusing to bargain with the union on and after December 4, 1974.

77. 223 NLRB No. 98 (1976); 227 NLRB No. 70 (1976). Members Fanning and Jenkins applied the traditional unit standards and found the boiler operators constituted a separate appropriate unit. Chairman Murphy agreed with the result, indicating that she "would continue to find appropriate a traditional powerhouse unit or a maintenance department unit in a hospital or other health care facility." Member Penello, with whom Member Walther agreed in a separate concurring opinion, concurred that the boiler operations were an appropriate unit on the facts of the case. Member Penello distinguished his position in *Shriners Hosps. for Crippled Children, supra*, n. 40, and stated that a craft maintenance unit might be appropriate when considered "in light of all the criteria traditionally [examined] . . . Its establishment [did] not conflict with Congressional mandate against proliferation of bargaining units. . . ."

78. 567 F.2d 588 (1977).

79. The Third Circuit also had disagreed with the NLRB in *Memorial Hosp. of Roxborough v. NLRB*, 545 F.2d 351 (1976) and concluded that the board had improperly extended comity to a PLRB certification where the parties had, as in *Allegheny*, contested the underlying unit determination.

80. 239 NLRB No. 104 (1978), (Chairman Fanning, Members Murphy and Truesdale; Member Penello dissenting; Member Jenkins did not participate.)

81. 608 F.2d 965 (3rd Cir. 1979).

82. 606 F.2d 22 (2d Cir. 1979), 102 LRRM 2259.

83. 570 F.2d 213 (7th Cir. 1978).

84. *NLRB v. Mercy Hosp.*, 606 F.2d 22 (2nd Cir. 1979), 102 LRRM 2259, *denying enforcement* and *remanding*, 238 NLRB No. 1018 (1978), *cert. denied* April 14, 1980.

85. In this connection, other cases also were expected to be vehicles for board explication. Thus, on January 17, 1980, the Second Circuit in *Yonkers Gen. Hosp. v. NLRB*, granted the hospital's petition for review and remanded the case to the board for reconsidering in light of *Mercy Hosp.*

Similarly, other cases in the circuit courts of appeals or issued by the NLRB may be the subject of further action by the board, e.g., *Jewish Hosp. Ass'n of Louisville*, 245 NLRB No. 25; *Garden City Hosp.*, 244 NLRB No. 108; *St. Agnes Medical Center*, 247 NLRB

No. 155; *Carney Hosp.*, 243 NLRB No. 127; *Missouri Methodist Hosp. Ass'n*, 245 NLRB No. 109; *Kansas City College of Osteopathic Medicine*, 243 NLRB No. 169; *Fresno Community Hosp.*, 245 NLRB No. 170; *Grant Hosp.*, 246 NLRB No. 110; *Riverside Methodist Hosp.*, 246 NLRB No. 10; *Trinity Memorial Hosp. of Cuddahy*, 242 NLRB No. 52; *Mercy Medical Center*, 235 NLRB 1475.

86. It should be noted that in addition to the Third and Second Circuits, the Seventh Circuit also has rejected the board's decision. *NLRB v. W. Suburban Hosp.*, 570 F.2d 213, 216 (7th Cir. 1978); *Mary Thompson Hosp., Inc.*, 241 NLRB No. 119 (1979) 100 LRRM 1572; 242 NLRB No. 83 (1979) 101 LRRM 1186. In denying enforcement (March 5, 1980), the Seventh Circuit upbraided the board for its failure to follow the admonition of the court in *W. Suburban*. The Seventh Circuit stated "Such flagrant disregard of judicial precedent must not continue. Not only is the Board obligated under the principles of *stare decisis* to follow this court's decision in *W. Suburban*, but it also owes deference to the other courts of appeals which have ruled on this issue. Because of the Board's reliance on traditional community of interest standards and because the Board failed to consider the congressional admonition, we set aside and deny enforcement of its order."

87. *Newton-Wellesley Hosp.*, 250 NLRB No. 86 (1980).

88. As examples, the board cited *St. Catherine's Hosp. of Dominican Sisters of Kenosha, Wisconsin, Inc.*, 217 NLRB 787 (1975) (the board refused to find appropriate a unit of L.P.N.s and included them in a broad unit of technical employees); *Levine Hosp. of Hayward, Inc.*, 219 NLRB 327 (1975) (the board refused to find a "residual" unit of employees in favor of a nonincumbent union, but rather insisted upon a petition by the incumbent for the residual group, or a petition by another labor organization for the overall service and maintenance unit); *Duke Univ.*, 217 NLRB 799 (1975) (the board refused to find a separate unit of switchboard operators); *Kaiser Foundation Hosps.*, 219 NLRB 325 (1975) (the board refused to find a unit of pharmacists).

89. *Saint Anthony Center*, 220 NLRB 1009 (1975); *National G. South, Inc.*, 230 NLRB 976 (1977).

90. *Maple Shade Nursing Home*, 228 NLRB 1457 (1977).

91. *Divine Providence Hosp. of Pittsburgh*, 248 NLRB No. 78 (1980).

92. *Newton-Wellesley Hosp.*, 250 NLRB No. 86 (1980).

93. 217 NLRB No. 132 (1975), (Chairman Murphy and Members Fanning and Jenkins; Members Kennedy and Penello dissenting).

94. 217 NLRB No. 133 (1975), (Chairman Murphy and Members Fanning and Jenkins; Member Kennedy dissenting; Member Penello dissenting in part).

95. 218 NLRB No. 620 (1975).

96. *Mercy Hosps. of Sacramento*, 217 NLRB No. 131 (1975).

97. See also *St. Catherine's Hosp. of Dominican Sisters of Kenosha, Wisconsin, Inc.*, 217 NLRB 787 (1975); *Sisters of St. Joseph of Peace*, 217 NLRB No. 135 (1975).

98. See *Sisters of St. Joseph of Peace*, 217 NLRB 797.

99. Section 2(3) of the act. See also Section 14(a): "Nothing herein shall prohibit any individual employed as a supervisor from becoming or remaining a member of a labor organization, but no employer subject to this Act shall be compelled to deem individuals defined herein as supervisors as employees for the purpose of any law, either national or local, relating to collective bargaining."

100. Section 9(b) of the Act. See *Peninsula Hospital Center*, 219 NLRB 139 (1975). See also *The Wackenhut Corporation*, 223 NLRB 1131 (1976).

101. *Shop-Rite Foods, Inc.*, 247 NLRB No. 143 (1980). *Wallace Murray Corp.*, 192 NLRB 1090 (1971); *Arthur C. Logan Memorial Hosp.*, 231 NLRB 778 (1977). See infra, pp. 899–900 (Khar rule).

102. *Wallace Murray Corp.*, 192 NLRB 1090 (1971).

103. *Shop Rite Foods, Inc.*, 231 NLRB 778 (1977). The petition was filed 101 days prior to the expiration of the then-current three-year contract.

104. *Peninsula Hosp. Center,* 219 NLRB No. 21 (1975); *Beth Israel Medical Center,* 229 NLRB 295 (1977).

105. *General Cable Corp.*, 139 NLRB 1123 (1962), modifying *Pacific Coast Ass'n of Pulp and Paper Mfrs,* 121 NLRB 990 (1958). *See also Appalachian Shale Products Co.,* 121 NLRB 1160 (1958).

106. *Leonard Wholesale Meats, Inc.*, 136 NLRB 1000 (1962), modifying *De Luxe Metal Furniture Co.,* 121 NLRB 995 (1958).

107. *De Luxe Metal Furniture Co., supra,* n. 107.

108. The pertinent amendment to Sec. 8(d)(4) reads as follows:

> Whenever the collective bargaining involves employees of a health care institution, the provisions of this section 8(d) shall be modified as follows:
> (A) The notice of section 8(d)(1) shall be ninety days; the notice of section 8(d)(3) shall be sixty days; and the contract period of section 8(d)(4) shall be ninety days.

109. 218 NLRB 199 (1975).

110. Section 8(a)(3) of the Act provides, *inter alia:*

> That nothing in this Act, or any other statute of the United States, shall preclude an employer from making an agreement with a labor organization (not established, maintained, or assisted by any action defined in section 8(a) of this Act as an unfair labor practice) to require as a condition of employment membership therein on or after the thirtieth day following the beginning of such employment or the effective date of such agreement, whichever is the later, (1) if such labor organization is the representative of the employees as provided in section 9(a), in the appropriate collective-bargaining unit covered by such agreement when made.

Section 8(f) of the Act provides, *inter alia:*

> It shall not be an unfair labor practice under subsections (a) and (b) of this section for an employer engaged primarily in the building and construction industry to make an agreement covering employees engaged (or who, upon their employment, will be engaged) in the building and construction industry with a labor organization of which building and construction employees are members (not established, maintained, or assisted by any action defined in section 8(a) of this Act as an unfair labor practice) because (1) the majority status of such labor organization has not been established under the provisions of section 9 of this Act prior to the making of such agreement, or (2) such agreement requires as a condition of employment, membership in such labor organization after the seventh day following the beginning of such employment or the effective date of the agreement, whichever is later.

111. The union shop provision does not require union membership as a condition of initial employment, but requires that employees become members of the union after a specified grade period (under the act, 30 days generally or seven days in the construction industry, and continued membership during the life of the agreement. It should be noted that under the National Labor Relations Act, as initially enacted in 1935, a closed shop provision was permitted, namely, membership in the union as a condition of initial employment and continued membership thereafter. The closed shop provision was made unlawful in the amendments in 1947.

112. The agency shop specifically provides that instead of union membership, as required by the union shop, the obligation is that after the required grace period, the employee pay support money for services provided by the union as the collective bargaining agent; the "service fee" usually is equivalent to the initiation fees and periodic dues.

113. The maintenance-of-membership provision usually provides no obligation to join the union, but an obligation to remain a member once the employee becomes one.

114. *Union Starch & Refining Co.*, 87 NLRB No. 779 (1949), *enforced* 186 F.2d (7th Cir. 1951), *cert. denied* 342 U.S. 815 (1951).

NLRB v. General Motors Corp., 373 U.S. 734 (1963).

Local 1104, Communications Workers v. NLRB (N.Y. Tel. Co.) 540 F.2d 411 (2nd Cir. 1975); *NLRB v. Hershey Foods Corp.,* 513 F.2d 1083 (9th Cir. 1975).

115. *Mid American Health Servs., Inc.*, 247 NLRB No. 109 (1980).

116. Section 8(g) on strike notice requirements:

> A labor organization before engaging in any strike, picketing, or other concerted refusal to work at any health care institution shall, not less than ten days prior to such action, notify the institution in writing and the Federal Mediation and Conciliation Service of that intention, except that in the case of bargaining for an initial agreement following certification or recognition the notice required by this subsection shall not be given until the expiration of the period specified in clause (B) of the last sentence of section 8(d) of this Act. The notice shall state the date and time that such action will commence. The notice, once given, may be extended by the written agreement of both parties.

117. Section 8(d) as modified on employee status:

> Any employee who engages in a strike within any notice period specified in this subsection, or who engages in any strike within the appropriate period specified in subsection (g) of this section shall lose his status as an employee of the employer engaged in the particular labor dispute, for the purposes of sections 8, 9, and 10 of this Act, as amended, but such loss of status for such employee shall terminate if and when he is reemployed by such employer.

118. Section 8(d) as modified on bargaining notice requirements:

> Whenever the collective bargaining involves employees of a health care institution, the provisions of this section 8(d) shall be modified as follows:
> (A) The notice of section 8(d)(1) shall be ninety days; the notice of section 8(d)(3) shall be sixty days; and the contract period of section 8(d)(4) shall be ninety days;
> (B) Where the bargaining is for an initial agreement following certification or recognition, at least thirty days' notice of the existence of a dispute shall be given by the labor organization to the agencies set forth in section 8(d)(3).
> (C) After notice is given to the Federal Mediation and Conciliation Service under either clause (A) or (B) of this sentence, the Service shall promptly communicate with the parties and use its best efforts, by mediation and conciliation, to bring them to agreement. The parties shall participate fully and promptly in such meetings as may be undertaken by the Service for the purpose of aiding in a settlement of the dispute.

119. 227 NLRB 132 (1976).

120. *General Serv. Employees Union Local 73 (A-1 Security Service Co.)*, 244 NLRB 434 (1976); *Laborers' Int'l Union of North America, Local 652, AFL-CIO, (Richard Sewell Inc.)*, 238 NLRB No. 986 (1978).

121. 227 NLRB 1630 (1977).

122. *See also Long Beach Youth Center*, 227 NLRB No. 1630 (1977), *enforced* 591 F.2d 1276 (9th Cir. 1979) 101 LRRM 2501. In that case, 17 employees staged a work stoppage to protest working conditions; the union that was attempting to organize the employees was not responsible, nor did it encourage or sanction the stoppage. In addition to the arguments advanced in *Walker Methodist*, the employer argued that the 17 employees constituted a labor organization under the act and, therefore, a violation of Section 8(g) had occurred. The board rejected that contention, finding that the employees did not take any formal or informal steps to become a labor organization and the fact that they had signed authorization cards for the union indicated an intention not to form any other labor organization. The board concluded that the discharge of the 17 employees was in violation of the Act.

See also Kapiolani Hosp., 231 NLRB No. 34 (1977), *enforced* 581 F.2d 230 (9th Cir. 1978) where the board adopted the conclusion of the administrative law judge that the employer violated the act by discharging an employee who, while unaffiliated with any labor organization, refused to cross a picket line of a union that had complied with the notice requirements of Section 8(g). The administrative law judge, relying on *Walker Methodist*, found that the worker did not forfeit status as employee by failing to give the hospital a ten-day notice of her intention to honor the picket line. (Citing Long Beach Youth Center and Kapiolani Hospital) the following cases: *NLRB v. Rock Hill Convalescent Center*, 585 F.2d 700 (4th cir. 1978); and *Montefiore Hospital and Medical Center v. NLRB*, 621 F.2d 510 (2nd cir. 1980).

123. *Walker Methodist*, 227 NLRB 1630, 1632 (1977).

124. 243 NLRB No. 106 (1979).

124a. *Montefiore Hospital and Medical Center v. NLRB*, 621 F.2d 510 (2nd cir. 1980).

125. General Counsel Memo 74-49, ''Guidelines Issued by the General Counsel of the NLRB for Use of Board Regional Offices in Unfair Labor Practice Cases Arising Under the 1974 Nonprofit Hospital Amendments to the Taft-Hartley Act.''

126. 240 NLRB No. 39 (1979).

127. General Counsel Memo 74-49, *supra*, n. 125.

128. 240 NLRB No. 39 (1979).

129. 243 NLRB No. 6 (1979).

130. General Counsel Memo 74-49, *supra*, n. 125.

131. On October 27, 1978, the union sent a letter to the institution stating that it intended to engage in ''informational picketing'' on November 6, 1978. The institution received the letter on the morning of October 28, 1978. The union commenced picketing on the morning of November 6. The picketing had minimal impact on patient care at the nursing home.

132. Report of NLRB General Counsel for Fourth Quarter of 1978.

133. 222 NLRB No. 212 (1976).

134. 232 NLRB No. 443 (1977).

135. Where handbilling activity is not part of a strike, picketing, or other concerted refusal to work, such activity would be outside the proscriptions of Section 8(g).

136. 229 NLRB No. 1010 (1979).

137. The case presented an interesting set of events. A grievance meeting was scheduled for March 2, postponed to March 4, cancelled, and rescheduled to March 9, all at the instance of the employer. Despite the pendency of seven grievances, the employer sought to cancel the session again because of a more important meeting. The union learned that that meeting was cancelled because the employer had gone to a birthday luncheon. There followed a series of events in which the union representative and several union members sought to speak to the administrator after lunch, only to be told he was not in. They noticed a light in the administrator's office, and peering under the door, saw the shoes of a man walking around the room. One employee said: ''He's in there.'' The light then went out, whereupon the union representative ordered all the employees down to the office. Several minutes later, the administrator, without hat and coat, came through the front door of the nursing home, brushing snow from his trousers. He then called the union representative and agreed to hold the meeting. There was credited testimony of foot tracks in the newly fallen snow from the administrator's office window to the facility's front door.

138. Member Murphy concurred in the dismissal on the ground that the union's action was not a strike within the meaning of Section 8(g) and that the employees' sole purpose was to confront the employer personally to express their dissatisfaction with the latter's conduct on the ground that it was disruptive of the bargaining process.

139. *See Mastro Plastics Corp. v. NLRB* 350, U.S. 270 (1956); *Arlan's Dept. Store of Michigan*, 133 NLRB 802 (1967); *Dow Chemical Corp.*, 249 NLRB No. 129.

140. *CHC Corp.*, *supra*, n. 136.

141. *CHC Corp.*, *supra*, n. 136.

142. General Counsel Memo 74-49, *supra*, n. 125.

143. 240 NLRB No. 81 (1979). *See also Commercial Management Inc.*, 233 NLRB 665 (1977).

144. 146 NLRB 770 (1964), *enforcement denied* 344 F.2d 617 (8th Cir. 1965).

145. 165 NLRB 1062 (1967).

146. 219 NLRB 837 (1975). Two companion cases, *Mercy Hosp. of Laredo*, 219 NLRB 846 (1975), and *Casey & Glass, Inc.*, 219 NLRB 698 (1975), issued at the same time. *See also St. Joseph's Hosp.*, 243 NLRB No. 113 (1979) and *infra*, n. 147.

147. *NLRB v. Int'l Brotherhood of Electrical Workers Union No. 388 (St. Joseph's Hosp. of Marshfield, Inc.)*, 548 F.2d 704 (7th Cir. 1977), denying enforcement to 220 NLRB 665 (1975); *cert denied* 434 U.S. 837; *Laborers' Int'l Union of N. America, AFL-CIO, Local Union, No. 1075 (Mercy Hosp. of Laredo)* 567 F.2d 1006 (D.C. Cir. 1977), denying enforcement to 219 NLRB 846 (1975) and denying enforcement to *Lein-Steenberg*, 219 NLRB 837 (1975).

148. 246 NLRB No. 148 (1979).

149. 248 NLRB No. 30 (1980).

150. *Supra*, n. 146.

151. In so doing, the Court of Appeals for the District of Columbia agreed with the view of the Seventh Circuit, which also refused to apply Section 8(g) to picketing by a construction union on hospital premises. *NLRB v. Electrical Workers*, 548 F.2d 704 (7th Cir. 1977), *cert. denied* 434 U.S. 837, *supra*, n. 147. In that case, Hoffman Co. was constructing a laboratory building to be connected to the main hospital by a common wall and corridor. The union picketed a subcontractor with area standards picket signs on hospital property, directly across from the hospital building and adjacent to the employee parking lot. There was no allegation that any hospital employees ceased work or that the picketing had an adverse impact upon the hospital's operations.

152. 246 NLRB No. 148 (1979).

153. 248 NLRB No. 30 (1980).

154. *Moore Drydock Company*, 92 NLRB 547 (1950).

155. 243 NLRB No. 113 (1979).

In *St. Joseph Hospital*, the hospital was engaged in the renovation and conversion of one of its buildings into an administration building. The interior and exterior painting work was assigned to four of the hospital's regularly employed maintenance employees who had performed painting work in the past as part of their duties; they were not covered by any collective bargaining agreement. During the conversion, the other hospital buildings continued to provide health care services.

The Painters Union, without giving 10-day notices to the hospital or FMCS, picketed one of the two entrances with signs indicating that the hospital was unfair. The union advised the hospital that the purpose of its picketing was ''to advertise to the employees of [the hospital] assigned to perform paint work that the hospital is not signatory to a collective bargaining agreement covering such work.''

The board concluded that such picketing violated Section 8(g) of the act. In so concluding, it stated that Section 8(g) applied whether or not the activity related to bargaining or contractual disputes with the hospital, that the section was not limited only to disputes involving employees performing direct ''patient-related'' functions, and that the picketing was directed against the hospital, which was not a neutral as was the case in *Lein-Steenberg*.

156. *St. Joseph Hosp., supra*, n. 155.

157. *Lein-Steenberg* and *Mercy Hosp. of Laredo*, 567 F.2d at 1009 (D.C. Cir. 1977), n. 15, quoting Hoffman Company, 548 F.2d at 707, n. 5. See also *Henry C. Beck Co.*, 246 NLRB No. 148 (1979) at n. 13.

158. 243 NLRB No. 113 (1979).

159. 219 NLRB 846 (1975).

160. 246 NLRB No. 148 (1979).

161. 567 F.2d 1006 (D.C. Cir. 1977).

162. 548 F.2d 704 (7th Cir. 1977).

163. 248 NLRB No. 30 (1980).

In this case, the board extended the rule of *Henry C. Beck* to a union that was picketing at the entrance to the hospital against a construction contractor working on the premises since the institution had not established a reserved gate for the contractor and since there was no evidence that the union was attempting to unlawfully enmesh the hospital.

4. Legal Developments under the Health Care Amendments

G. ROGER KING and WILLIAM J. EMANUEL

BACKGROUND AND JURISDICTION

Congress amended the National Labor Relations Act (Act) in August 1974 to extend its coverage to nonprofit health care facilities. Prior to that time only proprietary health care institutions had been covered. Concurrent with extension of the Act, Congress adopted a number of special provisions applicable only to health care institutions that have become known as the Health Care Amendments of 1974 (Amendments).[1]

Specifically, the Amendments added Section 2(14)[2] to the Act, which extended the jurisdiction of the National Labor Relations Board (Board) to the following health care institutions:

[A]ny hospital, convalescent hospital, health maintenance organization, health clinic, nursing home, extended care facility, or other institution devoted to the care of sick, infirm, or aged person.

The Board announced the jurisdictional reach of the amendments in the case of *East Oakland Community Health Alliance, Inc.*[3] The Board held that any health care institution operating at the following dollar volumes would be subject to the Act's jurisdiction under the new Amendments:

1. $100,000 annual gross revenue for nursing homes, visiting nurse associations, and related facilities;

2. $250,000 for private nonprofit hospitals—identical to the standards for proprietary hospitals; and

3. $250,000 for other health care institutions, including health maintenance organizations and health clinics.

The board has continued to adhere to these jurisdictional standards and has continued to focus on the amount of income of the facility, not the source, of such revenue. For example, in *Mon Valley United Health Services, Inc.*,[4] the Board held that it would assert jurisdiction over an employer even though 45 percent of its revenue was derived from federal funds.[5]

In *Atwood Leasing Corp.*,[6] however, the Board declined jurisdiction over an outpatient medical clinic, finding that the gross annual revenue of the employer's corporations was below the $250,000 industry standard. The Board ruled that although its jurisdictional standard would have been met easily by including the gross revenues of all the physicians practicing at the clinic, those doctors did not exercise sufficient control over employment terms and conditions to qualify as joint employers.

The NLRB also has asserted jurisdiction over dental facilities[7] and family clinics engaged in providing abortions, vasectomies, gynecological care, and birth control counseling on an outpatient basis,[8] finding such entities to be "health care institutions" within the meaning of Section 2(14) of the Act. Mental care facilties also have been held by the Board to be health care facilities as defined by the Amendments.[9]

The board has held, however, that a medical laboratory testing human medical specimens,[10] and a diagnostic medical laboratory service testing human blood, body fluid, and tissue for hospitals, clinics, nursing homes, and individual physicians,[11] are not health care institutions within the meaning of Section 2(14) of the Act. In each case the Board interpreted the legislative history of the Amendments to apply only to patient care situations, and not to purely Administrative facilities related to health care. Blood banks also have been held to be outside the reach of the Amendments since they are not involved in direct patient care.[12]

Finally, in *St. Elizabeth Community Hospital*,[13] the board rejected a health care institution's jurisdictional argument that it should be exempt from the Act based on the religion clause in the First Amendment to the United States Constitution. In support of its contention, the hospital had relied upon *The Catholic Bishop of Chicago v. NLRB*,[14] in which the U.S. Supreme Court concluded that application of the act to parochial schools violated the free exercise and religious establishment clauses of the First Amendment.

The Board reaffirmed its position that health care facilities operated by religious entities or orders were subject to the act's jurisdiction after that decision when it held that a nursing home owned by a corporation that served as a regional representative of the Seventh Day Adventist Church and that operated church health care facilities in a four-state area could not be removed from the Act's jurisdiction because of a conflict with the religious establishment clause in the First Amendment.[15] The legislative history of the Amendments, the Board concluded, clearly evidences that Congress rejected a proposal that would have removed religious health care facilities from the Act's jurisdiction.[16] Further, the Board concluded that Congress regarded any "potential conflict between an employee's religious beliefs and collective-bargaining responsibilities" when it created Section 19 of the Act, which provides:

> Sec. 19. Any employee of a health care institution who is a member of and adheres to established and traditional tenets or teachings of a bona fide religion, body, or sect which has historically held conscientious objections to joining or financially supporting labor organizations shall not be required to join or financially support any labor organization as a condition of employment; except that such employee may be required, in lieu of periodic dues and initiation fees, to pay sums equal to such dues and initiation fees to a non-religious charitable fund exempt from taxation under Section 501(c)(2) of the Internal Revenue Code, chosen by such employee from a list of at least three such funds, designated in a contract between such institution and a labor organization, or if the contract fails to designate such funds, then to any such fund chosen by the employee.

Although the NLRB's position on this issue has yet to be tested thoroughly in the courts, it appears that Section 19 may be of particular assistance since the Supreme Court in the *Catholic Bishop of Chicago* case characterized this statute as "reflecting Congressional sensitivity to the First Amendment guarantees."

HEALTH CARE BARGAINING UNITS—PRE-1977

Probably the most important, and certainly the most litigated, aspect of the Amendments is the mandate of Congress that proliferation of bargaining units should be prevented in health care institutions. Ironically, this subject was not dealt with in the statutory changes. However, in both the Senate and House committee reports, Congress stated that "[d]ue consideration should be given by the Board to preventing proliferation of bargaining units in the health care industry."[17]

Most of the important NLRB decisions interpreting this congressional directive were decided prior to 1977 and were devoted to developing a basic unit structure in hospitals. The pre-1977 Board law can be summarized as follows.

Professional Employees

Because there had been a measure of prior bargaining history in separate registered nurse units in limited geographical areas—characterized by the Board as a "singular history of separate representation"—the NLRB bifurcated the professional segment of the hospital work force into a unit of R.N.s and a residual unit of all other professionals.[18] R.N.s and other professionals were combined into a single professional unit only on an extent of organization basis—i.e., if a union sought a unit of R.N.s, it was granted, notwithstanding the employer's argument that the other professionals must be included; but if a union sought an all-professional unit, including R.N.s, it was granted, even though the employer urged that two separate units should be found appropriate.[19] This doctrine was applied on a per se or automatic basis, with no exception for small hospitals employing only a few professionals other than R.N.s.[20] Separate groups within the "other professional" category—such as pharmacists and medical laboratory technologists— were denied separate bargaining units.[21]

Technical Employees

The Board surprised everyone by holding that technical employees were entitled to a separate unit if sought,[22] and that they must be excluded from a service and maintenance unit at a petitioning union's request.[23] Included in such technical units were all of the hospital's licensed practical nurses (L.P.N.s) and other employees whose job required specialized training or certification. An exception was announced for small hospitals employing only a few technical employees, the Board concluding that in these circumstances technicals should be included in a service and maintenance unit over the union's objection.[24] However, that exception was applied subsequently in only one reported case.[25]

Business Office Clericals

A separate bargaining unit was established for health care business office clericals, who were excluded from service and maintenance units.[26]

Service and Maintenance Employees

The Board held that a service and maintenance bargaining unit (all nonprofessionals excluding technicals, business office clericals, and guards) was appropriate.[27] However, frequent attempts were made to split off separate units of maintenance department employees or boiler operators. In most cases, the NLRB held a maintenance department unit inappropriate,[28] but there were several exceptions, including the approval of a boiler operator unit in one case,[29] but the Board found such a unit inappropriate in a later decision.[30]

Guards

Some hospitals employ "guards" as defined in section 9(b)(3) of the Act.[31] That section precludes the Board from including guards and nonguards in the same unit. Thus, a separate unit of guards is required if they seek to organize. The Board has held that mixed units of guards and nonguards established prior to the Amendments may be separated in a unit clarification proceeding.[32]

Exceptions

Exceptions from the basic structure just outlined were granted as a result of comity (deference) to a state agency bargaining unit determination,[33] prior bargaining history in the hospital,[34] or a stipulation or agreement of the parties.[35]

Only one court decision affecting hospital bargaining units was issued prior to 1977. In *Memorial Hospital of Roxborough v. NLRB*,[36] a Board decision permitting a separate maintenance department unit was reversed, in part because of the agency's failure to consider the Congressional nonproliferation mandate and in part because it granted comity to the unit determination of a state labor relations board. The court held that the board could not grant comity to state agency decisions in unit determination cases.

HEALTH CARE BARGAINING UNITS—POST-1977

Physicians

A separate bargaining unit subsequently was established by the Board for physicians employed by a hospital in *Ohio Valley Hospital Association*.[37] In a split decision, the Board majority excluded house physicians and emergency room doctors from a unit of all other professional employees, concluding that "within the hospital hierarchy, physicians are the pivotal employees and all other patient care employees are subject to their professional direction." The NLRB further based its finding of a distinct community of interest for physicians on the following factors:

1. the essential functions of physicians cannot be performed by other employees;
2. limited supervisory authority over physicians is confined to other physicians;
3. physicians have a high rate of compensation;
4. physicians are required to have extensive education, training, and skills; and
5. the Board desired to accord physicians the same separate unit status that it previously had provided for registered nurses.

The two dissenting Board members would have included the physicians in an all-professional unit.

In *Cedars-Sinai Medical Center*,[38] the Board was confronted with the unit placement of hospital interns and residents. However, it found it unnecessary to decide this question in view of its conclusion that interns and residents were primarily students and not "employees"[39] as defined in the Act.[40]

Pursuant to that case, the Board sought a federal court injunction to prevent the New York State Labor Relations Board from taking jurisdiction over interns and residents, arguing that federal law preempted the regulation of labor relations of such individuals even though they were not employees under the Act. In *NLRB v. Committee of Interns and Residents*,[41] the Second Circuit, reversing the district court's denial of an injunction, held that the preemption doctrine precluded the State Board from asserting jurisdiction. In a supplemental order, the court enjoined the State Board from asserting jurisdiction. The Supreme Court declined to view the case.[42]

The Board's decision that interns and residents were not employees was upheld in 1980 by the federal Court of Appeals in the District of Columbia.[43] Congress also has refused to overrule the Board's position.[44] Accordingly, residents and interns are subject to the Act but cannot require hospitals to bargain with them because of their classification as students.

In *Montefiore Hospital and Medical Center*,[45] the NLRB found appropriate a combined unit of physicians and dentists in an outpatient diagnostic and treatment center that functioned as part of a larger medical center. Although the employer sought a broader professional unit, the Board approved one confined to physicians and dentists because they were the only professional employees, and the only unrepresented classifications, in the outpatient center. The issue of whether the physicians should have been placed in a unit apart from the dentists was not raised by either party, and was not discussed by the Board.

Registered Nurses

The NLRB has continued to insist upon a division between R.N.s and other professionals. In *Texas Institute for Rehabilitation and Research*,[46] the employer argued for different treatment because it operated a rehabilitation center rather than an acute care facility. However, the Board rejected this contention and found a separate R.N. unit appropriate, over the employer's objection that the unit should include all other professionals.

Conversely, a unit of all professionals excluding R.N.s was found appropriate in *Samaritan Health Services, Inc.*,[47] although the employer contended that R.N.s should have been included. However, in a later case, *Allegheny General Hospital II*,[48] the Board changed the rationale for a separate R.N. unit, this time asserting that it applied traditional community-of-interest criteria in such cases, including area practice and patterns of bargaining. Thus, it appears that the Board has abandoned national bargaining history as the underpinning of the R.N. unit policy and will base future decisions on traditional community-of-interest criteria.

The Board's per se approval of R.N. units received a sharp rebuke from the Ninth Circuit in *NLRB v. St. Francis Hospital of Lynwood*,[49] where the agency refused to allow the hospital to introduce evidence in support of an all-professional unit. The Ninth Circuit reversed, holding that "the *per se* policy established in the Board's *Mercy* decision . . . is [in]consistent with the congressional directive that the Board give 'due consideration' to preventing undue proliferation of bargaining units in the health care industry and Congress's expressed approval of the trend towards broader units in this area." The court concluded "[f]rom the legislative history of the 1974 Amendments . . . that Congress sought to encourage the Board to find broader bargaining units in the health care industry rather than narrower ones." The court acknowledged that a separate R.N. unit might be appropriate under some circumstances, but stressed that "a demonstration, not a mere presumption, of a disparity of interests between registered nurses and other hospital employees" would be necessary to justify such a decision."

The Board's rigid policy of finding a separate R.N. unit appropriate applies only when a petitioning or intervening union seeks such a unit. When a petitioning union seeks a combined unit of R.N.s and other professionals, and no other union seeks a separate R.N. entity, the combined group is held appropriate,[50] even though the employer seeks a separate R.N. unit.[51]

The Board has included in an R.N. unit both on-call registered nurses[52] and graduate nurses (graduates of an accredited nursing school who have not taken or passed the registered nurse examination).[53] Nurse practitioners (registered nurses with additional education and responsibilities) also were included in an R.N. unit,[54] although in another case physician extenders (specialized R.N.s with advanced training) were included in a residual professional unit while other R.N.s were excluded.[55]

In *St. James Hospital*[56] the Board held that a residual professional unit not composed of registered nurses or physicians may include R.N.s who are not working on patient floors but who review charts to determine whether hospitalization is necessary under Medicare and Medicaid guidelines. The Board stated that while its separate unit status policy regarding R.N.s was based upon "a basic tie to the nursing profession, amounting to a community of interest," the nurses in question were serving as utilization review coordinators with primarily administrative duties. Accordingly, placing such individuals in a unit other than an all-R.N. group did not contravene its basic bargaining unit polity in health care facilities with respect to that category of professionals.

Further, in *Mt. Airy Psychiatric Center*[56a] the Board found an all-professional unit to be appropriate that included registered nurses and other professional employees—pharmacists, occupational therapists, social workers, and special education teachers. The Board based its decision on the fact that a unit of only registered nurses would include nine professional employees in other job classifications and create the possibility of a residual professional unit for such individuals. Such a bargaining unit the Board concluded would not be in keeping with the intent of the Amendments to avoid unit fragmentation.

The NLRB in 1980 reaffirmed its policy of finding a separate unit of R.N.s appropriate[57] and it remains to be seen what fate such a policy will have in the courts.

Other Professionals

The board took another look at whether pharmacists should be entitled to a separate unit in *San Jose Hospital and Health Center, Inc.*,[58] where the union introduced testimony regarding national bargaining history in pharmacist units. The Board was not sufficiently impressed by this evidence to change its policy, and held that the pharmacists could have an election only in a unit that included all other professionals, excluding R.N.s.

Technical Employees

The Board continues to approve separate technical units or will exclude technical employees from a service and maintenance unit if desired by the petitioning union, notwithstanding the employer's argument that the two groups should be combined. However, technical employees will be combined with service and maintenance employees if requested by a petitioning union, even if an employer argues that under Board policy there should be two separate units.

This was the result in *Memorial Medical*,[59] where the agency granted a combined unit, although the employer contended that licensed vocational nurses (L.V.N.s), who are regarded as technical employees, should be excluded. The same result was reached in *Appalachian Regional Hospitals, Inc.*,[60] and in *Allegheny General Hospital II, supra.* Similarly, when a

union sought to represent licensed practical nurses only, the Board ruled, and was supported by the Sixth Circuit Court of Appeals, that such a unit was inappropriate. A separate unit for technical employees (laboratory, x-ray, EKG, and operating room technicians as well as L.P.N.s) was approved, however.[61]

A unit of technical employees excluding L.P.N.s was approved by the Board in *Pontiac Osteopathic Hospital*.[62] However, the L.P.N.s in that case already were represented in a separate unit. The Board reached the same result in a similar but more complicated factual setting in another case.[63] There it excluded L.P.N.s from a combined two-facility technical unit because of prior bargaining history in an L.P.N. unit in one of the two jointly owned facilities.

Business Office Clericals

The Board seemed to create an exception from its normal policy for small hospitals in *Appalachian Regional Hospitals, Inc.*,[64] where business office clericals were included in a service and maintenance unit at the union's request and over the employer's objection. The employer contended that, consistent with the agency's standard policy, there should be a separate unit for those clericals. However, because of the hospital's small size, and the higher than normal degree of functional integration that the Board inferred from these circumstances, a combined unit was found appropriate. It is unclear whether the decision would have been the same if the employer had argued for a combined unit and the union had sought separate ones. However, the Board intimated that the result would have been different under those circumstances, as it mentioned that no union had indicated a willingness to separately represent the business office clericals. Thus, this case, as in the professional and technical areas, has an aroma of extent of organization decision making by the Board.

In *NLRB v. Mercy Hospitals of Sacramento, Inc.*,[65] the Ninth Circuit denied enforcement of a Board order that refused to accept the agreement of the parties as to placement of clerical employees. (The Supreme Court declined review of the Ninth Circuit action.) The parties had stipulated to a service and maintenance unit and a separate all-clerical unit. The Board set it aside, holding that business office clericals must be in a bargaining unit separate from other clericals. The court held that the Board's refusal to accept the stipulation was improper. This case is significant in that it acknowledges the importance of the nonproliferation mandate set by Congress. It also is significant in that it reinforces the trend of judicial resistance to arbitrary decisions of the NLRB in determining hospital bargaining units.

The *Mercy Hospitals* decision does not, however, address the Board's fundamental policy of establishing a separate unit for business office clericals and excluding them from a service and maintenance unit. Following remand, the Board issued a supplemental decision directing an election in the stipulated units.[66]

Because of the operational and functional integration existing in most hospitals, the NLRB has had difficulty drawing a precise line between business office clericals and other hospital clerical employees. The business office clerical definition was applied to medical records department employees in two cases, with conflicting results, although in both instances the employees appeared to work in a separate office and their basic duties (maintaining medical records) were essentially the same.[67] The same definition was applied, again with conflicting results, in two cases involving admitting clerks, although in both situations the employees worked in an admitting office and their functions appeared to be essentially the same.[68] In a later case, the Board found patient admitting clerks and patient record clerks not to be business office clericals but rather, because of their substantial patient contact, held that they should be included in a service and maintenance unit along with other nonprofessional employees.[69]

Accordingly, although unit placement of clerical employees may vary somewhat, the NLRB appears to remain substantially committed to a separate bargaining unit for business office clerical employees and inclusion of all other clerical employees in service and maintenance units.

Service and Maintenance Employees

The Board continued to equivocate in the area of maintenance department and boiler operator units. Separate maintenance department units were rejected in *Northeastern Hospital*[70] and *Peter Bent Brigham Hospital.*[71] In *Mercy Center for Health Care Services,*[72] the Board found that a maintenance department unit was inappropriate but approved a unit of boiler operators. Maintenance department units were held appropriate, however, in four other cases.[73]

Other appellate courts have joined the Third Circuit's decision in *Roxborough* in reversing the Board on separate hospital maintenance unit decisons.

In all of the cases, the courts based their reversals, in part if not wholly, on the Congressional directive to avoid unit proliferation in the health care industry.[74]

One court admonished the Board for embarking "on an erratic course in making bargaining unit determinations"[75] and suggested future determinations be more in keeping with the intent of Congress.

St. Vincent's Hospital v. NLRB[76] is of particular significance as it constituted the first direct judicial attack on the Board's maintenance unit policy. After noting the Congressional concern for potential fragmentation of bargaining units in hospitals, the Third Circuit concluded that the NLRB had "failed to heed that admonition"[77] and refused to enforce the agency's determination that a separate unit of four boiler operators was appropriate.

St. Vincent's also is of critical importance as it is the first decision in which a court of appeals interpreted in definitive terms the Congressional mandate against proliferation of bargaining units. Although the case arose in the context of a separate unit of boiler operators, the scope of the decision is much broader because it prohibits reliance by the Board on traditional unit factors and establishes the Congressional mandate as the standard to guide the NLRB in unit determination cases involving health care facilities. Other appellate courts subsequently have adopted this position. The Third Circuit specifically refused enforcement of the Board order in *Allegheny General Hospital II*[78] that had found a separate hospital maintenance unit to be inappropriate.[79] The court held that it had "no intention of reappraising" its position in this area and stated its displeasure with the Board on the issue by concluding that "the Board is not a court nor is it equal to this court in matters of statutory interpretation. Thus, a disagreement by the NLRB with a decision by this court is simply an academic exercise that possesses no authoritative effect."

The Second Circuit Court of Appeals also disagreed with the board's decision in *Allegheny II.* In *NLRB v. Mercy Hospital Ass'n,*[80] the court, in response to the NLRB's theory on legislative history, stated "Congress was expressing concern not only that health care institutions be spared the egregious unit proliferation of the construction trades but that less extreme unit fragmentation arising from application of usual criteria could also impede effective delivery of health care services."

The NLRB attempted to persuade the Supreme Court to review the *Mercy Hospital Ass'n* decision but the Court refused to hear the appeal.[81] The Board thereafter stated its intention to reconsider the service and maintenance unit question in health care facilities. However, as of the end of 1980, it had not issued any new guidelines in this area and a substantial legal disagreement remained between it and the courts on this issue.

SECTION 8(g)—THE 10-DAY STRIKE NOTICE

Section 8(g)[82] of the Amendments establishes a notification procedure with which a labor organization must comply before a strike or other concerted work stoppage may take place. In an effort to ameliorate the threat that unannounced and unanticipated work stoppages pose to the uninterrupted delivery of health care services,[83] Section 8(g) requires that a labor organization provide the health care institution and the Federal Mediation and Conciliation Service (FMCS) with written notice specifying the date and time of any strike, picketing, or other work stoppage at least ten days in advance of the planned activity. If the strike follows bargaining for an initial contract after certification or recognition of the labor organization, the notice may not be given until expiration of an earlier 30-day notice required by Section 8(d)(B) of the act.

A failure to comply with Section 8(g) can carry with it two consequences. First, a strike or work stoppage in derogation of 8(g)'s notice requirement constitutes an unfair labor practice.[84] Second, a related amendment to Section 8(d) provides that union members who engage in activity regulated by Section 8(g) that is not preceded by a proper notice lose their status as employees protected by the Act. Thus, an employer generally may terminate such employees and not run afoul of the Act.[85]

The Board has adopted and steadfastly maintained a "literal" or "plain meaning" approach to 8(g)'s construction. In most instances this approach has led to a broad construction of the section, although in construing the term "labor organization" it has led to a narrow reading.

Construction Picketing Cases

One of the most significant developments in this area has been the appellate courts' refusal to accept the Board's broad, literal construction of the phrase "any strike or picketing . . . *at* a health care institution" that included picketing by nonhealth care employees directed at similar employees performing work at health care institutions.

This issue was first before the Board in 1975 in *United Association of Journeymen and Apprentices of the Plumbing and Pipefitting Industry of the United States and Canada, Local 630 (Lein-Steenberg).*[86] Lein-Steenberg had been retained by a hospital to perform construction work at the hospital. One of the subcontractors hired by Lein-Steenberg, Taylor, was nonunion and had a continuing dispute with Local 630.

Without giving a ten-day notice, Local 630 conducted area standards picketing at the gate that had been reserved for Taylor. It was stipulated that the reserved gate picketing in no way blocked the access of hospital employees to the facility and that none of the institution's work had been disrupted.

Thus, the Board was asked to determine if the phrase ". . . all picketing . . . *at* a health care institution" encompassed all picketing occurring on the property of the facility or only disputes directed against the institution itself. The Board concluded that a violation of the Act had occurred. It held that in enacting Section 8(g), Congress was concerned primarily with protecting the public against the disruption of the delivery of health care services. Consequently, the Board felt health care institutions were to be accorded special consideration by providing them with advance notice of any type of picketing and work stoppages.

Relying on its decision in *Lein-Steenberg*, the Board also found two other similar instances of nondisruptive, reserved gate picketing that were not preceded by ten-day notices to be violative of 8(g).[87]

All three of the NLRB's decisions, however, subsequently were denied enforcement by the courts. In *NLRB v. International Brotherhood of Electrical Workers, Local 388*[88] the court first applied the Board's literal meaning construction and found it wanting because it led to ambiguous results.

In order to determine the proper construction to be given the section, the court conducted its own review of 8(g)'s legislative history. Like the Board, the court was impressed by Congress's desire to protect the public from disruption of health care services. However, it reasoned that the harm from which Congress was protecting the public was the increase in concerted activities that could be expected on the part of health care employees who formerly were outside the Act's purview, rather than from increased activity by nonhealth care employees who historically had enjoyed the Act's protection. Thus, there was no reason for Congress to extend 8(g) to nonhealth care employees.

Relying heavily on the Seventh Circuit's decision in *Local 388*, the D.C. Circuit Court also denied enforcement of the Board's position in *Laborers' International Union of North America, Local 1057 vs. NLRB.*[89] Quoting liberally from the Seventh Circuit's analysis in *Local 388*, the D.C. Circuit was similarly convinced that the Board's plain meaning approach to construing Section 8(g) led to ambiguous results and therefore rejected its application.

The Board has subsequently withdrawn from its previous position with respect to 10-day notices in construction picketing cases and has adopted the position articulated by the courts.[89a] It will continue, however, to issue complaints in construction picketing cases if the picketing is directed at a hospital in general even if the union is not seeking to represent health care employees.[89b]

Unrepresented Employees

Prior to 1977, the NLRB did not have occasion to consider how broadly it would construe the term "labor organization" or whether it would require unrepresented employees to serve 8(g) notices before engaging in concerted work stoppages. However, the General Counsel of the Board indicated shortly after the Act's Amendments passage that based on comments made by Senator Robert A. Taft, Jr. during the debate,[90] strikes, picketing, and concerted work stoppages of unrepresented employees might require an 8(g) notice.[91]

The Board announced its position in *Walker Methodist Residence and Health Care Center, Inc.*,[92] holding that 8(g) applies only to labor organizations and does not require a notice before the concerted activities of unrepresented health care employees. In *Walker*, two unrepresented nurses' aides left their work post for approximately 15 minutes until their supervisor could meet with them in order to receive a grievance that they had prepared. Neither had served the employer with a ten-day notice prior to their work action. The employer subsequently discharged both employees for unauthorized absences from their work posts, and argued that their failure to give an 8(g) notice deprived them of whatever protection the Act otherwise would have given their work stoppage.

The Board again adopted a plain meaning construction of the statute and held that 8(g) applied only to the acts of "labor organizations"[93] and not to unrepresented employees.

It cited its earlier plain meaning cases and reiterated that this was the approach it always had adopted in construing 8(g) and that its literal interpretation of the term "labor organization" was consonant with the section's legislative history. The Board stated that the primary evil that Congress sought to eliminate—the interruption of health care services—was not posed by the activities of unrepresented employees. Rather, it held only strikes by unions raise the specter of jeopardizing the delivery of health care services because such strikes are larger, are likely to last longer, and are accompanied by picket lines.

Since *Walker*, the Board consistently has refused to require unrepresented employees to give 8(g) notices prior to any concerted work stoppages. For example, in *Mercy Hospital Ass'n, Inc.*,[94] six unrepresented nurses aides walked off their jobs to protest alleged understaffing and subsequently were terminated by the employer. Relying on *Walker*, the agency held that since the employees were not represented by a union the work stoppage was not that of a labor organization, and thus they were not required to give an 8(g) notice prior to walking off their jobs.

Probably the most extreme example of the NLRB's steadfast refusal to depart from its literal interpretation of "labor organization" is found in its opinion in *Long Beach Youth Center, Inc.*[95] Seventeen unrepresented employees met to draw up a list of written demands to present to management. They also carried out a "sick-in" to protest working conditions. No 8(g) notice preceded this work stoppage, and several of the employees subsequently were terminated by the employer.

The Board again relied on *Walker* and held that 8(g) applied only to picketing or concerted work stoppages carried out by employees who were formally represented by labor organizations. Furthermore, the Board rejected the argument that the 17 employees who had met previously to discuss their grievances and how to present them to management were nonetheless not a labor organization as that term is defined in Section 2(5) because they had not formally designated themselves as a labor organization, had not selected one of their number as their representative for purposes of presenting grievances to management, and had not signed authorization cards to be represented by a labor union rather than represent themselves. On appeal the court upheld the Board's position.[96]

The NLRB's construction of "labor organization" also was upheld by the court in *Kapiolani Hospital v. NLRB*.[97] There an unrepresented ward clerk was discharged when she failed to report to work because she refused to cross a picket line set up by the hospital's striking registered nurses. The employer unsuccessfully argued that the clerk's failure to give an 8(g) notice prior to her absence deprived her of any protection of the Act and made her discharge lawful.

The Board again relied upon *Walker* in *Villa Care Inc., d/b/a/ Edmonds Villa Care Center*.[98] There, several nurses' aides spontaneously left their posts, demanding extra pay for working while understaffed. The employer refused, explaining that the nurses' aides now were represented by a union (certified only days earlier) and only it could bargain for pay increases. When two aides refused to return to work, they were terminated. The Board held that the walkout did not lose its protected status despite failure to give ten-day notice; since negotiations had not yet begun, no labor organization was involved. It found no evidence that the union was connected in any way with the walkout, and treated the aides as if they were unrepresented. The Board also ordered the nurses' aides reinstated on the theory that their requests were consistent with union demands and past employer practice.

The Board and one court have held that the Section 8(g) notice does not apply to picketing activity of unrepresented physicians. The case, *Montefiore Hospital v. NLRB*,[99] involved two part-time physicians employed by the hospital who walked out without giving notice and joined in a sympathy strike with service and maintenance employees. The hospital discharged the physicians for taking part in the strike and for failing to provide a ten-day notice pursuant to Section 8(g). The Board and court rejected the hospital's argument that the physicians were required to provide a ten-day notice since they were not represented by any union. The court also rejected the hospital's argument that strikes without notice by physicians should be unprotected because of the special medical risks they might present to patient care.

The court did uphold the discharge of the physicians, however, based on their conduct on the picket line, which included giving false advice to the public that prospective patients could not be properly treated by the hospital. The court specifically found that their "misconduct went beyond the limits of fair persuasion and honest appeals to the public . . ." and ". . . were deceptive and aimed at evoking a submissive, unreasoned, misinformed reaction from those whose cooperation they sought." Accordingly, the physicians lost the Act's protection of their otherwise legitimate concerted activity. Similar arguments might be developed in the future by a hospital to focus upon strike misconduct of other health care employees, thereby causing them to lose their statutory protection.

Nondisruptive Concerted Activities

The Board's literal meaning construction of 8(g) has led it to adopt a broad per se rule, subjecting any picketing by a labor organization to 8(g)'s notice requirements, irrespective of whether the picketing disrupts the hospital's activities.

In *District 1199, National Union of Hospital and Health Care Employees (First Health Care Corporation)*[100] one union had begun picketing a hospital pursuant to a proper 8(g) notice. The officers of a second union joined the picket line in sympathy for an hour and a half, but failed to precede their picketing with an 8(g) notice. The Board found that the term "any picketing" as used in 8(g) encompassed various forms of such activity, including even a brief, nondisruptive

sympathy picket line. Therefore, it held that the union's failure to provide an 8(g) notice in advance of its picketing violated the Act.

The Board carried this per se interpretation even further in 1977 in *District 1199, National Union of Hospital and Health Care Employees (United Hospitals of Newark)*.[101] In that case, during the course of negotiations, the union organized a demonstration by several of its members in a show of support for its negotiating committee. The employees who participated did so during their off hours and did not block access to the hospital and in no way disrupted the facility's work. The demonstrating employees carried placards that bore such messages as, "We demand a union contract," "We need decent wages," and the like. No 8(g) notice had been given prior to this demonstration.

The NLRB held that Congress had designed Section 8(g) to minimize the threat of disruption of health care services and that any form of picketing carried with it such a risk. Thus, the Board concluded that Congress intended to subject all kinds of picketing to Section 8(g) irrespective of whether such picketing caused a work disruption.

The Board also has concluded that a union council was required to give ten days' notice before picketing to protect a hospital using its own unorganized employees to perform certain painting work.[102] The Board held such picketing potentially disruptive of the hospital's operations and rejected the argument that the 8(g) notice requirement applied only to work stoppages "which derive from contractual disputes."

Procedural Requirements for a Valid Notice

The Congressional committee reports accompanying the Amendments stated that a labor organization could decide unilaterally to start its picketing or strike activity later than the time set in the ten-day notice, but any extension beyond 72 hours of the notice time was unreasonable, and even within the 72-hour grace period, a union must give at least 12 hours' notice of the exact time the picketing or strike is to commence.

In *Federal Hill Nursing Center*[103] the union gave the employer written notice that picketing would begin on July 5 at 6 A.M. However, the picketing did not begin until July 8 at 2:30 P.M. The home was not given any notice of a delay nor was there any agreement between the parties regarding the delay. The Board found that the union had violated Section 8(g) because it did not begin its picketing within the 72-hour period after the ten-day notice had been expired, but did so 80½ hours after the notice date.

In another procedural case, the NLRB held that compliance with the intent of the statute was achieved even though the letter from the union giving notice of the strike was not received by the hospital until after the strike began.[104] The Board found the delay in receipt of the notice was the fault of the Postal Service and that the hospital had received actual advance notice elsewhere, thus providing it with an adequate opportunity to make patient care plans.

In *District 1199-E, National Union of Hospital and Health Care Employees (Greater Pennsylvania Avenue Nursing Center)*,[105] the board held that a union does not violate Section 8(g) when it merely threatens to strike before the expiration of the ten-day notice period. The Board reasoned that 8(g) requires the notice only just before a labor organization engages in picketing or strike activity; it does not prohibit threats of such activity before the expiration of the ten-day period.

Flagrant Unfair Labor Practices

At the time Section 8(g) was enacted, both houses of Congress recognized that there would be certain exemptions from its notice requirements that were not set forth in the section's express language. For example, both committees stated that the ten-day notice requirement would be excused in the event of flagrant unfair labor practices on the part of the employer.[106]

The parameters of this exemption were explored by the NLRB in *District 1199-E, National Union of Hospital and Health Care Employees (CHC Corporation)*.[107] There the employer's nursing home administrator repeatedly had cancelled grievance meetings with the employees' union representative and at one point hid to avoid meeting with him. When the union representative learned that the administrator was hiding in the building, he called the employees off the floor to the administrator's office, and the workers left their posts for 5 to 15 minutes while waiting to meet with the executive. The employer subsequently filed an unfair labor practice charge, claiming that the work stoppage violated Section 8(g) because it had not been preceded by a ten-day notice.

The Board held that the section does not sanction blatant disregard for the bargaining process and that such a disregard excuses the need for any notice prior to a union's protest of the employer's conduct.

The Board also held that although in its 8(g) analysis it generally was concerned with the threat of harm rather than the actual harm resulting from a strike, when there was egregious wrongdoing by the employer it would consider whether the union's conduct had resulted in any harm. As no patient had been harmed by

the short work stoppage in this case, the Board assessed no liability against the union.

Finally, in *Local 144, Hotel, Hospital, Nursing Home and Lodge Service Employees Union (Brooklyn Methodist Church Home)*,[108] the union picketed a health care center without first providing an 8(g) notice. The union claimed that the employer had committed massive violations of the Act by refusing to hire its members, thereby exempting it from 8(g)'s notice requirement. The Board held that the nursing home had committed no unfair labor practice because its refusal was fully justified by its preexisting agreement with another union.

Preemption

Section 8(g) also has played a role supporting the theory that the amendments preempt any state jurisdiction over health care employees, particularly state no-strike laws.

A year after the Amendments' enactment, the NLRB announced in *In Re: State of Minnesota*[109] that through its establishment of Section 8(g)'s prestrike notice requirements and the other provisions, Congress intended to permit strikes by health care employees. Thus, the Board concluded that the Minnesota state law that forbade strikes by health care employees was preempted, and refused to cede its jurisdiction over nonprofit health care institution employees to the Minnesota state agency that formerly had held sway.

However, in 1976 a New York court granted the state's attorney general an injunction enjoining a threatened strike of nursing home employees on the basis of New York legislation that prevented strikes by not-for-profit health care institution employees. *State of New York v. Local 1115, Joint Board Nursing Home and Hospital Employees Division*.[110] In an extensive opinion the state court concluded that New York law had not been preempted by the 1974 Amendments.

In response, the NLRB sought to enjoin the state from proceeding with the enforcement of the injunction. In *NLRB v. State of New York*[111] a federal district court granted the Board the injunction. The court reasoned that the Amendments granted health care employees the right to strike, limited only by the notice requirements of 8(d) and 8(g), and therefore the conflicting New York legislation had been preempted.

SECTION 8(d) NOTICE AND BOARDS OF INQUIRY

The Amendments established special time periods for filing Section 8(d)[112] notices. Under the amendments, any party desiring to terminate or modify a bargaining agreement in the health care industry must serve written notice of such intent on the other party at least 90 days before the expiration of the agreement[113] and give notice to the Federal Mediation and Conciliation Service (FMCS) and any appropriate state mediation agency within 30 days after each 90-day notice.[114] In the case of initial contract negotiations, "at least thirty days' notice of the existence of a dispute" must be given to the FMCS and any such state agency.[115]

Upon receipt of such a notice, the FMCS is required to contact the parties in an effort to achieve a settlement through mediation and conciliation. Parties to a dispute also can be required to participate in mediation at the direction of the FMCS.[116] If in the opinion of the FMCS, a threatened or actual strike or lockout affecting a health care institution will, if permitted to occur or continue, "substantially interrupt" the delivery of health care in the locality, the director may appoint a board of inquiry (BOI). The BOI must be appointed within 30 days after the 60-day notice to FMCS required by 8(d)(3) (or within 10 days after the 30-day notice to FMCS required by 8(d) in an initial contract negotiation). The BOI is required to investigate and issue a written report to the parties within 15 days of its establishment. The report is not binding on the parties.[117]

Two major issues have arisen as to the discretion of the FMCS's director in appointing a BOI:

1. What is the time frame in which a BOI must be appointed?
2. What is the scope of the judicial review of the director's discretion in determining that a strike or lockout would "substantially interrupt" the delivery of health care and thus warrant the appointment of a BOI?

The FMCS has taken the position that in a contract renewal dispute a BOI can be appointed either within 30 days of receipt of the 8(d) notice or within 30 days after the last day permitted for giving such a notice, whichever is later.[118] In a contract renewal dispute, this would permit the FMCS to appoint a BOI either no later than 30 days before the contract's expiration or within 30 days of actual receipt of the notice.

The FMCS also contends that under Section 213 its director has wide discretion in determining whether the appointment of a BOI is necessary, and that that discretion is subject only to very limited judicial review.[119]

In *Affiliated Hospitals of San Francisco v. Scearce*[120] the court enjoined the FMCS from proceeding with the appointment of a BOI because it had failed to establish the board within 30 days of the union's notice that an agreement had not been reached with the health care institutions. After reviewing Section 213's legislative history, the court held that a BOI must be appointed within 30 days of an 8(d) notice and that the director has no power to name one after that period.

However, in *Sinai Hospital of Baltimore, Inc. v. Scearce*,[121] the district court upheld the FMCS's view that it could appoint a BOI within 30 days of the last possible day on which an 8(d) notice could be given, even if that date was more than 30 days after the notice actually was served. Furthermore, the court held that under Section 213 it could make only a very limited review of the director's discretion in appointing a BOI.

However, appellate courts have held consistently that the FMCS must appoint a BOI within 30 days after receipt of an 8(d) notice. For example, in *Affiliated Hospitals*[122] the Ninth Circuit concluded that a BOI must be appointed within 30 days of an 8(d) notice.

In *Sinai Hospital of Baltimore, Inc. v. Scearce*[123] the Fourth Circuit held that the FMCS could appoint a BOI more than 30 days after receipt of an 8(d) notice. After reviewing the congressional debates, the court concluded that the FMCS director must appoint a BOI within 30 days of receipt of an 8(d) notice and that nothing in the legislative history pointed to a contrary conclusion.

However, the FMCS's view that its director's discretion is subject to limited judicial review has met with better success in the courts. In *St. Elizabeth Hospital v. Horvitz*,[124] the court upheld the broad discretion of the director to appoint BOIs, stressing "the great need for speed in this difficult area of labor relations" and that "neither judicial review of the substantive decision nor a full and formal administrative record should be required or expected, nor . . . [is] such . . . anticipated by the Statute."

The limited scope of judicial review of the director's discretion was again reaffirmed in *Sinai Hospital v. Scearce*.[125] In that action the hospital argued that the director had abused the discretion of that office in appointing a BOI because: (1) the director had appointed a BOI without finding that there was a threatened or actual strike or lockout; (2) if such strike or lockout occurred it would not substantially interrupt the delivery of health care in the locality; and (3) no impasse had been reached in the negotiations between the parties. The hospital particularly stressed the fact that any strike or lockout at its facility would have minimal impact on the community in that its 507-bed complement was very small compared to the 8,422 beds that were available in the metropolitan area. Notwithstanding these facts, the court rejected the hospital's position and expressed agreement with the *St. Elizabeth* conclusion that the scope of judicial review is very narrow under Section 213.

THE ALLY DOCTRINE

The Ally Doctrine is a legal doctrine developed from Board case law that defines the rights of third parties who provide assistance to an employer who is involved in a labor dispute. This doctrine states that where during the course of a labor dispute, a secondary employer performs work that, but for the existence of such labor dispute, would have been performed by the striking employees of the primary employer, the secondary employer loses his status of a neutral, and the labor organization involved is entitled to extend its economic activity to the secondary employer.

During the debates prior to the passage of the Amendments, Congress stated specifically that the Ally Doctrine exception to Section 8(b) (4)'s[126] proscription against secondary boycotts would be narrowed in the event of a strike against a health care institution. In identical language, the reports of both houses of Congress read:

> It is the sense of the Committee that where such secondary institutions *accept the patients of a primary employer* or otherwise provide life-sustaining services to the primary employer, *by providing the primary employer with an employee or employees who possess critical skills such as an EKG technician,* such conduct shall not be sufficient to cause the secondary employer to lose its neutral status . . . .[127] (Emphasis added.)

Congress thus intended to permit a neutral hospital to accept the patients of a primary employer and not thereby lose its status as a neutral.

Consistent with this legislative history, the General Counsel of the NLRB in his memorandum issued in 1974 shortly after the Amendments' enactment[128] stated that a hospital would not lose its neutral status if it accepted patients from, or supplied critical care help to, the struck institution. However, a neutral hospital would lose that status if it supplied noncritical personnel or if it not only accepted patients but also greatly expanded its noncritical staff in the process.

A memorandum issued by the Board's Division of Advice[129] significantly narrowed this exception to the Ally Doctrine, stating that a hospital could maintain its status as a neutral only if it accepted critically ill patients or those in potential need of immediate medical attention.

In the case before the Division of Advice, the union had struck a multihospital group. One of the hospitals had closed its infant intensive care unit and had made arrangements to have critically ill patients treated at another institution. Moreover, during the strike 46 pregnant women who were treated by doctors associated with the struck hospitals were admitted by their doctors to another hospital. The union threatened to picket both "neutral" hospitals, and the Division of Advice was asked to determine whether such picketing would be permissible under 8(b) (4).

The Division recognized that Congress's exception to the Ally Doctrine was applicable in this instance and that the union's threatened picketing would be unlawful. However, ignoring both Committee reports, the Division relied on a single statement made by Senator Harrison Williams (D., N.J.)[130] during the congressional debates and concluded that a neutral hospital could retain its status only if it accepted critically ill patients or those in need of immediate medical attention.

Thus, the NLRB's General Counsel's office now apparently views the Ally Doctrine exception as being dependent on the urgency of the medical needs of the patients who are transferred from the primary to the neutral hospital. This conclusion is of doubtful validity. As noted, Congress plainly intended to permit a hospital to accept all patients from a struck hospital without regard to the urgency of their medical needs and not thereby jeopardize its status as a neutral. Indeed, the Committee reports' only reference to "critical" was the statement that a neutral hospital could provide a struck hospital with employees who possess "critical" skills as well as accept the struck hospital's patients without losing its neutral status.

HEALTH CARE SUPERVISORS

Background

The NLRB's approach in determining whether health care employees are supervisors was established prior to the Amendments with respect to proprietary hospitals in *Doctor's Hospital of Modesto, Inc.*[131] Initially, the Board found that floor head nurses were supervisors within the meaning of Section 2(11) and therefore could not be included in a unit with other professional nurses.[132] However, it reserved judgment on charge nurses and certain other professional nurses, and permitted them to vote subject to challenge. In its second decision, the Board held that charge nurses and other nursing positions were not supervisory under the Act.[133] The authority exercised by charge nurses in informing other, lesser-skilled employees of work to be performed for patients, and ensuring that such work was done, was found to be incidental to their professional skills and without more, not an exercise of supervisory authority in the interest of their employer. This holding was distinguished from the prior determination that head nurses, in addition to performing their professional duties and responsibilities, also could make effective recommendations affecting the job and pay status of the employees working under them.

The appellate court agreed with the finding that nurses are highly trained professionals who occasionally use independent judgment did not necessarily make them managers or supervisors. Deferring to the NLRB's expertise, the court enforced the Board's order.

The Board was further encouraged in its approach when Congress considered the Amendments. Various groups representing health care professionals had urged Congress to amend Section 2(11) to exclude professionals from the definition of "supervisor." This was intended to ensure that registered nurses, physicians, and other professionals would not be denied protection of the Act because their professional duties required occasional direction of other employees with respect to patient care. In reporting out the bills, the Senate Committee on Labor and Public Welfare and the House Committee on Education and Labor both said they had studied the definition of Section 2(11) with respect to health care professionals and concluded that existing Board decisions obviated the need for such an amendment. The committees noted:

> [T]he Board has carefully avoided applying the definition of "supervisor" to a health care professional who gives direction to other employees in the exercise of professional judgment, which direction is incidental to the professional's treatment of patients, and thus is not the exercise of supervisory authority in the interest of the employer.

> The Committee expects the Board to continue evaluating the facts of each case in this manner when making its determinations.[134]

These are the only legislative statements directly relating to the identification of supervisors in the health care context, in which many persons of varying skills and tasks work together to provide patient care.

Subsequent to the passage of the Amendments, the Board continued to follow the policy of *Doctor's Hospital*. However, recognizing the need for apparent consistency, the NLRB asserted that aside from professional considerations, the traditional standards for determining supervisory status would continue to be applicable to health care professionals.[135] Later Board decisions suggest, however, that this assertion was not entirely candid.

For example, it is well established that an employee need possess only one of the factors enumerated in Section 2(11) in order to qualify as a supervisor.[136] However, Board decisions during the postamendment period suggest that with respect to health care institutions, some of the factors specified in Section 2(11) are more important than others, and that their absence would preclude a finding that a particular employee is a statutory supervisor even if other enumerated factors are present. For example, the Board evinced particular concern with whether alleged supervisors participated in the hiring process and effectively recommended the employment of applicants. Often, persons lacking this authority were found to be employees rather than supervisors even though they could issue oral reprimands or effectively recommend more serious discipline, promotion, and wage increases.[137] One Circuit Court has agreed with the Board's approach of focusing on particular types of "supervisory" authority.[137a]

The Board also was skeptical about the lack of authority to call in off-duty employees, modify or revise work schedules, or authorize overtime.[138]

Furthermore, subsequent to the Amendments, the traditional standards that the NLRB did apply to health care professionals appeared to be changed or modified from their original meaning, with incongruous results. For example, the Board had developed a rule that when an alleged supervisor supervised other employees only on certain types of jobs, 50 percent or more of work time would have to be spent on the jobs requiring the exercise of supervisory authority in order to qualify such person as a supervisor.[139] When this requirement, which had been developed in a special factual setting, was applied to health care cases, it developed into the very difficult rule that supervisory functions over nonunit employees would be counted under Section 2(11) only if they consumed more than 50 percent of the alleged supervisor's time. At the same time, the Board insisted that R.N.s be placed in a single unit, L.P.N.s in a technical unit, and nurses' aides and orderlies in yet a third unit. Thus, R.N.s inevitably would spend much of their time supervising "nonunit" employees; yet many of those supervisory functions would be virtually ignored by the Board.[140] In so restricting its analysis, the Board has made it quite difficult for any R.N.s or L.P.N.s other than high-level supervisors to qualify as supervisors under Sections 2(11) and 9.

During the postamendment period, the NLRB also began to extend to licensed vocational nurses (L.V.N.s) and licensed practical nurses (L.P.N.s) the standards it had developed to ensure that professional employees would not be found to be supervisors based on direction incidental to professional responsibility. L.V.N.s—who often are completely in charge of patient care in nursing homes and, pursuant to those responsibilities, direct aides and orderlies—were found not to be supervisors if they lacked authority to hire or fire other L.P.N.s or if they spent less than 51 percent of their time performing supervisory functions over nonunit employees.[141] This extension was somewhat surprising in light of the fact that Congress did not mention L.V.N.s as one of the professional groups that traditionally exercise direction over other employees as part of professional patient care. Furthermore, the Board refused to include L.V.N.s in the same unit as R.N.s because of the assertedly technical nature of the L.V.N.s' job as compared with the professionalism of the R.N. Nevertheless, the Board applied to L.V.N.s its "professional" standards rather than those used in settings not involving patient care.

Recent Decisions

Several recent cases clearly reveal the NLRB's deviation, in the patient care context, from its rule that any one of the factors enumerated in Section 2(11) will accord supervisory status. In *McAlester General Hospital* (1977),[142] the Board found that R.N.s acting as charge nurses were not supervisors even though their performance evaluations of employees—including staff nurses—were the sole determinants of pay increases. The Board held that because the point score rather than the supervisor's stated recommendation was determinative of whether an increase was given, the wage increase was not based on the charge nurse's judgment.

In *Turtle Creek Convalescent Center, Inc.* (1978),[143] the Board concluded that charge nurses were not supervisors. It held that they did not participate in the hiring process and apparently did not make effective recommendations for discharge.

In a 1980 case, *Exeter Hospital*,[144] the Board enumerated four functions required of a charge nurse to accord supervisory status. To be a supervisor, a charge nurse must prepare work schedules and hear and grant requests for time off; entertain grievances and administer discipline verbally and in writing; give recommendations for promotion that will be accepted without interference from the director of nursing; and evaluate performance of other nurses as the sole basis

for merit increases. Only if all four functions are present will a charge nurse be given supervisory status.

In the fourth case, *Pine Manor Nursing Home* (1978),[145] the Board decided that L.P.N.s who were authorized to discipline nurses' aides by warning and suspension, and whose recommendations for discharge of aides were routinely followed, nevertheless were not statutory supervisors. The primary reason was that L.P.N.s took no part in the interviewing or hiring process. The Board also pointed out that final decisions about terminations and serious discipline were made by the director.

In contrast, the Board found in *Associated Hospitals of the East Bay*[146] that nursing care coordinators (N.C.C.s) were supervisors. Again, the primary reason was the fact that N.C.C.s interviewed prospective employees and made effective recommendations about their hire. Although six out of the 90 recommendations were overruled by the director, this success rate was found to be sufficient to constitute effective recommendation. In addition, the nursing care coordinators were primarily responsible for evaluating other nurses.

Thus, in the health care context, nurses rarely will qualify as statutory supervisors unless they possess—and exercise—the authority to effectively recommend hiring.

In *A. Barton Hepburn Hospital*,[147] the NLRB found that an inservice education assistant was not a supervisor even though the person conferred with the personnel director prior to the hiring of nursing aides. Although she made recommendations on their hiring, the Board said that even if she did effectively recommend such hiring, her duties with respect to nurses aides, who are not in the unit in which the inservice assistant would be placed, assumed a very minor portion of her time—less than 50 percent. The Board therefore concluded that in these circumstances the inservice education assistant would not be a supervisor: "The Board has stated that, 'we shall exclude . . . only those . . . [professionals] who supervise other employees in the unit or who spend more than 50 percent of their time supervising non-unit employees.'"[148]

The Board also continued to apply its "professional standards," however described, to analyze the supervisory functions of L.V.N.s and L.P.N.s. In *Greenpark Care Center*,[149] the L.P.N.s were responsible for instructing aides and orderlies, assigning tasks to them, transferring them to other floors, evaluating their performance, and initiating warning slips. L.P.N.s also were consulted in discharge cases. However, primarily because they did not interview, hire, or make the final decision to discharge employees, the Board disregarded these other factors that in cases that did not involve professionals engaged in patient care would certainly indicate supervisory status. It pointed out that the L.P.N.s' evaluations of aides and orderlies were not discussed with the workers and there was no evidence that the evaluations actually affected their employment status. Although L.P.N.s had the authority to transfer employees, the Board seemed to find it significant that the R.N.s were informed of the transfers. All of these duties were found to be fundamentally related to patient care.

Similarly, in *Pine Manor Nursing Home,*[150] the NLRB again declined to find that L.P.N.s were supervisors within the meaning of the Act. The L.P.N.s directed nurses' aides through oral and written instructions. More importantly, the collective bargaining agreement specifically authorized the charge nurses to reprimand, suspend, and discharge the aides. Certain L.P.N.s testified that they were authorized to discipline aides by warnings and suspensions and their recommendations on discharges were followed routinely.

The Board concluded, however, that the L.P.N.s played no part in interviewing or hiring, and that the final decision to terminate was made by the director of nurses. The Board held that the L.P.N.s' disciplinary activities were limited to minor matters and that serious conduct breaches were referred to the director. Of particular significance was the fact that several L.P.N.s testified that, notwithstanding the collective bargaining agreement or the testimony of other witnesses, they did not have the authority to issue written warnings without consulting with the director. Thus, the Board concluded that although the union contract specifically authorized L.P.N.s to reprimand, suspend, and discharge aides, the employer in reality never had granted such power, and the L.P.N.s had not exercised it.[151] The Board also found that the temporary transfers did not require independent judgment by the L.P.N.s and that the instructions regarded patient care and were routine in nature.

Finally, supervisory nurses' participation in an organization or association does not automatically disqualify that entity from becoming a labor organization under the Act. In *Sierra Vista Hospital, Inc.,*[152] the NLRB ruled that R.N. supervisors could belong to and be actively involved in the leadership of a nurses' labor organization so long as their participation did not create "a clear and present danger to the bargaining integrity of the organization." Two factors were given as determining whether a conflict of interest existed sufficient to disqualify the organization as a bargaining representative:

1. The Board will look at the degree of participation in the labor organization generally, focusing in particular on the number of supervisors in positions of authority.
2. The Board will look at the particular institution and determine whether the facts are such that the participation of the third party employer's supervisors disqualifies the labor organization at that particular institution. The Board's rationale was founded on the "strong public policy favoring the free choice of a bargaining agent by the employees."

Sierra Vista has withstood a number of challenges since it was announced in 1979. Generally the Board has reiterated its position and found that the participation of supervisors was either minimal or insulated from the collective bargaining process.[153] In only one case has the employer succeeded in meeting its heavy burden of proof and demonstrated sufficient supervision to disqualify the labor organization.[154] There, an in-house "subcommittee" chaired by supervisors attempted to bargain for all R.N.s. The Board found insufficient precautions to insulate the bargaining process from the supervisors' conflict of interest.

NOTES

1. Pub. L. 93-360, 88 Stat. 395, 396, 397.
2. 29 U.S.C. § 152 (14).
3. 218 NLRB 1270, 89 LRRM 1372 (1975).
4. 227 NLRB 728, 94 LRRM 1676 (1977).
5. *See also, Mon Valley United Health Servs., Inc.,* 238 NLRB No. 129, 99 LRRM 1332 (1978).
6. 227 NLRB 1668, 94 LRRM 1629 (1977).
7. *Jack L. Williams, D.D.S.,* 219 NLRB 1045, 90 LRRM 1188 (1975), *enforced,* 538 F.2d 337 (9th Cir. 1976). The $250,000 gross annual revenue standard is applicable to dental facilities.
8. *See, e.g., Charles Circle Clinic, Inc.,* 215 NLRB 382, 87 LRRM 1736 (1974); *Planned Parenthood Ass'n of Miami,* 217 NLRB 1098, 89 LRRM 1198 (1975).
9. In *Resident Home For the Mentally Retarded of Hamilton County, Inc.,* 239 NLRB No. 2, 99 LRRM 1443 (1978); *Mental Health Management, Inc.,* 237 NLRB No. 980, 98 LRRM 1504 (1978), and *Mon Valley United Health Servs., Inc., supra,* n. 5.
10. *Boston Medical Laboratory, Inc.,* 235 NLRB No. 170, 98 LRRM 1113 (1978). *See also, Center for Laboratory Medicine, Inc.,* 234 NLRB No. 56, 97 LRRM 1224 (1978).
11. *Damon Medical Laboratory, Inc.,* 234 NLRB No. 55, 97 LRRM 1225 (1978).
12. *San Diego Blood Bank,* 219 NLRB 116, 89 LRRM 1593 (1975); *Sacramento Medical Foundation Blood Bank,* 220 NLRB 904, n. 3, 90 LRRM 1604 (1975).
13. 237 NLRB 1040, 99 LRRM 1052 (1978).
14. 440 U.S. 490, 100 LRRM 2913 (1979).
15. *Mid American Health Servs.,* 247 NLRB No. 109, 103 LRRM 1234 (1980). *See also Bon Secours Hosp.,* 248 NLRB No. 19, 103 LRRM 1375 (1980), and *St. Anthony's Hosp. Syst.,* 252 NLRB No. 12, 105 LRRM 1350 (1980).

16. An amendment that would have accomplished this objective was introduced by Senator Sam Ervin (D., N.C.). It was rejected. S. Rep. 6963, 120th Cong. (daily ed., May 2, 1974).

17. S. Rep. No. 93-766, 93d Cong., 2d Sess. 5 (1974); H.R. Rep. No. 93-1051, 93d Cong. 2d Sess. 7 (1974).

18. *Dominican Santa Cruz Hosp.*, 218 NLRB 1211, 89 LRRM 1504 (1975); *Mercy Hosps. of Sacramento, Inc.*, 217 NLRB 765, 89 LRRM 1097 (1975).

19. *Valley Hosp.*, Ltd., 221 NLRB 1239, 90 LRRM 1061 (1975), amending 22c NLRB No. 21g 9c LRRM 1411 (1975).

20. *Morristown Hamblen Hosp. Ass'n*, 226 NLRB 76, 1193, LRRM 1166 (1976); *Victor Valley Hosp.*, 220 NLRB 977, 90 LRRM 1341 (1975); *Bishop Randall Hosp.*, 217 NLRB 1129, 89 LRRM 2822 (1975).

21. *Kaiser Foundation Hosps.*, 219 NLRB 325, 89 LRRM 1763 (1975); *Mercy Hosps. of Sacramento, Inc.*, *supra*, n. 18.

22. *Barnert Memorial Hosp. Ass'n*, 217 NLRB 775, 89 LRRM 1083 (1975).

23. *Newington Children's Hosp.*, 217 NLRB 793, 89 LRRM 1108 (1975).

24. *Mt. Airy Foundation*, 217 NLRB 802, 89 LRRM 1067 (1975).

25. *Illinois Extended Care Convalescent Center*, 220 NLRB 1085, 90 LRRM 1387 (1975).

26. *Sisters of St. Joseph of Peace*, 217 NLRB 797, 89 LRRM 1082 (1975); *St. Catherine's Hosp.*, 217 NLRB 787, 789, 89 LRRM 1070 (1975); *Mercy Hosps. of Sacramento, Inc.*, 217 NLRB 765, 769-70, 89 LRRM 1097 (1975).

27. *Newington Children's Hosp.*, *supra*, n. 23.

28. *Mercy Center for Health Care Services*, 227 NLRB 1814, 94 LRRM 1534 (1977); *Sutter Community Hosps.*, 227 NLRB 181, 94 LRRM 1450, (1976); *Anaheim Memorial Hospital*, 227 NLRB 161, 94 LRRM 1058 (1976); *Greater Bakersfield Memorial Hosp.*, 226 NLRB 971, 93 LRRM 1386, (1976); *Paul Kimball Hosp., Inc.*, 224 NLRB 458, 92 LRRM 1342, (1976); *St. Joseph Riverside Hosp.*, 224 NLRB 270, 92 LRRM 1340, (1976); *Baptist Memorial Hosp.*, 224 NLRB 199 (1976); *Riverside Methodist Hosp.*, 223 NLRB 1084, 92 LRRM 1033 (1976); *St. Vincent's Hosp.*, 223 NLRB 638, 91 LRRM 1513, (1976); *rev'd on other grounds*, 567 F.2d 558 (3d Cir. 1977), 97 LRRM 2119; *Jewish Hosp.*, 223 NLRB 614, 91 LRRM 1499, (1976); *Metropolitan Hosp.*, 223 NLRB 282, 91 LRRM 1429, (1976); *Shriners Hosps. for Crippled Children*, 217 NLRB 806, 89 LRRM 1076 (1975).

29. *St. Vincent's Hosp.*, 223 NLRB 638, 91 LRRM 1513 (1976), *rev'd*, 567 F.2d 588 (3d Cir. 1977), 97 LRRM 2119.

30. *Paul Kimball Hosp., Inc.*, 224 NLRB 458, 92 LRRM 1342 (1976).

31. Section 9(b)(3) of the act, as amended, 29 U.S.C. § 159(b)(3).

32. *Peninsula Hosp. Center & Peninsula Gen. Nursing Home*, 219 NLRB 139, 90 LRRM 1034 (1975).

33. *Memorial Hosp. of Roxborough*, 220 NLRB 402, *rev'd* 545 F.2d 351 (3d Cir. 1976); 90 LRRM 1369 (1975). Prior to the passage of the Amendments, private nonprofit health care institutions in some states were subject to state labor laws.

34. *Bay Medical Center, Inc.*, 231 NLRB No. 107, 96 LRRM 1619 (1977); *Bay Medical Center, Inc.*, 218 NLRB 620, 89 LRRM 1310 (1975).

35. *Otis Hosp., Inc.*, 219 NLRB 164, 89 LRRM 1545 (1975); *Otis Hosp.*, 222 NLRB No. 47, 91 LRRM 1255 (1976), enf. 545 F.2d 252 (1st Cir. 1976), 93 LRRM 2778.

36. 545 F.2d 351 (3d Cir. 1976), 93 LRRM 2571.

37. 230 NLRB 604, 95 LRRM 1430, (1977).

38. 223 NLRB 251, 91 LRRM 1398, (1976).

39. Section 2(3) of the act, as amended, 29 U.S.C. § 152(3).

40. *See also, Kansas City Gen. Hosp. & Medical Center, Inc.*, 225 NLRB 108, 93 LRRM 1362 (1976).

41. 566 F.2d 810 (2d Cir. 1971), 96 LRRM 2342.

42. 435 U.S. 904, 97 LRRM 2809 (1978).

43. *Physician's House Staff Ass'n. v. Fanning*, ___ F. 2d ___, (D.C. Cir. 1980), 104 LRRM 2940.

44. H.R. 2222 96th Cong., 1st sess. (1979).

45. 235 NLRB No. 29, 97 LRRM 1474 (1978).

46. 228 NLRB 578, 94 LRRM 1513 (1977).

47. 238 NLRB No. 56, 99 LRRM 1558 (1978).

48. 239 NLRB No. 104, 100 LRRM 1030 (1978).

49. 601 F.2d 404 (9th Cir. 1979), 101 LRRM 2943.

50. *Valley Hosp.*, Ltd., 221 NLRB 1239, 91 LRRM 1061 (1975).

51. *Family Doctor Medical Group*, a professional corp., 226 NLRB 118, 93 LRRM 1193 (1976).

52. *Newton-Wellesley Hosp.*, 219 NLRB 699, 90 LRRM 1090 (1975).

53. *Carl H. Neuman, M.D.*, d/b/a *Lydia E. Hall Hosp.*, 227 NLRB 573, 94 LRRM 1105 (1976).

54. *Rockridge Medical Care Center*, 221 NLRB 560, 90 LRRM 1721 (1975).

55. *Kaiser Foundation Health Plan of Colorado*, 230 NLRB 438, 95 LRRM 1376 (1977).

56. 248 NLRB No. 131, 104 LRRM 1007 (1980).

56a. 253 NLRB No. 139, 1061 LRRM 1071 (1981).

57. *Newton-Wellesley Hosp.*, 250 NLRB No. 86, 104 LRRM 1384 (1980); *see also* Brookwood Hosp., 252 NLRB No. 107, 105 LRRM 1331 (1980), and *Frederick Memorial Hosp.*, 254 NLRB No. 2, 106 LRRM 1102 (1981)..

58. 228 NLRB 21, 96 LRRM 1391 (1977).

59. 230 NLRB 976, 95 LRRM 1478 (1977).

60. 233 NLRB No. 85, 96 LRRM 1528 (1977).

61. *NLRB v. Sweetwater Hosp. Ass'n.*, 604 F.2d 454 (6th Cir. 1979), 102 LRRM 2246.

62. 227 NLRB 1706, 94 LRRM 1417 (1977).

63. *Bay Medical Center, Inc.*, 218 NLRB 620, 89 LRRM 1310 (1975); *enforced, NLRB v. Bay Medical Center*, 588 F.2d 1174, (6th Cir. 1978), 100 LRRM 2213.

64. 233 NLRB No. 85, 96 LRRM 1528 (1977).

65. 589 F.2d 968, (9th Cir. 1978), 98 LRRM 2800; *cert. denied.* 440 U.S. 910 (1979).

66. 244 NLRB No. 34, 102 LRRM 1016 (1979).

67. *Central Gen. Hosp.*, 223 NLRB 110, 91 LRRM 1433 (1976); *St. Luke's Episcopal Hosp.*, 222 NLRB 674, 91 LRRM 1359 (1976).

68. *Southeast Louisiana Hosp. Ass'n.*, d/b/a/ *Lake Charles Memorial Hosp.*, 226 NLRB 849, 93 LRRM 1420 (1976); *St. Luke's Episcopal Hosp.*, 222 NLRB 674, 91 LRRM 1359 (1976).

69. *National G. South, Inc.* d/b/a/ *Memorial Medical*, 230 NLRB 976, 95 LRRM 1478 (1977).

70. 230 NLRB 1042, 95 LRRM 1464 (1977).

71. 231 NLRB No. 132, 96 LRRM 1546 (1977).

72. 227 NLRB 1814, 94 LRRM 1534 (1977).

73. *Allegheny Gen. Hosp.*, 230 NLRB 954, 96 LRRM 1022 (1977); *Trinity Memorial Hosp. of Cudahy, Inc.*, 230 NLRB 855, 95 LRRM 1414 (1977); *Hebrew Rehabilitation Center for the Aged*, 230 NLRB 255, LRRM 1279 (1977); *McLean Hosp.*, 234 NLRB No. 54, 97 LRRM 1322 (1978).

74. *Long Island College Hosp. v. NLRB*, 566 F.2d 833 (2d Cir. 1977), 96 LRRM 3119; *St. Vincent's Hosp. v. NLRB*, 567 F.2d 588 (3d Cir. 1977), 97 LRRM 2119; *NLRB v. W. Suburban Hospital, Inc.*, 570 F.2d 213 (7th Cir. 1978), 97 LRRM 2929; *NLRB v. Mercy Hospital Ass'n.*, 606 F.2d 22 (2d Cir. 1979); 102 LRRM 2259; *cert. denied*, ___ U.S. ___ (1980); *Mary Thompson Hosp. v. NLRB*, 621 F.2d 858 (7th Cir. 1980), 103 LRRM 2739.

75. *W. Suburban Hosp.*, 570 F.2d 213 at 216 (1978).

76. 567 F.2d 588 (3d Cir. 1977), 97 LRRM 2119.

77. *Id.* at 589.

78. 239 NLRB No. 104, 100 LRRM 1030 (1978).

79. *Allegheny Gen. Hosp. v. NLRB*, 608 F.2d 965 (3d Cir. 1979), 102 LRRM 2784.

80. 606 F.2d 22 (2d Cir. 1979), 102 LRRM 2259.

81. ___ U.S. ___ (1980), *cert. denied,* 64 L. Ed. 2d 248 (1980).

82. 29 U.S.C. § 158(g) reads in full:

> A labor organization before engaging in any strike, picketing, or other concerted refusal to work at any health care institution shall, not less than ten days prior to such action, notify the institution in writing and the Federal Mediation and Conciliation Service of that intention, except that in the case of bargaining for an initial agreement following certification or recognition the notice required by this subsection shall not be given until the expiration of the period specified in clause (B) of the last sentence of subsection (d) of this section. The notice shall state the date and time that such action will commence. The notice, once given, may be extended by the written agreement of both parties.

83. *See,* S. Rep. No. 93-766, 93d Cong., 2d Sess. 4 (1974); H.R. Rep. No. 93-1051, 93d Cong., 2d Sess. 5 (1974).

84. *See,* S. Rep. No. 93-766, 93d Cong., 2d Sess. 4 (1974); H.R. Rep. No. 93-1051, 93d Cong., 2d Sess. 5 (1974).

85. *See, e.g., Casey and Glass, Inc.,* 219 NLRB 698, 89 LRRM 1779 (1975).

86. 219 NLRB 837, 89 LRRM 1770 (1975).

87. *Laborers' Int'l Union of North America, Local 1057 (Mercy Hosp. of Laredo)* 219 NLRB 846, 89 LRRM 1777 (1975); *Int'l Brotherhood of Electrical Workers, Local 388 (Hoffman Co.);* 220 NLRB 665, 90 LRRM 1390 (1975).

88. 548 F.2d 704 (7th Cir. 1977), 94 LRRM 2536; *cert. denied,* 434 U.S. 837 (1977), *denying enforcement* of 220 NLRB 665 (1975).

89. 567 F.2d 1006 (D.C. Cir. 1977), 96 LRRM 3160; *denying enforcement* to both *Laredo Hosp., supra,* n. 87 and *Lein-Steenberg, supra,* n. 86. Judge Wilkey dissented but filed no opinion.

89a. *See, Painters Local No. 452 (Henry C. Beck Co.),* 246 NLRB No. 148, 103 LRRM 1002 (1979); and *Laborers' Intl. Union of North America, Local 1253, AFL-CIO) St. Mary's Hospital of Roswell, Inc.),* 248 NLRB No. 30, 103 LRRM 1526 (1980).

89b. *Bricklayers and Allied Craftsmen, Local 40 (Lake Shore Hosp.),* 252 NLRB No. 30, 105 LRRM 1317 (1980); and *Orange Belt District Council of Painters and Allied Trades (St. Joseph Hosp.),* 243 NLRB No. 113, 101 LRRM 1456 (1979).

90. Senator Taft stated:

> Clearly employees acting without a labor organization or in derogation of a representative would have no greater rights or fewer obligations, for example, under 8(g) than those of a labor organization. It would not be protected activity for employees acting without a labor organization to engage in a work stoppage or picket without giving the required notice.

120 Cong. Rec. S 6941 (daily ed. May 2, 1974).

91. *See,* Office of The General Counsel, NLRB Memorandum 74-79 (August 20, 1974), § III.J.

92. 227 NLRB 1630, 94 LRRM 1516 (1977).

93. "Labor organization" is defined in § 2(5) of the Act, 29 U.S.C. § 152(5):

> The term "labor organization" means any organization of any kind, or any agency or employee representation committee or plan, in which employees participate, and which exists for the purpose, in whole or in part, of dealing with employers concerning grievances, labor disputes, wages, rates of pay, hours of employment, or conditions of work.

94. 235 NLRB No. 97, 98 LRRM 1077 (1978).

95. 230 NLRB 648, 95 LRRM 1541 (1977), *enforced* 591 F.2d 1276 (9th Cir. 1979), 101 LRRM 2501.

96. *Id.*

97. 581 F.2d 230 (9th Cir. 1978), *enforcing* 231 NLRB No. 10, 96 LRRM 1035 (1977). *See also, NLRB v. Rock Hill Convalescent Center,* 585 F.2d 701 (4th Cir. 1978), 99 LRRM 3157 and *Mercy Hospital Ass'n., Inc.,* 235 NLRB No. 97, 98 LRRM 1077 (1978).

98. *See also, NLRB v. IBEW, Local 388 (Hoffman Co.),* 548 F.2d 704 (7th Cir. 1977), 94 LRRM 2536; *cert. denied,* 434 U.S. 837 (1977), 96 LRRM 2514.

99. *Montefiore Hosp. and Medical Ctr. v. NLRB,* 621 F.2d, 510 (2d Cir. 1980), 104 LRRM 2161.

100. 222 NLRB 212, 91 LRRM 1097 (1976) *enforcement denied, NLRB v. Dist. 1199, Nat'l. Union of Hosp. and Health Care Employees,* No. 76-407 (2d Cir. November 23, 1976) (unpublished). The Second Circuit issued no written opinion. Instead, at the close of oral argument, the court stated that the union's violation was *de minimis* and that it therefore would not enforce the Board's order.

101. 232 NLRB No. 67, 96 LRRM 1404 (1977).

102. *Painters Dist. Council (St. Joseph Hospital)* 243 NLRB No. 113, 101 LRRM 1456 (1979).

103. 243 NLRB No. 6, 101 LRRM 1346 (1979).

104. *Bio-Medical Applications of New Orleans, Inc.,* 240 NLRB No. 39, 100 LRRM 1300 (1979).

105. 227 NLRB No. 26, 94 LRRM 1083 (1976).

106. S. Rep. No. 93-766, 93d Cong., 2d Sess. 4 (1974); H.R. Rep. No. 93-1051, 93d Cong., 2d Sess. 6 (1974).

107. 229 NLRB 1010, 95 LRRM 1214 (1977).

108. 232 NLRB No. 5, 97 LRRM 1108 (1977).

109. 219 NLRB 1095, 89 LRRM 1785 (1975).

110. 95 LRRM 2337 (S.Ct. N.Y. 1977). *But see, N.Y. v. Local 144, SEIU,* 410 F. Supp. 225 (S.D.N.Y. 1976).

111. 436 F. Supp. 335 (E.D.N.Y. 1977), *enforced,* F. Supp. 98 LRRM 2307 (E.D.N.Y. 1978).

112. 29 U.S.C. § 158(d).

113. 29 U.S.C. § 158(d)(A). A 60-day notice period applies for all other industries covered by the act. 29 U.S.C. § 158(d)(1).

114. *Id.*

115. 29 U.S.C. § 158(d)(B).

116. 29 U.S.C. § 158(d)(C).

117. 27 U.S.C. § 183(a) [Section 213(a) of the act].

118. *See,* Fishgold, "The Role of the Federal Mediation and Conciliation Service - Notice Provisions and Other Legal Problems of FMCS," in ABA Labor Relations Section, *Labor Relations Law Problems in Hospitals and the Health Care Industry* 209, 213 (1977).

119. *Id.*

120. 418 F. Supp. 711, (N.D. Cal. 1976), 93 LRRM 2307; *aff'd,* 583 F.2d 1097 (9th Cir. 1978), 99 LRRM 3197.

121. 93 LRRM 2885 (D. Md. 1976), *rev'd,* 561 F.2d 547 (4th Cir. 1977).

122. 583 F.2d 1097 (9th Cir. 1978), 99 LRRM 31971; *(per curium), aff'g,* 418 F. Supp. 711 (N.D. Cal. 1976).

123. 561 F.2d 547 (4th Cir. 1977), 96 LRRM 2355 *rev'g,* 93 LRRM 2885 (D. Md. 1976).

124. 97 LRRM 3105 (N.D.N.Y.), *appeal dismissed,* 582 F.2d 1271 (2d Cir. 1978).

125. 100 LRRM 2157 (D. Md., 1978), affirmed, 621 F.2d 1267 (4th Cir. 1980), 104 LRRM 2171.

126. 29 U.S.C. §158(b)(4).

127. S. Rep. No. 93-766, 93d Cong. 2d Sess. 5 (1974); H.R. Rep. No. 93-1051, 93d Cong., 2d Sess. 7 (1974).

128. Office of the General Counsel, NLRB Memorandum 74-49 (August 20, 1974) § VI A.

129. Office of the General Counsel, Division of Advice, NLRB Memorandum, *Loma Linda Univ. Medical Center,* Case Nos. 31-CC-820, 31-CG-7, *Memorial Hosp. Medical Center of Long Beach,* Case Nos. 31-CC-821, 31-CG-8 (September 2, 1977).

130. The Board quoted Senator Williams as follows:

> . . . it was the intention of the committee to modify the Ally doctrine in order to permit a neutral hospital to . . . accept [the primary] hospital's critically ill patients so that a continuity of medical treatment might be maintained.

120 Cong. Rec. S12 105 (daily ed. July 10, 1974).

131. 183 NLRB 950, 76 LRRM 1784 (1970), *supplementing* 175 NLRB 354 (1969), *enforced sub nom., NLRB v. Doctor's Hosp. of Modesto, Inc.,* 489 F.2d 772 (9th Cir. 1973), 85 LRRM 2228.

132. The floor head nurses directed the activities of eight licensed vocational nurses (L.V.N.s) and nurses' aides. They independently allocated the workload for their wings, assigned each auxiliary employee to particular patients, and directed them as to how and when particular procedures should be performed. The head nurse also decided whether probationary employees would be transferred or discharged, and could request the transfer of auxiliary personnel. Finally, head nurses evaluated the work of the employees working under them, which were used by the director of nurses in deciding whether to grant wage increases.

133. In its supplemental decision, the Board determined that the obstetrics unit supervisor and the recovery room head nurse were supervisors within the meaning of the Act, but overruled challenges to the votes of the charge nurses, relief charge nurses, floor nurses, and staff nurses.

134. S. Rep. No. 93-766, 93d Cong., 2d Sess. 6 (1974); H.R. Rep. No. 93-1051, 93d Cong., 2d Sess. 7 (1974).

135. *Sutter Community Hosps. of Sacramento, Inc.,* 227 NLRB 181, 192, 94 LRRM 1450 (1976); *Trustees of Noble Hosp.,* 218 NLRB 1441, 1442, 89 LRRM 1806 (1975); *Wing Memorial Hosp. Ass'n,* 217 NLRB 1015, 1016, 89 LRRM 1183 (1975); *Doctor's Hosp.,* 217 NLRB 611, 612, 89 LRRM 1525 (1975).

136. *See, e.g., Vic's Shop 'N Save,* 215 NLRB 28, 32, 88 LRRM 1478 (1974); *Illini Steel Fabricators, Inc.,* 197 NLRB 296, 297, 80 LRRM 1582 (1972); *Nation-Wide Plastics Co., Inc.,* 197 NLRB 996, 999, 81 LRRM 1036 (1972). *See also, NLRB v. Monroe Tube Co., Inc.,* 545 F.2d 1320, 1324 (2d Cir. 1976), 94 LRRM 2020:

> Section 2(11) of the Act provides as follows: The term "supervisor" means any individual having authority, in the interest of the employer, to hire, transfer, suspend, lay off, recall, promote, discharge, assign, reward or discipline other employees, or responsibility to direct them, or to adjust their grievances, or effectively to recommend such action, if in connection with the foregoing the exercise of such authority is not of a merely routine or clerical nature, but requires the use of independent judgement.

137. *See, e.g., Doctor's Hosp;, supra* n. 135 (Member Kennedy dissenting); *St. Mary's Hosp., Inc.,* 220 NLRB 496, 90 LRRM 1316 (1975).

137a. *Misericordia Medical Center v. NLRB,* 623 F.2d 808 (2d Cir. 1980), 104 LRRM 2666.

138. *See, e.g., Doctor's Community Hosp.,* 220 NLRB 977, 90 LRRM 1341 (1975); *Trustees of Noble Hosp., supra* n. 135.

139. *Westinghouse Electric Corp.,* 163 NLRB 723, 726-727, 64 LRRM 1440 (1967), *enf'd.,* 424 F.2d 1151 (7th Cir.), 74 LRRM 2070, *cert. denied,* 400 U.S. 831, 75 LRRM 2379 (1970). In that case, the alleged supervisors were engineers who might be considered professionals, and the employees allegedly supervised were craft employees. The employer manufactured electric generating equipment. When the equipment was sold to customers, the employer either (1) provided technical advice to the customer's employees, who installed the equipment themselves, or (2) installed the equipment for the customer, with the employer's own labor. In the former case, the engineers acted as technical advisers but did not directly supervise the persons providing the labor. In the latter case, the engineers directly supervised the persons doing the labor. While the NLRB said that it would exclude as supervisors only those engineers spending 50 percent or more of their working time performing supervisory duties, it was clear from the discussion that the Board actually was concerned with the percentage of time spent on the supervisory as opposed to the technical advice jobs, and not with the percentage of time spent on strictly supervisory activities.

140. Although the "50 percent rule" has been applied occasionally to nonhealth care cases, it primarily has affected the health care industry because there, more than any other industry, employees with varying skill levels and functions work together within a single organization at structure. It should be noted that had the Board applied this rule to its initial decision in *Doctor's Hosp. of Modesto, Inc., supra,* n. 131, it would not have concluded that head nurses were supervisors.

141. *See, e.g., Pinecrest Convalescent Home, Inc.,* 222 NLRB 13, 91 LRRM 1082 (1976).

142. 233 NLRB No. 92, 96 LRRM 1524 (1977).

143. 235 NLRB No. 52, 98 LRRM 1407 (1978).

144. 248 NLRB No. 56, 103 LRRM 1441 (1980).

145. 238 NLRB No. 217, 99 LRRM 1323 (1978).

146. 237 NLRB No. 130, 99 LRRM 1069 (1978).

147. 238 NLRB No. 10, 99 LRRM 1230 (1978).

148. 99 LRRM at 1232.

149. 231 NLRB No. 104, 96 LRRM 1066 (1977).

150. 238 NLRB No. 217, 99 LRRM 1323, enf'd., 578 F.2d 575 (5th Cir. 1978), 99 LRRM 2156.

151. In evaluating supervisory status, the Board often has resolved evidentiary conflicts by finding that employees who clearly exercise supervisory functions are supervisors but that others who do not exercise their apparent authority in the same job position are employees. *See, e.g., Texas Inst. for Rehabilitation and Research, supra,* n. 46. This approach often results in findings that depend on the effectiveness of persons clearly intended to be supervisors. *Cf. NLRB v. Brown & Sharpe Mfg. Co.,* 169 F.2d 331 (1st Cir. 1948), 22 LRRM 2363. (It is a person's *power* to act as an agent of the employer in relations with other employees that establishes status as a supervisor.)

152. 241 NLRB No. 107, 100 LRRM 1590 (1979).

153. *Abington Memorial Hosp.,* 250 NLRB No. 98, 104 LRRM 1429 (1980); *Lodi Memorial Hosp. Ass'n, Inc.,* 249 NLRB No. 121 (1980); *Oak Park Community Hosp.,* 249 NLRB No. 120 (1980); *Farber, Sidney, Cancer Inst.,* 247 NLRB No. 1, 103 LRRM 1132 (1980); *Healdsburg General Hosp.,* 247 NLRB No. 30, 103 LRRM 1135 (1980); *Baptist Hosp. Inc. d/b/a Western Baptist Hosp.,* 246 NLRB No. 25, 102 LRRM 1394 (1979); *Lancaster Osteopathic Hosp. Assn., Inc.,* 246 NLRB No. 96, 102 LRRM 1645 (1979).

154. *Exeter Hosp.,* 248 NLRB No. 56, 103 LRRM 1441 (1980).

5. Appropriate Bargaining Units in Health Care Institutions

LAURENCE P. CORBETT

INTRODUCTION

Upon receipt of a National Labor Relations Board (NLRB) "Petition for Recognition," an employer looks directly to the description of the proposed unit and then to the estimated number of employees in it to ascertain what group the petitioner is seeking to represent. Section 9(b) of the National Labor Relations Act (NLRA) gives the NLRB the authority to define appropriate bargaining units. The section states that the board's purpose in making unit determinations is to ensure the employees "the fullest freedom in exercising their rights guaranteed by the Act." The first task of the NLRB is to determine the scope of the bargaining unit—that is, which job classifications should be included or excluded. Then the board must decide the composition of the unit—that is, which employees are to be excluded (e.g., supervisory, confidential, managerial, and/or guards).

Prior to the 1974 Health Care Amendments to the NLRA, health care institutions had recognized labor unions primarily to the extent of organization among their employees. In some states, such as California, institutions were forced to fashion their own bargaining units in the absence of any state labor relations laws, while in other states, such as New York, which has a "Little Wagner Act," the law was of no help in unit determinations. So it was that employee groupings were recognized, not based on any community-of-interest standard but rather depending on the aggres-siveness of the union involved and the amount of employee support it received. Accordingly, a patchwork of bargaining units developed before 1974. This situation prompted one well-known New York hospital administrator to state that, carried to its logical extreme, a large urban hospital could have different unions carve out some 45 separate and competing bargaining units covering each craft or specialty in an institution.

Aware of hospitals' legitimate concerns regarding a proliferation of bargaining units, the Senate Committee on Labor and Public Welfare made specific recommendations relating to the application of the NLRA to health care institutions. The committee was convinced that the NLRB's standard approach to bargaining units in other industries might lead to numerous units of employees, each seeking to outdo other hospitals in negotiations, with resulting disturbance and interference with patient care. In a deliberate attempt to prevent this from happening, the committee recommended:

> Due consideration should be given by the Board to preventing the proliferation of bargaining units in the health care industry.[1]

The Senate committee expressed its confidence that once the NLRB determined the scope of the unit, it could apply its traditional standards to establish the group's composition. For example, the report noted

587

that the board previously had determined that a health care professional who gives direction to other employees in the exercise of professional judgment incidental to the treatment of patients is not a supervisor within the meaning of the NLRA.[2] As a matter of strategy, the board delayed issuing any unit determinations from the effective date of the amendments in August 1974 to May 1975.

SCOPE OF THE BARGAINING UNIT

Background

The NLRB evaluates several factors in resolving unit determination issues. Its primary concern is whether the petitioned-for unit groups together employees who have substantiated mutual interests in wages, hours, and conditions of employment.[3] The ultimate issue, therefore, is whether the employees in question share a similar community of interest. The board is not concerned with whether the petitioned-for unit is *the only* appropriate unit, but rather whether it is *an* appropriate unit. Thus, an employer may have more than one appropriate unit for purposes of collective bargaining. Among the factors considered by the NLRB are: the nature of the employee's skills and job duties, common supervision, interchange and contact among and between groups of employees, the extent of union organization, benefits and pay rates, and bargaining history. Generally, the agency decides unit determination questions on a case-by-case basis in which decisions turn on the particular facts involved and in which the other enumerated factors are given appropriate weight.

Health Care Industry

Some nine months after the health care amendments were enacted, the board issued its first rulings on unit determinations under the new law—eight decisions on the same day covering a variety of issues in order to give guidance in fashioning appropriate units in the industry: *Mercy Hospitals of Sacramento,*[4] *Barnert Memorial Hospital Center,*[5] *St. Catherine's Hospital,*[6] *Newington Children's Hospital,*[7] *Sisters of St. Joseph of Peace,*[8] *Duke University,*[9] *Mount Airy Foundation,*[10] and *Shriner's Hospital for Crippled Children.*[11]

After weighing the congressional admonition to avoid undue proliferation of bargaining units, the board determined that, generally, there were five appropriate bargaining units: registered nurses (*Mercy*); a residual unit of professional employees, excluding registered nurses (*Mercy*); service and maintenance employees, including hospital clericals who work in locations other than the central business office (*Newington Children's Hospital*); office clerical employees working in the central business office (*St. Catherine's Hospital*); and all technical employees (*Barnert Memorial Hospital*). Two years later, the board added a sixth unit by indicating that one composed of house physicians and emergency room doctors would be appropriate (*Ohio Valley Hospital Association*).[12] However, the NLRB has varied from this six-unit formula when, for example, as in *Bay Medical Center,*[13] bargaining history indicates that a different unit may not be inappropriate. The courts, as noted *infra,* have not always agreed with these unit determination decisions and have admonished the board for its failure to weigh properly the congressional intent to avoid unit proliferation.

Registered Nurses

In *Mercy* and the cases that followed, the NLRB consistently has granted registered nurses a bargaining unit separate from other professional employees. According to the decision, registered nurses, unlike other professionals, are required to be on duty 24 hours per day seven days per week; their patient care duties and responsibilities cannot, by law, be delegated to other employees. In addition, they are required to pass a national licensing examination and maintain a state license to practice. Finally, and perhaps the determining factor, registered nurses have a history of separate representation that the board stated it had recognized prior to 1974.

> The Board itself has, in the past, recognized the separate interests of registered nurses and has routinely established separate nurses' units for collective bargaining purposes . . .[14]

Subsequently, the board in *Methodist Hospital of Sacramento*[15] and *St. Francis Hospital of Lynwood*[16] adopted the position that regardless of the factual situation at an individual hospital, registered nurses are "entitled" to separate representation in their own unit.

The circuit courts have rebuked the board for this per se rule that registered nurses are the only appropriate unit. In *NLRB v. St. Francis of Lynwood Hospital,*[17] the Ninth Circuit Court stated that the per se rule granting nurses a separate unit was incompatible with the congressional aim of avoiding unit proliferation. The court said that there would be situations where registered nurses should be included in a unit with other professional employees.

In *Newton-Wellesley Hospital,*[18] the board adhered to its position that a separate unit of registered nurses was appropriate. Nevertheless, it did back away from its position that registered nurses were per se an appropriate unit and conceded that, "A *per se* rule could result in the Board's giving insufficient attention to the Congressional admonition and could permit the splitting of professional or other employees into separate units regardless of whether the particular circumstances warrant it."

Other Professional Employees

Section 2(12) of the NLRA, *infra*, defines "professional employee," and Section 9(b) provides that the board shall not decide that any unit is appropriate if it includes professional employees and those who do not meet that definition unless the majority of professionals vote to be included in such a unit. In health care institutions, the NLRB has found appropriate a hospitalwide unit of professional employees excluding registered nurses and physicians *(Mercy)*. Although the board did not minimize the differences between various groups of professional employees, it decided that to give each group a separate unit would unduly proliferate the number of bargaining entities. The board relied heavily on the absence of any history of separate representation for those professional employees *(Mercy)*.

Maintenance and Service Employees Unit

In *Barnert*, the NLRB concluded that a separate unit of service and maintenance employees was appropriate. It noted the similarity in wage rates, job functions, educational requirements, and benefits among this group of employees. It concluded that employees in those areas shared a distinct and separate community of interest different from technical employees and business office clerical employees. (For a discussion on the placement of boiler room operators see the next section on NLRB conflicts with the courts.)

Office Clericals

Without reference to the aim of avoiding unit fragmentation, the board applied its industrial analysis and granted employees in the central business office a separate unit. However, clerical employees who work outside of the business office (ward clerks, laboratory clerks, etc.) were included in the service and maintenance unit *(Mercy)*. The board stated that it had long recognized that the interests of office clerical employees differed markedly from those of clerical workers in production areas *(St. Catherine's Hospital)*.

Technical Employees

Also in *Barnert*, the board established a hospital-wide unit of all technical employees. It noted that such a unit normally was held to be appropriate in the industrial sphere. The NLRB found that technical employees in the health care setting had specialized training, skills, education, and job requirements that distinguished them from service and maintenance employees on the one hand and professionals on the other. In determining whether employees are in the technical employee category, the board stated:

We apply the Board's standard criteria that technical employees are those who do not meet the strict requirements of the term professional employee as defined in the Act but whose work is of a technical nature involving the use of independent judgment and requiring the exercise of specialized training usually acquired in colleges or technical schools or through special courses.[19]

In *St. Catherine's*, the NLRB rejected a separate unit for licensed practical (vocational) nurses and included them in the technical employees bargaining unit. Despite this general proposition of including L.P.N.s in the technical unit, the board has allowed them on at least one occasion to have a separate unit *(Bay Medical Center)*.[20] In that case the board based its decision on the fact that L.P.N.s had a long and separate history of representation. The court, in upholding the board, found that the policy against unit proliferation was outweighed by the policy against disrupting existing collective bargaining relationships.[21] In *Pine Manor, Inc.*,[22] the board allowed licensed practical nurses to have a self-determination election as to whether they would be included in the service and maintenance unit or a separate unit of their own. The board carefully limited that decision to the facts of that case. There, L.P.N.s were the only technical employees of the employer.

House Physicians and Emergency Room Doctors

In *Ohio Valley, supra*, the board excluded house physicians and emergency room doctors from a residual unit of professional employees. Although there was no petition for a unit of such professionals, the board stated that by any community-of-interest standard, physicians constituted a class unto themselves. It noted that physicians had unique and extensive educational training and skills that set them apart from other employees.

In excluding doctors from the professional unit here involved, we are not unmindful that the Board has been admonished by Congress to avoid undue proliferation. . . . However, we consider this general caveat in connection with our unit determination pertaining to registered nurses and concluded that because of their special community of interest, that caveat did not preclude the Board from placing them in a separate unit or excluding them from an otherwise professional unit when requested.[23]

CONFLICT BETWEEN THE NLRB AND COURTS

As noted, there has been considerable conflict between the circuit courts and the NLRB over unit placement in health care institutions. Generally, the board gives greater weight to its traditional community-of-interest standards, whereas the courts tend to give more consideration to the congressional directive against proliferation of units. The unit question raised by the stationary engineers is illustrative of this point.

Originally, in *Shriner's Hospital,* the board rejected a separate maintenance unit for engineers. However, in *Kansas City College of Osteopathic Medicine,*[24] the NLRB found that the powerhouse engineers in the hospital were supervised separately, located apart from other employees, performed a specialized function, and did not interchange with other personnel. The board did not state that a service and maintenance unit was inappropriate, only that the facts in this case supported the conclusion that the powerhouse employees were an appropriate unit in and of themselves. Two years later the U.S. Court of Appeals for the Third Circuit came to an opposite conclusion in *St. Vincent's Hospital v. NLRB,*[25] a case involving boiler room operators on the ground that a separate unit was contrary to the congressional admonition to avoid proliferation of bargaining units in the health care field.

The circuit courts consistently have rejected granting separate bargaining units to maintenance or stationary engineers. *NLRB v. West Suburban Hospital* (1978),[26] *Memorial Hospital of Roxborough v. NLRB* (1976),[27] and *Long Island College Hospital v. NLRB* (1977).[28]

As a result of these court reversals, the NLRB reconsidered its decision in *Allegheny General Hospital I* (1977),[29] which was on appeal to the Third Circuit— the court that had reversed *Roxborough* on the same issue. Notwithstanding the court's construction of the

congressional mandate against proliferation of units, the majority of the board clung to its view that Congress did not intend to preclude reliance on traditional community-of-interest criteria applicable in the industrial sector. The majority reasoned that Congress was opposed to the proliferation of units in the health field to the extent that craft skills and job functions had been recognized for separate units in the construction industry but defended this approach in health care institutions as prevention of proliferation and in *Allegheny General Hospital II,*[30] it confirmed its decision in *Allegheny I, supra.* Indeed, even the Supreme Court's denial of certiorari in *Long Island College Hospital, infra,* which left standing the Third Circuit's reversal of the board, has not altered the position of the board's majority. *Garden City Hospital* (1979).[31]

MULTIEMPLOYER AND MULTIHOSPITAL BARGAINING UNITS

Multiemployer Units

Many employers, including some health care institutions, deal with labor organizations on a multiemployer basis. Thus, a group of employers becomes, in effect, one for the purposes of collective bargaining. Moreover, in order to establish a valid multiemployer bargaining unit, there must be an unequivocal manifestation by the employer members that they intend to be bound in future collective bargaining by group and not by individual actions. *York Transfer & Storage* (1953).[32]

Once a multiemployer bargaining association is established, any petitioned-for bargaining unit must be associationwide and encompass similar employees for each employer. A petition for recognition that does not encompass an association-wide unit may be dismissed. *St. Luke's Hospital* (1978),[33] *Samuel Merritt Hospital* (1975).[34] In *St. Luke's,* the board dismissed a petition limited to technical employees at a single hospital. St. Luke's was a member of a multiemployer bargaining association, and the board concluded that any unit must encompass all technical employees in all member hospitals. In *Merritt,* the NLRB regional director found inappropriate a unit limited to nursing instructors at the hospital's school of nursing. Merritt, too, was a member of a multiemployer association, and the regional director held that because there were continuing education instructors at other member hospitals, any unit must include such nurse instructors at other member hospitals.

Multilocation Units of a Single Employer

Another form of unit is multiplant, in which two or more separate geographical locations of the employer are regarded as a single unit. In *Mercy,*[35] the general hospital, Mercy General, and an acute care facility, Mercy San Juan, were located 13 miles apart. The record established substantial functional and operational integration between the two. They were operated by a single corporation and a single governing board. Each facility had a separate personnel department but both were subject to uniform personnel and labor relations policies, including common personnel forms, classifications, wage scales, and benefit programs. There was evidence that, although medical services differed somewhat between the two hospitals, interchanges of supplies, equipment, and support personnel took place regularly among several of the services performed at both institutions. The two also shared many internal and centralized services such as laundry, receiving, purchasing, data processing, billing, and accounting. In view of these factors, which established functional and operational integration between the two institutions, the NLRB determined that they constituted a single bargaining unit.

UNIT DETERMINATIONS BY STATE AGENCIES AND STIPULATIONS OF THE PARTIES

State Unit Determinations

Before the 1974 amendments, several hospital units had been certified by state agencies pursuant to state labor relations statutes. In other cases, health care units had been established by mutual agreement of the parties. However, despite the argument that hospitals were "predominantly local in character," the NLRB refused to cede to its jurisdiction over health care institutions to state agencies under Section 10(2) of the NLRA.[36]

Where state agencies had established health care units prior to 1974, the board has generally extended comity to their unit decisions, even when the units were in conflict with the board's basic approach *(Long Island College Hospital,*[37] *West Suburban Hospital*[38]*).* However, in these cases and others where the board's extension of comity has conflicted with the congressional admonition, the courts have refused to grant enforcement to the board's orders *(Memorial Hospital of Roxborough, supra).*[39] Notwithstanding the courts' rulings, the NLRB has continued to adhere to its position on comity *(Allegheny II, supra).*[40]

Stipulated Units

A stipulated unit is one to which all parties, including the board, have agreed and to which they all have stipulated. Consistent with its comity approach, the board gives effect to stipulated units even though they do not conform to the initial unit decisions of May 1975. *Otis Hospital, Inc.* (1975),[41] *Southwest Community Hospital* (1975).[42] True to form, the courts disagreed and, in *Mercy Hospitals, supra,* the Ninth Circuit Court overturned a stipulation that differed from the standard unit of business office clericals.

COMPOSITION OF THE BARGAINING UNIT

Statutory Exclusions from the Unit

Questions of scope and composition frequently overlap, and there is no easy distinction. Generally, however, questions of composition concern which employees are eligible to vote in any representation election and which are not eligible.

Some employees are excluded by statute: Section 2(3) of the NLRA excludes those who work for public sector employers (including federal and state governments, subdivisions, and Federal Reserve banks), agricultural laborers, domestic servants for a family or person in the home, an individual employed by parent or spouse, an independent contractor, an individual working as a supervisor, and an individual whose employer is subject to the Railway Labor Act.

Independent Contractors

The NLRB uses the common law "right of control" test to ascertain if an individual is an independent contractor or an employee. If the recipient of the services in question has a right to control not only the end to be achieved but also the means to be used in reaching such result, the individual performing the services is an employer. In *National Freight, Inc.* (1964),[43] the high degree of supervision over the owner-drivers of leased trucks placed them in employee status. A broader application than the common law master and servant relationship was reached by the board and approved by the Supreme Court in *NLRB v. Hearst Publications* (1944).[44] In that case, employees who worked for wages or salaries under supervision were compared with independent contractors who undertook a job for a price, decided how the work would be done, and relied upon the profit arising out of the job instead of wages for work performed. If the employees in question are found to be independent contractors, they are excluded from the bargaining unit.

Relatives of Management

The exclusion of an individual because the person is employed by a parent or spouse has been expanded by the NLRB to close relatives of the employer. An employee who was a close relative of a corporate management officer was excluded in *International Metal Products Co.* (1953),[45] as was the son of a major stockholder in a closely held corporation in *Foam Rubber City* (1967).[46]

Supervisors

Individuals found to be supervisors under Section 2(11) of the act are excluded from any bargaining units:

Section 2(11) The term 'supervisor' means an individual having authority, in the interest of the employer, to hire, transfer, suspend, lay off, recall, promote, discharge, assign, reward, or discipline other employees, or responsibly to direct them, or to adjust their grievances, or effectively to recommend such action, if in connection with the foregoing the exercise of such authority is not of a merely routine or clerical nature, but requires the use of independent judgment.

The NLRB has applied this definition to the health care field as Congress recommended[47] by continuing the policies it has developed in other industries over the years. The NLRB has not regarded a professional who gives direction to other employees as a supervisor if such direction is purely incidental to the treatment of patients, *Wing Memorial Hospital Association* (1975).[48] Head nurses who recommend wage increases, settle grievances, and assign work have been held to be supervisors in *Presbyterian Medical Center* (1975),[49] while charge nurses and team leaders engaged primarily in patient care with the responsibility for clinical direction, but not employee supervision, have not been classified as supervisors, *Trustees of Noble Hospital* (1975).[50] To be a supervisor within the meaning of the act, an employee must exercise one or more of the functions listed in Section 2(11). However, an employee does not lose supervisory status even if that authority is exercised only infrequently. In borderline cases, the NLRB will use secondary criteria to decide whether an employee is a supervisor: whether the individual and fellow workers consider the person to be a supervisor, *Gerbes Supermarket, Inc.* (1974);[51] the individual attends management meetings, *Typog-*

raphers Local No. 101 (1975);[52] the individual receives a higher wage rate than fellow workers, *Electrical Workers Local 901* (1975);[53] the individual receives benefits different from those of fellow workers, *Transworld Airways* (1974).[54] An employee does not become a supervisor because of sporadic and infrequent assumption of supervisory duties, *Complete Auto Transit, Inc.* (1974).[55]

Exclusions from the Unit by Decision

Managerial Employees

Managerial employees have been excluded from the act's coverage by NLRB and the courts. They are not defined in the NLRA but have been determined by the board to be employees who formulate and effectuate management policies by expressing and making operative the decisions of their employer and those who have discretion in the performance of their jobs, independent of their employer's established policy. *NLRB v. Bell Aerospace, Division of Textron, Inc.* (1974).[56] In this connection, management trainees have been held to be managerial employees. *Curtis Industries Division of Curtis Noll Corp.* (1975).[57]

Confidential Employees

Although the statute does not provide a definition of "confidential employee," the board has found confidential only those who "assist in a confidential manner an individual who determines, formulates, and effectuates management's labor relations policies." *B.F. Goodrich Co.* (1956),[58] *Minneapolis-Moline Co.* (1949).[59] Of critical importance in determining confidential status is the individual's access to confidential labor relations matters. The board has been reluctant to find employees to be confidential and, consequently, gives a narrow construction to its definition. *Clover Fork Medical Services, Inc.* (1972).[60]

Guards

Section 9(b)(3) of the NLRA provides that the board shall not decide any unit is appropriate if it includes, together with other employees, any individual employed as a guard to enforce against employees and other persons any rules to protect the property of the employer or to protect the safety of persons on the employer's premises. While the board applies a statutory prohibition against certifying single units of guards and nonguards, it also holds that guards or watchmen who are not responsible for enforcing an employer's rules do not come within the statutory prohibition. *Shattuck School* (1971).[61] Prior to the health care amendments, units established in hospitals included guards as defined in Section 9(b)(3). The board has indicated it will follow traditional policy in *Peninsula Hospital Center* (1975),[62] whose guards were removed from two preamendment combination guard/nonguard units by a unit clarification petition. As in the case of professional employees under Section 9(b)(1), it is not impermissible for the parties voluntarily to establish a unit of guards and nonguards so long as the NLRB is not called upon to determine the unit. *NLRB v. J. J. Collins' Sons, Inc.* (1964).[63]

Miscellaneous Eligibility Questions

Full-time and regular part-time employees usually are included in any bargaining unit and casual employees are excluded. Distinguishing between regular part-time employees and casual workers is not always an easy matter. Generally, the NLRB has looked to whether the circumstances of the individuals' employment gave them a community of interest with "regular" employees with respect to wages, hours, and working conditions. *Georgia Pacific Corp.* (1972),[64] *Myers Bros. Inc.* (1975).[65] Typically, students who work only during summer vacation or individuals who do not work a set number of hours over a definite period of time have been regarded as casual employees and have been excluded. If an employee performs a dual function, i.e., works for the same employer in one job classification that is included in the scope of the unit and one classification that is excluded, the individual is included in the unit only if the greater portion of the work time is spent at the job classification within the unit description. *Nu Life Spotless* (1974),[66] *Adelphi University* (1972).[67]

Employees who are on layoff, leave of absence, or vacation status and have a reasonable expectation of returning to work are included in the bargaining unit and are eligible to vote in any representation election. Conversely, employees who resigned or are discharged after the cutoff date for voter eligibility in a representation election are not eligible to vote, despite the fact that their names may appear on this eligibility list. *O & H Farms* (1971),[68] *Cato Show Printing Co.* (1975).[69]

Religious Objections

Catholic sisters who perform bargaining unit work have been excluded from professional units in many Catholic hospitals. This determination is based upon possible conflicts of interest in the case where a sister on the staff of a hospital is included in the unit of employees of a facility that is owned, managed, and operated by her religious order. *St. Rose de Lima* (1976).[70] In one case, the board gave more weight to the community of interest in working conditions that a member of a different religious order shared with lay persons than to the fact that the institution was operated by a religious order. *St. Anthony Center* (1975).[71] Congress took this situation into consideration with respect to the obligation to join a union and pay union dues. The health care amendments provide in a new Section 19 that established tenets or teachings of a bona fide religious body or sect that historically has held conscientious objections to joining or financially supporting a labor union may pay the equivalent of an initiation fee and dues to a 501(C)(3) nonreligious charitable fund.

Interns and Residents

Interns and residents are not included in any bargaining unit as the NLRB has found that they are not "employees" within the meaning of the act. *Cedars-Sinai Medical Center* (1976).[72] Since they were not under the NLRA, a house staff union in New York sought to compel the New York State Labor Relations Board to assert jurisdiction over residents and interns. Without reaching the question of whether they were "employees," the U.S. Court of Appeals for the Second Circuit held that the state agency did not have jurisdiction because it was the intent of Congress to bring all labor relations of all nonprofit hospitals within the exclusive jurisdiction of the NLRB. *NLRB v. Committee of Interns* (1977).[73] The U.S. Court of Appeals for the District of Columbia in reversing its own previous decision, *Physicians National House Staff Association v. Murphy* (1979),[74] held that the board's decision that house staff are not employees was not reviewable. *Physicians National House Staff Association v. Johnson H. Fanning* (1980).[75] The sum of these decisions is that interns and residents are not "employees" within the meaning of the NLRA and are not subject to state jurisdiction because Congress has preempted any state jurisdiction by the 1974 health care amendments. Thus, they find themselves in a no man's land without recourse to either state or federal labor laws.

CONCLUSION

The scope and composition of appropriate bargaining units in health care institutions are by no means settled, since differences continue to persist between the NLRB and the courts. The scope of the unit represents the most serious division, with the board following its traditional community-of-interest formula and the courts giving much weight to the congressional mandate against proliferation of bargaining units. Health care institutions can have some influence on the determination of appropriate units if they keep in mind the criteria examined and used by the NLRB. Elements influencing the board in such decisions are similarities in skills, jobs, training, education, compensation, benefits, hours, working conditions, degree of common supervision, interchange and contact among the employees in the work locations, and prior bargaining history.

In general, health care institutions are against proliferation of bargaining units for the reasons discussed. However, as a practical matter in some instances, hospitals recognize a small organized group, such as a unit of stationary engineers, to avoid a variety of pressures from such employees as well as the time and expense of resisting organization of larger units that might follow. On the other hand, if the institution's preference is indeed for broad units, it must give careful attention to all of the elements supporting such units in the light of board determinations that a group of employees can be included in more than one appropriate unit. By way of comparison, there is considerably less difference between the NLRB and the courts in the composition of units because both appear to be satisfied that the criteria applicable in other industries are appropriate for health care institutions.

NOTES

1. S. Rep. 93-766, 93 Cong., 2nd Sess. 5 (1974).

2. Idem.

3. *Fifteenth Annual Report of the NLRB,* 39 (1950).

4. *Mercy Hosps. of Sacramento,* 217 NLRB 765, 89 LRRM 1097 (1975).

5. *Barnert Memorial Hosp. Center,* 217 NLRB 775, 89 LRRM 1083 (1975).

6. *St. Catherine's Hosp.,* 217 NLRB 787, 89 LRRM 1070 (1975).

7. *Newington Children's Hosp.,* 217 NLRB 793, 89 LRRM 1008 (1975).

8. *Sisters of St. Joseph of Peace,* 217 NLRB 797, 89 LRRM 1082 (1975).

9. *Duke Univ.,* 217 NLRB 799, 89 LRRM 1065 (1975).

10. *Mount Airy Foundation,* 217 NLRB 802, 89 LRRM 1067 (1975).

11. *Shriner's Hosp. for Crippled Children,* 217 NLRB 806, 89 LRRM 1076 (1975).

12. *Ohio Valley Hosp. Ass'n,* 230 NLRB 604, 95 LRRM 1430 (1977).

13. *Bay Medical Center,* 218 NLRB 620, 89 LRRM 1310 (1975).

14. *Mercy Hosps., supra,* n. 4, at 767.

15. *Methodist Hosp. of Sacramento, Inc.,* 223 NLRB 1509, 92 LRRM 1198 (1976).

16. *St. Francis of Lynwood Hosp.,* 232 NLRB 32, 97 LRRM 1297 (1977).

17. *NLRB v. St. Francis of Lynwood Hosp.,* 601 F.2d 404 (1979), 101 LRRM 2943.

18. *Newton-Wellesley Hosp.,* 250 NLRB No. 86, 104 LRRM 1384 (1980).

19. *Barnert, supra,* at 777.

20. *Bay Medical Center, supra,* n. 13.

21. *Bay Medical Center v. NLRB,* 588 F.2d 1174 (1978), 100 LRRM 2213.

22. *Pine Manor Inc.,* 238 NLRB No. 217, 99 LRRM (1978).

23. *Ohio Valley, supra,* at 605.

24. *Kansas City College of Osteopathic Medicine,* 220 NLRB 181, 90 LRRM 1189 (1975).

25. *St. Vincent's Hosp. v. NLRB,* 567 F.2d 588 (1977), 97 LRRM 2119.

26. *NLRB v. W. Suburban Hosp.,* 570 F.2d 213 (1978), 97 LRRM 2929.

27. *Memorial Hosp. of Roxborough v. NLRB,* 545 F.2d 351 (1976), 93 LRRM 257.

28. *Long Island College Hosp. v. NLRB,* 566 F.2d 833 (1977), 96 LRRM 3119.

29. *Allegheny Gen. Hosp.,* 230 NLRB 954, 196 LRRM 1022 (1977).

30. *Allegheny Gen. Hosp. II ,* 239 NLRB No. 104, 100 LRRM 1030 (1978).

31. *Garden City Hosp.,* 244 NLRB No. 108, 102 LRRM 1146 (1979).

32. *York Transfer & Storage,* 107 NLRB 139, 33 LRRM 1078 (1953).

33. *St. Luke's Hosp.,* 234 NLRB 130, 97 LRRM 1099 (1978).

34. *Samuel Merritt Hosp.,* 20-Rd-13073 (1975).

35. *Mercy Hosps., supra,* n. 4.

36. *In Re: State of Minnesota,* 219 NLRB 1095, 89 LRRM 1785 (1975).

37. *Long Island College Hosp.,* 228 NLRB 83, 94 LRRM 1438 (1977), *enf. denied* 566 F.2d 883, 96 LRRM 3119.

38. *W. Suburban Hosp.,* 227 NLRB 1351, 94 LRRM 1704 (1977), *enf. denied* 570 F.2d 213 (1978), 97 LRRM 2929.

39. *Memorial Hosp., supra,* n. 27.

40. *Allegheny II, supra,* n. 30.

41. *Otis Hosp., Inc.,* 219 NLRB 164, 89 LRRM 1545 (1975).

42. *Southwest Community Hosp.,* 219 NLRB 351, 90 LRRM 1116 (1975).

43. *National Freight, Inc.,* 146 NLRB 144, 55 LRRM 1259 (1964).

44. *NLRB v. Hearst Publications,* 322 U.S. 111, 14 LRRM 614 (1944).

45. *International Metal Products Co.,* 107 NLRB 65, 83 LRRM 1055 (1953).

46. *Foam Rubber City,* 167 NLRB 623, 66 LRRM 1096 (1967).

47. *S. Rep. No. 93-766, supra,* n. 1.

48. *Wing Memorial Hosp. Ass'n,* 217 NLRB 1015, 89 LRRM 1183 (1975).

49. *Presbyterian Medical Center,* 218 NLRB 1266, 89 LRRM 1752 (1975).

50. *Trustees of Noble Hosp.,* 218 NLRB 1441, 89 LRRM 1806 (1975).

51. *Gerbes Supermarket Inc.,* 213 NLRB 803, 87 LRRM 1762 (1974).

52. *Typographers Local No. 101,* 220 NLRB 1173, 90 LRRM 1523 (1975).

53. *Electrical Workers Local 901,* 2210 NLRB 1236, 90 LRRM 1439 (1975).

54. *Transworld Airlines,* 211 NLRB 733, 86 LRRM 1434 (1974).

55. *Complete Auto Transit, Inc.,* 214 NLRB 344, 87 LRRM 1352 (1974).

56. *NLRB v. Bell Aerospace, Div. of Textron, Inc.,* 416 U.S. 267 (1974), 85 LRRM 2945.

57. *Curtis Indus., Div. of Curtis Noll Corp.,* 218 NLRB 1447, 89 LRRM 1417 (1975).

58. *B. F. Goodrich Co.,* 115 NLRB 722, 37 LRRM 1383 (1956).

59. *Minneapolis-Moline Co.*, 85 NLRB 597, 24 LRRM 1443 (1949).

60. *Clover Fork Medical Servs., Inc.*, 200 NLRB 291, 82 LRRM 1035 (1972).

61. *Shattuck School*, 189 NLRB 886, 77 LRRM 1164 (1971).

62. *Peninsula Hospital Center*, 219 NLRB 139, 90 LRRM 1034 (1975).

63. *NLRB v. J. J. Collins' Sons, Inc.*, 332 F.2d 523 (1964), 56 LRRM 2375.

64. *Georgia Pacific Corp.*, 195 NLRB 258, 79 LRRM 1263 (1972).

65. *Myers Bros. Inc.*, 218 NLRB 441, 89 LRRM 1386 (1975).

66. *Nu Life Spotless*, 215 NLRB 357, 88 LRRM 1403 (1974).

67. *Adelphi Univ.*, 195 NLRB 639, 79 LRRM 1545 (1972).

68. *O & H Farms*, 192 NLRB 53, 77 LRRM 1721 (1971).

69. *Cato Show Printing Co.*, 219 NLRB 739, 90 LRRM 1139 (1975).

70. *St. Rose de Lima*, 223 NLRB 1511, 92 LRRM 1181 (1976).

71. *St. Anthony Center*, 220 NLRB 1009, 90 LRRM 1405 (1975).

72. *Cedars-Sinai Medical Center*, 223 NLRB 251, 91 LRRM 1398 (1976).

73. *NLRB v. Comm. of Interns*, 556 F.2d 810 (1977), 96 LRRM 2342.

74. *Physicians Nat'l House Staff Ass'n v. Murphy*, 591 F.2d 1, (C.A.D.C. 1979), 100 LRRM 3045.

75. *Physicians Nat'l House Staff Ass'n v. Johnson H. Fanning*, _____ F.2d _____ (1980), _____ LRRM _____ .

6. Strikes, Solicitation, and Bargaining: The National Labor Relations Board Applies the Act to the Health Care Industry

SAUL G. KRAMER and WANDA L. ELLERT

In 1974, Congress passed the Health Care Amendments that placed nonprofit health care institutions under the jurisdiction of the National Labor Relations Board.[1] The NLRB now exercises its authority over all health care institutions that have a substantial impact on commerce[2] and that have gross annual revenues of $250,000 or more (except for nursing homes, which need have only $100,000 in such revenues).[3]

Congress was concerned to prevent undue disruption of health care services when it extended the coverage. The public interest required special restrictions for activities that otherwise would be permissible in private sector disputes. Some of these restrictions are expressly provided in the amendments themselves. Other limitations have evolved from the legislative history of the amendments and the interpretation and application of traditional labor relations law to the unique needs of the health care industry.

There are three major areas that have been accorded special treatment: (1) notice and mediation of strikes, picketing, and work stoppages; (2) when and where union solicitation and distribution of literature may be prohibited; and (3) what constitutes an appropriate bargaining unit. Additional areas of unique concern to health care employers, although not given any differential treatment by the NLRB, are strike problems, including patient welfare; strike duration; strike preparations and employee communications to patients concerning a strike; the supervisory status of employees and their participation in a bargaining organization; and mandatory bargaining subjects.

NOTICE OF STRIKE, PICKETING, OR STOPPAGE

Actions Requiring Notice

Section 8(g) of the amended National Labor Relations Act (NLRA) requires a labor organization to give ten days' written notice to a health care employer and the Federal Mediation Conciliation Service (FMCS) before engaging in "any strike, picketing, or other concerted refusal to work." Failure to give the notice is an unfair labor practice and injunctive relief may be sought. Furthermore, under Section 8(d) of the act, workers who participate in a strike for which proper notice has not been given lose their protected status as "employees" and may be discharged. The notice provision has been strictly interpreted as applying to any strike, picketing, or work stoppage at a health care institution.

For example, one union that had given proper notice was on strike and picketing at a hospital. A second union, which did not represent any employees at the hospital, engaged in "sympathy" picketing for about an hour and a half. The NLRB held that the second union also should have given notice.[4]

This rule applies, however, only when a labor organization is involved. The NLRB ruled there was no notice required where 17 employees staged a simultaneous stoppage because a union that was attempting to organize the workers was not responsible for and did not encourage the stoppage.[5]

Neither is any notice required from a nonhealth care union prior to picketing or striking a nonhealth care employer at a hospital or nursing home as, for example, when a construction union pickets a contractor doing work on hospital premises.[6] However, the cases to date have involved picketing confined to a gate reserved for the sole use of construction workers. It is not clear what the board's position would be if there were no reserved gate and a hospital's regular employee and delivery entrances were picketed by a nonhealth care union engaged in a dispute with a nonhealth care employer.

If the hospital is in any way a target of the picketing, though, the notice must be given. The Painters Union violated the act when, without providing a ten-day notice, it picketed a hospital's two main entrances with signs indicating that the institution was unfair to painters and was using nonunion help to perform painting work.[7] The hospital was explicitly a target of the picketing, and although a contractor was performing renovation work on the building, the painting was done by the hospital's regular maintenance employees. In the *Painters* case, the board rejected the union's arguments that notice was not necessary because the picketing was only "informational," the dispute did not relate to direct "patient-related" functions, and health care services were not disrupted.

The NLRB has given some indication that notice would not be required: (1) if the strike, picketing, or stoppage is in response to a "serious" or "flagrant" unfair labor practice committed by the employer; or (2) if notice has been given and the strike, picketing, or stoppage is initiated early because the employer engages in activities that would "undermine the bargaining relationship that would otherwise exist."[8] Congressional committee reports on the health care amendments indicate that the kind of activities that might "undermine the bargaining relationship" and justify an early walkout would include the stockpiling of supplies in anticipation of a long strike and the addition of large numbers of new personnel.[9] While an employer may take steps to ensure the maintenance of health care services, advance notice of a strike is not intended to allow the institution to try to establish a bargaining advantage before its onset.

The board also has taken the position that a union that during the course of negotiations threatens to strike need not give the Section 8(g) notice.[10]

Sufficiency of Notice

The notice required is a full ten days prior to the onset of picketing, which may not begin until the 11th day. The NLRB counts the date of receipt of a notice as the first day, and the day before the onset of the activity as the last. Therefore, a union violated the ten-day notice requirement of Section 8(g) when it picketed a nursing home on the tenth day after the home received a certified notice. Notice was received on October 28 and picketing commenced on November 6.[11]

The union also failed to give the FMCS proper notice of its intent to picket, having been mistaken in the assumption that placement in the mails ten days prior to picketing was sufficient notice to the agency. Extra time must be allotted for mail delivery.

Nor can a labor organization delay the start of picketing or a strike too far beyond the time indicated in the notice. A union that failed to start picketing until 80½ hours after the time stated in its notice of intent to do so was found to have violated the notice requirements of the act.[12] Congressional history indicates that while a union may unilaterally extend the time to strike or picket, any extension beyond 72 hours would be unreasonable, and even within the 72-hour extension, at least 12 hours' notice of the actual start should be given. The NLRB stated that any delays in beginning a strike or picketing "will be viewed in light of (1) the circumstances causing the union to delay its actions and (2) why the union could not give the health care facility notice of the new scheduled date and time. . . ."

Actual written notice under Section 8(g) may not be required if there is "substantial compliance" with the provisions. Even though a kidney center did not receive the written notice of intent to strike, where it had actual notice of the impending walkout, the employer was not prejudiced by the lack of written word and the union had made reasonable efforts to give the proper alert, the union was in substantial compliance with the notice requirements of the act.[13]

After failing to reach agreement on a collective bargaining contract, the union sent to the center and the FMCS by certified mail the required ten-day notice of intent to strike. The FMCS received its notice and telephoned the center to inform it. The letter to the center, however, did not arrive until well after the strike had begun, about a month and a half after it had been sent. The delay was due to insufficient postage and the failure of the Postal Service to follow its normal procedure of either delivering a letter with postage due or returning it to the sender.

The NLRB found that the union had acted reasonably, that the kidney center had expected the strike and had made arrangements for it, and that under the circumstances it would be unduly harsh to deprive strikers of their employee status because of a technicality.

Other Notice Requirements

There are other special notice requirements in the amendments.[14] Ninety days' written notice must be given to the other party prior to a proposed termination or modification of a contract, and 60 days' written notice to the FMCS and appropriate state agencies. A contract will continue in full force for 90 days after the initial notice or until its expiration date, whichever is later.

Thirty days' written notice must be given to the FMCS and to any government mediation or conciliation agency of the existence of a dispute concerning an initial agreement.

FEDERAL MEDIATION AND CONCILIATION

The amendments provide for mandatory mediation by the FMCS, and give its director the authority to establish an impartial board of inquiry if the dispute will "substantially interrupt" health care services.[15]

In August 1979, the FMCS issued new regulations to give the parties to collective bargaining disputes in the health care industry the option of having some input into the selection of any board of inquiry that the service might appoint.[16] The regulations contain other provisions under which the agency will "defer to the parties' own privately agreed-to fact-finding or arbitration procedure and decline to appoint a Board of Inquiry" as long as certain conditions are met. Both of the procedures would be at the option of the parties.

Under prior regulations, the board of inquiry was appointed without consultation with the parties. The new procedures permit the parties jointly to submit a list of arbitrators or other individuals acceptable to both sides. The list must be submitted at least 90 days before expiration of a contract or, in an initial contract situation, before the required statutory notice of the dispute to the FMCS. The agency will "make every effort" to choose the inquiry board from that list.

The list may be for a particular dispute or for all future disputes, for particular parties or for a group of employers and unions. Names may be ranked in order of preference, and if desired the parties may even submit one specific individual if that person agrees to be available for the inquiry time period.

The deferral procedure had been used in the past by the FMCS on an informal basis but now has become a formal policy. Parties at times have preferred to use their own fact-finding or arbitration procedures for a variety of reasons, including the avoidance of the time constraints of the statutory procedure, the control

gained over selection of a third party neutral, or a desire for binding arbitration.

Under the new regulations, the FMCS will defer to the parties' own procedure if they agree to it in writing and if the procedure includes a prohibition on strikes, lockouts, and changes in conditions of employment during the proceedings as well as for final and binding written awards by impartial arbitrator(s) selected by a fixed and determinate method.

The FMCS has conducted a two-and-one-half-year impact study of health care bargaining, the results of which were released in the summer of 1979.[17] The study covered bargaining from August 1974 through December 1976, and concluded, *inter alia:*

- The negotiating parties at large health care institutions generally expect fact-finding boards to be appointed, and thus tend to defer real bargaining until such a board is chosen. The boards often are named before the parties have narrowed their positions, so the boards are hampered in their efforts to make useful recommendations. Furthermore, without the crisis of a strike deadline, the boards encounter resistance to settlement suggestions. Consequently, the use of the boards has not altered the "11th hour" or "crisis atmosphere" of many health care negotiations. The study therefore recommends that fact-finding boards be appointed closer to contract expiration dates than in the past.

- A major bargaining influence is the role of third party payers. Management often claims an inability to pay and there is a tendency toward perfunctory bargaining and extended negotiations.

- The expanded coverage of the act has led to a "new wave of organizing activity, with unions winning about 60 percent of health care elections, but this is likely to level off to the 50 percent national average for all industries."

HEALTH CARE INDUSTRY STRIKE PROBLEMS

The NLRB has considered a number of other issues of special interest to health care employers faced with a strike, involving the protection of patients, the permissible duration of a strike, preparations for a walkout, and employee communications to patients.

The welfare of patients was at issue when a New York state court granted a preliminary injunction against a threatened strike at 20 nursing homes in Nassau and Suffolk counties. The state of New York had requested the injunction after the commissioner of health issued orders prohibiting the strike in the interest of protecting the public health.

The NLRB obtained a federal district court injunction against the state to prevent it from restraining the strike. The court ruled that federal law preempts state law as to the right to strike.[18]

However, even though the state could not prohibit a strike or peaceful picketing at a health care institution, the court pointed out that the state retained the power to act "when it appears that the lives and health of nursing home residents are threatened . . . , to take whatever reasonable steps are necessary to protect the residents from the effects of strike activity."[19]

The duration of certain types of picketing was limited by the NLRA even before the health care amendments. Picketing for the purpose of recognition and organization is permissible only for a "reasonable period of time not to exceed thirty days."[20] While no special provision was added for health care institutions, the NLRB has indicated that where patient care could be affected, picketing could be restricted to less than 30 days. "[R]elevant factors would include the nature of the illnesses being treated at the picketed institution and the effects of the picketing on the institution's ability to treat its patients."[21]

After receiving the ten-day notice of a strike, a hospital may properly attempt to determine whether employees intend to participate so it can determine the need for replacements.[22] The employees must be clearly informed that they are free to make their own decision and that no reprisals will be taken. But conducting individual interrogations, in which some employees who refused to answer were told it was assumed they would strike and their jobs would be in jeopardy, was found to be an unfair labor practice.[23] The key is whether the employer observes the safeguards of informing employees of the purpose of the inquiry and the right to respond freely without threat of reprisal.

The NLRB has determined twice that hospital employees were engaged in protected activity when they communicated to patients about strike activities. In one instance, two picketing doctors had discouraged patients from seeking treatment at a struck health care clinic.[24] The doctors were not represented by a labor organization but actively sympathized with a strike by District 1199 at the clinic where they worked in a teaching and consulting capacity as "preceptors" to residents. Although they gave no advance notice, the two doctors refused assignments and joined the picket line when the strike began.[25] While on the picket line, the doctors identified themselves as such to patients, informed them that there was a strike, that normal facilities were not available, and that they would be

better off seeking treatment at a facility where there was no strike.

The two doctors were discharged for their actions, and although they were reinstated later with the discharges converted to suspensions, their applications for full-time positions at the hospital and their requests for admitting privileges were denied.

The NLRB reasoned that pickets often "attempt to discourage . . . third persons from availing themselves of the service or product provided by the targeted establishment," that such attempts are protected under the act, and that physicians should not be treated any differently than nonphysicians.

The Second Circuit Court of Appeals reversed the board on this issue, ruling that while an appeal to patients to turn away out of sympathy with the strike would be permissible, the doctors' "deceptive" statements that competent treatment could not be obtained was "grossly improper" and "would have fully justified" permanent discharge.

In the other case, a hospital was found to have violated the act by discharging a nurse who spoke to a patient suffering from phlebitis concerning the adequacy of care in the event of a scheduled strike. The hospital contended that the nurse had initiated the conversation concerning the upcoming strike and had suggested the patient's well-being would be jeopardized by the absence of sufficient personnel. The nurse testified that it was the patient who had inquired about the strike, and that she, the nurse, had only reassured the patient that sufficient arrangements were being made for personnel. The nurse was one of the employees who intended to, and did in fact, go on strike.

The administrative law judge credited the nurse's testimony because the hospital did not present either the patient or her deposition at the hearing. Although the judge did not hold that the hospital terminated the nurse out of any antiunion animus, he did find that she was engaged in "protected activity" at the time of her alleged professional misconduct and could not be terminated if she was not, in fact, guilty of the misconduct. The activity was "protected" because the patient, according to the nurse, had challenged the propriety of the employees' decision to strike and the nurse was entitled to defend that decision.[26]

One other sensitive problem in health care strikes is the extent to which a hospital may accept patients from or supply services, including skilled employees, to a struck institution without losing the protective status of a "neutral" employer. An employer who becomes an "ally" of another struck employer becomes a legitimate target of picketing by the striking employees.

The congressional committee reports on the amendments indicate that institutions accepting the patients of the primary employer "or otherwise providing life-sustaining services" such as employees with critical skills should not lose this neutral status.[27]

However, the NLRB general counsel has advised that a neutral hospital will become an ally unless it limits its aid to the acceptance of critically ill patients or those in need of immediate medical attention, and to the supply of critical staff.[28] This would appear to be at odds with the congressional reports, which indicate that any patient could be accepted.

SOLICITATION AND DISTRIBUTION

General NLRB Approach

In general, the NLRB, with the approval of the Supreme Court, has declared that a rule barring union solicitation or distribution of literature by nonemployees at any time on the employer's premises is presumptively a valid rule.[29] There are two important exceptions: (1) if the union cannot reach the employees by other reasonable means;[30] and (2) if the rule is enforced selectively, discriminating against union activity.[31] Because of the latter exception, it is preferable for an employer to prohibit solicitations by all outside groups, although it may be permissible to allow very limited exceptions.

With respect to solicitation and distribution by employees, the NLRB, with court approval, has adopted these general presumptions: (1) it is valid to prohibit solicitation and distribution during working time, and to prohibit the distribution of literature in working areas; (2) it is not valid to prohibit solicitation during nonworking time, wherever it is, and it is not valid to prohibit the distribution of literature in a nonworking area during nonworking time.[32]

The Rules and the Health Care Industry

In the health care industry, the issue has been whether the special concerns for patients and their visitors justify broader no-solicitation/no-distribution rules.

A landmark decision in this area is the *Beth Israel Hospital* case decided by the Supreme Court in August 1978.[33] The hospital's rule barred solicitation and distribution of literature in any area to which patients or visitors had access. The Court held the rule invalid because there was only a remote potential for disruption of patient care by solicitation in the cafeteria and coffee shop, which were included in the ban.

The Court stressed the "critical significance" of the fact that only 1.56 percent of the cafeteria's patrons were patients and 9 percent were visitors. Several concurring justices expressed reservations about generally applying rules developed in the factory context to health care facilities, noting the unusual situation at Beth Israel where the cafeteria was patronized primarily by employees.

After *Beth Israel,* the lower courts attempted to apply its precedent to other hospitals. In November 1978, the Tenth Circuit struck down a no-solicitation rule that encompassed the hospital cafeteria even though 90 to 95 percent of the patients were ambulatory and took their meals there.[34] The court noted that the cafeteria was divided into two sections, one for employees and one for patients. The court applied a "balancing" test, weighing "the likelihood of disruption of patient care" with "the extent of the interference with union organizational activities." Here the court said there was no evidence that the patients "suffered upset or experienced disruption of tranquility" because of the solicitation, so there was no basis for prohibiting it.

In December 1978, the Tenth Circuit again held invalid a no-solicitation rule that included the hospital cafeteria and parking lot.[35] There was no proof of "special circumstances" to justify a ban in the cafeteria, the court said, where the hospital relied on conclusory testimony from an administrator and did not call any doctors as witnesses.

The NLRB had issued an order limiting the ban on solicitation to "immediate patient care areas." The court found the order too vague and instructed the board to make specific findings and conclusions as to the treatment areas and corridors to be protected.

The District of Columbia Circuit took a somewhat different approach. Prior to *Beth Israel,* that circuit had sustained the right of a hospital to ban solicitation and distribution of literature on the hospital premises, except for a small employees' locker room.[36]

After *Beth Israel,* the Supreme Court asked the District of Columbia Circuit to reconsider its earlier decision but only as to that portion dealing with the hospital cafeteria.[37] The Supreme Court let stand the lower court's ruling that permitted a ban on solicitation in the corridors.

In January 1979, on reconsideration, the circuit court suggested that a hospital might be able to have such a rule during peak hours of operation, but not at other times.[38] The court remanded the case to the NLRB to determine whether nonemployee use of the cafeteria was of a sufficient magnitude at times to warrant a no-solicitation rule during those periods. The NLRB also was to consider whether such a rule would be unreasonable during times when employee use of other facilities was most likely.

In June 1979, the Supreme Court had before it another hospital solicitation and distribution case, *Baptist Hospital*.[39] The NLRB position was that no-solicitation rules in other than "immediate patient care areas" were presumptively invalid unless a hospital could prove that disruption to patient care would necessarily result if solicitation and distribution were permitted. The Supreme Court held that the NLRB lacked substantial evidence to support its order enjoining a no-solicitation rule in corridors and sitting rooms on floors with either patients' rooms or operating and therapy rooms, where doctors testified that union solicitation in the presence or within hearing of patients could have adverse effects on their recovery.

The Court found that the hospital had successfully rebutted the board's presumption with the doctors' testimony, and further noted that

... the experience to date raises serious doubts as to whether the Board's interpretation of its present presumption adequately takes into account the medical practices and methods of treatment incident to the delivery of patient-care services in a modern hospital.[40]

However, the Court upheld the board's determination that union solicitation should be permitted in the hospital cafeteria, gift shop, and lobbies on the first floor. The Court noted that the hospital presented no clear data on the frequency of patient use of the first floor facilities, and that patients must have special permission to take meals in the cafeteria.

NLRB General Counsel's Guidelines

In response to the Supreme Court's criticism of the board's interpretation of "immediate patient care areas," the NLRB's general counsel's office issued guidelines to the board's regional directors proposing a broadening of the board's restrictions on solicitation rules in health care facilities.[41] The guidelines are intended to aid the regional directors in their reconsideration of a series of no-solicitation cases that were remanded to them by the board to receive additional evidence consistent with *Baptist Hospital*. The general counsel cautioned that the board might "adopt a far different approach from that proposed," and that regional officers therefore should concentrate on compiling extensive records to aid and support the NLRB in determining its policy.

The guidelines propose that the definition of patient care areas where no-solicitation rules are presump-

tively lawful be expanded to "include such places as corridors adjacent to patients' rooms, operating rooms and treatment areas; sitting rooms on patient floors accessible to or used by patients; and elevators or stairways used substantially to transport patients."

As to nurses' stations, the guidelines suggest that physical layout will be an important factor in determining whether they are within the "patient care area" category. Accordingly, it is recommended that evidence be adduced on "the extent to which patient treatment is given in the nurses' stations; the proximity of the stations to patient rooms or sitting areas; the physical separation of the stations from surrounding patient care areas; whether there are interior partitions that separate working from non-working areas within the station; whether employees take their breaks in the stations; and whether other types of nonwork related activities are permitted there."

"Public access areas," such as cafeterias, gift shops, lobbies, vending machine areas, and pharmacies, would continue to be places in which solicitation is presumed valid, as would be "working areas to which only employees have general access," such as kitchen, laundry, housekeeping, and medical records, and also "nonworking areas to which only employees have access," such as locker rooms, lounges, and parking lots.

As to the areas in which no-solicitation rules are presumed unlawful, the guidelines direct the regions to determine whether an employer might successfully rebut the presumption, taking into consideration "the actual use and the physical layout of each area of the health care facility" to ascertain whether patients might be disturbed or their care disrupted if solicitation were allowed in the area. Factors include the "nature of the services rendered in each area," "problems caused by the movement of patients or emergency equipment," "physical separation of the area," and "whether an area of predominantly public or employee use also has an important patient-care function."

"Most importantly," the guidelines state, the regions "should assess the extent to which the employer has provided its employees with alternative locations and means by which they can communicate with each other and where organizational activity could be meaningfully conducted." If so, a ban on solicitation in a presumptively invalid area could be lawful where "the employer establishes that considerations of patient care outweigh the need for additional solicitation areas." As an example, the guidelines suggest that if solicitation is allowed in the cafeteria where breaks are taken, vending machine areas, major portions of the main lobby, exterior grounds, and areas where only employees have access, solicitation might be prohibited in areas such as offices and laboratories where a ban would otherwise be presumptively unlawful.

Consistent Enforcement of Solicitation Rules

It is important to remember that an otherwise valid no-solicitation rule may be invalid if it is enforced selectively. The importance of enforcing solicitation rules consistently is illustrated by the case of a hospital that prohibited the "wearing of medallions and identification other than professional and hospital" pins. The NLRB found the rule to be invalid as to union buttons since United Fund buttons had been permitted.[42] The Sixth Circuit Court of Appeals asked the NLRB to reconsider its determination in light of two earlier board decisions involving union buttons at nursing homes.[43]

In one of those earlier decisions, the NLRB held that a ban on buttons, as well as any other adornments such as jewelry, was appropriate in the "special circumstances" where employees are in direct contact with elderly, ill patients.[44] The rule had been instituted and enforced prior to a union organizing campaign.

In the other case, the NLRB held that a rule against the wearing of union buttons was improper where others, such as "Smile" and "Jesus Saves" buttons, were permitted and the rule against union buttons was not adopted until an organizing campaign began.[45]

On remand in the first case, the board modified its broad order that the hospital refrain from maintaining and enforcing its rule against union buttons and required only that it not discriminate against its employees by applying and enforcing its dress code unequally.[46] The hospital must then permit union buttons in the same circumstances and to the same extent it has allowed other buttons to be worn.

APPROPRIATE BARGAINING UNIT

Unit Proliferation

Before a union representation election can be held, the NLRB must determine which employees are to be included in the bargaining unit. The NLRB chooses *an* appropriate unit, not necessarily the *most* appropriate, on the basis of a number of factors, including: (1) mutuality of interest in wages, benefits, and working conditions; (2) commonality of skills and supervision; (3) frequency of contact with other employees; (4) interchange and functional integration; and (5) practice and patterns of bargaining. Using these criteria, the board decides whether there is a sufficient "community of interest" among employees to justify their inclusion in a single unit.

In enacting the health care amendments, Congress admonished the board to avoid the proliferation of bargaining units in this industry.[47] The concern was that unit fragmentation would lead to jurisdictional disputes and work stoppages. The NLRB has had to consider this additional factor in determining appropriate bargaining units in these institutions.

The NLRB has taken the position that it can apply its traditional criteria to the health care industry so long as it avoids units for each job classification or craft of the sort it has established in the construction industry. Using this method, the board has determined the following to be appropriate employee units: (1) registered nurses; (2) physicians; (3) all professionals, excluding registered nurses and physicians; (4) service and maintenance; (5) technical; and (6) office clericals. In addition, it has found smaller units of maintenance employees or boiler operators appropriate where they have a "separate identifiable community of interest."[48]

Several of the courts of appeals have overturned the board's unit determinations for failing to give proper weight to the congressional directive to avoid a proliferation of bargaining units.

The Ninth Circuit refused to enforce an NLRB bargaining order for a unit composed solely of registered nurses where the board would not allow the hospital to present evidence that the appropriate unit should include all professional employees.[49] The court found that an irrebuttable presumption in favor of R.N. units was "arbitrary and capricious" in view of the congressional admonition against undue proliferation. The hospital therefore must be afforded an opportunity to present evidence on the propriety of the unit.

The court further concluded that the board's community-of-interest test for determining the appropriate bargaining unit is not sanctioned by the legislative history. The court suggested that the board should demonstrate a "disparity of interests" between R.N.s and other hospital employees to justify a separate unit but did not define "disparity of interests."

The Second Circuit also has held that the NLRB did not give a proper weight to the congressional admonition against undue unit proliferation when it certified a separate unit for a hospital's maintenance department employees. The board's analysis rested solely on its traditional "community-of-interest" criteria, with only a conclusory statement that the congressional directive did not "preclude the appropriateness of a maintenance unit." The court remanded the case to the board for reconsideration in light of the congressional concern. The board was directed to balance its traditional "community-of-interest" factors against the public interest in preventing fragmentation in this industry.[50]

The Seventh Circuit overturned a board certification of a unit composed only of hospital maintenance workers,[51] and the Sixth Circuit, while upholding a unit of technical employees including licensed practical nurses, cautioned that it would expect the rest of the hospital's nonprofessional employees to be covered by a single service and maintenance unit.[52]

The Third Circuit rebuked the NLRB for operating "outside the law" by its refusal to "apply the law announced by the federal judiciary" and denied enforcement of the board's bargaining order for a unit of hospital maintenance and housekeeping employees.[53]

The board had deferred bargaining unit determination to a state agency and had concluded that its traditional standards for determining bargaining units would have produced the same result. The board declined to follow prior decisions by the Third Circuit holding that the NLRB should not so defer in health care cases and that the board's traditional standards for determining appropriate health care bargaining units were inapplicable in light of the congressional directive to avoid the undue proliferation of such units. In so doing, the board stated that it was "respectfully disagreeing" with the court.

The court reprimanded the board: "Congress has not given NLRB the power or authority to disagree, respectfully or otherwise, with the decisions of this court."

At present, then, there is a conflict between the NLRB and the courts as to what is an undue proliferation of bargaining units in the health care industry. The NLRB probably will continue to certify smaller units, especially in the service and maintenance group, in the absence of a definitive Supreme Court ruling. Health care employers probably will continue to appeal these certifications to the courts.

Interns and Residents

In 1976 the NLRB held that interns and residents were not "employees" but were "students," and hence were outside the protection of the act.[54] In April 1979, a divided three-judge panel of the Court of Appeals for the District of Columbia Circuit overturned the NLRB, ruling that the health care amendments and their legislative history demonstrate a clear congressional intent to include interns and residents under the act.[55]

However, in July 1980, the court reheard the case sitting *en banc* and reversed to uphold the NLRB's

position.[55a] Therefore, at present, interns and residents remain outside the protection of the act.

Earlier, in December 1979, the House of Representatives rejected by a vote of 227 to 167 a bill to extend coverage of the NLRA to include hospital interns and residents. A major factor in the bill's defeat appeared to be congressional concern with containing hospital costs.

SUPERVISORY EMPLOYEES

Who Is a Supervisor?

Supervisors are required under the act to be excluded from a bargaining unit. In general, the NLRB has held that the test for determining whether a health care professional employee is a supervisor for purposes of the act is whether, in addition to giving directions to other employees in the exercise of professional judgment, the individual also exercises supervisory authority in the interest of the employer. A professional employee who gives direction to other employees in the exercise of professional judgment incidental to patient treatment is not exercising supervisory authority in the interest of the employer.[56]

In practice, the NLRB has taken a narrow view of who is a "supervisor" in a health care institution, and indicia of supervisory status that would be sufficient in nonhealth care situations often are not sufficient to establish that status in a hospital or home. For example, where L.P.N.s instructed aides and orderlies, assigning tasks, evaluating performance, giving warning slips and initiating transfers, the board nevertheless ruled they were not supervisors since they did not interview, hire, or make the final decision on discharge.[57] Similarly, where L.P.N.s were authorized to discipline nurses' aides by warning and suspension, and their recommendations for discharge of aides were routinely followed, the NLRB held that the L.P.N.s were not supervisors because they did not participate in interviewing or hiring and did not make final decisions as to termination and serious discipline.[58] Charge nurses[59] and head nurses[60] also have been found not to be supervisors in similar circumstances.

Thus it appears that the NLRB would find few nurses to be statutory supervisors unless they exercise the authority effectively to recommend hire and discharge.

By contrast, head nurses were found to be supervisors under the act where they: (1) effectively recommended the hire, discharge, and transfer of employees in their units; (2) independently assigned work and determined long-term scheduling for vacation days and personal leave; (3) periodically evaluated employees whose retention or promotion depended "almost primarily" on those appraisals; (4) issued warning notices and processed grievances; (5) received substantially higher salaries and more vacation time than R.N.s; (6) spent a minor portion or none of their working time on direct patient care; and (7) prepared management reports evaluating their unit and attended regularly scheduled supervisory meetings.[61] Furthermore, it was noted that if the head nurses were employees instead of supervisors, the supervisor-to-employee ratio would range from 1:50 to 1:134, as opposed to 1:5 to 1:26 with the head nurses as supervisors. Assistant head nurses also were found to be supervisors because they spent a substantial amount of time performing supervisory functions in the absence of the head nurses.

An inservice education assistant, however, was held not to be a supervisor and was included in a bargaining unit of registered nurses.[62] Although this assistant recommended applicants for hire as nurses' aides, the evidence was that the individual recommended almost everyone who applied and the personnel director made the hiring decisions. Furthermore, this assistant's hiring duties required relatively little of the work time and related solely to nurses' aides, who were not part of the bargaining unit. Employees exercising supervisory authority over nonunit workers will be excluded from the unit as supervisors only if they spend more than 50 percent of their time supervising those employees. If the education assistant had exercised supervisory authority over registered nurses, the 50 percent figure would not have had to be met because the unit consisted of registered nurses.

Because the board is inclined to segregate R.N.s, L.P.N.s, and aides and orderlies into separate bargaining units, many R.N.s and L.P.N.s exercising supervisory authority will do so with regard to employees in a different bargaining unit, and therefore will not be "supervisors" under the act unless they can meet the 50 percent test.

Supervisor Participation in Bargaining Organizations

A conflict-of-interest issue arises when a labor organization seeking to be certified as an employee bargaining agent has participating members who are supervisors. In the health care industry, this issue often is raised when nurses' associations seek to represent employees as bargaining agents. In the past, the NLRB resolved the problem by making certification as a bargaining agent contingent upon the nurses' associ-

ation's delegation of bargaining authority to a local autonomous chapter controlled by nonsupervisory employees.

In 1979 the NLRB abandoned that position.[63] Now the burden is on the employer to establish that the participation of supervisory employees in the affairs of the organization seeking certification presents a "clear and present danger" of a conflict of interest interfering with the collective bargaining process. The employer may raise such conflict-of-interest issues in NLRB representation election proceedings.

Subsequent to this shift in policy, the board ruled that there was no threat to the collective bargaining process where a Kentucky nurses' association had some officers who were supervisors. None of the supervisors were employed at the hospital where an election was sought, the bylaws restricted collective bargaining committee membership to nonsupervisory nurses, and the local unit formulated its own demands and selected a negotiating committee from its ranks. This, the board found, was sufficient to "insure that the collective-bargaining process is insulated at all levels from supervisory participation or influence." Accordingly, an election was ordered.[64]

MANDATORY AND PERMISSIVE BARGAINING SUBJECTS

The Supreme Court has ruled that bargaining items relating to "wages, hours, and other terms and conditions of employment" are mandatory subjects for discussion; the parties are obligated to bargain on these subjects, and are not required to compromise their position.[65] Other subjects that may be raised in bargaining negotiations, but are outside the scope of mandatory matters, are termed permissive subjects and may not be insisted upon by a party to the point of an impasse in negotiations, thereby interfering with the settlement of mandatory issues.

The unionization of professional employees has been marked by an increased emphasis in collective bargaining negotiations on subjects that traditionally have been thought of as management prerogatives, particularly in policy areas. The issue then arises whether employee demands in these areas are mandatory or permissive subjects for bargaining.

Organized professional health care employees have evidenced the same desire for some kind of role in the decision-making structure as have nonhealth professionals such as teachers, professors, engineers, and police. A study of bargaining contracts in hospitals before the health care amendments revealed that 73 percent of those involving professionals and 52 percent of those for technical units, but only 16 percent of those for nonprofessionals, provided for joint study committees.[66]

Whether the establishment of such committees is a mandatory or permissive subject of bargaining will turn on the jurisdiction and authority of the committee. A few cases in the university context may provide some illumination as to what would be the board's position in the health care industry. In one case the NLRB indicated that faculty participation in the selection of a division chairman is a mandatory subject.[67] The general counsel's office reached the same conclusion on participation in tenure and promotion decisions.[68] On the other hand, the general counsel's office ruled that faculty participation in the appointment of deans and other administrative personnel was a nonmandatory subject because such positions were outside the bargaining unit.[69]

A college was not required to bargain with a union over a "governance" proposal dealing with faculty committees and covering "the selection and duties of committee officers, the composition of the committees, a provision for the establishment of new committees, and preparation of agendas for faculty meetings" because some of the subjects in the proposal were nonmandatory, the NLRB advised.[70] The "subject of delegation to a group, such as a faculty senate or committee structure, of the power to negotiate concerning wages, hours, or other conditions of employment . . . would appear to be inherently *permissive* in nature."[71]

Subjects that were in the proposal but were mandatory in nature included items setting forth the duties of unit employees, how their duties were to be performed, and "the extent of required participation of unit employees" on the committees.

As yet the NLRB has not made many significant determinations on mandatory vs. permissive bargaining subjects in the health care industry. However, as a history of bargaining develops under the amendments it appears likely that this issue will arise with respect to the particular concerns of organized health care professionals.

The NLRB has determined that a nurse participating in an ad hoc patient care committee report on problems with cleanliness, staffing levels, and ratio of staff to patients was engaged in concerted protected activity because these subjects were related to conditions of employment.[72] Therefore, the hospital could not discharge her for her role in the report. The inference is that if these subjects are related to working conditions so that efforts to criticize or improve them were protected, they also would be mandatory for bargaining purposes.

A subject that apparently is not mandatory in health care industry bargaining is interest arbitration. A union that insisted to the point of impasse on an interest arbitration clause, providing for arbitration of any issues on which the parties could not reach agreement during negotiations for a new contract, was found to have violated the act.[73] The expired contract between the union and the hospital employer contained an interest arbitration clause, which the hospital proposed be deleted from the new contract. The parties were able to reach agreement on all other terms of a new contract but the union refused to drop the interest arbitration provision.

The NLRB found the interest arbitration clause to be nonmandatory. The First Circuit Court of Appeals agreed, citing decisions by the Fourth and Fifth Circuit Courts (in the context of other industries) holding that an interest arbitration provision bears only a remote relationship to terms or conditions of employment, so that bargaining is not required.

The court also rejected union arguments that a state law providing for arbitration of grievances or disputes not settled in health care industry bargaining and congressional concern (in enacting the health care amendments with the avoidance of strikes or work stoppages) justified an exception for the health care industry. The court observed that "to add to the list of subjects which the parties may insist on to impasse would, in our view, tend more to frustrate than to further the congressional objective of avoiding impasse situations in the health care field."

The board also has ruled that a health care clinic violated the act by refusing to consider a union proposal to limit the right of the clinic to use volunteers, so that bargaining unit employees would not be displaced.[74] This ruling is consistent with the NLRB's position in other industries that preservation of bargaining unit work is a mandatory subject of bargaining, at least where the work will be performed under similar conditions in essentially the same place.[75]

CONCLUSION

The dual purpose of the health care amendments—to ensure the collective bargaining rights of employees while maintaining adequate patient care services—has given the NLRB a unique responsibility. The board's response generally has been one of caution and reluctance to depart from the standards it has evolved in other industries. As a result, the board has found itself in fundamental disagreement with the courts on vital issues, in particular as to what are appropriate health care bargaining units and when and where no-solicitation rules may be enforced.

The courts, then, rather than the NLRB, are leading the way in formulating a new body of labor relations law suited to the special needs of the health care industry. Most of this developing body of law relates to organizing issues. As the number of established bargaining relationships increases, it can be expected that there will be more cases dealing with other matters.

The next few years should bring significant expansion in the evolution of health care labor relations law. It will be of particular interest to see whether the tension between the courts and the NLRB over the proper balance to be struck continues and, indeed, expands into new substantive areas.

NOTES

1. 29 U.S.C. §§ 152(2), 152(14), 153(c), 158(d)-(e), 158(g) (Supp. V, 1975), *amending* 29 U.S.C. § 151-68 (1970).

2. *Bio-Medical Applications of San Diego, Inc.*, 216 NLRB 631 (1975).

3. *East Oakland Community Health Alliance, Inc.*, 218 NLRB 1270 (1975).

4. *First Healthcare Corp.*, 222 NLRB 212 (1976), *enforcement denied sub nom.*, *NLRB v. Dist. 1199, Nat'l Union of Hosp. and Health Care Employees*, No. 76-407 (2d Cir. November 23, 1976). Although there is no written opinion, the court stated on the record that the violation was *de minimus*.

5. *Long Beach Youth Center, Inc.*, 230 NLRB 648 (1977), *aff'd*, 591 F.2d 1276 (9th Cir. 1979). *See also Mercy Hosp. Ass'n, Inc.*, 235 NLRB 681 (1978); *Walker Methodist Residence and Health Care Center, Inc.*, 227 NLRB 1630 (1977).

6. *NLRB v. Int'l Brotherhood of Electrical Workers Local 388*, 548 F.2d 704 (7th Cir.), *cert. denied*, 434 U.S. 837 (1977); *Laborers' Int'l Union of North America, Local 1057 v. NLRB*, 567 F.2d 1006 (D.C. Cir. 1977); *Painters Local 452*, 246 NLRB No. 148 (1979).

7. *Painters Dist. Council*, 243 NLRB No. 113 (1979).

8. *See The Dow Chemical Co.*, 244 NLRB No. 129 (1979), concurring opinion of Member Truesdale; General Counsel's Monthly Report, January 24, 1975; General Counsel's Memorandum 74-79 (August 20, 1974). *See also Cedarcrest, Inc.*, 246 NLRB No. 131 (1979), where the administrative law judge found that the employer was not a health care employer and therefore was not entitled to Section 8(g) notice; however, the judge concluded that even if the employer was a health care institution, its unilateral 50 percent wage cut was clearly a "serious" and "flagrant" unfair labor practice excusing notice of the strike.

9. *See* S. Rep. No. 93-766, 93d Cong., 2d Sess. 4-5 (1974); H. Rep. No. 93-1051, 93d Cong., 2d Sess. 6 (1974).

10. *Dist. 1199-E, Nat'l Union of Hosp. & Health Care Employees*, 227 NLRB 132 (1976); *Dist. 1199, Nat'l Union of Hospital and Health Care Employees (Elm Hill Convalescent Home, Inc.)*, 4 AMR ¶ 10,080 (1976).

11. *Retail Clerks, Local 727 (Devon Gables Health Care Center, Inc.)*, 244 NLRB No. 90 (1979).

12. *Dist. 1199-E*, 243 NLRB No. 6 (1979).

13. *Bio-Medical Applications of New Orleans, Inc.*, 240 NLRB No. 39 (1979).

14. *See* Section 8(d) of the act.

15. LMRA Section 213.

16. 29 CFR Part 1420.

17. "Impact of the 1974 Health Care Amendments to the NLRA on Collective Bargaining in the Health Care Industry," Federal Mediation and Conciliation Service Office of Research, 1979.

18. *NLRB v. State of New York*, 436 F. Supp. 335 (E.D.N.Y. 1977), *aff'd without opinion*, 591 F.2d 1331 (2d Cir. 1978), *cert. denied*, 440 U.S. 950 (1979).

19. *Id.* at 339.

20. Section 8(b)(7)(C).

21. General Counsel's Memorandum 74-49 (August 20, 1974).

22. *Preterm, Inc.*, 240 NLRB No. 81 (1979).

23. *Id.*

24. *Montefiore Hosp. and Medical Center*, 243 NLRB No. 106 (1979), *rev'd in part and enforced in part*, No. 79-4156; 4184 (2d Cir. 1980).

25. This reaffirmed the board's earlier position, noted *supra* at n. 5, that the notice of intent to strike required by Section 8(g) of the act applies only to labor organizations, not to individuals. Therefore, the doctors were not required to give advance notice before striking.

26. *Alexander Linn Hosp. Ass'n*, 244 NLRB No. 60 (1979).

27. S. Rep. No. 93-766, 93d Cong. 2d Sess. 5 (1974); H. Rep. No. 93-1051, 93d Cong., 2d Sess. 7 (1974).

28. Office of the General Counsel, Division of Advice, NLRB Memorandum, *Loma Linda Univ. Medical Center*, Case Nos. 31-CC-820, 31-CG-7, *Memorial Hosp. Medical Center of Long Beach*, Case Nos. 31-CC-821, 31-CG-18 (September 2, 1977).

29. *See, e.g., NLRB v. Babcock & Wilcox Co.*, 351 U.S. 105 (1956).

30. *See NLRB v. Babcock & Wilcox Co., supra*, 351 U.S. at 112; *Solo Cup Co.*, 172 NLRB 1110 (1968), *rev'd on other grounds*, 422 F.2d 1149 (7th Cir. 1970).

31. *See Republic Aviation Corp. v. NLRB*, 325 U.S. 793, 803 n.10 (1945).

32. *See, e.g., Republic Aviation Corp. v. NLRB, supra, Walton Manufacturing Co.*, 126 NLRB 697 (1960), *enforced*, 289 F.2d 177 (5th Cir. 1961); *Stoddard-Quirk Manufacturing Co.*, 138 NLRB 615 (1962); *The Rose Co.*, 154 NLRB 228 (1965).

33. *Beth Israel Hosp. v. NLRB*, 437 U.S. 483 (1978).

34. *NLRB v. National Jewish Hosp. and Research Center*, 593 F.2d 911 (10th Cir. 1978).

35. *NLRB v. St. Joseph Hosp.*, 587 F.2d 1060 (10th Cir. 1978).

36. *Baylor Univ. Medical Center v. NLRB*, 578 F.2d 351 (D.C. Cir. 1978).

37. *NLRB v. Baylor Univ. Medical Center*, 439 U.S. 9 (1978).

38. *Baylor Univ. Medical Center v. NLRB*, 593 F.2d 1290 (D.C. Cir. 1979).

39. *NLRB v. Baptist Hosp., Inc.*, 99 S. Ct. 2598 (1979).

40. *Id.*

41. General Counsel's Memorandum 79-76 (October 5, 1979).

42. *Baptist Memorial Hosp.*, 225 NLRB 525 (1976).

43. *NLRB v. Baptist Memorial Hosp.*, 583 F.2d 906 (6th Cir. 1978).

44. *Evergreen Nursing Home*, 198 NLRB 775 (1972).

45. *Ohio Masonic Home*, 205 NLRB 357 (1973), *aff'd, Ohio Masonic Home v. NLRB*, 511 F.2d 527 (6th Cir. 1975).

46. *Baptist Memorial Hosp.*, 242 NLRB No. 103 (1979).

47. *See, e.g.*, 120 Cong. Rec. 12944-45 (1974), remarks of Senator Taft.

48. *See Allegheny Gen. Hosp.*, 239 NLRB No. 104 (1978).

49. *NLRB v. St. Francis Hosp. of Lynwood*, 601 F.2d 404 (9th Cir. 1979).

50. *NLRB v. Mercy Hosp. Ass'n*, 102 LRRM 2259 (2d Cir. 1979).

51. *NLRB v. W. Suburban Hosp.*, 570 F.2d 213 (7th Cir. 1978).

52. *NLRB v. Sweetwater Hosp. Ass'n*, 604 F.2d 454 (6th Cir. 1979).

53. *Allegheny Gen. Hosp. v. NLRB*, 102 LRRM 2784 (3d Cir. 1979).

54. *Cedars-Sinai Medical Center*, 223 NLRB 251 (1976).

55. *Physicians Nat'l House Staff Ass'n v. Murphy*, 85 LC ¶ 11,205 (D.C. Cir. 1979).

55a. *Physicians National House Staff Association v. Fanning*, 89 LC ¶ 12,117 (D.C. Cir. 1980).

56. *Samaritan Health Servs., Inc.*, 238 NLRB No. 56 (1978).

57. *Greenpark Care Center*, 236 NLRB 753 (1977).

58. *Pine Manor, Inc.*, 238 NLRB No. 217 (1978).

59. *Methodist Home v. NLRB*, 596 F.2d 1173 (4th Cir. 1979).

60. *Misericordia Hosp. Medical Center*, 246 NLRB No. 57 (1979).

61. *A. Barton Hepburn Hosp.*, 238 NLRB No. 10 (1978).

62. *Id.*

63. *Sierra Vista Hosp., Inc.*, 241 NLRB No. 107 (1979).

64. *Western Baptist Hosp.*, 246 NLRB No. 25 (1979). *Accord, Healdsburg Gen. Hosp.*, 1980 CCH NLRB ¶ 16,659 (1980); *Sidney Farber Cancer Inst.*, 247 NLRB No. 1 (1980).

65. *NLRB v. Wooster Div. of Borg-Warner Corp.*, 356 U.S. 342 (1958).

66. H. A. Juris, *Collective Bargaining in Hospitals*, 28 Lab. L.J. 504 (1977).

67. *Kendall College*, 228 NLRB 1083 (1977).

68. *The Cooper Union for the Advancement of Science and Art*, Case 2-CA-13602, Advice Memo, September 26, 1975.

69. *The Cooper Union for the Advancement of Science and Art*, Case 2-CA-13602, Region 2 dismissal letter (April 23, 1975); *St. John's Univ.*, Case 29-CB-1858, Advice Memo, January 17, 1975.

70. *Endicott College*, 4 AMR ¶ 10,219 (March 18, 1977).

71. *Id.* at 5277. (Emphasis in original.)

72. *Misericordia Hosp. Medical Center*, 246 NLRB No. 57 (1979).

73. *NLRB v. Massachusetts Nurses' Ass'n*, 557 F.2d 894 (1st Cir. 1977).

74. *Preterm, Inc.*, 240 NLRB No. 81 (1979).

75. *See, e.g., Fibreboard Paper Products Corp. v. NLRB*, 379 U.S. 203 (1964); *NLRB v. Wm. J. Burns Int'l Detective Agency, Inc.*, 346 F.2d 897 (8th Cir. 1965).

7. No-Solicitation/No-Distribution Rules

LAURENCE P. CORBETT

INTRODUCTION

At the first appearance of union organizing leaflets on the automobile windshields in a hospital parking lot or in the wastebaskets of its cafeteria, the following questions immediately arise:

1. Is it too late to ban outsiders from organizing on the premises of the hospital subject to the National Labor Relations Act?
2. Or, can the hospital terminate or discipline employees who are identified as engaging in organizational activities within the institution?

Generally, a health care institution may promulgate rules that restrict the time and place of solicitation and the time and location of the distribution of literature. However, there is no simple answer as to exactly what activity may and may not be prohibited at a health care institution, since many National Labor Relations Board (NLRB) and court decisions in this area turn on a particular set of facts. The 1974 Health Care Amendments to the National Labor Relations Act (NLRA) do not contain any special provisions limiting either union solicitation or distribution of union literature. However, both the NLRB and the courts have allowed health care institutions to promulgate and enforce a no-solicitation/no-distribution rule that is more restrictive than those allowed in other industries under the act.

The NLRB considers several questions in determining the validity of a health care institution's no-solicitation/no-distribution rule:

1. Is the activity subject to limitation either union solicitation or distribution of union literature?
2. Are the individuals involved employees or nonemployees?
3. Is the activity being limited to nonworking time?
4. Is the activity being limited to nonwork areas?
5. If the rule is found to be valid on its face, was it promulgated for discriminatory reasons or applied in a discriminatory fashion?

An employer's liability for an invalid rule or discriminatory promulgation or enforcement of a valid rule may be significant. For example, if the no-solicitation/no-distribution rule is too broad, any discipline of employees for violation of the rule may be found to be an unfair labor practice and the employee may be made whole for any loss sustained. Or, in a representation election that the union has lost, the results may be set aside and a new election directed. Thus, it is important that the health care institution know what activity can and cannot lawfully be prohibited.

609

EMPLOYEES

Solicitation

The General Rule

Historically, solicitation has been afforded different treatment from distribution of literature. The NLRB and the courts have reasoned that because distribution of union flyers, pamphlets, and other literature may pose a litter problem for an employer, it may be limited to a greater degree than solicitation. Although solicitation generally is oral in nature, both the NLRB and the courts have extended it to encompass handing out and signing union authorization cards. *Rose Co.*, (1965).[1]

In a landmark decision, *Republic Aviation v. NLRB (1945)*,[2] the U.S. Supreme Court ruled that an employer may prohibit solicitation only during working time. In defining working time, the Court did not include rest periods or lunch periods, despite the fact that these may be paid for by the employer. Obviously, working time did not apply to employees who were permitted to be on the premises before their shift began or after their shift ended. In *Essex International (1974)*,[3] the NLRB has found invalid rules that broadly prohibited solicitation during all nonwork hours, since they may be construed to include paid rest and lunch periods.

The general rule established by the NLRB and the courts has been to disallow a rule that restricts solicitation to nonworking areas. Exceptions to the rule have been made in the case of a department store's right to prohibit solicitation on the selling floor at any time (*Meier & Frank Co.*, 1950)[4] and a restaurant's right to prohibit solicitation at any time in customer access areas (*McDonald's Corp.*, 1973).[5] Health care institutions contended there should be an exception for patient care. In recognition of special circumstances in this field, the NLRB and the courts have made an exception to the general rule by allowing institutions to prohibit solicitation during nonworking time in "patient care areas."

Health Care Institution Exception to the General Rule

In its first major decision addressing health care institutions, the NLRB permitted a hospital to prohibit solicitation during nonworking time in immediate patient care areas, "such as patient rooms, operating rooms and places where patients receive treatment, such as x-ray and therapy areas." *St. John's Hospital and School of Nursing, Inc.*, 1976.[6] The NLRB reasoned that solicitation in those areas, even on non-

working time, might be unsettling to the patient and interfere with the hospital's primary function of patient care. However, the board struck down that part of the hospital's rule that prohibited solicitation in all work areas or areas where patients might have access. It reasoned that solicitation in areas such as the cafeteria and lounges would not affect patient care adversely. "On balance, the interests of patients well enough to frequent such areas do not outweigh those of employees to discuss or solicit union representation."[7]

Three U.S. Supreme Court decisions provide guidance for interpreting the NLRB's "patient care areas" concept, otherwise known as the "*St. John's* rule." *Beth Israel Hospital v. NLRB* (1978)[8] held that employees on nonwork time cannot be prohibited from solicitation in the hospital's cafeteria or coffee shop, both areas being primarily used by employees and not by patients. The Court was influenced by the past practice of using the hospital's cafeteria for a variety of purposes and by the fact that there were only a few other areas, such as employee locker rooms and restrooms, where employees would be allowed to solicit. In so holding, the Court endeavored to strike an appropriate balance among the rights of employees to engage in organizational activity and the interests of patients and the hospital in undisturbed patient care.

In its second decision, the Court allowed the health care institution to prohibit solicitation in areas such as hospital corridors and hallways accessible to patients. *Baylor University Medical Center v. NLRB* (1978).[9] Although, as in *Beth Israel*, there remained a few areas in which to solicit (the cafeteria issue was remanded to the lower court for reconsideration), the Court in *Baylor* found that the NLRB's presumption in favor of solicitation was not supported by any evidence that this activity in such areas would not affect patient care adversely. To the contrary, the evidence showed that congestion in the corridors impeded the operation of the medical staff and annoyed patients and visitors, and that the hallways were used for treatment and served as the only available waiting rooms.

Finally, in *NLRB v. Baptist Hospital, Inc.* (1979),[10] the Court was confronted with a no-solicitation rule that prohibited solicitation in the hospital's lobbies, cafeteria, gift shop, corridors, and sitting rooms accessible to patient's rooms. The NLRB had found that all these areas were not "immediate patient care areas," and there was no demonstrated likelihood that solicitation there would disrupt patient care or disturb patients. With respect to corridors and sitting rooms on floors having either patients' rooms or operating and therapy rooms, the Court reversed the board and found that immediate patient access to such areas, and possible adverse effects on patient recovery, gave the hospital the right to prohibit solicitation there. In connection with patient access areas, the Court, in reviewing the NLRB record, appeared to be influenced by the testimony of three witnesses, two physicians and a hospital administrator, who gave detailed information relating to the incidence of patient access and testified to the adverse effect union solicitation would have on patients. On the other hand, the Court found that the hospital had presented no clear evidence of the frequency with which patients used the cafeteria or gift shop or visited the lobbies on the first floor. The Court noted the testimony of the hospital's witnesses that solicitation in public areas such as the cafeteria would be unlikely to have a significant adverse impact on patients or patient care. Thus, the Court found that portion of the rule invalid. In expressing the opinion of the majority of the court, Justice Powell stated:

> [T]he Board [bears] a heavy continuing responsibility to review its policies concerning organizational activities in various parts of hospitals. Hospitals carry on a public function of the utmost seriousness and importance. They give rise to unique considerations that do not apply in the industrial settings with which the Board is more familiar. The Board should stand ready to revise its rulings if future experience demonstrates that the well-being of patients is in fact jeopardized.[11]

Further insight into the Court's reasoning is expressed in the concurring opinion of Justice Blackmun:

> I join the Court's opinion and its judgment. I write only to underline what is plainly said in the opinion, *ante,* at 15-16, and n.16, that these hospital cases so often turn on the proof presented. What may be true of one hospital's gift shop and cafeteria may not be true of another's. And I continue to have difficulty perceiving any rational distinction between the Board's recognition that solicitation is inappropriate in a department store, see *Beth Israel Hospital v. NLRB,* 437 U.S. 483, 511-512, and nn. 2 and 3, 98 LRRM 2727 (1978) (Powell, J. concurring opinion); *id.,* at 508 (concurring opinion), and its contrary presumption with respect to the retail shop (usually operated on a non-profit basis) and cafeteria in the hospital. The admonition contained in the last paragraph of n.16 of the Court's opinion [quote from Powell's decision], cannot be overemphasized.[12]

Baptist stands as the sum of the Court's decision on union solicitation by employees on nonworking time and provides a guide for the establishment of a rule.

The Court approves the *St. John's* exception prohibiting solicitation in patient rooms, operating rooms, and places where patients receive treatment, such as x-ray and therapy areas. As for the broader interpretation of "immediate patient care areas," the Court suggests a case-by-case approach in which the institution has the burden of proving by medical and other evidence that a specified area is used by or accessible to patients to the extent that union solicitation would disrupt health care operations or disturb patients.

In addition to the controversial areas such as cafeterias, lobbies, and coffee shops, there are working areas within hospitals to which there is no patient access, such as laundry, kitchen, maintenance department, and the business office. In striking a balance between the interests of the employees in organizational activity on the one hand and patients' care on the other, it appears the courts and the NLRB will apply the usual rule allowing solicitation in nonpatient areas such as those mentioned above, as well as employee locker rooms and restrooms; will apply the *St. John's* exception strictly to immediate patient care and treatment areas; and will apply patient access tests on a case-by-case basis to the locations that remain.

Distribution of Literature

General Rule

An employer may establish a no-distribution rule that prohibits distribution of literature during working time and during nonworking time in work areas. *Stoddard Quirk* (1962).[13] The board supported a stricter rule for distribution in working areas than for solicitation, citing, among other factors, the employer's legitimate interest in keeping the work areas free from litter and in maintaining cleanliness, order, and discipline.

Health Care Institutions

It has not been determined whether health care institutions may prohibit distribution in areas where the NLRB and the courts have allowed solicitation. For example, can distribution take place in the lounges, coffee shop, and cafeteria? The NLRB has not addressed the issue. It has intimated, however, that it will apply the same general analysis to distribution of literature as it used in determining what areas may be off limits for solicitation. In *Medical Center Hospitals* (1979),[14] the NLRB, following the Supreme Court's analysis in *Baptist,* found unlawful a ban on employee distribution on nonworking time at such locations as the outside walkway and driveway of a hospital used by patients, visitors, and employees. Thus, it would seem that a health care institution may be able to limit distribution in all working areas on the basis of a litter problem and, if the evidence supports it, in nonworking areas where distribution would interfere with patient care.

Other Solicitation–Distribution Activities by Employees

Union Insignia

A related form of solicitation occurs when employees wear union buttons, insignia, badges, lettered T-shirts, or arm bands. The NLRB and the courts have found that an employer may not prohibit employees, absent "special circumstances," from wearing union buttons and insignia during work time. *Republic Aviation, supra,* provided that the need for maintaining production and discipline did not call for their prohibition. *Floridian Hotel of Tampa, Inc.* (1962).[15]

However, in *Evergreen Nursing Home* (1972),[16] the NLRB upheld the employer's prohibition against allowing employees to wear any unnecessary adornments on their uniforms during work time. The board found that the union buttons in this case fell within the "special circumstances" rule: the union buttons were large and conspicuous, the employees were in direct contact with elderly patients whose reactions to the buttons were unpredictable, the employer had an interest in protecting patients from something that might upset them, and the rule against wearing unnecessary adornments had been in effect and enforced long before the union's organizing drive began. Thus, a rule of reason may apply in prohibiting employees with patient contact from wearing provocative emblems or buttons with the potential of disturbing patients. However, it is unlikely that the NLRB will uphold a prohibition of standard union buttons or insignia.

Bulletin Boards

An employer may establish a rule that reserves bulletin boards for official government and hospital material and prohibits use by employees for any purpose. *Stanley Furniture Co.* (1979).[17] However, the employer must enforce the prohibition in a nondiscriminatory fashion and not have been motivated to promulgate the rule in response to the knowledge of a union's organizing drive. Thus, if a health care institution permits the use of bulletin boards for a variety of employee messages with prior approval by the hospital, any prohibition against posting union material

would be unlawful. *Liberty Nursing Homes, Inc.* (1978).[18]

NONEMPLOYEES AND OFF-DUTY EMPLOYEES

Nonemployees

Solicitation and Distribution

An employer may prohibit the distribution of union literature by nonemployees on the employer's premises if reasonable efforts through other available channels of communication will enable the union to reach workers and if the employer does not discriminate against the union by permitting access to other nonemployee groups. *NLRB v. Babcock & Wilcox* (1956).[19] Thus, if other channels of communication, such as newspapers, television, and radio, as well as off-premises locations to distribute, are available to union organizers, a health care institution may promulgate a rule that prohibits nonemployee union organizers from distributing or soliciting on the institution's premises.

Although the NLRB and the courts in an industrial setting have maintained that the no-access rule be applied strictly to all nonemployee organizations, the board has allowed limited exceptions to health care institutions. In *Rochester General Hospital* (1978),[20] the board upheld the prohibition on nonemployee union organizers despite the fact that the hospital had permitted access to the Red Cross and volunteers' fund-raising drives. It reasoned that such activities assisted the hospital in carrying out its health care functions and responsibilities.

Off-Duty Employees

An employer may not prohibit off-duty employees from coming onto its premises to distribute union literature or solicit union membership unless it has established a rule generally prohibiting them from entering the premises before working hours, after working hours, or on their days off. The NLRB, in *G.T.E. Lenkurt* (1973),[21] equated the status of such off-duty employees with nonemployees and upheld a rule denying off-duty workers access to the premises for any purpose. *Tri-County Medical Center* (1976)[22] tightened the *Lenkurt* decision by requiring the employer to communicate the order to all employees, specify limitation of access to the interior of the plant and work areas, and apply the rule uniformly to all off-duty employees seeking access to the plant for any and all reasons. In *M Restaurants, Inc.* (1975),[23] the board determined that a prohibition against employee solicitation after the shift was discriminatory and the rule thus was invalid because off-duty employees were permitted to remain on the premises after their shift for other purposes. While justifiable business reasons may permit the enforcement of no-access rules in some areas, hospital parking lots generally do not have factual considerations that warrant prohibition against access by employees. *Presbyterian Medical Center* (1977).[24] Consequently, employees who are off duty may make use of hospital parking lots for union solicitation and distribution of union literature.

CONCLUSION

Solicitation and distribution rules are not established by operation of law. Such rules have to be in writing, posted conspicuously, and communicated to the employees. It is more desirable to have promulgated the rules prior to organizing efforts by a union because the communication of no-solicitation/no-distribution rules after an organizing drive begins could be construed by the NLRB as discriminatory and thereby make the rules unenforceable. *Tekform Products Co.* (1977).[25] This does not mean that if the union commences organizing, the hospital should settle for no rule at all.

As an assistance to NLRB regional directors, the general counsel of the board, in the fall of 1979, issued an interpretive memorandum as a guide to disputed cases involving solicitation and distribution. (*CCH Labor Law Reporter*, ¶ 9208).[26] He urged careful consideration of the following factors in such cases: (1) the nature of the services provided in each area, (2) problems caused by the movement of patients or emergency equipment, (3) physical separation of the area in question from patient-oriented areas, and (4) whether an area of predominantly public or employee use also has an important patient care function.[27] (*CCH Labor Law Reporter, supra*, at p. 15936).

According to the general counsel, solicitation or distribution may be banned under the *St. John's* rule in patients' rooms, operating rooms, and treatment rooms. The ban also is extended to all corridors or patient sitting rooms located adjacent to such patient and treatment rooms and to elevators and stairways used frequently to transport patients. A ban on solicitation/distribution in working areas, such as the kitchen, laundry, supply rooms, housekeeping department, and medical records department, to which only institutional employees have normal access, is presumptively invalid as is a ban in nonworking areas such as locker rooms, lounges, restrooms, and parking lots, to which only employees have access. Treated on a case-by-case basis are nursing stations and public access areas such as cafeterias, vending machine areas, pharmacies, gift shops, lobbies, entranceways, exterior grounds, and walkways.

The NLRB general counsel indicates full awareness of the fact that a ban will be upheld if the evidence shows patients frequenting those areas would be disturbed by union solicitation and if the employee solicitors have adequate alternative channels of communication to other workers. In the general counsel's opinion, the board would have the burden of proving that union solicitation on nonwork time in immediate patient care areas would not adversely affect patients or disrupt patient care. As to all other areas, other than those for immediate patient care such as those for employees only, public access, and patient access, the burden would be on the hospital to show how solicitation would affect patients adversely and disrupt patient care.

From the foregoing, it is clear that employees may solicit for a union where a ban on solicitation is invalid because patients do not have access to such areas. The right to solicit in other areas is decided on a case-by-case basis and depends upon the facts, as in the case where ambulatory patients mix with the public and could be disturbed by union activity. In the event solicitation is permissible, it can take place only on the nonworking time of those soliciting and of those being solicited. Such nonworking time includes rest periods, meal periods, and the time employees are permitted under a nondiscriminatory rule to be on the premises before and after their work shifts. Employees may distribute union literature where solicitation is permitted on nonworking time, except that there is precedent to further restrict distribution if it causes litter or disorder.

Nonemployees, including those who are off duty and who cannot go into a hospital because of a nondiscriminatory rule, are treated alike and can be prohibited from soliciting for the union and distributing union literature in a health care institution. The nondiscriminatory rule, however, must apply to all outsiders and all employees in terms of nonworking time use of the facilities, with a narrow exception for health agencies and volunteer efforts that complement a health care institution's operations. Nonemployees of course can distribute literature on the public sidewalks adjacent to hospitals but may be prohibited from distribution in hospital parking lots, depending upon the enforceability of state trespass laws.

The NLRB and the courts have made progress in defining at what time and at what places solicitation/distribution can occur lawfully. Health care institutions can establish rules governing such activity, provided they are not discriminatory on their face or in practice. In promulgating a rule covering the controversial areas of patient access, detailed evidence of the frequency of patient use and expert medical testimony regarding the effect of solicitation/distribution on patients will be needed to support the validity of the rule.

Indeed, health care institutions have the tools, provided they know how to use them, to protect patients from disturbance and annoyance and patient care from disorder and disruption caused by union solicitation and distribution activities.

NOTES

1. *Rose Co.*, 154 NLRB 228, 229 n. 1, 59 LRRM 1738 (1965).

2. *Republic Aviation v. NLRB*, 324 U.S. 793, 16 LRRM 620 (1945).

3. *Essex Int'l*, 211 NLRB 749, 86 LRRM 1411 (1974).

4. *Meyer & Frank Co.*, 89 NLRB 1016 (1950).

5. *McDonald's Corp.*, 205 NLRB 404, 84 LRRM 1316 (1973).

6. *St. John's Hosp. and School of Nursing v. NLRB*, 557 F.2d 1368, 95 LRRM 3058 (10th Cir. 1977).

7. *St. John's, supra*, at 1511.

8. *Beth Israel Hospital v. NLRB*, 437 U.S. 483, 98 LRRM 2727 (1978).

9. *Baylor Univ. Medical Center v. NLRB*, 578 F.2d, 35, 97 LRRM 2669 (1978), *cert. denied* in part and *remanded* in part, 439 U.S. 9, 99 S.Ct. 299 (1978).

10. *NLRB v. Baptist Hospital, Inc.*, ____ U.S. ____, 99 S.Ct. 2598, 101 LRRM 2556 (1979).

11. *Beth Israel Hospital, supra*, 437 U.S. at 508, quoting *Beth Israel, supra*, 554 F.2d at 481.

12. *Baptist Hospital*, Justice Blackmun.

13. *Stoddard Quirk*, 138 NLRB 620, 51 LRRM 1110 (1962).

14. *Medical Center Hospitals*, 244 NLRB No. 116, 102 LRRM 1105 (1979).

15. *Floridian Hotel of Tampa, Inc.*, 137 NLRB 1484, 50 LRRM 1433 (1962).

16. *Evergreen Nursing Home*, 198 NLRB No. 775, 80 LRRM 1825 (1972).

17. *Stanley Furniture Co.*, 244 NLRB No. 96, 102 LRRM 1065 (1979).

18. *Liberty Nursing Homes, Inc.*, 236 NLRB 456, 99 LRRM 1435 (1978).

19. *NLRB v. Babcock & Wilcox*, 351 U.S. 105, 38 LRRM 2001 (1956).

20. *Rochester General Hosp.*, 234 NLRB 253, 97 LRRM 1410 (1978).

21. *G.T.E. Lenkurt*, 204 NLRB 921, 83 LRRM 1684 (1973),

22. *Tri-County Medical Center*, 222 NLRB 1089, 91 LRRM 1373 (1976).

23. *M Restaurants, Inc.*, 221 NLRB No. 48, 90 LRRM 1494 (1975).

24. *Presbyterian Medical Center*, 227 NLRB No. 135, 94 LRRM 1695 (1977).

25. *Tekform Products Co.*, 229 NLRB No. 111, 96 LRRM 1036 (1977).

26. *CCH Labor Law Reporter*, ¶ 9208, p. 19208.

27. *CCH Labor Law Reporter, supra*, at p. 15936.

8. How to Act or React to a Union Organizing Drive: What You Can Do

NORMAN METZGER

Reprinted with permission from *The Health Care Supervisor's Handbook,* by Norman Metzger, published by Aspen Systems Corporation, Germantown, Md. © 1978.

After almost three decades in the field of labor relations, I have come to the conclusion that what upper management does or doesn't do, what labor lawyers retained as consultants for institutions do or do not recommend, what the board of trustees believes should be the basic philosophy of the institution—all of these are not as significant as the effect of the first-line supervisor on employees' desire or lack of desire to take collective action. *More employees vote for or against their immediate supervisor than vote for or against the top administration, the board of trustees, or consultants.* It is at the day-to-day level of intercourse between the first-line supervisor and the employees that the institutional lifestyle impacts upon the rank-and-file employee; that impact is critical in a union organizing compaign. *Unions rarely organize employees; rather it is the administration's poor employee relations record (uppermost in that grouping is the first-line supervisor) that drives employees into unions.*

Management failure is the root cause of the majority of successful union campaigns. Management failure can include a lack of understanding of employee needs; a lack of competitiveness of salaries and fringe benefits; a lack of clear and usable communication lines; a lack of sound personnel policies; a lack of a formal and understandable grievance mechanism; a lack of appropriate and acceptable working conditions; the presence of arrogant, insensitive, overworked, and harried supervisors.

It is also patently clear that institutions that provide all the benefits and conditions of a union shop—with all the protection inherent in a union contract, such as seniority provisions, grievance and arbitration mechanisms, promotional opportunities—will not become unionized. It is the absence of these conditions plus the presence of insensitive management that *drives* employees into unions.

WHY PEOPLE JOIN UNIONS

There is a myth that outside rabble-rousers and militants, often corrupt or radical in their politics, are responsible for organizing of employees. Lloyd Reynolds gives us some idea why people join unions by stating:

The decision to join is by no means strictly a natural decision. It is probably more like a religious conversion than like deciding to buy a pair of shoes. The worker does not estimate whether the results he will get from the union will be worth the dues he pays. He is confronted with an emotional appeal and urged to take part in a social and political crusade and he finally decides to accept. Moreover, the decision to join is usually not an individualistic decision. The first few workers (in a hospital) who join the union have to make up their own minds. After a nucleus has been secured, however, the growth of the union develops into a mass movement. Most of the workers join because others have done so and hold-outs are gradually brought into line by the pressure of social ostracism (in the hospital).[1]

We often look at unions as a movement. The fact is that most union members do not view the union as a movement, but rather as a means to an end—as a limited purpose, economic institution. What they are looking for is what they cannot presently find in the institution. It is a matter of unfulfilled needs.

[Let us review earlier material.] We found that there is a marked relationship between worker morale and how much employees feel their boss is interested in discussing work problems with the work group. *Their boss is you*. We found that when the supervisor treats subordinates as human beings, there is greater group loyalty and pride. Employees with group loyalty and pride do not need unions to fill their needs. We also learned that by seeing problems through the eyes of the workers, the supervisor can translate employee needs to top management and thereby help arrive at policy decisions that are realistic and satisfy both administration and employees. Policies arrived at in this way will not drive employees into the arms of union organizers. It was also noted that the basic employee desires are for "full appreciation of work done," "feeling in on things," and "sympathetic help on personal problems." When an employee does not feel appreciated, is not in on things (does not know what is going on and most important, does not know about the things that affect his daily work life), or cannot look to his supervisor for empathy, *then that employee will look elsewhere*. The union stands ready to listen, to promise, to take up the battle for unfulfilled employee needs.

We also [found] the major dissatisfiers in the work area: company policy, administration, supervision, salary, interpersonal relations, and working conditions. These were compared to the major satisfiers: what the employee does, recognition, responsibility, advancement, and achievement. By improving managerial practices and by proper utilization of both people and technology, the supervisor can increase the satisfaction and productivity of employees. *Satisfied and fulfilled employees are not receptive to union organizers*.

THE UNION ORGANIZER

The typical union organizer has a natural affinity for people, is a good listener, and knows how and at what level to communicate. Chaney and Beech[2] point out some interesting facts about union organizers and sketch this profile:

1. He or she has a natural capacity to like people. A union organizer is a warm, gentle, outgoing person who communicates well and relates effectively to all types of people.
2. He or she has the ability to adapt to the immediate surroundings and warm up to people very quickly.
3. He or she is patient with people. The union organizer realizes that nonunion employees are not immediately sold on organization. Therefore, the organizer makes an ongoing effort to sign up or convince all employees of the values of unionism and collective action.
4. Many labor relations experts have depicted organizers as a combination missionary, salesperson, psychologist.

Elliot Godoff, who was an especially effective organizer and trainer of organizers, once told me that he had developed a staff that knows how to approach people. His people no longer talk simply about wages and benefits; they establish a rapport with the workers on a much higher level. They know when to raise the key issue of employee rights. They show workers how to establish their rights, how to meet with management as equals, how to protect themselves as individuals, and how to win identity within the hospital as important human beings. He added that the organizer who merely tells the worker, "You earn twenty cents less than workers at X hospital and, therefore, you should organize," is out of the picture. Management is more sophisticated; they know more about the union than they did before; their approach is different. He thought that his organizers had kept up with this change.

Let me quote from an interview that I was fortunate to have with Mr. Godoff.

I think that you will probably get reports from the management in the areas where we work that we don't operate the way we did years ago. You are not going to see circulars floating around and a lot of excitement in the very early stages. Some of our best organizers really work for a period of weeks or months to build an organizing committee, and that means that not a single person has yet signed the card or has made any commitment in terms of paper or materials—simply developing a *very close relationship with people* on the following ratio. If it is a hospital, let's say with a thousand workers, then we will aim for a minimum of a sixty-man or woman organizing committee with whom we are going to meet periodically, raise issues, raise questions, get all the vital information about the hospital—the number of people in the units, the division of the departments, how many in each department, the ethnic division, the character of the supervision, who is the son of a bitch among the supervisors that we can hit the hardest—and then to orient them on a question of rights, rights, rights and rights. We say management can give you wage increases, management can give you benefits, management can do a lot of things, but one thing they are not going to give you is rights. When that becomes something that workers feel—it may be very abstract, it may be very vague—but when they feel rights, they will tell you: I haven't got rights; I want rights. And each one imagines it in his own way, but that becomes the greatest strength that the union can muster in any situation.[3]

Now let us look at what one union sets down as a guide for union organizers.[4] Nicholas Zonarich, organizational director of the Industrial Union Department, AFL-CIO, states:

The organizer has two immediate objectives when he makes his first contacts with the workers at the plant. He is looking for leadership for his compaign and information about the specific problems and complaints of the employees.

There is no blueprint for meeting individual workers and gaining their confidence—conversations can be started in restaurants and bars, through "leads" passed on by other union members, and by acquaintances made through social affairs. If there is any rule at all, it is that contacts are *not* made by suddenly appearing at a plant gate with a leaflet urging employees to sign a union authorization card and mail it to a post office box.

Most organizers are interested primarily in meeting the type of employee who is respected by his fellow-workers and who has influence inside the plant. Getting to know a few of these employees is more important—at this stage—than meeting the maximum number of workers.

Once a potential plant leader has been contacted, it is important to win his confidence and trust. Time spent in developing this leader, answering his questions about the union, and explaining the benefits of collective bargaining will be well worthwhile after the organizing campaign

gets underway and this leader becomes a union spokesman inside the plant.

Articulate and respected leaders inside the plant are vital to any campaign, but the representative must use his own judgment in selecting the right people. He must be sure that they are not known as chronic "gripers" or "soreheads" and that they are not motivated simply by a desire for revenge or a driving personal ambition.

In the "perfect" campaign, the organizer will find a leader for every group in the plant—a woman for the female workers, leaders within minority, racial, and national groupings, and spokesmen for the various departments and shifts. Since the "perfect" situation rarely exists, the staff man must develop a leadership group as representative as possible.

Both Godoff and Zonarich make some interesting points to which I direct your attention. Godoff said they look at "the character of the supervision, who is the son of a bitch among the supervisors that we can hit the hardest." Zonarich points out that the organizer must be sure that the leaders are not known as chronic "gripers" or "soreheads" and that they are not motivated simply by a desire for revenge or driving personal ambition. The union is looking for bona fide constituents to use in the organizing drive. Yes, they will latch on to the petty gripes and perceived injustices, but they are also looking closely for supervisors who are an easy mark—those who are not employee-centered, who have not built up group loyalty.

YOUR EMPLOYEES ARE RATING YOU

There is no question that the first-line supervisor is the person most dramatically affected by the organization of employees. The institution itself may be exposed over the years to restrictions on management rights, increased wages, and increased fringe benefits, but in the final analysis the real impact of unionization is felt at the day-to-day level of supervisor-employee intercourse.

The first-line supervisor must understand the key role he or she plays during the organizational drive. The union is keenly interested in and often extremely aware of the day-to-day supervisor-employee relationship, especially the issues of fairness and consistency. If the employees believe that they are not being treated fairly by their supervisor, they will be more interested in the union's carefully presented approach in the area of employee rights. If the supervisor has played favorites—has handled similar cases in different ways for different employees—then that supervisor and that institution are more vulnerable to the organizers' demand for collective power to enforce such consistency and fairness. Employees look carefully at their supervisor's behavior in similar situations, looking for consistency in more cases than looking for the actual punishment. As we have learned earlier, a sympathetic ''no'' may be more effective than a harsh ''yes.'' Similarly, a sympathetic ''no'' in one situation will be compared to the ''yes'' of the prior situation for the test of consistency. If your decision has been different in what may appear to be similar cases, it is important that you make the difference acceptable by sharing the underlying facts of both situations. But beware: if the underlying facts are similar and you still have reached a different decision, you must explain your reasons.

When groups of employees are faced with the choice of voting for or against the union, they often think in terms of their relationship to their supervisors. Critical to that relationship is a supervisor's integrity. How you are perceived by your employees when they are in the voting booth is often a reflection of your actions over the years. Have you truly represented the workers to the management and the management to the workers?

Several suggestions that can produce group loyalty and high productivity (and most important, reflect favorably on your integrity) should be reviewed at this time:

1. Keep employees informed about developments.
2. Recommend pay increases where they are indicated.
3. Keep your people posted on how well they are doing.
4. Take the time to listen, empathetically, to employee complaints and grievances.
5. Permit employees to discuss work problems with you.
6. Recommend employees for promotional opportunities.
7. Don't take all the credit; share the product of your department's labor with all participating and productive members of the team.
8. Display consistent and dependable behavior.
9. Discipline in private.
10. Help employees improve and broaden.
11. Treat all members of your department as equals.

Labor unions capitalize on management mistakes. The need for unionization is created by the management rather than the union. If the management (and that includes the first-line supervisor) does not understand or care about employee needs, the union wins

the election. It is evident that institutions and supervisors have become increasingly sophisticated and aware of what drives employees into unions.

HOW UNIONS HAVE FARED IN ELECTIONS

During the first ten months of the health care industry's inclusion under the National Labor Relations Act (July 1974-April 1975), health care unions won 59.7 percent of the elections as compared with a win record in industry of 47.4 percent. It was clear that the health care industry was more vulnerable to unionization than were other industries at that time. But in the next twelve months (May 1975-April 1976), health care unions won only 58 percent of the elections as compared with a win record in industry of 47.2 percent—a movement, although not dramatic, toward fewer union wins.

In the period from April 1976 through January 1977, 281 elections were conducted in the health services industry. The unions won 132 of these, a win record of only 47 percent. This latest statistic shows the reversal of a trend in which unions were more victorious in the health services industry than in other industries. I believe that we have stopped playing the part of Brutus who looked to the stars for the cause of his misfortune. Rather we have adopted the view of Pogo, ''We have met the enemy and they are us.'' We have looked into ourselves for the root causes of employee unrest and collective action. We have been more pragmatic about our approaches to employee relations, and it is showing.

WHAT YOU CAN AND CANNOT DO DURING A UNION ORGANIZING DRIVE

A committee of the American Bar Association and a committee of publishers and associations included in a declaration of principles that writers who deal with any subject that has or may have legal overtones shall declare that they are not engaged in rendering legal service. *If legal service or other expert assistance is required, the services of a competent professional should be sought.* There is no question that when a union approaches an institution that institution should have sound labor relations and, if necessary, legal advice. But in the final analysis a simple dose of common sense would suffice.

You, the first-line supervisor, will be on the firing line in such a situation. You will have to know what is and is not permissible as far as the National Labor

Relations Act is concerned. But given the pressures of the moment and the supervisor-employee relationships that have developed over the years in your department, it may seem strange to deal with legalities at such a time.

Let's refer then to the overall common-sense approach that has been complicated by legal interpretations. There are three basic proscriptions when dealing with employees during a union organizing campaign:

1. Don't threaten them. (I suggest that you not threaten them at other times as well and, therefore, this warning may seem a little redundant in a book on positive employee relations.)
2. Don't promise them any reward for staying out of the union.
3. Don't interrogate them, especially about their preferences. Never ask, "Are you for the union or are you against the union?"

When and if the union approaches employees in your institution, there will be a great deal of pressure put upon supervisors to deliver a vote for management. Ideally, there will be a complete and open discussion of the pros and cons of unionization led by the top management of your institution, directed toward supervisors at every level. You will be tempted to put pressure on the employees to vote against the union. The National Labor Relations Board (NLRB) has set up general guidelines for managerial behavior during a union organizing drive. You may not threaten employees with the loss of their jobs or reduction in their wages; you may not use threatening or intimidating language. Of course, even common sense directs you not to threaten employees in the exercise of their right to support a union.

Although you cannot personally urge an employee to convince other workers to oppose the union, you may tell employees that when a union enters an institution, problems must be directed toward the shop steward, eliminating the one-to-one discussion between employee and the supervisor. You can share with employees the disadvantages of belonging to a union: paying dues and initiation fees, the possibility of loss of income due to strikes, the necessity for picket line duty. Without using threatening language, you may tell employees that the administration does not want a union and that the institution does not need a union.

You cannot promise increased wages, promotions, or benefits if employees reject the union. You can tell the employee that a union will out-promise an employer, but in the final analysis, the union cannot guarantee anything. It must bargain with the employer, and in order to attain benefit levels, must reach agreement with the employer. You may remind the employees of their present benefits and compare these benefits with those in unionized institutions.

Supervisors may not ask employees their personal opinions about the union or what they believe are the feelings of other employees. You cannot call employees away from their work areas into your office to urge them to vote against the union. You cannot systematically visit the homes of employees to urge them to vote against the union.

You, as a supervisor, can tell employees that they do not have to sign union authorization cards and, indeed, do not have to speak to union organizers at their homes if they do not so desire. You can speak to employees individually or in groups at the employees' work station, in the employee cafeteria, or in other areas where employees are accustomed to being. Remember, it is illegal to ask employees what they think about a union, or how they intend to vote, or if they have signed cards or attended union meetings. But it is permissible for you to tell employees why a union is not necessary in your institution. You may continue to operate normally and continue to discipline and discharge as the situation requires, but not for the sole reason that the employee is involved in union activities—although employees are expected to work at their assignments during working hours.

SOLICITATION AND DISTRIBUTION[5]

Many supervisors find themselves perplexed and anxious to take immediate action when employees in their departments come to work wearing buttons that urge employees to vote for a specific union. The following two cases involve hospitals and the issue of union button wearing.

In the first case, *St. Joseph Hospital,*[6] the National Labor Relations Board *reversed* an administrative law judge's decision in favor of the hospital and its longstanding dress code against employees who wore union buttons. The buttons said, "Vote for Health Care Division, LIUNA, AFL-CIO." The judge had earlier ruled that the action of the hospital was legal in shielding its patients from controversial issues, but the National Labor Relations Board, who reviewed the administrative law judge's decision upon appeal by the union, said under the dress code employees were permitted to wear other buttons such as those designed to observe hospital week and doctor's day as well as a St. Patrick's Day button saying, "Kiss me, I'm Irish." Thus, the Board concluded, the dress code as applied by the hospital merely prohibited the wearing of union insignia and was not designed to protect the patients.

Rather the rule was intended to thwart the union-organizing campaign. The hospital was therefore ordered to cease the discriminatory enforcement of its dress code.

In the second case, *Baptist Memorial Hospital*,[7] the NLRB *sustained* an administrative law judge's decision that the hospital had violated the act by prohibiting its employees from wearing union buttons. The decision observed that such prohibition served no legitimate hospital purpose, because the wearing of United Fund pins was permitted. Therefore, the judge concluded, "The prohibition against wearing union buttons was designed to thwart the union-organizing campaign of the State, County and Municipal Employees Union." The NLRB concurred with the judge's decision and said that discriminatory application of the hospital rule against wearing insignias *other than professional and hospital pins* was a violation of the act and unlawful.

These two decisions point out that the National Labor Relations Board will rule *against* a hospital's rule that permits the wearing of any buttons or insignia other than professional hospital insignia and at the same time prohibits the wearing of union buttons or insignia. If your hospital wishes to legally prohibit employees from wearing union buttons or insignia, it must strictly enforce a rule that authorizes the wearing of professional and hospital pins and insignias only.

What we should understand from the Board's decisions in this area is that the key question is whether the employer's rule is for purposes of efficiency or safety and is nondiscriminatory in nature—that is, is not directed solely against the union's organizing campaign.

The issue of solicitation is most complex. Solicitation includes the attempt by union organizers (employees or nonemployees) to sign up employees and distribute union campaign material. In general, an employer cannot prevent union organizational activities outside working hours even though the activities take place on the employer's property. This rule was first pronounced by the NLRB and approved by the Supreme Court:

> . . . Time outside working hours, whether before or after work, or during luncheon or rest periods, is an employee's time to use as he wishes without unreasonable restraint, although the employee is on company property. It is therefore not within the province of an employer to promulgate and enforce a rule prohibiting union solicitation by an employee outside working hours, although on company property. Such a rule must be presumed to be an unreasonable impediment to self-organization and, therefore, discriminatory in the absence of evidence that special circumstances make the rule necessary in order to maintain production or discipline.[8]

It has also been held that lunch hours and rest periods are not "working time" despite the fact they may be short or irregularly scheduled and even though employees may be paid for the periods. Past decisions have indicated that an employer can impose a no solicitation rule during working hours so long as the rule is reasonable, necessary for productive operations and not discriminatory. If the rule is valid on its face but is applied in a discriminatory way, or is used as a lever to prevent the workers from exercising their lawful right to organize, the NLRB will call for its elimination.[9]

Another key question is should hospital cafeterias and vending machine areas be off limits to union solicitation or the distribution of union campaign material? The American Hospital Association (AHA) asked the court to justify additional restrictions on employee solicitation and distribution in order to maintain the tranquil atmosphere essential to a hospital's primary function of providing high quality patient care. The opinion appeared in a brief to a most interesting case, *St. John's Hospital and School of Nursing*.[10]

> . . . All areas of the hospital to which patients have access must be areas which the hospital is entitled to regulate. Additionally we submit the special circumstances which the duties owed to patients and visitors place upon the employer and the employee . . . extend beyond "strictly patient care areas." *They extend throughout the hospital to areas where patients and visitors have access.*

The American Hospital Association maintains that the patient—removed from familiar surroundings and anticipating pain, discomfort, the unknown, and the use of procedures and practices he or she simply does not understand—needs to have considerable and thoughtful support from all personnel involved in the delivery of health care. The AHA asserts that any disruption in that setting (which would include union organizing activities) creates patient anxiety, unrest, or emotional stress.[11] The court ruled that the hospital had the right to prohibit solicitation in its cafeteria and gift shop, both of which are open to the public. The court concluded that the hospital maintains the same commercial interest in its cafeteria and gift shop as is held by the management of retail stores and restaurants located in other types of establishments. The hospital does not lose its right to prohibit solicitation in those facilities, "simply because its public cafeteria and gift shop is a part of the hospital complex rather than a shopping mall or a drive-in restaurant." Of course, *this case pertained only to St. John's.* In a recent Supreme Court ruling [*Beth Israel Hospital v. NLRB,* No. 77-152 (June 22, 1978)], the Justices unanimously upheld a decision of the NLRB that the Boston hospital could not bar solicitation and distribution of literature in its cafeteria and coffee shop. Although the NLRB has barred such activity in public restaurants, the Court noted that 77 percent of the cafeteria's customers at the hospital were employees, making it "a natural gathering place for distribution of union material." It should be noted that four of the nine Justices agreed with the result, but challenged the general application to hospitals of a 1945 industrial ruling that employer interference with distribution of union literature is presumed to be illegal absent special circumstances. This should give you some idea of the complex nature of the solicitation question. Since this area is highly technical, hospital administration would do well to retain labor counsel.

PERMISSIBLE AND IMPERMISSIBLE CAMPAIGNING

We will once again review what is and is not permissible regarding management action during a union organizing campaign. Various decisions of the National Labor Relations Board in this area have established legal distinctions that govern the rights of management to speak freely when combating a union organizing drive. The following checklist is not all inclusive but is presented to encourage your institution to take a stand during such a period. It cannot be said too often that taking a neutral position or taking no position at all during a union organizing campaign is tantamount to agreeing to the organization of your employees. If the hospital is against recognizing a union, it can and should:

1. Explain the meaning of union recognition and the procedure to be followed.
2. Encourage each member of the bargaining unit (those employees who will be permitted to vote in a union election) to actually cast their ballot in the election.
3. Communicate to employees that they are free to vote for or against the union, despite the fact that they have signed a union authorization card.
4. Communicate to all employees why the administration is against recognizing a union.

5. Review the compensation and benefits program, pointing out the record of the administration in the past.
6. Point out to employees statements made by the union which the administration believes to be untrue, and communicate its own position on each of these statements.
7. If there is a general no solicitation rule, prevent solicitation of membership by the union during working hours.
8. Continue to enforce all rules and regulations in effect prior to the union's request for recognition.
9. Send letters to employees' homes stating the administration's position and record and the administration's knowledge of the union's position in other hospitals.
10. Discuss the possibility of strikes when unions enter hospitals; discuss the ramifications of such a strike.
11. Discuss the impact of union dues and in general the cost of belonging to a union. Point out to the employees that the union can promise the employees anything, but it can deliver on promises only with the agreement of the administration.
12. Discuss with employees, individually at their work areas, the position of the institution.
13. In response to the union's promises during the preelection period, point out to employees that if the hospital were to meet these demands it might be forced to lay off workers. (This statement can be made as long as the administration points out that it would be an involuntary action and a consequence of a union's demands.)

Of course the hospital *cannot* and *should not* engage in the following activities during the union organizing drive:

1. Promise benefits and threaten reprisals if employees vote for or against the union, or have supervisors attend union meetings or spy on employees to determine whether or not they are participating in union activities.
2. Grant wage increases or special concessions during the preelection period unless the timing coincides with well-established prior practices.
3. Prevent employees from wearing union buttons, except in cases where the buttons are provocative or extremely large.
4. Bar employee union representatives from soliciting employee membership during *nonworking*

hours when the solicitation does not interfere with the work of others.

5. Summon an employee into an office for private discussion of the union and the upcoming elections. (This does not preclude an employee from coming in voluntarily to discuss these things.)
6. Question employees about union matters and meetings.
7. Ask employees how they intend to vote.
8. Threaten layoffs because of unionization or state that you will never deal with a union even if it is certified.
9. Hold meetings with employees within the 24-hour period immediately preceding the election.[12]

There is much that the employer can say and do during the union organizing campaign. In a health care facility as discussed above, no solicitation and no distribution rules can be enforced if properly constructed and properly administered without discrimination per se against the union and in the interest of maintaining patient care. As we shall see, it is essential that as many qualified members of the employee body—those who are included in the bargaining unit—vote at a time of an election. It has been shown that employees who are eligible to vote but do not vote in the union election would probably vote *against* the union; on the other hand, employees who favor unions will come out to vote. So, as a supervisor you should encourage all employees in your department who are eligible to vote to do so.

It is essential to differentiate between communications that are threatening or carry promises of reward and those designed to bring management's position honestly and forthrightly to all eligible employees. As to the question of free speech, the National Labor Relations Board judges each case on its own merits. The essential element is the "total context" which will determine whether the communication was coercive, threatening, or contained promises. Employees should be told that signing a union authorization card is not equivalent to a vote for the union; the voting will be by secret ballot and an employee can make a *final* decision at that time, notwithstanding the fact that he or she has signed a union authorization card. In an election conducted by the National Labor Relations Board, the marking of ballots is decisive, not the presentation of signed authorization cards.

I repeat an important point made earlier, that I do not contend to render legal service in reviewing this critical and complex area of union organization. If legal service or other expert assistance is deemed necessary by your institution, the services of a competent professional should be sought.

THE BARGAINING UNIT

The bargaining unit is defined as employees who will vote in an election to determine whether or not they wish to be represented by a union. Appropriate bargaining units are determined by the National Labor Relations Board. The health care industry, only recently included under the Taft-Hartley Act, had special problems that were addressed in the deliberations of the congressional committees considering the inclusion of the health care industry in 1974. One of the considerations of the committee was stated in the congressional report:

. . . Due consideration should be given by the (National Labor Relations) Board to prevent the proliferation of bargaining units in the health care industry.

Congress recognized the difficult burden that would be thrust upon health care institutions if various employee groups could form into separate bargaining units, thereby forcing the hospital to negotiate contracts with dozens of unions. The issue of an appropriate bargaining unit is a complex one, but in general you may be dealing with units of:

- service and maintenance employees,
- registered nurses,
- guards,
- technical employees,
- business office clericals,
- MDs, and
- other professionals.

One thing is clear—you, as a supervisor, are *excluded* from the provisions of the act. Therefore, the administration need not recognize a bargaining unit of supervisors; the board may not certify a labor organization seeking to represent supervisors.

Once the bargaining unit is determined, the board will ascertain whether there is an appropriate "show of interest." This show of interest is displayed by the union presenting union authorization cards for at least 30 percent of the bargaining unit employees. Remember, however, although this 30 percent figure will enable the union to obtain an election under National Labor Relations Board auspices, the union needs much more support than that to win the election. (We will cover this later in this article.)

THE ELECTION PROCESS

Once having determined that there is a "show of interest," the NLRB will set an election date and determine the time and place for the election. Usually the election will be held on hospital premises. The voting place is determined by mutual agreement between the employer and the union, but final determination is made by the board itself. Present at the polling area is an NLRB representative who is directly responsible for conducting the election. In addition, the union provides an *observer* and the hospital provides an *observer*. The hospital's observer may not be a supervisor.

Within seven days after the NLRB regional director has approved an election, the board is provided with a list of all eligible employees. This list contains the names and addresses of all unit employees. Generally, employees are eligible to vote if they are on the employer's payroll for the period immediately prior to the date on which the election is held. In addition, employees who are engaged in an economic strike and have been permanently replaced are still eligible to vote if the election is held within twelve months of the strike. Employees who are on layoff status but have a "reasonable expectation of reemployment" in the near future have been deemed eligible to vote. Those who have been discharged for cause or who have quit between the date the election was set and the actual voting day are ineligible unless such employees have been discriminatorily discharged.[13]

Employees have the opportunity to vote in secret. They mark a simple ballot *yes* or *no* on the question of whether they wish to be represented by the specific union petitioning. *A union must receive a majority of the valid ballots cast in order to be certified.* If 50 percent plus one employee of the employees who voted in the election cast their ballots in favor of the union, the union will become the certified representative of the bargaining unit for the purposes of collective bargaining.

A simple illustration will underscore the importance of getting out the vote. If a bargaining unit of 500 service and maintenance employees at your institution is involved in an election, the union must receive a majority of the valid ballots cast. If only 400 of these employees actually vote, the union need only receive 201 votes. As you can plainly see, if 201 out of 400 voting employees cast their ballots for the union, the union will be certified to represent all 500 employees in the bargaining unit. The 100 employees who did not vote have no effect on the outcome of the election. Remember, many presidents of the United States have been elected by a majority of the votes cast, but by a significant *minority* of the eligible electorate. *So go union elections.*

KEY POINTS IN A UNION ORGANIZING DRIVE

1. More employees vote for or against their immediate supervisor than for or against top management, the board of trustees, or consultants.
2. Unions rarely organize employees; rather, it is administration's poor record in employee relations that drives employees into unions.
3. Institutions that provide all the benefits and conditions of the union shop will not become unionized.
4. There is a marked relationship between worker morale and the extent to which employees feel their boss is interested in discussing work problems with their work group. If the boss—*that's you!*—is not interested, workers will discuss those problems with outside groups—*in some cases, unions.*
5. Employees who feel group loyalty and pride do not look outside to unions for need fulfillment.
6. Improved managerial practices and the supervisor's attention to the best utilization of people and technology can increase job satisfaction and productivity. *Satisfied and fulfilled employees do not look to unions.*
7. Unions are looking for bona fide issues to use in the organizing drive. Although they will latch on to petty gripes and perceived injustices, they often look for supervisors who are vulnerable. Such supervisors are usually not employee-centered, have not built up group loyalty, and are not interested in employee needs.
8. Labor unions capitalize on management mistakes.
9. You should not threaten employees or promise them any reward for staying out of the union. Do not interrogate them about their preferences during a union organizing drive. These are unfair labor practices.
10. You can tell employees how the institution feels about unionization. You can share with them the employee disadvantages of belonging to a union.
11. You cannot call employees away from their work areas into your office in order to urge them to vote against the union.

12. You should tell employees that they do not have to sign union authorization cards or speak to union organizers if they do not so desire.

13. You should inform employees that even though they have signed a union authorization card, *they can change their mind* and vote any way they wish at the time of an election.

14. You should encourage each member of your department who is in the bargaining unit (those employees eligible to vote) to actually cast a ballot in the election.

15. You should continue to enforce all rules and regulations in effect prior to the union's request for recognition.

16. You should keep top management apprised of day-to-day developments during the union organizing campaign. You will be the person closest to the employees at that time. Your perception of trends is critical to administration planning.

17. Recent statistics indicate that unions win only 47 percent of elections in the health care industry. This is a reversal of earlier statistics obtained during the first year of the industry's coverage under the Taft-Hartley Act. The reversal indicates a more sophisticated and concerned management approach toward employee needs.

NOTES

1. Lloyd Reynolds, *Labor Economics and Labor Relations* (Englewood Cliffs, N.J.: Prentice-Hall, Inc., 1956), p. 60.

2. Warren H. Chaney and Thomas R. Beech, *The Union Epidemic* (Germantown, Md.: Aspen Systems Corporation, 1976), pp. 45–46.

3. From an interview with Elliot Godoff conducted by Norman Metzger on February 29, 1972. The late Mr. Godoff was executive vice president/organization director of District 1199, Drug and Hospital Union.

4. *A Guidebook for Union Organizers,* Industrial Union Department, AFL-CIO, Distributed by Master Printers of America, Washington, D.C.

5. *See* update on the issues of solicitation and distribution in prior articles (Articles 3, 4, 6, and 7 of Part III).

6. *St. Joseph Hospital,* 225 NLRB 28, 16 CA 6019, Fort Worth, Tex., June 30, 1976.

7. *Baptist Memorial Hospital,* 225 NLRB 69, 26 CA 5743, 5781, 5875, Memphis, Tenn., June 30, 1976.

8. *Republic Aviation v. NLRB,* 324 U.S. 793, 65 S. Ct. 982.

9. *Ground Rules for Labor and Management during Organizing Drives* (Englewood Cliffs, N.J.: Prentice-Hall, Inc., 1970), p. 22.

10. *St. John's Hospital and School of Nursing, Inc. v. NLRB,* CA 10, 82 LC, paragraph 10,021.

11. Brief of the American Hospital Association, amicus curiae, *St. John's Hospital and School of Nursing, Inc. v. NLRB,* ibid.

12. Norman Metzger and Dennis Pointer, *Labor Management Relations in the Health Service Industry: Theory and Practice* (Washington, D.C.: Science and Health Publications, Inc., 1972), pp. 143–144.

13. Dennis Pointer and Norman Metzger, *The National Labor Relations Act: A Guidebook for Health Care Facility Administrators* (New York: Spectrum Publications, Inc., 1975), pp. 72–73.

9. Maintaining Nonunion Status

CHARLES L. JOINER

Excerpted with permission from "Management's Response to the Union
Phenomenon" in *Hospital Progress*, May 1978, © 1978
The Catholic Health Association.

Maintaining nonunion status is largely dependent upon what managers do to prevent the need for a union. This view is based on the philosophy that unionization is preventable if management is doing enough of the "right things." When management actions do not support a positive employee relations climate, workers may find it necessary to seek external help and, in some situations, they deserve help from a union.

This argument may be supported further by the fact that union organizers typically do not attempt to organize an employee group until workers themselves have sought union assistance. Union elections seem to suggest that employees really are voting for or against management instead of for or against a particular union. Based on these premises, this article seeks to help health care managers by identifying issues important to good personnel relations and the maintenance of nonunion status.

To provide a sound basis for prevention of unnecessary problems it is essential to understand the historical perspective of the underlying issues, including employee perceptions of the need for unionization. The purpose of the article, therefore, is accomplished through a review of labor law history and trends, an overview of the fundamental causes of friction between management and labor, a summary of reasons health care employees give for joining unions, an analysis of criteria used by union organizers to evalu-ate health care institutions and, finally, specific recommendations for establishing a preventive management program and maintaining nonunion status. Since knowledge of the legal framework is essential to any manager who desires to avoid foolish mistakes in the implementation of a well-conceived program, it is appropriate to review labor law history and trends first.

LABOR LAW HISTORY AND TRENDS

The National Labor Relations Act (NLRA) is the foundation for the labor laws of the United States. The NLRA (the Wagner Act) was adopted in 1935 and has been amended by the Taft-Hartley Act of 1947, the Landrum-Griffin Act of 1959, and Public Law 93-360 (the Health Care Amendments) in 1974.

The Wagner Act authorized the formation of the National Labor Relations Board (NLRB) to administer the provisions of the act. The Wagner Act encompassed all institutions that had an impact on interstate commerce. The status of nonprofit health care institutions was left to the interpretation of the courts. Proprietary institutions and nursing homes were considered within the jurisdiction of the act. Since by definition governments are not employers, federal, state, and municipal hospitals were specifically exempted from the jurisdiction of the act.[1]

Under the protection of the Wagner Act, unions flourished in virtually all types of industries. This rapid growth created a host of problems regarding the regulation of union-management relations. Industries had to contend with many jurisdictional strikes caused by disputes between competing unions. Some labor leaders, because of their new and unbridled power, refused to bargain in good faith.[1] The Wagner Act proved to be inadequate to curb these and other abuses of the bargaining process. Therefore Congress in 1947 passed the Labor Management Relations (Taft-Hartley) Act. It is this legislation that has become the backbone of the nation's labor laws.[1]

The Taft-Hartley Act amended the Wagner Act by listing specific unfair labor practices. It also specifically exempted nonprofit health care institutions from coverage under the act. The status of other types of health care institutions did not change.

In 1959, Taft-Hartley was amended by the Labor-Management Reporting and Disclosure (Landrum-Griffin) Act. Among its many provisions, this act requires employers, including voluntary nonprofit health care facilities, to submit a report to the U.S. Secretary of Labor detailing the nature of any financial transactions and/or arrangements that are intended to improve or retard the unionization process.[1]

Until 1967, the courts on a case-by-case basis determined which proprietary health care institutions and nursing homes had an impact on interstate commerce and thus came under the NLRA. As a result of several court cases, the National Labor Relations Board (NLRB) in 1967 issued guidelines for selecting those facilities: proprietary health care institutions with an annual gross revenue of at least $250,000 and nursing homes, regardless of ownership, with an annual gross revenue of at least $100,000.[1]

With voluntary hospitals comprising the largest sector of the health care industry, it was only a matter of time until they too would fall under the NLRA. Their shift in status occurred in 1974, when Congress passed P.L. 93-360 to amend the act. These amendments extended the coverage of the labor laws to include all health care institutions under nonpublic ownership and control. They defined a health care institution as any "hospital, convalescent hospital, health maintenance organization, health clinic, nursing home, extended care facility, or other institution devoted to the care of sick, infirm or aged persons."

Only about 20 percent of the total nonpublic health care labor force of approximately 1.6 million workers is now unionized.[2] However, because of their declining rate of growth among blue-collar laborers, labor unions are renewing their interest in the organizable group of white-collar workers in the health care industry.[3,4] Attempts have been made in recent years to modify the Taft-Hartley legislation to favor union organizational campaign strategies. Under the administration of President Reagan, the fate of these efforts was uncertain.

The legislative background and prospects certainly point to difficult times for health care managers seeking to stay nonunion. For a realistic perspective on maintaining nonunion status, management should have a good understanding of the fundamental causes of labor problems. Reasons for labor-management friction are summarized next.

CAUSES OF LABOR-MANAGEMENT PROBLEMS

Fundamental differences between the goals and objectives of management and labor create friction that cannot be totally explained in terms of higher wages, shorter working hours, or better working conditions. Two fundamental causes of such friction are: (1) the issue of management rights and (2) the issue of efficiency vs. human value. Management always will assert its right to prescribe certain modes of action or levels of desired productivity in order to justify its existence or that of the organization. Yet labor unions question whether management should have complete power over the work force. This is a point of conflict. Organized labor attempts to shift the locus of control by seeking to obtain a voice for employees about working conditions and terms of employment.

The question of management's right to govern is paralleled by the question of human value vs. efficiency. If management is to achieve its stated goals and objectives, it must maintain efficiency through increased productivity and cost containment. On the other hand, the union seeks to improve its members' standard of living. Neither side may be totally right nor totally wrong in its demands, and unfortunate circumstances often trigger open conflict. For example, management may wish to improve the existing fringe benefits package for employees but may be prevented from doing so because of pressures to contain costs. Evidence of this type of conflict is mounting almost daily, especially as new crises (e.g., malpractice insurance) arise and cause even greater cost increases.

With an understanding of the fundamental causes of labor problems, administration can begin developing its philosophy for a preventive management program by reviewing research on employee reasons for joining unions. The following analysis summarizes findings from a selected number of such studies.

WHY EMPLOYEES JOIN UNIONS

The desire to unionize is thought to be centered on three issues: wages, employee dissatisfaction with work benefits, and the organization. However, other factors have contributed to the increased activity in the health care industry. Over the last two decades social turmoil has precipitated civil rights legislation and stimulated changes in the attitudes and social conscience of many individuals. The idea of being represented by a union is not considered as unprofessional as it once was.[5, 6] The health care industry is just beginning to feel the effects of this turmoil, and the passage of P.L. 93-360 only served to release the pent-up emotions of the industry's workers and union leaders. The recent labor reform efforts are further evidence of labor's continuing struggle to swing the pendulum in its favor.

In an attempt to identify why some health care workers seek union representation, 11 publications were sampled. Table 9-1 outlines the findings of the search. While not all-inclusive, the data do show that money and fringe benefits are not always the only issues to employees. Other, less tangible factors such as poor communication, poor supervision, bad working conditions, and inconsistently enforced personnel policies carry considerable weight.

The less tangible issues may be just as important to employees. One reason workers frequently mention for joining unions is that management "does not treat them fairly, decently, or honestly." Employees view management as fair, decent, and honest if it recognizes the needs of individuals and treats them with dignity. Issues such as wage disputes, respect, and recognition for loyalty and service to the institution are related to the individual need to be recognized and to be treated fairly. A specific example is employees' feeling that management offers no educational opportunities for upgrading their skills as a means to career mobility.[15] Unless these opportunities are available, employees often believe that they are locked into dead-end jobs.

Generally, the reasons health care personnel give for joining unions may be grouped into two broad categories: (1) poor communication and (2) perception of poor treatment. Almost all of the reasons are related in some way to communication problems (e.g., little upward communication) or employees' belief that they are not receiving fair treatment on specific work-related issues. As a generalization, employees may consider the union alternative when they perceive a prevailing attitude that management does not consider meeting employee needs as a primary goal of the institution. Administrators should find an interesting relationship between why employees join unions and what the union organizer looks for (next section). Although this study does not include a correlation analysis, some relationships are evident between the findings of the two.

WHAT THE UNION ORGANIZER LOOKS FOR

Before actually considering some of the kinds of things union organizers look for, it should be understood that they typically get involved only after employees have asked for help. Employees usually try to resolve their problems internally before seeking outside help. In other words, if a union organizer is involved, it is likely that pro-labor activity has progressed to a serious level.

Table 9-1 Reasons Health Care Employees Join Unions

	Publication*										
Issue	5	7	8	9	10	6	1	11	12	13	14
Poor communication	x	x	x	x	x	x	x	x	x	x	x
Personnel policies	x		x			x	x	x	x	x	x
Supervision	x	x	x	x		x	x		x		x
Fringe benefits			x	x			x	x	x	x	x
Work conditions		x	x	x	x			x	x		x
Grievances	x	x	x					x			x
Job security	x	x	x		x	x	x				x
Human dignity	x			x	x		x				x
Shift differentials		x	x								x
Wages	x	x	x	x	x	x	x	x	x	x	x

*Derived from a sampling of studies in 11 publications. For the name of the study and publication information, see NOTE of the same number at the end of this article.

There is no blueprint the administrator can use to determine how a union organizer will evaluate the institution. The method of evaluation depends upon the organizing team sent into the area and the team's previous experience or success. Its tactics may vary considerably, depending upon the contacts from employees and how management addresses the situation. However, the organizer may concentrate in certain areas, including the following.

Employee Loyalty by Work Shift

Normally, the first shift is the most loyal to the organization, the second shift less loyal than the first, and the third the least loyal. This probably is because new employees usually start on the second or third shift. They may seldom or never see top management, and the supervisory force usually is smaller. Thus, there often is no one who can provide consistent supervision, e.g., answering employee questions about personnel policies or benefits. These employees tend to feel overlooked and forgotten. They are more susceptible to the pleas of the union organizer, who usually is available on the later shifts.[7, 8, 16, 17]

Female-Male Employee Ratio

Women historically have been less interested in unions than have men. In the past, many women worked to supplement the family income, but this has changed rapidly.

Nursing personnel, a majority of whom are women, are increasingly recognizing the need to organize in order to improve their status. The American Nurses' Association is attempting to upgrade and negotiate conditions of employment for its membership. Other professional organizations, such as the American Society of Hospital Pharmacists, American Society of Medical Technologists, National Association of Social Workers, and American Dietetic Association, are, also, actively seeking more voice in the representation of their members.[3,5,18,19,20]

Work Environment

Employees want clean working and eating environments and expect management to provide them. If the health care institution allows the work environment to deteriorate, employees may think that the institution does not care much about them.[8]

Wage Rates

Traditionally, the health care employee has subsidized health care institutions with low wages. This is an injustice to the employee who must compete daily in the retail market for goods and services. In addition, the institution must have fair and regular wage differentials. Failure to update these differentials will cause a compression effect between the new employees' base pay and the tenured employees' level.[4, 8, 11, 16, 17]

Incentive Pay

In areas where an incentive pay program has been implemented, employees may complain that some of the rates, or daily quotas, are too high. High quotas obviously breed dissatisfaction if management engineers do not respond by reexamining the quotas periodically.[17]

Overtime Practices

Problems arise in this area when overtime is scheduled for employees without their consent. Management thinks that the worker would like to earn extra money for overtime, but this often is not the case. Overtime can be very disruptive to the employee's family life and leisure time. The union organizer will exploit this fact and force management to hire additional workers. Inequities in the distribution of overtime is another aspect of the problem.[5,17]

Seniority

While management may prefer to recognize the skill and health of a worker in assigning a new job, it must not overlook the employees' view of seniority. Seniority to them is job security. If management takes the time-honored seniority concept away completely, it is asking for employee dissatisfaction and unionization. This may be particularly true in geographical areas where unionization already is well entrenched.[17]

Promotion Policy

When a new job opens up or an employee leaves, present personnel should be given an opportunity to apply for the position. A good job-posting policy can be extremely helpful. Health care institutions also should have education/training programs available to assist employees' vertical or lateral movement.[21]

Job Transfers

Most often it is the ambitious employee who would like to be promoted to a more convenient shift or a different job. Research has shown that supervisors many times sabotage the promotion of ambitious employees. The supervisor does not want to lose a good worker or have to train a new one. Such practices should be avoided. Frequently, the best employees are those who have worked up the organizational ladder.[17]

Fringe Benefits

Research has revealed that most managements underrate the value of fringe benefits to the employee. And, as employers continue to increase the benefits portion of total compensation, the benefits package is likely to increase in relative importance to employees. With the news media and the next-door neighbor discussing the benefits of union representation, it is foolish for health care management to neglect to establish a good benefits program *and* to adequately explain to employees the benefits the institution offers.

Discipline and Grievance Procedures

If the institution does not provide employees with written rules about what is not allowed and what is and to what degree, some supervisors may abuse their authority to reprimand. The grievance procedure serves as a safety valve for employees to release their frustrations about their supervisors or other problems of a major nature. Management should develop and implement a procedure that employees will use internally instead of resorting to an outside agency to settle disputes. Management also should review the procedures periodically to make sure they are serving workers' needs. For example, many grievances are either about or under the direct control of the employees' immediate supervisor. In these cases, the employees probably will not use the procedure unless there is some provision to circumvent that superior.[12,17,22]

With an understanding of why health care personnel join unions and some of the criteria by which labor organizers evaluate an institution, management should begin the process of assessing its employee relations climate as well as planning its strategy for maintaining nonunion status.[8,17]

A PREVENTIVE MANAGEMENT PROGRAM

Assessing an institution's employee relations climate and implementing a program to prevent unionization is a process for which a myriad of management responses are possible. Each institution must carefully design a strategy that is both practical and suited to its own particular situation. Recognizing the significant relationship between the reasons given by employees for joining unions and what an organizer looks for, there is substantial reason to believe that the primary reasons for unionization do include ''communication problems'' and the perception by employees of ''unfair treatment.''

Therefore, a preventive management program should be designed with a primary emphasis on improving communication and dealing with employees and related problems in an honest and fair manner. This emphasis is detailed in several ways in the following recommendations for establishing a preventive management program. These recommendations are an outgrowth of previously described employee-related issues and could serve as the general framework within which each management team builds its own strategy.

Nonunion Policy

If a health care institution intends to be nonunion, it should give careful consideration to the development and publication of such a policy. Good labor counsel should be consulted to assist in the development of an up-front nonunion policy and to advise the best alternatives for communicating the policy to all who wish to work at the institution. All prospective employees should be informed in the screening process and given written evidence of the institutional position regarding unions along with other significant policies. The prospective employee then has the choice of whether or not to work for a nonunion institution. This, in itself, should be an indication of fair treatment. Management also should consider publishing the nonunion policy in the employee handbook for reference during orientation and other worker group meetings.

Personnel Selection

Management must have effective policies and procedures regarding selection of new employees. Prevention of labor-management problems begins with the proper matching of personnel to specific jobs. A good wage and salary program including job analyses, job descriptions (with performance objectives), and job evaluation is essential to this matching process. If good procedures are used for selecting on the basis of both the individual's qualifications and the requirements of a specific job, the result is likely to be a better fit for the institution and the employee. Concurrently, the institution is likely to avoid many communication and morale problems. A fair wage and salary system provides at least a basis for establishing an objective employee evaluation system.

Employee Attitude Assessment

Employee attitude surveys, when conducted properly, can provide much valuable data to management at normal costs. The method chosen should be simple to implement and should require concise employee responses. The result should be an accurate assessment of the topics surveyed, clearly differentiating between positive and negative attitudes.

Attitude surveying should be done on a planned, periodic basis so that employees perceive continual concern for their needs and management keeps abreast of fluctuations in worker attitudes. If this procedure is combined with efforts to obtain upward communication through formal or informal channels at all levels of the institution, the result should be a positive change in the attitudes of employees and the development of a management system for dealing with personnel problems before they become sore spots. Once attitudes are assessed and problems identified, management should be ready to take corrective action, including an appropriate training program.

Probably the single most important part of the attitude measurement analysis process is communication with the employees about (1) purpose, (2) how the data will be analyzed and used, (3) confidentiality of the individual responses, (4) feedback concerning the findings, and (5) what changes, if any, they can expect as a result of their participation in the survey. Management should be careful not to make many promises that cannot be fulfilled, but should make a strong effort to do whatever is possible to improve employee relations.

In summary, if management asks employees to take valuable time to participate in a survey, it is extremely important for them to feel that administration values their input and is doing what it can to meet their needs.

Employee Training

Administration should examine its role and responsibilities in training employees as a function of management rather than as a staff function. If this self-examination indicates that management is assuming little, if any, responsibility for employee training, it is very likely that this is related directly to workers' perceptions of poor treatment. For employees to perceive fair, honest, or decent treatment, top management must make the commitment to assume responsibility for training and must transmit it down through all levels to first-line supervisors. This is necessary, for example, before management can develop an adequate performance appraisal and reward system that employees will consider equitable.

Once management makes the commitment to assume its training responsibility, it must determine what type of training program it will implement. The following questions may provide evaluative insight into employee needs:

1. Are employee functions and responsibilities agreed upon and clear?
2. Do employees have the ability (technical training and experience) to do what is expected?
3. Do job descriptions contain specific performance objectives?
4. Do employees know what performance standards are being used to evaluate their work?
5. Is there a positive relationship between employee performance and reward?

Management implementation of an appropriate training program should have positive effects on employee attitudes and productivity and should be a major asset in eradicating the dead-end job syndrome.

Employee Value Systems

Management should recognize the different types of value systems that exist among various employee groups. They frequently represent a wide diversity of value systems in both professional and nonprofessional categories. Research has identified as many as seven different employee value systems varying from tribalistic to existentialist.[23] Some examples of ways to respond to the myriad of value systems and needs include flexible work scheduling, earned time programs, methods of job enrichment, and a cafeteria approach to fringe benefits. The bottom line is that management must develop a variety of imaginative ways to respond to the needs of multiple employee "families."

First-Line Supervisors

Management must recognize the importance of first-line supervisors in preventing serious labor problems. The logic is simple. First-line supervisors represent all of management in the operational contact with nonsupervisory personnel. If these supervisors do not have good management skills, the institution is inviting unionization. Frequently, the first-line supervisor problem is manifested by the number of grievances filed involving situations that are either about or under the direct control of the immediate supervisor. Management should evaluate the effectiveness of first-line supervisors' employee relations skills carefully and regularly. When deficiencies are found, management should either assist the supervisor through training or terminate the person, depending on the individual's past record and potential.

Performance Appraisal

The institution should establish a performance appraisal policy that reflects a management attitude of developing employees to their potential. If management behavior indicates anything other than this philosophy, workers are likely to perceive poor or unfair treatment by supervisors. Performance appraisal must be done on an honest and regular basis to be effective in improving morale and productivity of all employees.

Management's avoidance of an honest appraisal of the nonproductive employee simply demonstrates to all workers that the reward system is inequitable or that the laggards receive the same rewards as those who are productive. This can be interpreted logically by productive employees as evidence that the nonproductive actually are rewarded more than the productive in relation to their effort. If this attitude prevails, management very likely is "teaching" its employees to move toward mediocrity and union thinking. The implementation of a good performance appraisal system depends largely upon the management skills of the first-line supervisors. In other words, the appraisal system used is not nearly so important as the people (managers) who implement it. The best system is as weak as the people who operate it.

Disciplinary Policies and Procedures

Management must take great care in applying disciplinary policies and procedures consistently. Consistent and fair application normally can prevent unnecessary employee relations problems and grievances.

One basic principle is that management should have just cause for imposing discipline. While the definition may vary from case to case, there are several basic tests that can be applied to determine whether just cause exists for disciplining employees:

1. Was the disciplinary rule reasonably related to efficient and safe operations?
2. Were the employees properly warned of potential consequences of their conduct?
3. Did management conduct a fair investigation before applying the discipline?
4. Did the investigation produce substantial evidence of guilt?
5. Were the policies and procedures implemented consistently and without discrimination?
6. If a penalty resulted, was it related to the seriousness of the event as well as the past record of the employee? Or, in other words, did the "punishment fit the crime"?

Some form of grievance procedure should be viewed as a part of any prevention program since it is intended to provide a mechanism to allow employees to complain formally about a perceived problem without the fear of subjective reprisal. Although any grievance procedure is subject to problems of interpretation and application, there are some basic factors that can be applied equally in evaluating the system from the employees' perspective:

1. The procedure should be written so that all employees can understand the mechanics of filing a grievance, as well as where they can go to ask questions about any step of the system.
2. When employees file grievances, they expect prompt action. Promptness is one of the most important aspects of a grievance settlement and failure to resolve the problem with reasonable speed is likely to lead to adverse employee feelings.
3. The first-line supervisor typically is the first step in a grievance procedure except when that individual is perceived to *be* the problem. When this kind of situation prevails, employees need to know that they have some recourse in the grievance procedure without going through the first-line supervisor. However, the employees should take every reasonable step to solve the problem with the immediate supervisor before going to someone else with the grievance.

When employees realize that a fair grievance procedure is available and when management is doing what it can to prevent unnecessary problems, the end result should be a decreased number of complaints, fair and objective processing of those that are filed, and an employee feeling that management is concerned about employee needs.

Wages

The health care institution should be very careful to stay competitive with regard to wages and at least annually should compare its rates to similar institutions in the same geographical area. Frequently, wage survey data can be found that apply to the local area, but if this is not the case management should conduct its own survey. Even a sample survey of representative jobs will help keep the institution abreast of trend information. Of course, certain shortage points will have to be dealt with on a case-by-case basis and possibly more frequently than every year. While competitive wages are a necessary condition in any preventive management program, it should not be concluded that being competitive in wages is sufficient for maintaining nonunion status.

As has been indicated, wages is only one of many factors that may enter into employee decisions to seek union help. It should be recognized that health care no longer is as far behind other industries in wages as it was 15 or 20 years ago. Management also should be cognizant of the fact that wages may not be the major motivating factor for a significant portion of employees in a given institution. Although there may not be a great deal that management can definitively conclude from research regarding wages as a motivating factor, the folly of relying totally on competitive wages to prevent unionization can be illustrated best by a review of wage structures in institutions that have had union elections recently.

In summary, the absence of competitive wage levels (particularly in times of double-digit inflation) is a potentially severe problem, but the presence of good wage levels is not sufficient, in itself, to prevent unionization. This is particularly true in multidimensioned institutions that employ a diverse group of employees with a variety of value systems.

CONCLUSIONS

Maintaining nonunion status is an attainable goal. Whether or not it will be achieved is related directly to the behavioral dedication of management in demon-strating its concern for meeting employee needs in a fair and equitable manner. Although the material in this article is not all-inclusive and is not intended to represent a formula to guarantee nonunion status, it is suggestive of management practices necessary to prevent communication problems and to avoid employee perceptions of unfair treatment.

While the unionization process is highly situational, and in some locations may be essentially inevitable, a positive nonunion philosophy and program usually should obviate the need for a labor organization. When employees do not perceive a need for union assistance, the probability is slim that they will elect one and begin paying union dues.

NOTES

1. J. S. Rakich, "Hospital Unionization: Causes and Effects, *Hospital Administration*, Winter 1973, p. 10.

2. D. D. Pointer and L. L. Cannedy, "Organizing of Professionals," *Hospitals, JAHA* 48, no. 6 (March 16, 1974): 70–73.

3. D. D. Pointer and Norman Metzger, *The National Labor Relations Act—A Guidebook for Health Care Facility Administrators* (New York: Spectrum Publications, Inc., 1975), p. 272.

4. K. A. Reed, "Preparing for Union Organization," *Hospital Topics* 48, no. 4 (April 1970): 30–32.

5. E. S. Stanton, "The Charleston Hospital Strikes," *Southern Hospitals*, March 1971, p. 39.

6. D. E. Phillips, "Taft-Hartley: What to Expect," *Hospitals, JAHA* 48, no. 13 (July 1, 1974): 18a–d.

7. M. Goodfellow, "If you aren't listening to your employees, you may be asking for a union," *Modern Hospital* 113, no. 4 (October 1969): 88–90.

8. ————, "Keeping Your Employees' Morale Up Takes More Than Money," *Hospital Financial Management* 28, no. 11 (November 1974): 24–29.

9. A. A. Imberman, "Communications: An Effective Weapon Against Unionization," *Hospital Progress* 54, no. 12 (December 1973): 54–57.

10. H. L. Lewis, "Wave of Union Organizing Will Follow Break in the Taft-Hartley Dam," *Modern Healthcare* 1, no. 2 (May 1974): 25–32.

11. R. A. Milliken and G. Milliken, "Unionization-Vulnerable and Outbid," *Hospitals, JAHA* 47, no. 20 (October 16, 1973): 56–59.

12. R. E. Sibson, "Why Unions in the Hospital," *Hospital Topics* 43, no. 8 (August 1965): 46, 48, 54.

13. E. S. Stanton, "Unions and the Professional Employee," *Hospital Progress* 55, no. 1 (January 1974): 58.

14. Norman Metzger and D. D. Pointer, *Labor-Management Relations in Health Services Industry: Theory and Practice* (Washington, D.C.: Science and Health Publications, Inc., 1972), p. 360.

15. D. D. Pointer, "How the 1974 Taft-Hartley Amendments Will Affect Health Care Facilities," *Hospital Progress* 55, no. 10 (October 1974): 68–70.

16. "How to win the labor tug of war," *Modern Healthcare* 2, no. 3 (September 1974): 58, 59, 68.

17. M. Goodfellow, "Checklist: How The Union Organizer Rates Your Institution," *Risk Management*, December 1972, pp. 1–6.

18. Norman Metzger, "Labor Relations," *Hospitals, JAHA* 44, no. 6 (March 16, 1970): 80–84.

19. D. R. Matlack, "Goals and Trends in the Unionization of Health Professionals," *Hospital Progress* 53, no. 2 (February 1972): 40–43.

20. —————, "Goals and Trends in the Unionization of Health Care Professionals," *Hospital Progress* 53, no. 2 (February 1972): 40–43.

21. C. L. Joiner and K. D. Blayney, "Career Mobility and Allied Health Manpower Utilization," *Journal of Allied Health*, Fall 1974, pp. 157–161.

22. R. Clelland, "Grievance Procedures: Outlet of Employee, Insight for Management," *Hospitals, JAHA* 41, no. 18 (August 1, 1967): 60.

23. Charles L. Hughes, "Making Unions Unnecessary," *Executive Enterprises Publications Co.* (New York, 1976), p. 43.

10. You Can Keep Your Hospital Nonunion If:

ROBERT T. LYONS and ROGER W. WILLIAMS, SR.

What must be done by managers and supervisors to preserve the right to manage in a union-free environment?

The right to manage is a delicately balanced relationship with nonunion employees. It is a conditional right, not an absolute one. It is conditioned by applicable statutory law. It also is conditioned by the character, style, and effectiveness of the management process itself. And ultimately, it is conditioned by the way employees interpret and evaluate the quality of life that exists under their current managerial process.

A hospital must be regarded as a social system with a complex pattern of individual and group interrelations. The elements in this system must be looked upon as interdependent parts of a whole with two major sets of problems:

1. There are problems of external balance (including economic issues) and of doing the functional job the organization was set up to do. These problems can be assessed in terms of cost, quality of patient care, and technical efficiency.
2. There are problems of internal equilibrium. These chiefly involve the maintenance of a kind of social organization in which individuals and groups, through contributing their services to the common enterprise, can obtain the personal satisfaction that makes them willing to cooperate and eager to accomplish.

The kind of social organization that exists within an institution is related intimately to the effectiveness of the total enterprise. A great deal of attention and scientific development is lavished on economic or external problems. On the other hand, internal or sociological problems frequently are ignored, leaving vast stores of productive energy and social satisfaction untapped.

THE BASIC ELEMENTS

The elements that must be considered in understanding a health care institution as a social system may be outlined as:

1. The technical organization: the physical environment in which people work.
2. The human organization: the people who do the work, who must be considered first as *individuals*, each with unique conditioning, motivation, attitudes, problems, and demands to make on the job. Then, as a further delineation of the social organization with its various levels of "we" and "they" groupings, it involves:

   - A formal operation established by management and made up of certain patterns of interaction shown in the formal organization flow charts and certain ideas and beliefs based on the economic logics of cost and efficiency.

635

- An informal operation established by the people themselves, also involving certain patterns of interaction not shown on an organization chart, and certain ideas and beliefs based on a logic of sentiments that expresses the values residing in the interhuman relations of the different individuals and groups within the institution.

The limits of collaborative effort are determined far more by the informal than by the formal organization of the health care entity.

The social organization and the individuals and groups that comprise it tend to achieve a state of equilibrium such that any changes in one part of the system are accompanied by changes in other parts. The system will react against changes, whether positive or negative, unless:

- changes in the technical organization are introduced at such a rate and in such a way as to permit the slower-moving social organization to adjust to them, and
- the effect of any change on the informal organization and its codes and sentiments is considered fully.

The human problems of management must be reformulated in the light of this approach. The conventional breakdown into problems of fatigue, working hours, physical conditions of work, grievances, salary incentives, efficiency, etc., are not adequate. Each problem can be understood only in terms of the entire social situation in which the problem arises. The major human problems of management may be restated as:

- *Problems of changes in the social structure.* Changes of a technical nature and in the formal organization must be made in such a way as to bring about a minimum dislocation of the social equilibrium.
- *Problems of control and communication.* There must be a two-way street involving employees, supervisors, technical staff, professional staff, and management. The effects of the informal organization and the potential pitfalls in maintaining this condition must be recognized.
- *The problem of the individual's adjustment to the structure.* Each person's relation to the total social situation must be a matter of constant interest to management. Through proper orientation to changes, adequate supervision, and personal counselling, the individual's equilibrium must be maintained.

Where there is significant disruption in this equilibrium, either within the individual or the group, there will be discontent and dissatisfaction. It is at this point that individuals begin to look for something or someone to restore this sense of equilibrium. As a last resort, the dissatisfied individual sometimes seeks out a third party, or outside party—a labor organization.

Experience has shown that where wage and benefit levels are competitive, employees ordinarily will not seek or accept the involvement of a union *if* the character of daily interaction among people reflects a just reconciliation of human values with economic values.

TEN REQUISITES FOR GOOD RELATIONS

The following basic requirements are felt to be essential to good employee relations. No claim is made that these ten characteristics constitute the only way to compartmentalize the requisites of union-free management. Neither is it claimed that all of these requisites can be met fully by one level of management alone; some of them require the assistance and support of every level of management.

Periodic comparisons of the relationships that exist at a health care institution with these requirements of good employee relations will bring to light specific soft spots and shortcomings that may exist. If administration corrects them, it will continue to enjoy the right to manage in a union-free environment.

Basic Requirement One

The administrator creatively "manages" the effort toward sound employee relations with the same concern and initiative that the executive manages the effort toward excellence in patient care.

In large measure, this basic requirement will be met *if*:

1. The administrator functions as head of a "community" in which the aspirations of employees, as individuals, are justly reconciled with the aspirations of the community as a whole through plans and policies that are thoughtfully conceived and fairly administered.
2. The administrator sets a good example by reconciling human values with economic values in all personal dealings with subordinates.
3. The administrator regularly is visible to an ever-widening number of employees at all levels of the work force (not just a select few), in a

friendly and easy-to-approach manner, eager to know and be known by all fellow citizens in the hospital community.

4. The administrator keeps a constant managerial eye on such sensitive functions as personnel policy development and revision, complaint handling and its procedures, supervisory selection and training, organizational planning as correlated with employee goals and aspirations, all phases of policy or practice, etc., that impact directly on relations with employees.

5. The administrator functions as the core communicator of the mind and conscience of management, reaching out to infect the entire institutional community with a desire to achieve—but always in a manner consistent with the balanced best interests of patients and employees alike.

6. The administrator sincerely listens to all levels of the hospital community with an open mind and a willingness to consider change when it is in the balanced best interests of patients and employees alike.

7. The administrator periodically evaluates the tone and character of the overall climate in the institution, then takes positive steps to correct and strengthen those facets of hospital affairs requiring it.

Basic Requirement Two

All levels of supervisory management reflect a proprietary concern for the well-being and fair treatment of employees, consistent with hospital policy and what is "right" in the balanced best interests of patients and employees alike.

In large measure, this basic requirement will be met *if*:

1. Persons who are selected or promoted to higher level positions (including first-level supervisory jobs) are qualified by reason of temperament, social skill, intelligence, and technical know-how and are not retarded in this progress by improper reasons, such as race, sex, or ethnic background.

2. New, first-level supervisors are given concentrated coaching in the skills of directing people as well as training in the administration of hospital policy and practice.

3. Supervisors and department heads continually evaluate their own supervisory performance as to how they relate to employees and take prompt remedial and corrective action when required.

4. All levels of supervisory management are held accountable for maintaining sound relations with employees to the same degree that they are accountable for providing quality care for patients.

5. All levels of supervisory management make the established complaint procedure work effectively, encouraging employees to use it when necessary and taking the initiative to assist employees in the exercise of their rights of appeal.

6. All levels of supervisory management work to create an in-hospital environment where the dignity and uniqueness of employees, as individuals, is acknowledged daily by friendly, courteous, and responsive contacts by management representatives.

Basic Requirement Three

The personnel director effectively impacts as a humanizing influence on the processes and conscience of management rather than being simply a passive and compliant functionary.

In large measure, this basic requirement will be met *if*:

1. The personnel director has adequate and competent staff sufficient to provide the quality and breadth of service employees rightfully expect and sufficient to be able to periodically step off the playing field to do the planning, programming, and evaluating necessary to have a creative impact on the broader needs of the institution as a whole.

2. The personnel director provides periodic opportunities for all levels of supervisory management to formally evaluate existing hospital policy and practice and to formally participate with the hospital director in the formulation of new or revised policies and practices.

3. The personnel director functions as the servant and facilitator of justice, rather than as its administrator and enforcer, in all matters pertaining to employee discipline, complaint handling, and the application of the institution's policy and practice.

4. The personnel director makes it "my business" to know about and critically evaluate all phases of supervisory practice insofar as each phase has an impact on relations with employees.

5. The personnel director functions as a persuasive advocate of ordered and reasonable change where it is warranted and can be accomplished within the bounds of existing procedures.

6. The personnel director spends sufficient time (five to ten hours each week) out on the floors where the action is, relating as friend to all but

playing favorites with none, and listening critically to everything that is said but acting prudently on whatever is said.

Basic Requirement Four

Personnel policies and practices are designed and administered fairly in the balanced best interests of patients and employees alike.

In large measure, this basic requirement will be met *if*:

1. All levels of supervisory management are (a) furnished with a current, up-to-date policy manual covering all areas of hospital policy and practices, and (b) trained in the correct interpretation and application of these elements.
2. Current policies are reviewed critically with supervisory management on a regularized schedule to evaluate the fairness and effectiveness of existing policy statements and to determine what revisions or new policies may be needed.
3. Current policies and practices are communicated adequately to employees via handbooks, bulletin boards, small group employee meetings, etc., so that all workers may know their rights as well as the hospital's intentions and so that its actions and interpretations may be understood—even appreciated.
4. Current policies and practices are administered fairly and consistently by all levels of management.
5. Policy and practice are not looked upon by management as an immutable force but rather as a living process of governing relations with employees and hence subject to change as new circumstances emerge.

Basic Requirement Five

Effective, continuing communication with employees is viewed by management as a necessary condition, rather than an optional or peripheral one, to the pursuit of sound personnel relations.

In large measure, this basic requirement will be met *if*:

1. All levels of supervisory management are encouraged and effectively prepared to function as the principal interpreters of the institution to employees and, conversely, the principal interpreters of employees to the administration.

2. The administrator periodically holds two-way, participative meetings with all levels of supervisory management to exchange views on plans, programs, problems, and goals with respect to both the human and operational affairs of the institutional community.
3. The administrator regularly (every six to eight weeks) and effectively conducts two-way communication sessions with representative small groups of nonsupervisory employees, at least once a year addresses the entire hospital community on appropriate subjects of interest to employees, and periodically (at least four times each year) issues a timely and newsworthy letter to employees at their homes.
4. The administrator and the executive staff jointly plan and creatively prepare for the conduct of each group meeting to determine how best to enrich and improve the sessions.
5. The personnel director communicates with supervisory management by periodic, planned group meetings, newsletter, bulletins, etc. The director also communicates with employees by judiciously prepared answers published in response to employee questions asked in small group meetings conducted by the administrator, and by locally prepared articles for the hospital newspaper.
6. Both the administrator and the personnel director use each daily contact with nonsupervisory employees and members of supervisory management to build two-way bridges of understanding, concern, and loyalty between the individual and the institutional community.

Basic Requirement Six

Employee complaints and their fair, orderly resolution are looked upon by management as positive opportunities to achieve justice and improved relations with workers rather than as time-consuming annoyances to be dealt with as matters of secondary importance.

In large measure, this basic requirement will be met *if*:

1. A clearly defined appellate-type complaint procedure is designed, implemented, communicated, and adhered to as the formal vehicle of justice in the hospital community.
2. The final appeal step of the established complaint procedure terminates at a management level no lower than the administrator, and possibly with a grievance review committee composed of equal

representation from employees, management, and a neutral outside party.

3. All levels of supervisory management are given periodic training in sound techniques of complaint investigation, complaint discussion with employees, and complaint response.

4. The personnel director devises and maintains effective reporting procedures to be able to monitor the progress and status of complaint handling at all steps of the procedure.

5. The personnel director functions as a neutral service agent and facilitator of justice, assisting both employees and line management representatives to assemble pertinent facts and to interpret and apply pertinent policies and procedures correctly rather than acting as a direct functionary and minister of justice in the disposition of complaints.

6. The administrator periodically monitors the complaint-handling process by insisting on appropriate reports from and reviews with the personnel director regarding all aspects of this most sensitive employee relations activity.

Basic Requirement Seven

Continuing education, training, and development of the entire hospital community are recognized as necessary—not optional—requirements in the effective pursuit of efficiency and sound relations with employees.

In large measure, this basic requirement will be met *if*:

1. Supervisors and the management group are trained properly in:

   - the skills and techniques of job instruction
   - policy interpretation and application
   - the economic facts of life regarding hospital income and operating costs
   - human relations skills and complaint-handling techniques
   - operating objectives, plans, and programs
   - employee benefits and their proper application
   - performance planning and evaluation techniques
   - counseling techniques, including career planning
   - affirmative action and equal employment opportunity.

2. Nonsupervisory employees are trained (and/or educated) properly by supervisory management in:

   - job methods and skills (via on-the-job training, inservice programs, etc.)
   - hospital policy, practices, and rules
   - hospital organization and objectives
   - inservice educational and career opportunities available

3. Each human resource development activity is prepared to fulfill a need within the health care institution—organizational, departmental, or individual—and employees participate in the identification of needs when appropriate.

Basic Requirement Eight

All phases of wage and salary administration are carried out by a management determined to do the right thing voluntarily, consistent with established wage policy, plans, and practices.

In large measure, this basic requirement will be met *if*:

1. Management keeps abreast of wage trends in its own labor market area and promptly makes appropriate corrections when necessary to stay competitive.

2. Comprehensive, clearly defined job classifications that advocate the principle of equal pay for equal (or comparable) work are established.

3. Jobs are reevaluated promptly and honestly whenever changes in their content occur, and appropriate retroactive pay adjustments are made to incumbents whenever a position is upgraded in consequence of such reappraisals.

4. Production standards are set fairly and revised honestly in accordance with changes in methods, materials, and working conditions.

5. Merit increases are granted objectively on the basis of demonstrated job performance and not on such other unrelated criteria as attitude, relations with others, or attendance factors that should be dealt with through other corrective measures.

6. All levels of supervisory management exercise a sincere concern for fair wage and salary administration and honestly reexamine the soundness of their judgments when called into question by employees.

Basic Requirement Nine

Established benefit programs and policies are administered in a manner consistent with the intentions of the health care institution and the good will of employees and are communicated in a manner intended to achieve reasonable personnel understanding and appreciation.

In large measure, this basic requirement will be met *if:*

1. Benefit administrators view their direct contacts with employees as opportunities to generate worker good will and understanding rather than merely to administer and control the application of benefit plans and policies.
2. Benefit administrators assume a proprietary concern for ensuring the complete and timely application of benefits supported by vigorous follow-up measures where necessary in the interests of hospital and employees alike.
3. Personnel directors regularly monitor the awarding of benefits to be sure that such plans and policies are being interpreted and applied properly.
4. Members of supervisory management are given continuing training and education in the elements and levels of benefits so they can function effectively as supporting merchandisers of the hospital's benefits as well as facilitators of justice in behalf of employees when benefit applications are called into question.
5. Administrators and personnel directors will look for, and carry out, effective means to improve employee understanding and appreciation of benefit plans and policies via employee meetings, newspaper articles, benefit statements, contests, posters, etc.
6. Administrators and personnel directors promptly convey to employees information relative to any problem areas and/or inequities that may arise under existing benefit plans and policies as well as information pertaining to benefit trends in the local labor market.

Basic Requirement Ten

All levels of line and staff management assume proprietary concern for creating and maintaining a quality of life throughout the hospital community that is responsive to the reasonable aspirations of employees and the economic aspirations of the institution.

In large measure, this basic requirement will be met *if:*

1. Continuing managerial supervision is given to improving various hospital service activities such as the cafeteria, dispensary for employees, medical service for employees, parking facilities, etc.
2. Continuing managerial supervision is given to correcting and/or eliminating unsafe or unreasonable job conditions, unreasonable periods of extended overtime, unreasonable work schedules, adverse working conditions resulting from poor temperature control, poor ventilation, excessive noise, poorly maintained washroom facilities, etc.
3. Management fosters and supports wholesome social and recreational activities among employees.
4. The suggestion system is administered effectively and creatively, with full awareness of its high potential as a cost-saving and motivational device.

A sincere and continuing commitment to these basic requirements will establish a high level of immunity against any union organizing attempts. Administration should make them a "living experience," and employees for the most part will not feel the need for an outside party to represent them. There always will be change in a hospital organization as in any other social structure, but any resultant disruption to employees' equilibrium will be at a minimum when these requirements become an integral part of the daily life at the health care institution.

SUGGESTED READINGS

David Sirota, "The Myth and Realities of Worker Discontent," *Wharton Quarterly,* Spring 1974, pp. 5–9.

Mary B. Yelito, "Make Employee Communication a Two-Way Street," *Medical Laboratory Observer,* July-August 1974, pp. 28–31.

Nathaniel Stewart, "Change Requires Employee Support," *Nation's Business,* August 1959.

Richard L. Epstein, "The Grievance Procedure in the Non-Union Setting: Caveat Employer," *The Employee Relations Law Journal* 1, no. 1 (Summer 1975): 120–127.

Richard E. Walton, "How to Counter Alienation in the Plant," *Harvard Business Review* 50, no. 6 (November-December 1972): 70–81.

Fritz I. Roethlisberger and William J. Dickson, *Management and the Worker* (Cambridge, Mass: Harvard University Press, 1939), pp. 292–328.

John W. Riday, "Measuring Employee Morale," *Journal of the American Bankers Association* LXIII, no. 2 (July 1970): 35–36, 90.

Samuel E. Oberman, "The Hidden Costs of Unionism," *Journal of the American Bankers Association* LXVI, no. 3 (September 1973).

11. The Method behind the Madness, or, Know Your Adversary

WARREN H. CHANEY and THOMAS R. BEECH

The five largest and most active unions in the health care field are the American Federation of State, County, and Municipal Employees; the Service Employees International Union; the National Union of Hospital and Health Care Employees (all three are affiliates of the AFL-CIO); the Teamsters; and the American Nurses' Association (ANA). In addition, there are other professional associations similar to the ANA that are actually quasi-unions, since they express the views of the members and are making demands for collective bargaining rights. At their convention in June 1974, in San Francisco, the ANA passed an emergency resolution supporting the strike of 4,000 nurses in the area.[1]

The unions are more than eager to provide the necessary help in organizing labor in hospitals. The massive numbers employed represent considerable dues income to unions. In the authors' immediate Houston area, union representatives have distributed handbills to over sixty hospitals and have held National Labor Relations Board (NLRB) scheduled elections at nine health care facilities. Unions are dedicated to win the war against management.

THE BARGAINING ELECTION PROCESS—AN OVERVIEW

The bargaining unit determination and election processes are set in motion after a petition for an election has been filed with the NLRB. This petition can be filed by an employee, a group of employees, or an individual of a labor organization acting on behalf of the employees. The NLRB requires such petition to be supported by a showing of interest from at least thirty percent of the employees sought to be represented. Upon receipt of the petition, the NLRB conducts an investigation and may hold a hearing to determine:

1. if jurisdiction can be asserted under the act,
2. whether sufficient interest on the part of the employees has been demonstrated,
3. if an election is being sought in an appropriate unit,
4. whether the union named in the petition is qualified to participate in an election, and
5. whether there are any existing barriers against holding an election.[2]

Sometimes elections are the result of an agreement between the employer and union representative. If neither can agree to have the election, the NLRB has the authority to order a representation hearing and order an election to be conducted under the direction of the NLRB regional office. In such an election several guidelines are followed.

1. More than one union may appear on the ballot.
2. Eligibility to vote is determined by a previous payroll roster of the employees.

641

3. The election is usually held on the employer's premises in an area easily accessible by employees and at a time opportune for the employees.
4. The NLRB supplies the ballot upon which is listed all options, i.e., choice between union(s) and no union.
5. Each party may have observers at the polling place and challenge any employee's right to vote.
6. Ballots are tabulated by the NLRB at the conclusion of the voting period, in the presence of observers. A majority of the votes cast are required for union representation. If more than one union was on the ballot and the vote was split, a runoff election would be held.
7. Within five days of the announcement of results, both parties can challenge the election on the grounds that: (a) the manner in which the election was held was illegal; (b) the employer or union intimidated employees; (c) false promises or misrepresentations were made; and (d) reproductions of the official ballot were misused as campaign literature.[3]

Should the union lose the election, the union must wait at least one year before petitioning for another election in the same unit.

Because the health care industry is relatively new territory for unions, the recent expansion in collective bargaining agencies in hospitals is expected to continue in even greater proportions. It is clear that unions have one terrific advantage over hospital management—experience. Due to their experience, unions will know exactly how to approach hospital employees, persuade them to unionize, and utilize available alternatives in the event of unfair labor practices. Management, on the other hand, will be forced to learn from its mistakes, mistakes which could well be hazardous to the hospital.

THE UNION ORGANIZER

Good union organizers are active practicing "psychologists." The organizer's expertise is human relations; and in such a field, unorganized working men and women are the raw materials to be refined by the professional union organizer through group action.

Basic Tools of a Union Organizer

Three primary personality tools make a successful union organizer, and a good practitioner usually is amply talented in all three. First, he/she needs a native quality and capacity to like people. This is more than just back slapping, telling jokes, and having beer with the boys. A union organizer is a warm, gentle, outgoing person who communicates and relates effectively to all types of people.

Second, he/she needs the ability to adapt to the immediate surroundings. A union organizer, as the lizard which changes colors, must adapt to his immediate surroundings and not feel superior or out of place among any group of employees. He has the tendency to warm up to people very quickly, usually within ten or fifteen minutes after meeting a new prospect.

Finally, patience with people is his *forte*. A union organizer is a patient person. Nonunion employees are rarely completely sold on the idea of union organizing or unionism in the first discussion. The union organizer realizes this and considers it an ongoing effort to sign up or convince all employees about the values of unionism and collective action.

Union Organizing Strategy

Regardless of the union, the organizer has one primary advantage over his opposition in health care administration: he is a trained fighter. He has been to war many times and has lost some, but won many. The majority of union organizers have come up through the ranks. It is a grave error to underrate the casual dress and slang language. Beneath the innocent or unpolished exterior lurks the mind of a well-organized trained soldier.

The bargaining units of the AFL-CIO and the Teamsters represent the most sophisticated union threat. The ANA and other such associations are still fighting among themselves as to the degree of "union" they want to be. They lack the experience of the older, more established unions; and they lack the track record.

Each union carefully trains its organizers and usually has a detailed guidebook to cover almost every conceivable situation. It is worthwhile to look at the union adversary and determine the specific campaign strategy being used in your facility. Union organizing attempts primarily incorporate one or more of three steps.

STEP 1: The Hospital Survey. Background information is a necessary part of any campaign. Unless the organizer has a thorough understanding of the hospital, its policies, its key people, its problems, etc., a formalized strategy cannot be developed. Consequently, the first step is to do a "target" survey.

Initially, the organizer spends several hours simply observing the facility, talking to cafeteria employees, workers in housekeeping, nurses, and so on. From such conversations the organizer attempts to determine the number of employees per shift; employee breakdown by sex, age, race, etc.; what eating and drinking facilities are nearby; available transportation facilities for the employees; and special problems the facility might face.

The second part of a survey involves establishing contact with the existing labor movement in the community. Here the organizer determines the labor position of the mass media; the labor history of the organization; names of employees who are active in community work such as churches, civic groups, and politics (these persons often make good initial contacts); names of former employees who belonged to a union; a general idea of wages, conditions, and problems; community relations with the target facility; community reaction to organized labor; and meeting dates and places for local union groups.

STEP 2: Selecting the Employee Leaders. Having completed his initial survey of the facility, the organizer is now ready to make his first contact with the employees of the health care facility. Most union organizers are primarily interested in finding the employee who is respected by his/her fellow workers and who has informal influence within the health care facility. These are the workers that the organizer will depend on for "internal leadership" and information about the specific problems and complaints of the employees.

The labor organizers court potential internal leaders. The benefits of the union are explained, and an attempt is made to build up the trust of the leaders. The organizers try to get leaders for every faction within the organization; for the women, the men, the minority groups, etc. They create committees and encourage mass participation.

The importance of in-house employee organizers cannot be overemphasized. As a Teamsters' Union organizing training manual states,

> . . . the real job of organization will take place inside the plant or shop from day to day and hour to hour under the nose of the foreman or supervisors. The organizer can only implement and give general directions from the outside. The basic job of bringing people together for the common cause can only be successfully done by the group itself under the day to day leadership of key contacts within the plant.[4]

STEP 3: Showing the Union Presence. In Step 3 the union will begin actively to distribute handbills and/or begin seeking authorization card signatures for the purpose of forcing an election. The purpose of this first handout distribution is little more than to show union presence. Such leaflets tend to be general in nature and are usually prepared by the union's international or national office.

Once the "internal leaders" begin bringing the organizer the signed union authorization cards, the organizer dramatically steps up the campaign by seeking the trouble spots, evaluating internal leadership, determining the area in which to build additional support, and determining the best areas for the key supporters within the health care facility.

Demand for Recognition

Early in a campaign the union usually will send a telegram, letter, or even the organizer in person demanding recognition as the official bargaining unit for the health care employees. This demand for recognition usually asserts that:

1. the union has been officially designated as the exclusive bargaining agent by the majority of employees in the bargaining unit,
2. the union is prepared to begin immediate bargaining with management.
3. the union is prepared to present its authorization cards to management or to a third party to validate its claim of majority representation, and
4. the employer should beware of violating its "employees" statutory rights guaranteed under the National Labor Relations Act.

The purpose in sending this demand is to seek voluntary recognition without an election. Failing that, the demand is reflected in the official petition for an election filed to initiate the National Labor Relations Board's election procedures. Health care supervisors should be aware of the dangers in this demand for recognition, however.

An unwary administrator can accept the demand without question (out of fear or uncertainty) and become saddled with a union. Labor counsel should be consulted first. Usually, labor counsel will send a standard letter to the union stating that the hospital doubts that the union represents an uncoerced majority of employees; the hospital believes that the best method for determining the true wishes of the employees is through the secret ballot; the hospital has no knowledge of the method by which the union solicited authorization cards and, thus, cannot accept their validity (management should be certain not to examine the cards or to agree to a third party examination); and the hospital recommends that the union file an election petition with the NLRB, which has jurisdiction over such activities.

Union Authorization Card

The typical union authorization card simply authorizes the union to act as an employee's agent for purposes of collective bargaining with the hospital.

In addition, the card serves four other important purposes. The first one is to satisfy the NLRB's thirty percent showing of interest requirement. In other words, the union must obtain a thirty percent show of interest by signed authorization cards or employees' signatures on a petition to file with the NLRB to hold a secret ballot election (conducted by the NLRB).

Second, the authorization cards are usually a reliable barometer of the employee sentiment within the hospital. Third, authorization cards are useful for an internal purpose. Union organizers are judged by their productivity, measured by the number of new authorization cards that the union organizer reports to his superiors. This, of course, makes it tempting to the union organizer to forge or persuade employees to sign cards without regard to the employees' real interest in the union.

Fourth, a hospital can be ordered by the NLRB to bargain with the union, even if the union lost the election. This can happen if fifty percent or more of the employees have signed authorization cards *and* the employer/hospital commits serious unfair labor practices, which tend to preclude the possibility of conducting a second election.

Having failed to get management to agree voluntarily to collective bargaining, it now becomes necessary to carry the campaign toward an election. The majority of effort is spent on encouraging those that signed the cards to actually vote for the union. Inside the health care facility the prounion employees try to persuade the other employees to support the effort. Participation is the key word in a union organizing attempt. The organizers create all types of committees (whether they need them or not). A union training manual states, "there is always room for more help in a campaign. Participation demonstrates to the individual worker that he/she is helping to build his or her union and to generate enthusiasm for the union within the plant."[5] Committees include, but are not limited to:

1. membership (accumulate potential members, names, groups);
2. publicity (to discuss union information within the facility);
3. distribution (mimeographing, handing out pamphlets, maintaining mailing lists, etc.);
4. strategy (works with organizer in developing tactics and strategies for the campaign effort); and
5. community (to explain the need for the union to the community and to try to get its support).

Another primary purpose for getting as many inside workers as possible on committees is to prevent management from claiming that the union activity is the result of "outside agitation," or to protect from the attack that it is the work of "a minority of disgruntled employees."

OTHER MAJOR UNION TACTICS

Meetings

The major reason for union meetings is to achieve a large turnout, thereby demonstrating solidarity, strength, and enthusiasm and getting the union's message over to the greatest number of employees at the same time.

Because publicly announced meetings always run the risk of being poorly attended, the early meetings are scheduled mostly by word of mouth. Once scheduled, the organizer spares *no* effort in filling the meeting hall. Beer, drinks, etc. are usually the fare. The ploy is "come on over and just hear what we have to say. Even if you don't like it, you can have all the free beer you can drink." Once there, the employee tends to think all the others in attendance are prounion.

The meetings are carefully *staged* with speakers instructed to keep their talks brief and with time always scheduled for a question and answer period. Union promises are seldom specific; they tend to be more general with an emphasis on "we can do it if we stick together." Such meetings always have "good" contracts from other health care institutions available to show "what can be done." Sometimes these contracts stretch the imagination. The authors once discovered that a 500-bed hospital in a high rent area of Philadelphia (recently organized) was the "contract" model used by the union organizing a poor 150-bed unit in a low cost of living area in Texas. The employees were impressed that wages were thirty percent higher. Of course, investigation later showed that the cost of living in Philadelphia was higher by about the same percent.

Before the meeting adjourns, the organizer attempts to secure additional authorization cards. Employees who will take cards and distribute them are encouraged to do so. The organizer notes each member there and tries to schedule a house call as he is introducing himself.

House Call

The house call is considered to be one of the most important tactics in a union organizing campaign. The employee is visited at home, and it is in this environment that the generalities accompanying a union campaign can be dropped. The individual's complaints and problems can be discussed and an explanation given on "how the union can help." It is here that more specific promises can be made. The union member making the house call attempts to get the relationship on a buddy basis . . . making it us (union and employee) against big, old, powerful-autocratic them (management).

Telephone Campaign

In large bargaining units it becomes necessary to limit house calls somewhat and become more dependent upon the telephone. Teams of volunteer callers are set up, and the routine follows the same essential pattern as the house call.

Publicity

Publicity is used as a weapon in every organizing campaign. Publicity efforts include handbills, advertising in the mass media, news releases, union movies, mail sent to homes of the employees, and other such material.

In most of the publicity, the emphasis is on the emotional appeal. Use of such words as dignity, security, justice, fear, threats, self respect, etc., are often used.

Union handbills all have three points in common: (1) they have some type of eye-appealing attraction (usually a cartoon) to get attention; (2) one or (at most) two issues are discussed briefly; and (3) a method of settling the problem (vote union!) is at the bottom of the handout. Sometimes a cartoon can be redrawn and used by management against the union with great success. In one campaign the authors were waging, the union distributed an anti-management handbill. Pictured on the front was a poor hobo with his hand out for a dime saying, "and management said I didn't need a union." The authors redrew this by adding a flag (held up by the hand sticking out) which read "on strike." Needless to say, the union did not appreciate the changes in its own handout.

Warning the Employees

Warning the employees is a favorite ploy of unions. They seek to tell in advance what the hospital will say and do. Obviously, having so much experience (health care management is at a disadvantage here), the union organizer knows specifically what the hospital will say and do; that they will become nicer, will start stating the reasons for employees not needing a union, and so on. Consequently, when the hospital begins to take such predictable measures, the employee is led to think, "Well, if the union was right about this, it must be right about other things." The key to management, here, is to do the unexpected, to take the offense, and to tell the employees what the union is going to do.

ELECTION DAY ACTIVITY

The NLRB will set aside any election if an election speech is made to massed assemblies of employees on hospital time within twenty-four hours before the scheduled time for starting the election. The union, however, still works hard on the last day. They are still out trying to "talk up" the union with employees on a one-to-one basis. They also work to turn out the vote. A committee is usually appointed to watch who has and has not voted. Phone calls are made, and others provide cars for those needing transportation to the polls.

If the union organizer feels (usually the day before the election) that the outcome of the vote will be close or that he might lose, he will increase his challenge of certain voters (those most likely to vote nonunion). Such votes are then placed in a separate envelope and are counted separately (and at a later time). The result of such a ploy is to throw the election outcome into uncertainty. This has certain advantages when the organizer is working to unionize several institutions and does not want a loss on the record for the union at that particular time.

AFTER THE ELECTION

If management wins by a large vote, it is unlikely that the union will file objections to the election. If the majority vote is narrow, however, then objections are almost a certainty.

The union will usually contrive a story for the employee supporters if they lose—that management used unfair labor practices, fired employees for union activities, and so on. Again, the purpose is to make the election loss appear more as a strategic withdrawal than an actual defeat.

WHAT A UNION VICTORY MEANS TO YOU

If the union wins the election and negotiates a collective bargaining agreement with your hospital, you are the one who will have to deal with the union on a daily basis, with the union steward, with the grievances and arbitrations, with the complaints, with the slowdowns, and with the harassment.

As a supervisor your main function is working with employees and making daily decisions about each one. These decisions can involve discipline, discharge, promotion, overtime, work schedules, transfers, job assignments, and any number of others. The point is that in a nonunion status these decisions remain yours and the hospital's and should relate to the overall purpose of a hospital: quality patient care. With a union, however, your actions in all these areas can be the subject of union challenge. To make matters worse, the union steward, an employee picked by the union, is most often an employee with whom you are least able to get along on a day to day basis. Specifically, you will find your management rights drastically limited in these four areas.

Discipline. A union will severely curtail your authority to discipline employees. With a union contract, disciplinary actions such as reprimands or suspensions must first be taken up with the union steward, and perhaps even the business representative of the union. At the time of your action the union will examine your management record for any pattern of employee discrimination or favoritism. Additionally, the union makes discharge, as a form of discipline, a near impossibility.

Promotions. Management authority to promote employees based on job competence and ability to learn is virtually eliminated. Seniority or time in service becomes the main and sometimes only yardstick for measuring an employee's eligibility for performance. In fact, the hospital's refusal to promote a long service employee must have a detailed written justification.

Work scheduling and assignments. The scheduling of work and the assignment of job tasks is vastly com-

plicated by union presence. Job descriptions must be followed to the letter. No task can be given an employee without that task being presented in a formally prepared and negotiated job description. For example, a delivery truck, too large to fit an unloading ramp, recently pulled up to a major unionized hospital in New York City containing badly needed beds for an intensive care unit. Because of its size the truck had to be located away from receiving. The receiving department employees refused to work in other than their designated area, and housekeeping personnel refused to unload because it was not in their job description. Consequently, the unloading of twenty electric beds and all components was accomplished by the supervisors from various departments, including housekeeping, maintenance, nursing, personnel, and administration.

Strikes, walkouts, slowdowns, and sick-ins. The stoppage of work in a health care facility represents a real threat to management and the welfare of patients whom the hospital is dedicated to protect. Strikes, walkouts, slowdowns, or other types of work stoppages can be called by the union for just reason, little reason, or no reason at all—the latter two seeming to be the most predominant. Should a strike occur, the health care facility is literally shut down. The simple delivery of a unit of blood from an outside source becomes a major problem. Violence and sabotage can happen, as evidenced by health care union strikes in such states as New York, Illinois, and California—to name only a few. The only way to avoid such problems is to remain nonunion.

The purpose of this article has been to demonstrate the dynamics of the adversary in a war, which, for nicety, is called a labor union campaign. Obviously, it is to the hospital's best interest to know the tactics of its adversary before developing its own campaign to win the war.

NOTES

1. Dennis Dale Pointer, "How the 1974 Taft-Hartley Amendments Will Affect Health Care Facilities, Part 1," *Hospital Progress* 55, no. 10 (October 1974): 68–70.
2. *Ibid.,* p. 176.
3. *Ibid.,* p. 178.
4. "Some Notes For Trade Union Organizers" (President's Address, Central States Conference on Teamsters, International Brotherhood of Teamsters, 1974).
5. *Guidebook for Union Organizers* (AFL-CIO, Industrial Union Department, 1972).

● DEDICATED
  TO YOUR JOB

Dedication to your job
is an obvious
necessity!

If you weren't
dedicated, you would
not be in the health
care profession!

You care -- that's why you
do what you do! You are dedicated
to do your job

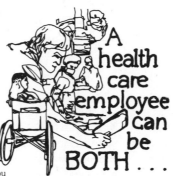

A health care employee can be BOTH . . .

● RESPONSIBLE
  TO YOURSELF

RESPONSIBILITY to
yourself is obviously just
as important!

You must look out for your
own needs -- your own goals
in life in in your work!

You must be responsible for
the welfare of yourself
and your family

If you want to be both DEDICATED TO YOUR JOB AND RESPONSIBLE
TO YOURSELF, then perhaps you should take a serious look at
one of the fastest growing labor organizations for health
care employees, the Hospital and Nursing Home Division of
Retail Clerks International Association.

Throughout the United States, thousands of employees in nursing
homes and hospitals have decided that they no longer wish to be
"second class" citizens when it comes to wages, hours, and
conditions of work. They have seen how the cost of living has
skyrocketed while their pay remains low -- and they have done
something about it!

The Federal Law now protects your right to form a Union and
your right to have a union contract without fear of coercive or
discriminatory action being taken against you by your administrator or supervisors.

Attached you will find a postage-paid, pre-addressed authorization
card. By filling out and mailing this card, you are taking the
first step toward having the true job security and increased
benefits of a union contract that so many of your fellow employees
in nursing homes and hospitals already enjoy.

These cards are confidential and WILL NOT BE SEEN by your
employer!

Fill out and mail your card today! If you want more information
please call 694-5541.

HOSPITAL & NURSING HOME DIVISION

RETAIL CLERKS UNION, LOCAL NO. 455 AFL-CIO
4615 NORTH FREEWAY, SUITE 300
HOUSTON, TEXAS   77022

CLERICAL WORKERS ARE THE UNSUNG HEROINES OF EVERY HOSPITAL

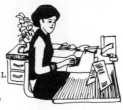

Usually tucked away behind the scenes, its the clerical workers who do all of the paperwork without which any hospital would shut down in confusion inside of 24 hours.

From the accounting office to the switchboard to the supply section, these "paper slingers" keep the administrative wheels turning; they keep the cash flowing and the mails moving. They are the oil that keeps the health machine in working order.

Without a competent, experienced clerical force, any hospital would be in big trouble--in fact, it would be out of business. But while that's the case, hospital administrators will be the last to admit it. Because if they did, hospital clerical workers would be enjoying better wages and benefits than they do today.

It's sad but true that Hospital wages are low--very low. And hospital clerical employees sufer

as much, if not more, than all other hospital employees. Without a union, hospital clerical workers, just like the other employees in the hospital, just don't get a fair shake.

There's a union in town that can help make things a lot better. It's the union that represents more health care clerical workers than any other union in the country. The name is Service Employees International Union, AFL-CIO--a union of more than one-half million members, with 200,00 of those members working in the health care industry.

SEIU local unions from New York to California and virtually all points in between have negotiated collective bargaining agreements that bring recognition to hospital clerical workers--recognition in terms of money,

in terms of benefits like vacations, holidays and health plans, and just plain recognition of your integral role in the life of the hospital.

Hospital clerical workers care about people-- that's why they work in hospitals. Isn't it time you cared about yourself just a little. Start caring today -- check out what SEIU, the nation's largest union of hospital workers, can do for you. Mail the attached card today and get started toward a better deal for yourself right away.

AUTHORIZATION FOR REPRESENTATION

LOCAL 47, SERVICE EMPLOYEES INTERNATIONAL UNION, AFL-CIO

I hereby authorize Local 47, Service Employees International Union, AFL-CIO, to represent me for the purpose of collective bargaining with my employer, and to negotiate and conclude all agreements respecting wages, hours and other terms and conditions of employment. I understand that this card can be used by the Union to obtain recognition from my employer without an election.

NAME _____ DATE _____

EMPLOYEED AT _____

JOB TITLE _____ DEPT. OR DIV. _____

DATE HIRED _____ HOURS PER WEEK _____ HOURLY WAGE RATE _____ SHIFT _____

HOME ADDRESS _____ CITY OR TOWN _____ ZIP _____

SIGNATURE _____ PHONE _____

READ BEFORE SIGNING

LOOK WHAT'S HAPPENING TO YOUR HOSPITAL...

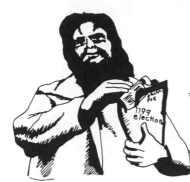

**The <u>Professional Unit of 1199</u> Organizing Committee (medical technologists, pharmacists, social workers, physical therapists, etc) have filed a petition with the National Labor Relations Board to have a secret ballot election for the purposes of collective bargaining.

**The <u>Technical Unit of 1199</u> (LPN's, technicians, etc.) are revising a petition to be filed with the N.L.R.B. for the same purpose.

**Since Nov. 19, 1973, the engineering and maintenance employees of Newport Hospital have enjoyed all the benefits of 1199 membership -- comprehensive medical benefits, significant pay increases, democratic grievance procedure, and full seniority & pension rights.

****

JOIN LOCAL 1199 TODAY!

Don't Be Left Out In The Cold!

Technical, professional and maintenance employees all know the value of organization. They know that behind the door meetings with Mr. Healy will not guarantee their hard earned right to job security and better working conditions. They know that only an organization run by and for hospital employees like 1199 can defend and preserve these rights.

Now the Newport Hospital administration makes all the decisions while YOU do all the work. As members of 1199, employees and administrators sit down as equals to negotiate the <u>employees</u> working conditions. During negotiations, decisions are made after BOTH sides have had their voices heard

Now, only one side has the final work.

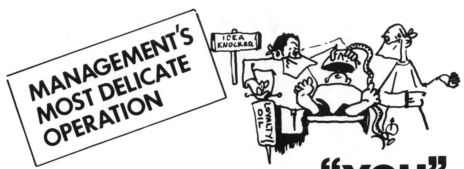

...TAKING THE "YOU" OUT OF "UNION"

If management of Arlington Memorial Hospital has their way, YOU and YOUR fellow employees will NEVER receive the benefits of a GUARANTEED UNION CONTRACT.

Regardless of what Management says, REMEMBER, its YOU and YOUR families wages and working conditions, as outlined below, that will be IMPROVED through a UNION CONTRACT!

.....LIVING WAGES   .....FULL PAID HOLIDAYS

.....EMPLOYER PAID INSURANCE   .....PENSION PROGRAM

WITHOUT A UNION

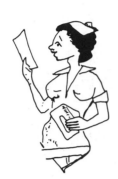

Whose Voice IS Speaking? FOR YOU

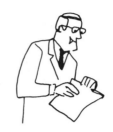

THE HOSPITAL ADMINISTRATOR

TO ALL EMPLOYEES
ARLINGTON MEMORIAL HOSPITAL

What can a Union do for you? It can help you negotiate improvements in
your wages, hours and other conditions of employment. -- Why not have
your employment benefits guaranteed in a signed contract.

DO YOU WANT OPEIU LOCAL 277'S
BARGAINING PROGRAM FOR
YOU?

BENEFITS NEGOTIATED BY OPEIU
AT ANOTHER HOSPITAL
ARE MUCH HIGHER THAN
YOURS!

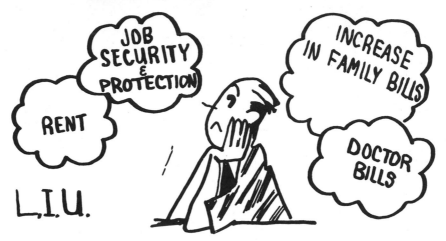

BELOW IS A TEST TO SEE IF YOU NEED
UNION HELP

Please Circle
One

		YES	NO
1.	Do you need a better living wage?	YES	NO
2.	Do you need job security?	YES	NO
3.	Do you need company paid insurance?	YES	NO
4.	Do you need protection from an abusing boss?	YES	NO
5.	Do you need cost of living increases in pay?	YES	NO
6.	Do you need a system of retirement?	YES	NO

IF YOU'RE IN THE HEALTH CARE FIELD AND YOU HAVE ANSWERED

THE ABOVE QUESTIONS YES-YOU NEED A UNION--AFL-CIO LOCAL 1199

ST. JOSEPH'S FOUND <u>GUILTY</u>

On September 19, 1975 the National Labor Relations Board issued a decision in which St. Joseph's Hospital was found guilty of violating your right to a fair election in the following ways.

LYING

In a letter sent to all employees shortly before the election, and signed by Sister Miriam Regina, the hospital claimed that 1199 contract provided for a single flat rate of pay of $2.40 and $2.50 per hour. This of course is not true and the National Labor Relations Board said that it was clear that the statements made by the Hospital were materially false and misleading and substantially misrepresented the wage rates negotiated and won by the Union in other areas represented.

THREATENING EMPLOYEES

In the weeks before the election, dietary employees were questioned by their supervisor about their views on the union. The N.L.R.B. said such questioning was objectionable. The hospital also had a rule forbiding employees from distributing union literature anywhere on the property and asking employees to tell management if they saw any employee break this rule. The N.L.R.B. said that such a rule was not valid.

1199 believes that the majority of service and maintenance employees at ST. Joseph's want a UNION. We believe that a fair election would prove this. The election held on April 17 was NOT FAIR. BECAUSE OF THE LIES AND THREATS ON THE PART OF THE HOSPITAL, YOUR RIGHTS WERE VIOLATED AND THE FEDERAL GOVERNMENT HAS FOUND THE HOSPITAL GUILTY.

Your right to a fair election will be protected. Things have not at all improved at St. Joseph's without a union as you all know. Stick with 1199 and you will win.

"THE DOUBLE DEALER UTTERETH LIES" (Proverbs, XIV, 25)

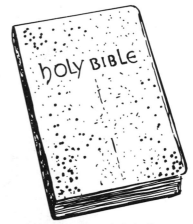

"A righteous man hateth lying"
(Proverbs, XIII, 5)
"A poor man is better than a liar"
(Proverbs, XIX, 22)
"He that speaketh lies shall not escape" (Proverbs, XIX, 5)
"A lying tongue hateth those that are afflicted by it" (Proverbs, XXVI, 28)
"With lies ye have...strengthened the hand of the wicked" (Exekiel, XIII, 22)

IT'S A SIN TO TELL A LIE!

ST. JOSEPH HOSPITAL FOUND <u>GUILTY</u> OF MAKING FALSE AND MISLEADING STATEMENTS OF AN UNLAWFUL NATURE BY THE NATIONAL LABOR RELATIONS BOARD!

If Newport Hospital Can Do This to Us, When Will YOU BE NEXT??

RESIGNATION: 1 LPN

FIRED: 1 Medical Technologist

RESIGNATION: 6 Nurses, due to overwork and understaffing.

"Forced resignation" is the hospital game to get rid of loyal employees who buck the Newport Hospital administration and demand a voice in THEIR hospital. Sometimes the hospital administrators are not so subtle. Sometimes they out and out fire a work, like the woman in the lab.

Now Mr. Robert J. Healey, deputy director of Newport Hospital can freely hire, fire and harass YOU, the unorganized worker. And because you are not united within an organization that can and will protect your needs and problems as working people, the administration can step on you.

What has Healey done since he came to Newport Hospital?

HEALEY PROGRAM FOR NEWPORT HOSPITAL:
Workers are not being replaced when they quit or retire.
Foreced retirement when a worker reached 65 years.
Speed ups on the job.
Forced resignations.
No democratic grievance procedure.
No representation.
Closed door meetings.
Harrassment
****
Want to see an end to The Healey program? Join one of the 1199 Organizing Committees and you'll see some fast improvements. Workers who have already joined are employees like yourself who want to put a stop to the Healey way of doing things.

How Can You Join 1199?

If you want to join 1199 National Union of Hospital and Health Care Workers, or if you just want to get more information about us, attend a very important meeting:

> SUNDAY, February 8, 1976
> Newport Motor Inn
> 1 P.M. or 7 P.M.

LPN's and other workers at Women and Infants' Hospital will talk about their experience with 1199.

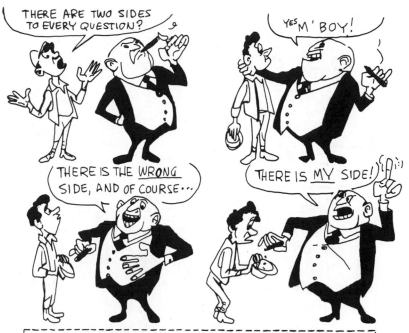

SPEAK UP WITH 1199!

JOIN 1199 today! We'll see that your side is heard because we:

- are organized and led by health care workers
- know and understand the problems of hospital workers
- are experienced and skilled in organizing hospital workers and in negotiating contracts
- can help you organize and win a contract at your hospital that will enable you and your family to keep up with today's cost of living

WE'RE THE ONES TO HELP YOU HELP YOURSELF

ATTENTION! Important Meeting! ATTENTION!

Join us in a frank discussion with several 1199 members in Rhode Island. Find out about how 1199 has improved both their working conditions and patient care

      ***WHEN: Sunday, February 8, 1976
      ***TIME: 1 P.M. & 7 P.M.
      ***PLACE: Newport Motor Inn

Having problems at the hospital? Need more information on 1199? Call (collect) 881-1225, or contact anyone on the organizing committees.

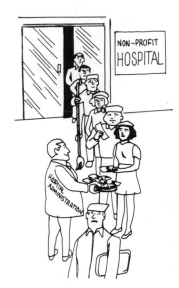

Yes, you. You and your fellow hospital employees contribute millions of dollars each year to the support of the nation's hospitals. How?

Through your low wages. Long hours. Poor working conditions.

Through your lack of a decent health care plan.

Through the lack of a decent retirement plan.

You (like all hospital employees) help to provide a vital service to the American people. You share in maintaining an important and necessary function in the life of every community in the nation.

Yet all the statistics show that you are among the lowest paid workers in your community--when you aren't actually _the_ lowest.

Recent figures show that unorganized hospital workers lag 60 cents an hour (often more) behind the average American worker. When you multiply that by the number of hospital workers it mounts into the millions.

In effect, your low wages and poor working conditions are a forced contribution. Its a subisdy from those who can lease afford it for the benefit of those who can afford it far easier.

You can end this forced charity--as hundreds of thousands of hospital workers have--by joining SEIU. If you're interested in learning more about SEIU and what it can do for you, mail the attached card.

----------------(TEAR OFF AT DOTTED LINE AND MAIL. NO STAMP NECESSARY.)----------------
HOSPITAL WORKERS ORGANIZING COMMITTEE

SERVICE EMPLOYEES INTERNATIONAL UNION, AFL-CIO

YES, I'd like to know more about how SEIU can help me get higher wages and better benefits.

__ Please send me more information.

__ I will help form an SEIU Committee. Please have a union representative contact me.

My name is: ....

My address is: ....Zip...........Phone.........

I work at: ....

Address: ....

SIGNED: ....

ARE YOU MAKING ENOUGH MONEY?

ENOUGH TO FEED YOUR FAMILY THE WAY YOU'D
   LIKE TO?
ENOUGH TO TAKE CARE OF ALL YOUR BILLS?
ENOUGH TO LIVE WHERE YOU'D LIKE TO?

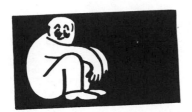

THE ODDS ARE YOU'RE NOT. HOSPITAL PAY
HAS ALWAYS BEEN BAD, AND TODAY INFLATION
MAKES A BAD SITUATION WORSE.

   THERE'S A WAY TO GET A BIGGER PAY-
CHECK--AND BETTER BENEFITS AND TREAT-
MENT ON THE JOB, TOO. IT'S CALLED
SERVICE EMPLOYEES INTERNATIONAL UNION,
AFL-CIO--THE NATION'S LARGEST UNION
OF HEALTH CARE WORKERS.

   THE ODDS ARE THAT SEIU'S HALF-MILLION
MEMBERS IN THE UNITED STATES AND CANADA
ARE LIVING BETTER LIVES THAT YOU ARE.
WHY? BECAUSE WHILE THEY HAVE UNION
CONTRACTS THAT GUARANTEE REGULAR WAGE
INCREASES, YOU DON'T.

   IF YOU WANT A CHANCE TO WIN BETTER
WAGES AND BENEFITS FOR YOURSELF AND
YOUR CO-WORKERS, VOTE FOR THE AFL-CIO'S
SEIU--THE LARGEST UNION OF HEALTH CARE
EMPLOYEES IN THE NATION. UNLESS, OF
COURSE, YOU DON'T THINK YOU NEED THE
MONEY.

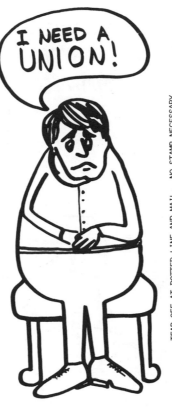

TEAR OFF AT DOTTED LINE AND MAIL. NO STAMP NECESSARY

AUTHORIZATION FOR REPRESENTATION

LOCAL 47, SERVICE EMPLOYEES INTERNATIONAL UNION,
AFL-CIO

I hereby authorize Local 47, Service Employees International Union, AFL-CIO to
represent me for the purpose of collective bargaining with my employer and to
negotiate and conclude all agreements respecting wages, hours and other terms
and conditions of employment I understand that this card can be used by the
Union to obtain recognition from my employer without an election.

NAME _____   DATE _____

EMPLOYED AT _____

JOB TITLE _____   DEPT. OR DIV. _____

DATE HIRED _____   HOURLY WAGE RATE _____   SHIFT ___

HOME ADDRESS _____   CITY OR TOWN _____   ZIP ___

SIGNATURE _____   PHONE _____

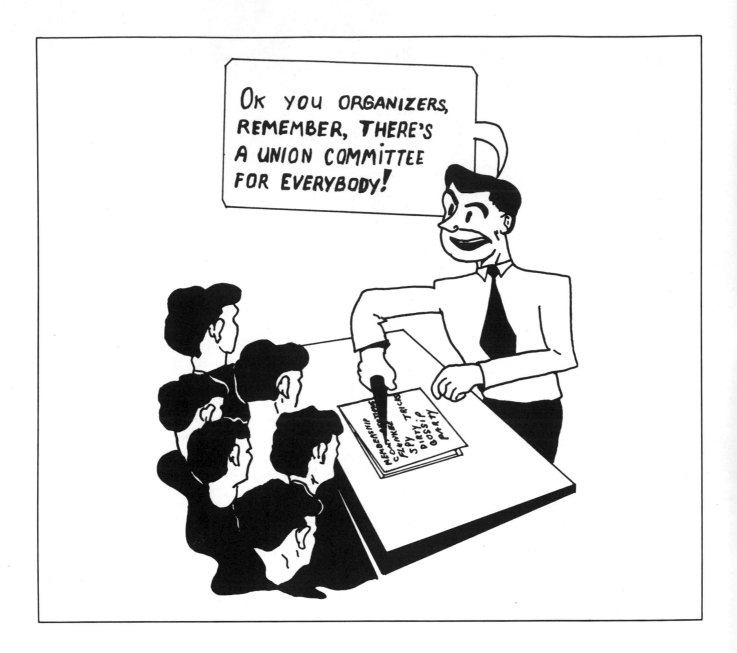

12. How to Deserve What's in Store for You, or, Bad Management

WARREN H. CHANEY and THOMAS R. BEECH

Reprinted with permission from *The Union Epidemic*, by Warren H. Chaney, Ph.D., and Thomas R. Beech, J.D., published by Aspen Systems Corporation, Germantown, Md., © 1976.

Many experts say that no single identifiable cause exists for employees to be receptive to union organizational attempts. It is rather when employees' general feelings about their jobs and working environment are negative that they are responsive to a union's effort. So the real problem is to uncover and consider the employees' subjective perceptions about the hospital. In other words, supervisors too often have an unrealistic sense of their employees' true feelings and actual desires.

All hospitals do not have the same problems that could lead to a union organizing drive. For instance, the discharge of a popular employee in the dietary department of one hospital leads to union organizing activities among all the dietary employees. In other words, the employees themselves may actively seek out the union organizer or make a trip to a local union hall to discuss organizing a particular hospital's employees. Yet in another hospital a layoff or cutback of any employees could result in the remaining employees becoming concerned enough about their job security to seek out a union organizer, or the failure to grant an expected wage increase could cause a union organizing drive.

In other situations, the union organizer just shows up to try and generate employee dissatisfaction and seeks to actively organize a particular hospital's employees. In Houston, Texas, the Teamsters Union made an active citywide solicitation of almost all the hospitals in the area to find the degree of dissatisfaction that existed. They easily gained seven hospital elections by merely getting employees to return mailed authorization cards enclosed in standard brochures.

In other areas of the country, the union can gain major advances in the hospital community by organizing only one major institution in the community. After that successful organizing drive they will spend whatever time necessary to obtain a contract with improved benefits. That contract can then be used as an organizing device for all other hospitals in the community.

Many hospital administrators believe the strongest motivation in all union organizing campaigns is the employees' desire for more wages. However, this simply is not the cause in many, many cases. Over thirty years ago, when the Congress of Industrial Organizations was a very militant organization, they stated, "Workers organize into labor unions not alone for economic motives but also for equally compelling psychological and social reasons."[1]

MERE SIZE OF HOSPITALS CREATES SPECIAL PROBLEMS

Long ago in the mass production industries, such as automobile production and steel mills, it was discovered that the coldness and impersonality of large plants caused workers to feel alienated from their jobs and not a part of any team. Unions have always

659

thrived on this atmosphere and have used it as the basis for mounting an organizing drive.

The same problem is faced in any large health care institution. The union takes advantage of the situation by pointing to the institution as being large and rich with a low wage scale. Hospitals must be aware that their pay scales rank lower than much of the industrial sector. The unions will certainly use this in their arguments; but even more importantly, they will exploit employee alienation.

The larger institution or hospital is also more likely to have internal fragmentation among various working groups. Employees disassociate themselves from the institution itself or the hospital that employs them and instead, identify with fellow employees in a specialty or subspecialty. In hospitals with fifteen or twenty x-ray technicians, it is natural for these employees to cluster together for socializing as well as working purposes. They are going to develop loyalty to the group rather than to the hospital.

Such fragmentation is often reinforced by the hospital itself, particularly since it has to stress job specialization. Employees respond to these specialization requirements by protecting their specialty and emphasizing its importance over other positions or jobs within the hospital. Thus, a very real danger for hospitals lies among its technical and professional employees. A union will have a special appeal to represent their common interests, which they consider separate from others in the hospital.

THE ANSWER IS COMMUNICATION

There is only one sure answer, and that is communication. Administrators and supervisors should talk to their employees on every floor and every shift on a regular basis to find out about their problems and their actual feelings. Supervisors, administrators, and department heads need to be visible to their employees, visible on the floor. They should not wait until the union campaign starts for their subordinates to see them and talk to them for the first time.

Supervisor's Role in the Communication Process

Supervisors in most plants or industrial organizations are clearly designated. But in the hospital community, especially large multipurpose facilities, the lines of supervisory authority are often blurred. Regis-

tered nurses direct the work of the licensed practical nurses (LPN), aides, and orderlies. On other occasions, the LPNs will direct the work of the aides and orderlies. This overlapping can cause confusion and anxiety on the part of the employees. In one recorded case, the LPNs of the hospital were in direct charge of evaluating the aides and orderlies working for them; and in an organizing campaign, certain prounion LPNs threatened the aides or orderlies with bad ratings if they did not assist in getting the union in the hospital.

Supervisors in hospitals are often well educated in modern health care techniques and training methods; but they rarely receive any training in the human relations side of health care supervision, which is another problem in hospitals. As a result, many hospital supervisors are excellent at the technical aspects of their jobs but are too insensitive to their subordinate employees.

The other side of the same problem is that lower level supervisors in a hospital might empathize so closely with employees that the supervisor will actually assist the union organizing campaign, or even openly attend union meetings. Such conduct certainly justifies the termination of such supervisors.

Communications Audit

The day of the attitude survey is about over. Historically, attitude surveys produced only symptoms and opportunities for negativism. The communications audit, therefore, has been developed to discover interruptions in the flow of both informal and formal communication channels. It is possible, through a communications audit, to see the communications network within the health care institution and to pinpoint basic problems, not external symptoms.

In some large hospitals, isolation and alienation become the rule rather than the exception. In the authors' experience, communication audits have revealed that workers often feel like a third hand, useful, but not necessary. The employee feels powerless as an object being controlled and manipulated by other persons in an impersonal work system. If such a worker feels that the system cannot be changed he/she becomes prime bait for unionization.

It is beyond the scope of this article to go into the specific techniques of the audit, but there are a number of excellent references available in the libraries, or one might consider using the services of an independent consultant specializing in such an area. Beyond the communications audit and consultants there are a number of ways by which you can now open channels of communication.

IMPROVING COMMUNICATIONS

Review Your Communications

Take a look at your communications to your employees. These include your policies, your memos, your bulletin board messages, and so on. Do they read like a Department of Health, Education, and Welfare regulation? If so, it is no wonder that employees do not understand hospital policies. Do your communications reflect the "feel" of the organization or do they reflect stagnation? Do they inform or preach? Are they meaningful or meaningless? Do they consider the human interest or take the employee into account? Most importantly, do they encourage feedback?

Encouraging Feedback

A major problem in most health care organizations is the lack of employee feedback. It is interesting to note that in most of our advanced technological computer systems, over sixty-five percent of the system functions to check its own reliabilies. Sadly in management, we often tell the employee as little as possible and as firmly as possible. If we want feedback, and you should, you must:

1. Listen to all the employee is saying. Do not interrupt to explain or justify your action. If you ask for employee feedback, the burden is on you to listen and try to understand.
2. Request more information from employees. When you do have an opportunity to get more information or feedback from an employee, you can help the process by simply saying, "That is really helpful. Can you tell me more?" Or, "Is there anything else I should know?"
3. Make employee feedback a way of life. If the feedback is negative. accept it as being an honest reaction of the individual employee providing it. Express and acknowledge your appreciation for the employee discussing it with you. Do not use it as an excuse to "jump down the employee's throat."

Broadcast—Don't Just Receive

All too often management is guilty of receiving all the communications upward and never reversing the flow by broadcasting. Employees are interested in what management has to say, particularly its reaction to current problems and issues facing employees or the hospital. Naturally those at the top should be informed as to what is going on, but they should never forget to furnish employees with their side of the "two-way street" of communications.

Face to Face Communication

It is a fact that for maximum understanding, face to face communication is the most effective. Too often supervisors become "desk jockeys" and sit behind their two-penned desks, nursing stations, or executive office doors and issue directives, never getting to the floors where the action is.

In all communications, supervisors should use as many channels as they possibly can. If the employee can hear it, see it, touch it, taste it, or even smell it, the communication is going to be more effective. When messages can stimulate multiple senses, the receiver has a variety of reinforcing signals that help greatly to reduce message interference. For example, an employee hearing a message from his/her boss and seeing it in writing has twice the opportunity for confirmation of message content.

Reduce Status Awareness and Social Distance

One of the major barriers to communication in health care is the perceived necessity to maintain social distance and status by imposing such barriers as artificial titles. Status differences are always going to be with you, but if you are to have effective communications and substantially reduce the chances for unionization you need to try to reduce status symbols. How many times have you heard, "Why, if I let my people call me by my first name they wouldn't have any respect for me." If you have a prestigious title this tends to be even more ominous. The end result is that the supervisor is seen as a "title" not a person, and who wants to go to a title with a problem?

We can learn from union organizers by the way they work. They consistently approach the employee on an informal basis, always using their first name, and often with the result that they get more production out of them in a short campaign than a supervisor can get out of the same individual in a year. Respect is not conferred with a title; it must be earned.

Get to Know Your Employees

Getting to know your employees is not only a primary necessity for effective communications but for good management as well. In the authors' experience it has been the rare individual who knows his/her employees on a first name basis. Many say they do but in reality don't. You might want to give yourself the following test:

1. What are the first names of all employees that work for you?
2. What is the name of each employee's spouse?
3. How many children does each have, and what grades are they in?
4. What major illnesses have occurred in the employee's family recently?
5. What hobbies does each of your employees have?
6. What educational or vocational courses has each of them taken?
7. Where does each of the employees live? (Not by street address or number, but in what section of town.)
8. How long does it take for each to get to work, and how does each get to work?

If you took the above quiz and did not know the answers to at least 5 or 6 questions about each employee under your supervision then you are a prime target for a union because you don't really know your employees. Do not make the fatal error of falling back on the lame excuse of "well, I don't know names, but I can remember faces." Research has indicated this isn't the case. One of the authors recently conducted an experiment using fifty executives attending a "memory training" seminar. Photographs of employees who had worked for the managers, many working currently, were flashed on the screen together with faces of employees that worked elsewhere. Also included were faces of people with whom the group had been in conference three weeks earlier. The conferees were asked to name the people shown on the projection screen. If they were unable to name them then they were to identify faces that were familiar. The group failed miserably. The average manager could only name those with whom he/she was having current contact and only by the last name. In addition, they often identified faces they had never seen as being a "face I could never forget."

The point is to care enough to know your employees. If you don't, the union will.

IMPROVING SUPERVISION

The employee in a health care facility is represented by his/her immediate supervisor. In every case when a hospital goes union, considerable blame can be placed at the feet of poor supervision. For example, many of the barriers to effective communication can be overcome only with the help of effective supervisory participation. There are four primary ways to improve supervision.

Develop a Good Selection Procedure

The selection of personnel for a health care organization is a difficult process that involves the matching of the abilities, aptitudes, interests, and personalities of applicants against the specifications of the job. Management should use every possible tool to get the right person on the right job. Such tools include development of current and accurate job specifications and job descriptions. Management also needs data about the applicant for the position, whether the applicant is coming from within or outside of the hospital. Such data can be obtained from the application form, references (that have been validated), background checks, credit reports, validated personality tests, and in-depth interviews with the applicant.

It is important to match the right person with the right job. If you put a good person in a mediocre job, you can count on developing a mediocre person.

Provide Sound Supervisory Training

Unfortunately, too much time is devoted to skills training in hospitals as opposed to supervisory human relations training. When supervisory training is offered it is too often the same timeworn material. It will tell us in what block a person is or should be and what kind of carrot will motivate (actually manipulate) an employee to pull a cart. Seldom is a health care periodical or piece of management literature published without reference to the two-factor theory, the one that says basically, "money doesn't motivate." Yet such research has been proven to be wrong and full of methodological error time and time again—which just goes to show that things are often said because they can be said well, not because they are based on fact.

Good management training teaches a manager how to manage in the present situation as well as in the future. Discussion of the X and Y theory, the managerial grid (which is the same thing) is a good training aid, but it will seldom develop good supervisory personnel.

On the other hand, communication skills and interpersonal skills training can offer supervisory management the opportunity to develop. It is interesting to note that Transactional Analysis (TA), which is thought to be new but is really as old as Aristotle, has been of immense use in management development. TA is a practical and useful system of understanding interpersonal relationships. In reality it is simplified psychology and, as clinicians are finding out, more effective than classical psychology. It is easy to learn and provides a positive communication tool that is immediately usable. It increases a supervisor's on-the-job effectiveness by providing better insights into personalities and transactions that occur among people. Most important, it is a nonthreatening approach to self evaluation and offers a method for not only analyzing people scripts but scripts of organizations as well.

Unfortunately, there are too few qualified people to teach TA in organizations. There are many who try after reading books such as, *I'm OK—You're OK, Born to Win, Games People Play*, etc. These popular books all give an excellent, though superficial, insight into TA but fail to provide the requirements for teaching in a management development situation. The health care manager should watch for the "instant consultant" or the "mini-shrink," who claims to be a management consultant in everything. This, of course, would apply to any consultant who would be considered to be hired to work in your organization. It is sometimes better to pay a little more and get quality than to skimp and get a union.

Management training is extremely vital. If in-house capability is not present, and often it is not due to the prohibitive cost, then consider outside sources such as local universities, qualified consultants, or attend top-notch seminars that are periodically offered by quality organizations such as the American Management Associations, Aspen Systems Corporation, etc. Remember that good management is a skill that must be developed. Few people are born with the natural ability necessary to supervise effectively.

Develop Good Supervisory Evaluation

The supervisor who does not listen, does not talk, does not develop his/her people, and does not care will stay that way unless corrected in a formal evaluation. Such a supervisor is a liability to any organization. Surprisingly there are many hospitals that still have no form of supervisory evaluation, or if they do, it is more perfunctory than practical in nature. A supervisor should receive a rating on a minimum of every six months, but the standard is more likely once a year or not at all.

Maintain High Supervisory Involvement

Getting supervisors into decision-making is essential. To do this involves keeping the supervisors (at all levels of management) informed as to the status of the current operations, providing sources of two-way communications, and periodically getting them involved in the decision-making and goal-setting processes.

The benefits are several. A manager who is part of the decision-making process has more invested in reaching that decision, as does a manager who takes part in the setting of a goal. He has more invested in the achievement of that goal. By the same token, a manager who is involved in creativity has more invested in the outcome of what is created.

DEVELOP A GOOD GRIEVANCE PROCEDURE

Employees who feel helpless to change their working situation are fertile territory for unionization. They feel they are the victims of the system, and management is the persecutor. A union organizer then convinces them that the union can be the liberator by promising the installation of a grievance procedure whereby employees can be guaranteed a fair deal in a management/labor conflict. Every health care organization will benefit if it develops and uses a grievance procedure before any union activity commences. The authors have noted that in many successful unionization campaigns, the hospital did not have or did not use such procedures.

To be effective a grievance procedure should include:

1. A simple written account of the grievance procedure.
2. Varying steps of appeal (usually three is sufficient) through which the employee can seek redress for his/her perceived unfair treatment.
3. Alternate routes of appeal which can be taken by an employee should he/she feel the need to bypass an immediate supervisor. Ordinarily the personnel department is the alternate route. Figure 12-1 presents an example of a grievance system that might exist in a hospital for the nursing department.
4. A time limit must be set for each step, so management is prohibited from delaying the processing of a complaint. This requires the grievance system to have total support of all management, to avoid the possibility of it becoming just a formality for approving management actions. The grievance (large or small) must be acted on in all cases. This is necessary for the system to build integrity.
5. An appeal mechanism for both management and employees. If an employee is turned down on the

Figure 12-1 Nursing Department Grievance Procedure

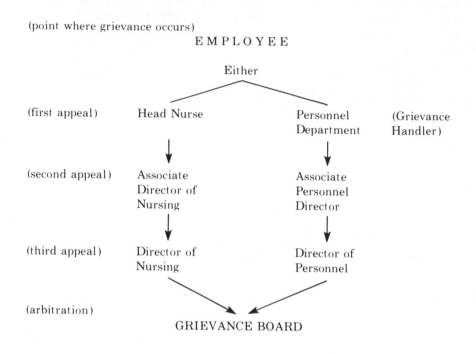

initial appeal or if management feels that the decision was truly unfair, each should have the right to continue on to the next appeal.

6. A final review board for arbitration, containing employees as well as management personnel. True representation must be provided. If employee representation is not provided, then employees usually view the whole grievance process as a mere rubber stamp for the supervisor.

In small organizations a grievance committee or a board of neutral individuals (individuals without vested interest in the outcome) could substitute for a formal grievance procedure. Sometimes an "open door" policy can be used effectively, whereby any employee is free to talk to any level of supervision and express grievances. Though the "open door" policy sounds great and is widely advertised to employees by many managers, especially around union election time, it seldom works. Managers too often feel "bound" to support their supervisors, and they should to a certain extent. Consequently, the final decision process for resolving grievances is best left in the hands of those further removed from the questioned action, and those without vested interests.

DEVELOP GOOD EMPLOYEE EVALUATION AND SALARY ADMINISTRATION POLICIES

Often in a union election campaign, the union will raise complaints about the hospital's pay and promotion policies. Employee evaluation is frequently never done or poorly done. The problem here, of course, is that many hospitals have never faced the responsibility for employee evaluation.

Much of the time an employee is rated on the basis of personality traits, which have little to do with job performance. To compound this problem, job performance is seldom related to pay, so the basic problem becomes evident. The employee is supposed to get paid for the work he/she performs; there should be a connection between pay and work. If there isn't, a natural discrepancy and bad morale most likely will result. The following is a summary of steps of a pay evaluation procedure that the authors have used with great success in various organizations.

1. With input from the employee, develop performance requirements. Both the employee and supervisor should determine how well the employee is expected to do his/her duties.

2. When finalized, discuss the performance requirements with the employee and adjust them periodically, upon mutual agreement, as needed.

3. Observe and discuss current employee performance.

4. The employee's performance should be evaluated against his/her performance requirements.

5. The results of the evaluation must always be discussed with the employee.

6. Action should be taken as a result of the evaluation. Such action could be corrective or advisory in nature, or a raise of pay if justified.

Additional elements that serve to make a good pay-evaluation program include a period of evaluation not less than once a year, with twice or three times being even better. Expectations should be known by both parties (supervisor and employee) and agreed upon in advance of the evaluation. Ordinarily it is good to develop these in writing for the benefit of the employee, as well as the supervisor, and to get consenting signatures.

An appeal process should be available to any employee who is dissatisfied with his evaluation. Ordinarily this can be the grievance procedure system. It is a good idea to get the evaluation commented on or reviewed by the next level of supervision. Any discrepancy between levels of supervision should be reconciled, which is best done by the remaining levels of management. Finally, there should be a written performance review, which should contain positive as well as any negative areas. When negative evaluative criteria are present, corrective action should be given. Such corrective action is best developed by the immediate supervisor and the employee together.

The performance evaluation, when done correctly, can be a powerful tool for employee development. It can also become one of the mainstays for preventive unionism.

DEVELOP FAIR JOB PROMOTION AND JOB TRANSFER POLICIES

Most of the major corporations in the United States long ago recognized the importance of fair job promotion and job transfer policies. They recognized that it is important for an employee not only to know his/her present status within the organization but also the opportunities available within the organization. One method to accomplish this is through job posting.

Job posting is a system whereby all available jobs are posted on a bulletin board. Employees are given this opportunity so they can indicate that they might have an interest in a particular job. Personnel screens the applicants and refers those who are qualified. Each applicant is then notified regarding his/her application for the job and the final action that was taken.

Such a procedure provides the worker with the opportunity of applying for any new position with the same privileges as an "outsider." As often happens, we look outside our organizations for replacements without considering those inside. It is too easy to say, "we do not have anyone qualified." It is more honest to admit that we may be too lazy to even look.

Frequently, the causes of unionism include the lack of clarity and enforcement of management policies relating to the promotion and job transfer. Sometimes these policies seem "hit and miss." This gives the employee a feeling of hopelessness, which is increased if he/she sees better jobs going to "newcomers" who are not necessarily the best qualified. It is important for managers to realize that often good employees are not recommended for promotion because their first line supervisor does not want to lose good people. Management must wage a campaign to win the loyalty of its employees and to turn its "lip service" actions into actual practice.

CONSIDER A RESTRUCTURING OF THE ORGANIZATION

Without a doubt, the structure of an organization influences the relationships within that organization. As health care facilities grow in size, they tend to become impersonal, leaving the employee feeling like a pawn in a huge game of chess. He/she feels far removed from the decision-making process and from those controlling his/her welfare. Oddly enough the same feeling is engendered in managers. With both management and nonmanagement feeling isolated it is no small wonder that communication problems exist and that unionization attempts begin. There are a number of ways management can reduce these dilemmas. The organizational structure of the health care facility might need to be restructured to reduce possible built-in conflicts.

Try Job Enrichment/Enlargement

Job enrichment or enlargement procedures are high-sounding names, which might make a hospital supervisor feel the expert services of the most qualified management consultant or industrial engineer available are required. Such is not the case. Some methods of job enlargement/enrichment are within the realm of every supervisor:

1. Removing some of the management controls over people without removing accountability. By doing this, personal achievement is stimulated within the employees.
2. Providing additional authority, thus giving an employee more opportunity to make decisions. This means increasing job freedom within the job itself. The motivators of responsibility, achievement, and recognition are powerfully stimulated when job freedom is increased.
3. Increasing employees' accountability for their own work.
4. Giving employees a whole natural unit of work to do when possible. Make them responsible for doing it. In many ways we have become too mass-production-minded. The Vega automobile plant realized that in 1972 when their workers went on strike to rebel against mind-confining jobs, e.g., attaching 8,000 bolts to a fender per day. The more complete a job a worker can do, the more achievement-oriented that worker will tend to be.
5. Making informational or periodical reports and the like available to the employee. In this way the employee is made to feel "in on things."
6. Introducing new and more difficult tasks to employees from time to time. These should be tasks that have not been previously handled by the employee, stimulating growth and learning.
7. Assigning specific or specialized tasks to employees from time to time to help them become experts in an area. This not only stimulates growth and learning but motivates the employee for advancement as well.

Job enrichment/enlargement is an excellent way to build up worker morale by increasing the number of intrinsic rewards gained from work activity. Such rewards gained from the work itself are far more satisfying than a supervisor's "pat on the head."

Reduce the Number of Levels of Supervision

Considerable research has proven that professional organizations function better when the management hierarchy is limited. There is no magic number of people who can or should report to a supervisor. You often hear the number "ten," but that is just a myth. The number depends largely on the jobs being done by the employees, the communication required between supervision and employees, and the strengths of the supervisors.

Obviously, if there are ten employees all doing totally separate jobs and each requiring approval of the supervisor, even that number could be too many. On the other hand, if twenty people are doing similar jobs and a minimum amount of actual supervision of activities is required, then the number of employees within the span of management can be increased.

SUMMARY

If unions are promising better working conditions, increased benefits, and wages and employees feel that they can only get these needs fulfilled by voting union, why doesn't management fulfill the promises first?

Unions realize that if there are no problems in communications and if management follows sound practices, they do not have a very good chance of organizing. The organizers spend a considerable amount of their time seeking out the problems in health care organizations to exploit management's weaknesses or management's failures. If unions promise employees that they have the remedy for management's failures, then it is only logical to assume that management can implement that remedy and do it first.

Specifically, this article has recommended that the health care facility: (a) consider a communications audit to determine its current problems in communications; (2) improve communications through review and feedback, maintaining open communication by both broadcasting and receiving, using multimedia communication, and reducing status awareness and social distance; (3) get to really know your employees as individuals; (4) improve supervision through good selection, training, evaluation, and involvement; (5) develop fair grievance procedures; (6) develop good employee evaluation and salary administration policies, as well as good job promotion and transfer policies; and (7) consider restructuring the organization through job enlargement and reduction of the management hierarchy.

In summary, though these suggested remedies might appear to be defensive, they should represent those things we would want to do, not because we fear any union, but because we are interested in the employee and the enhancement of health care that will benefit the patient as a result of the mature development of all the organization's supervisors and employees.

NOTE

1. C. S. Golden and H. J. Ruttenberg, *The Dynamics of Industrial Democracy* 3 (Cleveland, University of Ohio Press, 2d. ed., 1942) p. 314.

13. Negotiating the Collective Bargaining Agreement

RALPH F. ABBOTT, JR., BRIAN E. HAYES, JAY M. PRESSER,
MARTIN E. SKOLER, AND JAMES N. TRONO

Reprinted with permission from *Health Care Labor Manual,* Vol. 1, by Skoler & Abbott, P.C. attorneys at law, Springfield, Mass. (Martin E. Skoler, Ralph F. Abbott, Jr., Brian E. Hayes, Jay M. Presser, and James M. Trono; (Editor-In-Chief, Brian E. Hayes) published by Aspen Systems Corporation, Germantown, Md., © 1974.

INTRODUCTION

Following an election in which a union has been certified as the exclusive bargaining agent of employees in an appropriate unit, the health care employer's legal obligation under federal law and many comparable state laws is to *bargain in good faith* with the union. There may be no more complex or important administrative task for the health care facility than negotiating a labor agreement, especially a first agreement.

The stakes at the bargaining table are high. A poorly negotiated contract may deprive management of flexibility and authority necessary to make the institution viable. A wage bargain that is poorly conceived or miscalculated may make the institution's patient-care costs unreasonably high and threaten its very survival.

The collective bargaining process, complex and closely regulated by law, might be understood most readily by studying some commonly asked questions:

1. How should the management team be chosen?
2. What preparations should be made before bargaining begins?
3. What are the mechanics of the collective bargaining process with respect to the time, place and length of sessions? What are desirable sessions? What are desirable ground rules? What information must be shared with the union?
4. What should the health care executive know about the composition and strategies of the union bargaining team?
5. What is "good faith" bargaining? What subjects *must* the employer bargain about, and what subjects may the employer refuse even to discuss with the union?
6. What significant differences are there between a first contract and successor contracts?
7. How can the union's wage and benefit demands be "costed out" in order to understand their long-term impact on the facility's budget?
8. What contract clauses are uniquely important for the health care institution to protect its managerial flexibility?
9. What contract clauses will the union view as uniquely important to its self-interest?
10. How can trade-offs or compromises be achieved?
11. How can a union's unrealistic proposals be disposed of?
12. How should the management negotiating team treat strike threats?
13. What kinds of notes or records should be kept of negotiations? Should tape recordings be made? Should there be a verbatim transcript?

LEGAL ASPECTS OF THE BARGAINING OBLIGATION

Collective bargaining is usually defined as the bilateral *process* of reaching an agreement between an agent representing employees and an employer with respect to wages, hours, and other terms and conditions of employment. The opposite of collective bargaining is individual bargaining between employee and employer: The employer is legally free to make unilateral changes in employment conditions whenever it likes and the employee is free to negotiate the best deal he can for himself.[1]

The Wagner Act of 1935 significantly changed the structure of American labor-management relations. That law established a framework for statutory collective bargaining, requiring the parties to deal with each other, and established the National Labor Relations Board (NLRB) to police compliance with the law. Between 1935 when the Wagner Act was passed and 1947 when the Taft-Hartley Act was passed, the NLRB began, on a case-by-case basis, to give substance to the bargaining obligation created by the law. The Taft-Hartley Amendments of 1947 confirmed many of the NLRB's early decisions that defined and applied the statutory duty to bargain. In particular, Congress added a new section to the law in 1947, Section 8(d), which defines the obligation to bargain in good faith. It is:

> the performance of the mutual obligation of the employer and the representative of the employees to meet at reasonable times and confer in good faith with respect to wages, hours, and other terms and conditions of employment, or the negotiation of an agreement, or any question arising thereunder, and the execution of a written contract incorporating any agreement reached if requested by either party, but such obligation does not compel either party to agree to a proposal or require the making of a concession . . .

This definition of good faith bargaining can be more easily understood by examining its seven major elements: *First*, the duty to bargain in good faith applies to *both* parties, employers and unions. *Second*, it requires the parties to meet at "reasonable times." This language has been interpreted to mean that the parties must not only meet at a reasonable hour of the day, but also that they must spend a reasonable amount of time in the bargaining process. It is illegal, for example, for one party to impose an arbitrary time limit on bargaining of one hour a week. *Third*, the parties are required

to "confer in good faith." What is "good faith"? Hundreds of NLRB decisions provide answers in different factual settings. But "good faith" might also be understood more readily by looking at two dimensions: one objective and the other subjective. These will be discussed below. *Fourth*, the parties are required to bargain about three kinds of subjects: "wages, hours, and other terms and conditions of employment." These subjects are extremely broad and elastic. Subjects that come within these three categories are called *mandatory* subjects of bargaining. It is illegal for a party to refuse to discuss a mandatory subject. But all other subjects are discretionary; a party may but is not legally obliged even to discuss them. *Fifth*, if the parties reach an agreement, they must reduce their agreement to writing at either party's request. *Sixth*, the obligation to bargain in good faith does *not* require either party to agree with the other or to make a concession or even to make counterproposals. *Seventh*, whenever collective bargaining involves employees of a health care institution, certain notices must be served upon the other party prior to the start of the actual bargaining,[2] upon the Federal Mediation and Conciliation Service, and any appropriate state or territorial agency during the course of the bargaining.[3]

These seven aspects of the duty to bargain should be carefully reviewed by the novice negotiator. In labor law, as in most phases of the law, ignorance of one's legal obligations is no excuse.

The seventh aspect of collective bargaining, which involves the notice requirements imposed on both parties, will be fully discussed below. The new health care amendments changed the existing law contained in Section 8(d) of the Act with respect to such notices, and it is imperative that a health care administrator acquaint himself with the new amendments.

Initial Contract Negotiations

Where a union has been certified as a bargaining agent by the NLRB, the parties usually will then engage in collective bargaining for the first time. In the event the parties cannot reach agreement, a new provision in the law, Section 8(d)(B),[4] requires a union to give at least 30 days' written notice of the existence of a dispute to the Federal Mediation and Conciliation Service (FMCS) and any appropriate state or territorial labor agencies. The new Section 8(d)(C) requires the FMCS, upon receipt of notice of an initial contract dispute involving a health care institution, to promptly communicate with the parties and attempt by mediation conciliation to bring them to agreement.[5] Such meetings are not discretionary; the parties are mandated to participate fully and promptly.[6] Apparently, any party in a health care institution dispute who refused to participate fully and promptly in mediation meetings undertaken by the FMCS would be refusing to bargain and would be violating either Section 8(a)(5) or 8(b)(3) of the Act.[7] It should be stressed that while the duty to participate in mediation is mandatory, any solutions or suggestions put forth by the mediator are not binding on either party.[8]

Another aspect of the 30-day notice to the FMCS is its relation to Section 8(g) of the Act which calls for a 10-day notice to the health care institution of an intent to strike or picket that institution.[9] Section 8(g) makes it clear that the 10-day pre-strike or picketing notice is to be read in tandem with the Section 8(d)(B) 30-day notice to the FMCS requirement, thereby imposing a 40-day period before a strike or picketing can commence after an impasse in initial contract negotiations. (*See* Chapter 7 of the Volume of *HCLM* from which this is reprinted for a detailed discussion of Section 8(g).)

Under the new Section 213 of the Act, if within 10 days of the notice to the FMCS, the Director of the FMCS determines that a threatened strike would interrupt the delivery of health care in the affected locality, he may convene a Board of Inquiry to determine the facts and to make a recommendation for settlement.[10] If such a board is convened, it must make its report within 15 days.[11] During this entire period, the parties must continue bargaining and mediation and only if no agreement is reached within the 30 days of filing the notice with the FMCS may a union then file its 10-day notice of intent to strike or picket.

Figure 13-1, developed by the FMCS, reflects the notice requirements for health care institutions which are applicable to the negotiating of an *initial agreement*.

Contract Renewal Negotiations

Any party desiring to change or modify a labor agreement involving employees of a health care institution must serve written notice of such intention upon the other party to the contract 90 days (instead of the usual 60-day requirement for other industries) prior to the actual or proposed termination or modification date.[12] While neither the law, nor its legislative history, makes it clear to whom at the institution a union must send the 90-day notice, it is the General Counsel's opinion that such notice should be served on someone who has been designated to receive the notice or through whom the institution will actually be notified.[13]

Figure 13-1 Initial Agreement Notice Requirements

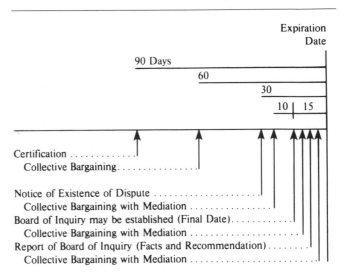

Sixty days prior to the expiration of the agreement (instead of the normal 30 days), the party desiring the change must give written notice to the Federal Mediation and Conciliation Service (FMCS) and any appropriate state or territorial agencies.[14] Thereupon, the mandatory mediation will begin shortly thereafter.

Another facet of the new law is that if within 30 days after notification to the FMCS, the director of the FMCS determines that a threatened strike would interrupt the delivery of health care in a locality, he may set up a Board of Inquiry to determine the facts in dispute and to make a recommendation for settlement.[15] The director's decision to set up a Board of Inquiry is discretionary and is subject only to limited judicial review.[15a]

The timing of FMCS's appointment of a Board of Inquiry has been challenged successfully by a group of private nonprofit hospitals. The hospital's view, that FMCS cannot appoint a Board of Inquiry unless it does so within 30 days of actual receipt of notice of the dispute, was upheld by the Fourth Circuit Court of Appeals. The court issued an injunction barring the Board of Inquiry from convening in this case. The court agreed with the hospital that Board of Inquiry appointments must be made within thirty days of receipt of notice. FMCS had argued that the thirty-day period extends from the last permissible day on which FMCS must be notified (60 days prior to the expiration of the contract), not from the day on which FMCS actually receives notice.[16] In a similar case, the Ninth Circuit Court of Appeals agreed with this interpretation of the LMRA.[17]

The Board of Inquiry must issue its report within 15 days of its establishment and the parties to the dispute are required, except by mutual agreement, to maintain the status quo from the time of the establishment of the board until 15 days following the issuance of the report.[18] Again, it should be noted that the Board of Inquiry, if convened, cannot force a given solution on either party but may only make recommendations for settling the dispute in a prompt, peaceful, and just manner.

As to the 10-day notice of intent to strike or picket a health care institution provided for by Section 8(g), it is clear from the legislative history that such a notice may be given before or after the commencement of the final ten days of the conciliation period where one party wishes to terminate or modify an existing agreement.[19] Thus in a contract renewal situation, the union could serve a 10-day notice at the same time as a 90-day notice or during the 90-day period.

The FMCS has prepared a second chart (Figure 13-2) reflecting the notice requirements for health care institutions involved in *contract renewal* negotiations.

ATTITUDES IN BARGAINING: WHAT IS "GOOD FAITH"?

The most complex and subtle requirement of the federal law is that the parties negotiate in "good faith." The National Labor Relations Board and courts have said that a good faith attitude is one in which one has *an open mind* and a sincere desire to reach agreement. This is a highly subjective determination that can be made only by a careful survey of the external and surrounding circumstances.[21]

Figure 13-2 Contract Renewal Notice Requirements

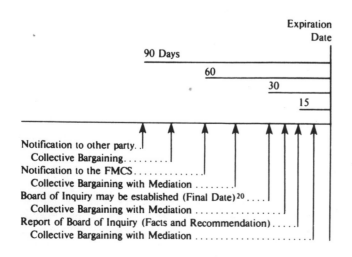

To take a clear example, a party would violate the bargaining obligation of Section 8(a)(5) by refusing to engage in rational dialogue about the issues in dispute. The National Labor Relations Board and the courts have said that discussion and exchange of views about the issues are so fundamental to the processes of collective bargaining that an out-of-hand rejection of a proposal is itself evidence of bad faith.[22] Hence, an intransigent insistence by one party that its offer be accepted or the other's rejected—without discussion—is an unfair labor practice.

Although one ingredient of good faith bargaining is a willingness by each party to discuss the other's proposals, *mere discussion* is not enough. Many NLRB decisions have dealt with "surface" or "shadow" bargaining in which one party (usually the employer) engages in extensive discussion but never reaches agreement on anything.[23] The failure to reach agreement or to make a concession alone does not constitute bad faith bargaining. But, in combination with other factors, unwillingness to reach common ground on any significant issue might be viewed—in a totality of the circumstances—as convincing evidence that a party's attitude lacks requisite good faith. For example, in negotiating an initial contract, if an employer refused to reduce to writing and to put into a contract the employer's own personnel rules and practices, the board has frequently ruled that the employer's attitude indicated bad faith.[24]

The board has also found bad faith in the following circumstances: the employer comes to the bargaining table unprepared to negotiate;[25] the employer delays making counterproposals in an extended period of time or otherwise engages in dilatory tactics;[26] the employer presents offers to the union that require union relinquishment of most bargaining rights;[26a] the employer fails to appoint a negotiator who has authority to reach agreements;[27] the employer reneges on prior commitments;[28] the employer undermines the union's bargaining team by refusing to allow uncompensated leave for an employee bargaining for other units;[28a] or the employer undermines the union's authority by dealing directly with employees.[29]

The Board and a circuit court recently ruled that an employer's "bonus" payment to non-striking workers was indicative of bad faith bargaining.[29a]

It bears reemphasis that the failure to reach agreement with the union is not itself unlawful, for there may be many reasons why an employer, bargaining in good faith, might fail to reach agreement. The union's position might be unreasonable for example, and the law does not require an employer or a union to sacrifice its basic economic interests or abandon any legitimately held economic position in order to reach an accommodation. Similarly, a union may strike to achieve its objectives, no matter how excessive they may be, and an employer may lockout employees or force them to strike over unreasonable management positions.

The line between subjective good faith bargaining and bad faith bargaining is often very thin. Each case is unique; no automatic formula can ensure an employer that its conduct will be regarded as lawful at the bargaining table.

Especially important to management is the question of its right to negotiate a strong management rights clause. May an employer *insist* on such a clause to the point of impasse? In the leading *American National Insurance Company* case of 1952, the employer proposed a management rights clause which would have reserved to management complete authority over promotions, discipline, and work schedules. The NLRB ruled that management insistence upon this clause proved that management lacked good faith. But the Supreme Court disagreed. It held that the employer's proposing and insisting upon that clause was not in itself a violation of the Act.[30]

If an employer may insist to the point of impasse on a strong and broad management rights clause, may it similarly present the union with a complete bargaining package from which it refuses to budge? Such bargaining posture is popularly known as Bulwarism, a form of tough take-it-or-leave-it bargaining usually associated with the General Electric Company and its former vice-president, Lemuel C. Bulware. In a major case that examined G.E.'s bargaining tactics in 1960, the NLRB and the U.S. Court of Appeals in New York ruled that G.E.'s *total pattern* of conduct in the 1960 negotiations reflected an unwillingness to view the union's proposals with an open mind.[31] Legal experts regard this case as highly exceptional and unique. Many legal observers believe that take-it or leave it bargaining is not condemned as such, but that the case indicates a determination to examine carefully the total pattern of an employer which pursues such a negotiating strategy.

Providing Information to the Union in Negotiations

The NLRB and the courts have said that collective bargaining ought to focus on *rational* decision making. Thus, if an employer takes a bargaining position based on information in its sole possession, and if the union asks to examine that information to enable it to engage in intelligent bargaining, the employer may be obliged to provide that information to the union.[32]

What kind of information is the union legally entitled to demand? In general, it is entitled to information that might aid it to perform its duties as bargaining agent in negotiating or administering the contract.[33] A union is not entitled to demand information which it already possesses, nor may it make a demand for the purpose of embarrassing or harassing the employer.[34] The NLRB has approved requests for information relating to present and past wage rates, fringe benefits, job categories, and various types of relevant information about employees in the bargaining unit.[35] The guiding principle is that an employer may not withhold information in its exclusive possession that might aid the union in the responsible performance of the union's bargaining obligation.

The Supreme Court's leading decision on the subject is the *Truitt Manufacturing Co.* case. There an employer pleaded financial inability to grant a union's wage demands. The union then asked for the opportunity to examine the employer's financial records to verify the employer's claim. When the employer declined this request, the union processed a refusal to bargain charge which was, ultimately, sustained by the U.S. Supreme Court, which commented:

Good-faith bargaining necessarily requires that claims made by either bargainer should be honest claims. This is true about an asserted inability to pay an increase in wages. If such an argument is important enough to present in the give and take of bargaining, it is important enough to require some sort of proof of its accuracy. And it would certainly not be farfetched for a trier of fact to reach the conclusion that bargaining lacks good faith when an employer mechanically repeats a claim of inability to pay without making the slightest effort to substantiate the claim.

* * * *

We do not hold, however, that in every case in which economic inability is raised as an argument against increased wages it automatically follows that the employees are entitled to substantiating evidence. Each case must turn upon its particular facts. The inquiry must always be whether or not under the circumstances of the particular case the statutory obligation to bargain in good faith has been met.[36]

In a more recent decision the high court agreed with the NLRB that an employer's duty to bargain includes an obligation to grant a union's request for "relevant" information during the life of the contract to enable the union to act intelligently in processing grievances.[37]

Some employers have avoided the risk of having to supply a union with that financial data which would be required under the rule enunciated in the *Truitt* case by carefully phrasing their bargaining positions in terms of an *unwillingness*—as distinguished from an inability—to grant the union's proposed wage increases.

Frequently cases involving requests for information arise during bargaining, but, long before the legal dispute over the union's demand for information is satisfied, the parties compromise their differences and execute a new labor agreement. Does the execution of the collective bargaining contract wipe out or waive the union's right to such information? No. An unfair labor practice proceeding might be litigated long after the contract itself has been finally consummated.[38]

The U.S. Supreme Court has held that an employer may lawfully refuse to disclose to a union the aptitude test questions and individual scores of employees who have not authorized the release.[39] The union had maintained that it needed the tests and scores to properly process promotion grievances. The Court pointed out that the employer had promised confidentiality of scores and that release of actual test questions would impair the future use of the test. The Court's decision reversed the NLRB's decision that the employer had violated its duty to bargain.

SUBJECT MATTER OF NEGOTIATIONS

As indicated earlier, the Labor Act does not require parties to bargain over all subjects, only over those that fit within the three broad categories of "wages, hours, and other terms and conditions of employment" (Section 8(d)). Subjects that fall within these categories are known as "mandatory" or "statutory" subjects of bargaining, and it is illegal for either party to refuse to negotiate about them. Subjects that fall outside these categories are known as "permissive" or "discretionary" subjects.[40] The parties *may* but are not legally obliged to bargain these subjects. It is, moreover, illegal to precondition negotiations on agreement upon a permissive subject or to bring negotiations to an impasse because of insistence upon a permissive subject.[41] Furthermore, it is unlawful for a union to strike or for management to lock out employees over permissive subjects.[42]

In a 1978 case, for example, the NLRB ruled that an employer violated its bargaining obligation by insisting to the point of impasse on its proposal to change the scope of the bargaining unit that had been officially certified by the NLRB. The scope of a bargaining unit, the NLRB reasoned, is not a mandatory subject of

bargaining because it does not fall within the prescribed bargaining subjects of "wages, hours and other terms and conditions of employment."[43]

The list of *mandatory* subjects is long, and it includes most of the traditional and familiar issues in American labor relations. The subject of *wages* includes, for example: hourly rates,[44] salaries, piecework[45] and incentive rates,[46] overtime,[47] shift differentials,[48] holidays,[49] vacations,[50] severance pay,[51] bonuses (except for genuine gifts),[52] pensions,[53] insurance,[54] welfare plans,[55] profit-sharing plans,[56] stock purchase plans,[57] rents for employer-operated housing,[58] the price of food in employer-operated cafeterias,[59] and employee discounts.[60]

The subject of *hours* includes: length of the work day;[61] days of work, including Saturday and Sunday work;[62] and work schedules, including the number, length and hours of shifts.[63]

More complex is the third and elastic category—"other terms and conditions of employment." It includes the following examples: seniority,[64] union security arrangements,[65] grievance procedures and arbitration,[66] workloads,[67] productivity standards,[68] union access to the employer's premises,[69] vacations and holidays,[70] subcontracting,[71] performance of bargaining unit work by supervisors and others,[72] promotions,[73] layoffs,[74] mandatory physical examinations,[75] health and safety matters,[76] compulsory retirement,[77] management rights,[78] employee rules,[79] no-strike obligations,[80] the physical, logistical and other arrangements for negotiations,[81] and "zipper" clauses.[81a]

The U.S. Supreme Court has endorsed a consistently applied NLRB policy and ruled that the prices of food served in an employee cafeteria and in vending machines are within the meaning of "terms and conditions of employment" and are, therefore, mandatory subjects of bargaining.[82] The Court held that, because the employer had retained the right to review and control the prices, it violated Section 8(a)(5) by refusing to bargain over the prices. The Court left open the question of whether the inauguration of in-plant food services where none already exists is a mandatory subject of bargaining.

In *Medicenter, Mid-South Hospital*,[83] the NLRB held that a requirement that employees submit to a polygraph test as a condition of continued employment was a mandatory subject of bargaining.

The permissive or discretionary subjects include *everything else*. In practice, the most familiar of these subjects include the following examples: changes in the certified bargaining unit,[84] inclusion of supervisors and other persons in the bargaining unit who have been excluded by the NLRB in a unit decision,[85] naming as a party to the collective bargaining agreement someone other than the certified union,[86] performance bonds,[87] internal union affairs,[88] the use of a union label,[89] employer contributions to industry promotion funds,[90] the settlement of unfair labor practice charges,[91] and management's right to go out of business completely.[92]

Union recognition is not a mandatory subject of bargaining. An employer planning to move to a new location who insisted to the point of an impasse on including a clause in the contract calling for termination of recognition of the union at the time that it ceases operations at its nursing home violated Section 8(a)(5) of the LMRA.[93]

It is also well established that a decision to file a lawsuit or petition for review of a Board order is not a mandatory subject of bargaining.[93a] Obviously such a lawsuit does not affect the working relationship, but rather concerns itself with the relationship between the union and the employer. Thus, in a more recent case, a union violated Section 8(b)(3) when it struck over an employer's refusal to withdraw a petition for court review of a Board order concerning pension contributions.[93b]

The issue whether "interest arbitration" (whereby a neutral party resolves deadlocked contract issues for the parties) is a mandatory or permissive subject of bargaining was decided by the Board in late July 1975.[94] The majority of the Board agreed with the Administrative Law Judge who ruled that interest arbitration clauses are nonmandatory subjects of bargaining. However, the Conference Report on the new Section 213[95] appeared to encourage "interest arbitration" in the health care field.

In its first decision dealing with interest arbitration in the health care field, the NLRB ruled that the Massachusetts Nurses Association violated the Act by bargaining to impasse on this nonmandatory subject of bargaining.[96] The parties remain free to agree voluntarily on an interest arbitration provision.

SELECTING A NEGOTIATOR

Negotiating a labor agreement differs in many respects from negotiating other kinds of contracts. Not only does it require specialized knowledge of the subject matter of labor-management relations, but it also requires an understanding of and sensitivity to the dimension of labor relations.

A question commonly asked by health care institutions is whether it is desirable to engage the services of an outside, professional negotiator, such as a management lawyer.

Many large profit and nonprofit employers have in-house, staff resources for labor negotiations and do not need outside consultants. Smaller institutions which lack in-house staff resources often find that it is sensible to engage the services of a management attorney to serve as chief negotiator. While lawyers frequently make good negotiators because of their experience and training, not all lawyers are equally skilled in labor negotiations. For this reason it is prudent to inquire about the background and reputation of management lawyers in the community before making a selection. Moreover, it seems obvious that a management negotiator who has had bargaining experience in the health care field would be a better choice—all other things being equal—than one who has not. There are also a number of nonlawyers who have expertise in negotiations. The advantage of engaging a lawyer is that he will be professionally qualified to represent the institution in the event that any circumstances at the bargaining table lead to unfair labor practices before the NLRB or litigation in the courts.

It is generally believed that the single, most important labor contract that the institution will ever negotiate is its *first* collective bargaining contract, for this establishes the environment and attitudes that will shape future relations between the parties. Moreover, experience proves that language which the parties insert in their initial contract often becomes deeply imbedded in their collective bargaining relationship and hard to eliminate. Therefore, the chief negotiator at the bargaining session for the first contract plays a very important role.

The role of the chief negotiator is one that varies. In most cases, the chief negotiator is the *only* member of the management team who actually speaks for management in negotiations. Thus, he is not only the head of the management team, but he is the one who articulates authoritatively management's point of view on the issues. To perform his assignment effectively, he must be someone who can work harmoniously with the other members of his team, who enjoys the respect of the union's negotiators, who has a reputation for integrity and fairness, and who is known to keep his word.

CHOOSING THE MANAGEMENT TEAM

The first step management must take before bargaining begins is selecting its negotiating team. Because of occasional efforts by unions in the 1930s and 1940s to interfere with management's choice of its own negotiators, Section 8(b)(1)(B) of the Taft-Hartley Act expressly prohibits such union interference.[97]

It is almost always desirable for management to be represented by a *team,* rather than by a single negotiator. It may be essential, for example, to have more than one witness who can prove what was said and done at the bargaining table. Several heads, moreover, are usually better than one in devising strategies and analyzing the strategies of the other side. Further, a single negotiator is unlikely to be as knowledgeable about the complex personnel practices and technology of the modern health care facility as is a carefully selected team.

Every bargaining team should have a "chief negotiator," the principal spokesperson for management. If he is knowledgeable and experienced, he will guide management's team with the skill and sensitivity of a surgeon in an operating room. It is he who should do *all* of the talking for management, except when he believes it advisable to encourage discussion by other members of the team. He is usually the chief strategist as well as the main spokesperson for management.

Other members of the team should normally include the chief administrator or his assistant, the chief personnel officer and such other representatives of the institution as may be needed to advise the chief negotiator on issues that are likely to arise. Of course, management has the right to expand and contract its bargaining team as circumstances require. On one day it may be desirable to have the institution's chief financial officer at the bargaining table, but the same may not be true another day. Often the negotiating team should be advised by a *separate* committee of staff representatives, who can react intelligently and quickly to the negotiation team's reports of the progress made at the bargaining table.

Members of the management team must be prepared to make a *major* commitment of time, for the process of labor contract negotiations is enormously time consuming. It may consume whole weeks of an executive's time. The team must also be capable of exercising restraint, patience and a sense of humor in the face of angry provocation, for bargaining often becomes heated and unpleasant. A few union negotiators have been known to deliberately provoke and insult management negotiators as a method of proving to the union's rank-and-file negotiating team that the union is "tough."

While management's team should include key representatives of the institution, it should not be too large. Rarely, for example, should the management team be larger than four or five persons. The larger the bargaining team, the less manageable it becomes and the more likely it is that disagreements will occur between members of the team. Large bargaining teams also increase the risk that "leaks" of confidential strategies might occur and the possibility that the institution's staff time might be wasted.

PREPARING FOR NEGOTIATIONS

Collective bargaining, contrary to popular misconceptions, is not simply a table-pounding, name-calling confrontation. On the contrary, often it is in the nature of a quiet discussion—a dialogue related to specific, relevant data that both parties prepare before bargaining. Even when bargaining is heated and emotional, its focus is usually on specific data and substantive arguments.

The data that should be collected before negotiations depends, of course, on the issues in controversy. Typically, management collects the following kinds of data before negotiations begin.

1. *Cost of Living.* The Consumer Price Index (C.P.I.), prepared by the Bureau of Labor of the U.S. Department of Labor, is issued monthly. It is widely regarded as the most reliable monitor of changes in the cost of retail goods and services. These data are commonly discussed at the bargaining table as grounds for considering whether employees are entitled to increased wages in order to stay even with inflation. Information about the C.P.I. is available from regional offices of the Bureau of Labor Statistics or from the U.S. Department of Labor's excellent monthly magazine, *The Monthly Labor Review.*

2. *Comparability.* Perhaps the single most important factor in wage negotiations is "comparability," which simply means wage comparisons. Labor and management usually agree in principle that an employer should not be expected to pay wages that are significantly lower or higher than wages paid by similar employers for the same kind of work in the community. For this reason, it is customary for negotiators to look with great interest at data bearing on comparative wages.

How does one establish what comparative wages are? A comparison can be made by referring to reliable and relevant wage surveys. They are published by the U.S. Department of Labor and state agencies. Large employer associations also conduct wage surveys, and individual employers commonly conduct their own.

A wage survey is a statistical study of wages (and/or benefits) paid to workers in a defined job classification or industrial classification at a given point in time. In the case of unionized employers, it may be easy to determine their wage rates by examining their collective agreements. A second and more common method is to circulate a questionnaire among employers.

3. *Ability to Pay and Other Economic Data.* A third type of information concerns the economic status of the institution. If the institution's economic future looks bleak, when bargaining this fact ought to be emphasized as a factor favoring wage restraint, because the ability of an employer to pay is always relevant to wage negotiations.

There are many sources of data that may be helpful to the institution in painting an economic picture of the institution's future. Trade associations normally have useful economic data. State and regional associations similarly may also have data of a background nature that can be used in bargaining. Moreover, state and federal governments publish great volumes of economic data that might be helpful in exploring questions bearing on the institution's future.

4. *Productivity and Related Matters.* In a period when health care institutions are under great pressure to provide more and better quality services at an affordable cost to the public, management must be conscious of employee *productivity,* usually defined as output of employees per man-hour input.[98] While there are a number of basic approaches to productivity, such as worker incentives, technological innovation and the like, increases in productivity often result from improved management. At the bargaining table, management should be conscious of the impact that any contract clause might have on productivity.

Management should also consider, when preparing its position for collective bargaining, whether barriers to improved productivity were erected under an old contract or under existing practices.

Productivity bargaining is in an early stage in the United States, but in Europe, particularly in England, productivity bargaining has recently received much attention. Experts have identified a number of approaches to higher productivity, principal among which are these:

a. New technology or automated procedures to supplement or substitute for handwork.
b. Incentive systems to encourage employees to produce either greater quantity or better quality.
c. Rearrangement of existing work patterns that might result in higher productivity.
d. New personnel policies and strategies to elevate employee morale (such as rearranging the work week through flex-time or flex-day and the like) and to diminish absenteeism and turnover rates.

The difficulty of productivity measures in the health care industry should not be underestimated. The former executive secretary of the National Commission on Productivity, Leon Greenberg, has commented on the difficulty of measuring the intangible quality of services in the health care industry.

The reason frequently given for nonmeasurement of . . . [health care services] is that there is no definable, quantifiable unit of output. The more likely reason is that there is often more than one way to identify or define output of an establishment and it is difficult to make a choice. Another important factor is that each unit of output is often subject to a wide band of quality, and the quality is difficult to evaluate and measure.

Health care service is the result of inputs from a variety of sources—doctors, hospitals, druggists, drug manufacturers. If all of them were to be included in the input part of the productivity ratio, what would the output be? In this case it might be logical to use the population death rate as an inverse measure of health care but then we would have to consider the impact of pollution, public health services, diet, and other factors.

It is useful to make a distinction between the measurement objectives of the economist or sociologist and those of the administrator of a particular service. The former may be concerned with an output measure which reflects service to the community at large. The administrator can sharpen and pinpoint his attention to examination of what his particular service unit is required to do.

The hospital administrator may be able to develop such measures of output as patient-days of hospital care. Different types of patient requirements would require different types of care. So the output measurement system would require different weights for different illnesses, operations, accidents, and other service requirements.

This measure is not foolproof. If surgical procedures change so that for some types of operations a patient is discharged two days earlier, the output per man-hour for that operation and postoperative care may decline! The most intensive care is usually given in the first few days of hospitalization, the final days or periods of recovery requiring fewer hours of nursing and other care. If the hospital stay is reduced, the number of hours of patient care is reduced, but the average number per patient-day will rise.[99]

Active or Passive Management Strategies

When collective bargaining was still new to American industry in the late 1930s and early 1940s, there was a tendency for management to regard labor negotiations as a reactive process: that a union would make contract demands and management would react to those specific demands. The process was viewed as one in which management's role was solely to limit union penetration into the rights of management, while management itself was rarely an active party seeking positive gains for itself.

The philosophy of management towards bargaining has undergone significant changes. In particular, sophisticated management negotiators increasingly advocate that management take the initiative and design strategies to help achieve defined managerial objectives. According to this activist view, management can profitably view the bargaining process as one through which a more productive and efficient work environment can be achieved.

Anticipating the Union's Proposals

In designing a management strategy for bargaining, it is useful to anticipate the union's demands so as to have maximum time to plan responses. To do so requires understanding the process by which a union formulates its demands and to learn to differentiate between union demands which should be taken seriously and those that have political significance for the union, but which will soon be forgotten at the bargaining table because they are not high among the union's priorities.

A union is a political organization whose officers must respect the wishes of the membership or run the risk of being thrown out of office. For this reason, the union's collective bargaining proposals—especially at the outset of bargaining—reflect the diverse interests of each of the union's internal constituencies. For example, the union may heed the wishes of older members nearing retirement by making proposals to improve the institution's retirement program. But, at the same time, the union may respect the needs of its younger members, who typically are less concerned with retirement benefits than with current income by proposing direct wage increases. Similarly, unions find ways to satisfy their highly skilled members as well as their unskilled members.

A union normally does not sort out priorities between diverse membership groups at the outset of bargaining. Instead, it will put all of its demands from every membership interest group on the bargaining table, never expecting to gain most of its demands. By putting *everything* into its initial contract demands, the union looks good politically to every member. Then, when bargaining eliminates the union's insubstantial demands, it can blame management for its failures.

Because a union's initial demands are not only highly political but are also likely to be inflated as well, management must be sensitive in evaluating each demand's *real* significance.

By anticipating the union's demands, management will be better prepared to respond at the bargaining table, for the union's initial demands are merely that, *viz.,* demands. They are almost always subject to modifications in the bargaining process. Hence, the more time management has to consider the union's proposals, the more likely it is that management might fashion satisfactory counterproposals.

Receiving the Union's Demands and "Costing Out"

Parties design their own procedures for collective bargaining. In some cases, the parties prefer to exchange bargaining demands by mail, well in advance of their first, formal meeting. However, that is the exception, rather than the rule. More common is the practice of calling a first session at which the union alone submits its proposals. That meeting is perfunctory. It does, however, bring the parties together and gives them an opportunity to size each other up. It also gives the union's rank-and-file bargaining committee a sense of how the bargaining process will proceed. Typically, therefore, the first bargaining session lasts only a few minutes.

Having received the union's demands, management will then begin the systematic process of evaluating and "costing out" union proposals. For purposes of analysis, it is customary to divide contract proposals into two major categories: noneconomic and economic.[100]

A union's noneconomic proposals will normally cover the whole range of the parties' relationship. Some of these will be of particular concern to employees, such as equal distribution of overtime. Others will be of greater interest to the union as an organization, such as union security. In evaluating a union's noneconomic proposals, management should carefully determine whether any proposals seek to penetrate too far into areas of traditional management decision-making and which management will choose to oppose as a matter of principle, without regard to the merits of the union's proposals. In this respect experienced negotiators are sensitive to the first suggestion of union efforts to penetrate these areas, however innocent or reasonable the union's proposal may seem, for it is hard to stop bargaining about management prerogatives once the process begins. Ultimately, the question that management must ask concerning *each* noneconomic proposal is whether it can be granted without sacrificing legitimate needs and objectives of the institution.

Impact of Union's Economic Demands on Nonbargaining Unit Employees: "Extension Costs"

The first step in evaluating a union's economic demands requires determining how many employees will be *indirectly* affected by the union's demands. Of course, all employees in the bargaining unit will be directly affected by any contract negotiated with the union. Granting wage or benefit increases to unionized employees almost always results in a moral and practical obligation to grant identical increases and benefits to employees outside the bargaining unit, including professionals, supervisors, and administrators. The failure to extend such economic benefits to unrepresented employees may result in severe employee dissatisfaction with a concomitant worsening of morale, and also it may lead them to seek union representation.

The question that an institution evaluating a union's economic demands must consider, therefore, is this: If one or more of the union's economic demands are granted, what would the *extension* cost be? For example, would granting a 5% wage increase to a union that represents 100 nurses require the institution also to grant a 5% wage increase to 1,000 other employees? If so, the cost of granting the nurses' request for 5% would not be 5% of the nurses' payroll, but 5% of the total payroll.

The same may also be true of fringe benefits. If the institution agrees to a third week of vacation after 10 years of continuous employment to a union that represents nonprofessional employees, how can the institution decline to extend that vacation benefit to its supervisors, professional employees and administrators? Hence, in computing the cost of the third week of vacation after 10 years' employment, the institution must count the present and potential number of bargaining unit employees who will become eligible for that benefit, and realistically it must also count the institution's other employees to whom that benefit may be extended. For example, in a unit of nonprofessional employees where turnover is quite high, the cost of granting a third week of vacation after 10 years' continuous employment might be extremely low because few employees in that category accrue 10 years of service. But, if the institution extends that identical benefit to its professional and administrative employees, where the turnover is low, the real cost of granting that benefit could be prohibitive. *A note of caution: Management is entitled to consider the cost of extending negotiated benefits to unrepresented employees. But management should not deny a union proposal on the sole ground that management would be obliged to extend the benefit to unrepresented employees.* The union is legally entitled to bargain only for employees in the bargaining unit. If management were to reject a proposal on the ground that the cost of extending that benefit is too costly, management might be guilty of refusing to bargain in good faith. Simple prudence dictates that management should take into account any extension costs, but it should refrain from discussing this matter at the bargaining table.

Data Needed to Cost Out the Union's Proposals

In order to understand the financial impact of the union's proposals, management can collect several kinds of data. These data will vary from one set of negotiations to another. If the union makes proposals to improve a retirement plan, for example, management must know how many employees are currently participating in its retirement plan, how many will become eligible to participate, how many have actually retired, and how many are likely to retire during the term of the contract.

It may also be necessary to know the age and sex of employees in the bargaining unit. Suppose, for example, that the union proposes that employees be granted a three-month leave of absence with pay in the event of pregnancy. Obviously management would need to know how many of its employees are female and of child-bearing age in order to make a reasonable estimate of the cost of that benefit.

Computers and Costing Out

So many variables are taken into account in costing out a union's contract proposals that some sophisticated employers assess the cost of union proposals by programming computers to weigh the stated variables. Moreover, some major firms are now relying on mathematical models as the basis for assessing union proposals. The use of computers and models in collective bargaining is still relatively new, but there is every indication that computers offer great promise for more accurate costing-out assessments. An institution which has access to computer time might advantageously consider ways to use computers to analyze and store data.[101]

Management's Responses and Counterproposals

Management's responses to the union's bargaining proposals usually consist of two parts: first, a reaction to each of the proposals made by the union; second, management's own counterproposals.

The law requires management to give the union *some response* to every proposal. In the early stages of bargaining, management often tries to find *some* areas of immediate or potential agreement simply to demonstrate its good faith. But those demands that involve excessive costs or that threaten managerial authority should be firmly rejected or set aside for later consideration.

Responding to the union's initial proposals requires that attention be paid to both style and substance. As a matter of style, in order to comply with the Taft-Hartley Act, management should make clear its willingness *to discuss any proposal* that concerns wages, hours, and working conditions. Hence, even though management may initially turn down a union proposal, management should never refuse to discuss it for a reasonable period of time, to listen to the union's reasons for advancing it, and to state fully and accurately management's reasons for rejecting it.

Management may also wish to offer counterproposals, although it is not required to do so. These may be in the nature of proposals that differ significantly from the union's, but which deal with the same subject matter. To take an obvious example, management probably will wish to propose a strong management rights clause and a so-called "zipper" clause.[102]

Upon receipt of management's responses and counterproposals, the union will then react to them. The process goes back and forth in what is known as the "give-and-take" of the negotiations, until at some point the parties either reach an agreement or reach an impasse.

The Reservation Concerning Reaching Agreement on Single Issues

It is usually in management's interest to state clearly and unequivocally at the outset of bargaining that management will not give *final* agreement on any single issue until the parties reach full agreement on an entire contract. This is an important reservation. If management agrees to be bound on each issue as it is negotiated, management loses flexibility to withdraw from its agreement on one issue in exchange for agreement on another. It also risks bargaining in bad faith if it later withdraws from final agreement on a single issue. Unions frequently insist on the same res-

ervation, which is popularly phrased as "no agreement on anything until full agreement on everything."

The Reservation Concerning Contract Ratification by the Union's Membership

No law requires a union to submit the terms of a new collective bargaining contract to its members for "ratification," but it is a tradition that runs very deep in the American labor movement and is required by most union constitutions. Experienced union negotiators are careful to state at the outset of bargaining their reservation that *any* agreement reached by the parties will be subject to ratification by the union's members.

Typically management does not need such a reservation concerning ratification, for it is usually a simple matter for management's negotiators to keep their principals informed of the status of bargaining. Moreover, it is assumed that management negotiators have secured authority in advance of their entering into any final agreement, whereas it is normally not possible for union negotiators to secure advance approval from their members.

Notes, Transcripts and Recordings of Negotiations

It is important that good notes of negotiations be kept for two main reasons: first, to use in the grievance procedure and arbitration where proof of contract history may be helpful; second, to use in NLRB proceedings where questions of bad faith may be raised.

Each party usually takes its own notes and records in bargaining. Ordinarily, where no unlawful conduct of the employer is involved, the NLRB has held that a stenographic transcript of the bargaining sessions may be made by the employer over the union's objections.[103] In recent years, however, a question has arisen over the use of the tape recorders. In response, the NLRB has held that an employer violates its Section 8(a)(5) duty to bargain in good faith if it insists upon the use of tape recorders throughout negotiations over the vigorous objections of the union.[104]

The NLRB reconsidered its long-standing position in 1978 on the insistence by one party upon the use of a court reporter or a tape recorder over the other party's objections. Reversing a number of its earlier decisions, the Board ruled in the *Bartlett-Collins Company* case[105] that neither party may insist, to the point of impasse, upon use of a court reporter or a tape recorder in bargaining. This decision appears, however, to permit a party to take detailed personal notes or even to bring a stenographer to the bargaining table to take verbatim notes, provided that the stenographer is not a court reporter who officially certifies the notes.

The *Bartlett-Collins* decision was cited in a recent NLRB decision where it was ruled that tape recordings of negotiations could not be admitted into evidence at a Board hearing where the employer recorded the negotiations without the union's knowledge. The Board explained that to allow such recordings into evidence would inhibit free expression during negotiations and would fly in the face of the Board's reasoning in *Bartlett-Collins*.[106]

Countless arbitration cases have been decided on the basis of minutes of negotiation meetings that proved the parties' purpose in agreeing upon particular words or phrases.

Minutes of negotiations should be carefully filed and kept indefinitely, for it is not uncommon for such minutes to become relevant in an arbitration proceeding twenty or thirty years later.

Techniques and Strategies of Bargaining

Collective bargaining may be more of an art than a science. A good negotiator usually is patient, impersonal, well-informed, tough-minded and determined to achieve the best possible results without unnecessarily antagonizing the other side. He bears in mind that negotiating the contract is only the first step in developing a relationship between a health care institution and a union. Hence, it may be short-sighted to negotiate a contract that is so wholly favorable to management that the institution's relations with the union deteriorate and create hostility and strain. Unions must be able to show some gain for their members as a political necessity, and robbing the union of credit will force it into a hostile mood. Experienced negotiators refine their skills and strategies over a period of years, and one cannot hope to become an expert negotiator by reading a book. There is simply no substitute for experience, practice, and keen observation. There are, however, several guiding principles that are followed by experienced negotiators.

1. *Keep objectives clearly in mind.* However tempting it may be to reach a hasty agreement or to become deeply involved in controversies over a single issue, experienced negotiators understand that it is the *long-term* and overall objectives that must be pursued. They do not let attention to details obscure their ultimate objectives.
2. *Avoid unnecessary involvement in personalities.* Experienced negotiators are aware that it is easy

to become personally antagonistic to negotiators on the other side. However tempting it might be to defend one's honor and to lash out against one's counterpart, professional negotiators never allow their personalities to become an issue in the bargaining process. There are countless examples of negotiators who failed to achieve their objectives because they became enmeshed in personal disputes. Some union representatives use the strategy of "rattling" their opponent in an effort to achieve a short-term tactical advantage. There is little to be gained from this tactic, but some union negotiators believe they strengthen the will of their members when they belittle management and make slashing personal attacks.

Timing of Proposals

The most important factor in negotiating strategy is *timing*. Timing is as important to a negotiator as it is to an actor.

How does one know what the right time is to make a proposal or a counterproposal?

Timing should be guided by the unfolding drama of the bargaining process. At the outset of the bargaining, for example, when the parties feel out each other's point of view, the relationship tends to be formal and stiff. As the parties better understand each other's proposals and establish a more personal bond which results from working together, the stiffness of the early sessions may turn into a more friendly and cooperative mood. As the environment warms up, proposals can be made in the spirit of cooperation and compromises are more likely to be accepted, than at an earlier point, when relations are formal and mistrustful.

Of course, collective bargaining has no rigid cycles. While the initial stages tend to be formal and the later stages tend to be more cooperative, the opposite might also occur.

The point remains: Timing is crucial. Each negotiator must make the most sensitive and careful assessment as to when his best offer should be laid on the table. Nothing can be more damaging to a party's bargaining position (or more humiliating to its negotiator) than to have its last and best offer brushed aside as inadequate.

SUBSTANTIVE CONTRACT PROVISIONS

Management Rights

Collective bargaining always impinges on managerial freedom. Before collective bargaining, management is free to take any lawful personnel action unilaterally. After collective bargaining, management normally may act only bilaterally with respect to personnel matters. As a practical matter, therefore, health care management should plan to protect those areas of decision-making that it does not wish to give up or to compromise. Management may lawfully bargain for the retention of its traditional managerial powers, and some reason that management rights are "reserved" and are never given up in collective bargaining unless they are *explicitly* compromised.

While the "reserved rights" theory is widely accepted in management circles, it is less accepted by arbitrators and courts. Management is safer with clear, unambiguous and unmistakable management powers in the collective bargaining contract itself.

Management negotiators do not agree as to the best way to protect traditional managerial powers. There are two major kinds of "management rights" clauses: the short-and-comprehensive management rights clause and the long-and-detailed management rights clause.

The short clause, in a single sentence or two, provides that management reserves all powers which have not been explicitly limited by the contract. Theoretically this clause should protect managerial freedom and reserve to management all rights that have not been expressly limited. In innumerable arbitration and NLRB cases, however, this clause was not sufficiently positive to protect management.[107] For example, a traditional problem in labor relations concerns whether management may subcontract bargaining unit work. If the contract does not expressly limit management's right to subcontract, does a short, comprehensive management rights clause protect management's rights to subcontract? Some arbitrators and boards have held that it does; others have held that it does not. There can be no doubt that management would have a better case in arbitration, before the NLRB and in the courts if it had an express contract provision granting management the right to subcontract. It is hard to negotiate such an explicit subcontracting clause, however. Even unions which might agree, in principle, to management subcontracting rights find it politically impossible to acquiesce to an express subcontracting clause. For this reason, management often finds that the best protection it can negotiate is the short-comprehensive clause.

By contrast to the short-comprehensive management rights clause, the detailed management rights clause attempts to define each of the areas of management activity which is expressly preserved for management alone and which may not be abridged by the remainder of the collective bargaining agreement.

Typically, the long-and-detailed management rights clause begins with a declaration that *all* rights of management which have not been expressly limited are reserved to management, followed by a detailed listing of those matters as to which management may act in its discretion. Prominent among the matters for which management may wish to preserve unilateral decision-making authority are the following: services that the institution will provide; the hours that the institution will operate; methods of operating and providing services; selection and assignment of personnel to perform services; subcontracting various kinds of work; determination of work assignments and methods; promulgation of rules and regulations; and determination of work standards.

This list is merely typical, for it could easily be expanded with dozens of other matters which management might choose to preserve for itself. But, there is an ever-present risk in negotiating a long-detailed management rights clause. The risk is that the inadvertent omission of a specific reservation of power might be interpreted by an arbitrator as an intentional relinquishment of that power. Still the strength of such a management rights clause is that it unmistakably identifies those specific rights of management that cannot be abridged. Most health care employers have a firm idea of those aspects of management which should be specifically protected in a collective bargaining agreement. In most cases, therefore, it is not impossible for management to draft a highly satisfactory detailed management rights clause.

Union Security

The subject of union security—involuntary membership in or fee payments to a labor organization—is one which has historically been controversial in past decades. This controversy has largely abated in the private sector although debate over its suitability to the private nonprofit and public sectors continues.

The advantages of union security clauses to labor organizations are undeniable. Such a clause typically gives a union reasonable assurance that its income will be continuous during the life of the contract. Moreover, it virtually guarantees that management will not attempt to undermine the union's status through deprivation of income. Because union security clauses are of prime importance to unions, they expect management to extract some price at the bargaining table in exchange for agreement to such a clause.

From management's point of view, whether or not to agree to a union security clause may be extremely complex. Large employers often begin a collective bargaining relationship by categorically refusing to acquiesce in demands for union security. This position is most common when management believes that its long-time employees should not be required to join a union as a condition of employment. There are few large, national employers today which continue to oppose all forms of union security. In fact, some employers readily agree to union security, for they believe that there are advantages to dealing with a secure, stable, and responsible union. When a union is insecure and believes that its very survival is threatened by management, a union's customary response is to act with exaggerated aggressiveness. Moreover, if a union has no regular source of income, it must constantly organize employees in the work force, and the union may believe that it must prosecute every grievance to arbitration and to exhibit other forms of militancy. Such behavior may be costly to management. By contrast, unions that are secure and believe that management does not challenge their right to exist in the workplace tend to be more responsible and mature in processing grievances. Additionally, secure unions are less prone to strike, for they have no need to prove their strength.

The Taft-Hartley Act regulates union security arrangements in great detail. The maximum form of union security permitted by the Act is a union shop clause, which requires employees to join a union. The employee would be required to join no sooner than the 31st day following the date on which the contract is executed or the 31st day following initial employment, whichever is later. Actually, the law requires no more of an employee than he pay regular and uniform monthly dues and a uniform initiation fee.[108] The law does not require employees to attend union meetings or otherwise to participate in union affairs *as a condition of employment*. There is a complex body of the law dealing with the right of unions to enforce their rules internally and through the courts. Most important to management is that under the Taft-Hartley Act unions may not require of employees any more than payment of uniform dues and initiation fees.

The main forms of union security in the United States are these: the closed shop; the union shop; the agency shop; maintenance of membership; the modified union shop; and the check-off.

Section 19, Religious Exemption

The new health care amendments contain a new Section 19, which provides that an employee of a health care institution who is a member of and adherent to teachings of a bona fide religion, body, or sect which has historically held conscientious objections to joining or supporting labor organizations shall not be required to join or financially support any labor organization as a condition of employment.[109] Congress, however, in anticipation of any "free rider" problems, provided that such employees may be required, in lieu of periodic dues and initiation fees, to pay equal sums to a nonreligious charitable fund.[110] Section 19 provides that the employee may choose from three such nonreligious, tax-exempt charitable funds designated in a contract between the health care employer and the union. If no such designation is made in the contract, the employee may designate his own non-religious tax-exempt fund.

Closed Shop

Prior to the 1947 amendments to the Wagner Act, the closed shop was lawful. A closed shop contract requires that an applicant for employment must be a member of a union *prior to employment*. In other words, under a closed shop contract, an employer may employ only members of a particular union. Congress was sharply critical of closed shop arrangements, for in many cases closed shops had the effect of excluding persons from a work force entirely if the union denied them membership. That was the situation in a number of crafts. In fact, some unions operated their closed shops so as to exclude from their crafts all but the first-born sons of members.

Congress condemned the closed shop in 1947 as an arrangement which not only gave the unions excessive power over admission to a craft or industry, but which also, in Congress' opinion, resulted in discrimination against members of minority groups. Section 8(a)(3) of the Taft-Hartley Act, therefore, made the closed shop illegal. No employer or union in interstate commerce may today enter into a contract under which employees must be a member of a union as a condition of employment. There is one exception to this general statutory prohibition against closed shop agreements and that applies to so-called "prehire" agreements applicable solely to the building and construction industry under Section 8(f) of the 1959 Landrum-Griffin Amendments.

Union Shop

Under a union shop employees are required by contract to become union members within a stated number of days after their initial employment or execution of a contract. Section 8(a)(3) of Taft-Hartley provides that the *shortest* period within which an employee may be required to join is 30 days following his initial hire or following execution of a collective bargaining contract, whichever is later. A contract which requires employees to become union members sooner than the 31st day is unlawful on its face, even though it may in fact be lawfully administered. Even though a contract may be lawful on its face, it might still be unlawful if its administration has the effect of requiring employees to join a union before the 31st day.

The phrase "union membership" in a union shop clause is somewhat misleading, for the Supreme Court has interpreted the obligation under Section 8(a)(3) to mean that unions may require employees to pay uniform dues and initiation fees. Unions may not, as a condition of employment, require employees to swear loyalty, to attend meetings, or to engage in any other form of membership activity.

Agency Shop

The agency shop (not to be confused with the Section 19 religious exemption) is a variation of the union shop. It provides that employees, who choose not to join a union voluntarily, must pay the union an "agency service fee" in exchange for the union's collective bargaining services."[111] The agency shop was first designed by the late Chief Justice Rand of the Canadian Supreme Court and for many years was called the "Rand Formula."[112] In substance, it is a compromise between the union shop and a so-called "open shop" under which employees have no obligation whatever to the union.

Courts have found the agency shop an attractive way to protect the rights of Jehovah's Witnesses and members of other religious groups who for theological reasons cannot become union members. Also, because of the "special humanitarian character of health care institutions."[113] Congress enacted the religious exemption (Section 19), which, as already noted, provides an alternative solution for an employee whose religion forbids union membership.

What is the lawful amount of the service fee? That question has been answered both under the federal law and under the law of a number of the states. The National Labor Relations Board and the federal courts have held that the service fee charged by unions must be "proportionate" to the actual cost of providing collective bargaining services. As a practical matter, that means that a union may not charge more for a service fee than it charges its own members for regular monthly dues, nor may it set the amount of the service fee as high as regular monthly dues in those cases.[114]

The Eighth Circuit affirmed the NLRB's decision that discharge based on a contractual agency shop clause was unlawful where a union treated a nonmember as "delinquent" if his service fee was not paid within ten days after it was due whereas a member was not considered "delinquent" until ninety days after his dues payments were due. The Board and court ruled that the union committed an unfair labor practice by causing a hospital to discharge a nonmember under the circumstances of this case. They rejected the union's argument that the longer, ninety-day grace period for members was an allowable membership benefit.[115]

Maintenance of Membership

The form of union security called "maintenance of membership" was devised during World War II. Under such a clause, employees who are members of the union when the collective bargaining contract is signed must maintain their membership in good standing for the life of the contract. All other employees, however, are free to remain outside the union. Commonly, a maintenance of membership clause requires any employee who voluntarily joins the union during the life of the contract to maintain his membership in good standing. The advantage of the maintenance of membership clause is that it assures the union that present members must continue their membership and dues payments, whereas to management it offers the advantage that persons who are not currently members of the union will not be required to join.

Modified Union Shop

The modified union ship takes various forms. In its most familiar form it requires *newly hired* employees to become members of the union 31 days after their initial employment, but it does not require current employees to become union members. It, thus, has the advantage of excluding all employees of the employer at the time the contract is signed from any obligation to join and pay dues to the union, whereas new employees—who should be advised upon their employment of this clause—must join the union and maintain membership in it.

Check-Off

The check-off is a contract arrangement under which employees authorize their employer to deduct dues from their wages each month which are to be transmitted to the union. The check-off is lawful, provided that an employee has executed a written authorization for the automatic deduction, and provided further that the employee is given an opportunity at least once each year to revoke his dues deduction authorization.

Unless the employee provides his employer with a *written* authorization for the check-off, the employer would violate Section 302 of the Taft-Hartley Act, a criminal provision, by transmitting any sums to the union. In the automobile industry and in several other industries, employers charge unions a fee to cover the administrative costs of deducting employees' dues and transmitting them to the union.

If an employer and a union have a recognition agreement which does not contain a union security provision, the employer will violate the LMRA by requiring employees to sign dues check-off authorization cards on behalf of the union.[116]

The Supreme Court has held that Section 302 provides that employees may revoke their authorization at two distinct times: (1) on the anniversary of the authorization and (2) at the termination of the collective bargaining agreement, whichever comes sooner.[117] This statutory right may not be nullified by a new contract between union and employer negotiated before the expiration of the old collective bargaining agreement. Employees still have the right to revoke their dues check-off authorization at the original date of the earlier contract.[118]

The check-off is an arrangement that may accompany any of the forms of union security discussed above. Whenever employees wish to belong to the union voluntarily or are required to join or pay a fee to the union voluntarily, they may choose to participate in a check-off arrangement so that their dues are deducted automatically. Most employers which have established collective bargaining relations with unions have agreed to the check-off.

Open Shop

The open shop describes the absence of any form of union security. Employees are not required to join or to pay dues or fees to a union, and there are no check-off arrangements.

Right-to-Work Laws

Approximately 20 states, principally in the Southeast, have "right-to-work" laws—laws that prohibit compulsory union membership. These laws have been enacted under the authorization of Section 14(b) of the Taft-Hartley Act which allows the states to prohibit union membership as a condition of employment. Thus, even though federal law permits parties to enter into a union shop agreement, this agreement is illegal under state law in the so-called "right-to-work" states.[119]

No-Strike, Lockout Clauses

The assumption that underlies a collective agreement is that the parties will live amicably during the contract's term. The single most common provision of any collective bargaining agreement, therefore, is one guaranteeing that during the life of the agreement the union will not call, condone, or authorize a strike and the employer will not lockout employees.

A typical no-strike clause provides:

The union agrees for the life of this contract that it and its agents will not call, encourage, authorize, condone, or support any strike, work stoppage, picketing, or other form of work interruption against the employer. The employer agrees that for the life of this contract it and its agents will not lockout any employees.

Historically, the problem has not been with lockouts, but with strikes. A strong no-strike clause helps assure the employer of employment stability during the life of the contract. The employer may sue the union for damages (or invalidate the contract entirely) if the union violates its no-strike promise.

A complex body of law deals with the interpretation and enforcement of no-strike clauses. Most of the cases concern whether an employer may sue for damages and/or secure an injunction against a strike. In a series of leading cases, the Supreme Court has held that an employer may secure an injunction in the federal courts against an illegal work stoppage in breach of contract, and it may also sue a union for money damages for an illegal strike—provided that the grievance-arbitration provision of the contract does not require the employer to submit grievances of contract violations to the arbitration procedure. If, on the other hand, the contract authorizes and requires the employer to file grievances over alleged contract violations, then the employer may not seek an injunction or damages for a strike in violation of the contract.[120]

In addition, unless the no-strike, no-lockout clause specifically restricts a union's right to engage in sympathy work strikes, the employer may be left without recourse in the federal courts.[121]

The Seventh Circuit Court of Appeals, however, has refused to enforce a Board ruling that an employer was guilty of § 8(a)(1) and (3) violations when it discharged certain employees because of their participation in a sympathy strike.[121a] The court arrived at its decision even though the contract's no-strike clause did not specifically restrict the union's right to engage in sympathy strikes. The court noted that a no-strike clause need not contain the specific term "sympathy strike" in order to constitute waiver of the union's right to engage in such protected activity.[121b] That court went on to state that while the general language of a broad no-strike clause, standing alone, will probably not suffice to prohibit sympathy strikes, the courts must follow controlling principles of contract interpretation and examine the contract as a whole.

Seniority

The issue of seniority always arises in collective bargaining. (For a discussion of the equal employment ramifications of seniority, see Chapter 9 of the volume from which this article is reprinted.) The union's position typically is that seniority should be the sole factor to govern promotions, layoffs, shift preferences, and other matters. Management generally prefers to minimize reliance on seniority in favor of reasonable reliance on merit, skill, and experience. The outcome of bargaining over seniority is usually a reflection of the parties' relative power. Most employers readily agree to permit seniority on a facility-wide, departmental, or classification basis to govern layoff procedures. In health care institutions, due to the diverse functions and skills involved, employees who are least senior in a given classification are usually laid off first. Such arrangements are based on the premise that junior employees ought not to have preference over senior employees in periods of economic adversity. This is good personnel practice, for it rewards senior employees for their loyalty to the institution. But management should protect itself from any overly rigid application of seniority in layoffs by insuring that those workers who remain are capable of performing the necessary work.

A more serious problem with respect to seniority concerns its application to job promotions within the bargaining unit. Management normally wishes to promote employees who have demonstrated skill, loyalty, and dependability. Unions, on the other hand, prefer to make seniority the governing criterion. A compromise that is favorable to management provides as follows:

Where applicants for a new job or for promotion have *relatively equal* ability, then seniority will govern.

This is known as a "relative ability" clause, in which management may select the more skilled of two or more job applicants, without regard to their seniority. Under this clause it is only when two applicants have substantially equal ability that the principle of seniority will govern.

On the other hand, a compromise that is regarded as more favorable to unions provides as follows:

Seniority will govern matters relating to job assignment and promotion, provided that the senior applicant has sufficient ability to perform the job in question.

This is called a "sufficient ability" clause. It differs profoundly from a "relative ability" clause. Under a "sufficient ability" clause, the senior applicant must be granted the job provided only that he has sufficient ability—usually meaning the bare *minimum* ability—to perform the job in question.

If there are two applicants for a job vacancy, both of whom can perform the job but the junior of whom is distinctly more skilled, management could choose the junior applicant under a "relative ability" clause. But, under a "sufficient ability" clause, management would be obligated to promote the senior employee because he has the minimum capability to perform the job.

As a matter of sound personnel policy, management must be sensitive to seniority, whether or not there is a contractual obligation, for employees accept the principle of seniority as the basis for preference in many aspects of the employment relationship. In other words, even in unorganized institutions, employees as a subgroup respect seniority, and, in turn, expect management to treat seniority as a valuable and earned basis for preferences within the institution.

The union normally prefers to make promotions subject to so-called *strict* seniority. A strict seniority clause, which few employers agree to, gives management no discretion whatever to reject applicants for promotion but instead management is bound to follow the single test of years on the job.

Superseniority clauses which grant union stewards broad preferential rights and are not on their face limited to layoff and recall rights are presumptively unlawful, since they tie job rights to union activism. The burden of rebutting that presumption (*i.e.*, establishing justification) rests on the shoulders of the party asserting their legality.[122]

Furthermore, a court has held that the mere maintenance of a superseniority clause without any showing of actual use of the clause violates the NLRA.[122a] In the same case, however, the union was able to justify the inclusion of the clause by demonstrating that it provided union stewards with greater accessibility to coworkers.[122b]

A divided Board extended its *Dairylea* holding in 1977, holding that a contract granting superseniority to union officers for purposes of layoff and recall is presumptively valid even if those officers do not perform steward-type functions.[123]

The Board, however, has drawn the line short of granting superseniority rights to *all* union officials.[123a] The Board in 1979 reconsidered the *Dairylea* line of cases and was unable to articulate a clear majority position as to the legality of such a clause. Two of the three majority members would look to whether the union officers were stewards or actually engaged in contract administration. The third Board member found the clause lawful, but held that its application was unlawful based upon the specific facts of the case.

The two dissenting members continued to unsuccessfully argue, as they had in *Dairylea,* that superseniority clauses should not be restricted.

Grievance Procedures and Arbitration

Unions usually seek to negotiate a multistep grievance procedure under which they may challenge violations of the collective bargaining agreement. The final point in a grievance procedure is normally binding arbitration. By agreeing to arbitration, the institution agrees that disputes as to the meaning or application of the contract would be resolved by a neutral third party. In Chapter 6 of the volume from which this article is reprinted, the various kinds of grievance procedures and the various types of arbitration arrangements that are familiar in American industry are discussed in some detail. In this discussion, therefore, we simply indicate that contract negotiations over grievance procedures are customary and should be expected.

The first guide to the negotiation of a grievance-arbitration clause is that management normally wishes to make the *scope* of the grievance and arbitration clause as narrow as possible. In other words, management normally tries to limit the matters that the union may arbitrate. By contrast, unions normally wish to make the scope of the grievance-arbitration clause as broad and hospitable as possible.[124]

The HMO and Collective Bargaining

The Health Maintenance Organization and Assistance Act of 1973 (P.L. 93-222) was designed to encourage the delivery of comprehensive prepaid health services to employees. The Act contemplated that HMOs would operate in open competition with other, more conventional modes of health care delivery and payment. Congress wished to encourage what it considered to be a superior and cost-effective health care delivery system.

Services Offered by the HMO

Subject to statutory restrictions, an HMO must provide each enrolled member with unlimited basic health services which the law defines as:

physician services (including consultant and referral services by a physician);

inpatient and outpatient hospital services;

short-term outpatient hospital services;

medically necessary emergency health services;

short-term outpatient evaluative and crisis-intervention mental health services;

medical treatment and referral services for alcohol and drug abuse or addiction;

diagnostic laboratory services and diagnostic and therapeutic radiologic services;

home health services; and

preventive health services.

An HMO must also provide a full range of supplemental health services to its members. Supplemental health services are defined in law as:

services of facilities for intermediate and long-term care;

vision care not included as a basic health service;

dental services not included as a basic health service;

mental health services not included as a basic health service;

long-term physical medicine and rehabilitative services (including physical therapy); and

prescription drugs prescribed and provided by the HMO in the course of providing a basic or supplemental health service.

HMO members may voluntarily contract with the HMO for the entire range of supplemental health services offered or for one or more specific service.

Ordinarily, the HMO must provide its members with the opportunity to contract for each supplemental health service listed above. However, if the health manpower needed to offer a specific service is not available in the HMO's service area, then the HMO is not required to provide that particular service.

Payment for Services

Basic health service payment.— Each HMO member receives basic health services in return for a basic health service payment which must be fixed, uniform, and prepaid on a periodic basis. These payments are to be determined by the HMO according to a community rating system[125] and may be supplemented by additional nominal payments, known as copayments, levied for specific basic health services. The amount of the basic health service payment is not affected by the kind of service or the number of services which may be used by a member during a particular time period.

Copayments.—Copayments are levied by the HMO at the time a health service (such as a physician's office visit) is rendered. The HMO must set the amount of an individual copayment according to the Secretary's prescribed regulations. However, the copayment cannot exceed 50 percent of the total cost to the HMO of providing that specific basic health service to a given group of members. Nor can it exceed, in the aggregate, 20 percent of the total cost to the HMO of providing all basic health services to a given group of members.[126]

Copayments may not be charged if they would prevent a member from seeking health care. They are not to be used as devices to reduce utilization of health care services. Rather they are intended only as a marketing device to enable an HMO to purvey its services on a competitive basis with other health care providers.

Supplemental health service payment.—Members contracting for optional supplemental health services pay a supplemental health service payment. Like the basic health service payment, the supplemental payment is prepaid, fixed, uniform, and determined according to a community rating system.[127]

Dual Choice

Section 1310 of the Act requires that an employer who has twenty-five or more employees covered by the Fair Labor Standards Act (FLSA) and who contributes to the cost of the employees' health insurance, must offer to contribute the same amount to a federally qualified HMO in the vicinity where the employees reside as an alternative to the employer's existing health benefits plan. In view of the Supreme Court's decision in *National League of Cities v. Usery*,[128] which invalidated extension of the FLSA to state and local governments, it would appear that state and local government employers may not be required to offer the HMO option to their employees.

The implementation of this dual choice mandate awaited the adoption of regulations by the Department of Health, Education & Welfare (HEW) to resolve the question of how health benefits, which are a condition of employment and a subject of mandatory collective bargaining under the National Labor Relations Act, were to be treated. A literal reading of the dual choice

provisions of the HMO Act permitted inclusion of the HMO option by an employer's unilateral action.

HEW issued regulations effective in November 1975, which deal with this provision and clarify the employer's obligations to employees represented by a collective bargaining agent.[129]

HEW considered public comments on this issue and consulted with the National Labor Relations Board and the Department of Labor. Consistent with the overwhelming majority of the comments, HEW concluded that the employer's obligation is satisfied if the offer is made to the bargaining representative in accordance with the requirements of the NLRA.

Should the employer and the bargaining agent agree to include an HMO in the health benefits plan offered to the represented employees, the option would, of course, be presented to the employees. However, even if the union should reject the option, the employer's obligation to his represented employees would be satisfied.

Under 42 C.F.R. 110.805 and 42 C.F.R. 110.806, the offer of the health maintenance organization alternative, the selection of supplemental health services, and copayment levels is subject to the collective bargaining process for represented employees.

Under C.F.R. 110.802(a)(4), the regulations apply in each calendar year to an employer which has received a written request for inclusion in its health benefits plan from one or more qualified HMOs that operate in an area in which any eligible employee resides.

With respect to a collective bargaining agreement, C.F.R. 110.802(b) requires that the HMO request be received 90 days in advance of the expiration or renewal date of the collective bargaining agreement. If a collective bargaining agreement has provided for changing wages, hours, or conditions of employment during its term, it shall be treated as renewable, for purposes of this subpart, at the time provided for renewal.

Section 110.802(b) recognizes the additional time needed to prepare brochures, design enrollment and coverage change forms, arrange corresponding payroll deduction accounts and procedures, plan for a communication strategy, and allow for enrollment.

Thus, the HMO request for inclusion in the health benefits plan must be received at least 180 days prior to the expiration or renewal date of an employer-employee contract or a health benefits contract. Where the health benefits available to an employee are governed by both a collective bargaining agreement and a health benefits contract, the HMO's request for inclusion must satisfy both the 90-day and 180-day requirements.

Unrepresented Employees

For those employees not represented by a bargaining agent, the offer of the HMO option must be made directly, and the selection of copayment levels and supplemental health services for eligible employees must be made through whatever decision-making process exists with respect to the existing health benefits plan.

There are other clauses which usually are included in a collective bargaining agreement. The Appendix to the volume from which this article is reprinted contains additional materials which will be helpful in determining the content of such clauses.

UNILATERAL CHANGES IN WORKING CONDITIONS

Generally speaking, an employer may not make unilateral changes—changes made by management without bargaining—but must submit proposed changes to the exclusive bargaining agent of its employees for negotiation. While the NLRB approaches problems of unilateral changes in working conditions on a case-by-case basis, and while it should be remembered that each case has its own factual profile, several general principles have been articulated by the Board and courts.

First, an employer may not normally make changes in wages, hours, and working conditions without the union's agreement while collective bargaining is in progress. Changes that are made during collective bargaining are usually regarded as unfair labor practices which violate Section 8(a)(5) of the Act.[130]

Second, an employer may normally make unilateral changes in wages, hours, and working conditions *after a total impasse* has been reached in bargaining, provided that those changes the employer seeks to make have first been offered to and rejected by the union.[131]

It is often difficult to establish when an impasse (meaning a deadlock) has been reached in bargaining; it is a factual question in each case. Generally speaking, an impasse is reached when after extensive good faith bargaining it becomes obvious that there are irreconcilable differences in the parties' positions with respect to one or more issues. Since it is not always clear when such a bona fide stalemate has been reached, an employer should always seek competent legal advice before instituting any unilateral changes in wages, hours, or working conditions.

Third, an employer may *not* make unilateral changes even after a total impasse, *if* the impasse has been produced by the employer's own illegal conduct, such as illegally refusing to supply relevant information.[132]

Fourth, an employer may *not* make unilateral changes after an impasse if the benefits that the employer wishes to confer upon employees unilaterally *exceed* those offered to the union at the bargaining table[133] or were never offered to the union in bargaining at all.[134]

An impasse does not terminate the duty to bargain, but merely suspends it.[135] Nor is an impasse difficult to end; almost any change in circumstances can terminate the suspension of the duty to bargain. One party's willingness to make concessions[136] or to totally accept prior proposals[137] may terminate an impasse. Also, a change in the business climate may signal the end of an impasse.[138] Again, as in the onset of an impasse, there are no hard and fast rules by which an employer can determine when an impasse has terminated, and competent legal advice should be sought before choosing a course of action.

Fifth, an employer that is a successor (i.e., an employer who has purchased the assets of the original employer and engages in substantially the same business, at the same location, and employs the same employees) to the original employer may *not* make unilateral changes without bargaining with the union.[139] A more detailed explanation of the rights and obligations of a successor employer is discussed in Chapter 4 of the volume from which this article is reprinted.

NOTES

1. It is common to think of collective bargaining as a recent development in American economic history, but in fact unions and employers have negotiated agreements of various types and purposes since the late 18th century. Not until the 20th century, however, did the American labor movement and the institution of bilateral collective bargaining, as we know them, take a well-defined form. While there are countless works of labor history, there are few historical studies of the institution of collective bargaining, the best of which is *Milton Derber, The American Idea of Industrial Democracy, 1865-1965* (1970).

2. U.S.C. § 158(d)(A).

3. *Id.*

4. 29 U.S.C. § 158(d)(B).

5. 29 U.S.C. § 158(d)(C).

6. *Id.*

7. Office of the General Counsel Memorandum 74-49 (August 20, 1974) at 21.

8. *See, e.g.,* Kent Nursing Home, 69 LA 771 (1977), where a fact finder made recommendations following a bargaining impasse for the terms of a successor contract.

9. 29 U.S.C. § 158(g).

10. 29 U.S.C. 183. *See, e.g.,* St. Elizabeth Hosp. v. Horvitz, _____ F. Supp. _____, 97 L.R.R.M. 3105 (N.D.N.Y. 1978), where the court held that the FMCS Director has broad discretion in appointing Boards of Inquiry.

11. *Id.*

12. 29 U.S.C. § 158(d)(A).

13. Office of the General Counsel Memorandum 74-49 (August 20, 1974) at 20.

14. 29 U.S.C. § 158(d)(A).

15. 29 U.S.C. § 183.

15a. *See* Sinai Hosp. of Baltimore, Inc. v. Horvitz, et al. _____ F.2d _____, 104 L.R.R.M. 21717 (4th Cir. 1980), in which the court determined that the decision to set up the Board was not subject to judicial review since the Board's recommendations are advisory and do not substantially affect negotiating rights.

16. Sinai Hosp. v. Scearce, 561 F.2d 547, 549, 96 L.R.R.M. 2355 (4th Cir. 1977).

17. Affiliated Hosp. v. Scearce, _____ F.2d _____ 99 L.R.R.M. 3197 (9th Cir. 1978).

18. *Id.*

19. S. Rep. No. 93-988, 93d Cong., 2d Sess. 5 (1974) (Conference Report).

20. As indicated at notes 16 and 17, *supra,* the Fourth and Ninth Circuit Courts of Appeal have held that the final date for the establishment of the Board of Inquiry is 30 days from the date the FMCS actually received the notice of the dispute, not 30 days from the last permissible date the FMCS must receive the notice (60 days prior to the expiration of the contract) as indicated in the chart.

21. *See, e.g.,* NLRB v. Montgomery Ward & Co., 133 F.2d 676, 12 L.R.R.M. 508 (9th Cir. 1943).

22. *See* NLRB v. Highland Park Mfg., 110 F.2d 632, 6 L.R.R.M. 786 (4th Cir. 1940).

23. *See* Globe Cotton Mills v. NLRB, 103 F.2d 91, 4 L.R.R.M. 621 (5th Cir. 1939).

24. *See* Irvington Motors, 147 N.L.R.B. 565, 56 L.R.R.M. 1257 (1964), *enforced,* 343 F.2d 759, 58 L.R.R.M. 2816 (C.A. 3, 1965).

25. *See* NLRB v. Exchange Parts, 339 F.2d 829, 58 L.R.R.M. 2097 (5th Cir. 1965).

26. *See* Solo Cup Co., 142 N.L.R.B. 1290, 53 L.R.R.M. 1253 (1963), *enforced,* 332 F.2d 447, 56 L.R.R.M. 2383 (4th Cir. 1964).

26a. Brownsboro Hills Nursing Home, Inc. 244 N.L.R.B. No. 47, 102 L.R.R.M. 1118 (1979).

27. *See* NLRB v. Fitzgerald Mills, 313 F.2d 260, 52 L.R.R.M. 2174 (2nd Cir. 1963).

28. *See* San Antonio Machine Corp. v. NLRB, 363 F.2d 633, 62 L.R.R.M. 2674 (5th Cir. 1966).

28a. NLRB v. Indiana & Michigan Electric Co., No. 77-1685, 101 L.R.R.M. 2470 (7th Cir. 1979).

29. *See* Medo Photo Supply Corp. v. NLRB, 321 U.S. 678, 14 L.R.R.M. 581 (1944).

29a. NLRB v. Rubatex Corp. No. 78-1341 (4th Cir., June 29, 1979).

30. NLRB v. Am. Nat'l Ins. Co., 343 U.S. 395, 30 L.R.R.M. 2147 (1952).

31. General Electric Co., 150 N.L.R.B. 192, 57 L.R.R.M. 1491 (1964), *enforced,* 418 F.2d 736, 72 L.R.R.M. 2530 (2nd Cir. 1969), *cert. denied,* 397 U.S. 965, 73 L.R.R.M. 2600 (1970).

32. NLRB v. Truitt Mfg. Co., 351 U.S. 149, 38 L.R.R.M. 2024 (1955).

33. *See* J.I. Case Co. v. NLRB, 253 F.2d 149, 41 L.R.R.M. 2679 (7th Cir. 1958).

34. *See* Albany Garage, 126 N.L.R.B. 417, 45 L.R.R.M. 1329 (1960).

35. *See* NLRB v. Item Co., 220 F.2d 956, 35 L.R.R.M. 2709 (5th Cir. 1955).

36. NLRB v. Truitt Mfg. Co., n. 32, *supra.*

37. NLRB v. Acme Industrial Co., 385 U.S. 432, 64 L.R.R.M. 2069 (1967).

38. The parties may even reach agreement on a contract during the trial on the unfair labor practice.

39. Detroit Edison Co. v. NLRB, _____ U.S. _____, 100 L.R.R.M. 2728 (1979).

40. NLRB v. Wooster Div. of Borg-Warner Corp., 356 U.S. 342, 42 L.R.R.M. 2034 (1958).

41. *Id.*

42. *Id.*

43. Newport News Shipbuilding and Dry Dock Co., 236 N.L.R.B. No. 218, 98 L.R.R.M. 1475 (1978).

44. Dicten & Masch Mfg. Co., 129 N.L.R.B. 112, 46 L.R.R.M. 1516 (1960).

45. Tex-Tan Welhausen Co. v. NLRB, 419 F.2d 1265, 72 L.R.R.M. 2885 (5th Cir. 1969), *modified,* 434 F.2d 405, 75 L.R.R.M. 2554 (5th Cir. 1970).

46. Providence Journal Co., 180 N.L.R.B. No. 103, 73 L.R.R.M. 1235 (1970).

47. Braswell Motor Freight Lines, Inc., 141 N.L.R.B. 1154, 52 L.R.R.M. 1467 (1963).

48. Smith Cabinet Mfg. Co., 147 N.L.R.B. 1506, 56 L.R.R.M. 1418 (1964).

49. Singer Mfg. Co., 24 N.L.R.B. 444, 6 L.R.R.M. 405 (1940), *enforced,* 119 F.2d 131 (7th Cir. 1941).

50. *Id.*

51. NLRB v. Adams Dairy, 322 F.2d 553, 54 L.R.R.M. 2171 (8th Cir. 1963), *vacated,* 379 U.S. 644, 58 L.R.R.M. 2192 (1965), *on remand,* 350 F.2d 108, 60 L.R.R.M. 2084 (8th Cir. 1965), *cert. denied,* 382 U.S. 1011, 61 L.R.R.M. 2192 (1966).

52. Century Elec. Motor Co., 180 N.L.R.B. No. 174, 73 L.R.R.M. 1307 (1970).

53. Windemuller Elec., Inc., 180 N.L.R.B. No. 106, 73 L.R.R.M. 1111 (1970).

54. Connecticut Light & Power Co. v. NLRB, 476 F.2d 1079, 82 L.R.R.M. 3121 (2nd Cir. 1973).

55. Sylvania Elec. Prods., Inc. 127 N.L.R.B. 924, 46 L.R.R.M. 1127 (1960).

56. Kruger Co., 401 F.2d 682, 69 L.R.R.M. 2425 (6th Cir. 1968).

57. Richfield Oil Corp., 110 N.L.R.B. 356, 34 L.R.R.M. 1658 (1954), *enforced,* 231 F.2d 717, 37 L.R.R.M. 2327 (D.C. Cir.), *cert. denied,* 351 U.S. 909, 37 L.R.R.M. 2837 (1956).

58. NLRB v. Hart Cotton Mills, Inc., 190 F.2d 964, 28 L.R.R.M. 2434 (4th Cir. 1951).

59. Ford Motor Company v. NLRB, _____ U.S. _____, 101 L.R.R.M. 222 (1979).

60. NLRB v. Central Illinois Public Service Co., 324 F.2d 916, 54 L.R.R.M. 2586 (7th Cir., 1963).

61. Weston & Brooker & Co., 154 N.L.R.B. 747, 60 L.R.R.M. 1015 (1965).

62. Long Lake Lumber Co., 160 N.L.R.B. 1475, 63 L.R.R.M. 1160 (1966).

63. Smith Cabinet Mfg. Co., Inc., 147 N.L.R.B. 1506, 56 L.R.R.M. 1418 (1964).

64. Cone Mills Corp., 156 N.L.R.B. 370, 61 L.R.R.M. 1052 (1965).

65. *See, e.g.,* NLRB v. Wooster Div. of Borg-Warner Corp., 356 U.S. 342, 42 L.R.R.M. 2034 (1958).

66. *See* Hilton-Davis Chemical Co., Div. of Sterling Drug, Inc. and Local 342, Int'l Chemical Workers Union, 185 N.L.R.B. 241, 75 L.R.R.M. 1036 (1970).

67. Beacon Piece Dyeing & Finishing Co., 121 N.L.R.B. 953, 42 L.R.R.M. 1489 (1958).

68. Ozark Trailers, Inc., 161 N.L.R.B. 651, 63 L.R.R.M. 1264 (1966).

69. *See* NLRB v. Arkansas Rice Growers Cooperative Assn., 400 F.2d 565, 69 L.R.R.M. 2119 (8th Cir. 1968).

70. Zaleskie v. Singer Mfg. Co., 24 N.L.R.B. 444, 6 L.R.R.M. 405 (1940).

71. Fibreboard Paper Products Corp. v. NLRB, 379 U.S. 203, 57 L.R.R.M. 2609. Generally an employer may temporarily subcontract, without bargaining, during the course of a strike. However, *see, e.g.*, Alexander Linn Hosp. Ass'n, 244 N.L.R.B. No. 60, 102 L.R.R.M. 1252 (1979) in which the *long-term* subcontracting of all electrocardiogram (EKG) and stress testing work without bargaining with the union violated Section 8(a)(5) although it was done during a strike. Since the subcontract would, very possibly, extend beyond the duration of the strike it was a mandatory subject of bargaining.

72. Crown Coach Corp., 155 N.L.R.B. 625, 60 L.R.R.M. 1366 (1965).

73. Houston Chapter, Associated Gen. Contractors, 143 N.L.R.B. 409, 53 L.R.R.M. 1299 (1963), *enforced*, 349 F.2d 449, 59 L.R.R.M. 3013 (5th Cir. 1965) *cert. denied*, 382 U.S. 1026 (1966).

74. Laclede Gas Co., 173 N.L.R.B. 243, 69 L.R.R.M. 1316 (1968).

75. LeRoy Mach. Co., 147 N.L.R.B. 1431, 56 L.R.R.M. 1368 (1964).

76. Gulf Power Co., 156 N.L.R.B. 622, 61 L.R.R.M. 1073 (1966).

77. Inland Steel Co., 77 N.L.R.B. 1, 21 L.R.R.M. 1316, *enforced*, 170 F.2d 247, 22 L.R.R.M. 2505 (7th Cir. 1948), *cert. denied*, 356 U.S. 960 (1949).

78. NLRB v. Am. Nat'l Ins. Co., 343 U.S. 395, 30 L.R.R.M. 2147 (1952).

79. Miller Brewing Co., 166 N.L.R.B. 622, 61 L.R.R.M. 1073 (1966).

80. Lloyd A. Fry Roofing Co., 123 N.L.R.B. 647, 43 L.R.R.M. 1507 (1959).

81. Borg-Warner Co., Borg-Warner Controls Div., 198 N.L.R.B. No. 93, 80 L.R.R.M. 1790 (1972).

81a. Union Hosp. Ass'n, N.L.R.B. Ad. Mem., 102 L.R.R.M. 1677 (1979), issued by NLRB Associate General Counsel Harold J. Datz. *See also, infra*, n.102.

82. Ford Motor Company v. NLRB, _____ U.S. _____, 101 L.R.R.M. 222 (1979).

83. 221 N.L.R.B. No. 105, 90 L.R.R.M. 1576 (1975).

84. Local 428, Operating Engineers, 184 N.L.R.B. 976, 74 L.R.R.M. 1705 (1970).

85. Pittsburgh Plate Glass Co., 427 F.2d 936, 74 L.R.R.M. 2425 (1970).

86. NLRB v. Wooster Div. of Borg-Warner Corp., 356 U.S. 342, 42 L.R.R.M. 2034 (1958).

87. NLRB v. F.M. Reeve & Sons, Inc., 47 L.R.R.M. 2480 (10th Cir. 1960), *cert. denied*, 366 U.S. 914 (1961).

88. Am. Seating Co. of Miss., 176 N.L.R.B. 850, 71 L.R.R.M. 1346 (1969), *aff'd*, 424 F.2d 106, 73 L.R.R.M. 2996 (5th Cir. 1970).

89. Kit Mfg. Co., 150 N.L.R.B. 662, 671, 58 L.R.R.M. 1140 (1964), *enforced*, 365 F.2d 829, 62 L.R.R.M. 2856 (9th Cir. 1966).

90. Local 964, Carpenters, 181 N.L.R.B. 948, 74 L.R.R.M. 1081 (1970), *aff'd*, 447 F.2d 643, 78 L.R.R.M. 2167 (2nd Cir. 1971).

91. Palm Beach Post Times, Div. of Perry Publications, Inc., 151 N.L.R.B. 1030, 58 L.R.R.M. 1561 (1965).

92. NLRB v. Transmarine Navigation Corp., 65 L.R.R.M. 2861 (9th Cir. 1967).

93. Jewish Center for Aged, 220 N.L.R.B. No. 21, 90 L.R.R.M. 1222 (1975).

93a. Peerless Food Products, Inc., 231 N.L.R.B. 530, 96 L.R.R.M. 1048 (1977).

93b. Operating Engineers, Local 12, 246 N.L.R.B. No. 81, 102 L.R.R.M. 1636 (1979).

94. The Columbus Printing Pressmen & Assistants' Union No. 252 (R.W. Page Co.), 219 N.L.R.B. No. 54, 89 L.R.R.M. 1553 (1975).

95. S. Rep. No. 93-988, 93rd Cong., 2d Sess. 5 (1974) (Conference Report).

96. Mass. Nurses Ass'n, 225 N.L.R.B. No. 91, 92 L.R.R.M. 1478 (1976).

97. Section 8(b)(1)(B): "It shall be an unfair labor practice for a labor organization or its agents—(1) to restrain or coerce . . . (B) an employer in the selection of his representatives for the purposes of collective bargaining or the adjustment of grievances. . . ."

98. *See* L. Greenberg, *A Practical Guide to Productivity Measurement* (1973).

99. *Id.* at 40-41.

100. *See* M.H. Granof, *How To Cost Your Labor Contract* (1973).

101. *See The Impact of Computers on Collective Bargaining* (A.J. Siegel, ed. 1969).

102. A "zipper" clause is one which typically provides that *all* matters agreed upon by the parties have been incorporated in their written contract and that there are no other written or oral agreements of any kind. Some "zipper" clauses go even further to provide that the parties have discussed all relevant subjects and that during the life of the contract neither party will have any obligation to engage in negotiations over any subject. A "zipper clause" is a mandatory subject of bargaining. Union Hosp. Ass'n, N.L.R.B. Ad. Mem., 102 L.R.R.M. 1677 (1979). The NLRB General Counsel has indicated that a properly worded zipper clause forecloses any obligation to bargain over union demands midterm in the contract. Report of the General Counsel for Fourth Quarter of 1978, 101 L.R.R.M. 191 (1979).

103. Allis-Chalmers Mfg. Co., 106 N.L.R.B. 939, 32 L.R.R.M. 1585 (1953).

104. Architectural Pottery, Architectural Fiberglass Div., 165 N.L.R.B. 238, 65 L.R.R.M. 1331 (1967).

105. Bartlett-Collins Co., 237 N.L.R.B. No. 106, 99 L.R.R.M. 1034 (1978). *See* HLCM Current Comment Number 19.

106. Carpenter Sprinkler Corp., 238 N.L.R.B. No. 139 (1978).

107. *See, e.g.*, Proctor Mfg. Corp., 131 N.L.R.B. 1166, 48 L.R.R.M. 1222 (1961).

108. Union Starch and Refining Co., 87 N.L.R.B. 779, 25 L.R.R.M. 1176 (1949), *enforced*, 186 F.2d 1008, 27 L.R.R.M. 2342 (7th Cir. 1951), *cert. denied*, 342 U.S. 815, 28 L.R.R.M. 2625 (1951).

109. 29 U.S.C. § 169.

110. *Id.*

111. *See* NLRB v. General Motors Corp., 373 U.S. 734, 53 L.R.R.M. 2313 (1963).

112. Ford Motor Co. of Canada, 1 L.A. 439 (1946 I.C. Rand, arbitrator).

113. S. Rep. No. 93-988, 93d Cong., 2d Sess. 4 (1974) (Conference Report).

114. *See* J.J. Hagerty, Inc., 153 N.L.R.B. 1375, 59 L.R.R.M. 1637 (1965).

115. NLRB v. Hosp. Employees, Local 113 (Mounds Park Hosp.) _____ F.2d _____, 97 L.R.R.M. 2160 (8th Cir. 1977).

116. River Manor Health Related Facility, 224 N.L.R.B. No. 38, 93 L.R.R.M. 1069 (1976).

117. Felter v. Southern Pacific Co., 359 U.S. 326, 79 S.Ct. 847, 3 L.Ed.2d 854, 43 L.R.R.M. 2876 (1959).

118. NLRB v. Local 527, 523 F.2d 783, 90 L.R.R.M. 3121 (5th Cir. 1975). The NLRB, citing this ruling, has held that check-off authorization is a contract between employer and employee. The procedure for revoking a dues check-off authorization cannot be modified without the individual assent of each affected employee. Cameron Iron Works, Inc., 227 N.L.R.B. No. 56 (1976).

119. Ala. Reomp. Code 1958, Tit. 26 § 375.

Ariz. Const. Art. 2, § 35; Ariz. Rev. Stat. Ann. §§ 56-1301–56-1308.

Ark. Const. Amend. No. 34; Ark. Rev. Stat. Ann. § 101-1.
Fla. Const. Art. 1, § 6.
Ga. Code Ann. §§ 54-901–54-908.
Iowa Code Ann. §§ 736A.1–736A.8.
Kan. Const. Art. 15, § 12.
La. Act 397 (1956) (coverage only for agricultural workers).
Miss. Const. Art. 7, § 198-A; Miss. Code Ann. § 6984.5.
Neb. Const. Art. 15, §§ 13–15; Neb. Rev. Stat. §§ 48-217–48-219.
Nev. Rev. Stat. §§ 613.230–613.300.
N.C. Gen. Stat. §§ 95-78–95-98.
N.D. Cent. Code § 34-01-14.
S.C. Code Ann. §§ 40-46–40-46.8.
S.D. Const. Art. VI, § 2; S.D. Code §§ 17.1101, 17.9914.
Tenn. Code Ann. §§ 11412.8–11412.13.
Tex. Rev. Stat. Ann. Art. 5207A, §§ 1–5.
Utah Code Ann. §§ 34-34-1–34-34-17.
Va. Code Ann. §§ 40.1-58–40.1-69.
Wyo. Stat. Ann. §§ 27-245.1–27-245.8.

It should be noted that in 7 states—Arizona, Florida, Kansas, Nevada, North Dakota, South Dakota, and Texas—an agency shop arrangement may be permissible. However, competent counsel should be sought before entering into such an agreement.

120. *See generally, The Developing Labor Law* 495-496 (C.J. Morris, ed. 1971).

121. *See* Gary-Hobard Water Corp., 210 N.L.R.B. 742, 744, 86 L.R.R.M. 1210 (1974); Keller-Crescent Co., 217 N.L.R.B. 685, 691, 89 L.R.R.M. 1201 (1975); and Local 18, Operating Engineers, 238 N.L.R.B. No. 58, 99 L.R.R.M. 1307 (1978).

121a. W-I Canteen, Inc. v. NLRB, _____ F.2d _____, 102 L.R.R.M. 2447 (1979).

121b. *See* NLRB v. Rockaway News Supply Co., 345 U.S. 71 (1953).

122. Dairylea Cooperative, Inc., 219 N.L.R.B. No. 107, 89 L.R.R.M. 1737 (1975, *enforced sub nom.* NLRB v. Teamsters, Local 338, _____ F.2d _____, 91 L.R.R.M. 2929 (2d Cir. 1976); Teamsters Local v. NLRB, _____ F.2d _____, 102 L.R.R.M. 3080 (D.C. Cir. 1979).

122a. NLRB v. Teamsters Local 443, No. 78-4195 101 L.R.R.M. 2622 (2d Cir., June 6, 1979).

122b. *Id.*

123. U.E. Local 623, 230 N.L.R.B. No. 59, _____ L.R.R.M. _____ (1977).

123a. American Can Co., 244 N.L.R.B. No. 78, 102 L.R.R.M. 1071 (1979), *modifying* 235 N.L.R.B. No. 102, 98 L.R.R.M. 1012. The case involved the retention of a union trustee and guard, with less seniority than a number of other employees, during a layoff.

124. "Arbitrability"—the promise to arbitrate—is one of the most complex and controversial issues in labor-management relations law. *See* P. Prasow and E. Peters, *Arbitration and Collective Bargaining: Conflict Resolution in Labor Relations* (1970).

125. *See* section 1302(8) of P.L. 93-222 for a statutory definition of the term, "community rating system."

126. *See* pages 31-32 of the conference report on P.L. 93-222 (S. Rep. 93-621) for a more detailed discussion of the legislative intent regarding copayments.

127. The preceding sections on Services and Payment were quoted in their entirety from S. Rep. No. 14, 93d Cong., 2d Sess. 2, 3, (1974).

128. Nat'l League of Cities v. Usery, 426 U.S. 833, 22 Wage & Hour Cas. 1064 (1976).

129. *See* Chapter 12 of the volume from which this article is reprinted for a copy of the regulations.

130. NLRB v. Katz, 369 U.S. 736, 50 L.R.R.M. 2177 (1962).

131. *See* NLRB v. U.S. Somics Corp., 312 F.2d 610, 52 L.R.R.M. 2360 (1st Cir. 1963).

132. *See* Palomar Corp. and Gateway Service Co., 192 N.L.R.B. 592, 78 L.R.R.M. 1030 (1971).

133. *See* Falcon Tank Corp., 194 N.L.R.B. 333, 78 L.R.R.M. 1587 (1971).

134. *See* Sioux Falls Stock Yards Co., 208 N.L.R.B. No. 4, 85 L.R.R.M. 1095 (1974).

135. Phillip Carey Mfg. Co., 140 N.L.R.B. 1103, 52 L.R.R.M. 1184 (1963).

136. Webb Furniture Corp., 366 F.2d 314, 63 L.R.R.M. 2163 (4th Cir. 1966).

137. Idaho Fresh Pak, Inc., 215 N.L.R.B. No. 115, 88 L.R.R.M. 1207 (1974).

138. Kit Mfg. Co., 138 N.L.R.B. 1290, 51 L.R.R.M. 1224 (1962.)

139. L.A.X. Medical Clinic, Inc., 248 N.L.R.B. No. 112, 104 L.R.R.M. 1092 (1980).

14. Union Security Arrangements

DENNIS D. POINTER and NORMAN METZGER

Reprinted with permission from *The National Labor Relations Act* by Dennis D. Pointer, Ph.D., and Norman Metzger, published by Spectrum Publications, Inc., New York, © 1975.

TYPES OF UNION SECURITY AGREEMENTS

Once a union has been certified as the collective bargaining agent for the employees in a health care facility, one of its primary aims is to obtain a contractual provision that gives it (the union) maximum protection as to its continued existence in that institution. It, therefore, attempts to bargain some form of compulsory union membership. These provisions are called union security arrangements. There are five major forms of union security:

1. closed shop;
2. union shop;
3. modified union shop;
4. maintenance of membership shop; and
5. agency shop.

Closed Shop

A closed shop requires applicants for employment to be members of the union before they can be hired. This form of union security was usually accompanied by a union hiring hall provision. The union is notified of the employment needs of the employer and forwards applicants to fill the jobs. A sample closed shop clause follows:

The health care facility shall hire only applicants for employment who are members of the union.

The union shall furnish such applicants for employment provided that, however, if the union is unable to fill such request, the health care facility may hire applicants who are not members of the union, but such applicants must become members of the union immediately upon being hired.

Under Section 8(a)(3), the closed shop is declared illegal.

Union Shop

The great majority of collective bargaining agreements contain a union shop clause. This type of union security provides that all employees in the bargaining unit must join the union within a specified period of time after hire, usually at the end of a probationary period. Under the Act, any union shop agreement must provide new employees with a minimum of thirty days in which to become members of the union. It is an unfair labor practice to allow nonmembers less than thirty days to join a union. It is also illegal to maintain a requirement that a nonmember must state his intent to join before thirty days of employment. A sample union shop provision follows:

All employees on the active payroll at the time of the signing of the contract who are members of the union shall maintain their membership in the union in good standing as a condition of continued

691

employment. All employees on the active payroll as of the time of the signing of the contract who are not members of the union shall become members of the union within thirty (30) days after the effective date of the contract. All employees hired after the effective date of the contract shall become members of the union no later than the 30th day following the beginning of such employment and shall thereafter maintain their membership in the union in good standing as a condition of continued employment.

Under the union shop arrangement, if an employee fails to join the union within the prescribed period of time (thirty days or longer), the union may request the discharge of such an employee.

Modified Union Shop

A modified union shop arrangement provides an option to employees currently on the payroll. Those who are members of the union must maintain their membership, but those who have not joined the union need not join. As to new employees, they must join the union within a specified period of time after hire—again, usually after the probationary period. This form of union security is a compromise which protects current employees who do not wish to join the union. The movement from a modified union shop to a union shop is sometimes effected by a clause which states that after a certain percentage of employees have joined the union, all those remaining out must join the union.

Maintenance of Membership

A more permissive union security arrangement is a maintenance-of-membership arrangement. In the maintenance-of-membership shop, members of the bargaining unit are not required to become members of the union to keep their jobs, but those employees who do decide to join the union must maintain their membership in the union for a specific length of time: either one year or for the duration of the contract. This is called an "escape" period. It clarifies the time when union members may drop out of the union without losing their jobs. The following is a typical maintenance-of-membership clause:

Any employee who is a member in good standing of the union at the end of thirty (30) days from the date the provision becomes effective or who thereafter joins the union during the term of this agreement shall remain a member of the union in

good standing as a condition of employment with the health care facility.

It is clear under this agreement that nonmembers have no duty to join the union.

Agency Shop

The agency shop was a comparatively rare form of union security which had a rebirth as a counterposition of unions to right-to-work laws. Section 14(b) gave state "right-to-work" laws precedence over union shop provisions of the Act. It stated:

Nothing in this Act shall be construed as authorizing the execution or application of agreements requiring membership in a labor organization as a condition of employment in any State or Territory where such . . . is prohibited. . . .

Right-to-work laws outlawed mandatory or compulsory union membership. Under an agency shop requirement, the employee can join or not join the union and can remain a member or drop out, but all employees in the bargaining unit represented by the union must pay a service fee to support the union as a condition of employment. This service fee is usually equal to the amount paid by union members for dues.

The Supreme Court, in *NLRB v. General Motors Corp.*[1], upheld union security provisions calling for an agency shop. The Court stated in its decision that Congress, in passing the Taft-Hartley Act, did not intend to make the union shop the only valid union security device, but, rather, meant to limit the union's power to obtain discharge for any reason other than nonpayment of dues. The Court held that the agency shop is "the practical equivalent of union 'membership' as Congress used the term in the proviso to 8(a)(3)" and is therefore legal.

Right-to-work laws have been enacted in twenty states. Fourteen states have provided for such arrangements by statute: Alabama, Georgia, Iowa, Louisiana, Nevada, North Carolina, North Dakota, South Carolina, South Dakota, Tennessee, Texas, Utah, Virginia and Wyoming. In the case of Louisiana, the statute applies only to agricultural workers. Six states provided constitutional amendments dealing with the right to work: Arizona, Arkansas, Florida, Kansas, Mississippi and Nebraska.

The absence of any form of union security is generally referred to as an open shop. Under the open shop, employees can join or not join the union as they see fit and can remain in or drop out of the union without losing their jobs.

ARGUMENTS ABOUT MANDATORY UNION MEMBERSHIP

Specific forms of union security are not mandated items which employers must incorporate in a collective bargaining agreement. The employer must bargain over the form and extent of a union security provision across the table. Labor leaders in presenting their arguments in favor of compulsory union membership base their position primarily on the so-called "free rider" inequity. The "free rider" employee, labor leaders argue, reaps all the advantages hard won by the union in their negotiations with the institution, yet is not required to support the union.

Regardless of the type of union security agreement, all employees (even those that do not belong to the union) are covered by conditions of the contract if they are part of the bargaining unit. If the employees are given the option to remain out of the union, they are nonetheless covered by all provisions of the collective bargaining agreement including the grievance procedure; however, they may not attend meetings and may not vote on union issues. Union leaders maintain that the philosophy of compulsory union membership is rooted in a basic democratic principle: the rule of the majority. It is their position that given a free choice, employees will join the union but that usually they remain out because of fear of reprisal or promise of reward by the employer.

Management, in defending its position for optional membership across the table in collective bargaining, usually does so on the basis of the inherent right of the individual to make choices and therefore to withhold his membership from any organization. It is well to note that in actual practice, there are some advantages to management in agreeing to a compulsory union security provision. Too often when the employees are given an option to join or not join the union, only the most militant and outspoken critics of management join the union and their views are not modified by those of more conservative employees. Additionally, in a modified union security arrangement, the union continues its drive to enroll employees and often undertakes this activity during the normal workdays throughout the year.

In summary, the position of the union in support of its argument across the negotiating table for compulsory union membership is based on its need to continue its existence and to service the employees effectively; it maintains that in order to do this it must have financial support from all employees. Its argument is bolstered by its very presence at the negotiating table which was established by majority rule. Union leaders maintain that since a majority of the employees voted for the union, all employees in the bargaining unit should be required under the compulsory union security clause to join the union. This, they further state, will reduce strife and factionalism.

On the other side of the table, employers, in negotiating union security agreements, state that compulsory union membership is an undemocratic mechanism. They wish to insure freedom of choice. Employers maintain that their position in support of a lesser form of union security is not part and parcel of an attempt to undermine the union. They further state that forcing employees to join the union when they do not wish to will not contribute to more harmonious or responsible labor relations. In fact, employees who are forced to join a union under a compulsory union security arrangement often are resentful and may indeed terminate their employment.

UNION SECURITY DISCHARGES

Section 8(a)(3) of the Act forbids the discharge or suspension of an employee under a union shop contract for loss of membership in good standing in the union except where such loss of membership is caused by the employee's failure to pay or tender payment of his union dues and initiation fee. It also forbids the discharge of an employee under a union shop contract if the employee was denied membership in the union on the same terms and conditions as all other employees who are members of the union.

The Board has ruled that union membership must be available on a fair and nondiscriminatory basis. It has further stated that any requirement for membership in addition to dues and an initiation fee may not be used as a basis for the nonmember's discharge even if such requirement is fair and nondiscriminatory. Where an employee tendered the requisite money to the union but refused to attend meetings or take an oath of loyalty, the Board found both the institution and the union guilty of unfair labor practices for discharging the employee for nonmembership.

It is clear that after an employee joins a union, he can only be discharged for violation of a union shop agreement on the basis of his failure to tender his dues to the union.

CHECKOFF

The checkoff is an arrangement included in a collective bargaining agreement under which the dues and initiation fees of members of the bargaining unit are deducted from employee payroll checks by the employer and forwarded to the union. It is illegal to automatically checkoff union dues. In order to legally effect a checkoff arrangement under provisions of the Act, the employer must obtain written authorization cards from each employee.

Section 302(c) of the Act authorizes an employer to deduct union dues from the employee's pay and forward such funds to the union only on the basis of an authorization card signed by the employee—such authorization cannot be irrevocable for more than one year or the duration of the existing collective bargaining agreement providing for the checkoff, whichever is the shorter period. The term "dues" has been interpreted to include initiation fees and general assessments uniformly leveled. A sample checkoff clause follows:

1. Upon receipt of a written authorization from an employee, the health care facility shall, pursuant to such authorization, deduct from the wages due said employee each month, starting not earlier than the first pay period following the completion of the employee's first thirty (30) days of employment, and remit to the union regular monthly dues and initiation fees, as fixed by the union. The initiation fee shall be paid in two (2) consecutive monthly installments beginning the month following the completion of the probationary period.

2. Employees who do not sign written authorizations for deductions must adhere to the same payment procedure by making payments directly to the union.

3. The health care facility shall be relieved from making such "checkoff" deductions upon (a) termination of employment, or (b) transfer to a job other than one covered by the bargaining unit, or (c) lay off from work, or (d) an agreed leave of absence, or (e) revocation of the checkoff authorization in accordance with its terms or with applicable law. Notwithstanding the foregoing, upon the return of an employee to work from any of the foregoing enumerated absences, the health care facility will immediately resume the obligation of making said deductions, except that deductions for terminated employees shall be governed by paragraph 1 hereof. This provision, however, shall not relieve any employees of the obligation to make the required dues and initiation payment pursuant to the union constitution in order to remain in good standing.

4. The health care facility shall not be obliged to make dues deductions of any kind from any employee who, during any dues month involved, shall have failed to receive sufficient wages to equal the dues deduction.

5. Each month, the health care facility shall remit to the union all deductions for dues and initiation fees made from the wages of employees for the preceding month, together with a list of all employees from whom dues and/or initiation fees have been deducted.

6. The health care facility agrees to furnish the union each month with the names of newly hired employees, their addresses, social security numbers, classifications of work, their dates of hire, and names of terminated employees, together with their dates of termination, and names of employees on leave of absence.

7. It is specifically agreed that the health care facility assumes no obligation, financial or otherwise, arising out of the provisions of this Article, and the union hereby agrees that it will indemnify and hold the health care facility harmless from any claims, actions or proceedings by any employee arising from deductions made by the health care facility hereunder. Once the funds are remitted to the union, their disposition thereafter shall be the sole and exclusive obligation and responsibility of the union.

Some institutions attempt to negotiate checkoff clauses in exchange for an arrangement which will reimburse the institution for the cost of operating such a program. In addition, a safeguard commonly found in checkoff provisions in collective bargaining agreements is a clause which clearly states that the union will assume responsibility for dues collection if the employee's earnings are curtailed. This is a guarantee that the union will relieve the institution of any legal liability growing out of improper deduction of union dues by the institution. No matter what shape or form the union's demand for a checkoff provision takes, the employer has a duty to bargain concerning the dues checkoff. This position was clearly stated by the Board.[2]

Although the checkoff is at times a controversial negotiating item and is often resisted by institutions, some employers feel that by agreeing to a checkoff provision they prevent the disruption and hostility which may develop from continuous activity on the part of union officers and delegates in their duties to collect dues.

RELIGIOUS OBJECTIONS AND UNION SECURITY

Section 19 was added to the Act by the 1974 amendments stating that

Any employee of a health care institution who is a member of and adheres to established and traditional tenets or teachings of a bona fide religion, body, or sect which has historically held conscientious objections to joining or financially supporting labor organizations shall not be required to join or financially support any labor organization as a condition of employment; except that such employee may be required in lieu of periodic dues and initiation fees, to pay sums equal to such dues and initiation fees to a nonreligious charitable fund exempt from taxation under section 501(c)(3) of the Internal Revenue Code, chosen by such employee from a list of at least three such funds, designated in a contract between such institution and a labor organization, or if the contract fails to designate such funds, then to any such fund chosen by the employee.[3]

This section holds that employees of health care facilities who object on religious grounds to joining or financially supporting a labor organization shall not be required to do so as a condition of employment. It is important to note that this exclusion applies only to employees of health care facilities as defined in the Act. To be eligible for the exclusion the employee must be a member of a bona fide religion, body or sect that has historically held an objection to joining or financially supporting labor organizations. In lieu of union dues and fees the employee may be required to make payments to a nonreligious charitable fund. Designation of the funds can be made by the employer and union pursuant to the collective bargaining agreement.

NOTES

1. *NLRB v. General Motors Corp.*, 373 U.S. 734, 53 LRRM 2313 (1963).
2. *U.S. Gypsum Co.*, 94 NLRB 112, 28 LRRM 1015 (1951).
3. Pub. L. 93-360 § 19, 88 Stat. 395 et seq.

15. Guidelines to Productivity Bargaining in the Health Care Industry

MYRON D. FOTTLER and WILLIAM A. MALONEY

Reprinted with permission from *Health Care Management Review*, Vol. 4, No. 1, Winter 1979, published by Aspen Systems Corporation, Germantown, Md. © 1979.

Health care managers will become increasingly concerned with productivity in the years ahead as cost containment becomes a major environmental reality. While the Carter Administration proposal for a nine-percent limitation on the annual increase in hospital costs does not appear likely to pass Congress soon [Ed. note: It did not.], similar proposals appear likely to continue to be made. The reasons are obvious. The public has become convinced that it is spending too much for health care and receiving too little. The era of ''open-ended'' funding which has characterized the past does not appear likely to continue in the future. One method of dealing with this new situation is to generate more output from existing resources, i.e., to increase productivity.

Productivity is a subtle concept, particularly in the context of health organizations whose primary purpose is to provide services rather than goods. Productivity in the health sector is difficult to measure, difficult to conceptualize and difficult to realize.

There are basically two approaches to raising productivity. First, there are unilateral management changes with respect to capital investment, new technology, work organization, work scheduling or work rules.[1] The second approach is productivity bargaining which occurs in the context of a collective bargaining relationship.

Collective bargaining has increased dramatically in recent years. More than 25 percent of the nation's hospitals have some sort of bargaining agreement with their employers, compared to only three percent in the early 1960s.[2] These figures are much higher in urban areas, on the east and west coasts, in highly unionized areas and in areas where health institutions had been legally required to bargain prior to 1974.[3]

While a number of factors both stimulate and inhibit collective bargaining,[4] the most important stimulant has been the 1974 amendments to the Taft-Hartley Act which removed prior exemptions for and constraints on organization and collective bargaining by nonprofit health care institutions. The term *health care institution* is defined broadly to include any hospital, convalescent hospital, HMO clinic, nursing home, extended care facility or other institution devoted to the care of the sick, infirm or aged persons.[5] The predicted increase in union organizing has occurred,[6] and unions are now winning 62.5 percent of elections in hospitals, 57.8 percent in nursing homes, and 60.7 percent in other health care facilities.[7] The trends are obvious. An increasing proportion of the health care industry will engage in some form of collective bargaining in the future.

The *potential* conflict between the growth of collective bargaining and the increasing concern for productivity should be obvious. A natural opposition of interests can develop between managers of health care facilities who are under pressure to decrease costs while increasing the quantity and quality of service, and labor unions or professional associations who are under pressure from their membership to improve wages, fringe benefits, working conditions and job security.

As more and more health care employees become unionized, collective bargaining increasingly will become the means by which labor costs, including the direct costs of earnings, fringe benefits and retirement benefits, are determined. While disputes exist over the extent to which collective bargaining actually changes the distribution of power in health care wage-setting processes, prevailing opinion is that it reduces somewhat the influence of management in the wage-setting process.[8] With rising labor costs, health care management has difficulty in calibrating increases in labor costs with revenue and expenditure trends.

The noneconomic impact of labor unions on health institutions is somewhat unclear. An earlier study by Miller and Shortell concluded that unions had a generally *neutral* effect on patient care during the 1961–67 period studied.[9] Studies by Osterhaus showed the impact of unionization on management of health care organizations in the following ways: more attention and emphasis is given to the personnel-industrial relations functions, employee participation in management is increased, communications between management and employees is improved and coalition bargaining with many unions is just beginning.[10–12] More recently, a study by Becker provides evidence that collective bargaining stabilizes employment by reducing turnover.[13] Also, health care unions evidently tend to place more emphasis than management on wages, grievance procedures and the application of seniority to promotions and layoffs.[14] Yet a case study of collective bargaining by nurses indicated that there has been little, if any, impact on quantity or quality of employee productivity as a result of collective bargaining.[15]

The most reasonable conclusion from these studies is that collective bargaining probably has had a mixed impact on employee productivity and varies greatly from situation to situation. The specific impact may depend on how management deals with the union and the nature of the eventual relationship which develops.

Productivity bargaining is one method of linking the interests of management and the employee representative so that the potential positive aspects will be maximized and the negative minimized. For purposes of the present analysis, *collective bargaining* will include negotiations between professional associations and management as well as the more traditional union-management negotiations. The term *labor union* will also refer to professional associations which engage in such negotiations as well as labor organizations representing primarily nonprofessionals.

SOME DEFINITIONS

Productivity, or more accurately, productivity increase, means more output per unit of input, not merely more output. Such output should be of acceptable quality. Productivity is a relational concept involving both outputs and inputs. The inputs include *all* resources used in a productive effort, such as capital, labor, land, space, supplies and materials.

Productivity bargaining has been defined by various authors as follows:

The negotiation and implementation of formal collective bargaining agreements which stipulate changes in work rules and practices with the objective of achieving increased productivity and reciprocal worker gains.[16]

A method of negotiation in which changes in wages are tied to changes in work with the object of reducing or stabilizing unit costs, resulting in a mutually agreed share of the benefits between management and labor.[17]

When unions and management bargain over work practices in the expectation that both workers and the employer will benefit from changes agreed upon—in essence, that management will offer certain incentives to its work force in return for anticipated increases in the latter's productivity.[18]

From these definitions, it is clear that productivity bargaining involves two distinct issues: the first is the negotiation of changes in traditional or existing rules and practices; the second is the sharing of the savings accruing from the resultant increased productivity. This sharing of the savings is inseparable from the negotiation of various changes. Productivity bargaining is therefore the negotiation of a formal collective agreement which details specific changes in work rules and practices and the distribution of the resultant savings. It is a means by which an employer *already engaged in collective bargaining* with his employees may modify existing collective bargaining agreements to eliminate constraints on individual or group productivity.

The conventional collective bargaining agreement defines the rights and responsibilities of management and labor that will maintain the traditional approaches to achieving output goals. Occasionally, the traditional agreement may incorporate minor or quite significant productivity changes, but these are not seen by the parties as fundamental goals aimed at changing the overall productivity of the organization.

However, in productivity bargaining agreements, change and efficiency are the basic objectives. The agreement may change basic occupational roles and relationships, including new combinations, elimination or unique rearrangements of occupations. Therefore, when management engages in productivity bargaining as opposed to collective bargaining, it is introducing new and highly unstable questions concerning union jurisdiction, job rights, status, promotion opportunities and established customs and traditions.

Productivity bargaining can be distinguished from informal bargaining, traditional collective bargaining and various productivity improvement schemes. The formal nature of the negotiations, the written agreement and the sharing of savings distinguish productivity bargaining from the informal, shop-level bargaining that allows labor agreements to be made more workable. It is also distinguishable from traditional collective bargaining even though both can be viewed as the negotiation of a wage-effort agreement. The wage side of the relationship is concerned with the total amount and forms of compensation to be paid to an individual for the performance of a specific job; the effort side of the relationship is concerned with the individual's input and output, i.e., the productivity of the individual.

Historically, collective bargaining has primarily focused on the wage side of the relationship. Union leaders have concentrated on increasing the level of total compensation, and employers have attempted to minimize these increases. The effort side of the relationship has generally been ignored or relegated to a low priority with the exception of union attempts at negotiating work rules to preserve employment opportunities. Unlike traditional collective bargaining which emphasizes the *wage* side, productivity bargaining emphasizes the *effort* side of the wage-effort bargain. It attempts to offset present and future increases in compensation with increases in productivity to stabilize or reduce unit labor costs. Productivity bargaining is also distinguishable from other joint productivity improvement schemes because it considers the institutional relationship between the parties. Both parties bargain over the institutional schedule of rules which govern the work place where these rules, depending upon the point of view, either protect the worker's rights or inhibit productivity by constraining management.

Productivity bargaining consists of two distinct phases. Phase I is the negotiation for the removal of constraints on productivity that have been developed through collective bargaining and the necessary quid pro quo for these changes. In a sense, it is a "negative" action involving the removal of hindrances to productivity. Phase II is the negotiation of practices which motivate the employees to increase their pro-

ductivity from the previous artificially low level. This includes economic and noneconomic approaches and can be viewed as a "positive" action. In order to have true productivity bargaining, Phase I must precede Phase II. Since productivity improvement schemes involve only Phase II, they cannot be considered productivity bargaining.

The PAR System

An example is the Participation-Achievement-Reward (PAR) system proposed by Schultz and McKersie.[19] This plan attempts to improve productivity by establishing an area of collaboration between labor and management where that collaboration is to be accomplished *without* adverse effects to the local union or to collective bargaining between the union and management. It illustrates the second phase of productivity. The PAR approach, because of the inviolability of the collective bargaining agreement, cannot be viewed within the definitions of productivity bargaining that have previously been discussed. In addition, attempts at increasing productivity through the payment system by means of incentives, whether individual or group, cannot really deal with the primary objectives of traditional productivity bargaining of worker flexibility and free assignment of manpower.

The PAR approach attempts to motivate workers, individually and collectively, to increase productivity within the existing institutional framework of rules, not by changing these rules or practices. Even though the PAR approach may result in a change in the employees' behavior so that productivity increases, its potential for gain is greatly enhanced when Phase I of traditional productivity bargaining is used to remove any institutional constraints on productivity increases. Without such prior changes in institutional constraints, the potential for productivity increase is often limited.

Unit Labor Cost Bargaining

Productivity bargaining may be a misnomer. A more appropriate name may be unit labor cost bargaining. Even though its emphasis may be on the effort side of the bargain, productivity bargaining does not ignore the wage side of the relationship. The wage side influences unit labor costs as does the effort or productivity side of the bargain. Productivity bargaining looks at the wage side of the wage-effort bargain in two areas. As pointed out in the definitions of productivity bargaining, it looks first to the wage side of the bargain to determine the compensation increases, the quid pro quo, required to obtain changes in the work rules and practices on the effort side. Second, productivity bargaining examines pay practices to determine those that are outmoded and in need of change.

Although many of the changes reported in the literature are just common sense, they were not done until a special productivity effort was made. For example, in the construction industry, some local unions have agreed to work Saturday at straight-time pay to make up for days lost during the week because of inclement weather. This is a change from the prior pay practice of requiring double-time for work performed outside of the normal work hours of 8:00 a.m. to 4:30 p.m., Monday through Friday. The unit labor cost is reduced even though there has been no change in productivity. The definitions of productivity bargaining cited above accurately describe the process if work rules and practices are viewed broadly to include pay practices.

It is imperative that productivity be viewed in the broadest context and not simply as output per man-hour in order to attain the full potential of productivity bargaining in a health care environment. McKersie has discussed four factors that influence productivity: (1) the duration of effort, (2) the intensity of effort, (3) the effectiveness with which the effort input of workers is combined with technology and other resources and (4) the overall efficiency with which these inputs are translated into usable outputs of acceptable quality.[20] Thus productivity bargaining is concerned with the negotiation of changes in work rules and practices that negatively affect any of these four factors. Examples are easily seen: excessive absenteeism or tardiness, formal or informal limitations on employee output, excessive staffing, etc.

A natural subject for productivity bargaining would be the scheduling of manpower. For example, if the demand for a given health service varies throughout the week or year, it should be possible to match the availability of manpower to the exigencies of demand. Such a plan would require considerable analysis of operations, as well as direct consideration of employee needs. Some employees may like staggered work patterns, others may not. Productivity bargaining should put it all together into a workable plan.

THEORY OF PRODUCTIVITY BARGAINING

Productivity bargaining is accurately described by Walton and McKersie's model of integrative bargaining which is defined as "the system of activities which is instrumental to the attainment of objectives which are not in fundamental conflict with those of the other party and which therefore can be integrated to some degree."[21] It is a *variable* sum game in which both parties can gain, although not necessarily equally, rather than the *fixed* sum game of traditional bargaining. The fundamental premise upon which integrative bargaining is based is the joint problem-solving process. Walton and McKersie's model, depicted in Figure 15-1, consists of three distinct, but interrelated, steps: (1) recognition and definition of the problem, (2) search for alternative solutions to the problems and their consequences, and (3) an evaluation of the alternatives against some criteria for acceptance or rejection.[22]

The recognition and definition of the problem require the parties to jointly explore areas of concern and the factors underlying them to identify mutual problems. The parties, in this step, must expand their discussions to reach the problem rather than simply discussing the symptoms of the problem. For example, management may be faced with declining patient days which result in the employees facing the possibility of layoffs. The institution's loss of revenue and the workers' potential layoffs may be perceived by each as independent problems, but in reality, they may be symptoms of a single problem: the employer's inability to compete with alternative sources of care, due to a variety of reasons.

In order for the remainder of the integrative bargaining process to be effective, the parties must reach a consensus definition of the specific problem. If the parties reach agreement on the definition of a general problem but attempt to solve different specific problems, the integrative potential of the bargaining process is lost and the bargaining quickly deteriorates into fixed sum traditional bargaining.

At this point, it is also necessary to set forth the constraints with which possible solutions must be compatible. These may include existing needs and demands, compatibility with higher level planning such as HSAs, present and projected levels of patient care in total and by category, existing facilities, occupational licensing requirements and other legal constraints on innovative manpower utilization patterns, economic resources and timing. After considering these factors, redefining the problem may be necessary.

Alternative Solutions

Once the problem has been defined, the second step is to search for alternative solutions to the problem and the consequences of these alternatives. Many alternative solutions are not obvious and finding them requires imagination, invention and creativity on the part

Figure 15-1 The Integrative Bargaining Model

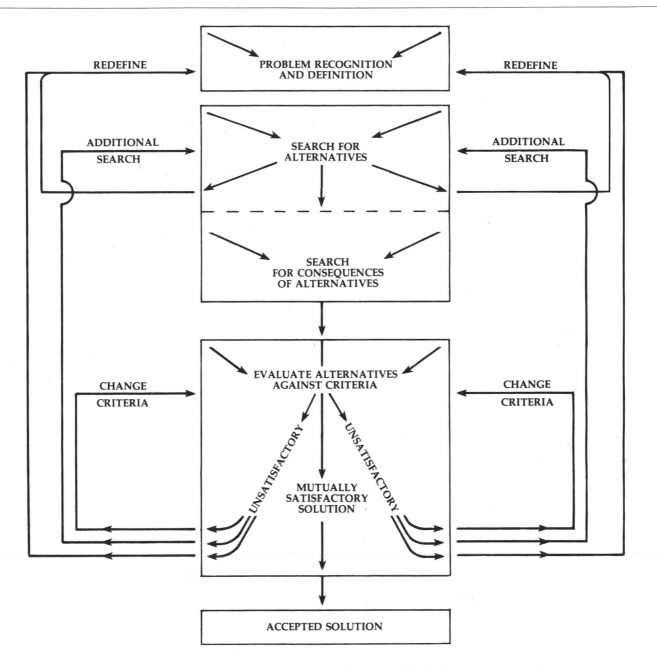

of both parties. The parties must now allow themselves to enter into this step of the process with preconceived notions or formulated solutions to the problem because of the limitations that would be placed on the search process. To facilitate the search for alternatives, it may be beneficial to establish special study committees on particularly difficult problems to con-

duct a fact-finding study of the problem and develop alternative solutions to the problem. The effectiveness of the problem-solving process is directly related to the scope of the search process. If the parties are unable to discover alternative solutions, the model provides for feedback to the first step to allow for redefinition of the problem.

The search for solutions to the problem entails an analysis of work rules, arrangements and pay practices to determine those that are restricting productivity and/or elevating unit labor costs. Solutions, for example, could include such changes as elimination of coffee breaks and changes in staffing requirements. Each of these solutions will carry with it consequences or payoffs for both the employer and the workers. For management, there will be the positive consequence of potentially increased productivity and, thereby, an improved ability to compete.

On the employees' side, the consequences of each alternative are initially negative. The changes that are made typically require the workers to give up rights and benefits developed under the old system of rules. To alleviate these negative consequences, the parties must agree on the quid pro quo necessary to make the changes. This normally involves a change in financial compensation either in the form of increased wages, a lump sum payment, employer guarantees of some level of income or improved noneconomic benefits relating to working conditions or job security.

The Creative Decision-Making Process

The search for alternative solutions and their consequences may be approached through what has been labeled the creative decision-making process, which involves the following five steps:[23]

1. *saturation:* becoming thoroughly familiar with a problem as well as ideas and activities akin to the problem;
2. *deliberation:* mulling over these ideas, analyzing them, challenging them, rearranging them and evaluating them from several viewpoints;
3. *incubation:* relaxing, turning off the conscious and purposeful search and letting the subconscious mind work;
4. *illumination:* receiving a sudden insight or bright idea which appears to have promise for solving the problem;
5. *accommodation:* clarifying the idea, putting it on paper, getting the reaction of others and reframing and adopting it.

Ideally, the various approaches developed through creative decision making will be analyzed in very specific terms during the final stage of accommodation. Each approach should be stated in terms of who, what, how, when and where. Once solutions have been developed, the parties must assess each to determine the positive and negative consequences of such an action.

Ideally, both parties would receive large positive payoffs from the implementation of each solution, but it is possible to receive either a positive *or* a negative payoff.

The final step of the process requires the evaluation of the alternatives against criteria established by each party for acceptance. Possible selection criteria might include total cost, expected results, cost effectiveness, risk, effect on job security of present employees, political costs and benefits and timing. The selection criteria are then applied to the possible approaches.

There are four possible courses of action during the evaluation process. First, the parties may agree that the payoffs of an alternative meet the criteria for acceptance and therefore the alternative is a mutually satisfactory solution. A second course of action is to change the criteria if none of the alternatives measures up to the original acceptance criteria, thus allowing a previously rejected alternative solution to become a mutually satisfactory one. If none of the alternatives is acceptable, a third course of action is to require an additional search for additional alternatives. Finally, if none of these courses of action is feasible, the parties may have to redefine the problem and begin the problem-solving process again.

If and when the payoffs from any of the alternative solutions meet its acceptance criteria, management may respond by improving the economic package or noneconomic benefits in order to gain the employees' and the union's acceptance of the solutions. The noneconomic benefits might include providing additional opportunities for continuing education and job upgrading, job rotation, job enrichment, flexible hours and days of work, hours reduction, recreation programs and special recognition programs on either an individual or a group basis. For professional employees, the noneconomic benefits might also include educational leave and attendance at conferences.

Like most theoretical discussions, this section of the article offers few practical guidelines for the conduct of productivity bargaining in health care settings. Developing highly specific and detailed criteria is outside the scope of this article. However, a brief discussion of some elementary and cautionary considerations is appropriate and is the subject of the following section. These are based on experience in other industries and in other countries.

SOME POTENTIAL PROBLEMS

Health care managers must recognize that the introduction of productivity bargaining does not necessarily alter preexisting bargaining or power relationships between labor and management, but it does expand the number and nature of issues upon which the bargaining power of the parties is tested. The utility of productivity bargaining is closely related to the configuration of bargaining power between labor and management. In extreme situations, where management dominates labor or labor dominates management, productivity bargaining does not appear to be a particularly useful managerial tool. In the first situation, few incentives exist for management even to engage in productivity bargaining because unilateral changes may be imposed by management without trading off "premium" wage increases or other benefits, thereby increasing unit costs. Conversely, where labor has traditionally dominated management, few incentives exist for labor to engage in the work rule tradeoffs upon which productivity bargaining is based.

Before the parties can move to productivity bargaining, there must be a strong underpinning of true collective bargaining. Without that base, there is no foundation to build on for future mutual trust. Job and income maintenance guarantees are also prerequisites for achieving employee cooperation in changing work methods. Only then can the worker approach the proposed changes secure in the knowledge that the productivity program will not threaten his or her livelihood. When and where management takes the employees' and the union's concerns into account, much less difficulty is usually encountered in improving work practices and methods. When these concerns are not considered, there may be long delays in realizing anticipated productivity increases at best, and chaos at worst.

There are no quick and easy steps for health care managers and unions to follow in negotiating over established interests and prerogatives which involve transforming their existing patterns of relations, even though both parties might see the promise of mutual benefit. If past experience in other industries is any guide, external pressure for productivity improvement or some kind of crisis is required. Among the most important factors external to the bargaining relationship in health care might be federal or state government pressure for cost containment, similar pressure from funding agencies such as Blue Cross, increased competition, loss of revenue or various other changes in government legislation or regulation. The existence of a formalized outside constituency that requires a mechanism for accountability is itself a strong incentive for productivity bargaining.

The threat of potential job loss will motivate the individual worker and/or the bargaining representative to participate in productivity bargaining which may result in saving the job. Likewise, management will have

similar motivations to prevent deficits and other negative outcomes. The level of the parties' motivation influences the exchange of information which is necessary to develop a consensus definition of the problem(s) facing the parties. The more the parties are motivated, the more information they will exchange and the more effective will be the process.

Management Commitment

Strong management commitment is required to overcome apathy, keep the communications flow open and avoid a cyclical or long-term reduction of enthusiasm after the initial good feeling. Ideally the program should be initiated only after the executive director and board of directors have established positive support for the program and clearly defined the role of productivity bargaining in achieving the institution's mission. Subsequently, the executive director should be prepared to spend substantial blocks of his own time dealing with the bargaining agent for the employees, various department heads and other members of management.

The health care manager should also be prepared for negative reaction. Some managers and some employees tend to emphasize the potential problems of a particular proposal rather than the potential benefits. Several work procedures may have to be changed, employees may have to be retrained, the union might file a grievance, other disruptions may occur and some of the proposals may be incompatible with existing legislation and regulation. Convincing these individuals to experiment with new ways of thinking and new approaches to problems will not be easy. But one of the primary jobs of a manager is to solve problems, not to walk away from them.

The attitudinal and behavioral changes required of managers, union officials and employees in general are difficult to achieve. There is little reason to expect rapid development of the cooperation needed to move in a comprehensive manner in bargaining over productivity. The attitudes of managers are often more difficult to change than those of employees. For many managers, any admission that things can be done better is tantamount to acknowledging that they were not doing their jobs properly before. Yet without such recognition, it is unlikely that any lasting changes in how work is done will be brought about.

Most managers proceed from the premise that all authority in the employment relationship is vested in the employer except as limited by law, certain historical practices and the collectively negotiated agreement. This attitude affects the potential for cooperative relationships with the union. To the extent management views its relationship with the union in terms of power or legalities, rather than as a partnership in managing the institution, it will have great difficulty in engaging in productivity bargaining.

The traditional protective role of unions may constitute a barrier to union participation. Most unions do not perceive their duty as cooperation with or participation in management. Also, some potential political costs may emanate from such participation. While the union's duty to protect and advance the interests of its members may at times necessitate the utmost cooperation with management, at other times it may require opposition to management. Although unions have objectives directly at odds with those of management, joint consultation over productivity is both possible and desirable, and in some cases has been quite successful. The inherent limitation is that in the final analysis, collective bargaining is a power relationship.

Although both labor and management have a responsibility to create the necessary conditions for productivity bargaining, management has a special obligation to create the mutual trust which will enable the union to withdraw from a strictly protective posture with respect to existing work practices and the collective bargaining contract. Such trust may be slow in coming and difficult to achieve.

According to a Louis Harris poll conducted for the National Commission on Productivity, only 20 percent of American workers believe productivity increases benefit employees and nearly 60 percent believe that for productivity to increase, machines must replace people and employees must lose their jobs.[24] Productivity is thus viewed with distrust and concern since for many it is just another name for speed-up, layoffs and a general reduction in employee security.

These concerns must be allayed from the very beginning by guarantees against any layoffs or pay cuts resulting from the proposed changes. Such guarantees are basic conditions for effective productivity bargaining. If job changes require the abolition of certain jobs, such abolition should not be made in one sweeping gesture, but rather gradually, allowing attrition to curtail the number of positions. The establishment of formal retraining programs and the encouragement of transfers to areas of greater need may also prove helpful.

Guarantees against income loss can be achieved by "red circling" wage rates which appear to be out of line with the redefined functions of a particular position. This would assure present employees that they would not suffer any cut in earnings, although new employees could be paid at the newly established lower wage levels.

Another potential problem from the management perspective is the possibility of the costs of productivity bargaining exceeding the benefits. Increases in output per labor hour are not desirable per se. The cost to the employer of the employment and income guarantees plus any payments accruing to the employees from increased productivity must be less than the benefits accruing to the employer from increased productivity if the unit labor cost is to remain constant or be reduced. Unless this is true, the productivity gain is completely negated. In fact, productivity gains may be dysfunctional if they are accomplished by too-rapid increases in the price of inputs—largely labor costs.

The union practice of demanding a premium salary in exchange for productivity increases contributes to upward pressure on unit labor costs and makes managerial recognition of the possible tradeoffs between cost and service increases particularly relevant. One of the most serious problems with the city of New York's Productivity Program has been the failure of management to accurately estimate the future costs and benefits of productivity agreements. The result has been rising unit labor costs.[25]

Management has to be extremely careful in designing the method by which the quid pro quo is calculated. A detailed discussion of the various methods such as "buy out," "incentive formula" and "gain sharing" is beyond the scope of this article.[26, 27] The important point is that whatever method is chosen should not cost the organization more than the benefits of the productivity increase.

Output and Productivity Measurement

The measurement of output and productivity is the final potential problem. The measurement of the output of health services is difficult, but not impossible. However, productivity bargaining cannot be effective if the parties are unable or unwilling to develop appropriate measures. Obviously, providing rewards based on productivity increases is impossible if such increases are not measured.

The usual macro-type measures, such as patient days or the employee-to-patient ratio, are deficient for productivity bargaining purposes because they are affected by many factors other than employee productivity. These must be supplemented by more precise measures at the departmental level if valid indications of productivity are to be found.

Since health care organizations provide so many functions, there is a need for a number of measures to be defined by function and department. A list of such measures for hospitals is shown in Exhibit 15-1. These

Exhibit 15-1 Possible Performance Measures for Hospitals

Department	Performance Measure
Anesthesiology	Number of patients; hours of administration and use
Basal metabolism	Number of tests
Blood bank	Number of 500 cc units prepared for transfusions
Central supply	Dollar value of processed requisitions
Delivery rooms	Number of deliveries
Dietary	Number of meals served
Electrocardiology	Number of examinations
Housekeeping	Hours of service rendered to various departments
Inhalation therapy	Number of hours oxygen is administered
Laboratory	Number of tests
Laundry	Pounds or pieces of laundry processed
Nursing	Hours or days of service
Occupational therapy	Hours of teaching supervision
Operation of plant	Thousands of pounds of steam produced, plus pounds of ice produced, plus kilowatt-hours of electricity produced
Operating room	Number of operations, hours of use
Pharmacy	Dollar value of prescriptions and requisitions processed
Physical therapy	Number of treatments
Postoperative recovery room	Number of patient hours of service
Radiology/diagnostic	Number of films taken, plus number of fluoroscopic exams
Radiology/therapeutic	Number of x-ray treatments plus number of radium implementations plus number of treatments by radioactive elements

Source: Reprinted with permission from N. Williams, *The Management of Hospital Employee Productivity* (Chicago: American Hospital Association), © 1973.

performance measures provide baseline data for labor and management as they attempt to increase productivity.

Such measures constitute a beginning, but require some adjustments before they are useful for productivity bargaining. For example, one laboratory test may take five times as long to run as another. Since there are typically multiple outputs within a given depart-ment or functional area, some system of weighting is needed. The joint development of such a weighting system is both complex and necessary if productivity bargaining is to be successfully implemented.

Adjustments will also have to be made to factor in qualitative considerations. For those functions which deal directly with patient care, various measures of quality such as patient access, patient comfort and continuity of care will need to be developed.

Productivity bargaining only contributes when the ultimate output is maintained or improved as a result of the increase in productivity, not when volume alone is simply increased. The data for such measures can be developed through the use of patient satisfaction questionnaires, supplemented by patient charts, audit of the medical record and data on staff turnover and waiting time.[28]

In order to facilitate the introduction of productivity bargaining into the organization, initial attention should be focused on departments and services where output is relatively easy to measure and adjust. Typically, these functional areas will not be involved with direct patient care. For example, New York City's Health and Hospital Corporation has an agreement that has provided handsome benefits for all concerned. As a result of engaging in productivity bargaining with their employees, they have produced an agreement that doubled the number of Medicare and Medicaid claims processed daily in exchange for a $500 per year productivity raise per affected employee. The resultant increased speed of claim processing has increased collection by more than 200 times the total cost of the salary increase. Previous delays had caused the loss of some state and federal reimbursements.[29] However, this favorable experience occurred in claims processing where productivity measurement is relatively easy, rather than in a function involving direct patient care. This approach suffers because employees may not be able to control their output because they can only process as many claims as require processing. Employee productivity, as measured by claims processed per day, is influenced as much by the flow of claims as it is by the intensity and duration of the worker's effort. Productivity is also limited since a person is able to physically process only a finite number of claims.

Since the performance indicators listed in Exhibit 15-1 measure output rather than output per unit of input, they also have to be related to some measures of input. If these performance measures are not related to inputs, the parties will not be able to take into account McKersie's fourth point: efficiency with which inputs are translated into outputs of acceptable quality. The problem is that the traditional measure of labor productivity, labor hours, may not always be a valid input measure. For example, if a health facility is staffed to meet peak demand, there will be overstaffing during part of the work period. Consequently, a labor hour of input during a peak period may produce a much higher output than a labor hour of input during a slack period. This may occur without any difference in the effort or efficiency of personnel employed during each period. Therefore the parties must develop input measures which recognize the unique aspects of health care if the results of productivity bargaining are to be accepted by the affected employees.

IMPLICATIONS OF PRODUCTIVITY BARGAINING

The adoption of productivity bargaining in any health care organization will not be easy. There will be many problems which must be overcome and adaptations which must be made. Many decision-making areas, such as the distribution of rewards and recognition, may be already preempted by law, rules and regulations. Performance measures are often lacking and difficult to develop. Opposition to such an innovative approach is likely on the part of individuals identified with both management and labor. None of these potential problems will necessarily destroy the value of productivity bargaining, although they may limit realization of its full potential. Solution of such problems is one of the primary jobs of a manager.

Where collective bargaining already exists, the alternative to not adopting productivity bargaining is continuation of decision making based heavily on relative bargaining power. Such traditional relationships tend to set wage levels on the basis of "comparability" with wages and benefits in other health organizations, or "cost-of-living" increases. Within a given job category, wage rates have often been primarily based on tenure or seniority. All of these traditional criteria undermine any attempt to relate wages to productivity and consequently fail to utilize the motivational potential of wages.

Health care organizations should have two major objectives: to provide quality patient care and to efficiently use financial resources. These are the basic objectives of effectiveness and efficiency. Since wages and benefits often constitute 60 to 65 percent of total operating costs, labor expenditures are ultimately related to the efficient use of financial resources. Total labor costs are a function of staff size, wage rates employee benefits and employee turnover.

When traditional collective bargaining approaches are used, all of these labor costs could be considerably higher than they might be with a productivity bargaining program. The effectiveness of the employees' work effort remains considerably below potential and either more staff are required or the quality of patient care declines and the institution's objectives for effectiveness and efficiency remain unmet. The cost of a decision *not* to engage in productivity bargaining could be high indeed.

One of the chief virtues of productivity bargaining is its ability to highlight "sacred cows" and other impediments to increased effectiveness and efficiency. The beneficial results of productivity bargaining might include one or more of the following: increased employee productivity (quantity and quality), improved results from volunteer workers, more effective crime prevention through improved security techniques, lower administrative costs of operation and a reduction in wasted effort or waste of any asset. As mentioned previously, whether or not the value of such potential benefits exceeds the potential costs should be evaluated for each specific situation.

The need and potential for productivity bargaining in the health care industry are perhaps greater today than ever before because of several recent trends. Among the most important of these are the growth of collective bargaining in health care, the existence of multiple unionism and the desire for "comparability" within a given organization and the increasing external pressures for accountability and productivity. In addition, the 1980s may be a decade of "close-ended" funding rather than the traditional "open-ended" funding. The beginnings of this trend can already be seen in the reimbursement limitations that various states have imposed on providers under the Medicaid program. The introduction of a national health insurance program should accentuate this trend.

Forward-thinking health care managers should anticipate the future now by fully exploring the potential benefits as well as the problems of productivity bargaining where traditional collective bargaining relationships already exist. Where it appears feasible, they should experiment with the concept by matching it to the requirements and circumstances of their own institutions. Health care managers should have one objective in common with labor unions, i.e., to obtain a greater return which can be shared by both. Productivity bargaining is one of many tools which can facilitate this sharing process. The prospects for true productivity bargaining hinge in large part on increased appreciation by both managers and union officials of their interdependence.

NOTES

1. C. P. McLaughlin, "Productivity and Human Services," *Health Care Management Review* 1, no. 4 (Fall 1976): 47.

2. C. L. Hobart, "Collective Bargaining with Professions: Conflict, Containment, or Accommodation," *Health Care Management Review* 1, no. 2 (Spring 1976): 7.

3. M. D. Fottler, "The Union Impact on Hospital Wages," *Industrial and Labor Relations Review* 30, no. 3 (April 1977): 342.

4. L. B. Osterhaus, "Factors Stimulating or Inhibiting Unions," *Hospital Progress* 48, no. 7 (July 1967): 78.

5. E. C. Farkas, "The National Labor Relations Act: The Health Care Amendments," *Labor Law Journal* 29, no. 5 (May 1978): 259.

6. J. C. Hyatt, "Organizing Workers in Nonprofit Hospitals Begins: Move Likely to Boost Wage Costs," *The Wall Street Journal,* July 29, 1974, p. 20.

7. K. Demarko, J. W. Robinson, and E. C. Houch, "A Pilot Study of the Initial Bargaining Demands by Newly Organized Employees of Health Care Institutions," *Labor Law Journal* 29, no. 5 (May 1978): 275.

8. Fottler, "The Union Impact on Hospital Wages," p. 342.

9. J. D. Miller and S. M. Shortell, "Hospital Unionization: A Study of the Trends," *Hospitals, JAHA* 43, no. 16 (August 16, 1969): 16.

10. L. B. Osterhaus, "The Effect of Unions on Hospital Management," *Hospital Progress* 48, no. 7 (July 1967): 48.

11. _____ , "Union-Management Relations in 30 Hospitals Change Little in Three Years," *Hospital Progress* 49, no. 2 (February 1968): 72.

12. _____ , "The Industrial Relations System in the Hospital Industry," *Personnel Journal* 47, no. 5 (May 1968): 72.

13. B. Becker, "Hospital Unionism and Employment Stability," *Industrial Relations* 17, no. 1 (February 1978): 96.

14. Demarko, Robinson, and Houch, "A Pilot Study," p. 275.

15. Hobart, "Collective Bargaining," p. 7.

16. C. A. Newland, "Personnel Concerns in Government Productivity Improvement," *Public Administration Review* 32, no. 6 (November-December 1972): 808.

17. E. J. Robinson, *Productivity Bargaining and the Engineering Industry* (London: Engineering Employers Federation, 1969), p. 1.

18. A. Kleingartner and R. E. Azevedo, "Productivity Bargaining and Organizational Behavior," in J. Goldberg et al., eds., *Collectivity Bargaining and Productivity* (Madison, Wis.: Industrial Relations Research Association, 1975), p. 119.

19. G. P. Schultz and R. B. McKersie, "Participation-Achievement Reward Systems (PAR)," *Journal of Management Studies* 10, no. 2 (May 1973): 141.

20. A. B. McKersie, "An Evaluation of Productivity Bargaining in the Public Sector," in J. Goldberg et al., eds., *Collectivity Bargaining and Productivity* (Madison, Wis.: Industrial Relations Research Association, 1975), p. 45.

21. R. E. Walton and R. B. McKersie, *A Behavioral Theory of Labor Negotiations* (New York: McGraw-Hill Book Co., 1965), p. 5.

22. Ibid., pp. 137–139.

23. W. H. Newman and C. E. Summer, *The Process of Management* (Englewood Cliffs, N.J.: Prentice-Hall, Inc., 1964), p. 280.

24. National Commission on Productivity, *Second Annual Report of the National Commission on Productivity* (Washington, D.C.: U.S. Government Printing Office, 1973), pp. 95–103.

25. R. D. Horton, "Productivity Bargaining in Government: A Critical Analysis," *Public Administration Review* 36, no. 4 (July-August 1976): 407.

26. McKersie, "An Evaluation of Productivity Bargaining," p. 45.

27. Kleingartner and Azevedo, "Productivity Bargaining," p. 119.

28. A. R. Kovner and H. L. Smits, "Point of View: Consumer Expectations of Ambulatory Care," *Health Care Management Review* 3, no. 1 (Winter 1978): 69.

29. National Commission on Productivity, *Employee Incentives to Improve State and Local Government Productivity* (Washington, D.C.: U.S. Government Printing Office, 1975), p. 79.

16. Multiemployer Bargaining

THOMAS A. HELFRICH

INTRODUCTION

Justice Goldberg once noted that:

Today, between 80% and 100% of the workers under union agreements are covered by multi-employer contracts in such important industries as men's and women's clothing, coal mining, building construction, hotel, longshoring, maritime, trucking and warehousing. Between 60% and 80% of unionized workers are under multiemployer pacts in baking, book and job printing, canning and preserving, textile dyeing and finishing, glass and glassware, malt liquor, pottery and retail trades.[1]

Although in the aggregate, the preponderance of collective bargaining agreements are negotiated on an individual employer basis,[2] even when all industries are viewed as a whole multiemployer bargaining remains a prominent feature of the labor relations landscape.[3]

Indeed, in a number of respects multiemployer bargaining is the most significant innovation by which employers and unions have structured the union/management relationship. Thus, it has been argued that multiemployer bargaining results in "unnecessarily" high wage (cost) structures and reduces competition by impeding entry of new firms into an industry and by creating "stultifying uniformity." Its critics point out that while it generally results in fewer strikes, those that do occur have the great destructive potential to paralyze not only the struck industry but others that are directly and indirectly connected with it.[4] However, despite its critics, numerous advantages to such a structure on both public policy and pragmatic labor relations grounds have been cited by various commentators;[5] on a number of occasions Congress has declined to enact bills directly aimed at restructuring or prohibiting multiemployer bargaining.[6]

Working Definitions

An employer association arises when one or more employers join together to develop a common bargaining front against a labor union representing the employees of each. The employers agree to be bound by the decisions of the group in cases where the association acts as their collective representative in matters of contract bargaining and administration. The employers delegate authority to bargain with the union to the association, which acts as a common spokesman.[7] No special legal form or organization is necessary to fit this definition; in practice, the full gamut is run from loose federations organized on an ad hoc basis to formal incorporated organizations.

A basic premise of this procedure for bargaining is the voluntary consent of the employers and the union to bargain on a multiemployer basis. A multiemployer bargaining relationship or unit exists where a union has consented or agreed to bargain with an employer association in the exercise of the latter's authority as the *collective* representative of the employers.[8] The parties have the intention of reaching a joint agreement as to the terms and conditions of employment for the employees of the otherwise several employers and for whom the union is the exclusive bargaining representative.[9]

Reasons for Multiemployer Bargaining

Employers form employer associations because they perceive it to be to their individual and hence collective advantage. Such an association is a protective device by which employers in an industry respond in an effort to counteract the actual or potential imbalance of collective bargaining power that otherwise would result when a union, which has organized all or a substantial segment of an industry, is pitted against a single concern that in many instances may not have the wherewithal to match a strong well-financed labor organization. In addition to the benefits that accrue from pooling financial and labor relations resources, such an association has various tactical labor relations advantages such as retarding or eliminating the ability of a union to divide and conquer the employers by whipsaw and other tactics. In a general economic sense, employers often benefit through the reduction or virtual elimination of wage costs as an element of competition.[10]

Logically, it would seem that if employers joined together to bolster their bargaining power to the detriment of the union, the union, if free to do so, would decline to enter such a relationship. There are at least two answers:

1. People act on the basis of their *perceptions* of reality and each side may conclude—based upon its view of the economic and political situation—that multiemployer bargaining increases its own bargaining power.
2. There are objectives in addition to relative bargaining strength, labor relations and otherwise, that lead a party to engage in joint bargaining; for example, the desire of a union to standardize wages, working conditions, and employment practices in the industry.

It is axiomatic that since the economic and technological conditions in an industry are subject to change, and decision makers come and go, the same parties may arrive at different judgments over time as to the wisdom of entering, continuing, or discontinuing

the multiemployer bargaining relationship; this fact provides the basic grist for the balance of this article.

The sections that follow explore the basic legal foundations of employer associations and multiemployer bargaining. The broad parameters within which such arrangements remain lawful are touched upon to establish an overall framework, although they are not examined at length since the major legal check, antitrust restriction, is a vast topic in itself. The basic objective is to develop, from a collective bargaining point of view, the manner in which Congress, the National Labor Relations Board (NLRB or board) and the courts have defined employer associations, multiemployer bargaining, and the legal obligations that arise from them:

1. the legal elements for determining when an employer association and a multiemployer bargaining relationship are formed
2. the rights and obligations that arise as a result
3. activities by either side that may constitute legally proscribed conduct
4. the circumstances under which it is legally permissible to withdraw from multiemployer bargaining

CONGRESSIONAL AND COURT POSITIONS

Congress has declined to adopt various proposals aimed at eliminating multiemployer bargaining. In fact, public policy has long been in the opposite direction. The NLRB and courts generally have chosen a position of protecting and encouraging this bargaining practice as an instrument of federal labor policy. Thus, in *Buffalo Linen Supply Co.* (1957),[11] the Supreme Court held that nonstruck members of a multiemployer bargaining association, engaged in joint negotiations, could use the lockout as a defensive measure against selective strikes by the union in order to protect the group orientation of the bargaining. The Court recognized as legitimate the interests of employers in (1) preserving multiemployer bargaining as a means of counteracting the bargaining strength of the union, and (2) avoiding the competitive disadvantages resulting from nonuniform contractual terms.

Buffalo Linen afforded the Court the opportunity to comment on the rationale behind, and development of, multiemployer bargaining:

. . . Multiemployer bargaining long antedated the Wagner Act. . . . This basis of bargaining has had its greatest expansion since enactment of the

Wagner Act because employers have sought through group bargaining to match increased union strength [so that today] approximately four million employees are now governed by agreements signed by unions with thousands of employer associations. At the time of the Taft-Hartley amendments, proposals were made to limit or outlaw multiemployer bargaining. These proposals failed of enactment. They were met with a storm of protest that their adoption would tend to weaken and not strengthen the process of collective bargaining and would conflict with the national labor policy of promoting industrial peace through effective collective bargaining.

The debates over these proposals demonstrated that *Congress refused to interfere with such bargaining because there was cogent evidence that in many industries the multiemployer bargaining basis was a vital factor in the effectuation of the national policy of promoting labor peace through collective bargaining.*[12] (Emphasis added.)

Since *Buffalo Linen* the federal courts have continued to recognize that bargaining on a multiemployer basis is an important element of national labor policy. Thus, such negotiating generally is regarded as legally appropriate unless, in a particular instance, the activities of the parties result in a combination or conspiracy in restraint of trade. Through the enactment of the Clayton Antitrust Act[13] and the Norris-LaGuardia Act,[14] Congress repeated its desire to create a broad labor exemption to the Sherman Antitrust Act, which had been interpreted as outlawing many of the normal forms of union activity.[15]

In *U.S. v. Hutcheson* (1941) the Court held that a determination of whether union conduct violates the Sherman Act is to be made by reading the Clayton and Norris-LaGuardia Acts together:

So long as a union acts in its self interest *and does not combine with nonlabor groups,* the licit and the illicit under §20 [of the Clayton Act] are not to be distinguished by any judgment regarding the wisdom or unwisdom, the rightness or wrongness, the selfishness or unselfishness of the end of which the particular union activities are the means.[16] (Emphasis added.)

It is of obvious import to those concerned with multiemployer bargaining that management is, of course, a "nonlabor" group. In several subsequent cases[17] the Court explored the implications of this restriction to the labor exemption.

In *Pennington*[18] the Court noted that while the Clayton and Norris-LaGuardia Acts permit a union, as such, to operate in the ordinary manner without violating the Sherman Act, neither act expressly deals with arrangements between unions and employers. In deciding the case the Court applied the *Allen-Bradley*[19] doctrine that when unions participate with a combination of employers to eliminate competition among themselves and prevent competition from others, such activity is not included within the Clayton and Norris-LaGuardia exemptions. Thus, the Court had no difficulty in finding that an agreement between the United Mine Workers and the employer association designed to drive nonassociation coal operators out of the market was beyond the labor exemption from antitrust liability.

However, a more difficult question was presented by a term of the collective bargaining agreement that required the union to obtain the same wages and benefits from nonassociation employers. The Court noted that the employers in the association could not finance the increase demanded by the union unless they quickly mechanized mining operations. However, rapid mechanization would prove uneconomical unless the output of certain nonassociation mines was curtailed. The government contended that a clause in the union/association agreement whereby the UMW was bound to obtain the same wage increases in its negotiations with nonassociation employers, and a commitment by the union to insist on such increases irrespective of an employer's ability to pay, evidenced a combination of labor with a nonlabor group to limit industry production by driving economically marginal firms out of business. The Court found that such a conspiracy, if proved, violated federal antitrust law.

The Court rejected the union's contention that the agreement was exempt from antitrust restrictions merely because it concerned wages—a mandatory subject of bargaining. Although the Court agreed that involvement of a mandatory subject of bargaining was relevant in determining the scope of the labor antitrust exemption, it stated that there were limitations on what a union and an employer could do in the name of wages. The obligation to bargain under the act, the Court declared, does not mean that the agreement reached can disregard other laws.

The Court made clear that a union is free to make a wage agreement with employers in multiemployer bargaining and thus eliminate the wage element from competition among the employers in the group without violating the antitrust laws. As a matter of its own unilateral policy, the union also may seek the same wages from other employers. But, the Court ruled, the union loses the protection of the exemption where it binds itself to a further agreement with one set of employers to impose the same or another wage scale on other employers where the joint object of management and labor is to reduce or eliminate competition. This conclusion was founded on a two-pronged rationale:

1. As a matter of labor policy, the union does not properly serve the interests of the employees it represents outside the multiemployer unit by binding itself to seek the set scale, despite its legitimate aim to obtain uniform labor standards. Its duty to bargain requires that it retain the flexibility to treat each bargaining situation based upon the individual circumstances and the needs of the employees involved in the situation.
2. The policy of the antitrust laws is plainly opposed to union/employer agreements seeking to impose labor standards outside the bargaining unit.

Thus, where it can be shown that the wage agreement incorporates a stipulation that the union is obligated to impose that same term on employers outside the unit, the union and the employers run the risk of exceeding the labor exemption. But it remains significant that through the vehicle of multiemployer bargaining, the employers, when they reach agreement with the union, also can agree among themselves on industrywide wages, notwithstanding the "indirect" restraint to competition that results.

FORMING AN EMPLOYER ASSOCIATION

Legal Test for Multiemployer Bargaining

The definition of an employer association achieves its greatest labor relations significance when combined with the multiemployer bargaining definition. This creates the legal circumstances under which the rights of the individual employer and the union to unilaterally insist on individual bargaining are superseded by a new duty of both to bargain on a multiemployer basis and to be bound by the outcome of such negotiating.[20] The statutory obligation to bargain in good faith now includes the duty of the employer to bargain through its association instead of as an individual employer.[21] Of course, there are the concomitant rights of both sides to insist on the performance of the other's newly created duty.[22]

Thus, a union commits an unfair labor practice when it insists on negotiating individually with a member of the association and illegally restrains or coerces "an employer in the selection of his representatives for the purpose of collective bargaining"[23] where it exerts

strike pressure to gain the employer's agreement to an individual contract.[24] An individual employer is bound by the collective bargaining settlement otherwise properly negotiated by the association, whether or not it individually agreed to it,[25] and commits an unfair labor practice if it refuses to sign the agreement.[26]

Since these rights and duties do not arise unless and until the legal elements that form the multiemployer bargaining relationship come into being, it is important to establish the factors laid down by the NLRB and the courts that cause such a relationship to exist. There are five key elements:

1. The association is formed by the employers with the intention of establishing it as a common bargaining agent.
2. Exclusive bargaining authority is delegated to the association for the negotiation of terms and conditions of employment with a union representing employees of the several employers.
3. The employers agree among themselves that the delegated bargaining authority encompasses the power to bind them as a group to an agreement negotiated by the association and that the members will be bound by the group's decisions in the exercise of that authority.
4. These points are communicated to the union(s).
5. The union agrees or consents to such a negotiating arrangement.

Thus, the rule has long been established by the NLRB that the applicable test to determine whether multiemployer bargaining exists is:

Whether the members of the group have indicated from the outset an unequivocal intention to be bound in collective bargaining by a group rather than individual action, and whether the union representing their employees has been notified of the formation of the group and the delegation of bargaining authority to it, and has assented and entered upon negotiations with the group's representative.[27]

This rule has gained acceptance by the courts[28] and has been applied in a number of circumstances. The result is that the employers must exhibit an unequivocal intent to be bound on a group basis. There is no multiemployer bargaining where they merely designate a common negotiator that enters negotiations with the union with the understanding that it represents them in their several capacities but with each one reserving its individual right to ratify any agreement that may be reached.[29] Likewise, multiemployer bargaining does not arise where a group of independent companies merely follows the lead of an association in agreeing to contracts negotiated by it and this practice alone does not establish that they are part of the multiemployer bargaining relationship with the association.[30] However, the intention of an employer to be bound in multiemployer bargaining may be implied by its active participation in negotiations of a joint group,[31] and the employer need not be an actual member of the association.[32]

The consent of the union may be express or implied. In *Western States Regional Council No. 3 v. NLRB*,[33] there was no express consent or agreement. However, the Supreme Court sustained the finding of the board that the consent of the union was implied in fact from its conduct where it: (1) "responded favorably" to informal suggestions by employers regarding their creation of an association, (2) subsequently was given formal notice of the agreement among the employers to be bound by a labor contract negotiated by the association, and (3) with this knowledge entered into negotiations with the association's negotiating committee, making its—the union's—proposals to the association *qua* association and responding to its offers as group offers. This finding was sustained despite the fact that a copy of the agreement among the employers forming the association had not been made available to the union and that it was unaware that a 75 percent vote was required to authorize the association to reach agreement with the union; virtual unanimity would be required among the employers for ratification of an agreement (with the union). Only six employers comprised the association.

Legally Proscribed Conduct

Multiemployer bargaining may be established only by the voluntary consent of both the employers and the union(s) involved.[34] Indeed, it has been held that absent establishment of circumstances that meet such a test, the NLRB cannot compel an employer to join a multiemployer unit.[35]

Employer Conduct

It is well settled under the act that, absent the union's consent,[36] employers may not lawfully insist on multiemployer bargaining. In *NLRB v. A&P Stores, Inc.*,[37] the Second Circuit held that a lockout designed to force the union to accept multiemployer bargaining constituted conduct prohibited by the act.

In *San Diego Cabinets*[38] six employers historically bargained on an individual basis with the union. The individual agreements with each generally followed a pattern set by a local multiemployer association. The union notified each employer of its desire to negotiate a renewal contract on an individual basis, having completed its negotiation with the association. The employers responded that during the term of their expired contracts they had joined another employer association in the area that had been formed recently and had negotiated a collective bargaining agreement with a conference of unions of which the instant union was a member, and that they would bargain on a multiemployer basis only through the other association.[39] The board found that the union had joined the conference merely as an accommodation at a time when none of the employers involved was under contract with it, and that this did not constitute consent of the union to engage in multiemployer bargaining. Accordingly, the board ordered the employers to cease insisting on multiemployer bargaining and refusing to bargain on an individual basis.

Even though there is a history of multiemployer bargaining, an employer commits an unfair labor practice if it refuses to bargain separately with a union after the union has withdrawn unilaterally from multiemployer bargaining in a timely manner.[40] This rule is based on the premise that, to be legally binding, the multiemployer bargaining relationship must be founded upon the mutual consent of the parties where both sides are free to withdraw.[41]

Union Conduct

A union commits an unfair labor practice if it induces a strike, or threatens, coerces, or restrains an employer, where in either case it seeks to force or require an employer to join an "employer organization."[42] In *Frito-Lay v. Teamsters*[43] the court found that Congress intended to prevent involuntary multiemployer bargaining and held that the union violated the act when it struck with the object of forcing several employers to bargain as if they were an employer association. The case involved three employers with a long history of bargaining as an employer association that they had dissolved prior to the negotiations at issue. In the bargaining with each employer, the union insisted that the company accept one contract covering employees of all three companies, or three separate contracts with identical provisions. By striking, the union sought to compel acceptance of such a contract or contracts.

In an interesting case[44] the board found the union in violation of the act's prohibition against restraining or coercing an employer in the selection of a bargaining representative (§ 8(b)(1)(B)) by striking to compel several employers to rejoin an employer association.

However, the board refused to sustain the employers' charge that the union unlawfully refused to bargain by refusing to negotiate on an individual employer basis. Multiemployer bargaining had persisted over a number of years and originally was predicated on a board election and certification of an associationwide unit—the votes were tallied as if all employees worked for a single employer. On the theory that the only unit in which the employees had expressed the wish to bargain was the certified unit, and that they had not expressed a desire to be represented by the union in individual negotiations, the majority held that the union could lawfully refuse the request of the employers to bargain individually.

> Similarly, by these employers' actions of withdrawing from the Council they could lawfully resist Respondents' [the union's] demands that they return to the multiemployer unit. Consequently, the net result of our decision is that we cannot compel bargaining to take place herein unless one of the parties changes its position, and agreement is reached as to the unit appropriate for bargaining.[45]

Just as a union commits an unfair labor practice when it attempts to force an employer to bargain on a multiemployer basis, a similar result obtains where it seeks to compel an employer to abandon multiemployer bargaining once it has begun. Thus, the Seventh Circuit[46] upheld a board ruling that a union violated the act when it engaged in such conduct after negotiations had begun. In *Teamsters Local 1205 (New York Lumber Trade Association),*[47] the union was found to have violated the act by refusing to bargain with the association after negotiations had started, threatening to strike, striking various association members to force them to negotiate and sign individual contracts, and by signing individual contracts with some of the struck employers that had succumbed to the strike pressure.

WITHDRAWAL FROM MULTIEMPLOYER BARGAINING

General Principles: Reciprocal Application of the Law

In *The Evening News Association*[48] the NLRB enunciated its philosophy that the basic principles governing union and employer withdrawal from multiemployer bargaining should be the same:

If, as is apparent, the basis of a multiemployer bargaining unit is both original and continuing consent by both parties, the Board cannot logically deny the bargaining representative the same opportunity it allows employers of withdrawing from the multiemployer unit by withdrawing its consent to such unit.

. . . .

The rules for withdrawal from multiemployer bargaining units should be the same for unions as for employers because we perceive no material difference in the impact on the employing entity and on the union flowing from an employer's withdrawal from a multiemployer unit on the one hand, and the union's withdrawal, on the other hand. In either case, the withdrawing party forces the other to forego bargaining in the established multiemployer unit.

. . . .

The freedom of the parties involved to form and dissolve, to modify and adopt multiemployer units should be left intact.

Although one member dissented strongly from this approach, it has been followed by the board in its subsequent decisions in the area and this basic premise has gained wide acceptance among the Courts of Appeals.[49] In doing so, the courts have followed the general principle enunciated by the Supreme Court in *Buffalo Linen* ". . . that Congress intended . . . to leave to the Board's specialized judgment the inevitable questions concerning multiemployer bargaining which were bound to arise in the future."[50] Thus, the appropriate standard for the courts to apply upon review of the board's decisions regarding withdrawal from multiemployer bargaining is whether in so holding in a particular case, the board has acted without a rational basis or has abused its discretion.[51]

The fundamental purpose of the act to foster and maintain stability in bargaining relationships is the touchstone for analysis of the rules that have been developed in this area.

The Basic Rule

The basic test for determining whether withdrawal from multiemployer bargaining is permissible was enunciated first by the NLRB in *Retail Associates, Inc.* (1958).[52] Prior to negotiations, either an employer or a union that is a party to an established multiemployer bargaining relationship may withdraw unilaterally—without the consent of the other party—provided written notice evidencing an unambiguous intent to withdraw is given to the second party. Once negotiations have started, withdrawal is permissible only by mutual consent of the employer and the union, except that a party may withdraw unilaterally in the event of "unusual circumstances."[53] The Courts of Appeals have approved and followed this formulation.[54]

To be timely, notice must be given prior to the date set by contract for modification, or the date upon which negotiations were set to begin. Mere good faith will not excuse an employer that makes untimely withdrawal.[55] An employer who fails to pay dues to the association that the company can afford to pay, thereby causing expulsion from the group, remains in the multiemployer unit.[56] Similarly, an employer who discharges all union employees after negotiations have begun commits a refusal-to-bargain violation if it will not sign an agreement reached later by the association and the union, even though the NLRB general counsel has declined to bring charges as to the discharges, and even assuming the dismissals were proper.[57]

The Consent Exception

The general rule contemplates that withdrawal will be permitted after negotiations have commenced where the other party consents. That consent may be express or implied in fact. However, mere silence or inaction by the union following notification by an employer of its intention to withdraw does not rise to the level of consent since the union is under no legal duty to protest in any manner.[58] However, the union must take care to preserve its right to relief from the board because the Courts of Appeals have split on whether a new 8(a)(5) violation for refusal to sign the association agreement accrues each time a demand to sign is made.[59]

In *Hartz-Kirpatrick Construction Co., Inc.*,[60] the employer initially participated in the bargaining between the association and the union and was one of a number of employers that adamantly resisted a particular union demand comprising the major issue in the negotiation. At one point the parties adjourned *sine die* because of their disagreement on that matter. Some time later a strike ensued; when the negotiations resumed, that employer did not participate. Later, just 11 days before the association and the union reached and signed an industrywide agreement, the employer wrote the association unequivocally revoking its bargaining authority. It simultaneously gave written notice of this action to the union, declaring its intention not to be bound by any contract the association

might make subsequently. The union promptly responded by telegram that the employer's withdrawal was "untimely, illegal and in bad faith" but added "despite your illegal activities you will shortly be contacted to arrange a series of negotiations for a new contract with the union."

After the multiemployer contract was executed, a union business representative visited the employer, gave him a copy of the contract, but did not ask him to take any specific action when the employer commented that he did not think he could agree to all its terms. When the business representative made a second visit, the employer made clear that he had no intention of signing the contract. He then made several proposals that the business representative agreed to transmit to the union, although expressing his belief that there was "little hope" the proposals would be acceptable. However, before leaving, the business representative offered the employer two proposals that were not in the multiemployer agreement. Picketing commenced upon rejection of the employer's proposals and his refusal to change his position.

The NLRB held that the conduct of the union representative (e.g., transmitting the employer's proposals to the union and offering new proposals for the union) at the two meetings demonstrated acquiescence by the union in the employer's withdrawal and its implied consent to the employer's proposal to negotiate individually.[61]

Thus, when applied in the context of withdrawal from multiemployer bargaining, the concept of implied consent is a double-edged sword. A union that engages in individual negotiations with an employer after his untimely withdrawal, by implication consents to the withdrawal and may not hold the employer to the association contract. On the other hand, participation by an employer in multiemployer bargaining subsequent to an effective withdrawal may result in a holding that the employer by such conduct has become "rebound" to multiemployer bargaining. In *NLRB v. Associated Shower Door, Inc.*[62] the court found that the employer's withdrawal from multiemployer bargaining was justified under the "unusual circumstances" exception.[63] However, after the notice of withdrawal was served on the union, the employer took part in a subsequent multiemployer bargaining session and an association caucus. The court, agreeing with the board, held that this subsequent conduct amounted to a "retraction" of the employer's original withdrawal from the multiemployer bargaining, and "reestablish[ed], through either actual or apparent authority, an agency relationship with the representatives who had formerly represented the old multiemployer unit."[64] It also adopted the reasoning of the administrative law judge that the employer had, in fact, acquiesced to the union's rejection of its withdrawal, or retracted its own statement that it was withdrawing, in attempting to obtain the benefits of both worlds, namely, participation in multiemployer negotiations while silently reserving its right to insist on individual negotiations.

The 'Unusual Circumstances' Exception

As applied by the NLRB, the "unusual circumstances" exception from the general rule requiring consent by the other party is given a narrow construction in order to encourage stability of the multiemployer bargaining unit. Thus, the board takes the position that the exception should be limited to two general classes of cases:

1. extreme financial hardship threatening the existence of the employer as a viable business entity, and
2. fragmentation or dissipation of the multiemployer bargaining unit.[65]

Thus, for example, a mere strike by the union during multiemployer negotiations,[66] even a selective whipsaw strike,[67] does not fall within the exception. Nor does the agreement of the association to include illegal provisions in the contract permit withdrawal, at least where the provisions are not so pervasive as to preclude the enforceability of the remainder of the contract.[68]

A brief review of two cases where the board found exceptional circumstances demonstrates the determined rigor with which it has applied its standard so as to limit the instances where multiemployer bargaining may be subject to disruption by the unilateral withdrawal of either party.

In *Lingerie Corp.*[69] the employer was a debtor in possession that about three months before the date set for bargaining had filed a petition under Chapter XI of the Bankruptcy Act. The union had been "fully briefed" concerning the employer's serious financial condition, but refused the employer's request to modify a contract between the union and another concern that the employer proposed to join in partnership to improve his financial condition. He also asked the union to help him obtain contracting work but apparently the union's attempts in this regard failed. At about the time multiemployer bargaining began, the employer obtained an agreement from the bankruptcy creditors' committee to relocate his business outside

the local area.[70] Within a few days the employer "discovered" that joint negotiations had started and gave written notice of withdrawal to the association and the union. The union promptly "rejected" the employer's action.

In holding that the facts presented such unusual circumstances as to justify an untimely unilateral withdrawal, the board carefully noted that such result followed only because of "all the circumstances of the case," and by repetition emphasized that: (1) the employer's economic problems antedated the start of multiemployer negotiations, (2) he had withdrawn from the association in order to relocate his business outside the area, (3) he had unsuccessfully sought help from the union as part of his attempt to overcome the "difficult economic straights" he faced, (4) he occupied the status of debtor in possession, and finally, (5) his relocation intentions raised issues "inherently more amenable" to individual negotiations as opposed to a multiemployer basis.

In applying the multiemployer bargaining fragmentation or dissipation test, the board has shown that by "dissipation" or "fragmentation" it means just that. Thus, the mere withdrawal of a few employers is insufficient.[71] In *Connell Typesetting Company*[72] a multiemployer bargaining unit had been in existence more than 25 years at the time negotiations began with the Printing Industries Association of Kansas City, Inc. (PIA). After protracted bargaining, the union struck 22 of the 36 employers, including the four respondents. In the ensuing 12 months a series of successive individual employer-union negotiations resulted in "interim agreements" that were to be superseded by whatever agreement ultimately was reached with PIA (the union and PIA continued negotiations as to the other association members).[73]

At the point where only 13 of the original 36 employers with fewer than 18 percent of the original 209 employees remained in the multiemployer bargaining unit, four employers rescinded the PIA's bargaining authority and advised the union to this effect, stating they would not be bound by any agreement subsequently made with PIA. The union promptly rejected these positions, advising the employers that it would consider them bound by any such agreement (which was reached later during the pendency of the proceeding).

The board found that under *Retail Associates* the unilateral employer withdrawals were justified by the exceptional circumstances of the case. It noted that while it was true that the employers signing the interim agreements remained obligated to sign the PIA agreement, and to that extent remained part of the multiemployer unit, practically speaking they were removed from contesting the remaining issues at the bargaining table. As their collective strength was thus removed, in practical effect they had "withdrawn from further bargaining as to this contract."

The Board is always concerned as to stability in the collective bargaining relationship. However, in our opinion, this unit has, with the consent of the Union, been so reduced in size and strength that it would be unfair and harmful to the collective bargaining process to require Respondents to continue in a unit merely because the Union, which consented to the withdrawal of so many others, is unwilling to consent to their withdrawal. In these unusual circumstances we conclude that Respondents were not required to remain within the multiemployer bargaining unit.[74]

The unusual circumstances exception has been a source of controversy between the NLRB and several Courts of Appeals, the courts generally following a less stringent view of circumstances that justify unilateral employer withdrawal from multiemployer bargaining once negotiations have commenced.[75] This exception is the focal point of an argument over whether a bargaining impasse justifies unilateral withdrawal from multiemployer bargaining by an individual employer. The board steadfastly adheres to the view that it does not,[76] notwithstanding the contrary view of six of the seven Courts of Appeals that have considered the question.[77] Thus, an individual employer who contemplates withdrawal under such circumstances will be confronted with a sure unfair labor practice finding from the board, albeit on a basis that has not been favored in the courts; enforcement of that order, therefore, will be questionable. Moreover, the problems that normally accompany a situation of this nature are compounded by the fact that, as a legal matter, the existence of an impasse itself is an issue of fact involving a complex judgment[78] about which the minds of impartial people may, and often do, differ.[79]

CONCLUSION

The foregoing discussion makes clear that multiemployer bargaining has endured, and will continue to do so, as a permanent fixture of collective bargaining in the United States. Notwithstanding this fact, in particular cases its perceived usefulness by an employer or group of employers, or union, or both, will come and go. This brings the close of this discussion full circle to the point where it opened.

NOTES

1. *Local 189 Amalgamated Meat Cutters v. Jewel Tea Co.*, 381 U.S. 676 (1965), citing Reynolds, *Labor Economics and Labor Relations* (3d ed. 1959), p. 170.
2. William J. Abelow and Norman Metzger, "Multiemployer Bargaining for Health Care Institutions," *The Employee Relations Law Journal*, no. 3 (Winter 1976): 391.
3. For example, a New York State survey shows that there are in excess of 565 multiemployer bargaining associations party to more than 980 different collective bargaining agreements; these account for slightly less than half of the total unionized work force in the state. New York State Department of Labor, *Employer Associations Engaged in Collective Bargaining in New York State* (Albany, N.Y.: Division of Research and Statistics, 1965).
4. H. W. Davy, *Contemporary Collective Bargaining* (1959).
5. *See* Davy, *id.*, pp. 93–95, and Abelow and Metzger, *supra*, note 2, p. 404.
6. *Amalgamated Meat Cutters*, *supra*, note 1.
7. Readers should distinguish the multiplant bargaining model in which a single employer with facilities at separate locations bargains a single agreement with a union or unions representing its employees in separate plants.
8. The legal elements for creation of such a relationship and its connection with the definition of an employer association are examined in depth in the section on the formation of the employer association.
9. It is important to distinguish this from the concept of appropriate bargaining unit where, in certain circumstances, the NLRB finds that, for the purposes of certification and election, the employees of legally separate employers, which may or may not be engaged in multiemployer bargaining, together constitute a single appropriate unit for the holding of an election. The way in which the board applies its rules to guide its determination in such matters is beyond the scope of this article. *See generally Electric Theatre*, 156 NLRB 1351, 61 LRRM 1269 (1966).
10. *See* analysis beginning with *U.S. v. Hutcheson* for a general discussion of the antitrust implications.
11. *NLRB v. Truck Drivers Local Union No. 449 (Buffalo Linen Supply Co.)*, 353 U.S. 87 (1957).
12. *Id.*, 353 U.S. at 94 (footnotes omitted).
13. 38 Stat. 730 (1914), as amended, 15 U.S.C. §§15,17,26 (1970), 29 U.S.C. §52 (1970).
14. 49 Stat. 70 (1932), 29 U.S.C. §§101-15 (1970).
15. *United States v. Hutcheson*, 312 U.S. 219 (1941).
16. *Id.*, at 232.
17. For example, *see Ramsey v. United Mine Workers*, 401 U.S. 302, 915 S.Ct. 658 (1971); *Local Union No. 189, Amalgamated Meat Cutters v. Jewel Tea Co.*, 381 U.S. 676, 85 S.Ct. 1596 (1965); *United Mine Workers v. Pennington*, 381 U.S. 657, 85 S.Ct. 1585 (1965); *Allen-Bradley Co. v. Local Union No. 3, IBEW*, 325 U.S. 797, 65 S.Ct. 1533 (1945).
18. *Id.*
19. *Supra*, note 17.
20. *Plumbers Local 638 (HV & AC Contractors' Ass'n, Inc.)*, 170 NLRB 385, 67 LRRM 1615 (1968); *Intergraphic Corp. of America*, 160 NLRB 1284, 63 LRRM 1205 (1966).
21. *Id.*
22. *Id.*
23. NLRA, Section 8(b)(1)(B).
24. *Painters Local 1238 (Northwest Floor Covering Ass'n)*, 183 NLRB 41, 74 LRRM 1700 (1970).
25. *NLRB v. John J. Corbett Press, Inc.*, 401 F.2d 673 (2d Cir. 1968), 69 LRRM 2480.

26. *Id.*

27. *The Kroger Co.*, 148 NLRB 569, 573; 57 LRRM 1021 (1964); *see also Van Erden Co.*, 154 NLRB 496, 499; 59 LRRM 1770 (1965).

28. *Komatz Construction, Inc. v. NLRB*, 458 F.2d 317 (8th Cir. 1972), 80 LRRM 2005; *Western States Regional Council No. 3, Int'l Woodworkers v. NLRB*, 398 F.2d 770 (D.C. Cir 1968), 68 LRRM 2506; *NLRB v. Johnson Sheet Metal, Inc.*, 442 F.2d 1056 (10th Cir. 1971), 77 LRRM 2245; *Tennessee Products and Chemical Corp. v. NLRB*, 423 F.2d 169 (6th Cir. 1970), 73 LRRM 2725.

29. *Santa Barbara Distributing Co.*, 172 NLRB 665, 69 LRRM 1001 (1968).

30. *Shoe Industries of Southern Mass.*, 81 NLRB 224, 23 LRRM 1320 (1949).

31. *Quality Limestone Products, Inc.*, 143 NLRB 589, 53 LRRM 1357 (1964).

32. *Bunker Hill & Sullivan Mining and Contracting Co.*, 89 NLRB 227, 25 LRRM 1544 (1950).

33. *Supra*, note 28. The case involved a lockout by unstruck employers in response to a whipsaw strike by the union after a deadlock had developed. Based upon the finding that there was multiemployer bargaining, the court sustained the board's holding that the employers' action was lawful under *NLRB v. Truck Drivers Local No. 449 (Buffalo Linen)*, 353 U.S. 87 (1957).

34. *The Kroger Co.*, *supra*, note 27.

35. *NLRB v. Sklar*, 316 F.2d 145 (6th Cir. 1963), 53 LRRM 2005.

36. *The Evening News Ass'n*, 154 NLRB 1494, 60 LRRM 1149 (1965), *enf'd sub nom.*, *Detroit Newspaper Publishers Ass'n v. NLRB*, 372 F.2d, 569 (6th Cir. 1967), 64 LRRM 2403; *Hearst Consol. Publications, Inc.*, 61 LRRM 1011 (1965), *enf'd sub nom.*, *Publishers Ass'n of New York City v. NLRB*, 364 F.2d 293 (2d Cir. 1966), 62 LRRM 2722, *cert. denied* 385 U.S. 971, 63 LRRM 2527 (1966).

37. 340 F.2d 690 (2d Cir. 1965), 58 LRRM 2232.

38. 183 NLRB 1014, 76 LRRM 1703 (1970).

39. The contract between the other association and the conference had terms substantially more favorable to the employers than that negotiated by the local association with the union.

40. *Detroit Newspaper Publishers Ass'n*, *supra*, note 36; *Publishers' Ass'n of New York City v. NLRB*, *supra*, note 36.

41. The rules governing withdrawal from multiemployer bargaining are examined in detail in the section bearing that heading.

42. It is interesting to note in passing that at common law the object of inducing an employer to join, remain in, or withdraw from an employer association may have been improper *if* the employees did not reasonably believe that this membership or nonmembership would aid the collective interest of the workers. Restatement of Torts §793. The Restatement took no position in the case where the workers did so reasonably believe.

43. 401 F. Supp. 370, 90 LRRM 2757 (N.D. Calif. 1975), *aff'd.*, _____ F.2d _____ (9th Cir. August, 1980). The case involved an action pursuant to Section 303(b) of the act for monetary damages sustained as a result of a strike.

44. *Local No. 44 Plumbers' Union (Arnold and Jeffers, Inc.)*, 195 NLRB 225, 79 LRRM 1308 (1972), *enf'd sub nom.*, *NLRB v. Local 44, et al.*, 82 LRM 2687 (9th Cir. 1972).

45. 79 LRRM 1310.

46. *NLRB v. Local Union No. 103 (Associated Gen'l Contracting)*, 81 LRRM 2705 (7th Cir. 1972).

47. 191 NLRB 917, 77 LRRM 1880 (1971).

48. *The Evening News Ass'n*, *supra*, note 36.

49. *Pacific Coast Ass'n*, 163 NLRB 892, 64 LRRM 1420 (1967); *The Evening News Ass'n*, *supra*, note 36; *Hearst Consol. Publications*, *supra*, note 36; *NLRB v. Associated Shower Door Co.*, 512 F.2d 230 (9th Cir.), 88 LRRM 3024, *cert. denied*, 423 U.S. 893, 90 LRRM 2614 (1975); *Hi-Way Billboards, Inc.*, 206 NLRB 22, 84 LRRM 1161, *enf. denied on other grounds*, 500 F.2d 181 (5th Cir. 1974), 87 LRRM

2203; *Fairmont Foods Co.*, 196 NLRB No. 122, 80 LRRM 1172, *enf. denied on other grounds*, 471 F.2d 1170 (8th Cir. 1972); *Beck Engraving Co.*, 213 NLRB No. 13, 87 LRRM 1037, *enf. denied on other grounds*, 522 F.2d 475 (3rd Cir. 1975), 90 LRRM 2089.

50. *Supra*, note 11 at 96.

51. *Detroit Newspaper Publishers Ass'n v. NLRB*, *supra*, note 36.

52. 120 NLRB 388, 41 LRRM 1502 (1958).

53. *Id.*; *NLRB v. Beck Engraving Co.*, *supra*, note 49.

54. *NLRB v. Brotherhood of Teamsters, Local No. 70*, 470 F.2d 509 (9th Cir. 1972), 82 LRRM 2016, *cert. denied* 414 U.S. 821 (1973); *NLRB v. Dover Tavern Owners Ass'n*, 412 F. 2d 725 (3rd Cir. 1969), 71 LRRM 2542; *NLRB v. Tulsa Sheet Metal Works, Inc.*, 367 F.2d 55 (10th Cir. 1966), 63 LRRM 2217; *NLRB v. Paskesz*, 405 F.2d 1201 (2d Cir. 1969), 70 LRRM 2482; *NLRB v. Sklar*, *supra*, note 35; *NLRB v. Sheridan Creations, Inc.*, 357 F.2d 245 (2d Cir. 1966), 61 LRRM 2586.

55. *NLRB v. Tulsa Sheet Metal Works, Inc.*, *id.*

56. *NLRB v. Paskesz*, *supra*, note 54; *NLRB v. Dover Tavern Owners' Ass'n*, *supra*, note 54.

57. *NLRB v. John J. Corbett Press, Inc.*, 401 F.2d 673 (2d Cir. 1968), 69 LRRM 2480.

58. *Fairmont Foods Co.*, *supra*, note 49; *see NLRB v. John J. Corbett Press, Inc.*, *supra*, note 57; *but see NLRB v. Spun-Jee Corp.*, 385 F.2d 379 (2d Cir. 1968), 66 LRRM 2485.

59. *See NLRB v. Strong*, 386 F.2d 929 (9th Cir. 1967), 65 LRRM 3012; and *Int'l Union, United Automobile Workers v. NLRB*, 363 F.2d 702 (D.C. Cir. 1966), 62 LRRM 2361 (holding that a new cause accrues on subsequent demand), versus *NLRB v. Field & Sons, Inc.*, 80 LRRM 2534 (1st Cir. 1972) (which, following a contract law analysis, distinguished a failure to bargain or breach of a general duty imposed by the act from failure to perform a particular act, held that refusal to sign the agreement was of the latter type, and hence reasoned that a repeated demand by the union to the employer to sign did not result in accrual of a new refusal to bargain).

60. 195 NLRB 863, 77 LRRM 1536 (1972).

61. See *Fairmont Foods Co. v. NLRB*, *supra*, note 49.

62. *Supra*, note 49.

63. The court applied the impasse exception reviewed in the section on the "Unusual Circumstances" Exception *infra*.

64. *NLRB v. Associated Shower Door Co.*, 512 F.2d 230, 232-233 (9th Cir.), 88 LRRM 3024, *cert. denied*, 423 U.S. 893 (1975).

65. *NLRB v. Beck Engraving Co.*, *supra*, note 49.

66. *NLRB v. State Electric Serv., Inc.*, 477 F.2d 749 (5th Cir. 1973), 82 LRRM 3154.

67. *NLRB v. Beck Engraving Co.*, *supra*, note 49.

68. *NLRB v. Tulsa Sheet Metal Works, Inc.*, *supra*, note 54.

69. *U.S. Lingerie Corp. and U.S. Lingerie Corp., Debtor In Possession*, 170 NLRB 77, 67 LRRM 1482 (1968).

70. The union was one of the ten largest creditors but was not on the committee and did not assent to the arrangement.

71. *NLRB v. Beck Engraving Co.*, *supra*, note 49.

72. 212 NLRB No. 140, 87 LRRM 1001 (1974).

73. Some employers signed "final" contracts, that is, withdrew from the multiemployer unit with the union's consent; one employer had withdrawn with the consent of all parties and won a decertification election.

74. 87 LRRM 1004.

75. Contrast the approach taken by the board with *NLRB v. Siebler Heating & Air Conditioning, Inc., et al.*, 563 F.2d 366 (8th Cir. 1977), 96 LRRM 2613 and *NLRB v. Unelko Corp.*, 478 F.2d 1404 (7th Cir. 1973), 96 LRRM 2613.

76. *Hi-Way Billboards, Inc.*, 191 NLRB No. 37, 84 LRRM 1161 (1973), *enf. denied NLRB v. Hi-Way Billboards, Inc.*, 500 F.2d 181, 87 LRRM 2203.

77. *NLRB v. Beck Engraving Co.*, 522 F.2d 475 (3rd Cir. 1975), 90

LRRM 2089; *NLRB v. Hi-Way Billboards, Inc.,* 500 F.2d 181 (5th Cir. 1974), 87 LRRM 2203; *Fairmont Foods Co. v. NLRB,* 471 F.2d 1170 (8th Cir. 1972), 82 LRRM 2017; *NLRB v. Independent Ass'n of Steel Fabricators, Inc.,* 582 F.2d 135 (2d Cir. 1978), 98 LRRM 3150; *H & D, Inc. v. NLRB,* 105 LRRM 3070 (9th Cir. 1980). *See NLRB v. Associated Shower Door Co.,* 512 F.2d 230, 232 (9th Cir.), 88 LRRM 3024, *cert. denied,* 423 U.S. 893, 90 LRRM 2614 (1975) (dictum). For the board's response *see Charles D. Bonanno Linen Serv., Inc.,* 243 NLRB No. 140 (1979), *enf'd. NLRB v. Charles D. Bonnano Linen Service, Inc.,* 630 F. 2d 25 (1st Cir. 1980).

78. "Whether a bargaining impasse exists is a matter of judgment. The bargaining history, the good faith of the parties in negotiations, the length of the negotiations, the importance of the issue or issues as to which there is disagreement, the contemporaneous understanding of the parties as to the state of negotiations, are all relevant factors to be considered in deciding whether an impasse in bargaining existed." *Taft Broadcasting Co.,* 163 NLRB 475, 64 LRRM 1386, 1388 (1967), *enforced,* 395 F.2d 622 (D.C. Cir. 1968), 67 LRRM 3032. *Fairmont Foods Co. v. NLRB, supra,* note 49.

79. Thus, in two of the cases where the impasse exception was applied, the NLRB could not sustain its contention that its finding of no impasse was supported by substantial evidence, and in one case the question was remanded because the court doubted that the board's initial finding of no impasse would pass muster.

17. Multiemployer Bargaining—The Minnesota Experience

IRVING PERLMUTTER

Collective bargaining on a multiemployer basis is not a new phenomenon. A few units date back to the early 1900s.[1]

Bargaining by groups of employers with labor unions is conducted on an industrywide, regional, or local basis, with the most common being local or citywide units.[2] The growth of employer groups organized for collective bargaining purposes paralleled the growth of union power in the 1930s and 1940s and now includes a significant portion of the American labor force.[3] Its use in the hospital field, however, has been confined largely to metropolitan areas where labor unionization was manifested early, notably in the San Francisco Bay area, in New York City, and in the Twin Cities of Minneapolis and St. Paul. As labor unionizing activities increase at health care institutions in other large cities, employer groups are likely to explore the merits of multiemployer bargaining.

There are several arrangements for structuring multiemployer bargaining units.[4] An organization created to conduct the collective bargaining in behalf of its members, such as the League of Voluntary Hospitals in New York City, is one arrangement.[5] Other associations, such as Health Manpower Management, Inc., (HMMI) in Minnesota, may evolve to cover a broader geographic area and to provide a wider range of employee relations services. In yet another example, a state hospital association may agree to provide labor relations expertise as part of its statewide general ser-

vices program. It also is possible for a group of institutional employers simply to agree to meet together for the sole purpose of negotiating a uniform contract with a specific union. Finally, employers who sign identical contracts at the request of a union, even in the absence of an employer association, may be viewed as participants in a multiemployer unit.

THE BASIC REQUIREMENT: CONSENT

The fundamental basis of multiemployer bargaining is consent. For purposes of certification by the National Labor Relations Board (NLRB), a multiemployer unit will not be found to be an appropriate entity over the objection of either party.[6] Once all parties agree to bargain on a multiemployer basis nothing more is required than for all employer members to express unequivocal intent to be bound in future contract negotiations by group, rather than individual, action. This intent can be found either in the express delegation of authority to the multiemployer group or where there has been a substantial history of participation in the group bargaining process.[7]

It is the early unionization of the hospitals in Minnesota, coupled with a pioneering state labor relations act and an active hospital association, that combined to provide the Minnesota experience in health care collective bargaining on a multiemployer basis.

The hospitals in Minnesota have enjoyed a long history of cooperation. The Minnesota Hospital Association was organized in 1917 to provide a forum for the discussion of mutual concerns of these institutions throughout the state.[8] On the local level, the hospitals in the Twin Cities had organized two separate city councils prior to 1917 for the same purpose.[9] Failure to combine the two city councils, despite several attempts, was based largely on rivalry between the two cities.[10] Nevertheless, representatives of both groups met regularly to discuss wages and personnel policy matters. Undeterred by the lack of formal organization, the combined group called itself the Twin Cities Joint Hospital Council.

An illustration of some of the earliest developments in this multiemployer bargaining system's history is found in the resolutions adopted by this council. For example, in 1947 representatives from 25 hospitals from both sides of the Mississippi River met to discuss the action to be taken in response to a request for recognition from the Minnesota Nurses' Association (MNA) to act as the bargaining agent for all general duty nurses. The council, in a series of resolutions,[11] agreed:

1. to recognize the MNA as the representative of the general duty nurses
2. to urge individual hospitals to accept a set minimum wage for these nurses
3. to appoint a committee to meet and confer with representatives of the MNA for the purpose of agreeing upon minimum standards of employment
4. to authorize a committee to agree to a shortened workweek and to develop a uniform grievance procedure
5. to urge the adoption of the policy that any agreement reached between the MNA and the committee be subject to ratification by the Twin Cities Joint Hospital Council before any individual hospital accepted the terms

As early as 1947, multiemployer agreements were being developed that provided for association approval without disturbing the autonomy of the individual hospitals.

THE PERIOD OF GROWTH

As the hospitals grew more complex, the activity of the councils increased. In 1952 the St. Paul Hospital Council hired its first full-time staff member and a year later the two city councils formally merged and became the Association of Twin City Hospitals. The association's program included public relations, third party payer negotiations, education and training, and labor relations.[12] By this time, the metropolitan area hospitals were extensively organized. In addition to the MNA, six hospitals in St. Paul and nine in Minneapolis had identical contracts with Local 113, Service Employees International Union (SEIU),[13] covering nonprofessional employees. Labor relations actively increased and soon became one of the most important functions of the association.

Over time the name of the association was changed, first to the Twin City Regional Hospital Council to respond to the structuring of the state hospital association into regional councils, and later to the Twin City Hospital Association (TCHA). The membership and the association changed very little.[14]

The members of the TCHA recognized the duplication of services that had developed between the state and metropolitan associations and in 1970 appointed a liaison committee to explore the possibility of merging the two. The state association, which included many small nonunionized hospitals, was unwilling to undertake the much-needed labor relations service. A decision was made to sanction two organizations, permitting the state association to continue its program of a full range of services except for labor relations. The TCHA was renamed Health Manpower Management, Inc., and was changed from a metropolitan council to a statewide service providing employee relations consultation and representation.[15]

HMMI currently has 68 members, including nursing homes, homes for children and for the aged, small hospitals in rural Minnesota, and hospitals in medium-sized and metropolitan areas. The type of membership varies in accordance with the level of service each receives.

There are 171 short-term general community hospitals with 24,000 beds in Minnesota. In addition to the 37 metropolitan hospitals in the Twin Cities, 18 are located in Rochester, Duluth, and St. Cloud. Sixty percent of the hospitals have fewer than 100 beds and 5 percent have more than 500.[16]

HMMI is managed by an executive director under the authority of an 11-member board. Nine of the members are elected from among the Twin City hospital administrators and two are appointed from among the directors of personnel. Ad hoc committees and negotiating teams are appointed from among the general membership.

In 1974, HMMI established a series of multiemployer units for the Twin City hospitals that historically had been party to the jointly negotiated, but separately executed, agreements. An assignment of bargaining rights was executed by the Twin City members attesting to their consent to bargain as a multiemployer unit and agreeing to abide by its majority decisions. Seven multiemployer contracts, affecting 28 hospitals and more than 20,000 employees, are covered by these agreements. Another 40,000 employees are affected indirectly as a result of pattern bargaining in single-employer agreements and as a result of nonunion hospitals' adoption of the wage rates and fringe benefits.

In Minnesota, most of the classic advantages of multiemployer bargaining can be observed.[17] Labor and management realize cost efficiencies in the negotiation process as well as in contract administration. For the hospital, whipsawing has been avoided; for the union, there is some protection from raiding by rival unions. The raiding protection is not absolute, however, as shown in the results of a 1980 election involving 1,500 licensed practical nurses (L.P.N.s) in 18 Twin City hospitals. The L.P.N.s, which had been represented by the Minnesota Licensed Practical Nurses' Association (MLPNA) since 1949, voted to be represented by Local 113 of the SEIU by a 2 to 1 vote.

LEGISLATION AND UNION GROWTH

The early development of the employer association and union strength in Minnesota followed the passage of the National Industrial Recovery Act (NIRA) in 1933. NIRA was aimed at alleviating mass unemployment by encouraging industrial development. Although the NIRA was declared unconstitutional two years later, the act established the rights of employees to organize and bargain collectively without employer interference, and the unions quickly accelerated their organizing activities.[18] Neither federal nor state industrial relations legislation provided adequate mechanisms for coping with the conflict arising from the organizing drives. In Minnesota, the National Guard was called upon in 1934 to maintain order during a dispute involving truck drivers and their employers and again in 1935 during the streetwear dispute. The unions—which later organized hospital employees—organized workers in the office and public buildings in the Twin Cities during this period of unrest (1933-1935).[19]

After the NIRA was declared unconstitutional, Congress enacted the National Labor Relations (Wagner) Act (NLRA), which further strengthened employee rights. The Wagner Act provided for representation elections and declared refusal by employers to bargain with employees to be an unfair labor practice.[20] Union organizing increased dramatically across

the nation and, in Minnesota, proceeded rapidly in the construction, public utilities, transportation, manufacturing, service, and food industries.[21]

The Minnesota Labor Relations Act

To cope with the conflict between employers and employees, the state legislature in 1939 passed the Minnesota Labor Relations Act (MLRA). The MLRA declared certain employee activities, such as seizure of property, sit-in strikes, acts to coerce other workers to join unions, and striking in violation of a collective bargaining agreement, to be unfair labor practices. A ten-day notice of intent to strike or to lock out was necessary. Voluntary arbitration was sanctioned. A division of conciliation was established to administer the part of the law pertaining to conciliation, arbitration, and employee representation cases.

The basic principle of the MLRA was the use of all voluntary means available for the avoidance of a labor dispute before a strike or lockout occurred. The first report by the labor conciliator, covering the period April 24, 1939 to June 30, 1940,[22] indicated a material reduction in strikes and a general improvement in labor relations. During the first 14 months of operation, 383 disputes affecting 30,042 employees were settled by conciliation. Twenty-five strikes were reported in 1939 affecting 2,996 employees compared to an average of 68 strikes affecting 15,865 employees during the preceding three years.

Section 7 of the MLRA, commonly referred to as the public interest clause, required the labor conciliator to refer contemplated strikes or lockouts that would affect the well-being of a community to the governor for appointment of a three-member fact-finding commission representing the public, labor, and industry. The commission was required to report its findings within 30 days. As the question of applicability of the MLRA to nonprofit hospitals surfaced, Section 7 proved to be the pivotal point.

Local 113, SEIU, had organized a unit of 125 janitors, laundry workers, firemen, and elevator operators at a Minneapolis hospital in 1937. The union began picketing and the hospital successfully appealed to the court for an injunction, which stalemated the union's quest for recognition. Immediately after the passage of the MLRA, Local 113 filed a notice of intent to strike the hospital. The labor conciliator barred the strike on the basis of Section 7. The commission appointed by the governor reported that these hospital employees had a right to strike, and the state's attorney general confirmed the commission's judgment. When the restraining order was lifted, the hospital appealed to the courts. It emphasized its public, charitable, and nonprofit attributes and argued that the MLRA was intended to deal only with industrial peace among commercial employers and their employees. The Minnesota state court's response was that the MLRA did not make an employee's right to bargain collectively dependent on the employer's type of operation. The court reasoned that inclusion of the public interest clause in the MLRA was sufficient indication that the legislature had contemplated the possibility of strikes such as those that might occur in hospitals.[23]

In reaching its conclusion, the court reviewed two similar cases in New York and Pennsylvania in which nonprofit hospitals were ruled exempt from the state labor codes. In each case, the hospitals were dependent on state or city funds and, unless excluded as a political subdivision of the state, were not otherwise specifically excluded. In this Minnesota case, however, despite acknowledgment that if the hospital were unable to operate the state would be obliged to carry the burden, the court viewed the clarity of the MLRA such that no weight could be given to these cases. Injunctive procedures were available in those states where the courts ruled the hospitals to be exempt from the state labor codes, but in Minnesota the court's findings left the charitable hospitals clearly vulnerable to strikes.[24]

During the war years, 1940 through 1945, Minnesota experienced the same decline in strike activity as was evident throughout the country. Local 113, however, continued an aggressive and successful campaign against the hospitals and, by 1945, had been recognized by 20 institutions and represented 5,000 nonprofessional employees.

Taft-Hartley and the Tydings Amendment

In 1947, Congress attempted to curtail the growing power of labor by passing the Taft-Hartley Act,[25] which was branded by unions as a "slave labor act."[26] The Tydings amendment to the Taft-Hartley Act excluded not-for-profit hospitals from federal jurisdiction.

In the same year Minnesota, with a comprehensive state law already in place, reacted to hospital organizing activities and the potential consequence of strikes by passing the Charitable Hospitals Act (CHA) over the bitter objection of labor.[27] The CHA amendment to MLRA provided that any unresolved dispute relating to wages and hours be submitted to mandatory binding arbitration at the request of either or both parties. Strikes and lockouts were prohibited. The CHA applied to all state, university, county, and municipal hospitals.[28]

The CHA did not halt union organizing activity in hospitals. In addition to the Minnesota Nurses' Association and Local 113, the operating engineers had evolved into two separate locals, one for each city's hospitals. The licensed practical nurses (MLPNA) organized units in 18 Twin City hospitals in the late 1940s, and in the early 1960s a unit of pharmacists and a separate unit of radiologic technologists were certified under the MLRA.

The growing strength of the unions and the absolute prohibition on strikes resulted in a constitutional challenge by Local 113. In 1953 the union indicated it would strike nine hospitals in the Twin Cities over union security. The court issued an injunction at the hospital's request, but the union appealed. It contended that the CHA was unconstitutional because it removed the union's right to strike without providing an adequate substitute. It argued that compulsory arbitration was an inadequate substitute, inasmuch as it was limited to "any unsettled issues of maximum hours of work and minimum hourly wage rates," and did not provide a dispute settlement mechanism for noncost items such as management rights and union security.

The state court[29] agreed that a broader interpretation of the restrictive language of the arbitration clause could be applied to items such as holidays and other benefits that affected employees' welfare but found no reason to determine that the legislature had acted in an arbitrary, capricious, or discriminatory manner in omitting noncost items. The court ruled that employees' constitutional rights had not been violated and that both parties had been treated equally by the no-strike, no-lockout provision.

The court reasoned that the legislative intent regarding the exclusion of the security clause may have been prompted by the knowledge that much of the work in hospitals was performed by members of religious and charitable organizations who, because of religious beliefs or otherwise, considered themselves ineligible for union membership. On the question of internal management, the court assumed legislative knowledge that issues bearing on the life or death of a patient are too vital a matter to be entrusted to anyone but the skilled medical technicians and staff members. Thus, the prohibition of strikes and lockouts and the provisions for compulsory arbitration withstood the challenge.[30]

A second, lesser challenge to the CHA came in the form of a work stoppage by the same union over a scheduling dispute in 1964.[31] The strike was enjoined after two days and the dispute was submitted to arbitration as provided in the CHA.

SINCE THE 1974 NLRA AMENDMENTS

At the point of passage of the 1974 amendments to the NLRA, Minnesota had enjoyed a 27-year history of labor-management relationships free of work stoppages during a period of growth in hospital union membership and in the industry. Only two work stoppages have occurred in the voluntary nonprofit hospital sector since 1947. The first strike resulted from the work scheduling dispute mentioned above and the second was a 1980 MNA contract dispute with a small suburban hospital, not party to the existing multiemployer bargaining agreement. The MNA action represented the first strike in its history and the first legal hospital strike in the state since 1947.

The restoration of the right to strike to hospital employees prompted Minnesota to petition the NLRB to cede its jurisdiction to the state, citing the success of the state's labor relations record under the CHA. The petition had the support of most hospital unions, the state hospital association,[32] and public officials. Congressional support, in addition to that of the Minnesota delegation, came from Senator Robert Taft (R., Ohio), who stated that

. . . the CHA has worked extremely well and is endorsed by the state AFL-CIO and the state hospital association and other interested groups in the state. Under these circumstances, it would certainly seem that the Board should consider ceding jurisdiction.[33]

Senator Harrison Williams (D., N.J.), chairman of the Senate Labor and Public Welfare Committee and a principal proponent of the 1974 amendments, indicated his support for the NLRB to accept the petition[34] and Congressman Frank Thompson (D., N.J.), chairman of the Subcommittee on Labor of the House Education and Labor Committee, stated that

. . . in my opinion, Minnesota occupies a totally unique position among states in its enactment and application of its state statute dealing with labor relations in nonprofit hospitals.[35]

These favorable opinions notwithstanding, the NLRB denied the petition on the basis that federal law preempted any inconsistent state regulation and concluded that it lacked the discretion to allow a single state to continue to operate under its own law.[36]

HMMI then adopted a policy of attempting to include contract clauses in its negotiated agreements that provided for interest arbitration as a means of resolving contractual disputes. Such clauses were included in the multiemployer bargaining agreements with the MNA, MLPNA, Minnesota Society of Radiologic Technologists, Local 113, and the Professional Employee Pharmacists of Minnesota. Other single-hospital agreements subsequently adopted similar clauses. Only Local 34 and Local 36 of the operating engineers, which had opposed the state's petition to the NLRB, refused to include such a clause in their contracts. The agreements barred strikes and lockouts for a period that at the time exceeded the term of the contracts by six to eight years. The last of these agreements expires in 1984 unless renewed by the parties.

THE NLRB AND MULTIEMPLOYER BARGAINING

The long history and extensive use of multiemployer bargaining has not met with widespread acceptance, and the resulting political controversies were not resolved by congressional action. Neither the Wagner Act nor the Taft-Hartley Act provided explicit language regarding multiemployer bargaining. The NLRB assumed that it was empowered to certify multiemployer units on the basis of the definition of an employer as described in the act as "any person acting as an agent of the employer."[37] Students of the labor legislative process can find strong and diverse opinions on the subject.

In its initial form, multiemployer bargaining was viewed as an effective method of giving employers, especially small companies, greater leverage in dealing with unions. It also permitted employees, particularly those in occupations where jobsites changed frequently, to benefit from uniform terms of employment.[38]

By the time the 1947 Taft-Hartley amendments were being debated, considerable opposition to multiemployer bargaining had surfaced and proposals to restrict it were introduced. The mood of Congress was influenced by growing public sentiment that unions had become too powerful. Economists pointed to the wage-price spiral as evidence that the growing union strength should be curtailed. Several congressmen advocated a prohibition of industrywide negotiation, charging that it was anticompetitive and had the propensity to magnify the impact of a strike. While the attempts to restrict multiemployer bargaining failed, the Taft-Hartley amendments remained silent on the issue, allowing the controversy to continue.[39]

In 1953, a proposal was introduced that would have restricted multiemployer bargaining by mandating that one union representing employees at one location would be ineligible to represent workers of a competing firm if the two concerns were less than 50 miles apart.[40]

Congressman Franklin Roosevelt, Jr. (D., N.Y.), in his "Don't Pulverize Labor" speech in the House of Representatives, urged Congress not to pass the amendment on the ground that it would destroy the delicate fabric of the institutional relationship between management and labor that had taken years to build.[41]

The Supreme Court Decision

Ultimately, it was the U.S. Supreme Court that recognized the importance of multiemployer bargaining and the authority of the NLRB to certify such units. In the 1957 *Buffalo Linen* case, the court observed:

At the time of the debates on the Taft-Hartley amendments, proposals were made to limit or outlaw multiemployer bargaining. These proposals failed of enactment. They were met with a storm of protest that their adoption would tend to weaken and not strengthen the process of collective bargaining and would conflict with the national labor policy of promoting industrial peace through effective collective bargaining. . . . the inaction of Congress with respect to multiemployer bargaining cannot be said to indicate an intention to leave the resolution of this problem to future legislation. Rather, the compelling conclusion is that Congress intended that the Board should continue its established administrative practice of certifying multiemployer units, and intended to leave to the board's specialized judgment the inevitable questions concerning multiemployer bargaining . . . .[42]

With respect to withdrawal from a multiemployer unit, the concept of consent also governs. If the parties agree, either party can withdraw at any time for any reason. In the absence of consent, rules have been established by the NLRB for withdrawal:

An employer can withdraw from a multiemployer bargaining unit at will, provided only that the withdrawal request is made before the date set by the contract for modification or before the agreed-upon date to begin the multiemployer negotiations, and the withdrawal is unequivocal.[43]

In a case in which an employer notified the union by a timely written notice of intent to withdraw but failed to advise the association and continued to attend all negotiating sessions, the NLRB did not permit the employer to withdraw on the basis that the action did not meet the test of unequivocal intent to withdraw.[44]

The NLRB also has permitted limited exceptions[45] to the withdrawal procedure by rulings that permitted an employer to withdraw under unusual circumstances, i.e., where the company's existence as a business is threatened[46] and where, upon bargaining impasse, the union proceeds to conduct separate negotiations with employers, thereby deliberately undermining the integrity of a multiemployer unit.[47]

Where Rulings Conflict

Two additional NLRB rulings providing for employer withdrawal have been met with conflicting court rulings. On the matter of whether an impasse within a multiemployer unit during negotiations is sufficient to justify unilateral withdrawal from the bargaining unit, the NLRB adheres to the doctrine that an impasse cannot be regarded as an unexpected event in that process and does not necessarily reflect a breakdown in the bargaining relationship.[48] The board has ruled consistently that an impasse does not permit unilateral withdrawal of an employer member of the association.[49] However, the circuit courts that have addressed this issue have uniformly held to the contrary: that a genuine impasse justifies withdrawal.[50]

On the question of a multiemployer association's disregard for a minority member's interest, the board has ruled that the employer's withdrawal is untimely if decided following the conclusion of contract negotiations. The courts, on the other hand, have reasoned that while mere dissatisfaction with the negotiated results does not justify untimely withdrawal, it may be justified in circumstances where the majority membership makes but a feeble attempt to protect and advance minority interests.[51] The courts have reasoned that multiemployer bargaining will work only when the interests of all parties are represented fairly.

Balancing the interests of all parties is among the most unpredictable aspects of multiemployer bargaining. In retrospect, multiemployer bargaining has worked in Minnesota, serving both unions and employers well. The success appears to be the result of a fortuitous set of circumstances, including early organization of the hospitals by a small number of unions, an employer association oriented to cooperative action, and, finally, a state labor relations act that provided a lengthy period during which conflict was resolved by arbitration. The maturity of this relationship provides some optimism for the future.

THE CHANGE IN HOSPITALS— AND THE FUTURE

Consideration of the use of multiemployer bargaining in settings with or without circumstances similar to those found in Minnesota requires recognition of the changing nature of hospitals. External pressures on hospital operations have resulted in increased competition and efforts to increase efficiency, primarily through merger and the use of new technologies.

As hospitals grow in complexity, the modern ones may be even more reluctant to surrender any portion of their autonomy and, in a multiemployer unit, each individual hospital must be willing to abide by the decision of the majority. In the same way, the modern hospital values its ability to be flexible according to its own priorities, but multiemployer bargaining tends to restrict the flexibility of the participating members.

Modern hospitals compete in other ways. The potential of significant losses in revenue due to an inadequate supply of skilled workers may cause intense competition for the available personnel supply and weaken the bonds holding employers to the multiemployer bargaining relationship.

The most serious consideration in the adoption of multiemployer bargaining is the impact of strikes. While it generally is agreed that strikes occur less frequently in multiemployer situations, it also is acknowledged that when they do occur, they usually are wider in scope, affect more employees, and are more difficult to settle. It is impossible to predict whether a strike will have the effect of bringing hospitals together to strengthen their position by developing systems of mutual aid or other alternatives, or whether it will have the opposite effect because of the differences in the way the walkout is perceived by individual hospitals. Much depends upon the specific precipitating incident and the people and issues involved.

To the extent that there is a history of a relationship, that history will have an influence on the perceptions of the parties. In a multiemployer bargaining unit with an extensive history of amicable settlements, the parties are likely to strive for early resolution of differences in order to avoid a strike in the first place, and the same history will tend to lessen the use of extreme action during the strike.

Not all the lessons learned in the past have applicability for the present or for the future. Multiemployer bargaining, depending as it does upon the consent of the parties, is a fragile concept and may require significant modification to cope with the changing times and the changing outlook of the parties as they evolve.

NOTES

1. Joseph Shister, ed., *Readings in Labor Economics and Industrial Relations* (New York: J. B. Lippincott Co., 1951), pp. 196–204.
2. Wilbert E. Moore, *Industrial Relations and the Social Order* (New York: The Macmillan Co., 1951), pp. 345–347.
3. Gordon F. Bloom and Herbert R. Northrup, *Economics of Labor Relations*, 8th rev. ed. (Homewood, Ill.: Richard D. Irwin, Inc., 1977), p. 211.
4. "Types of Bargaining Units," *Labor Law Guide*, Vol. 1 (Chicago: Commerce Clearing House, Inc., 1972), ¶ 3014–3015, p. 2012.
5. Norman Metzger and Dennis D. Pointer, *Labor-Management Relations in the Health Services Industry: Theory and Practice* (Washington, D.C.: Science and Health Publications, Inc., 1972), p. 330.
6. *Steamship Trade Ass'n of Baltimore, Inc.*, 155 NLRB 232, 60 LRRM 1257 (1965).
7. *Kroger Co.*, 148 NLRB 569, 57 LRRM 1021 (1964).
8. Clarence W. Palmateer, Jr., *Recommendations for the Organizational Structure of a Single Hospital Council for St. Paul and Minneapolis, Minnesota*, submitted to the faculty of the Program in Hospital Administration, University of Minnesota, to fulfill requirements of the Clerkship Course, P. H. 166, 1956, p. 1.
9. Ibid.
10. Ibid.
11. Minutes, Twin City Hosp. Council, September 29, 1947.
12. Palmateer, Jr., op. cit., p. 5.
13. This local, now Local 113, Service Employees Int'l Union (SEIU), was known first in Minnesota as the Public Building Service Employees and later as the Public Building Service and Hospital and Institutional Employees Union, AFL. It is referred to as Local 113 throughout.
14. Articles of Incorporation, Twin City Hosp. Ass'n, March 1964, recorded May 8, 1964, State of Minnesota, Book N-2, p. 60.
15. Minutes, Twin City Hosp. Ass'n, July 17, 1972.
16. American Hosp. Ass'n, *Hospital Statistics* (Chicago: American Hospital Association, 1979), p. 86.
17. Sylvestor Garrett and L. Reed Tripp, *Management Problems Implicit in Multiemployer Bargaining* (Philadelphia: Univ. of Pennsylvania Press, 1949), pp. 59–61.
18. F. Ray Marshall, Allan M. Cartter, and Allan G. King, *Labor Economics Wages; Employment and Trade Unionism*, 3rd rev. ed. (Homewood, Ill.: Richard D. Irwin, Inc., 1976), p. 413.
19. Harry L. Hanson, Labor Conciliator. *Biennial Report of the Div. of Conciliation, State of Minnesota* July 1952–July 1954, p. 1.
20. National Labor Relations Act of July 5, 1935, c. 372, 49 Stat. 449.
21. Lloyd J. Haney, Conciliator, *First Annual Report of the Div. of Conciliation, State of Minnesota*, August 1, 1940, p. 17.
22. Ibid, p. 16.
23. *Northwestern Hosp. v. Pub. Bldg. Serv. Employees Union, Local 113* and others, 208 Minn. 389, 294 N.W. 215.
24. *Jewish Hosp. of Brooklyn v. Doe*, 252 App. Div. 581, 300 N.Y.S. 111; *W. Penn Hosp. v. Lichliter*, 49 Dauph Co. Rep. (Pa.) 326, 1941.
25. Labor Management Relations Act, June 23, 1947, c. 120, 61 Stat. 136.
26. P.L. 93-360, August 25, 1974.
27. Minn. Labor Relations Act, Minn. Stats., Sec. 179.35–179.39 (Charitable Hosps. Act [CHA] of 1947).
28. In 1971, the CHA was amended to exclude university and state hospitals, which were then covered by the Public Employees Labor Relations Act (PELRA).

29. *Fairview Hosp. and Others v. Pub. Bldg. Serv. and Hosp. and Inst'l Employees Union, Local 113, AFL.* 241 Minn 523, 64 N.W. 2d 16, 1954.

30. Sec. 179.38 of the CHA relating to arbitration was amended in 1971 to include other terms and conditions of employment.

31. Children's Hosp., St. Paul, Fall, 1964.

32. *In Re State of Minnesota,* Memorandum of Minn. Hosp. Ass'n to NLRB in Support of Petition to Cede Jurisdiction, 1975.

33. *Congressional Record,* S. 7311, May 7, 1974.

34. *Congressional Record,* S. 12109, July 10, 1974.

35. *Congressional Record,* H. 6393, July 11, 1974.

36. *In Re State of Minnesota,* 219 NLRB No. 170, 89 LRRM 1785 (1975).

37. *Shipowners Ass'n of the Pacific Coast,* 7 NLRB 1002, 2 LRRM 377 (1938) and *Associated Shoe Industries of Southeastern Mass., Inc.* 81 NLRB 224, 23 LRRM 1320 (1949).

38. Bloom and Northrup, op. cit., pp. 211–214.

39. Marshall, Cartter, and King, op. cit. p. 359.

40. H.R. 2545, 1953, Committee on Education and Labor; Rep. Lucas, Texas, p. 2.

41. *Congressional Record,* H. February 19, 1953.

42. *NLRB v. Truck Drivers Local 449 (Buffalo Linen,* 353 U.S. 84 (1957)).

43. *Retail Associates, Inc.* 120 NLRB 388, 41 LRRM 1502 (1958)

and *Evening News Ass'n,* 154 NLRB 1494, 60 LRRM 1149 (1965).

44. *Interstate Construction Co.,* 229 NLRB 37, 95 LRRM 1277 (1977).

45. For examples, *see Sheridan Creations, Inc.,* 357 F.2d 245, 61 LRRM 2586 (2d. Cir. 1966); *W. E. Painters, Inc.,* 176 NLRB 964, 72 LRRM 1089 (1969); and *Serv-All Co., Inc.,* 199 NLRB No. 159, 81 LRRM 1495 (1972).

46. *U. S. Lingerie Corp.,* 170 NLRB 77, 67 LRRM 1482 (1968).

47. *Typographics Service Co.,* 238 NLRB 211, 99 LRRM 1649 (1978), *in accord, NLRB v. Associated Shower Door Co.,* 512 F.2d 230, 232-233 (9th Cir., 1975); *cert. denied* 423 U.S. 893 (1975) (dictum).

48. *Hi-Way Billboards,* 191 NLRB No. 37, 77 LRRM 1461 (1971); remand: 206 NLRB 22, 84 LRRM 1161 (1973).

49. *Florida Fire Sprinklers,* 237 NLRB 155, 99 LRRM 1078 (1978), and *Bonnano Linen Service, Inc.,* 243 No 140, 102 LRRM 1001 (1979).

50. For examples, *see NLRB v. Beck Engraving Co.,* 522 F.2d 475 (3d Cir. 1975), 90 LRRM 2089; *NLRB v. Hi-Way Billboards, Inc.,* 473 F. 2d 649 (5th Cir. 1973), 82 LRRM 2527; and *NLRB v. Hi-Way Billboards, Inc.,* 500 F.2d 181 (5th Cir. 1974), 87 LRRM 2203.

51. *NLRB v. Siebler Heating and Air Conditioning,* 563 F.2d 366 (8th Cir. 1977), 96 LRRM 2613.

18. Collective Bargaining by Nurses: A Comparative Analysis of Management and Employee Perceptions

JOAN R. BLOOM, G. NICHOLAS PARLETTE,
and CHARLES A. O'REILLY

Reprinted with permission from *Health Care Management Review*, Vol. 5, No. 1 (Winter 1980)
published by Aspen Systems Corporation, Germantown, Md., © 1980. The article is based on a
paper presented at the annual meeting of the American Public Health Association in 1978.

Current management literature says and reported studies seem to prove that:

1. Good managers try to foster honest organizational communication that flows upward, downward and across unit boundaries.
2. Good managers know that productive communication is dependent upon the listening skills of the participants, particularly those of the responsible executives; they know it is important to listen to not only what others are saying but also how they are saying it.
3. Good managers believe that the most productive individuals in the organization are motivated by a drive for autonomy and self-realization.[1]

If these tenets of good management are sound, and there is no evidence to the contrary, why do some managers of large health service complexes act as if these principles do not apply in the area of collective bargaining?

This seeming contradiction in the behavior of management became apparent during interviews with nurses and members of the management team in a county health service agency where a county-wide strike had recently been settled. Was it possible that there was so little communication between the disputing parties that their perceptions of the importance of issues had become distorted? Or could this apparent contradiction be due to differences in the expectations

that each party held as to the wants and needs of the other? Interviews with the nurses and management provided significant answers to these questions, answers that relate to the three basic models of management.

MODELS OF MANAGEMENT

With some bending and molding, administrative theories of leadership can be categorized as one of three models: (1) traditional model, (2) human relations model and (3) human resources model.[2] These models differ in the assumptions made, the expectations for the average worker and the implications each has for the role of the manager. Briefly stated, the traditional model assumes that work is inherently distasteful. What one earns is more important than what one does, and few want or can handle work that requires creativity, self-direction or self-control. The second model, the dominant theme of management theory during the last 50 years, emphasizes the similarity of needs among all organization members. While common needs are recognized, similar capabilities are not. In fact, managers are seen as the planners and doers while the workers are viewed as willingly cooperating with their superiors when their needs to feel useful and important are fulfilled.

The human resources model departs from the former models in several important ways. First, it views organization members not only as a supply of physical skill and energy, but also as an untapped source of creative ability with the capacity for responsible, self-controlled behavior. Second, as in the human relations model, the leader is urged to share information and decision making. Unlike the human relations model, however, the purpose of the human resources model is to improve decision making and efficiency of the organization rather than to improve morale and satisfaction. Finally, motivation for work is seen as intrinsic. Rewards flow from the workers' feelings of accomplishment and the knowledge that a job has been well done rather than from extrinsic motivators, such as increases in pay and fringe benefits or improvements in work conditions.

Management's Expectations

The research of Ray Miles and his colleagues indicates that in the health field, administrators hold not one, but two sets of attitudes.[3] When administrators consider their relationships with their subordinates, their leadership and supervisory attitudes lean toward those of the human relations model. When they consider their relationships with superiors, however, their attitudes are closer to those of the human resources model.

Expectations of Outside Experts

In addition, management's view of striking nurses has been affected by the collective bargaining process. Collective bargaining in the public sector is a relatively recent development. Perhaps management has had to rely on people outside the public sector for assistance in collective bargaining because it is so new. The outsiders' views of collective bargaining have emerged from legal interpretations of the Labor Relations Law as well as from previous experiences with labor negotiations, primarily in the industrial sector.[4] Typically, workers have been viewed as selling their labor for the highest possible price and economic benefits. Both management and labor negotiate issues toward these ends, including salaries and benefits, hours and other aspects of working conditions, job security and grievance handling. Therefore, collective bargaining is viewed as a means to improve the economic situation of the worker. In the public sector, as costs are not easily passed on, each bargaining issue is carefully weighed to determine its fiscal impact upon the institution. Issues without fiscal implications are not seen as equally important. Thus, this view of collective bargaining, brought to the health care industry by outside experts, reinforces the traditional model of management.

Nurses' Expectations

The nurses' definition of the situation, however, might be quite different from management's; thus, their reasons for striking and their assessment of the bargaining issues would not be congruent with those of management. Nurses' expectations have changed since World War II along with their education, salaries and ideology.

When the California Nurses' Association withdrew its no-strike pledge in 1968, the Economic and Security Program of the American Nurses' Association had been in effect for over 20 years with little improvement in the economic position of nurses relative to that of workers in occupations requiring similar education and responsibility. During this time, however, changes were taking place in nursing education. Between 1962 and 1972 half of the traditional three-year, hospital-affiliated nursing programs were phased out,[5] and an increasing number of students were attending collegiate nursing programs.

At one time nurses espoused Florence Nightingale's service ideal, which advocated the provision of quality nursing care by technically competent individuals and placed the needs of society before the personal needs and desires of the care provider. Now this ideal is slowly being replaced by professionalism ideology. In this ideology, characteristic of law, theology and medicine, the individual not only makes a strong commitment to the client and to technical expertise, but also assumes sole responsibility for clients and practices autonomously. This professionalism ideology is particularly evident among college graduates, which the majority of public health nurses are.[6]

Since 1968 nurses' salaries and other economic benefits have become competitive with those of individuals of similar education and job responsibility.[7] Today issues of autonomy and control rather than issues of economics have become foremost for many public sector nurses. In Maslow's terms, lower-level needs for security have already been met,[8] and nurses have become concerned about higher-level needs. The human resources model of management is consistent with the needs and expectations of professionalized employees such as nurses. They are capable and desirous of assuming responsibility and participating in organizational decision making.

As a result, the nurses' reasons for striking and their assessment of the bargaining issues may differ significantly from management's view of the situation.

STUDYING NURSES, MANAGEMENT AND COLLECTIVE BARGAINING

For the past several years, data have been collected on how nurses, predominantly public health nurses, view collective bargaining and its issues. In addition, key management personnel within public agencies and governmental jurisdictions have been interviewed to ascertain their views of collective bargaining in the public sector.

Collecting Data

Data have been collected from public health nurses and R.N.s in three large community health care agencies in California (work stoppages had occurred in two of them). The nurses were all county employees represented by locals of an international union. Data from one of these counties support the belief that collective bargaining among professional employees must be different from that traditionally carried on in labor negotiations in the industrial setting, and preliminary analyses of data collected from the other two counties further substantiate this belief.

In the county with complete results, there is a work force of 96 public health nurses, including first-line supervisors. Background information about the nurses and their attitudes toward professionalism, collective bargaining and the specific strike issues was collected by a self-administered questionnaire, which was mailed to the nurses. Ninety percent (89) of the questionnaires were returned and provide the sample for the analysis. Because of late returns, four of the questionnaires were not included in the analysis. Thus, the sample consisted of 78 staff nurses in three different grades and 11 supervisory nurses. The median age of the respondent was 35 years. Average tenure with the county was 7.5 years. As public health nurses, all had obtained a baccalaureate degree; 18 also had a master's degree. Most held, or at least espoused, values consistent with professionalism. Although there was high agreement between striking and nonstriking nurses as to the importance of bargaining with management, there was disagreement as to who should be negotiating for them. Those nurses who were older and from lower social class origins viewed the professional nurses' association as their bargaining agent, while those who were younger and from higher social class origins viewed the union as their bargaining agent.[9] These data are consistent with those of Aluto and Belasco, who studied registered nurses in general hospitals.[10]

At the same time, a series of interviews was conducted with ten members of management. Included were the public health nursing management team consisting of the director of nursing, her three assistant directors, the director of public health and the county managers most involved with the strike. In addition to participating in an open-ended interview, management and the nurses were asked to indicate how extensively each of 17 issues was thought to be a factor in the nurses' decision to strike. These 17 issues were compiled as a result of the preliminary interviews with members of the health department management team and 15 staff public health nurses. Each responded to this list of issues on a four-point scale ranging from "Not a factor at all in my (their) decision" to "A major factor in my (their) decision."

Testing Hypotheses

Two hypotheses had been formulated: (1) perceptions of key issues in the strike by management and by the nurses were not congruent and (2) management was primarily concerned with issues that had economic implications, while nurses were primarily concerned with issues related to professional control and autonomy. The first hypothesis was tested by calculating the percentage of nurses who felt that a particular issue was important in their decision to strike or not. The percentage of each group that stated that an issue was a factor in their decision is displayed in Exhibit 18-1. Also included in this table is the percentage of managers who stated that a particular issue was a factor in the nurses' decision to strike or not.

Spearman's Rank Order Coefficient of Correlation (Rho) was used to determine the degree of agreement between the perceptions of management and those of both the striking and nonstriking nurses. As indicated in Exhibit 18-1, little relationship existed between management and either group of nurses. (Rho between management and striking nurses is 0.17, and Rho between management and the nonstriking nurses is 0.15; both figures are significant.)

Most noticeable in Exhibit 18-1 is that the nurses who went on strike saw the issues differently from those who did not. These differences were statistically significant for 11 of the issues. When multiple significance testing is done, five percent of the tests would be expected to be statistically significant by chance, i.e., two to three tests. The results in Exhibit 18-1 indicate that 50 percent were significant. What is equally noticeable (and may have contributed to the walk-out) is that management at all levels in the county saw the issues which led to the strike differently from either

Exhibit 18-1 Factors Influencing Decision to Strike Or Not

	Percent Important			
	Nurses			Manage-ment
Collective Bargaining Issue	Strikers (n=45)	Non-strikers (n=40)	Total (n=85)	(n=10)
1. Inability to communicate my concerns effectively to *county management* through normal channels.	79	36*	61	42†
2. Inability to communicate my concerns effectively to *health department* management through normal channels.	67	31*	51	42
3. A belief in collective bargaining as a way to balance employee-management power.	75	31*	57	50
4. Authoritarian behavior on the part of management.	65	19*	45	28†
5. Support for the demands of all county union members, e.g., community workers, hospital R.N.s.	90	32*	66	50†
6. Support for other members of my public health nurse unit.	96	49*	76	57†
7. The union's attempt to gain power.	21	81*	47	85†
8. A belief that strikes are inappropriate for public health nurses.	33	72*	50	28§
9. The need for additional public health nurse slots in the county.	63	31*	49	42
10. "TOE" days (time off for education).	32	17	26	50§
11. The use of split codes (one position for two public health nurses).	57	26*	44	62§
12. Personal economic costs in terms of lost wages.	54	36	48	28†
13. Concern for job security.	52	36	45	14†
14. Pressure by public health nurses in the unit to either support or not support strike.	56	26*	43	85†§
15. A better pay increase.	44	31	38	75†§
16. Changes in grievance procedures.	29	14	23	28
17. Pressure by management to remain on the job.	27	9	19	28

*Chi square significance p < .01 (strikers and nonstrikers).
†Chi square significance p < .01 (management and striking nurses).
§Chi square significance p < .01 (management and nonstriking nurses).

the striking or nonstriking nurses. Management agreed with the nonstriking nurses on the importance of only one issue: both saw the strike as an attempt by the union to gain power.

There is little agreement between striking nurses and management on what the important issues were to the nurses. (Important issues were defined as those with 60 percent agreement within one of the three groups.) To nurses who went on strike, the important issues were (1) support for nurses in their own work unit and other county workers, (2) inability to communicate with management, (3) authoritarian behavior on the part of management and (4) a belief in collective bargaining as a way to balance employee-management power. The only economic issue that was important in the nurses' decision to strike was the need for more nursing positions, an issue that is also related to professionalism. Managers, on the other hand, agreed in their belief that nurses' concerns were economic: a pay increase and the use of split codes, that is, one position for two nurses. (The second issue also has practice/professional implications.) Managers were in even greater agreement that the union was trying to gain power and that the nurses were pressuring one another to go on strike. These attitudes may be understandable but certainly cannot increase management's ability to negotiate productively. None of these four issues was important to the nurses.

Identifying Predominant Factors

Statistical methods (principal component analysis with a varimax rotation) were used to decrease the 17 issues to a more manageable set. The results of the factor analysis are presented in Exhibit 18-2. This procedure identified consistencies in how the nurses responded to the issues. The four predominant factors that were identified and the issues subsumed are as follows:

1. *Factor 1—Problems with Management:* defined by communication problems (issues 1 and 2), the use of collective bargaining to balance manage-

Exhibit 18-2 Collective Bargaining Issues and Varimax Factor Loadings*

Collective Bargaining Issue†	Rotated Factor Loading			
	Factor 1	Factor 2	Factor 3	Factor 4
1. Inability to communicate my concerns effectively to *county management* through normal channels.	.90	.15	.18	.03
2. Inability to communicate my concerns effectively to *health department* management through normal channels.	.88	.08	.25	.07
3. A belief in collective bargaining as a way to balance employee-management power.	.75	.23	.17	.23
4. Authoritarian behavior on the part of management.	.75	.20	.18	.11
5. Support for the demands of all county union members, e.g., community workers, hospital R.N.s.	.43	.70	.15	.17
6. Support for other members of my public health nurse unit.	.29	.68	.20	.39
7. The union's attempt to gain power.	−.02	−.76	−.05	.11
8. A belief that strikes are inappropriate for public health nurses.	−.11	−.64	−.06	.13
9. The need for additional public health nurse slots in the county.	.33	.15	.73	−.17
10. "TOE" days (time off for education).	.20	.02	.67	−.07
11. The use of split codes (one position for two public health nurses).	.16	.19	.59	.27
12. Personal economic costs in terms of lost wages.	.12	−.04	−.06	.74
13. Concern for job security.	.21	−.16	.01	.60
14. Pressure by public health nurses in the unit to either support or not support strike.	−.11	.23	.19	.48
15. A better pay increase.	.36	.12	.28	.31
16. Changes in grievance procedures.	.49	.08	.39	.24
17. Pressure by management to remain on the job.	.31	−.06	.23	.39
Common factor variance accounted for:	59%	17%	14%	10%

*N = 85.

†Respondents were asked to indicate, on a four-point scale ranging from "Not a factor at all in my decision" to "A major factor in my decision," the extent to which the issue was important in the decision to strike or not.

Source: Reprinted with permission from "Changing Images of Professionalism: The Case of Public Health Nurses," by J. R. Bloom, C. A. O'Reilly, and G. N. Parlette, *American Journal of Public Health* 69, no. 1 (January 1979), pp. 43–46, © 1979.

ment power (issue 3) and authoritarian behavior by management (issue 4).

2. *Factor 2—Prounion Ideology:* defined by solidarity (issues 5 and 6), disagreement with the perceptions that the strike was a union attempt to gain power (issue 7) and inappropriateness of strikes for public health nurses (issue 8).

3. *Factor 3—Concern about the Conditions of Work:* defined by the desire for additional public health nurse slots (issue 9), time off for education (issue 10) and the use of split codes, that is, dividing one position between two nurses (issue 11).

4. *Factor 4—Personal Costs of Striking:* defined by concern for lost wages (issue 12), job security (issue 13) and pressure by other public health nurses to either support or not support the strike (issue 14).

Three issues were related to more than one factor. A pay increase (issue 15) and a changed grievance procedure (issue 16) were related to three factors—management, conditions of work and personal costs. Pressure by management not to strike (issue 17) was appropriately related to two factors—problems with management and personal costs.

Relationship between Nurses' Perception and Behavior

The congruency of the nurses' perceptions of the issues and their behavior was further tested by an analysis of the relationship between these variables. A statistical examination (regression analysis) was carried out for each of the four factor-based indices. (See Exhibit 18.3.) Only the first two indices explained the nurses' participation in the strike. Of these two indices, prounion ideology (factor 2) was more explanatory than were problems with management (factor 1).[11]

Contrary to the perceptions of management, neither a concern for working conditions (factor 3) nor personal costs (factor 4) appeared to be significant in predicting who would strike. While there was some agreement (60 percent or more) among nurses that problems with management were important, only half of the managers interviewed perceived this to be important, and nurses and management agreed on only one of the issues of factor 2. In summary, while the nurses who went on strike perceived problems with management to be the key area of concern, few of the managers were aware of this factor.

In addition, as part of the ongoing study, nurses were asked a series of questions to identify their attitudes toward collective bargaining. The responses of

Exhibit 18-3 Regression Results for Issues on Participation in Strike*

Independent Variables	Standardized Regression Coefficient	Simple Correlation	ΔR^2
Problems with management (factor 1)	.20†	.53	.28
Prounion ideology (factor 2)	.65§	.77	.36
Conditions of work (factor 3)	.08	.21	.01
Personal costs of striking (factor 4)	.07	.40	.00

*N = 85, F = 33.9, $p < .001$, $R^2 = .65$, $R^{-2} = .63$.
†$p < .01$
§$p < .001$

Source: Reprinted with permission from "Changing Images of Professionalism: The Case of Public Health Nurses," by J. R. Bloom, C. A. O'Reilly, and G. N. Parlette, *American Journal of Public Health* 69, no. 1 (January 1979), pp. 43–46, © 1979.

striking and nonstriking nurses can be seen in Exhibit 18-4. The point to be emphasized is that both striking and nonstriking nurses believed (96 and 83 percent respectively) that it was appropriate for nurses to organize and bargain with management. The main difference was that nonstrikers wished to be represented by the professional association rather than by the union. Both groups agreed (94 and 68 percent respectively) that collective bargaining allows nurses to have a voice in management decisions which affect them.

A NEW LOOK AT COLLECTIVE BARGAINING

Thus, the study showed that (1) the perceptions of the striking nurses differed from those of the nonstriking nurses for 11 of the 17 issues and (2) the perceptions of the striking nurses differed from those of management personnel on 8 of the 17 issues. While management felt that industrial sector bargaining issues such as wages and job security were the critical prob-

Exhibit 18-4 Attitudes toward Collective Bargaining

Attitude	Percent Agreement		
	Strikers	Non-strikers	Chi Square
Without collective bargaining we would not get our fair share of economic benefits.	91	56	12.4*
Collective bargaining allows me to have a voice in management decisions which affect me.	94	68	7.6†
Collective bargaining is a positive force for the nursing profession.	93	59	12.7*
Since I am automatically enrolled in the union, I see no reason to drop out.	50	3	19.1*
The union is the *only way* I have available to me to participate in management decision making.	59	8	21.9*
Collective bargaining by public health nurses is incompatible with professional standards.	4	42	15.4*
I feel the union is responsible to my personal inputs.	91	25	35.0*
I believe public health nurses should support the demands of other county employees in collective bargaining.	63	13	20.1*
I believe that it is appropriate for public health nurses to organize and to bargain with management.	96	83	2.5
I believe the union represents my professional interests.	83	15	37.4*

*$p < .001$
†$p < .01$

lems for the nurses, the nurses were more concerned about matters related to communication with management and participation in organizational decision making. The last two issues have important implications because they predicted strike behavior.

This is not the first time that it has been pointed out that management's view of its employees' concerns may differ from that of the employees[12] or that position in the organizational structure has been implicated as the cause of such differential perceptions.[13] The model of management internalized by management for its workers and the model internalized by the workers for themselves help explain the differential weight given issues by the disputing groups. But expectations may be especially incongruent in the health field when the worker is professionalized, such as in the case of public health nurses. When experts in labor relations, often from the industrial sector, are brought in to assist with the negotiations, an additional element of incongruity is added. The industrial sector viewpoint has strong appeal to the embattled manager confronting a work stoppage. Each demand can be simply defined in

terms of its cost implications, making it easier to understand than one couched in abstract terminology such as "quality of care." In addition, there is no threat of loss of influence or power such as that implied by demands for increased responsibility and freedom to practice as a professional.

Clearly public health nurses, as a professional group, see collective bargaining as useful to them individually and collectively. And other studies suggest that the same is true of hospital nurses.[14] The more the bargaining unit is seen to represent their professional interests, the more likely they will become members and take militant action. The disagreement among nurses is not whether they should organize, but what type of organization (professional association or union) should represent them. It is also clear that, because the more militant nurses are young and well educated, this trend will continue and in all likelihood be strengthened.[15]

The growth of organizing in the public sector has been phenomenal. Most enabling legislation has occurred within the last ten years with about ten states now having such legislation. In New York, for example, state and local governments have had enabling legislation only since 1967, yet about 90 percent of eligible public employees have organized. Across the country 65 percent of all municipal employees are represented by employee organizations, and more than one-third of all public employers are represented in exclusive bargaining units. Contrast this with 28 percent of all private employees in nonagricultural establishments who have organized and opted for collective bargaining.[16]

While there is still time, managers of health care agencies need to consider carefully whether the industrial labor relations model with its emphasis on economic issues is the right approach for the health care industry. Furthermore, they need to examine seriously the contribution of their own behavior to work stoppages, and whether, by focusing on the economic issues, they screen out fundamental issues and thereby increase the probability and duration of a strike.

NOTES

1. R. E. Miles, *Theories of Management: Implications for Organizational Behavior and Development* (New York: McGraw-Hill Book Co., 1975), p. 35.

2. Ibid., p. 34.

3. R. E. Miles, L. W. Porter, and J. A. Craft, "Leadership Attitudes Among Public Health Officials," *American Journal of Public Health* 56, no. 12 (December 1966): 1990–2005.

4. C. L. Hobart, "Collective Bargaining with Professionals: Conflict, Containment or Accommodation?" *Health Care Management Review* 1, no. 2 (Spring 1976): 7–16.

5. A. C. Twaddle and R. M. Hessler, *A Sociology of Health* (St. Louis: C. V. Mosby Co., 1977), p. 189.

6. J. R. Bloom, C. A. O'Reilly, and G. N. Parlette, "Changing Images of Professionalism: The Case of Public Health Nurses," *American Journal of Public Health* 69, no. 1 (January 1979): 43–46.

7. *Facts About Nursing 1974–75* (Kansas City, Mo.: American Nursing Association, 1976).

8. A. H. Maslow, "A Theory of Human Motivation," *Psychological Review* 50 (July 1943): 370–396.

9. Bloom, O'Reilly, and Parlette, "Changing Images of Professionalism," p. 45.

10. J. A. Alutto and J. A. Belasco, "Determinants of Attitudinal Militancy Among Nurses and Teachers," *Industrial and Labor Relations Review* 27, no. 2 (January 1974): 216–227.

11. C. A. O'Reilly, J. R. Bloom, and G. N. Parlette, "Professional Workers and Union Activity: The Impact of Individual and Contextual Factors on the Decision to Strike." Paper presented at annual meeting of the American Psychological Association, 1977.

12. Miles, Porter, and Craft, "Leadership Attitudes," pp. 1990–2005.

13. W. R. Scott et al., "Task Conceptions and Work Arrangements." Paper presented at annual meeting of the American Sociological Association, 1971.

14. Alutto and Belasco, "Determinants of Attitudinal Militancy," pp. 216–227.

15. *Facts About Nursing, 1974–75*.

16. J. F. Atwood, "Collective Bargaining's Challenge: Five Imperatives for Public Managers," *Public Personnel Management* (January-February 1976), pp. 24–31.

19. Collective Bargaining with Professionals: Conflict, Containment, or Accommodation?

CHRISTINE L. HOBART

Reprinted with permission from *Health Care Management Review,* Vol. 1, No. 2, Spring 1976, published by Aspen Systems Corporation, Germantown, Md. © 1976.

Collective bargaining in the health care industry has increased dramatically in the last few years. Present estimates are that 25 percent of the nation's hospitals have some sort of bargaining agreement with their employees. In the early 1960s only three percent of the hospitals were unionized. Now union activity has crossed all the occupational boundaries and levels in health care to encompass house officers, interns and residents, registered nurses, pharmacists, technologists, therapists, technicians, aides, orderlies, housekeeping and maintenance workers, engineers, laborers, and clericals.

The 1974 amendments to the Taft-Hartley law, the nation's labor relations arbiter, have intensified this activity. Large labor unions, sophisticated in organizing techniques and in the intricacies of the law have accelerated their efforts. Unions like the Service Employees International (SEIU), and the American Federation of State, County and Municipal Employees (AFSCME) have joined with the National Union of Hospital and Health Care Employees, formerly Local 1199 RWDSU, in the competition for the right to represent the 1.5 million employees in the 3,300 private hospitals that were brought under the jurisdiction of the law by these new amendments. These unions have indicated—and directly in the case of Local 1199—indicated that their common goal is one national union for all health care workers. The appeal of these unions has been mostly to the nonprofessional service workers, such as housekeepers, nursing aides, and orderlies.

EQUAL FEARS

These organizing drives have aroused the fears of management, and not without reason. Some union attempts at organization in New York City in the late fifties and early sixties, for example, were marked by strikes, slowdowns and other stratagems that resulted in reduced or withdrawn services, with serious impact on patient care. Managers of health care organizations do not want a recurrence of this situation. Beyond these difficulties lies the prospect, for the manager, of sharing the right-to-manage with "outsiders"—the bargaining representatives of his employees. The manager knows that these representatives are not held responsible in the end for the effectiveness and productivity of the institution, and he does not want to lose control.

There is another important group in health care whose fears have been similarly aroused by recent union activity—the professional employee. Unionization of professional and white collar employees generally has lagged behind that of the industrial worker in this country, but there have been some exceptions. As far back as 1946 the first attempts at organizing were made by the state affiliates of the American Nurses' Association (ANA). The registered nurses, the largest single occupational group in health care, originally endorsed collective bargaining as a means to improve their professional standing. Since that time the nurses have become the only serious contenders among

THE PARTICIPANTS: EMPLOYED PROFESSIONALS

Any single definition of a professional lends itself to a range of interpretations. This is particularly true in the health care field in which there are many new occupational groupings that are attempting to raise their status. The NLRA precisely defines professionals, supervisors, and management representatives for purposes of election unit determination as well as for exclusion from the Act's coverage. Professional employees are included and may elect separate units if they so desire. Supervisors and managers are excluded from the Act.

In the context of this article, the term *professionals* denotes those individuals with specialized training in a recognized discipline who make a significant number of independent decisions with respect to care of patients: registered nurses, residents and interns, skilled therapists, technologists and pharmacists.

Most of these professionals have their own associations whose purposes traditionally gravitate around issues of standards, certifications, continuing education, advancement of the discipline and job placement. With the increased involvement in health care by federal and state government, and the opportunities and challenges of enabling state and now national labor laws, government lobbying and collective bargaining for improvement of economic and working conditions have been added to the purposes of these associations.

The American Nurses' Association has been a forerunner in professional collective bargaining and a model for a type of professional unionism. It has an active membership of about thirty percent of 860,000 registered nurses in this country. The three major groups within the association are nurse-educators, nurse-managers and nurse-practitioners. About 80,000 nurses made up of practitioners and educators are under bargaining contracts, some of which date back to the late 1940's.

THE LAWS: NATIONAL AND STATE

The National Labor Relations Act (NLRA) was passed in 1935 and amended in 1947, 1959, and 1974. Since the 1947 amendments, the NLRA has been generally referred to as Taft-Hartley. It guarantees the right of employees to organize and to bargain collectively, through representatives of their own choosing, with their employers, or alternatively to refrain from all such activity. The Act limits activities of employers and unions so that employers may exercise their statutory rights. It seeks to serve the public interest by reducing interruptions in interstate commerce caused by industrial strife. The Federal Mediation and Conciliation Service (FMCS), an independent agency, was established by the 1947 amendments to assist in the process of free collective bargaining and to prevent or minimize strikes when they occur and the loss of work time.

The National Labor Relations Board (NLRB) has administered the Act from the beginning. Its two major functions are 1) to determine and implement, through secret ballot elections, the free democratic choice by employees as to whether they wish to be represented by a union and, if so, by which one, and 2) to prevent and remedy unlawful acts, designated as unfair labor practices, by either employers or unions.

The 1974 Amendments (Public Law 93-360) not only brought private health care institutions under Taft-Hartley provisions but also established certain special provisions in mediation and fact-finding. These were designed to ease the way for settling disputes and to avoid interruptions in the care of patients. For example, the new Section 8(g) of the Act prohibits a labor organization from striking or picketing a health care institution without giving a ten-day notice to the employer and to the FMCS. The FMCS also plays an active part in a special dispute-settling procedure set up by the amendments. As of January 1, 1976 FMCS had handled 2092 cases in the industry of which 1533 had been closed. Seventy work stoppages had taken place and 81 fact-finding boards were appointed under these special dispute-settling provisions.

In the 1930s many states enacted labor relations acts similar to the NLRA. Massachusetts was one of these and, in 1965, both registered and licensed practical nurses in private health care institutions were brought under the provisions of the state labor relations law with the important addition of compulsory arbitration to handle unresolved grievances between the parties in such facilities. A no-strike provision was also included. In 1966, nonprofessional employees in health care facilities were included under the act.

THE PROCESS: COLLECTIVE BARGAINING

National labor policy encourages and protects the process of collective bargaining in the United States. Section 8(d) of the NLRA defines the process as one requiring an employer and the representative of his employees to meet at reasonable times to confer in good faith about certain matters and to put into writing any agreement reached if requested by either party. The parties must confer in good faith with respect to wages, hours, and other terms of employment, the negotiation of an agreement, or any question arising under an agreement.

The written contract is the basic document outlining in detail the relationship between the parties and there can be no changes in the document except by mutual agreement. There are approximately 150,000 labor-management contracts in this country covering the organized 22 percent of the total labor force.

The important terms of the relationship cover such issues as salaries and benefits, hours of work and working conditions, job security, grievances and arbitration, management rights, and recognition—who is the employee representative and precisely what employees are covered by the terms of the agreement, participation in a professional association—usually known as union security, payroll deductions for membership fees, and sometimes maintenance of membership as terms of continued employment. Recently "agency fees" have appeared, service charges rather than membership fees for representation. In nurses' contracts the agency fee has to be voted in by the membership of the local unit.

There is some agreement that the labor-management relationship moves along a continuum which can be roughly described as beginning with a mutual attitude of complete opposition and moving toward an attitude of accommodation. The way stations between are neutrality, cooperation and consultation. Since labor relations are so decentralized in this country it is difficult to find common agreement on the identifying criteria for these way stations, or to predict the time span between stations; but there is general agreement that the conditions of accommodation are a worthwhile goal for both parties to the relationship.

THE SCOPE

Until such time as there is an attempt for a comprehensive and permanent collection of statistics, all national figures about collective bargaining in the health care industry are estimates; there has been no attempt to collect comprehensive statistics. Nevertheless, the following figures provide some idea of the segment of the health care industry that has been and might be affected by collective bargaining.

The health care industry employs over three million people, mostly in hospitals or hospital related institutions. For example, 57 percent of ANA members are hospital based. Prior to the enactment in 1974 of the Taft-Hartley amendments, nearly 20 percent of the hospitals (1,197) had some sort of collective bargaining covering about 300,000 workers. The amendments brought under its jurisdiction 1.5 million employees and 3,300 non-profit hospitals.

Most of the organized employees are nonprofessionals and are represented by trade unions, with the exception of the nurses. The largest unions are the Service Employees International Union (SEIU), American Federation of State, County and Municipal Employees (AFSCME), and the National Union of Hospital and Health Care Employees, formerly Local 1199.

---

health care professionals for the representation rights of workers *other* than R.N.s.

NURSES: INNOVATIVE BARGAINERS

It was not the numbers of organized nurses that convinced their competitors and interested their colleagues—by 1975 they had organized only about ten percent of the profession. It was their skill at adapting traditional bargaining techniques to new settings that made the nurses attractive as representatives to other groups. Other professionals have looked to this experience and the special nature of nurses' bargaining for guidance in their efforts which, to date, have been sparse.

Though the Nurses' Association has been considered seriously by unions, the nurses themselves fear the possible inroads of well financed and single-purpose unions, particularly among the general staff nurses—the "bedside" nurses who are just one of many levels and interests among the more than 860,000 ANA-member nurses. This diversity of membership sometimes blunts the Association's effectiveness as a professional union. At a minimum, the enabling structure of a typical state nurses' association (SNA) allows only a limited regional response to national organizing drives by other unions. Fears persist that the nurses and other professional workers may be taken over by unions whose only goals are economic improvement and security.

The mark of the nurse's relative standing on the scale of accepted professionalism depends on the ultimate authority the nurse holds over the treatment of a patient or a client. So, while management on the one hand fears the effect of unionism on the corporate right to *manage*, professionals on the other hand fear the effects of a hospital-wide union on their right to *manage patient care*. This fear increases as one ascends the hierarchy in both corporate management and in the occupation.

A LOOK AT "CENTRAL HOSPITAL"

Since the late 1960s most concern over the effects of collective bargaining in health care has centered on the initial organizing phase and the dramatic and episodic effects on the employee adversaries and the patient. Far less attention has been paid to the effects of this process on management functions over a period of time, and its effects on the interplay between the professional prerogatives, the manager's delegated authority, and the potentially eroding effects on both by a collective bargaining agreement. Until there are sufficient case histories for the study of bargaining relationships between employed physicians and hospital management, where these issues can be sharply drawn, the implications taken from a study of a ten-year bargaining relationship between employed nurses and hospital management are a good beginning.

A typical non-profit community general hospital— let's call it "Central Hospital"—provides an example of a ten-year bargaining experience between the hospital and a nurses' professional association, where the manager faces the uncertainties of a bargaining future with professional associations and/or unions. Nurses' bargaining at Central Hospital provides a picture far removed from the dramatic headlines of the 1974 California Bay Area nurses' strike, or for that matter the 1975 strike of interns and residents in New York and Chicago. The participants' initial fears have changed, some have been found unwarranted—and there have been some unexpected benefits.

TEN YEARS, TEN CONTRACTS

The circumstances surrounding the Central Hospital situation will sound familiar to anyone who saw the rising demand for, and spiraling costs of, health care in the late 1960s. The initiation of collective bargaining in this labor-intensive industry was bound to increase management's concern.

Central Hospital, founded in the late 19th century as a result of the voluntary efforts of concerned citizens, is a general hospital of 300 beds serving a community of 90,000 people near Boston, a national center for medical care. The community it serves has an industrial base, and the hospital is the second largest employer. Like many nonprofit institutions, in recent years Central's reliance on voluntary support has declined and its reliance on federal funding has increased.

The organization of the hospital is traditional: the administrator and his staff report to a volunteer board of directors and its president. The administrator's primary responsibility has been for financial and managerial matters and for the coordination of direct patient care with the medical and nursing services. The nursing service constitutes about 60 percent of the total hospital payroll and reports to the administrator through its director.

THE POST-WORLD WAR II ENVIRONMENT

Following World War II, changes in health insurance coverage played a major role in the development of hospitals across the country. State and federal funds replaced hospital resources in paying for services for the poor and the elderly. Medicare and Medicaid came into being and, with the vast increase in the use of medical services, came a critical shortage of health personnel. This shortage was felt most acutely in nursing care.

Partly as a result of these shifts in financing, the 1950s and 1960s saw a marked increase in the interest and activity of nurses, through their national and regional associations, and other occupational groups, in their right to organize to protect their interests and insure their economic security. In addition, registered and licensed practical nurses had come under the state labor law in 1965 for purposes of collective bargaining. The key amendment that aided the law's passage was the substitution of the right to strike for compulsory arbitration of unresolved grievances.

These developments, together with a lack of local nursing leadership, the inability of the individual nurse to have an impact on professional nursing matters, and unmet wage and benefits demands, provided sufficient basis for a hospital nursing staff of Central's size to become involved in protective organizing activities.

Central Hospital's nurses overwhelmingly elected the state nurses' association as their bargaining representative, initiating bargaining that led to the first written contract in the state between a health facility and a union. Between 1965 and 1975 there have been ten contracts, the first and the sixth of which were resolved by arbitration. The progression of these contracts delineates the bargaining relationship between the parties, and in the aggregate these ten contracts reflect the changes in that relationship over a decade.

MANAGEMENT FEARS

Since the focus here is on the management's response to the presence of professional associations as adversaries, let's first examine the fears of Central's managers in 1965.

1. **Costs:** An organized hospital has higher labor costs and in general is more expensive to operate than a non-union hospital.
2. **Management effectiveness:** A union contract limits managers' rights to manage, decreases flexibility and inhibits innovativeness. A contract increases a manager's workload, while tending to decrease productivity because of its protection of senior, marginal workers.
3. **Reordering of professional priorities:** Membership in a union decreases a professional's concern with professional standards as it increases concerns about economic improvements and security provisions.
4. **One union leads to another:** One professional union will open the hospital to other professional unions as well as non-professional unions. This increases fragmentation of patient care and brings on jurisdictional disputes.

If all of these fears were realized, patient care would be negatively affected.

In 1965, Central's management also feared the unknown. There were no models to follow in health care; there were no trained and experienced guides. Further, Central's managers accepted the conventional wisdom of American management: once you let a union get in, you can't get rid of it. Consequently,

strategy at Central was to prevent the union from forming if at all possible.

This suspicious atmosphere and negative attitude prevailed at Central Hospital when I began my study which formed the basis for my dissertation on the influences affecting collective bargaining between the Massachusetts Nurses' Association (MNA) and a group of hospitals.

Some sense of the charged atmosphere and the fears of both sides can be caught by the following excerpts from the campaign literature:

Central said: "Although we are not fully aware of the reasons for the institution of these actions, it is our sincere belief that collective bargaining is unnecessary and could be detrimental to both employees and patients alike. [Central] Hospital has a growing personnel program which provides equitable compensation, substantial fringe benefits, good working conditions and other sound practices for all its employees . . . . improvements in recent years were arrived at by mutual participation of all nursing groups, accomplished without third party interference and at no cost to you (i.e., union initiation fee, dues, assessments)."

MNA said: "The Economic Security Program was developed to assure professional nurses a voice in the determination of their conditions of employment. The reason that hospital management is opposed to this program is their objection to giving nurses an effective voice in discussing employment conditions. We are all aware that a nurse who is underpaid and overworked cannot adequately fulfill her professional responsibilities. The Economic Security Program is directed at securing for registered nurses job security and a level of salaries and benefits commensurate with their professional status."

In light of both the fears and aspirations of the parties at the beginning of the decade, what does a study of those contracts and the nature of the relationship they reflect show after ten years?

COSTS

Nurses' salaries did increase dramatically—from $90 a week in 1966 to $214 in 1975. Fringe benefits were also increased. The first three contracts resulted in salary increases of over 40 percent; the later contracts levelled off at about seven percent. It is still difficult to determine with any degree of accuracy to what extent the level of these increases is attributable to pattern setting by the large inner-city hospitals of Central's contiguous metropolitan area. However, Central does maintain a higher salary scale than the other hospitals in its immediate local area; they followed the wage increase pattern set by Central without equalling Central's absolute wage rates. Both the local and large inner-city hospitals have remained unorganized.

Due to an initial shortage of nursing personnel, high rates of staff turnover, and an increase in demand for beds, part-time nursing coverage increased. The ratio of part-to full-time nurses reached nearly 50 percent by 1969. However, the contracts reflected a disproportionate extension of full-time employee benefits, and the part-time nurses banded together to present their demands in negotiations. By 1975, there was no longer a shortage of nurses, demand for beds had decreased, the hospital's bed capacity had remained constant, nursing staff turnover had decreased markedly, but the ratio of part- to full-time nurses remained close to 50 percent and the disproportion in benefits had not been corrected.

There may have been an unexpected benefit from the presence of the nurses' union—the impact of publicity about the anticipated wage increase resulted in considerable public acceptance of an increase in room rates that followed the wage settlement.

MANAGEMENT EFFECTIVENESS

In general, the presence of the nurses' union at Central had a minimal direct impact on the hospital's administration. The key clauses in the Central contract affecting management's right to manage are as follows:

Management Rights—The management of the Hospital and the direction of the working force including the right to select and hire employees, the right to make temporary transfers, the right to suspend, discipline or discharge employees for just cause, the right to lay off employees for lack of work or other legitimate reasons and the right to promulgate reasonable rules and regulations are vested exclusively in the Hospital provided that such rights shall not be exercised so as to violate any provisions of this Agreement.

Grievance and Arbitration—The Hospital and the Association recognize that their principal obligation is that of patient care and that only by estab-

lished harmonious relationships can the best interest of the Hospital, the nurse, employees and the community at large be best served. It is the intent and purpose of this Agreement to promote orderly collective bargaining and the resolving of all differences, grievances, and disputes through the arbitration set forth.

Nurses' Committee—There shall be a Nurses' Committee not to exceed nine (9) members established by the Association which will meet periodically with the representatives of the Hospital to discuss matters of mutual interest.

These clauses have remained unchanged over ten years. The nurses have not tested management's ultimate authority or right to operate the hospital by pressing professional issues or definitions of patient care, either in negotiations or through the grievance procedure. The administration of the contract has been relatively free of grievances, and those that occurred were of a minor nature. Maintenance of the contract and the legal requirements resulting from the existence of a collective bargaining agreement increased administrative time and cost somewhat. As noted, two contracts went to arbitration, but never as tests of management's right to manage. However, the presence of the contract may have resulted in lost opportunities for management to make organizational and structural changes.

The bargaining situation was initially controlled by nursing supervisors and this may have added to the supervisors' power at a critical time when efforts should have been made by management to concentrate the power in a strong executive at the head of the nursing service. However, it may have been more advantageous to the administration to continue the status quo in nursing service by stabilizing the supervisors' alliance, at least in part through the bargaining agreement, than to attempt to transfer the power to an unknown director of nursing service.

There was no serious effort made by management to use the contract, specifically the consultative and collaborative possibilities present in the Nurses' Committee clause, as a positive force in preparing for and instituting procedures aimed at securing greater efficiencies or alterations in working conditions. Although the contract might have introduced new rules and encouraged inflexibility that could have deterred management from introducing new systems or eliminating inefficient practices, observations of Central's present physical and financial condition would argue to the contrary.

PROFESSIONAL PRIORITIES

Aside from the initial spur to organize and the euphoria resulting from the first contact, interest in the contract by the Association's members has been negligible. The bargaining atmosphere has been peaceful and conflict-free. Bargaining strategy has been in the hands of SNA representatives and only a few of the unit's membership. The pattern of negotiations was set in the first three contracts and has remained constant over the years: amicable tone, expeditious proceedings controlled by legal representatives for each party, and emphasis on issues that dealt almost exclusively with economic and security improvements. The nurses' professional concern for improving standards of patient care were not issues brought to the bargaining table, except as demands for improvements in working conditions can be considered euphemisms for these concerns.

Without exception there was a lack of active membership participation in the unit, except at the supervisory or faculty nursing ranks. The typical staff nurse assumed that the nurses' association was run for and by the educators of the nursing schools and the director of the hospital's nursing services, namely the supervisors of the staff nurses. Representation by the State Nurses' Association for purposes of collective bargaining was free for nonmembers of the association in the absence of a contract provision requiring mandatory membership or an agency fee for such services. Had management chosen to vest power in a single, strong executive at the head of the nursing service, she could have controlled the bargaining process with a strong hand, given the lack of interest by the membership-at-large. On the other hand, staff nurses should have realized that administration of the local bargaining unit theoretically would provide excellent training for future positions of influence and leadership. However, since neither training in leadership skills nor education for bargaining had been offered, these opportunities were overlooked by the staff nurses.

IMPLICATIONS OF TAFT-HARTLEY AMENDMENTS FOR PROFESSIONAL PRIORITIES

The posture of passivity and accommodation that has existed during the past ten years, particularly on the part of the general staff nurse, may soon give way to activism. The amendments to the Taft-Hartley law and a growing number of agency shop security provi-

sions in hospital contracts may produce some dramatic changes. In the past, membership in Central's local units has paralleled virtually the full range of the professional association's membership from supervisor to staff nurse, from nurse anesthetist to faculty instructor. Under the amendments to the Taft-Hartley law, this no longer will be possible.

In 1965 the initiators of bargaining at Central were the supervisors. Subsequently, they advanced in nursing management or entered specialty areas and were, therefore, removed from the bargaining unit even under the wider interpretation of the former state labor law. However, prior to the mid-1974 Taft-Hartley amendments, the separation of these nurses from the head and staff nurses could be a moot point worked out at each hospital according to local norms or experiences. Furthermore, all registered nurses could be represented by one professional association for a multitude of necessary functions such as certification, continuing education, placement, standardization, security and protection.

Now, under the Taft-Hartley amendments, supervisors are specifically excluded from the bargaining unit, and the issue of the nurses' association, as a management representative, dominating the nurses' unions is being tested before the NLRB repeatedly in the light of various state nurses' association structures.

One of the effects of the amendments has been to isolate local bargaining units to the extent that they are considering coalition with selected trade unions for protection from other raiding unions. This is the incongruous coming-to-fruition of the fear expressed earlier by the hospital. Furthermore, the increasing frequency of contracts specifying agency shops has compounded the incongruity of the situation. As the staff nurse becomes more isolated—by legislation rather than by choice—her representatives in bargaining become more influential in the board rooms of the nurses' associations as the service fees come rolling into their treasuries.

For example, Central Hospital's unit of nurses voted in the agency fee effective for all nurses hired after September 1974. In addition, five of the 30 private hospitals under contract in the state have an agency shop at present. With more hospital bargaining units voting for this form of union security, the additional income will increase the importance of the Economic and General Welfare Program (EGW), the nurses' euphemism for collective bargaining, as opposed to the other purposes of the professional association: nursing education and administration. Some of the real impact on Central's nurses will become evident as more association resources are put into the service and training of local nurses to handle more of their own negotiations and to formulate their own demands.

With training and opportunity there may well be a rejuvenation of interest by a larger proportion of nurses from the lower end of the nursing hierarchy. Consequently, the demands they formulate may be a continuation of the economic and security concerns of the earlier units, rather than demands affecting professional standards of care, such as those being formulated by other nursing groups in association and being tested in regulatory or legislative arenas.

INCREASED UNIONIZATION

Management's fear that organization by the SNA would spread to other Central employees was only partially justified. The Licensed Practical Nurses (L.P.N.s) did organize and are represented by their own association. For many years, the L.P.N.s retained the same legal firm as Central's R.N.s. Their contract was patterned after the nurses' negotiations; the formula was that the L.P.N.s should receive 80 percent of what the registered nurses received in every instance. If the nurses were eventually to be considered a benign presence at the bargaining table, the L.P.N.s were innocuous in the extreme.

There was little if any other union activity until the period surrounding the August, 1974, effective date of the Taft-Hartley law's coverage of private hospitals. Central withstood the organization drive of a non-professional union which sought to represent a combined ancillary unit of its employees. At present, the hospital has just completed a contract covering its maintenance employees with a trades council that the administration felt might be a lesser evil than a competing union.

In some respects, the management of Central was fortunate to be able to cut its collective-bargaining teeth on a professional association such as the nurses. With the experience gained over ten years and ten contracts, management learned to live with collective bargaining and even to gain some operational advantage.

BARGAINING THE '72 CONTRACT

The bargaining of the 1971–1972 contract is a case in point. This contract was arbitrated, repeating the experience of the first contract in 1966. However, in 1966 there was virtually no bargaining; all key items were unresolved and sent to arbitration. The initial advantage in arbitration favored the nurses. In contrast, in 1971 there was one key issue: whether the agency shop

was a bargainable issue. In addition, economic issues and union security were also submitted to arbitration, but these money items initially were bargained down in hopes of settlement on the agency shop. For the first time, management was testing the advantage of compulsory arbitration from *its* position. Whereas initially compulsory arbitration, the unique feature of the state labor law, was used indiscriminately, with experience it was used strategically and responsibly within the context of the bargaining relationship.

AT THE END OF A DECADE

Management has made a serious effort to learn from each contract negotiation. It appears to have applied that learning and sophistication in successful strategy formulation when faced with the possibility of organization from other unions, particularly those representing nonprofessional employees. Central's management has accommodated itself to what is clearly a long-term presence of the professional union.

During ten years the relationship between the management of Central Hospital and the Massachusetts Nurses' Association as representatives of the hospital's nurses has moved from complete opposition in 1965 to neutrality in 1975. The logical end of the spectrum will be a condition called accommodation through consultation. The way-stations between opposition and accommodation exist theoretically along a route travelled by all parties in negotiations. The length of stay at any one stop is determined by many factors—local conditions being an important one. Central moved with relative speed from complete opposition to neutrality; the weak form of unionism that the nurses represented was an important factor, a weakness caused primarily by the divided nature of the profession between nurse-managers, nurse-educators and nurse-practitioners.

1976: CONDITION OF NEUTRALITY

The condition of neutrality at Central is marked by relative ease between the parties and simplicity of administration, yet there is still a sense of detachment and aloofness between the parties. Possibly the lack of grievances and the protocols observed during the annual formal negotiations may account for this. The initial fears and mutual resentments have been replaced by the acceptance of a necessary process that is now imbedded in administrative routine. Strategy formulation and decisions are still made at high levels in both organizations; the rank and file staff nurse is not yet an active participant in, nor is she being trained to take over, the total bargaining. The personnel function of the hospital handles the greater portion of the administration of the contract and attends to the auditing and stabilizing responsibilities attendant upon its effective implementation.

The local hospital administrator has been able to benefit more from this process than his bargaining counterparts, the local nurses. He has become more able to control the organizational response to this type of bargaining than the nurses. They cannot change, with similar ease, the direction of their professional association.

IMPLICATIONS FOR HEALTH CARE MANAGERS

By placing more of the health care industry under a national labor law, the Taft-Hartley amendments have accelerated the need for studies of the effects of collective bargaining on managements, on employed professionals, and on patient care. It is heartening to know that such groups as the Institute of Medicine of the National Academy of Science and the American Public Health Association are proposing such studies.

Central Hospital has provided a site for viewing one hospital management's response to the presence of adversaries in the form of a professional association. The natural opposition of interests between these groups is highlighted if one remembers that managers of health care facilities are under pressure to decrease costs while increasing the quality and quantity of service, and simultaneously professional associations are under pressure from their membership—the employees of these same facilities—to protect the standards of the profession at the workplace.

The key to the direction that professional unionism will take lies within management's response to its challenge or presence. Management at Central found that, of all the fears expressed at the advent of professional unionism, only the one dealing with professional priorities is still unresolved ten years later. Wage and salary rates may be out of the hands of the local manager; management rights have not been eroded and a contract can become an avenue for consultation leading to increased organizational effectiveness; and managers experienced in bargaining increase their abilities in dealing with other forms of unionization.

PROFESSIONAL PRIORITIES

Understanding the unresolved professional priorities is not a simple task, but I believe that effort expended here by the manager will be rewarded. The nursing profession remains fragmented and highly differentiated, and the Taft-Hartley amendments will further segment it. Who speaks for the nurses at the workplace—the director of nursing services, a management representative, or the unit steward under the contract? These questions have not yet been answered, but individual managers can respond by recognizing the differentiation, understanding the implications of the federal legislation, and instituting organizational mechanisms by which the professional's knowledge can be utilized in balance with the professional's acceptance that management has ultimate responsibility to run the institution. It is this partnership, a type of collegiality, that should bring maximum returns in improved patient care.

20. House Staff Unionization

CARL W. VOGT and JOSEPH T. SMALL, JR.

INTRODUCTION

More than 61,000 medical interns, residents, and fellows (house staff or house officers) are enrolled in graduate medical education programs in more than 1,700 hospitals throughout the United States. The Physicians National House Staff Association (PNHA), as well as various local house staff unions, have engaged in collective bargaining for some house officers, primarily in New York City,[1] Chicago, Ann Arbor, Mich., and Los Angeles. In addition, the PNHA and some local unions have sought to represent medical interns, residents, and fellows enrolled in certain other teaching hospitals throughout the country.

This article discusses the legal framework for house staff organizational efforts, the current status of such efforts, and the potential impact of unionization upon the structure of graduate medical education.

HOUSE STAFF ORGANIZATIONAL EFFORTS

To understand the current status of house staff organizational efforts, it is important to draw distinctions between the various legal jurisdictions involved.

Organizational Efforts under Taft-Hartley

In 1974 the National Labor Relations Act (Taft-Hartley Act), which governs labor relations for private

sector employers, was amended to include private, not-for-profit health care institutions.[2] Shortly after the amendments became effective, numerous petitions for elections were filed by unions seeking to represent house staff enrolled in graduate medical education programs affiliated with private hospitals. After close factual analysis, the National Labor Relations Board (NLRB) concluded that house staff members are primarily students and, as such, are not entitled to unionize as employees under the act.[3] The NLRB's decisions were based upon legal precedent pertaining to graduate and undergraduate students in all educational disciplines.[4]

In particular, the NLRB determined that medical interns, residents, and fellows were engaged in programs of graduate professional education and that their activities were directly related to, and indeed constituted an integral part of, those educational programs. The board also recognized the fundamental distinction between the activities of house officers and those of hospital employees:

> [T]he mutual interests of the students and the educational institution in which the service is being rendered are predominantly academic rather than economic in nature. Such interests are completely foreign to the normal employment relationship and, in our judgment, are not readily adaptable to the collective bargaining process.[5]

The U.S. Court of Appeals for the District of Columbia Circuit in 1980 concluded that the NLRB's house staff decisions are not reviewable by the courts.[6]

Since the NLRB dismissed the initial election petitions, house staff union organizational efforts in private health care institutions have virtually ceased. Some private hospitals in New York have continued to bargain voluntarily over some issues with their traditional house staff unions, while others have withdrawn completely from any relationship.

Organizational Efforts under State Law

The PNHA has sought to bypass the NLRB's decisions both judicially and legislatively. First, it has attempted to organize medical interns, residents, and fellows in private hospitals under state law. In 1977, however, the U.S. Court of Appeals for the Second Circuit determined that the Taft-Hartley Act preempts state authority to regulate labor relations in private hospitals. *NLRB* v. *Committee of Interns & Residents.*[7] Second, the PNHA has lobbied Congress to amend the Taft-Hartley Act to specifically include medical interns, residents, and fellows within the statutory definition of "professional employee." On November 28, 1979, however, the House of Representatives, 227 to 167, rejected a bill (H.R. 2222) that would have accomplished this. In so doing, the House refused to reverse legislatively the NLRB's decisions holding that house staff are primarily students and not employees under Taft-Hartley.

Organizational Efforts in the Public Sector

House staff unions have attempted to organize medical interns, residents, and fellows at public hospitals owned and operated by state, county, or municipal governments. Where such state laws or local ordinances exist, the unions have invoked the authority of labor relations laws covering state and municipal employees. Some of these laws include house staff in their definitions of "employees." For example, some New York City hospitals have been negotiating with house staff unions under New York state law since the early 1970s. In addition, some house staff enrolled in programs affiliated with the University of Michigan have unionized under the jurisdiction of that state's labor relations statute for public employees.

In California, the PNHA filed an unfair labor practice charge under state law governing labor relations for University of California employees (the Berman Act), charging that the regents had failed to withhold union dues for house staff members at the university's five medical centers. In a proposed decision, issued on April 9, 1980, a hearing officer for California's Public Employment Relations Board dismissed the charge and ruled (as had the NLRB) that medical interns, residents, and fellows are students, not employees, and therefore are not susceptible to the deduction of union dues from their stipends. The proposed decision was appealed to the state board. In Los Angeles, meanwhile, house staff at the county hospital have been unionized for some time under local labor relations ordinances.

Organizational Efforts in the Federal Sector

House staff unions have attempted to represent medical interns, residents, and fellows enrolled in graduate programs in federally owned and operated hospitals. The PNHA, for example, has filed petitions with the Federal Labor Relations Authority (the authority) under the Civil Service Reform Act of 1978 to represent house staff at the Veterans Administration Medical Centers in Long Beach and Martinez, Calif., and Brooklyn, N.Y. Representation hearings have been held in the Long Beach and Brooklyn cases. The Long Beach and Brooklyn cases are still pending with the Federal Labor Relations Authority. A representation hearing has not yet been scheduled in the Martinez case because that case is subject to an agreed upon stay until the Federal Labor Relations Authority rules upon the Long Beach and Brooklyn cases.

In each of these cases, the issue is whether house staff are students or employees within the meaning of the law governing federal workers. Until final decisions are reached, the future of house staff unionization in the federal sector will remain uncertain.

THRESHOLD BARGAINING ISSUES

Jurisdictional Problems

Although private and public sector labor relations laws differ in some respects, the unionization of house staff under virtually any statute could raise certain threshold jurisdictional issues. For instance, it often is difficult, if not impossible, to determine when an individual intern, resident, or fellow is "employed" by a particular hospital within the meaning of various collective bargaining statutes. Typically, graduate medical education programs are conducted in affiliation with independent health care institutions, including medical schools and hospitals. Medical interns, residents, and fellows often rotate through many, if not all, such affiliated institutions during their educational programs. Moreover, individual house officers, enrolled in the same programs, may receive stipends from different institutions. In this context, it is difficult, if not impossible, to determine when and for how long a particular hospital may "employ" these individuals for purposes of collective bargaining.

As another example, affiliated hospitals and medical schools often are owned or administered by federal or local governments or by private organizations. Because most house officers rotate through affiliated institutions, jurisdictional disputes could arise among the federal, state, and local agencies attempting to regulate house staff-hospital labor relations under different laws. The PNHA contributed to the potential confusion by filing two election petitions, under different statutes, for the same house officers. The union filed two petitions under California state law to represent house officers enrolled in programs at the University of California's medical schools in Irvine and Davis. At the same time, it filed a petition with the Federal Labor Relations Authority to represent house officers at the Veterans Administration Medical Center in Long Beach, which is affiliated with the university's medical school in Irvine. House officers enrolled at Irvine rotate through the Long Beach Veterans Hospital and thus are potentially subject to conflicting federal and state jurisdictions.

Appropriate Unit Problems

As a final example of a threshold issue, hospitals could be presented with enormous problems regarding the determination of appropriate units for collective bargaining. Under most labor relations statutes, employees in an appropriate unit must show a "community of interest." Medical interns, residents, and fellows at many hospitals lack any such community of interest. Not only do house staff rotate for varying periods through different programs and affiliated hospitals and receive stipends from different sources, but within programs they rotate through various specialties. Typically, contacts between residents in different programs are minimal. Standards for supervision are different. Determinations of duty hours and program content are made by different program directors. In this context, a "community of interest" often is impossible to discern.

Bargaining under Taft-Hartley

A primary concern among medical educators is that collective bargaining may implicate medical education. For example, if house staff in private institutions were considered to be employees under the Taft-Hartley

Act, well-established legal precedent indicates that teaching hospitals would face the prospect of bargaining about matters involving substantive aspects of their graduate medical education programs. To the extent that laws governing federal, state, and local labor relations follow Taft-Hartley precedent, this prospect may be realized outside the private sector.

In this context, collective bargaining could present unique problems for hospitals. Under Taft-Hartley, for example, employers are required to meet with their employees' collective bargaining representatives at reasonable times and places and to bargain in good faith about wages, hours, and other terms and conditions of employment. These so-called mandatory bargaining subjects govern the fundamental relationship between employer and employees, and neither labor nor management can refuse to negotiate them. In addition, it is only over these subjects that labor and management can insist upon their respective positions to the point of impasse, which can result in a strike.

Under Taft-Hartley, house staff unions could insist upon bargaining about virtually all aspects of a teaching hospital's graduate medical education programs. It is well established, for example, that hiring is a mandatory subject of collective bargaining. Thus, the current practice of admitting graduate medical students into residency programs under the National Resident Matching Program[8] could be negotiable. Residents could insist, for instance, that a traditional union-type hiring hall system be established whereby a hospital would apply to a union to supply residents from the union's roster.

Clearly, hours of work under the act are a mandatory subject of collective bargaining. The flexibility of a clinical chairman or a program director to schedule graduate medical students so that the process of a particular disease might be followed, or to ensure adequate exposure to a variety of medically relevant circumstances, therefore could be bargainable.

The length of training programs and the duration of rotations also could be mandatory bargaining subjects. Although the Essentials* of an accredited residency prescribe the minimum criteria for accredited programs, including their minimum duration, program directors often adopt variations for particular programs or individuals. The full range of programmatic flexibility, including the number of clinical procedures to be performed, rotations, and even the Essentials themselves, could become part of the bargaining process.

---

*Essentials are published by the Liaison Committee on Graduate Medical Education and promulgate the standards for the board certification in residency programs.

It is well established that the termination of employees is a mandatory subject of bargaining. Thus, the manner in which interns, residents, and fellows are reappointed could be bargainable. Testing could become a mandatory bargaining subject. In fact, if medical interns, residents, and fellows were determined to be "employees" as a matter of law, the entire educational component of their "employment" could be construed to be a fringe benefit, no aspect of which would escape the requirements of mandatory bargaining.

Finally, an employer's agreement to submit grievances and contract disputes to binding arbitration is, under the act, the quid pro quo for a no-strike commitment by a union. Consequently, disputes over contractual terms such as terminations, rotations, work assignments, and hours could be subjected to grievance procedures and binding awards by outside arbitrators.

POTENTIAL IMPACT ON GRADUATE EDUCATION

From the foregoing it is clear why medical educators are concerned that unionization, particularly under the Taft Hartley Act or public employee laws that follow private sector precedents, could have a significant, wide-ranging, and irrevocable impact upon graduate medical education.

In addition to involving aspects of education in collective bargaining, unionization also could change the traditional structure of graduate medical education. First, the treatment of medical interns, residents, and fellows as employees would adversely affect the essential collegial relationship between house staff and hospital teaching faculties. As a matter of law, this would change from that of student-teacher to an adversarial, employee-employer relationship. In considering this possibility, the NLRB has observed:

The inevitable change in emphasis from quality education to economic concerns which would accompany injection of collective bargaining into the student-teacher relationship would, in our judgment, prove detrimental to both labor and educational policies.[9]

Most medical educators believe that medical interns, residents, and fellows lack the experience and judgment necessary to review meaningfully and to bargain collectively about the training decisions of a hospital's teaching staff. The collective bargaining process could limit the ability of the teaching staff to exercise its independent educational judgment and could cause a shift in emphasis from competent health care education to a predominant concern with the negotiated conditions of house staff relationships with hospitals and their faculties.

For example, it is undisputed that some of these individuals spend long hours in hospitals during certain parts of their graduate medical education. They must be exposed to the wide range of medical experience, including the treatment of numerous diseases, many of which require continuous observation to be understood. Unfortunately, medical emergencies do not always occur conveniently between the hours of 9 a.m. and 5 p.m., Monday through Friday. Thus, the length of a given work week for a medical intern, resident, or fellow is related directly to that student's educational program. Nevertheless, as noted, hospitals could be required to negotiate with house staff unions over the hours that these individuals were required to spend in the facility as a part of their educational programs.

Unionization could inhibit the ability of a hospital's faculty to accommodate the individual educational needs of these students. The teaching staff, as a result of unionization, would be required to deal with them on a collective basis. Most medical educators believe, however, that effective graduate medical education requires individual, rather than collective, treatment of students. Each of these persons possesses different abilities and educational backgrounds. A hospital's teaching staff is responsible for fashioning a training program to meet the needs of each student. Only through individualized treatment can each graduate medical student acquire the knowledge and skills necessary for the independent practice of medicine.

On the other hand, collective bargaining, as its name implies, is predicated upon "collective" treatment of all who are represented, and thus in many respects is the very antithesis of personal individualized education. Such collective treatment of house officers as "employees" could impede individualized medical training at teaching hospitals.

Finally, unionization could have a direct impact upon the accreditation of graduate medical programs. As a result of the collective bargaining process, medical interns, residents, and fellows could demand conditions in conflict with the minimum required educational standards. In such instances, hospitals would face an impossible choice. They would be forced to bargain over contract terms incompatible with the minimum standards or face the prospect of strikes and other job actions, as well as unfair labor practice charges.

CONCLUSION

The potential ramifications of house staff unionization are manifest. The manner in which the issues raised by unionization are addressed by teaching hospitals could have a direct and long-lasting impact upon graduate medical education.

NOTES

1. On March 17, 1975, the Committee of Interns and Residents (CIR), a union representing the house staff at a number of hospitals in New York City, called a strike. Three thousand medical interns, residents, and fellows at 11 voluntary hospitals participated. The strike, which arose in connection with collective bargaining between the League of Voluntary Hospitals and Homes of New York and the CIR for renewal of a collective bargaining agreement, lasted four days and received wide publicity as the first multihospital "doctors' strike" in the country.
2. Such institutions previously had been excluded from the coverage of this federal law.
3. *See St. Clare's Hosp. and Health Center,* 229 NLRB 1000 (1977); *Wayne State Univ.,* 226 NLRB 1062 (1976); *Kansas City Gen. Hosp.,* 225 NLRB 106 (1976); *St. Christopher's Hosp. for Children,* 223 NLRB 1032 (1976); *Univ. of Chicago Hosps. and Clinics,* 223 NLRB 1002 (1976); *Cedars-Sinai Medical Center,* 223 NLRB 251 (1976).
4. *See, e.g., The Leland Stanford Junior Univ.,* 214 NLRB 621 (1974); *Adelphi Univ.,* 195 NLRB 639 (1972).
5. *St. Clare's Hosp., supra,* at 1002.
6. *Physicians Nat'l House Staff Ass'n v. Fanning,* No. 78-1209 (July 11, 1980).
7. *NLRB v. Comm. of Interns & Residents,* 566 F.2d 810 (2d Cir. 1977), *cert denied,* 435 U.S. 904 (1978).
8. The National Resident Matching Program is a computerized matching plan used by virtually all accredited graduate medical education programs in teaching hospitals to select residents for their first graduate year. Graduating medical students register with the plan by submitting a signed agreement that confirms their understanding that they and the education programs will be bound by the matching results. Hospitals and program directors sign a similar agreement. Students are supplied with a directory of participating hospitals describing each one's accredited graduate medical education program. They then apply to the programs and the hospitals of their choice and list them with the matching program in their orders of preference. Each hospital submits a similar list. Each student and hospital then are matched, according to their respective preferences. Upon accepting a position, students receive from the hospital with which they are matched a letter of appointment for one academic year. In each successive year, students' reappointments are based upon evaluations of their individual performances.
9. *St. Clare's Hosp., supra,* at 1002.

21. The Board of Inquiry: A New Dimension in Private Sector Health Care Collective Bargaining

NANCY CONNOLLY FIBISH

INTRODUCTION

When Congress amended the National Labor Relations Act (NLRA) in 1974 to cover all employees in the private sector's health care industry, regardless of whether they are employed by profit- or not-for-profit institutions, it also enacted special provisions dealing with health care industry labor disputes. These special provisions provided for earlier notification periods for existing contracts that were required for other industries in the private sector, a special notification requirement for first contracts, mandatory mediation by the Federal Mediation and Conciliation Service (FMCS), a ten-day strike notice, and a special board of inquiry (BOI) procedure to be used by the director of the FMCS in resolving health care industry labor disputes.

Ever since their enactment, the BOI procedures—particularly the rigid time constraints they establish for the appointment of BOIs—have provoked mixed reactions among the industry's labor relations practitioners, including neutrals. Despite doubts about the usefulness of the BOI as a dispute resolution tool, the process has become an integral part of the way in which collective bargaining impasses are mediated. This article describes how this has come about.

THE HEALTH CARE INDUSTRY

Health care is a sizable industry, important to the nation's economy, and a major employer. Nationwide, expenditures for medical care account for approximately 10 percent of the gross national product (GNP) and are projected to reach between 11 to 12 percent by the end of this decade. Much of the expected growth will take place in the Sunbelt states, mainly because of major population shifts during the seventies from northern to southern states. These shifts were followed by a steady increase in the number of health care institutions in the South: major medical centers, general hospitals, nursing homes, and clinics. Because of the growing proportion of the elderly in the nation's population and in part because of Medicare, nursing homes and other health care facilities aimed at meeting the medical needs of this group are growing in all areas of the country.

The private sector of the health care industry employs close to 5,000,000 persons, excluding those engaged in producing pharmaceuticals and equipment. Although these employees are not highly unionized, there are pockets of well-organized areas in the Northeast, on the West Coast, and in some parts of the Midwest. Most new organizing efforts appear to be taking place in the South and in some portions of the Midwest.

Labor contracts in this industry tend to be of shorter duration (normally one to two years) than those in other industries in the private sector, so that renegotiations are more frequent. Not surprisingly, given the 1974 NLRA amendments, population shifts, and industry growth, FMCS caseload data reveal that approximately 30 percent of all negotiations in the industry involve first-contract situations—substantially higher than in other industries in the private sector. Since agreement is more difficult to reach in first-contract negotiations than in long-established collective bargaining relationships, mediators find it necessary to hold more meetings in health care negotiations than in other private sector disputes.

Although the major issues in health care bargaining are the same (wages and fringes) as those in other industries, the issues of patient care and continuing professional training are of some importance in negotiations involving units of nurses and other professional employees. The number of employees assigned to shifts (tours of duty) is a prevalent issue for all types of bargaining units in the industry. As is usual in most first-contract talks, union security, dues checkoff, and grievance and arbitration procedures play prominent roles.

Changes in health care funding in recent years have put increasing control over expenses, including labor costs, into the hands of third party payers and cost review commissions. The development of cost review agencies, whose purpose is to keep a watchful eye on expenditures, has been most apparent on the Northeast and West Coasts. Significant increases in public and private reimbursement funds have given third party payers control not only over reimbursement rates but over the method and timing of these payments to health care institutions. This control often gives them an offstage presence at the bargaining table, even though they are not a party to the negotiations. As has been pointed out, it may be necessary for the neutral to arrange to get the third party payers' representatives on stage and into discussions to clarify reimbursement formulas.

SPECIAL NOTICE AND TIME PERIODS

The health care amendments require either party to a collective bargaining contract desiring to terminate or modify that agreement to notify the other party at least 90 days and the FMCS at least 60 days before its expiration—as contrasted with the 60-day and 30-day notice requirements for the rest of the private sector. After receipt of this 60-day notice from either party, FMCS has 30 days to decide whether to appoint a BOI. In a first-contract situation, the union must give at least 30 days' notice of a labor dispute to the FMCS (no notice is required in the rest of the private sector). After receiving such a notice, the FMCS has ten days to appoint a BOI.

Once named, the BOI has 15 days to investigate the issues and make a written report of its findings of fact and its recommendations for settling the dispute. These recommendations are not binding on the parties.[1] During the 15 days of the BOI's investigation and report procedure and for 15 days after it issues its report, both parties must maintain the status quo in their bargaining relationship. The latter 15 days are designated to be used for further negotiations and mediation, based on the BOI recommendations, before a strike or lockout can take place. In both initial and renewal or reopener situations, the union must give the health care institution and the FMCS ten days' notice of its intent to strike.

It is important to note that the FMCS is using its best mediation efforts to bring the parties to agreement during the very same time period within which it must decide to appoint a BOI. It is equally important to understand the internal process and flow of information that takes place within the FMCS once a health care assignment is made to a field mediator.

Once assigned to a health care dispute, the field mediator's first task is to obtain basic information in order to make a personal evaluation of the situation. The field mediator obtains information on the nature of the facility (e.g., general hospital, clinic, nursing home, etc.); number of beds and percentage occupied; size and composition of the bargaining unit; type of work performed by the bargaining unit; identity and bargaining unit size of other unions, if any; prior bargaining experience of the union and management; special or unique services and/or facilities provided by the establishment (e.g., intensive care unit, shock trauma or burn centers, dialysis equipment); other establishments in the locality, if any, and their number of beds and special services; and other information relevant to the probable impact a work stoppage would have on the delivery of health care in the locality.

The mediator also is asked to comment on the status of negotiations, meetings held or planned, degree of FMCS involvement, and whether the appointment of a BOI would help or hinder the parties in reaching agreement. After considering these factors, including any circumstances that may be unique to a particular dispute, the mediator then is asked to make a recommendation regarding the appointment of a BOI.

The mediator's initial report is reviewed by the regional director, who then makes a recommendation to the FMCS director and to the health care coordinator in the agency's national office as to whether or not to appoint a BOI. All health care disputes are screened by the regional offices and the national health care coordinator. When necessary, discussions involving the general counsel and the director of arbitration services are held before the director makes a final decision.

The FMCS has had to develop its policy and procedures for administering the BOI appointments in the half-dozen years since adoption of the amendments in response to both the time constraints of the act and the parties' needs. In both initial and renewal contracts, the parties often have done little or no bargaining up to the time the statute provides for the director's unilateral appointment of a BOI. If contract talks have not progressed to a certain stage—or if the parties have negotiated down to a manageable number of issues but are at a sensitive point in their negotiations—the appointment of a BOI could be minimally helpful or even harmful.

To get around this dilemma, the FMCS has developed the technique of using a joint stipulation agreement between the parties by which they authorize the FMCS director to appoint a factfinder (FF) at a later date—for example, at the end of the contract if no new agreement is reached, or when a union serves a ten-day strike notice. Normally, such an FF operates under the same time limits and procedures as a BOI, unless the parties and the FMCS agree to others.

The FMCS has been flexible in tailoring the terms of the stipulation agreement to the needs of the parties so long as the terms are consistent with the intent of the statute. It has been the agency's experience that the parties generally have adapted to the timing of the FF appointment and have been able to make greater use of that neutral's recommendations in resolving their dispute than when a statutory BOI is interjected into the dispute at the wrong time. There also has been an increased number of FF appointments and a diminishing number of BOIs in the last several years. These appointment statistics are analyzed in the next section.

There are additional reasons for the agency's appointment of a BOI or FF other than those already discussed. The FMCS may believe that, in certain bargaining situations, the parties are not at a point where factfinding can reasonably be expected to provide them with recommendations for a settlement within the allotted time period. However, the factfinding period may "buy" needed calendar time for continuing their negotiations with informal assistance from the factfinder. During this period, the FMCS mediator, without violating confidentiality and without entering into the formal factfinding procedure, can cooperate informally with the factfinder in sifting and sorting the issues and alerting the BOI/FF to any political nuances involved.

If the parties still are unable to resolve their differences at the end of this factfinding period, or if a substantial number of issues remain open, the mediator—if it is thought that this technique will avert a strike and lead to a settlement—may persuade the parties to sign a stipulation for an extension or "new appointment" of an FF. In effect, the FMCS provides a mediation-factfinding umbrella in some situations that it believes is consistent with the intent of the statute.

TRENDS IN CASELOAD STATISTICS[2]

From August 1974 through March 1980, the FMCS recorded a cumulative total of 8,402 health care disputes cases closed and pending. Since one- and two-year contracts are the norm in this industry, the cumulative figure includes repeat negotiations during this period. The FMCS assigns every health care dispute to a mediator because of the "mandatory mediation" provisions of Section 8(d)(C) of the act and because it must decide whether a BOI/FF appointment is needed. Consequently, mediators have early and continuing contact with the parties even if they are not working with them directly at the bargaining table. The FMCS also extends mediation services to the parties both before the appointment of a BOI or FF and after the factfinding process has been completed. The combination of these factors, plus the high percentage of difficult first-contract negotiations in the industry, generally means that the mediator holds more joint sessions in health care disputes than in the rest of the private sector.

The combined total of BOI/FF appointments has leveled off in recent years. From September 1974 through March 1980, the FMCS recorded a cumulative total of 212 BOI/FF appointments out of the total of 8,402 assignments, which averages out to approximately a 2.5 percent appointment rate. In the first two years after the health care amendments were passed, the service appointed BOIs/FFs in a high proportion of health care disputes because it used as its basis for such action the standard of "potential impact on health care services in the event of a strike."

When the service introduced a new criterion into its decision making on naming BOIs—that is, whether a factfinder would help or hinder the bargaining process—the number of appointments declined substantially. From September 1974 through September 1976, the service appointed 115 BOIs/FFs, of which three-fourths were statutory BOI appointments and less than one-fourth were at the parties' written stipulation to the director. Over the last several years, not only has the total number of BOI/FF appointments declined but the number of stipulated FF appointments has increased in relation to the number of statutory BOI appointments. From October 1, 1976, to April 1, 1980, the service appointed only 97 BOIs/FFs, of which 41 were statutory BOIs and 56 were stipulated FFs. This decline can be attributed to several factors:

- Increasing sophistication on the part of the parties in finding ways to settle without the appointment of BOIs/FFs.
- Earlier efforts on the part of the field mediators to obtain a written stipulation from the parties, thus reducing the need for the FMCS to appoint a BOI in sensitive situations simply because the clock has run out, the parties are not at settlement, and a strike could have a serious impact. With the signed stipulation in hand, the parties tend to relax and get on with the bargaining. Often the signed stipulation never has to be activated by the field mediator and the regional office for the appointment of an FF.
- Greater selectivity and earlier timing on the part of the field mediators and regional offices in suggesting the appointment of a BOI/FF, as well as earlier discussion between the field and the national office about potential appointment situations.
- Finally, in situations where the FMCS does appoint, it appears that the factfinding recommendations are having greater acceptability with the parties. This may be the result in part of the growing practice of informal mediator-factfinder discussions about a dispute. Or it may be that the parties and the neutral, in becoming increasingly familiar with the factfinding procedure, also are growing increasingly resourceful in tailoring the procedure to the peculiarities of the bargaining situation.

How well is collective bargaining working? Have the amendments reduced work stoppages? If the FMCS strike figures are viewed in absolute numbers, the incidence of strikes has increased since 1974. However, when viewed against the total collective bargaining activity since 1974, the strike ratio has remained relatively stable. From August 1974 to October 1, 1976, the FMCS recorded 2,244 closed health care disputes, with 110 strikes; from October 1, 1976, to October 1, 1978, it listed 2,732 closed disputes and 131 strikes; from October 1, 1978, to April 1, 1980, there were 1,899 closed health care disputes, with 96 strikes.

On an annual basis, the strike rate has ranged from 4.2 to 5.5 percent of all health care cases. Table 21-1 shows total closed caseload, total strikes, and the strike ratio for health care disputes for FY '75 through the first six months of FY '80.

Table 21-1   Health Care Industry Strike Case Report

Fiscal Year	Total Health Care Cases* (Closed)	Total Strikes	Strike Ratio
8/74 to 7/1/75	719	32	4.5
7/1/75 to 10/1/76**	1,525	78	5.1
10/1/76 to 10/1/77	1,419	59	4.2
10/1/77 to 10/1/78	1,313	72	5.5
10/1/78 to 10/1/79	1,277	67	5.2
10/1/79 to 4/1/80	622	29	4.7
Aggregate	6,875	337	4.9

*These represent 6,875 out of 8,402 total health care cases, in which mediators closely monitored or actively participated in the resolution of the dispute from initial contact with the parties to termination of the dispute.

**The fiscal year was changed from July 1 to October 1 in 1976, which accounts for an additional three months of caseload statistics during this transition quarter.

NEW REGULATIONS ON BOIs AND FFs

Ever since the 1974 amendments, a number of entities in the health care industry have expressed to the FMCS a desire to have some input into the BOI selection process or to use their own private dispute-resolution procedures.[3] After considerable input from labor and management representatives, in July 1979 the FMCS published regulations in the *Federal Register*[4] that became effective August 1, 1979. The regulations have two major subparts: (1) a provision to allow the parties at their option to have some input, under certain specified procedures, into FMCS's selection of any possible BOI or FF; and (2) a statement of FMCS's newly stated policy of deferring to the parties' own private factfinding or arbitration procedures if they met the conditions specified in the new regulations.

These regulations do not really reflect anything new by way of the informal procedures under which the FMCS had operated during the first five years under the health care amendments. From 1974 to 79, through informal discussions between the parties and the FMCS in certain negotiations, the agency had concluded that some individuals would be more acceptable to the disputants as a BOI or FF and had tried to appoint them whenever possible. Similarly, there had long been instances where the parties had clauses in their contracts, or special written agreements drawn up during the negotiations, to go to private factfinding or interest arbitration if necessary, and the FMCS had deferred to those procedures. What is new about the

1979 regulations is that they now are a matter of public knowledge.

Submission of Lists

The first part of the new regulations provides that, if the disputants jointly want input into the FMCS's potential selection of a BOI/FF, they may at any time (at least 90 days prior to the expiration of a collective bargaining agreement or at any time before the notice required under Section 8(d) of the act for first-contract disputes) jointly submit to the FMCS a list of arbitrators or impartial factfinders who would be BOI/FF appointees acceptable to both sides. The parties may submit only one name, if they wish. The agency will make every effort to make its selection from that list, although it is not bound to appoint that individual.

These joint recommendations may be submitted by a particular set of parties for a particular dispute or for use in all future disputes. A group of health care employers and unions in a community or geographic area may submit a list of recommendations for use in all disputes between any two or more of these parties. The parties may jointly rank the individuals in order of preference.

Submission of a joint list of recommendations to the FMCS is a purely optional procedure that allows both sides to have some input into the BOI/FF selection process. Submission of such a joint list will not be viewed by the FMCS as evidence of the appropriateness or desirability of a BOI. In short, the submission of a joint list will not compel a BOI/FF appointment by the agency.

Deferral to the Parties

The second part of the 1979 regulations establishes a policy of FMCS's deferral to the parties' private factfinding and interest arbitration procedures so long as they satisfy the FMCS's responsibilities under the act and are consistent with it.

Specifically, the agency will defer to a *private factfinding procedure* if both parties have agreed in writing to this procedure and so long as it meets the following conditions:

1. It must be invoked automatically at a specified time (e.g., at contract expiration).
2. It must provide a fixed and determinate method for selecting the impartial factfinder(s).
3. It must provide that there can be no strike or lockout and no change in conditions of employment (except by mutual agreement) prior to or

during the factfinding and for at least seven days after the procedure is completed.
4. It must provide that the factfinder(s) will make a written report to the parties, containing the findings of fact and recommendations for settling the dispute, with a copy of this report to be forwarded to the agency. (The agency is empowered to pay for the services of those BOIs and FFs appointed by the FMCS. However, it cannot and does not pay for a factfinder appointed under the parties' own agreement.)

The FMCS will defer to the parties' private *interest arbitration procedure* and will decline to appoint a BOI/FF if both sides have agreed in writing to their own interest arbitration procedure and if the procedure provides that:

1. There can be no strike or lockout and no changes in conditions of employment (except by mutual agreement) during the contract negotiations covered by the interest arbitration procedure and during any subsequent interest arbitration proceedings.
2. The award of the arbitrator(s) will be final and binding on both sides.
3. There will be a fixed and determinate method for selecting the impartial interest arbitrator(s).
4. There will be a written award by the arbitrator(s).

Parties to a dispute who have agreed to either a private interest arbitration or factfinding procedure should jointly submit a copy of their agreed-upon procedure to the appropriate regional office of the FMCS as early as possible but at least before a BOI/FF is appointed.

These new regulations were developed by the FMCS to accommodate the stated needs of the parties while remaining faithful to its obligations under the NLRA. It is possible that these procedures will be modified again as the needs of parties in health care disputes change. In fact, since these regulations were published, the agency has had informal discussions with management and union negotiators as to how they may be modified.

CONCLUSION

The statutory BOI procedure has added a new dimension to health care negotiations. In some cases, it has put pressure on the parties to make progress early in their negotiations in order to avoid the unilateral appointment of a BOI by the FMCS; its time restrictions have prompted the agency to create the stipulated factfinding procedure to allow more flexibility in the timing of the appointment of a factfinder; and it has been the catalyst for the FMCS's deferral to private factfinding or arbitration.

The BOI/FF is, in fact, a mediating arm of the director of the FMCS. Such an appointment is one of a variety of mediation and conciliation services offered by the agency to the parties in health care disputes. It is intended to promote speedy resolution of any contract dispute between a private sector health care institution and its employees so as to avoid, or at least minimize, disruption to patient care.

NOTES

1. The BOI may be composed of one or more individuals, depending on the number of health care institutions and size of the bargaining units involved, the number of open issues, the complexity of the situation, etc. The appointees are not FMCS mediators but are private arbitrators or other qualified neutrals selected from the FMCS official roster maintained in its Office of Arbitration Services.
2. FMCS caseload statistics are given in fiscal, not calendar, years.
3. The reasons ranged from the parties' wish to avoid premature appointments and the time limits of the statutory BOI procedure to winning some measure of control over the selection of the third party neutral. Some parties preferred using interest arbitration rather than the nonbinding BOI/FF procedures of the FMCS if they could not settle their differences.
4. *Federal Register*, Vol. 44, no. 141, Friday, July 20, 1979, "Rules and Regulations," pp. 42683–42684.

22. Strike Two: Hospitals Down but Not Out

PAUL E. BRODY and JOSEPH B. STAMM

Reprinted with permission from *Health Care Management Review,* Vol. 3, No. 3, Summer 1978, published by Aspen Systems Corporation, Germantown, Md., © 1978.

Less than three years after New York City experienced its first hospital strike, a second walkout occurred. From July 7 through 17, 1976, District 1199, the National Union of Hospital and Health Care Employees, staged a strike which affected all member institutions of the New York City League of Voluntary Hospitals and Homes. Unlike the first strike where the hospitals were caught off guard, during the 1976 strike hospital management used contingency measures to minimize disruption of patient care and reduce the negative economic effect of the strike.

CONTINGENCY MEASURES

Contingency measures were implemented when a federal law preempted the National Labor Relations Act which sought to outlaw hospital strikes. These measures included:

1. stockpiling essential supplies;
2. categorizing patients into three classes: those able to be sent home, those who probably could be sent home and those who definitely required care;
3. consolidating patients into fewer wards; and
4. assigning to supervisors, professionals and volunteers remaining on the job all functions normally performed by the striking workers (virtu-

ally all employees except registered nurses and physicians).[1]

In addition, the Board of Health authorized the city's health commissioner to declare a health emergency, if necessary, to enable delivery and sanitation trucks to pass through the picket lines. This would allow hospital services to continue with minimal interference.

COMPARISON OF THE STRIKE'S IMPACT: A CASE STUDY

One of New York City's largest nonprofit voluntary hospitals with more than 1,000 beds was studied to determine (1) the actual gross and net dollars lost because of the strike, and (2) the effect of the first strike on hospital management in preparing contingency measures to minimize the negative economic effect and disruption of patient care.

Normal Operation Costs Saved

During the strike, the 1,000-bed hospital "saved" money by not paying salaries and employee benefits to the striking workers. In the 1976 strike this amounted to savings of $750,000 in salaries and $166,000 in fringe benefits not paid out to striking District 1199 employees. Comparable figures for the 1973 strike were

$400,000 and $70,000 respectively. Calculating the average *daily* savings for the strikes reveals daily savings of $83,000 in 1976, compared to $59,000 in 1973. (See Table 22-1.)

The percentage difference in the average daily savings can be attributed to a 22-percent salary and benefit package increase (accounting for 75 percent of the difference in savings between the two strikes), as well as an increase in the number of District 1199 workers.

Patient Revenues Lost

The major negative effect on the hospital during the strike was the loss of patient revenues that would have accrued under normal circumstances. Losses were felt in the emergency room (ER), outpatient department (OPD) and inpatient medical/surgical (med/surg) units.

In order to determine the loss of patient days and visits attributable to the strike and to control for possible seasonal effects, the number of patient visits to the hospital during the respective strike months (November 1973 and July 1976) were compared to the average number of visits in the three months prior to the strike and to the three months after the strike. In an effort to eliminate possible time trend effects, similar analysis was performed for the two years preceding each strike as measured by the percent difference for three months prior to and three months after the strike month for the years between 1971 and 1976. ("Strike month" refers to November for the years 1971 to 1973 and July for the years 1974 to 1976.) The results shown in Table 22-2 reveal several interesting developments.

1. The ER operated more effectively during the second strike than during the first one. This is evident by examining the percentages for the strike periods in 1973 and 1976. The difference indicates much less of a decline in ER visits in the 1976 strike. The difference is statistically significant (see discussion below).

Table 22-1 Average Daily Savings during the 1973 and 1976 Strikes

1973 Strike

$$\frac{\$400,000 \text{ salary} + \$70,000 \text{ fringe savings}}{8 \text{ paydays lost}} = \$59,000^*$$

1976 Strike

$$\frac{\$750,000 \text{ salary} + \$166,000 \text{ fringe savings}}{11 \text{ paydays lost}} = \$83,000^*$$

*Figures are rounded.

---

2. The OPD provided fewer services during the second strike. This too may be seen by the percentages for the 1973 and 1976 strikes as noted in (1) above.
3. The med/surg units operated at approximately the same level during the two strikes. Once again this is evident in the percentages in Table 22-2.
4. In general, the ER, OPD and med/surg units were used less during the respective strike month compared to the pre-three-month period and post-three-month period. However, during July 1976 the ER was used as much as the prior three-month period.

A major shift in priorities seems to have taken place in the second strike. During the first strike an attempt was made to operate all services in the hospital, but during the 1976 strike emphasis was on emergency care at the expense of preventive and acute self-limiting nonemergency care. Thus there was virtually no difference in the 1973 percentage change of utilization rates in these areas.

The hypothesis that a decrease in outpatient utilization would result in a concomitant increase in ER utilization was tested. The decrease in outpatient utilization was calculated as the difference between percentages of OPD visits during the 1973 strike period and those during the 1976 strike period (Table 22-2). Similarly, the increase in ER utilization was calculated as the difference between the ER percentages. The discrepancy between OPD and ER differences was tested by a student "t" test with two degrees of freedom. While strongly suggestive, the difference fell just short of statistical significance ($0.05 < p < 0.1$).

Student "t" tests were performed on actual data comparing the index, or strike month statistics, with the average of (1) the three months prior to and (2) the three months after the index month in question for all years between 1971 and 1976. These tests were performed for each of the index strike months independently.

The results indicate that for nonstrike years, the null hypothesis was sustained in each case, i.e., there was no difference between the strike month and the three months preceding and following the strike month. However, for the strike years, the hypothesis was rejected for the OPD and med/surg units in the 1976 strike as well as for the ER and med/surg units in the 1973 strike. (See Table 22-3.) This confirms the belief that there was a priority change from the OPD to the ER in the 1976 strike.

To determine the actual number of days or visits the ER, OPD and med/surg lost as a result of the strike, the following computations were made:

Table 22-2 Number of Patient Days/Visits and Percent Change during Strike Months Compared to Three Months Prior to and Three Months after Strike Months*

	Year					
	1971	1972	1973 (strike)	1974	1975	1976 (strike)
	ER					
3 Months Prior to Strike Month	−2,482 (−33.2)**	−359 (−7.0)	−1,067 (−21.7)	+97 (+2.0)	+827 (+17.3)	+21 (+0.5)
3 Months after Strike Month	+60 (+1.2)	+134 (+2.9)	−688 (−15.1)	−655 (−11.7)	+279 (+5.2)	−550 (−10.9)
	OPD					
3 Months Prior to Strike Month	+5,675 (+25.7)	+839 (+4.7)	−3,737 (−21.4)	−634 (−3.4)	−1,828 (−8.5)	−9,788 (−45.7)
3 Months after Strike Month	+213 (+1.2)	+908 (+5.2)	−3,895 (−22.1)	+397 (+2.3)	−1,713 (−8.4)	−8,611 (−42.5)
	Med/Surg Unit					
3 Months Prior to Strike Month	−17 (−0.1)	+67 (+0.3)	−2,917 (−11.6)	+859 (+3.4)	−142 (−0.5)	−2,373 (−8.5)
3 Months after Strike Month	−274 (−1.1)	+319 (+1.2)	−2,418 (−9.8)	+748 (+3.0)	+608 (+2.4)	−1,507 (−9.4)

*(−) indicates a percent decrease.
**This figure is nonrepresentative due to reorganization of the ER affecting total visits.

1. The combined average of the number of days/visits for the three months before and three months after the strike was calculated.
2. The actual number of days/visits during the strike month was subtracted from the calculated average.

Table 22-4 gives an example of calculating the number of days/visits lost in the med/surg unit in 1976. Table 22-5 shows the estimated number of days/visits lost for each service.

In order to quantify the loss of revenue, each service was broken down according to the percent of visits for each reimbursement category, i.e., Medicaid, Medicare, self-pay and Blue Cross, as recorded by the hospital under study. (See Table 22-6.)

An estimated $1,001,001.22 gross was lost in the 1976 strike as a result of a decrease in the number of visits made to the hospital. This represents a 70 percent increase over the 1973 figure of $588,935.34. (See Table 22-7.)

Additional insight into the effects of the strike can be gained by appropriately adjusting the difference in the length of the strike and the difference in the reimbursement rates.

Length of the Strike

The 1973 strike lasted eight days (Monday, November 5 through Monday, November 12) while the 1976 strike lasted 11 days (Wednesday, July 7 through Saturday, July 17). The 1976 figures were reconstructed to reflect 8/11 of the dollars lost for the ER and med/surg units. However, the strike affected the OPD only six days for 1973 and eight days for 1976 since these clinics do not operate on the weekends. Therefore, the 1976 OPD figures were reconstructed using a factor of 6/8. In addition, the 1976 per diem rates were converted into the 1973 rates to assure comparability. (See Table 22-8.)

Table 22-3 Results of Significance Tests for the Effect of the Strikes on the ER, OPD and Med/Surg Units

Service	1973 Strike	1976 Strike
ER	Significant (p<0.05)	Not significant
OPD	Not significant	Significant (p<0.01)
Med/Surg Unit	Significant (p<0.05)	Significant (p<0.05)

Table 22-4 Calculation for Estimating the Number of Days Lost in the Med/Surg Unit in 1976

$$\frac{26{,}485 \text{ (3 months average before} + 26{,}605 \text{ (3 months average after)}}{2} - 24{,}112 \text{ (number of visits in strike month)} = 2{,}433 \text{ days}$$

Once these figures were adjusted to allow comparable analysis, it was found that the hospital lost a total of $496,973.59 in the 1976 strike because of fewer patient days/visits. This reflected a 15.6 percent decrease from the 1973 strike loss of $588,935.43.

A comparison of the total dollars and days/visits lost in each category again illustrated the shift in emphasis away from the OPD to the ER and med/surg units during the 1976 strike.

Strike-Related Expenses

Overtime

During the strike efforts were made to operate the hospital as effectively as possible. Nonstriking employees were asked to fill the void by working additional hours. Two groups of personnel were utilized: administrative and other nonbargaining unit employees. The dollar amounts paid out to these employees for the two strikes are given in Table 22-9.

The additional salaries and fringe benefits paid out to nonbargaining unit employees in the 1976 strike were 20.5 percent less than those paid out in the 1973 strike. Converting these figures to reflect the 1973 strike (comparable length of strike and comparable pay scales), a 45.8 percent decrease in additional salary costs was evident. This was determined by (1) calculating the average cost per day for additional salaries, (2) converting the 1976 pay scale to the 1973 base scale, and (3) multiplying the average cost per day by the adjusted number of strike days (eight days).

The average additional cost for the 1973 strike was $96,000 ($770,000 ÷ 8 additional pay days) as compared to $56,000 for the 1976 strike ($612,000 ÷ 11 additional pay days). After adjusting the pay scales, the average cost per day would have been $46,000. (Figures are rounded.)

Table 22-5 Estimated Number of Days/Visits Lost Per Service

Service	1973	1976
ER Visits	877.5	264.0
OPD Visits	3,816.0	9,199.5
Med/Surg Unit Days	2,667.5	2,433.0

The difference in the dollar amounts paid out can be attributed to policy changes made during the second strike. During the first strike, all nonbargaining unit employees—administrative and nonadministrative personnel—were paid time and a half. Only nonadministrative personnel were so reimbursed during the second strike. Administrative personnel were reimbursed straight time.

The experience gained from the first strike is also evident when one examines other strike-related expenses incurred during the first strike but avoided during the second one. These additional expenses included food costs, outside security guards, and petty cash for supplies and equipment.

Food Costs

During the 1973 strike the hospital under review did not charge its employees for food consumed in the cafeteria. As a result, $25,000 of revenue that normally would have accrued was lost. An extra $25,000 was spent buying frozen foods for its employees who were served on paper goods and plastic tableware instead of regular dishes and tableware. In the 1976 strike the cafeteria operated as usual with employees paying for their meals.

Security Expenses

To augment security in the hospital, additional security guards were hired from the contract security service during the 1973 strike. An additional $55,000 had to be allocated for this service in order to maintain some sense of order in the hospital. In 1976 the hospital arranged special contingency measures in the event of a strike and thus no additional monies were spent for security. These measures included cooperation with the police department, which expanded the number of officers guarding the institution.

Supplies and Equipment

Estimated supplies and equipment expenditures, unlike those for security and food, were higher in the 1976 strike—$30,000 in 1976 compared to $10,000 in 1973. The bulk of this money was spent on buying assorted disposables for the med/surg units, the area on which the hospital placed its greatest emphasis. (A

Table 22-6 Total Dollars Lost per Reimbursement Category for the 1973 and 1976 Strikes

Reimbursement Category	% of Visits in Each Category	Number of Visits Lost in Month	Number of Visits Lost per Category	Rate per Category ($)	$ Lost per Category ($)
November 1973			ER		
Medicare	7.6		66.69	14.90	993.68
Medicaid	38.7	{ 877.5 }	339.59	19.65	6,672.94
Self-pay/others	53.7		471.21	5.80	2,733.91
Total	100.0		877.49		10,399.63
July 1976					
Medicare	9.4		24.81	29.51	732.14
Medicaid	35.2	{ 264 }	92.92	40.25	3,704.03
Self-pay/others	55.4		146.25	8.69	1,270.91
Total	100.0		263.98		5,707.08
November 1973			OPD		
Medicare	8.7		331.99	18.20	6,042.21
Medicaid	44.8	{ 3,816 }	1,709.56	49.94	85,375.42
Self-pay/others	46.5		1,774.44	5.75	10,203.03
Total	100.0		3,815.99		101,620.66
July 1976					
Medicare	11.7		1,076.34	29.47	31,719.73
Medicaid	42.6	{ 9,199.5 }	3,918.98	67.72	265,393.32
Self-pay/others	45.7		4,204.17	9.24	38,846.53
Total	100.0		9,199.49		335,959.58
November 1973			Med/Surg Units		
Medicare	32.0		853.60	172.50	147,246.00
Medicaid	18.9	{ 2,667.50 }	504.60	172.80	87,117.12
Blue Cross	32.7		872.27	170.00	148,285.90
Self-pay/others	16.4		437.47	215.48	94,266.03
Total	100.0		2,667.49		476,915.05
July 1976					
Medicare	38.6		939.13	253.00	237,599.89
Medicaid	13.3	{ 2,433.0 }	323.58	253.00	81,865.74
Blue Cross	33.2		807.75	278.00	224,554.50
Self-pay/others	14.9		362.51	318.10	115,314.43
Total	100.0		2,432.97		660,334.56

Total dollars lost in 1976 = $1,001,001.22
Total dollars lost in 1973 = $ 588,935.34

Additional dollars lost in 1976 = $412,065.88

(% of Visits in Each Category) × (Number of Visits Lost in Month) = (Number of Visits Lost per Category).
(Number of Visits Lost per Category) × (Rate per Category) = ($ Lost per Category).

Table 22-7 Calculation for Determining Percent Increase in Revenue Loss between the 1973 and 1976 Strikes

$$\frac{\$412,065.88 \ (\text{additional } \$ \text{ lost in 1976})}{\$588,935.34 \ (\text{total } \$ \text{ lost in 1973})} \times 100 = \% \text{ additional loss} = 70\%$$

Table 22-8 1973 and "Adjusted" 1976 Dollars and Number of Days/Visits Lost during the Strikes

Service	1973 Dollars	Number of 1973 Days/Visits	1976 Adjusted Dollars	Number of 1976 Adjusted Days/Visits
ER	10,399.63	878	2,213.61	192
OPD	101,620.66	3,816	179,606.97	6,900
Med/Surg Units	476,915.05	2,268	315,153.01	1,769
Total	588,935.34		496,973.59	

Table 22-9 Additional Salaries and Benefits Paid Out in the 1973 and 1976 Strikes (in Dollars)

Category	Year 1973	Year 1976
Additional Salaries Paid to Administrative Staff	320,000	290,000
Additional Salaries Paid to Other Nonbargaining Unit Employees	400,000	305,000
Additional Nonbargaining Unit Fringe Benefits	50,000	17,000
Total	770,000	612,000

fraction of the increase in expenditures was attributed to inflation.)

A comparable balance sheet of the two strikes reveals that although the 1976 strike lasted longer and although the hospital stood to lose more because of higher per diem rates, there was a 27.6 percent decrease in the cost of the 1976 strike. Also, once the strike was adjusted for duration and dollar changes in salaries and per diem rates, a 65.5 percent decrease in cost was evident. (See Table 22-10.)

Impact of the Strike

A comparison of the *gross* cost of the strike reveals that in 1976 the hospital incurred $277,000 less in costs

Table 22-10 Total and Adjusted Costs of the 1973 and 1976 Strikes (in Dollars)

	Year 1973	Year 1976	Year 1976 Adjusted
Expenses			
Loss of Income Due to Loss of Inpatient Days	477,000	659,000	315,000
Loss of Income Due to Loss of OPD Visits	102,000	336,000	180,000
Loss of Income Due to Loss of ER Visits	10,000	6,000	2,000
Additional Salaries Paid to Administrative Staff	320,000	290,000	173,000
Additional Salaries Paid to Other Nonbargaining Employees	400,000	305,000	182,000
Additional Nonbargaining Employee Fringe Benefits	50,000	17,000	10,000
Additional Security	55,000	—	—
Additional Food	25,000	—	—
Loss of Revenue from Cafeteria	25,000	—	—
Additional Supplies and Equipment	10,000	30,000	30,000*
Total	1,474,000	1,643,000	892,000
Savings			
Salaries Not Paid to District 1199 Employees	400,000	750,000	447,000
Savings on District 1199 Union Employee Benefits	70,000	166,000	99,000
Total	470,000	916,000	546,000
Gross Cost of Strike (Total Expenses—Total Savings)	1,004,000	727,000	346,000
(Change in Cost of Strike)		(27.6%)	(65.5%)

*No adjustments were made for additional supplies and equipment.

than in 1973, even though the 1976 strike lasted for three more days. The overall *net* cost, however, was higher for the 1976 strike. This was the result of a policy decision made by New York State not to adjust the reimbursement rates. Whereas in 1973 rate adjustments were made to offset some of the hospital's unforeseen strike losses, the state froze the 1976 reimbursement rate. This is clearly seen in Table 22-11.

This policy had an obvious devastating effect on the hospital. The gross cost of the strikes was $1,004,000 for 1973 and $727,000 for 1976. (See Table 22-10.) Subtracting the dollar amount of reimbursement from the gross cost of the strike, we find that in 1973 the hospital lost only $24,000 compared to $507,000 in 1976. (See Table 22-12.)

POSITIVE EFFECTS OF CONTINGENCY MEASURES

The contingency measures implemented at this major voluntary hospital had a positive effect. (However, caution must be exercised not to draw inferences to the entire hospital system for no claim is made that this is a wholly representative hospital.) These positive effects include:

1. The focus of attention turned to the treatment of patients most in need of medical care (ER and med/surg units) at the expense of preventive and

Table 22-11 Amount Reimbursed by Third Parties

Third Party	Dollar Amount Reimbursed	
	1973	1976
Blue Cross Appeal	330,000	——
Medicare Appeal	365,000	220,000
Medicaid Appeal	285,000	——
Total	980,000	220,000

Table 22-12 Gross and Net Costs of the 1973 and 1976 Strikes (in Dollars)

	1973	1976
Gross Cost of Strike	1,004,000	727,000
Reimbursement by Third Parties	980,000	220,000
Net Cost of Strike	24,000	507,000

acute self-limiting care. Thus one can see (Table 22-2) a significant drop-off in the number of outpatient visits during the strike month when compared to the three months prior to and three months after the strike. On the other hand the ER and the med/surg units operated almost at capacity.

2. Strike-related expenses (additional security, additional food costs and loss of revenue from cafeteria services) were totally eliminated during the second strike.

3. Overtime expenses were drastically reduced by instituting new procedures whereby administrative personnel were reimbursed straight time in place of time and a half.

The overall monetary effect of the contingency measures was a 27.6 percent decrease in the gross cost of the 1976 strike as compared to the 1973 strike. (The net dollar effect, however, was in reverse; the strike in 1976 cost $483,000 more than the 1973 strike. This was the result of New York State's decision to freeze reimbursement fees.) This is a remarkable achievement in view of the fact that the 1976 strike lasted three days more than the 1973 strike.[2]

NOTES

1. D. Bird, "Hospitals Girding for Strike Today," *The New York Times* (July 7, 1976), p. 1.
2. P. E. Brody and J. London, "How Costly Is a Strike?" *Hospitals, JAHA* 49 (September 16, 1975): 53–56.

23. The Role of the Mediator in Health Care Collective Bargaining

PAUL YAGER

The basic function of the mediator in labor-management negotiations is to assist the employee and employer representatives to meet their responsibilities to achieve a settlement. The health care industry presents some unique problems to mediators insofar as the employer cannot easily adjust the prices charged or the quality of the services provided when labor costs change as a result of labor-management negotiations.

Mediators know that most of the health care institutions, whether public, proprietary, voluntary, or some combination of those three, depend for much of their income on reimbursement from third party payers such as federal, state, and city government and the various insurance schemes such as Blue Cross for service contracts and other organizations for patient indemnity plans.

Mediators also know that government influence on the economics of the health care industry does not end at the cashier's window but also includes regulations that affect the number of beds available and the types of service provided. The civil servants who must exercise extreme care in the dispensing of public funds are committed to achieving maximum efficiency in the entire health care industry in order to minimize the burden on taxpayers. They exercise substantial influence on both the income of health care establishments and

the way in which such institutions function without having a direct role or responsibility in negotiations between employee and employer representatives.

Mediators also know that, however difficult the environment is for employers, the employees face the same vicissitudes in the economy as do workers at companies in other industries that may be more or less prosperous or more or less free to adjust prices after negotiations. The inability to pay because there are limits on health care institutions' income seldom convinces the employees that they should settle for less than their friends and neighbors who work in other industries. Therefore, the mediator in a health care dispute faces problems that are specific to that industry but that are not so remote from the mediator's experience in other industries that those problems inhibit the method of operation.

THE COMMITMENT TO THE ILL

Most participants in health care industry negotiations are highly sensitive to the commitment that they, their institutions, and their constituents have made to saving lives, treating the ill, and comforting the aged and infirm who are in their care. The participants and the mediator understand that the negotiations in this industry are conducted in an atmosphere that attracts a great deal of public attention, so the advocates on each side may feel restricted from maneuvering in negotia-

The comments expressed in this article are the personal opinions of the author and do not represent the views or policies of the Federal Mediation and Conciliation Service.

tions as freely as can their counterparts in other industries.

When all the factors that complicate negotiations in other sectors of the economy are added to the specific problems of the health care industry, the mediator must exercise extraordinary efforts to make an effective contribution toward settlement. Commentators debate whether mediation is art or science. In meeting the challenge of health care assignments, mediators must call upon all their personal resources and all the art *and* science at their command.

Since the mediator has no authority to compel any participant in collective bargaining to accept a particular settlement, the expert must enlist the support of the representatives of the parties. Since those representatives also are charged with the responsibilities of being keen advocates of the interests of their constituencies, it sometimes is difficult for them to indicate interest in settlement of various issues without also appearing to contradict themselves and thereby weaken themselves in their advocacy posture. The mediator on the other hand is charged with the responsibility to assist in achieving a settlement. In those circumstances, the mediator provides the balance between the parties' needs to advocate their interests keenly while simultaneously working to reach a settlement that serves the interests of everyone involved.

The mediator provides this balance in many ways. Techniques and procedures differ from dispute to dispute and mediator to mediator. Whatever the technique or procedure, the objective is the same: to help the representatives of the various interests involved to accommodate their conflicting needs to the realities of the economic and human environment in which they find themselves. No matter how restricted employers are by the limited resources available, they must face the fact that employees have needs and aspirations that must be satisfied. Wages, other economic benefits, and working conditions cannot be less generous in health care than in other sectors of the economy if qualified people are to be attracted to and remain in the industry. Therefore, the difficulties health care employers face in finding the resources to pay the personnel costs and to maintain humane working conditions cannot be an excuse for not meeting reasonable standards in the labor market.

RESPONSIBILITIES UNDER THE ACT

Congress has provided in Section 8(d)(C) of the National Labor Relations Act that employer and employee representatives in the health care industry must cooperate with the mediator's efforts:

. . . the Service shall promptly communicate with the parties and use its best efforts, by mediation and conciliation, to bring them to agreement. *The parties shall participate fully and promptly in such meetings as may be undertaken by the Service for the purpose of aiding in a settlement of the dispute.* [Emphasis provided.]

All this accomplishes, however, is to set the stage for meaningful negotiations. If either or both sides is determined to have a confrontation for whatever reasons, valid or not, they can frustrate every effort to reach agreement in order to precipitate such a situation. Fortunately, the proclivity for confrontations is minimal in the health care industry because all of its elements are responsive to the life-threatening nature of such situations.

The mediator assumes that representatives of the parties will cooperate. The mediator talks privately or jointly with these representatives. One of the first objectives is to establish a climate in which all the participants recognize their common responsibility to find a settlement. If such a climate is not established easily, the mediator continues to work to achieve it but does not allow the absence of a favorable climate to interfere with the mediation effort.

In the course of separate and joint discussions, the mediator helps the parties to understand each other's positions. This may be necessary when they have not been communicating directly with each other or may have been employing rhetoric that is so disturbing that the message is distorted and the other party cannot respond to the main thrust of the argument effectively. The mediator finds whether each side understands the other's real, not merely perceived, goals and objectives and makes sure that each side comprehends these points.

DEVELOPING AN AGENDA

The mediator may help the parties to develop an agenda so that discussion can take place in an orderly atmosphere. While this is being done, the mediator also may help the disputants establish priorities among the various issues so that each can indicate to the other which ones require the most serious consideration. During this stage of the negotiations, the mediator may help each side state the issues in terms that are more readily understood by the other and that also may indicate a basis for settlement.

As the agenda develops, the issues are clarified, and some priorities become evident, the mediator can help the participants deal with the substantive differences between them. By asking for clarification and illustration, by citing examples of resolution of a particular issue elsewhere, by requesting information about the costs and resources for meeting various proposals, the mediator helps the parties understand the dimensions of their problems better.

Sometimes what appears to be an unreasonably difficult problem in the early stages of negotiations may become more amenable to resolution when that problem is broken down into components. In moving back and forth between the disputants, the mediator may make suggestions about how a problem could be solved that are acceptable to the parties but that neither of them may have wanted to propose for fear of being misunderstood or that might not have occurred to them because they were so deeply involved in advocating a particular position that they did not think about a basis of accommodation on that issue. The mediator may suggest alternatives that do not occur to the parties.

Mediators can be helpful to the representatives when they are ready to modify their position on an issue but do not want to do it without some assurance that the new stance would be helpful toward achieving settlement. The mediator can help explore the prospects for progress without either party's making a commitment that might be regretted later if the exploration fails to develop a solution.

Some negotiators are concerned about when they should make certain moves and often delay too long, which gives the other side the impression of adamancy that really does not exist. The mediator can help each side analyze the dynamics of the bargaining and determine the best time for various moves.

As negotiations approach a deadline, the mediator may be able to help each side face the dilemma of choosing among the least evils. Sometimes it is important for various factions on each side to be satisfied, and the mediator may have to discuss the implications of that problem with the parties so that the proposals are designed and packaged to solve political as well as economic problems.

Mediators are neutral participants in collective bargaining negotiations whose services are provided to minimize the prospects of strikes where the parties are free to engage in economic warfare, i.e., strikes and lockouts. Being neutral, however, does not bar a mediator from asserting a considered opinion about the issues or the prospects. Mediators make such assertions in private when they believe it is important for the parties to have the benefit of the thinking of an experienced labor relations specialist in order to help them cope with their own problems.

DEADLINES—AND BEYOND

In the health care industry, many of the most difficult negotiations do not get resolved until the union gives the ten-day strike notice to the Federal Mediation and Conciliation Service and to the employer. The mediator can use the heightened tension that exists in the face of a deadline to illuminate the nature of the problems and the potential basis for settlement during the ten-day period. The mediator will schedule meetings even if the parties do not believe there is a need or even if they do not desire a session, because the mediator knows that without meetings and discussion and exploration and perhaps some shouting and table banging to precipitate catharsis, there may not be a settlement.

Sometimes even the best efforts by the advocates and the hard work of the mediator may fail to achieve a settlement. When a strike occurs, a mediator does not quit. The mediator calls meetings when appropriate and takes the responsibility for arranging a session when one of the parties requests it. The mediator can be helpful in dealing with the media when the advocates themselves want to avoid arguing about the merits of the issues in public. Even during a strike while the parties are testing their own resources to continue the confrontation, the mediator continues to explore and propose alternatives, to clarify issues, to package proposals, to meet specific problems, to counsel with both sides in order to help them end the dispute.

A mediator may suggest to each party, or to both, how they could settle some or all issues. Seldom does the mediator make a flat-out recommendation. Even less often does the mediator make a recommendation for settlement publicly. When such a recommendation is made privately or (in the rare case, publicly), it usually is put forward because the mediator is convinced that the parties' tactics or strategies prevent them from getting to that point themselves. The mediator is convinced, on the basis of experience and knowledge of the situation, that the recommendation would be a suitable basis for a settlement that thoughtful people could accept rather than prolong a confrontation.

In health care industry negotiations, mediators may, when appropriate, also help the disputants by enlisting the third party payers' representative in bilateral or even multilateral discussions when convinced such discussions are necessary to clarify or modify reimbursement formulas. Such discussions normally are not the mediator's responsibility, but most will not hesitate to go that route if it will help achieve a settlement.

Mediators respect the skills and dedication of the representatives of employees and employers. They know how difficult the tasks of the representatives are. Mediators show patience, imagination, tolerance, ingenuity, tirelessness, devotion, and many other valuable qualities when they are involved in handling an assignment.

But in spite of all the skills, efforts, and activities of a mediator, the responsibility for settlement remains with the parties. The representatives of the two sides should not hesitate to seek the assistance of a mediator when they recognize that that expert can enhance the negotiators' own efforts toward meeting their own responsibilities.

24. Grievance Procedures in Health Organizations

RICHARD PEGNETTER and SAMUEL LEVEY

INTRODUCTION

A collective bargaining relationship is sealed when labor and management conclude the negotiation of the contract. Its real impact and the success or failure of the relationship are determined by how the contract is administered. In the health care organization, this means the skill and effectiveness with which the various levels of management implement the contract and handle grievances.

The system for dealing with problems that arise under negotiated agreements is the contract grievance procedure. The use of formal grievance procedures to resolve what commonly are called rights disputes became popular during World War II.[1] The grievance procedure, which frequently ends in binding arbitration, represents a trade-off in collective bargaining for both labor and management:

1. For its part, the union gives up the right to strike over grievance disputes during the life of the contract. In return, the union[2] gets the contract protection of a grievance system that places ultimate decision-making power in the hands of an outside arbitrator, not under the unilateral control of management.
2. For its part, management gives up the unilateral right to impose its interpretation of the contract on the union in exchange for the union's obligation to not strike over grievances during the life

of the contract and, instead, to submit disputes to the grievance procedure.[3]

The acceptance of grievance procedures is almost universal in private sector labor relations. About 96 percent of all such contracts contain grievance procedures with arbitration. The practice also is accepted to a significant degree in both the public and private sectors of the health care industry. A 1977 study of hospitals found that 97 percent of their 817 contracts contained grievance systems, with arbitration as the final step in those procedures in 88 percent of the documents analyzed.[4]

Beyond the basic notion of peaceful dispute resolution, other important gains accrue to both health care management and employees under a systematic grievance procedure. The employees obviously gain a sense of fair treatment. They have a protected freedom to bring forward any claim that management has mishandled their rights under the contract and are represented by union officers who are available to help them understand the procedures and rights available.

Management also may realize significant benefits. While it is probable that more employee complaints will arise when a grievance procedure is in effect, an increase in such activity can hold significant communication advantages for the health care administrative team. Put simply, when an employee has a legitimate problem but is reluctant to bring it forward to a supervisor or to management, the complaint will not just disappear. Often, the discontent will grow and the employee will personally "adjust" the dissatisfaction by working a little less, will begin to experience attendance problems, or perhaps will even quit, thus necessitating a recruitment and retraining cost for the organization. On the other hand, if the employee felt encouraged by the presence of a formal grievance procedure and union representation to introduce the complaint to management, the problem could be identified and dealt with promptly and fairly. Even if the issue is not resolved in the employee's favor, the individual has had an opportunity to be heard and, if the procedure is administered properly, has seen the process give the grievance a thorough and even-handed hearing.

It is clear that grievance procedures are meaningful only if they work effectively. The purpose of this article is to identify the key elements and management concerns in maintaining a sound program of contract administration under a grievance procedure. To accomplish this end, the article is divided into five major sections.

The Management Team and Contract Administration focuses on the critical need for management to develop a team concept for the grievance procedure. Since all levels of management are involved in or touched by the settlement of contract grievances, the nature of a team system is analyzed.

The Contract Grievance Procedure evaluates the basic components of a formal grievance system. The role of each element in maintaining the integrity of the total system is discussed. These elements include the definition of a grievance and the time limits involved.

Principles of Handling Grievances reviews the basic steps for management when an employee raises a grievance. This section includes the methods of receiving and responding to grievances and the nature of management's investigation and evaluation of such complaints.

Examples of Grievance Problems uses two areas of contract grievances—discipline and transfers—to illustrate how health care management should approach the determination of employee complaints.

Monitoring Grievance Procedures examines the need for a system to maintain information about grievance activity. The role of this information in contract administration, the evaluation of supervisors, and future negotiations is identified.

THE MANAGEMENT TEAM AND CONTRACT ADMINISTRATION

Perhaps the most important effect of collective bargaining on the management of any health institution is the need for consistency in dealing with employees. This impact is generated by two aspects of a union contract. First, the implication of including any working condition in a collective bargaining agreement is that the issue or condition has been standardized. Consequently, if the contract provides that "in the event of a reduction in the work force, those employees with the least seniority within each job classification will be laid off first," then management is obligated to designate each employee's employment status according to the same measure. That is, if two employees are in the same classification and one must be laid off, the decision will be based only on the standard listed in the contract, namely, who is least senior. Thus all management decisions on layoffs across all job classifications must be made on the basis of the same standard, not with some managers determining layoffs by weighing seniority plus performance evaluations or other factors.

Second, once an aspect of working conditions has been written into the contract, it is the union's basic duty to see that there is enforcement of the terms standardized in the agreement. Thus, the union stewards and officers will be coordinating their activities across various departments and work areas in the health organization to police how management interprets and applies the contract. This means that a union with an effective contract administration program will monitor the actions of supervisors and managers so that, when necessary, employee grievances can be filed when rights standardized by the contract are violated. If the union fails in this responsibility, the terms of any contract become meaningless to the individual workers and they are likely to replace those union officers with more aggressive, effective representatives.

For administration, the net result of these two aspects of a union contract should be clear. Management must develop a systematized internal structure to provide for the implementation and administration of the contract. This plan must enable individual supervisors and managers to respond to grievances in an informed and consistent manner. Should such a structure not be developed and maintained, a skilled union negotiator soon would use managerial inconsistency to enlarge the parameters of the contract and dilute the protections for management's rights that had been won at the bargaining table.

Involvement

Part of developing a management team concept begins with the involvement of all key staff in the collective bargaining relationship. This involvement should begin with negotiation of the agreement itself. Many health care organizations have made the serious mistake of having three or four top staff officials solely responsible for the negotiations. Little or no input is solicited from and no information is given to supervisors and middle management officials as to progress. The results of this approach are multiple:

- First line and middle managers get their information about what is going on in bargaining from employees and the union, not their own executives, thus diminishing their status as part of management.
- Lower level managers tend to respond to the agreement as something imposed on them by an uncaring top management so their commitment to good contract administration will be minimal.
- The management negotiating team unknowingly may agree to language that causes expensive or disastrous impediments in some parts of the organization because no information was available about the impact of the language on first-line supervisors.

While this article does not prescribe a system for involving and updating various management constituencies in the negotiating process, it is evident that this is an important aspect of the team concept that carries over into contract administration.

A second focus for development of the management team occurs immediately after negotiations are finalized. The terms of the new contract must be distributed and explained to the management group. If it is a first agreement, the session or sessions should cover all of the provisions. If the negotiations only modified an existing contract, only the changes need review. This type of explanation is vital because of the nature of a collective bargaining contract. While many provisions are clear and straightforward, any negotiator knows that numerous clauses represent accommodation, necessarily general language, and understandings discussed during bargaining. The result is that contracts are laced with phrases such as *reasonable, insofar as practicable, whenever possible,* or *qualified employee.* If the intended meaning of such terms is not explained to the managers who must implement the contract on a daily basis, the result can be predicted readily; namely, the managers will make their own interpretations—and inconsistency will be inevitable.

The need for review of the new contract extends to staff managers as well as to supervisors. Staff managers' decisions can cause grievances and contract violations as quickly as those of direct supervisors. For example, if the chief of the maintenance engineering department decides that part of the ventilation system in a hospital wing should be expanded and hires an outside heating contractor to do the work, that manager might unknowingly have violated a contract clause on subcontracting that had been negotiated with the maintenance employees. The result could be an arbitration award ordering pay to the maintenance employees who had a contract right to the work done by the outside contractor. The point, is that, in different degrees, all management officials require at least a general knowledge of the terms of the contract. Instruction by the labor relations staff is the most effective way to transmit that knowledge and to minimize problems of contract administration.

Establishment of a Labor Relations Function

For purposes of contract administration, a labor relations office or function must be the hub of the grievance system. The labor relations function may be part of one person's job or require a full-time staff of several individuals, depending on the size of the organization. The critical element is to provide management of the health care institution with a centralized and immediate response mechanism for dealing with grievances. Equally important is that the individual(s) responsible for this function be well-versed in the principles of contract construction and administration and thoroughly familiar with the specific language of the agreement.

The role of a labor relations office is multifold. First, it provides support in contract administration to first-line managers, mainly supervisors. As is discussed later, a supervisor normally has a short time in which to respond to an employee grievance. The supervisor's response should be an affective and accurate interpretation or application of the contract. If the supervisor needs help in making some of these decisions, there should be an immediate and accessible source for guidance. Delay and confusion can result if multiple and varied sources of contract interpretation are used. A labor relations function that provides quick and decisive information to supervisors when needed will enhance the role and authority of those managers and make the individuals feel a supported part of the team.

Second, the creation of a central labor relations function can be a tremendous aid to ensuring consistency in contract administration. Any health care organization involves multiple departmental or functional areas. If a single labor contract covers the employees in more than one department, there is a potential for variation in the handling of grievances. The labor relations function can monitor the implementation of the contract across all departments to guard against inconsistency. The labor relations office then becomes a centralized clearinghouse for grievance activity and responses. This makes it difficult for variations in contract application to occur and provides management with an excellent shield against union efforts to whipsaw supervisors one against another on grievance matters.

Finally, the labor relations function must be assigned adequate authority for handling grievances. If department heads or supervisors are permitted to go their own way on grievances, against the decision of the labor relations office, the contract administration program soon will be rife with inconsistencies. At that point, a union with an effective grievance system will move to capitalize on the confusion and take several critical cases to arbitration, using management inconsistency in applying the contract as damaging evidence before the arbitrator.

Training for Contract Administration

As part of its preparation to maintain an effective grievance procedure, the management team should be given basic instruction in the principles of contract administration. The training should cover many of the areas treated in this article and, while first-line supervisors are the most critical group for instruction, all levels of management can benefit.

There are several reasons for this need for training. One is that the union normally provides similar training for its stewards. Supervisors often feel they are at a disadvantage in dealing with stewards on grievance matters if they are less familiar with the contract and its procedures. A common notion among supervisors, particularly under a new contract, is that a union steward has more time for and interest in becoming thoroughly familiar with the agreement than they do. Consequently, formal training in grievance handling is critical in alleviating concerns among supervisors and in making them feel equal to the task when they deal with union stewards.

A second reason for grievance training is the need to develop basic contract administration skills. While handling an employee grievance is not normally a complicated problem, it does require that the supervisor apply certain principles carefully. If the supervisor has not been instructed in the need for helping to maintain the integrity of the management grievance program or in the methods of investigating a complaint thoroughly before giving that significant initial response, a lax attitude and critical mistakes obviously can result.

A final reason for training stems from the arbitration mechanism at the end of the grievance procedure. If the grievance is not resolved internally and goes to arbitration, the supervisor and other management officials usually are the key witnesses in the hearing. Supervisors make much stronger witnesses when they understand the total process, feel confident in their ability to handle grievances properly, and understand the union's role. A supervisor thus equipped through training is much less likely to wilt under a union attorney's cross-examination on the witness stand.

The individual who provides training in grievance procedures is important only to the extent that the person's expertise is assured. The instruction can be provided by the labor relations office if it possesses the requisite skills in knowledge and teaching. Many health organizations prefer to use outside specialists to provide the training. This not only guarantees competence but an outsider often can enhance the importance of the grievance system in the eyes of supervisors and managers. Common sources for such training are the American Arbitration Association, the Bureau of National Affairs, the American Hospital Association, or the industrial relations department or business school of any major university. The programs typically last two days and cover both grievance procedures and arbitration.

Evaluation of Management's Performance

The members of the management team must be made aware that handling employee grievances constitutes a full-fledged part of their job function. As such, it should be made clear to them that their performance in contract administration will be evaluated.

A major reason for evaluation is to help ensure commitment to the contract administration program. Managers should be informed as to the standards of evaluation. This knowledge will demonstrate that contract administration is considered important by top administration. A frequent problem under a new contract relationship is that some managers tend initially to assign grievance handling the status of a minor, additional duty they will deal with if they can find time. This attitude soon produces lapses and inconsistency in management responses. Evaluation puts the management team on notice that grievance mistakes can be costly both to the organization and to the person responsible for the poor handling.

There are two basic tools for evaluating supervisors' grievance performance:

1. Information and observation that demonstrate that the supervisor is consistently following the basic rules of grievance investigation, response, and follow-up are highly useful. These rules are enunciated more fully in the later section on *Principles of Grievance Handling*. Much of this evidence should appear in the supervisor's grievance reports.
2. The quality of information and grievance decision making that appears are critically important when cases reach higher levels of appeal. The quality of a supervisor's performance in dealing with decisions before or below the written grievance level is analyzed through the monitoring system. This is discussed in the section on *Monitoring Grievance Procedures*.

In short, the team should know that individual managers are expected to be familiar with the language and intent of the contract, follow the principles of grievance handling in complaint investigation and response, and make consistent and effective decisions when the case falls within their jurisdictions.

THE CONTRACT GRIEVANCE PROCEDURE

There are many ways in which a contract grievance procedure can be written. While this section reviews some common aspects, the most important point is that every part of any grievance procedure is designed to serve a particular function. Specific functions can be lost or distorted if the management team does not identify and implement the formal grievance structure properly. A sample grievance procedure is provided in Appendix 24-A.[5]

Definition of a Grievance

A critical and essential building block for any complaint procedure is the concept of the term *grievance*. Put another way, this issue could be stated as a question: What can be grieved under the procedure? The most common approach is to define a grievance as an alleged violation, misinterpretation, or misapplication of the terms of the contract. Under this form of *closed* definition, if an employee has a complaint it will be given the title grievance only if it involves an issue in the contract. While management may decide to listen to complaints, only grievances may be taken into the

formal mechanism. If management fails to distinguish clearly that an employee problem is considered a grievance only when the issue is covered by the contract, the worker may become frustrated later when advised only then that administration has decided the matter is not grievable.

The reason for stressing the notion of contract grievance is significant. The terms of the contract represent areas where management has agreed to limitations on its authority. If issues not in the contract are grievable to arbitration because management has developed a practice of permitting any complaint to be grieved under the procedure, an arbitrator may end up expanding the contract beyond the clauses negotiated at the bargaining table.

Some contracts encourage such problems by using an *open* definition of a grievance: any contract matter or personnel policy that has caused employee dissatisfaction. Sometimes referred to as the clinical approach, this means that almost anything can become a grievance, whether or not the issue is in the contract. The recommendation here is that such open definitions of grievance should be avoided. At the very least, if an open definition is used, the arbitration clause should state emphatically that only grievances over issues covered by the contract can be submitted to arbitration.[6]

This emphasis on formal grievances is not intended to discourage supervisors from entertaining and dealing with employee complaints. Rather, the concern is that management always should distinguish carefully between contract matters and issues excluded from the contract in evaluating the manner in which to respond to employee complaints. Some complaints will qualify as grievances, others will not.

Procedures for Initiating a Grievance

The first part of a grievance structure is the manner in which an employee raises a grievance. Many contracts specify this aspect of the procedure in two parts: an informal stage and an initial formal stage. The informal stage usually involves a discussion of the issue between the supervisor and the employee. Part of the purpose of such a step is to resolve as many problems as feasible at the lowest possible level in the organization, namely, at the level of employee and supervisor.

The supervisor's role in receiving a grievance at this level is discussed later. However, it is important to note here that management should insist that some discussion take place at the informal stage to maximize the opportunity to adjust the grievance as quickly as possible. If the supervisor accepts a grievance at the next, or formal, stage without any employee-supervisor discussion, that step soon will atrophy and subsequent grievances will start with a written, formal filing. In some grievances, a discussion is not useful. For example, the grievance may be over a pay matter not controlled by the immediate supervisor. The point is that if the contract provides a grievance stage for informal discussion before the issue is formalized and put in writing, management can gain the value of such a negotiated step only if it insists that the informal stage procedure is followed regularly by employees and union.

Another issue at this pivotal first stage is union representation. Again, the contract procedure should specify the union role. A common practice is to state in the agreement that the employee, "with or without his or her union representative," will present the grievance to the immediate supervisor. Some contracts specify that the employee can initiate a grievance and not be present, instead sending the steward to see the supervisor. This second approach is not recommended. The presence of the union representative, if the employee chooses, can be a valuable aid in evaluating the grievance. But it may be very significant to have the employee, as well as the steward, present. This is reflected in the judicial system of due process. If the employee can observe the full discussion and treatment of the complaint at this initial stage, the individual often will understand and accept the adjustment of the grievance better. This acceptance may be minimized if the employee receives only an abbreviated version of what was discussed from the steward.

A common second part of the initial stage is the filing of a formal grievance if no informal resolution is achieved. This often means nothing more than reducing the grievance to writing and transmitting it to the immediate supervisor.[7] (A sample grievance form appears in Appendix 24-B.)

Multiple Grievance Steps

Most grievance procedures provide for multiple levels of review. These steps or levels normally move from the immediate supervisor to successively higher levels of management. (See Appendix 24-A for an example.) The union usually establishes a hierarchy of review that brings correspondingly higher levels of its own structure into the process.

The purpose of multiple steps in a grievance procedure is twofold:

1. The multiple levels often can add objectivity to management's assessment of the grievance. As a simple example, if the real problem in a com-

plaint situation is a personality clash between the supervisor and an employee, the former may have difficulty giving the grievance a fair and objective investigation and response. The case can be evaluated more objectively by management at a higher level in the procedure.

2. Some grievances involve issues beyond the scope of authority and knowledge of the supervisor who is the first management step in the process. Multiple steps and different authority levels permit more appropriate management decision making and help ensure through review of policy issues that may have widespread impact across many departments of the hospital or other health organization.

Procedural Time Limits

Grievance procedures usually include various time limits for different actions. The function of these time limits is to assure that both union and management treat grievance matters promptly. The first usually is the period in which an employee must initiate a grievance claim. At this point, the time pressure clearly is on the employee either to grieve a matter or forget it. The reason for the pressure is to have grievance issues raised quickly so they can be investigated effectively and decided. The more time that passes between the event and the decision to grieve, the greater the risk that information will be lost, events distorted, or the problem will increase in magnitude.

Management should insist that this initial time limit is enforced. If grievances are entertained as timely after the limit has long passed, when the employee finally decides to grieve all of the function of the time pressure obviously will be lost. If a practice of ignoring the time limit develops, management could well lose its right to claim that any grievance is untimely.

Once an employee files a timely grievance, the pressure swings more toward management. The contract procedure normally specifies a response time for management to reply officially to a written grievance. At this point, the union normally will insist on rigid adherence to the time limit. Many contracts provide that if management fails to reply within the time limit, the grievance can be taken, or will go automatically, to the next step of the procedure, and ultimately can reach arbitration. The role of the time limit for management replies is to avoid delays caused by executives' inattention to grievance matters and to attempt to ensure that cases are resolved as efficiently as possible to the benefit of both sides. Most contracts also specify time limits on union decisions to continue the grievance to the next step of the procedure.

Contracts commonly provide that the time limits can be waived by mutual agreement. This reflects the understanding that special problems may sometimes arise that need flexibility in handling. It should be stressed, however, that most unions will not lightly consent to waive the time limits for a management response. Unions also are sensitive to preserving the basic integrity of the total grievance system, including its time constraints.

The Arbitration Clause

The end point of most contract grievance procedures is arbitration. In addition to the role it plays in stimulating the acceptance of grievance procedures at lower or earlier levels, arbitration serves another function: it threatens both sides with loss of control in adjusting a grievance. When the parties settle grievances internally, they bilaterally control the outcome or result. When an issue goes to arbitration, the arbitrator takes over control of the outcome. The arbitration mechanism and procedure are discussed in detail in other articles in this book. The brief focus here is on elements of arbitration provisions common to grievance procedures.

1. Arbitration clauses normally are written so that either side can invoke the process unilaterally after the grievance procedure steps have been exhausted. This means that neither side can prevent a grievance from going before an arbitrator if no settlement is reached in the earlier steps.
2. The arbitration clause should specify how the arbitrator will be selected. A common practice is to stipulate an agency that maintains a list of qualified arbitrators, such as the American Arbitration Association or the Federal Mediation and Conciliation Service, and request a list of names—usually five or seven names. The parties then mutually select an acceptable arbitrator from the list, often by alternatively striking names till only one remains.
3. The clause should establish clearly the limits of the arbitrator's authority in reaching a decision. As indicated earlier, a common approach is to limit the arbitrator to deciding only issues within the terms of the contract. (The sample grievance procedure in Appendix 24-A illustrates a common arbitration clause on this point.) The clause also should state whether the award is binding on both parties or merely advisory in nature.
4. The clause commonly states a time period within which the arbitrator must issue an award and how the individual will be paid. A 30-day time limit is

typical, with each party paying half of the arbitrator's bill. The notion of equal shares of the bill and of mutual selection of the arbitrator are considered key factors in ensuring the individual's neutrality.

This brief overview is designed to identify the most critical elements to be included in a contract arbitration clause. Such protections avoid snags and delays for both parties in the event that arbitration is necessary. It should be stressed, however, that when management and the union have both established a sound program of contract administration, the parties can use the grievance system to resolve most disputes and there should be little need for third party intervention in the form of arbitration.

PRINCIPLES OF HANDLING GRIEVANCES

The general goal of a grievance procedure is to provide a system that will resolve most employee problems quickly, effectively, and at the lowest possible authority level. The achievement of this goal assumes that most grievances will be within the authority of the supervisor to decide and that these first-line managers will be trained to apply certain basic principles in handling employee complaints.

The first aspect of achieving the goal is beyond the scope of this article because it relates to the distribution of authority in the total organizational structure of various types of health institutions. However, a general comment can be made here. Evidence shows that organizations with extremely high levels of centralized authority in their structure have higher rates of grievance activity.[8] In other words, if supervisors, who usually are the first to confront a grievance, have little authority and are unable to make most initial decisions, then most grievances will be formalized and will rise to unnecessarily high levels in the structure. As stated earlier, supervisors normally lack the authority to deal decisively with all grievances. But, if they have virtually no authority to make initial decisions, the grievance process soon will produce frustration among both supervisors and the union.

The second aspect of the goal of grievance procedures is focused on the methods supervisors and managers use to receive and handle employee complaints. These methods can be divided into several major categories.

How to Receive a Grievance

The most basic rule in receiving a complaint is to be a patient and careful listener. The supervisor must permit and encourage the employee to give a full account of what the worker feels is a problem. This not only serves as part of the device to gather information about the issue, but also helps the individual sense that these problems or concerns are important to the health care organization.

After letting the employee describe the problem, the supervisor should ask any questions that seem appropriate. These might include aspects of location or time of an incident, the names of other employees, or sources of information used by the employee. It is imperative that any supervisor questions are asked in a nonthreatening manner. The purpose of this part of the procedure is to let the employee provide a review of that individual's version of the problem. This statement does not mean, however, that a supervisor should permit an employee to be abusive or threatening in the presentation of a complaint. This meeting is to provide a forum for discussion, not argument. The employee understandably may be heated or excited, but the supervisor's authority and position must be respected.

The supervisor should be prepared to avoid responding defensively during this discussion and should not be antagonized or resentful that a grievance is being raised. If such a reaction develops, not only will this be sensed by the employee and inhibit resolution, but equally important it will result in the supervisor's failing to collect and evaluate information objectively.

Many labor relations professionals also feel that, during the discussion, the supervisor should ask the employee how the problem might be solved. This can help the employee realize the difficulty of the supervisor's position or identify that a solution sought might be much simpler than had been anticipated.

Investigation of Grievances

The purpose of grievance investigation is to verify information received during the discussion with the employee and locate additional evidence that might be useful in resolving the problem. The information obviously will vary from grievance to grievance. A number of health care labor relations professionals have found it convenient to have the supervisor use a checklist or investigation report form to ensure thoroughness for this part of the process. Typical questions (with space left on the form for written answers by the supervisor) include:

- problem or issue raised by the employee
- section of the contract involved
- institutional personnel policy involved
- time, location, and date of incident

- timeliness of the grievance
- facts needed to evaluate the grievance
- work area and grade, job, or classification of the employee
- other supervisors involved in the grievance
- other employees involved in the grievance
- cause of the grievance
- special behavioral or political factors
- possible responses or solutions to the situation
- raising of this issue with other supervisors (if so, establishment of any precedent)
- transmission of decision to the grievant
- response of the grievant

It should be evident from this list that a good grievance decision should not and cannot be a quick or snap answer. A supervisor must try to avoid mistakes in initial decisions. As noted earlier, there are steps in the procedure by which the grievance may be appealed beyond the supervisor. The union's expected role is to scrutinize the supervisor's handling of the grievances and point out any errors and omissions in the initial decision. Avoidable mistakes caused by poor investigation not only reflect poorly on the supervisor but also may prove costly in time or money to the health care organization.

Following the investigation, the information should be evaluated to determine the decision. The evaluation should specify whether or not the decision is within the supervisor's authority. It obviously is important that the training, contract review, and explanation for the management team alerted supervisors to which areas require decision making at a higher level. Normally, most grievance decisions can be made at the supervisor level. Examples of how grievance information should be evaluated are given in the next section.

Responding to the Grievance

After the grievance decision has been made, the supervisor must transmit the outcome to the employee. Attention should be given to the time limits in the contract for this response. The contract also specifies whether or not the supervisor's answer must be in writing. These provisions should be followed. The approach taken in the supervisor's response will vary according to the type of issue involved and whether the grievance is granted or denied.

When the supervisor is wrong, the error should be admitted and the grievance should be granted. The supervisor should transmit this information in a manner that is direct, straightforward, and objective. If the granting of the grievance requires some action on the part of the supervisor, the grievant should be told what the adjustment is and when the action will be taken. The supervisor then should follow up to see that the adjustment is carried out.

Two common errors in granting a grievance should be guarded against. One is for the supervisor to take an overly apologetic or submissive posture in admitting a mistake. This can result in the complainant's feeling that the supervisor now owes the employee a special favor because of the error. The other is that the supervisor must not show resentment that the employee won the grievance. This may cause the employee to fear a reprisal and can add tension to both the employee-supervisor relationship and the union-management relationship.

When the supervisor denies the grievance, the same objective manner should be used. The supervisor should explain the denial and try to help the employee understand the reasons behind the decision.

There are several common problems to be avoided. The supervisor never should gloat over the fact that the employee lost the grievance. This attitude makes accepting the denial even more difficult for the employee, who might seek to retaliate, to get even, or to save face. The supervisor should not try to pass the buck in the decision to some other authority. If the supervisor indicates the personal feeling that the grievance should have been granted, but that it was denied because of hospital policy, then the integrity of the management team will be eroded in the eyes of the employee and the union. The supervisor should not engage in excessive sympathy with the employee over the denial. Some supervisors end up convincing themselves that, even though a policy was correct and applied fairly, they owe the employee some effort to make up for a grievance denial. Again, the best overall approach is to use a calm, objective manner and help the employee understand the reason for the denial.

If the grievance and response (denial) are transmitted on a written form, it should include a brief summary of the supervisor's position and the contract provision involved. A careless assumption that the grievant has stated the issue adequately and has noted an appropriate contract reference can be dangerous. It may prove costly to discover later at an arbitration hearing that the issue on which management prepared its case was not perfectly congruent with the issue the grievant stated when the complaint was filed.

The Role of the Union Representative

The basic function of the union steward is to assist employees with grievance problems. A well-trained union representative can help prevent grievances by investigating claims to determine whether or not they have merit and should be carried forward to management. A significant part of how the steward performs in interactions with the supervisor is provided in the collective bargaining agreement.

The contract normally specifies that an employee is entitled to union representation during the presentation of a grievance. The supervisor should respect this right and not react in an antagonistic manner to the steward's presence or participation in the discussion at the grievance meeting. On the other hand, the supervisor should insist on a reasonable demeanor from the steward. Threats and abuse are not part of the right to present a grievance.

The contract also frequently specifies in either a union rights section or in the grievance provisions that the steward will be given a reasonable amount of time to process a grievance. The supervisor should become familiar with the organization's policy and the contract language and should be equipped with answers to these questions: (1) Can the steward use work time to present and discuss grievances? (2) Can the steward use work time for grievance investigation? (3) In either case, is there a limit on the amount of time? (4) Must the steward get permission from the supervisor to stop work and deal with a grievance? Answering these questions usually is a simple task learned in the supervisor's labor relations training and contract familiarization program. The obvious need for consistency is not reexamined here.

Much of this section has focused on the supervisor's role in handling grievances. The section concludes with a brief note on dealing with the supervisor's decision at the second or third level. These are referred to as appeal stages, where the initial decision is reviewed. The concepts of greater objectivity or improving employee (and union) or supervisor understanding of the institution's labor relations policy on the issue involved are two major reasons for this appeal mechanism. Two major points should be noted regarding the treatment of grievances at these higher levels.

First, in addition to the type of information sought and used by the supervisor in making a grievance decision, two other kinds of material should not be ignored at the higher (or staff) level. These are notes and information about the bargaining history of the contract's language, and the awards of arbitrators who have dealt with the particular type of grievance issue in dispute, either under this contract or under similar ones. The bargaining history may provide vital information as to the intention and interpretation of the clause pertaining to the grievance. The use of arbitration award patterns can help managers retain an objective perspective in evaluating the grievance dispute and aid in identifying and weighing the type of evidence that arbitrators would stress if the case were not settled internally.

Second, management should be cautious concerning any temptation to trade grievances at these higher levels. That is, each grievance should be evaluated and adjusted on its own, individual merits. Many grievances that reach higher steps in the procedure will be settled by the parties, and management should never hesitate to make fair offers of settlement at these levels if it is appropriate.[9] But if management grants one grievance in exchange for the union's dropping another, two potential problems arise. The first is that the union may develop a habit of loading the mechanism with extra grievances just so it will have opportunities to trade. The second is that the agreed settlements, since they were trade-offs not based on their actual merits, may become part of precedent that over time distorts the language and intended meaning of the contract. This distortion may be difficult to explain to an arbitrator later or to correct at the bargaining table in future negotiations.

EXAMPLES OF GRIEVANCE PROBLEMS

This section uses two areas of contract administration to illustrate the kind of systematic evaluation of a grievance the management team should follow in making a decision: discipline and transfers. The focus is on weighing the information collected through the grievance investigation form and using it in reaching a decision.

Discipline

This is one of the most frequent areas of contract administration activity for many supervisors. Among unions, there is general acceptance of the fact that management has the right to implement a system of discipline. Hospital contracts reflect this acceptance to the extent that more than 80 percent contain discipline provisions.[10] The most prevalent notion is that, to be proper, discipline should be for just cause. This really is the cutting edge for a discipline decision by a supervisor or manager. When is there just cause for a particular employee to be disciplined?

To answer this question, management should weigh the information collected in the grievance investigation against the guidelines established for effective discipline. If the evidence does not meet any appropriate guidelines, that failing must be weighed in the final decision. It should be noted that in the event a discipline dispute goes to arbitration, the arbitrator normally applies such tests.

Forewarning

Did the health care institution give the employee forewarning that the action committed would be subject to discipline? To meet this test, the evidence should show that the employee had been instructed in the rules and regulations of proper and improper activity. If there was a list of rules, the evidence should demonstrate that the employee was given the list and, preferably, that the list was reviewed with the worker at some point. If a new, additional rule was involved, the evidence should show that it was transmitted to the individual or posted on an employee bulletin board near the work area. The only major exception to the need to show forewarning are the few universally accepted offenses such as the commission of a criminal act on the job (stealing, rape, etc.), insubordination, or coming to work intoxicated.

Common problems that would weaken management's position and may rule against disciplining an employee should be evaluated. Is the book of rules so extensive that even most supervisors would be unaware of much of the content? Is there evidence to show that supervisors commonly violate the rule and, therefore, create the impression for employees that it is not important?

Penalties

The issue of expected penalties is another aspect of forewarning. If the personnel policy or rules specify a certain penalty for a category of offense, then that should be the penalty imposed. If the contract contains a specific clause on discipline, it should be checked to determine whether a particular penalty is in order. For example, the contract may list a sequence of penalties that must be followed before a suspension can be imposed for certain types of offenses. The evidence should show that, if discipline is merited, the employee should not be surprised at the ensuing penalty.

Investigation

Was there a thorough investigation of the incident that led to the discipline, and substantial evidence to show that the employee violated the rule? The evidence should show that a proper investigation was made of the incident and that the employee's involvement clearly and knowingly violated the rule. The evidence should not be susceptible to the possibility that the employee was simply in the wrong place at the wrong time and not a true participant in violating a rule.

Enforcement

Has the institution been lax in its enforcement of a particular rule? Even if the employee clearly was aware of the rule, does the evidence show that management had never enforced it or imposed the penalty even though numerous, known violations had occurred in the past?

If an old rule is to be reactivated, the proper procedure is to reannounce the rule and restate the penalty, including a clear declaration that beginning at some specific point the rule will be enforced. The evidence should not show that management met, decided the rule was important and should be enforced, and then "announced" this policy by penalizing the first offender to serve as an example to other employees. The evidence should not show that rules and their enforcement are unclear or unpredictable for employees.

Even-Handed Application

Has the institution applied the rules and penalties evenly and without discrimination? The evidence should show that when two different employees commit the same offense, both are penalized and both receive the same penalty. This concern reflects the need in the investigation to check with other supervisors or the labor relations office. Variations in penalties are accepted as proper by employees and the union only if there is a variation in the degree to which a rule was violated or if there is a measurable difference in the background of the offenders, such as the number of previous offenses.

Progressive Discipline

Was the penalty used as part of an effort to promote "progressive" discipline? Progressive discipline involves the concept that discipline will be used to promote correct work behavior, not for purely punitive purposes. This means that the evidence in a discipline decision should show that for multiple offenses, increasingly harsher penalties were imposed for each succeeding offense. The evidence also should show that when an offense occurred, the employee was notified of the violation and given clear instructions regarding the improvements or corrections required. If the evidence shows that a supervisor collected five offenses on an employee in a secret notebook, never advised the individual of any of them, then used the total in a decision to fire the worker, the supervisor rather than the employee should probably be disciplined.

In short, health managers should use these questions to test the evidence collected during the investigation of an employee's discipline grievance. If the principle of sound discipline practices has been followed and the contract and rules have been applied in a consistent manner, this should be clear in the evidence and the grievance should be denied. On the other hand, if the evidence shows that management has failed one or several of the tests, the grievance should be settled by a modification or complete elimination of the penalty.

Transfers

Another issue common in health organization contracts is in-house employee transfers, often with seniority as a factor in the decision. Of the hospital contracts analyzed in a 1977 study, 65 percent provided for transfer rights with some use of seniority.[11] This discussion limits its focus to the determination of voluntary transfer grievances, i.e., where an employee seeks to be transferred to another position in the health care facility. Again, the approach of the manager or supervisor is to collect and evaluate information related to the grievance decision. This effort is pursued through a series of questions about the matter.

Language of the Contract

Does the contract contain provisions on employee-initiated transfers? If the contract is silent on this issue, information on practices on voluntary transfers should be sought from other supervisors and the labor relations staff. The absence of any practice means the first decision to permit voluntary transfers may carry significant precedent and should not be made by a single supervisor without consultation. More importantly, if the supervisor is dealing with a complaint that other supervisors permit voluntary transfers, this information must be verified and weighed in the response, even though no grievance is involved.

Employee Eligibility

If the contract does have such a clause, is the employee eligible to request a voluntary transfer? The clause normally indicates the criteria for eligibility, but not always clearly. As noted, a commonly used criterion is seniority. Having identified seniority as an eligibility factor, the supervisor should measure the employee's seniority as appropriate under the contract—that is, by department, by work group, or by years in the hospital, according to what the agreement requires. Sometimes the employee's measure of seniority varies from the determination used by the contract. The supervisor should identify the weight to be given seniority in the transfer decision. The employee might define seniority as total years of service in the hospital, while the contract might specify that seniority is determined by time in the department where the employee now works.

Another employee eligibility criterion is ability to perform the work in the new position. Again, the supervisor should pinpoint how the contract defines "ability." Does it mean certified or licensed, as in the case of a nurse or technician? Does it mean the employee must have completed a training program or passed a test? Does supervisor evaluation enter the determination of ability? Either by specific contract terms or by practices developed under the transfer clause by other supervisors, the measure of ability to perform the work must be applied. If the evidence shows that the employee meets the stated seniority criterion and clearly is within the criteria specified for qualification, and those are the controlling factors listed in the contract, then the grievance must be evaluated accordingly. If the evidence demonstrates that the supervisor has added personal criteria to prevent a transfer, the grievance should be sustained.

Transfer—or Promotion

Is requested assignment a transfer, as the employee claims, or is it actually a promotion? If the employee's transfer request was denied because the supervisor regarded the move as a promotion, not a lateral transfer, the evidence should support such a distinction. The contract should be checked to determine whether promotion is defined. If it makes such a distinction, the supervisor should note whether the same procedures are to be followed for both transfers *and* promotions. The evidence should verify which procedure the employee used.

Posting and Time Limits

What are the requirements for posting vacancies and the time limits for initiating a transfer request? If the contract or personnel policy provides that all vacancies will be posted for employees for a specified time before a position is filled, the evidence should verify that management followed the procedure correctly. The evidence should not show that management verbally advised just a few employees, who then applied and got the transfers, resulting in the vacancies' never being posted.

In a similar vein, the evidence should verify that the employee filed the transfer request in a proper and timely manner. If the contract stated that a written request should be filed, the evidence should show the veracity of the employee's claim that other supervisors had an established practice of accepting nonwritten transfer requests in spite of what the contract or personnel rule specified.

As in the example on discipline, the approach for evaluating a transfer grievance is the same. Management must investigate and analyze the complaint before responding. The facts of events and conditions must be collected and the contract and practices identified. Only then can a sound grievance decision be made.

MONITORING GRIEVANCE PROCEDURES

The monitoring of contract administration and grievance activity in many ways is equivalent to reading the pulse of the union-management relationships in the health care facility. The information developed through the monitoring program can serve a number of useful purposes for the management team.

One function of grievance information is to provide data for contract negotiations. If grievances on certain contract clauses appear much more frequently than on others, this may indicate areas where the union will seek changes in upcoming negotiations. Conversely, if certain parts of the contract are causing excessive grievances, the management team may want to initiate proposals for change. The absence of grievance activity may indicate that a particular provision is working effectively. This evidence of success may provide data that can be used to counter union bargaining demands to change workable parts of the agreement.

A second function of grievance information is to keep abreast of the contract administration program. Periodic reviews of grievance investigation forms, coupled with staff administrators' regular discussions with supervisors and department heads, can identify how well (or poorly) the contract is being implemented. Any problems of inconsistency or misinterpretation can be located and dealt with before serious patterns develop. The labor relations staff should closely track how grievances are being resolved at the first level of the procedure, not waiting to become aware of them when they are appealed to the second or third stage or to arbitration.

A third function of grievance monitoring is the development of information to aid in evaluating the labor relations performance of supervisors and managers. Grievance data can provide some measure of general skills in human resource management. However, as is noted later, the use of raw grievance frequencies without certain qualitative measures can be misleading information performance indicators for supervisors or managers.

For any of these three purposes, the measurement of grievance activity should have both quantitative and qualitative components. The reason for this two-phase measure is simple. Grievances can have a number of different causes. Consequently, a qualitative evaluation of such activity can identify the particular factor that may have caused or contributed to variations in grievance rates.

Contract Clauses

Perhaps the most obvious cause of many grievances is the content of certain contract clauses or how they are written. For example, the clause may have represented a bargaining compromise that is dissatisfying to certain employees. They might be using the grievance route to register their complaint. Or the clause might have ignored a critical need to define certain key terms. This oversight can generate disagreements as the parties implement the contract.

Union Internal Political Activity

Grievance rates can be influenced by union politics. If stewards are running for higher union office or seeking to be reelected, the number of grievances that they can claim they processed may become part of a political campaign tactic. This may produce a higher grievance rate in some parts of the institution.

On a similar note, if the union is being threatened with competition from another labor group, grievance activity can become a pawn in the organizing drive. The incumbent union may try to use the grievance rate to prove its value to members of the bargaining unit.

Approaching Negotiations

The grievance rate may change as the parties prepare to renegotiate the contract. The union may have decided that an increase in grievances prior to negotiations will be read by management as a sign of major employee unrest that should be softened by contract improvements. Or the union might see a need to grieve certain parts of the contract to generate evidence that those sections should be changed at the bargaining table. In either event, the result can produce grievance rates higher than normal.

Union Grievance Policy

Some unions have a policy of writing up all grievances so that records can be kept easily or so their higher officials at step two or three can control griev-

ance resolution. Such a policy may produce the appearance of a high grievance rate because those that are resolved easily are counted along with those that actually do represent deeper disagreement.

Steward Training

An effective union sees to it that stewards understand the contract and are trained in their role as grievance representatives. Trained stewards are knowledgeable in the methods of investigating and evaluating grievances to determine whether or not the complaint is meritorious. Stewards then screen certain grievances; if some stewards have not been trained well, they may feel that their role is to aggressively grieve all employee complaints, both meritorious and nonmeritorious. Again, a high grievance rate will result.

Change in Environment

A major change in the work environment can cause an increase in grievances. For example, if a staff cutback occurs in a department, the increased use of contract layoff procedures may generate grievances. Major changes in equipment or organization can produce an abnormal grievance rate in the affected areas.

Supervisor Attitude

Instead of adjusting to the demands of contract administration, supervisors may react improperly in one of two ways. First, some may feel their employees' selection of a union is a personal affront. They overreact and take a hard-line approach to dealing with grievances and the union representative. A high grievance rate then develops. Second, other supervisors may sympathize with employees or ignore contract administration. The result is no grievances because the supervisors are giving in to employee complaints or continuing to handle them in their own way.

This list of major causes in variation of grievance rates is not intended to be exhaustive; rather, the effort is to focus on qualitative aspects. These qualitative assessments should be used with quantity measures in the application of information from grievance monitoring. Thus, if two supervisors in the same department have highly different grievance rates, it may mean that one has poor human resource management skills. Or, both may be equally skilled managers but the steward for one supervisor is embroiled in a campaign to become president of the local union. Or, one supervisor properly implements the contract, which produces grievances, while the other gives in on every employee request and has no grievances. The point is that grievance monitoring can produce evidence on all three elements: bargaining data, evaluation of managers, and consistency in contract administration. But to be used properly in these functions, the causal factors of grievance activity also must be measured.

CONCLUSION

As a final note, much of the quality measure of grievances is a function of the types of measurement used in the monitoring system. It is critical that grievance investigation forms be evaluated for their thoroughness and perception of issues. Data on issues that were resolved without the filing of written grievances must be collected systematically. Periodic checks on how supervisors and managers are implementing the contract terms, even though no employee complaints were perceived, must be maintained. With this kind of comprehensive monitoring of the contract and grievance system, the management team will be constantly aware of the pulse of the collective bargaining relationship.

This article provides health managers with an understanding of the concept of grievance procedures. It should be clear that, when used effectively, a grievance system can be a valuable tool for administration and a critical part of a successful union-management relationship. The implementation of a grievance program is not complex, but it does involve effort and constant attention. The main elements in achieving the management grievance system goals that are such a vital part of contract administration can be summarized as follows:

1. develop a management team approach to contract administration
2. ensure involvement in understanding the contract terms at all levels of management
3. train supervisors in the proper methods of investigating and handling grievances
4. establish a program of evaluation of the grievance performance of the management team
5. organize a system for monitoring the grievance and contract administration activities under the labor agreement

NOTES

1. The term *"rights"* dispute simply means that the issue involves an employee's rights as provided in the contract. This is contrasted with an "interest" dispute where the issue is what the new terms of a contract under negotiation should be.

2. The term *union* is used to designate any employee organization with which the health care facility has a collective bargaining contract. This includes professional associations, such as nurses. Experience has shown that the grievance procedures in negotiated agreements and the principles of contract administration under all types of employee organization contracts, both professional and nonprofessional, are essentially the same.

3. This trade-off is viewed as such an essential element of labor contract law that the Supreme Court has held the presence of a grievance arbitration clause *implies* a no-strike pledge, even though the contract does not contain a no-strike clause. *Gateway Coal Co. v. United Mine Workers,* 414 U.S. 368, 85 LRRM 2049 (1974).

4. Hervey A. Juris, "Labor Agreements in Hospitals: A Study of Collective Bargaining Outputs," *Labor Law Journal* (August 1977), p. 508.

5. The sample grievance procedure is intended only as an instructional example. It is not provided as a model or preferred contract provision.

6. For an opposing view on this point *see* Archibald Cox and Derek Curtis Bok, *Labor Law,* 7th ed. (Mineola, N.Y.: Foundation Press, Inc. 1969), p. 503; or B. M. Selekman, *Labor Relations and Human Relations* (New York: McGraw-Hill Book Co., Inc., 1947), pp. 144–145.

7. It should be noted in relation to the grievance procedure mechanism itself that employees are not obligated to raise contract grievances through the union. Section 9(a) of the National Labor Relations Act provides that employees may take grievances forward on their own, without union representation, and have them adjusted by management. The statutory limitation on such grievance adjustments is that they must not be in violation of the terms of the agreement. Many public sector bargaining laws duplicate this employee right. Under the NLRA, the union must be permitted to be present and observe the individual grievance adjustment.

8. David Peach and E. Robert Livernash, *Grievance Initiation and Resolution: A Study in Basic Steel* (Boston: Harvard University, Graduate School of Business, 1974).

9. Offers of settlement made during prearbitration stages of grievance discussions generally are not admissible as evidence in arbitration proceedings. *See* Owen Fairweather, *Practice and Procedure in Labor Arbitration* (Washington, D.C.: Bureau of National Affairs, Inc., 1973), pp. 236–237.

10. Precise data on the prevalence of all types of clauses in union contracts, including grievance procedure provisions, can be found in *Basic Patterns in Union Contracts* (Washington, D.C.: Bureau of National Affairs, Inc., 1979).

11. Juris, op. cit., p. 508.

ADDITIONAL REFERENCES

Walter E. Baer, *Grievance Handling: 101 Guides for Supervisors* (New York: American Management Associations, Inc., 1970).

Earl R. Baderschneider and Paul F. Miller, *Labor Arbitration in Health Care: A Case Book* (Holliswood, New York: Spectrum Publications, Inc., 1976).

A. Elliot Berkeley and Ann Barnes, eds., *Labor Relations in Hospitals and Health Care Facilities* (Washington, D.C.: Bureau of National Affairs, Inc., 1976).

Frank Elkouri and Edina Aspen Elkouri, *How Arbitration Works* (Washington, D.C.: Bureau of National Affairs, Inc., 1973).

Sally T. Holloway, "Health Professionals and Collective Action," *Employee Relations Law Journal* 1 (Winter 1976): 410–417.

Hervey A. Juris, "Nationwide Survey Shows Growth in Union Contracts," *Hospitals, JAHA* 51, no. 6 (March 16, 1977): 122.

Thomas A. Kochan, *Collective Bargaining and Industrial Relations: From Theory to Policy and Practice* (Homewood, Ill.: Richard D. Irwin, Inc., 1980).

Norman Metzger, *Personnel Administration in the Health Services Industry* (Holliswood, New York: SP Books Division, Spectrum Publications, Inc., 1979).

Richard U. Miller, *Hospital Labor Relations* (Madison, Wis.: University of Wisconsin-Madison, Bureau of Business Research, 1980).

Ronald U. Miller, et al., *The Impact of Collective Bargaining on Hospitals: A Three Stage Study* (Madison, Wis.: University of Wisconsin, Industrial Relations Research Institute, 1977).

John B. Miner and Mary Green Miner, *Personnel and Industrial Relations: A Managerial Approach* (New York: Macmillan Publishing Co., Inc., 1977).

Dennis Dale Pointer, *Unionization, Collective Bargaining and the Nonprofit Hospital* (Iowa City, Iowa: The University of Iowa, College of Business Administration, Center of Labor and Business Management, 1969).

William S. Rothman, *A Bibliography of Collective Bargaining in Hospitals and Related Facilities, 1959-1968* (Ann Arbor, Mich.: The University of Michigan–Wayne State University, 1970).

——————— , *A Bibliography of Collective Bargaining in Hospitals and Related Facilities, 1969-1971* (Ann Arbor, Mich.: The University of Michigan–Wayne State University, 1972).

——————— , *A Bibliography of Collective Bargaining in Hospitals and Related Facilities, 1972-1974* (Ithaca, N.Y.: Cornell University, New York State School of Industrial and Labor Relations, 1976).

Maurice S. Trotta, *Handling Grievances: A Guide for Management and Labor* (Washington, D.C.: Bureau of National Affairs, Inc., 1976).

U.S. Department of Labor, *Impact of the 1974 Health Care Amendments to the NLRA on Collective Bargaining in the Health Care Industry* (Washington, D.C.: Government Printing Office, 1979).

Dale Yoder and Herbert G. Heneman, Jr., eds., *Employee and Labor Relations* (Washington, D.C.: Bureau of National Affairs, Inc., 1978).

SAMPLE GRIEVANCE PROCEDURE

I. A grievance is defined as a claim by an employee or group of employees that there has been a violation, misapplication or misinterpretation of the terms of the collective bargaining contract.

II. Procedures

Step 1. (a) An employee with a grievance claim will, with or without the Union Representative, first discuss the matter with his or her supervisor. This discussion must take place within 10 work days from the time at which the employee became aware of the event giving rise to the grievance claim.

(b) In the event that the above discussion fails to resolve the grievance, the grievance will be reduced to writing on the approved Grievance Form and submitted to the supervisor. The supervisor must respond to the grievance in writing within 5 working days of receipt of the employee's written grievance.

Step 2. If the grievance is not resolved at Step 1, within 5 working days of the supervisor's written response, the Union may appeal the decision of the supervisor to the aggrieved employee's department director in writing. The department director must provide the Union with a written response to the grievance within 5 working days.

Step 3. If the grievance is not resolved at Step 2, within 5 working days of the department director's written response, the Union may appeal the decision of the supervisor to the aggrieved Hospital Director for Employee Relations in writing. The Hospital Director must provide the union with a written response to the grievance within 5 working days.

III. Arbitration

A. In the event the parties are unable to settle a grievance satisfactorily within 5 working days of the completion of the above procedure, either party may, by written notice to the other party, submit the grievance to arbitration.

B. Within five (5) days after the date of notice of submission to arbitration the parties shall attempt to agree upon an impartial Arbitrator and if they have not been able to agree upon a mutually acceptable person, they shall forthwith jointly request the Federal Mediation and Conciliation Service to submit a list of five

(5) proposed Arbitrators. From this list the party requesting arbitration shall delete one (1) name and then the other party shall delete one (1) name, then they alternatively as above delete the other two (2) names. The remaining name shall be that of the impartial Arbitrator.

C. The impartial Arbitrator thus selected shall be contacted jointly by the parties and shall be requested to proceed as expeditiously as possible in hearing the case and rendering a decision.

D. The expense and fees for the services of an Arbitrator shall be borne jointly and equally by the Company and the Union.

E. The parties shall attempt to agree upon a submission of the question to be arbitrated. In the absence of such mutual agreement, the written grievance as submitted shall serve as the submission agreement of the parties.

F. The Arbitrator shall not add to or delete any part of this Agreement and his authority shall be limited to matters arising out of the application or interpretation of this Agreement.

IV. Miscellaneous

A. There shall be no lockout by the Hospital nor shall there be any slowdown, strike or suspension of work by the Union or its members during the period of this Agreement.

B. Any of the time limits specified in the above Grievance Procedure may be altered by mutual agreement between the parties.

GRIEVANCE FORM
COUNTY HOSPITAL

Grievance No. _____

Distribution: Union President
  Supervisor
  Grievance Chairperson
  Employee Relations Director

Department _____

Job Assignment _____

Name of Grievant _____

A. Date Cause of Grievance Occurred _____

B. Contract Article(s) violated _____

C. Statement of Grievance _____

_____

D. Relief Sought _____

_____

_____ _____
Employee Signature   Date

E. Received by Supervisor

_____ _____
Signature   Date

F. Disposition by Supervisor _____

G. Union Response

_____   _____
Signature   Date

H. Received by Department Director

_____   _____
Signature   Date

I. Disposition by Department Director ——————————————————————————

J. Union Position

_____   _____
Signature   Date

K. Received by Employee Relations Director

_____   _____
Signature   Date

L. Disposition by Employee Relations Director ——————————————————

M. Union Position

_____   _____
Signature   Date

25. Arbitration of Patient Abuse Grievances: Proposed Changes

JESSE SIMONS

Prepared for American Arbitration Association Labor-Management Conference, May 25, 1976.

THE BACKGROUND

A two-and-a-half year study by the New York State Department of Mental Hygiene of 57,400 patients, served by 60,500 employees, revealed in 1976 approximately 600 reported instances of patient abuse—about one victim per 100 patients over 30 months. This writer estimates that for each reported instance of patient abuse, two incidents went unreported, so it can be concluded that there probably were three incidents per 100 patients over that period.

This study further revealed that only a third of the employees charged with patient abuse were dismissed. Of the greatest significance is that when the department sought dismissal it failed in about 60 percent of the cases. This means that of those who actually committed reported and palpable acts of patient abuse, 60 percent continued in employment. The overwhelming bulk of these patients, in the author's experience, are so sedated or so psychologically depressed, infantalized, or cowed as to suggest they are virtually incapable of any aggression, not to speak of assault.

Thus 60 percent, at least 350 employees (assuming no repeaters), and possibly as many as 1,500, based on this estimate of unreported cases (one instance or three instances of abuse per 100 patients every 30 months) are free to abuse the retarded, brain damaged, senile, and otherwise mentally incapacitated in state and private institutions. This is more than sufficient grounds for support of the concept that a new and

distinguishable system of arbitration of patient abuse cases is necessary and desirable, one that not only will measure the level of proof against an employee but also will make some modest contribution toward determining all of the facts and the truth involving acts of patient abuse, as was proposed in the author's 1976 *Working Paper*.

Informal comments of those directly involved in the study indicate that patient abuse has decreased marginally since 1976, yet still is near the level in the study.

The Need for Modification

Arbitration in most instances is the critical point at which the final determination is made as to disposition of an employee charged with or discharged for patient abuse. As detailed later, the author believes that conventional arbitration procedures regarding grievances of employees charged with patient abuse need modification so that they can deal more effectively with this type of problem.

There is substantial precedent for this view despite the fact that there are some who regard arbitration of disciplinary disputes as a single, unitary procedure, virtually the industrial analogue of the judicial procedure of the criminal courts.

Assuming that there is value or validity in such an analogy, it cannot be accepted that the concepts, criteria, and procedures of the two processes are wholly identical or interchangeable. If it is dubious

791

that any useful purpose is served in comparing disciplinary arbitration to criminal courts, nonetheless it certainly is well worth noting that the underlying considerations of equity, justice, and due process that must inform any system of criminal justice nonetheless are subject to elaboration and variation depending upon the particular circumstances in which they are intended to function.

The procedures, practices, and standards applicable to the trial of an adult are not considered appropriate where the accused is a juvenile. The same citizen accused of the same crime will experience a considerably different trial if, being in military service, the individual is within the jurisdiction of a military rather than a civilian court, or if the offense is heard in a domestic court, etc. There are a variety of courts, all with procedural similarities and significant dissimilarities, the latter tailored to fit perceived needs.

Similarly, there exists a variety of systems of arbitration, each of which has aspects that are virtually identical, and each of which has unique and distinguishing features—i.e., conventional ad hoc private sector arbitration; permanent umpireships with their unique, informal consultation; panels of arbitrators who rotate; "instant" arbitration as used by the International Longshoremen's Association and the West Coast shipping industry; two dispute systems of arbitration under the National Railway Labor Act—Public Law Boards and Adjustment Boards; fire and police interest arbitration under state laws; arbitration of teacher tenure disputes under the New York State Education Law, and the just emerging system of arbitration under federal law of grievance disputes under Executive Order 1149 and the Civil Service Reform Act of 1978.

It is not possible to catalogue here the full range of differences in this incomplete list of procedurally distinguishable systems of arbitration. However, it is sufficient to note that each system corresponds to recognized needs; each was created to meet particular circumstances, often sui generis; each was fashioned and refashioned over the years to permit solutions to specific problems or types of problems.

A Lack of Enthusiasm

Recognizing this situation, and dismayed by the results of conventional arbitration for disposing of charges of patient abuse by employees, the author wrote the working paper describing the inadequacies perceived in conventional arbitration of patient-abuse disputes. It proposed a variety of modifications to be applied solely, and on an experimental basis, in arbitration of this type of case.

Under the auspices of the American Arbitration Association, this paper was circulated to some 75 labor and management representatives and attorneys actively involved in this area of health care, both private and public. Subsequently, a day-long conference was held. A summary of the comments was circulated to the participants.

Labor and management representatives, with virtual unanimity, stated in private (with considerably more vigor than in public) that proper disposition of patient-abuse charges was a critical problem, that something ought to be done, and that a solution must be found, but neither party publicly evinced enthusiasm for the innovations proposed in the working paper nor any real willingness to experiment in an attempt to effectuate needed changes.

In the September 1978 issue of the American Arbitration Association's *Arbitration Journal* there appeared an article that at the least acquiesced in, if it did not endorse, the existing system of arbitration under the New York Department of Mental Hygiene's collective bargaining agreement, one that, in the author's view, fails to produce the results both parties have stated they urgently desire.

This has prompted submission of the 1976 working paper for inclusion in this volume for two reasons: (1) to present another view, one believed to be more realistic of this aspect of the health care world; and (2) to again place before the labor-management community proposals that could constitute the basis for remedial action and, at the very least, provide a context for consideration of alternate and innovative measures to improve the results of conventional arbitration of patient-abuse charges. The working paper follows.

THE PROBLEM

Unimpeachable evidence exists of a patient assault in a mental hospital, a home for the brain damaged or mentally retarded, or a home for the aged. An employee is dismissed or otherwise disciplined. The employee files a grievance. The case is taken to arbitration. Most often the grievance is sustained for lack of proof that the grievant committed the assault.

The process of determining the truth and reaching a proper decision is fraught with difficulties unique to this problem in this type of work situation.

The particular limitations of each type of resident in these institutions that disqualify them as competent witnesses suggest the need (a) to reexamine the adequacy of present arbitral procedures common in these cases and (b) to explore modifications of existing methods to help meet the problems peculiar to these circumstances.

The first problem is ascertaining just how a patient received a physical injury. Rarely is a weapon involved, although occasionally there are such cases. More common is the trauma suffered by a patient who "fell" from a bed or table, or "stumbled" against an object or down a staircase. The point of contention invariably is whether the patient "fell" or was pushed, "stumbled" or was shoved.

A more difficult problem arises in cases of sexual molestation or assault. Evidence of bodily injury is not always apparent. The employee may—and often does—charge that the "abused patient is venting the fantasies of a sick or senile mind."

But even after it is established clearly that a patient was assaulted or injured and was not the victim of an accident, and assuming that it is proved beyond doubt that the patient was attacked or molested by a person, how can it be determined who the offender is: another patient, an employee, and if an employee, which one?

Under ordinary circumstances, the direct testimony of the patient (the offended party) would carry great weight. But in the unique setting under discussion—institutions that house people whose minds are of uncertain accuracy—patient testimony is of less than usual probative value. Even if other inmates support the testimony of the abused patient, their word is subject to the same kind of doubt.

Other employees who may have witnessed the events are another natural source of evidence. But experiences reveal that generally the professional esprit de corps is far too powerful for any of these to "snitch," to turn against a buddy. The result often is testimony that, with depressing unanimity, consists of denials of having seen or heard anything untoward.

Under these circumstances—lacking the necessary preponderance of evidence to prove employee misconduct—the arbitrator has little choice but to sustain the grievant (the employee) or, in the public sector, deny the employer's "intent to discipline."

One of Two Roles for Arbitrators

Enough cases arising out of efforts to discipline employees charged with patient abuse have accumulated to suggest that, while the rights of the employees are well protected (as they should be), the rights of patients remain totally unprotected in the arbitration process.

Indeed, the repeated failure of existing procedures to distinguish guilty from innocent employees and to punish miscreants becomes an unwritten license for some to continue their abuse of patients.

In cases of this kind arbitrators can choose one of two roles:

1. They can decide their sole object is to determine guilt or innocence under conventional arbitration procedure and practice and go no further. They can ask "what is the truth?" and then simply wash their hands of further responsibility. The parties may do likewise.
2. They may decide, however, that inherent in their basic responsibility is the need to go beyond present procedures to develop better ways of protecting patients who are abused. Labor and management may be equally interested.

If arbitrators, labor, or management do not concern themselves with the plight of the voiceless, helpless residents of these institutions, then who will? Repeated failures to ferret out miscreant employees become an unintended, but nevertheless inevitable, encouragement to abusive workers to continue to victimize their charges.

In any event, whatever the ethical or professional imperatives of arbitrators may be, and irrespective of whatever has impeded health care labor relations personnel and their union counterparts from developing a more effective means of dealing with this problem, it certainly would seem proper and timely to explore modifications of present methods:

1. to protect unprotected patients
2. to establish norms and standards for employees in these institutions
3. to make more meaningful dispositions of these types of grievances via arbitration

Abusers: Basically Two Groups

Employees who become involved with patient abuse by no means are all of one mold. They are propelled by a variety of impulses whose understanding should be utilized in coping with these problems. For purposes here, and in the absence of any definitive study in the area, there appear to be two categories.

The first group consists of those who are driven by neurotic or psychotic compulsions. Although this article makes no claim to specialized knowledge about mental disorders, it is fair to assume that employees who assault or molest defenseless patients and who do so out of passion or in cold blood or with casual disdain are sociopathic or psychopathic.

The second group is made up of those who commit patient abuse because an immediate situation has become too much for them. Confronted with repetitive incontinence, fecal smearing, vomiting, refusal to eat, or tossing of food, the exasperated employee slaps, pushes, or punches a patient. While any abusive behavior is highly objectionable and constitutes disciplinable misconduct, in these cases the misconduct is understandable and probably amenable to correction.

These two groups are quite distinct. They require different handling at two points, at least: in hiring and in subsequent disciplinary action.

As to the first group, institutions should make every effort to exclude such disturbed personalities from being placed in custodial roles over helpless people. Their very position of authority is bound to stimulate their worst compulsions, compulsions that will be aroused further by the feeling that objectionable acts are almost certain to go unpunished.

If such a compulsive is hired, and subsequently is found to be engaged in acts of patient abuse, it is the responsibility of management (with arbitral sanction) to remove such an employee from the institution where the individual can perpetrate injury on a patient.

As to the second group, it must be assumed that their employment after careful recruitment, interviewing, and reference checks does not necessarily qualify them for their custodial responsibilities. In most cases, their limited background, social condition, and educational exposure makes it desirable that they be given greater and regular indoctrination, briefing, and guidance for their assigned tasks.

Arbitration That Protects Both Sides

While improved recruitment, employment processes, and education can do much to raise the quality of custodial relations, it still will be necessary to reinforce such procedures with graduated corrective discipline where patients are abused.

In the case of either group—those who are disturbed personalities and those who are normal personalities in moments of stress—it is necessary to develop arbitral procedures that will result in proper disciplinary steps while fully preserving due process for employees.

At present, an employer must show just cause for a discharge or some other form of discipline and provide proof as measured by a "preponderance of evidence" for this action. The concept of "preponderance" falls short of the more exacting standard set by courts in criminal trials, namely, "proof beyond a reasonable doubt."

Much of the rationale for the less demanding type of proof used in arbitration relates to the less punitive character of arbitral decisions: reprimands, warnings, fines, suspension, and dismissal, all of which fall far

short of either incarceration or capital punishment.

While it may be argued that recent vesting legislation softens the blow of discharge, since the dismissed will be entitled to certain residual benefits, nevertheless the firing of an employee for patient abuse makes it extremely difficult for the person to find reemployment in the health care field or, perhaps, in any field requiring personal relations. For that reason, any modification of procedures to protect the patient against custodial abuse must be balanced by modifications in procedures to protect the employees against disciplinary abuse.

It is suggested that to make a just and factually founded decision, arbitrators should have access to a body of data that, even under ordinary proceedings, rarely is as complete as in criminal proceedings because management lacks a professionally trained investigative unit such as is at the disposal of law enforcement agencies. Indeed, in the arbitral system, the basic reason why the parties have accepted the test of "preponderance of evidence" is because in the absence of police, refined detection techniques, subpoenas, and possible perjury prosecution, arbitration often must be satisfied with lesser evidence for its findings.

But even such lesser evidence too often is absent in custodial cases because of reasons cited earlier. And yet, if there is no way to develop decisive data in these cases, then the discipline that is needed both to protect the patient and to correct the custodial employee becomes virtually impossible.

Expansion of Factors Needed

To maintain a balance between the right of such employees and of patients, it is imperative to find ways to ferret out the miscreants while protecting their rights fully. In effect, this means an expansion of factors on both sides of the equation: on the one hand, obtaining more information and insight; on the other hand, giving greater guarantees of due process.

In cases involving the unusual setting under discussion, it is suggested that the following measures be considered as profitable and prudent responses to a perplexing problem.

The kind of evidence to be admitted should be widened. At present, arbitrators accept not only direct testimony, but also hearsay, affidavits, depositions, grand jury indictments, and statements of district attorneys. This range could be extended to include:

- Rorschach and other psychological test results derived from all those who were in or around the site of the alleged patient assault

- polygraph test results of the same universe of witnesses
- previous employment histories of employees present or close to the scene of the disturbance

These data, with clues to the truthfulness, psychological impulses, behavior patterns, and prior employment records of those present, could serve a double purpose. First, these bits and pieces that usually are missing from the jigsaw puzzle may make it easier to know the otherwise unknown necessary to reach a just cause decision. Second, a better understanding of the assaultive employee (assuming that a finding of assault has been reached) would be useful to the arbitrator in setting a penalty. Such data would be submitted in the conventional matter. Such data, like evidence, would be subject to *voir dire;* the witnesses would be subject to cross-examination.

With these added factors on one side of the equation, it is proposed that factors be added to the other side. The reasons, as sketched earlier, are to enable the accused to defend themselves against a widened array of evidence, some of which would be considered "soft" and, in other types of hearings, not required or admitted; and also to give the accused every possible due process right where the penalty could carry grave consequences should it be dismissal.

THE SUGGESTED PROCEDURES

Therefore, the following procedures are suggested:

1. The employees should be entitled not only to written charges specifying in detail the nature, time, place, etc., of the offense, but also to prior disclosure of the evidence and data to be used in the arbitration.
2. The alleged miscreant should be assured adequate professional representation in the arbitration hearings.
3. A transcript should be made of the hearing, with copies to the parties and the arbitrator.
4. The arbitrator should be required to describe and delineate the findings that constitute the grounds for ultimate decision.

In addition, management might consider employing one person for each facility (with 1,000 or more residents) who is expertly qualified in interviewing to obtain information promptly from those in or near the scene of the assault. Such experts should be prepared to testify from written reports on the results of their interrogations.

Management also might well consider adopting the policy employed in hospital operating rooms where a tort occurs. Where no positive identification can be made as to who committed the tort, all those in the operating room are deemed responsible and culpable and all may be suspended on the ground that each has committed a suspendable act of misconduct by concealing knowledge of the tort. Thus, employees in the ward where the assault occurred, or in the vicinity, might be suspended because of their silence, on the ground that that silence makes them accessories to the patient assault. Such an approach might provide testimony that otherwise would not be forthcoming.

The Sociological Factors

Most of the facilities housing the type of patients discussed here are in rural areas. The bulk of the work force is drawn from the immediate vicinity, usually small towns or villages. Consequently, those employed usually have strong, lifelong ties, having gone to grammar and high school together and socialized with each other for many years. Experienced arbitrators expect a degree of employee reluctance to testify against fellow workers. In this work environment, for the sociological reasons stated, the degree of employee reluctance to testify against others is considerably greater than that normally encountered.

Many union leaders are sickened by the patient assault allegations against employees they represent. On occasion, they know or have a good idea, as do the employees generally, who the culprit is. Often the union and the employees tend to be passive out of a sense of solidarity, putting the onus on management to identify the culprit. More usually, a union is motivated by three factors: (1) acceptance of employees' "stories" (as in other kinds of grievances), (2) concern about rejecting any employee's claim to a hearing; (3) simply limited capacity to do its own investigation.

Many decent union officers and attorneys want to weed out those who commit assaults on residents or patients. It is possible that they might, after some exploratory discussions, agree on these procedures, or a portion of them, on an experimental basis so long as these modifications are limited to the narrow and specific circumstances described.

In time, union consent to changes in traditional arbitration procedure could be achieved if the modifications are presented objectively as being in the interest of all parties. Formal union agreement to establishment of these procedural changes is possible even in the face of some opposition among rank-and-file members provided the leadership describes why this information should be introduced into arbitration if emphasis is placed on the correlative additional due process rights described.

The Reaction of the Courts

If these proposed procedures were adopted, whether formally or informally, it is believed that the courts would hold unions blameless of a charge of unfair representation brought by employees penalized under them. This belief is grounded in the conviction that the courts will recognize that because of the peculiar circumstances of the victims of assault, there exists a need to strike a balance between the justice to which employees are entitled and the justice to which retarded, brain-damaged, mentally ill, and senile persons residing in these institutions are entitled.

While effectuation of these procedures by formal agreement between the parties is, of course, the preferred method, the goals sought here could be further assured if certain of the suggestions were made a written condition precedent to employment, or if they were enunciated unilaterally by the employer as a rule or regulation.

In most states generally, and New York state in particular, case law reveals that following the "trilogy," state courts have been extremely reluctant to vacate arbitration awards because of the nature or quality of the evidence accepted by arbitrators.

26. How to Select a Labor Arbitrator

ROBERT COULSON

Reprinted with permission from *Labor Arbitration—What You Need to Know,* 2d. ed., by Robert Coulson, published by the American Arbitration Association, New York, © 1978.

· The selection of the arbitrator is very important. The arbitration provision in the contract will ordinarily describe how this is to take place. While participating in the selection process, each party should strive for the best possible arbitrator.

Arbitrators are chosen in various ways. Many contracts contain a reference to the Labor Arbitration Rules of the American Arbitration Association. The description here will relate to the way arbitrators are chosen under that system.

A survey of AAA cases indicates many cases in which unions and employers have only one or two arbitrations during the year. Representatives of such parties find it difficult to become familiar with the relative abilities of individual arbitrators. In contrast, other practitioners constantly engage in labor arbitration, and come to know the arbitrators very well. A selection process that is appropriate for the experienced labor lawyer may not meet the needs of the novice.

A tripartite system was once popular. Parties now find it unnecessarily complicated. Now most parties seem to prefer a system where the entire case is presented openly to one impartial arbitrator. Employees tend to distrust "executive sessions," suspecting that deals and compromises take place. The trend in grievance arbitration is toward single neutral arbitrators.

No part of the arbitration clause is more important than how the arbitrator will be selected. The predictability of arbitration depends substantially upon the knowledge, experience and understanding which the arbitrator brings to the hearing. Careful consideration should be given to the selection process set forth in the collective bargaining agreement.

Most labor arbitration provisions guarantee to the parties the right to participate in the selection of an arbitrator. The facts and circumstances of the case and full information about available arbitrators must be carefully appraised by the parties before the selection is made. Hopefully, this process results in an appointment of the best available arbitrator. It is just here that the *ad hoc* system displays its strength.

A technique for suggesting appropriate names to parties in connection with specific cases is contained in the AAA Voluntary Labor Arbitration Rules. This system relies heavily upon the judgment of the tribunal administrators of the 23 AAA regional offices.

As the New York State Supreme Court has stated, "The AAA, through a long and active career, has gained an enviable reputation for the absolute impartiality of its conduct in all the various steps and phases of arbitration—so much so that it is commonly designated by the parties in contracts providing for arbitration."

The reputation of the AAA is based substantially upon the informed judgment of its regional directors and their staff, who keep abreast of the activities of labor arbitrators in their own area. They know which arbitrators are available, and what kind of cases they are best suited to handle. Parties may require an arbitrator with special expertise. The appointing agency must recognize these differences in submitting a list of arbitrators. A small union arbitrating a discipline case against a local job-shop may need a list of arbitrators quite different from the list provided when a large union brings a more complicated case against a national manufacturer. The personal judgment of the tribunal administrator is an important element in satisfying the needs of the parties.

The judgment of an impartial administrator can help the parties in selecting an appropriate arbitrator. Lists of labor arbitrators sent out by AAA offices reflect a professional judgment exercised on behalf of the parties.

Some contracts do not specify what happens if the parties are unable to agree on an arbitrator. In these cases it is sometimes necessary to go to court. However, if both parties are agreeable, a list can be obtained, since at any stage, parties to a labor dispute can turn to the AAA for help. But it usually avoids trouble if the AAA is specified in the collective bargaining contract.

SELECTING THE ARBITRATOR UNDER AAA PROCEDURES

Unless parties have selected a different method, the American Arbitration Association adheres to the following procedure:

1. Upon receiving a demand for arbitration, the AAA acknowledges receipt and sends each party a copy of a specially prepared list of proposed arbitrators. In drawing up this list, the tribunal administrator will be guided by the union's statement of the nature of the dispute. Basic information about each arbitrator is attached to the list. Where parties need more information about a proposed arbitrator, the AAA is glad to supply such information on the phone.
2. The parties cross off the unacceptable names, and state their preference as to those remaining.
3. When the lists are returned by the parties, the AAA determines which of the arbitrators is most acceptable. That arbitrator is then contacted. The arbitrator is asked for available dates, and whether there is any reason why he could not act with impartiality in a dispute between the parties. The Code of Professional Responsibility included in this book serves as a guide for arbitrators as to what should be disclosed.
4. Where parties are unable to reach a mutual choice from a list, the AAA will submit additional

lists, but only at the request of both parties. If the parties still fail to agree upon an arbitrator, the AAA is authorized to make an administrative appointment. In no case is an arbitrator appointed whose name was crossed out by either party.

Collective bargaining agreements sometimes provide for tripartite boards of arbitration, without setting time limits for appointment of the party-appointed arbitrators. Even there, the AAA system can be used to give force and effect to the wishes of the parties.

Where the collective bargaining agreement provides for selection of an impartial member of a board of arbitration "by the American Arbitration Association," lists are sent to the parties or to the party-appointed arbitrators, in accordance with the terms of the contract or the wishes of the parties.

ARBITRATOR LISTS

The AAA submits lists in accordance with the particular arbitration clause involved. In addition, the makeup of the list reflects what is known about the past preferences of the parties. The regional office staff know that their performance will be judged by the quality of the lists that they issue.

The AAA serves as an expediting agency, offering to parties those arbitrators who are most likely to be mutually accepted and withholding arbitrators who would be rejected. The AAA acts as an agent for both parties, seeking to calculate in advance what kind of arbitrators will be acceptable to both. By having this judgment made by a local representative, a sensitive and informed service can be provided.

All of this effort results in a list of names. Then the responsibility for the selection process shifts to the advocates. What do parties need to know about a particular arbitrator submitted on a list? What information is it useful for the AAA to supply? What must be obtained elsewhere?

SOURCES OF INFORMATION

A copy of each arbitrator's biography is mailed out with the list being submitted. Each AAA office is prepared to provide parties with additional, contemporary information about the arbitrator.

This information is only a portion of what the parties need to know about the arbitrators on the list. They may also want to study recent awards that the arbitrators have rendered, particularly on similar issues.

The AAA publishes the monthly *Summary of Labor Arbitration Awards*. The service has reported over

4,000 decisions since its inception in April 1959. The name of the arbitrator and the issues considered are listed in each case. The names of the parties and the location of the hearing are also included.

This service can be especially useful to a party wishing to find out what a particular arbitrator has previously written on similar issues. By using the cumulative index, decisions listed for that arbitrator can easily be located. The full text of those opinions which are of interest can then be obtained directly from the AAA.

Similar summaries are published for arbitration cases in the public sector. These are entitled *Arbitration in the Schools* and *Labor Arbitration in Government*.

COMMERCIAL SERVICES AND OTHER SOURCES

Other publishers also report arbitration awards. These opinions are acquired from various sources. Many are obtained from opinions filed with the Federal Mediation and Conciliation Service. In addition, publishers sometimes receive labor awards directly from arbitrators. Arbitration awards rendered by permanent umpires are also published. The AAA maintains an Award Bank on microfiche which contains awards rendered by AAA arbitrators or sent in by arbitrators to provide a sample of their work.

Several commercial services, catering to management representatives, report the opinions of employers and their counsel who have used a particular arbitrator in prior cases. Subscribers receive such information by paying an annual fee.

Management groups maintain clearing houses of information about arbitrators, as do several of the management-oriented law firms. When a member of the network uses an arbitrator, he is asked to fill out a report form which becomes part of the material on file.

In the same way, unions and labor-oriented law firms collect information available to certain union officials. Sometimes, these networks are administered by the education directors of the international unions.

Active practitioners will search out whatever networks of information are available for their use. There are ways to find out what the people on your side think of a particular arbitrator.

EVALUATING AN ARBITRATOR

Information about a particular arbitrator will be obtained primarily from parties who have used that arbitrator on prior cases. What do they say about the arbitrator's ability, philosophy, and impartiality?

Is the arbitrator competent to understand the particular kinds of issues that will be involved in the case? Does the arbitrator have general competence to sift facts in an adversary proceeding? Does the arbitrator have the engineering or technical background sometimes required on certain issues? The experience in the particular industry? Is he too legalistic or not legalistic enough? Does he have a particular philosophy which would make him suitable for the issues of the case? These are some of the questions that will be asked about the arbitrator who is being selected. The parties are not concerned with making positive or negative judgments of the man's philosophy; they are interested in winning the case.

Evaluating an arbitrator is a matter of opinion; expertise in this area varies from advocate to advocate. Many practitioners believe that their experience and judgment make it possible for them to match the issue to the arbitrator.

One unfortunate by-product of the system is that practitioners become hesitant to accept an unknown quantity. The tried-and-true arbitrators are used again and again. The new arbitrator does not get chosen.

Introducing relatively unknown arbitrators into the process is not easy, although the situation is not as hopeless as is sometimes claimed. New men and women are coming into the profession, and are being accepted. Some are being accepted with surprising speed. Looking at the matter statistically, we do find a fair proportion of relatively young arbitrators. A 1976 survey indicated that of the arbitrators who served on AAA cases, an increasing number were new to the profession.

Since the mechanism for the selection of labor arbitrators is entirely dependent upon the free choice of the parties, mutually exercised, it may be necessary for a significant change in attitude to take place before a flood of new and younger arbitrators enters the field. Over one hundred new arbitrators obtain appointments each year. Some go on to become widely accepted by the parties. A difficult challenge faces them, because the parties are conservative about their selection.

The conservatism of the advocates reflects pressures placed upon union agents and company personnel to obtain arbitrators who will render acceptable awards. The unknown quantity of a relatively new arbitrator is particularly frightening to a person who is under such pressures. It may be necessary for parties to instruct their representatives to take a chance on new arbitrators on appropriate cases. Only in this way can the problem caused by a narrow supply of arbitrators be overcome.

For its part, the American Arbitration Association is constantly seeking out both new arbitrators and qualified arbitrators already on the panel who are being under-utilized, considering their experience and potential acceptability. A particular effort is being made to recruit female and minority arbitrators.

HOW ARBITRATORS GET ON THE AAA PANEL

Over many years, the American Arbitration Association has created a roster of arbitrators for use in all kinds of labor arbitration cases throughout the country. Almost 2,800 labor arbitrators are now on the panel, although most of the work is done by less than 600 active arbitrators. Virtually every labor arbitrator in active practice in the United States is on the AAA list.

How are new names obtained? How are candidates screened by the AAA? And how is the quality of the panel maintained?

The AAA's officers and regional directors constantly search for persons who have a good potential for being accepted as labor arbitrators. Men and women who are being selected on an *ad hoc* basis by parties in their local area are one source of talent. Many arbitrators come from government labor relations agencies. Others teach industrial relations or labor law at universities, or have a strong academic background in these fields. We often will encourage a professor with industrial relations experience to file an application to the labor panel. Attorneys or other professionals with a knowledge of industrial relations frequently achieve acceptability.

Few experienced labor arbitrators also serve as advocates for labor or management. Such service tends to reduce potential acceptability as a neutral. Therefore, practicing advocates are not encouraged to apply to the AAA National Panel.

When a nomination is received from a reliable source, an invitation is issued. In a few cases, an initial investigation is made to determine whether it would be a waste of time to process the candidate's application. It serves no good purpose for anyone to recommend that an inexperienced or inappropriate person be invited to apply.

LABOR PANEL DATA SHEET

The candidate is required to fill out a Labor Panel Data Sheet. This document has two parts. One part requires information identifying the candidate, present and previous business affiliations, and professional licenses. Information about education and previous employment is requested. While most labor arbitrators have a thorough academic background, often including legal training, there are some who have not completed college. Most labor arbitrators have had some prior experience with practical industrial relations, but there are some who have never worked in the field. Many arbitrators are lawyers; over a third are not. Most lawyer arbitrators do not represent clients in labor relations; some do. In short, the guidelines are far from rigid. Exceptions are found to each of them.

The second part of the Data Sheet can be more relevant. Each candidate is asked to give the names of four union and four management references. Letters to these references produce comments as to the candidate's character and abilities. A few letters repudiate the applicant. Other references, not willing to make critical statements in writing, telephone the AAA and say that they cannot recommend the person who used their names. Sometimes reading between the lines there is indication of a reservation about a candidate. A frank discussion on the telephone with the writer of such a letter will often clarify the situation.

ADMITTANCE TO PANEL

A candidate may be admitted to the panel on the basis of the application form and letters of reference. The decision to accept candidates is made administratively by AAA staff.

In about one-third of the cases, the reference letters will indicate the need for further investigation. Such investigations are carried out by AAA regional offices, and may result in a decision not to place the arbitrator on the labor panel.

When a person is placed on the panel, a card is prepared which describes the arbitrator's history and background. A copy of this card is sent to those regional offices which are likely to issue the arbitrator's name on lists to the parties. The card of an arbitrator with limited acceptability may be sent to only one office. In other cases, cards may be distributed to several regional offices.

Arbitrators sometimes lose their acceptability. A chronic illness or advanced age may cause parties to distrust the arbitrator's judgment. Sometimes arbitrators encounter temporary personal problems: alcoholism, nervous breakdowns and the like. These problems may require that the arbitrator's name not be submitted on lists.

Where an arbitrator habitually overcharges parties or is unable to arrange a hearing within a reasonable time, AAA offices may stop sending out his name on lists. Sometimes, regional directors will be directed to use such an arbitrator with caution. The AAA's responsibility is to serve the interests of the parties by providing them with the best possible arbitrators.

In other situations, a regional office will not send out the arbitrator's name on certain types of cases. The AAA relies heavily upon the judgment of its local regional directors, who must weigh the acceptability of each arbitrator on their panel against the needs of the parties in the particular case. The regional office has responsibility for preparing lists for cases, for selecting the best names for the parties and the issues. Regional staff are expected to know their panel members' experience, expertise in special fields, availability for quick service, billing practices, and their record of acceptability for particular companies and unions. This knowledge can be converted into a practical benefit to parties when lists are issued on pending cases.

EXPOSING NEW ARBITRATORS TO THE LABOR-MANAGEMENT COMMUNITY

The AAA recognizes its duty to try to help new arbitrators become accepted by the employers and unions who might wish to use them. Often, these arbitrators are fully qualified: their problem is to be better known.

New arbitrators must be introduced to the attention of potential users. This can be done in a number of ways. The AAA's Department of Education and Training sponsors labor-management conferences: new arbitrators are invited to attend so that they may meet some of the practitioners in the field. Awards by new arbitrators are published in the *Summary of Labor Arbitration Awards*, and the other AAA monthly publications.

Frequently, the AAA has cooperated with other agencies in encouraging the use of a selected group of arbitrators. This has been done in areas where there is a shortage of practicing labor arbitrators. Such programs have been carried out in many cities. Participants accompany more experienced labor arbitrators to hearings and write practice awards. The local labor-management community participates in these programs, getting to know the new arbitrators.

What can a new labor arbitrator do to become more widely accepted in his profession? The arbitrator must be able to perform competently in those cases for which he or she is selected. The arbitrator must become known favorably throughout the labor-management community. This must be done on a personal basis. If possible, an arbitrator should join appropriate professional groups. It can also provide good

exposure to publish articles in *The Arbitration Journal* and other recognized publications.

We recently asked a number of newly successful arbitrators how they gained acceptability. This is what they said:

- Try to get on educational programs; meet as many labor professionals as possible; have a means of making a living while waiting to achieve acceptability.
- There is no real answer to this. Everyone must do his own thing. Those with sense, taste and restraint may have a better chance if exposed enough in the better forums.
- Meet other arbitrators and lawyers at bar association meetings, IRRA, etc. Attempt to become listed by state agencies.
- Become known to the parties on a personal and professional basis. Participate in and attend conferences, education programs, etc. Assuming that one has the attributes to become a mainstream arbitrator, the key to acceptability becomes exposure.
- Become known to the practitioners in the field either by government service, seminar or conference participation. Exercise patience and fortitude.
- Patience. Be professional, both in the conduct of the hearings and in the writing of opinions and awards.
- The following are most likely to be useful: go to a good law school and then get to know the local fraternity of labor lawyers through the Industrial Relations Research Association and other labor meetings; run hearings effectively and spend a lot of time on early awards, without billing for full time spent on preparation.
- Demonstrate knowledge in field.
- Must have experience in the field. Have an opportunity for exposure and be listed.
- Parties hesitate to use a person they do not know. Perhaps the answer, partially, lies with the Association. Sessions where parties and arbitrators meet should be scheduled.
- Internships are a good way to break in, but hard to find. Steel industry is an excellent starting point.
- Be well versed in the field of collective bargaining. Have knowledge of federal and state labor laws.
- Serve as a neutral in mediation and gain trust and confidence of parties.
- Serve an apprenticeship with a busy arbitrator.
- Get experience representing both labor and management. Serve as an ad hoc fact-finder or

mediator. Make contacts with labor and management representatives and neutrals, through such organizations as IRRA.

- The candidate should somehow acquire training and experience in the labor relations field; should demonstrate an active and sincere interest in being an arbitrator and should write well reasoned, concise and timely opinions when selected.
- A great deal of voluntary work in all industrial relations areas, i.e., schools, committees, speaking engagements.
- Get exposure and experience in arbitration through whatever means are available.
- Become an apprentice to a full-time arbitrator.
- Meet the people who appoint arbitrators. Successfully complete a comprehensive training course.
- Develop knowledgeability in the field and exposure to parties.
- Serve an apprenticeship with accepted arbitrators.
- Work as an apprentice with an established arbitrator.
- Should have exposure and acquire a reputation for being fair and knowledgeable.
- Attend and participate in professional meetings with labor and management groups and publish relevant articles.
- Have experience, preferably as a neutral, in labor relations for at least ten years.
- Gain exposure in non-arbitral setting. When selected for the first few cases, be firm, courteous and demonstrate knowledge, understanding and integrity. Permit full development of the parties' cases. Write up the parties' arguments fully and persuasively, whether they win or lose.
- A labor arbitrator needs contacts and acceptability by those who select arbitrators. Any activity that increases an individual's exposure to those who select arbitrators and builds confidence in that person's ability helps that person gain acceptance.
- Extensive experience in field should be a prerequisite. An apprenticeship is most helpful for a neophyte.
- Be seen and be heard from. Exposure is important to let people know who you are.
- Teach, lecture. Can get wonderful training, serving as mediator or fact-finder in public sector.
- Listing by agencies; exposure at seminars; improve knowledge of labor relations.
- Continued auditing of arbitral hearings with accepted arbitrators provides personal contacts with

both parties. The parties will not select a neutral that they haven't had a chance to meet.

- Before becoming an active candidate, obtain maximum experience in labor relations with either management or unions. Thereafter, activity in professional organizations.
- Prepare professionally. Make contacts—work with an experienced arbitrator.
- Should have either academic training in labor relations or experience in the field. Good idea to attend arbitration conferences to meet representatives of the parties.
- Need initial experience as advocate in labor relations.
- Develop a working relationship with other arbitrators. Make sure that awards are well reasoned and consistent with arbitral authority.
- Try to apprentice with an experienced arbitrator.
- Candidates must attend hearings with an arbitrator. The arbitrator should take time to teach the candidate how to arbitrate and expose the individual to the parties.
- Acquire training and skills; establish neutrality.
- Develop contacts with labor and management at conferences, teaching situations, and any other occasions. Study the literature intensively, so the initial cases will be well handled. Attend hearings with an experienced arbitrator, to learn procedure and the types of problems that can arise. In addition to AAA and FMCS, state and local agencies use mediators and fact-finders. Any appointments of this nature, or teaching assignments gain helpful exposure and experience.
- Establish an identity in labor relations, preferably as a neutral. Make availability known to practitioners who are in a position to select an arbitrator. Become a member on all possible panels of arbitrators.
- Patience is a must. A new entry must have another source of income for at least the first five years. Expertise in a specific field, such as pensions, insurance, or industrial engineering would be helpful as an opening wedge. Issues in the public sector, particularly in the field of education, require specialized knowledge. This field appears a little more open as many of the experienced arbitrators apparently avoid public sector disputes because of the legislated limit on per diem. A good working knowledge of industrial relations practices is helpful, plus an understanding of contractual language and its interpretation.
- Publish.
- Gain experience with a professional position in labor relations that will involve working out prob-

lems with labor relations practitioners. Over a period of time, this builds into a reputation and creates willingness on the part of others to accept a candidate as a neutral who has demonstrated a potential for understanding decisional factors.

- Practice labor relations for labor and management.
- The reputation of being completely objective, with an open mind and for deciding fairly and independently.
- Write good decisions, one at a time.
- Assuming appropriate education and experience, seek a neutral position (i.e., college teaching, government agency) from which to operate.
- The first imperative is to become acquainted with the people who make the decisions concerning who shall serve as arbitrator. If you are unknown to them, you are going to wait a long time for an appointment.

- Attend training sessions sponsored by various agencies. Work in personnel department for either company or labor organization.

The AAA serves the labor-management community by maintaining an excellent list of arbitrators, by submitting carefully selected lists in accordance with the arbitration clause in each collective bargaining contract, and by introducing new arbitrators whenever the parties agree to use them.

The AAA system assigns personal responsibility for the selection of names to local regional offices. Accurate and objective information as to panel members is supplied by the AAA. The dissemination of subjective opinions as to arbitrators is better left to partisan agencies.

By learning where to turn for information about arbitrators, the practitioner can do a better job of selecting the right arbitrator for the case. Nothing in labor arbitration is more important.

27. The Disclosure of the Clinical Records of Adverse Mental Patient Witnesses in Disciplinary Arbitrations: The Case for Disclosure

THEODORE RUTHIZER and ARTHUR C. HELTON

While the problem of patient abuse is indeed a serious one, the grave threat to reputation and livelihood faced by an employee who is charged with commiting such an act is an equally serious matter, particularly if the accusers are mental patients. Consequently, an attorney for a charged employee is virtually obligated to seek disclosure of the clinical records of an adverse mental patient witness in the disciplinary proceeding in order to challenge effectively the patient's competence and credibility during cross-examination. The employer usually opposes disclosure, asserting a physician-patient privilege and the requirements of confidentiality. The New York courts, however, grant disclosure and hold that an arbitrator does not commit arbitral "misconduct" for purposes of vacating an award by refusing to hear the patient witnesses in the absence of disclosure.

In civil service disciplinary proceedings, basic fairness and due process require that when a hospitalized mental patient is called to testify, the charged employee must be given the opportunity to challenge the individual's testimonial capacity and to impeach the patient's credibility. This is so because a mental patient's history and diagnosis may have a direct bearing on the factfinder's determination as to whether the person has the mental ability to perceive, remember, and narrate events accurately; can distinguish between fact and fantasy; is delusional or feels persecuted; and/or has made prior false complaints of a similar nature.

The New York Court of Appeals[1] has recognized the importance of such disclosure by holding that newly discovered evidence of the mental illness of a key witness compelled a new trial because it bore upon the issues of his credibility and his capacity to perceive and remember events accurately. In a civil service disciplinary case, Camacho v. Iafrate, the New York State Appellate Division, Second Department, adopted the same reasoning as to the need for disclosure and held that disclosure of clinical records to the accused employee's attorney is required in order to ensure full cross-examination of adverse patient witnesses.[2]

In Camacho, the Appellate Division affirmed an order directing "that the attorney for the accused employee may inspect the medical records of the patient . . . should the aforesaid patient be called as a witness in the arbitration proceeding." The order further provided for the production of the records in any event, the arbitrator to decide upon their use. In ordering disclosure, the lower court pointed to the gravity of the risks at stake in a civil service disciplinary proceeding and held that the confidential physician-patient privilege had been waived by the employer and patient in initiating the disciplinary action:

. . . the privilege has been waived both by the patient in initiating criminal and disciplinary proceedings and by the institution in further prosecuting the matter, based on the very information upon which discovery is sought (*Koump v. Smith*, 25 N.Y.2d 287, (i.e. plaintiff commencing civil proceedings), *Bremiller v. Miller*, 79 Misc.2d 244, 360 N.Y.S.2d 178). The logic of the *Koump* case is even more compelling when the privileged party desires not merely civil redress against the party requesting the information, but seeks to impose severe administrative and penal sanctions on the party requesting the information. . . .[3]

Nor can the *Camacho* decision be discounted on the ground that in addition to the disciplinary proceeding, a criminal complaint had been lodged. Such a distinction would simply ignore the fact that in *Camacho* the court required disclosure exclusively in connection with the disciplinary arbitration (and not a criminal prosecution). That a criminal complaint had been filed was not a relevant factor in the decision.

Indeed, such a purported distinction actually would support the claim for disclosure as it would underscore the gravity of the interests at stake in a disciplinary proceeding. The risks include the prospect of a tenured civil servant's being dismissed from the job, being effectively barred from future government employment,[4] and suffering the stigma of having been terminated for acts of "patient abuse," which would be likely to foreclose employment opportunities in the private as well as the public sector.

The *Camacho* decision, moreover, has now been endorsed (*Bell*) by the Appellate Division, First Department.[5] In the *Bell* case, the disciplinary arbitrator refused to hear the testimony of the mental patient witnesses absent disclosure by the employer of the clinical records that had been subpoenaed. The court found that the arbitrator's refusal to hear the evidence did not constitute arbitral "misconduct" and explained that "[t]he confidentiality accorded the hospital records of mental patients by the Mental Hygiene Law is not absolute. In a proper case, it must yield to the needs of justice."[6]

Indeed, numerous other courts have agreed with the rationale in *Camacho* and *Bell*, rejected the claim of physician-patient privilege, and required disclosure of hospital records in civil service disciplinary proceedings. In *Stewart v. Merges*,[7] the court held that the accused employee needed patient medical records in order to present an adequate defense to the disciplinary charges. In requiring disclosure, the court left it to the arbitrator to inspect the records and to determine which ones were relevant for disclosure to petitioners. The court also ordered disclosure in *DiMaina v. Dept. of Mental Hygiene*,[8] and found that by offering the patient's testimony the employer (and the patient) had waived any claim to the confidentiality of the

individual's records. The court noted that an arbitration proceeding is not public and that the patient's identity could be sufficiently protected by the arbitrator. In *Bremiller v. Miller*,[9] the court once more rejected the employer's privilege claim and ruled that disclosure was necessary to challenge the credibility and testimonial capacity of the patient-complainant.

Furthermore, the courts have not hesitated to require disclosure in analogous circumstances. In *Board of Education v. Butcher*,[10] the Appellate Division rejected a claim of confidentiality (of students' records) in a teacher disciplinary proceeding, explaining that "[a]ny degree of confidentiality accorded to the students' records must yield to the appellant's right to prepare his defense to the charges made against his reputation and his competence in the profession." In *Davis v. Alaska*,[11] the United States Supreme Court rejected a claim of confidentiality (of juvenile court records) holding that the right of confrontation is paramount to the state's public policy of protecting a juvenile offender. The Court emphasized that the cross-examiner must be "permitted to delve into the witness' story *to test the witness' perception and memory*"[12] [emphasis supplied].

In all of the decisions, the courts have recognized that fundamental fairness and due process mandate that when a tenured employee's livelihood and reputation are threatened by charges as serious as "patient abuse," no witnesses should be permitted to testify without subjecting themselves to scrutiny as to what effect their mental condition and character may have on their capacity to testify and on their credibility.[13]

Nor is there any question as to whom such disclosure is to be made. In *Camacho*,[14] the Appellate Division, without reviewing the patient records, specifically granted full disclosure of the information directly to the charged employee's attorney without need for inspection by either the arbitrator or the court. In the event that the patient witness was not called to testify, the court provided for production of the person's records to the arbitrator to supervise disclosure. Numerous courts have agreed with the *Camacho* decision and determined that it is the arbitrator, rather than the courts, who if necessary should supervise disclosure.[15] This is with good reason since the arbitrator is the trier of fact and therefore best equipped to appreciate and balance the varied interests involved in a discovery application in a disciplinary arbitration.

The authors do not quarrel with the very serious obligation to investigate and, if appropriate, discipline employees for acts of patient abuse. They do take issue, however, with any notion that to facilitate such investigations there must be a trade-off of the due process rights of employees in order to reduce the ''difficulties of proof'' by which the authorities otherwise would be encumbered. The understandable abhorrence with which patient abuse is viewed should not tempt responsible persons to discount an employee's right to adequate notice, an effective opportunity to challenge the adverse evidence, and the right to put the accuser to the test of proof.

NOTES

1. *People v. Rensing,* 14 N.Y.2d 210 (1964); also *see McWilliams v. Haveliwala,* 61 A.D.2d 1032 (2d Dept. 1978); *People v. Lowe,* 96 Misc.2d 33, 36 (Crim. Ct. of the City of N.Y. 1978); *People v. Maynard,* 80 Misc.2d 279, 288 (Sup. Ct. N.Y. Cty. 1974) [witness' mental condition ''raises the question of the accurateness, perception, truthfulness and susceptibility to suggestion . . .''].

2. *Camacho v. Iafrate,* 66 A.D.2d 799 (2d Dept. 1978), affirming ____ Misc. 2d ____ (Sup. Ct., Suffolk Cty. April 12, 1978), appeal dismissed, 46 N.Y.2d 709 (1979). The lower court decision in this case is unreported.

3. Ibid.

4. *See, e.g.,* Sec. 50(4) of the New York Civil Service Law.

5. *Civil Serv. Employees Ass'n, Inc. (Bell) v. Director, Manhattan Psychiatric Center,* 72 A.D.2d 526 (1st Dept. 1979).

6. Ibid.

7. ____ Misc.2d ____ (Sup. Ct., Dutchess Cty. January 3, 1978). The decision is unreported.

8. *DiMaina v. Dept. of Mental Hygiene,* 87 Misc.2d 736 (Sup. Ct., Albany Cty. 1976).

9. *Bremiller v. Miller,* 79 Misc.2d 244 (Sup. Ct., Dutchess Cty. 1974).

10. 61 A.D.2d 1011, 1012 (2d Dept. 1978).

11. 415 U.S. 308, 319 (1974).

12. Ibid., 316.

13. *Brown v. Ristich,* 36 N.Y.2d 183, 190 (1975), is not inconsistent with this position. Involved there was the issue of whether unsworn testimony by a mental patient may be received in a hearing. In particular, no issue was ever raised as to whether patient records should be disclosed. Indeed, the court explained that a foundation must be laid to show that the patient ''has the ability to observe, recall and narrate, i.e., be retained in his memory . . .'' 36 N.Y.2d at 189. Surely, in order to lay such a foundation, there must be disclosed significant information regarding the patient's mental condition.

14. *See* n. 2, *supra.*

15. *See, e.g., Stewart v. Merges* and *DiMaina v. Dept. of Mental Hygiene,* at nn. 7 and 8, *supra.*

28. The Jargon of Labor Arbitration: A Glossary

ROBERT COULSON

Reprinted with permission from *Labor Arbitration—What You Need to Know*, 2d. ed., by Robert Coulson, published by the American Arbitration Association, New York, © 1978.

1. *Ad Hoc* **Arbitrator.** An arbitrator jointly selected by the parties to serve on one case. Many employers and unions believe that decisions are more likely to be fair and equitable if the arbitrator is chosen on a case-by-case basis. If both parties are satisfied with the arbitrator's ability, they may select him again for another case. The *ad hoc* system enables the parties to retain their freedom of choice.

2. **Adjournment of Hearing.** The arbitrator has the power to postpone a hearing until another time, at the request of either party (see AAA Voluntary Labor Arbitration Rule 23). If the arbitrator unreasonably refuses to postpone a hearing, a losing party may have grounds for vacating the award.

3. **Administrative Agency.** An impartial private or governmental agency which maintains panels of labor arbitrators. Administrative and appointing services can be obtained by an appropriate reference to the agency in the collective bargaining contract. The AAA is the only private agency in the United States. The Federal Mediation and Conciliation Service and various state and local government agencies also issue lists of arbitrators.

4. **Administrative Appointment.** The designation of the arbitrator by an administrative agency. Sections 12, 13 and 14 of the Voluntary Labor Arbitration Rules provide for administrative appointments in the event of impasse. When parties have failed to agree on a mutual choice from a list submitted to them, the AAA may make the appointment. Under expedited arrangements, the parties may empower the AAA to make the appointment without a preliminary submission of lists.

5. **Advisory Arbitration.** A system under which an arbitrator is selected to render an award which recommends a solution to the dispute. Advisory arbitration has been used most frequently in public employment, often to help resolve bargaining impasses.

6. **Affidavit.** A statement in writing made upon oath, before a notary public or other authorized officer. Such statements are sometimes submitted and received as evidence in labor arbitration hearings. Section 29 of the Voluntary Labor Arbitration Rules states that "The Arbitrator may receive and consider the evidence of witnesses by affidavit, but shall give it only such weight as he deems proper after consideration of any objections made to its admission." Where the witness is available and could be cross-examined, the arbitrator may refuse to accept such an affidavit.

7. **Appeal.** A proceeding for obtaining a review of a decision. In arbitration, the right to an appeal is not available. An award may be challenged in court by a motion to vacate. In labor arbitration, such motions are generally based upon allegations that the arbitrator exceeded his authority.

809

8. **Appointment of Arbitrators.** Arbitrators are chosen by the parties in accordance with the procedures designated in the arbitration clause in their collective bargaining agreement. Most provisions call for the appointment of a single arbitrator. But some agreements still provide for the designation of "party-appointed arbitrators," who then select a single, neutral arbitrator to act as chairman. If the party-appointed arbitrators or the parties themselves are unable to agree upon an arbitrator, a court may make the appointment on the motion of one of the parties. The parties can avoid the necessity of going to court by designating an administrative agency in their contract.

9. **Arbitrability.** Does the moving party have a right to arbitrate the dispute? Procedural arbitrability often turns on whether specified steps have been carried out prior to the initiation of the arbitration. Substantive arbitrability concerns the scope of the arbitration clause. The arbitration agreement should describe the kinds of disputes it covers, and what prior steps must be completed before a party has the right to demand arbitration. Questions of arbitrability may be determined by an arbitrator or in court, depending upon the arbitration provision in the contract and the applicable law. Under Sec. 301 of the Taft-Hartley Act, arbitration will be required under an arbitration clause if the parties cannot be said "with positive assurance" to have excluded the subject from arbitration. *United Steelworkers v. Warrior & Gulf Nav. Co.,* 363 U.S. 574 (1960).

10. **Arbitration Clause.** That part of a collective bargaining contract which provides for the use of arbitration as the final step of the grievance procedure. A reference to the Voluntary Labor Arbitration Rules of the AAA establishes all the procedures necessary for arbitration.

11. **Arbitrator.** A person who is given the power to decide a dispute between parties. The labor arbitrator is usually selected because the parties have confidence in his ability to interpret collective bargaining agreements, and have faith in his impartiality. When selected, the arbitrator participates in a system of contractual self-government which the parties themselves have created. The arbitrator is insulated from legal responsibility for his actions. Under AAA administration, the arbitrator acts subject to the provisions of the Voluntary Labor Arbitration Rules or the Expedited Labor Arbitration Rules.

12. **Arbitrator's Authority.** The power of an arbitrator to hear and determine a dispute is derived from law and from the agreement of the parties. The extent of authority can be determined by examining the arbitration agreement.

In *Steelworkers v. Enterprise Wheel & Car Corp.,* Justice Douglas defined the authority of the labor arbitrator as follows: "When an arbitrator is commissioned to interpret and apply the collective bargaining agreement, he is to bring his informed judgment to bear in order to reach a fair solution of a problem. . . . Nevertheless an arbitrator is confined to interpretation and application of the collective bargaining agreement; he does not sit to dispense his own brand of industrial justice. He may of course look for guidance from many sources, yet his award is legitimate only so long as it draws its essence from the collective bargaining agreement. When the arbitrator's words manifest an infidelity to his obligation, courts have no choice but to refuse enforcement of the award." 363 U.S. 595 (1960).

13. **Award.** The decision of an arbitrator in a dispute. The arbitrator's award is based upon the testimony and arguments of both parties. In labor arbitration, the arbitrator's reasons are generally expressed in the form of a written opinion which accompanies the award. The opinion will analyze the evidence and the issues raised by the parties. In a growing number of cases, parties are requesting labor arbitrators to issue a summary award, disposing of the issue but dispensing with much of the *dicta*. This procedure can greatly reduce the cost of arbitration.

14. **Award upon Settlement.** An award made at the request of both parties, incorporating terms of a settlement made by parties.

15. **Back Pay Awards.** Under most arbitration clauses, an arbitrator may order reinstatement of an employee who has been discharged or suspended without just cause. The arbitrator may reduce the penalty by reinstating the grievant, without back pay, or may reduce back pay to the extent that the employee has been receiving compensation from another job or from unemployment compensation funds. Some contracts restrict the arbitrator's authority to fashion a remedy.

16. **Bias.** An arbitrator has a duty to disclose any facts or circumstances that might create a presumption of bias or might disqualify him from serving as an impartial arbitrator. Under Section 17 of the AAA Voluntary Labor Arbitration Rules, such a disclosure is required. The Code of Professional Responsibility for Arbitrators of Labor-Management Disputes is also applicable.

17. **Binding Effect of Arbitration Award.** An arbitrator's award is final and binding upon both parties. Labor arbitration awards may be confirmed in court. A judgment entered upon such an award may be enforced in other states. In practice, most labor arbitration awards are accepted by the parties; litigation is rare.

18. **Breach of Contract.** The failure to abide by the legal obligations of a contract. A labor grievance is an alleged breach of contract by the employer. But the union can file a claim under the grievance and arbitration procedure without abandoning its continuing rights under the contract. The United States Supreme Court has stated that "Arbitration provisions, which themselves have not been repudiated, are meant to survive breaches of contract, in many contracts even total breach. . . ." *Drake Bakeries v. Local 50, American Bakery & Confectionery Workers,* 370 U.S. 254 (1962).

19. **Brief.** A written statement in support of a party's position, which is submitted to an arbitrator either before or after the hearing. In labor arbitration, briefs are generally used to cite court decisions, prior arbitration awards and the language of the contract. The filing of such briefs tends to prolong the proceeding and to increase the costs of arbitration. Briefs should be used only when they are necessary for the arbitrator's understanding of the case. They are expensive to prepare and time-consuming to read.

20. **Challenge of Arbitrator.** A party in arbitration can challenge the impartiality of an arbitrator, with the aim of stopping his appointment or of removing him from office. This right is afforded by Section 17 of the Voluntary Labor Arbitration Rules of the AAA. In practice, such challenges occur very seldom in labor arbitration because the parties know the arbitrators and participate in the selection process.

21. **Closing Argument.** A statement customarily made by each party at the close of an arbitration hearing. The arbitrator will always allow the parties to make such a summation if they so desire, but may impose time limitations. Parties frequently use the closing argument to emphasize the points upon which they wish to base their case. Such a presentation leaves their position fresh in the mind of the arbitrator.

22. **Collective Bargaining.** Negotiation between an employer and an organization representing a bargaining unit of workers, to create or to make changes in a contract concerning the terms and conditions of employment. Once negotiated and set down in writing, this contract becomes a collective bargaining agreement. In such agreements, the arrangement for settling disputes concerning the interpretation or application of contract provisions is most frequently a grievance and arbitration procedure.

23. **Compensation of the Arbitrator.** The fee the arbitrator receives as remuneration for his services. Labor arbitrators in the United States are usually paid on a per diem basis, with reimbursement for travel expenses. The parties generally share such costs equally. When a list is sent to the parties by the AAA, the arbitrator's per diem is disclosed. The arbitrator charges the parties for the entire time he spends on their case. It is possible to reduce the cost of labor arbitration by expediting the hearing procedure, eliminating transcripts and briefs, and by permitting the arbitrator to file a summary award. Under the Expedited Rules of the AAA, labor arbitrators are expected to charge only for the hearing day, substantially reducing the overall cost to the parties.

24. **Compulsory Arbitration.** A system under which parties are compelled by law to arbitrate their dispute, sometimes found in statutes relating to bargaining impasses in the public sector. Laws in several states have adopted various forms of compulsory arbitration for employee groups such as policemen and firemen.

25. **Concurrent Jurisdiction.** A situation where one of the parties may be authorized to seek a remedy from the courts, from the National Labor Relations Board or from arbitration. For example, the collective bargaining agreement and the National Labor Relations Act may protect related rights. If a worker is discharged without just cause, his grievance may be subject to arbitration. But if he were discharged for union activities, he may have a right to file an unfair labor practice charge with the NLRB. A question may arise as to which tribunal should have primary jurisdiction. To cope with this conflict, the NLRB has determined, in the *Collyer* case, that the Board will withhold its jurisdiction in favor of arbitration if certain conditions exist. Where an award has been rendered on such a case by an arbitrator, the NLRB may defer to it.

26. **Confirming the Award.** A labor arbitrator's award can be converted into a judgment by a court. To complete this process, the winning party must make a motion before the court to have the award confirmed. If all legal requirements have been met, the court will enter judgment. This procedure is seldom necessary in labor arbitration, where parties customarily comply with the requirements set forth in the award.

27. **Death of an Arbitrator.** If a neutral arbitrator dies after being appointed, a successor must be mutually selected by the parties involved or by the administrative agency which appointed him. Section 18 of the Voluntary Labor Arbitration Rules provides for the replacement of an arbitrator.

28. **Default.** If a party fails to appear at an arbitration hearing, after due notice, the arbitrator may hear testimony and render an *ex parte* award. Under Section 27 of the AAA Voluntary Labor Arbitration Rules, an award may not be entered solely upon default. The arbitrator must require the party present to submit proof. Such an award can then be enforced in court.

29. **Delegation of the Arbitrator's Authority.** The authority of the arbitrator to decide a case cannot be delegated without the consent of both parties. The arbitrator should obtain the written agreement of the parties when he needs to consult outside experts to verify certain facts. The parties have selected the arbitrator for his ability to understand the case and to exercise his judgment. They do not expect him to rely upon the expertise of another person. Again, this subject is dealt with in the Code of Professional Responsibility.

30. **Delivery of Award.** The award is usually mailed to the parties at their last known address by a representative of the AAA or by the arbitrator. If there is no contrary provision in the arbitration clause of the contract or in the applicable rules, the award can be delivered personally or sent by registered or certified mail, or in any other manner prescribed by law.

31. **Demand for Arbitration.** The initial notice by one party to the other of an intention to arbitrate under the arbitration clause in their contract. This document may be in the form of a letter, as long as it contains the required information. The demand should identify and describe the grievance. It should contain the name of the grievant, the union and the employer, a copy of the arbitration clause, and a statement of the remedy or relief being sought. A copy of the demand should be sent to the opposing party, and another filed with the AAA.

32. **Deposition.** The taking of testimony under oath, to be used as evidence in an arbitration. Although arbitrators can order that such depositions be taken, the procedure is seldom necessary in labor arbitration. Testimony is given more weight if it is presented in person by the witness.

33. **Discovery.** A procedure invoked before a court trial to inform a party of the facts in a dispute in order to facilitate the attorney's preparation of his case. Discovery is seldom used in labor arbitration, where both parties have participated in the earlier grievance procedure. In rare situations, it may be necessary for adequate preparation. In these cases, discovery can be required by the arbitrator.

34. **Disqualification of Arbitrator.** An arbitrator may be disqualified for misconduct. The fact that an arbitrator failed to disclose a personal relationship with the lawyer for one of the parties might constitute sufficient grounds for disqualification. However, if the other party knows of the relationship and fails to object, he may have waived the right to challenge the award.

35. **Duty of Fair Representation.** The obligation of a union to safeguard the rights of all members of the bargaining unit. This duty is imposed by Federal labor law. Some union constitutions provide remedies for members who are dissatisfied with the union's handling of their grievances. The union's duty to represent its members in a fair manner does not require that every grievance be carried to arbitration. In the event of a failure to provide fair representation, both the union and the employer may be liable.

36. **Duty to Disclose.** The arbitrator must reveal any fact or circumstance detracting from his ability to render a fair and just award. When notified of his selection, the arbitrator should disclose anything of this nature. If anything develops later which was not previously known, the arbitrator should reveal it at once to the AAA administrator or to the parties. See the Code of Professional Responsibility.

37. **Enforcement of Arbitration Agreements.** Courts customarily enforce agreements to arbitrate. The most influential decision was *Textile Workers Union v. Lincoln Mills,* where the United States Supreme Court enforced an arbitration clause in a collective bargaining agreement, finding legislative support in Section 301 of the Taft-Hartley Act.

38. **Examination before Trial.** The examination of witnesses before the trial of a case. Most authorities consider this procedure to be incompatible with labor arbitration, where the grievance procedure gives both parties a prior opportunity to determine the circumstances of the case and to confront witnesses.

39. **Exclusionary Clause.** A provision in the collective bargaining agreement which states that specific subjects are excluded from the arbitration process.

40. Execution of Award. The signing of the award by the arbitrator, with whatever formalities may be required by law. Statutes differ as to their requirements. In some jurisdictions, the signature must be acknowledged. These technical requirements are known to each AAA regional office, so that awards issued in that state can be put in proper form.

41. Expert Witness. A person with special skills or experience in a profession or with a recognized knowledge of a technical area.

42. Federal Mediation and Conciliation Service (FMCS). An independent agency of the Federal Government, established under Title II of the Labor-Management Relations Act, 1947, to mediate and concilate labor disputes in any industry affecting commerce, other than in the railroad and air transportation industries. One of the major responsibilities imposed on the FMCS by the Labor-Management Relations Act of 1947 is the prevention of labor-management disputes. The FMCS provides governmental facilities for labor contract mediation. The FMCS also maintains a panel of arbitrators.

43. Functus Officio. An arbitrator who has completed his task by rendering an award has no further authority. The doctrine of "functus officio," as applied to arbitration, recognizes the termination of an *ad hoc* arbitrator's authority after rendering his award. Under most laws, only the parties or a reviewing court can authorize resubmission to the original arbitrator.

44. Grievance. A complaint, made on behalf of an employee by his union representative, against an employer, alleging failure to comply with the obligations of the collective bargaining contract. The grievance may result from disciplinary action against the employee. Any complaint relating to an employee's pay, working conditions or contract interpretation is generally considered to be a grievance. A grievance may also be a complaint which an employer has against the union.

45. Grievance Arbitration. The submission of labor grievances to an impartial arbitrator for final determination. Sometimes called arbitration of "rights." Grievances may involve a wide variety of issues. The arbitrator determines the meaning of the contract and clarifies and interprets its terms. Jurisdiction of the arbitrator is sometimes restricted to those disputes which involve the interpretation or application of the contract. Increasingly, arbitrators are required to resolve issues involving the application of various public labor laws, such as unfair labor practices and charges of employment discrimination. Arbitration, in most contracts, is the last step in the grievance procedure.

46. Grievance Procedure. The steps established in a collective bargaining contract for the handling of complaints made on behalf of employees. A grievance procedure provides a means by which a union or an individual employee can submit a complaint, without disrupting the production process or endangering the employee's job. The primary intent is to settle the dispute as soon as possible.

These procedural steps vary from contract to contract. For example, a grievance may be taken by the shop steward of the aggrieved employee to his supervisor. If no settlement is reached, it may be appealed through successive steps. The grievant may be represented by various union officials. Smaller companies tend to have shorter grievance procedures, consisting of two or three steps. In larger companies, or in multi-plant contracts, there may be grievance committees with union-management representation, followed by joint boards. These systems should be reviewed, from time to time, to assure that they are functioning properly.

47. Hearing. The presentation of a case in arbitration. The fundamental requirements for a valid hearing are that the arbitrator be present, that the persons whose rights are affected be given notice of the proceedings, and that the parties be heard, and allowed to present all relevant and material evidence and to cross-examine witnesses appearing against them. These rights are fully protected in the Voluntary Labor Arbitration Rules of the AAA.

48. Impartial Chairman. An arbitrator who is the impartial member of an arbitration board. Such a chairman may be appointed for the duration of the contract, in which case he is called a permanent chairman. The term is also used to designate the neutral member of an *ad hoc* arbitration board chosen by the mutual consent of the parties. In such a case, the other members of the tribunal may be party-appointed arbitrators, each having been chosen by one of the parties. Usually, it is understood that such persons are partisan.

49. Impasse. A deadlock in negotiations. When collective bargaining has failed to produce an agreement between the parties, the parties must decide whether to bargain further. Sometimes a strike is called to produce pressure for a settlement.

In some cases, the parties may be willing to use arbitration to help resolve some of the remaining issues. And in public employment, laws are being passed to require that the parties use a variety of settlement techniques, including mediation, fact-finding (with or without the power to make recommendations for settlement), cooling-off periods with various time limits enforceable by court injunction, or final and binding compulsory arbitration.

50. Individual Rights. Those rights which individual employees still retain despite the designation of a union as their exclusive bargaining agent. An employee may sue his union if he believes it has failed to represent him fairly, but the employee does not usually have an absolute right to have his personal grievance taken to arbitration. Although the union is the representative of all the employees, union interests rest with the majority. The union must be free to decide which grievances should be pursued.

51. Injunction. A court order restraining a person or an organization from performing an act which would result in serious injury to the rights of another person or group. An injunction may require a specific action. Any violation of an injunction is punishable as contempt of court. In rare instances today, injunctions may be used to order a union not to strike. They were issued more often before the passage of the Norris-LaGuardia Act in 1932, which limited the powers of federal courts to issue injunctions. A number of states adopted similar statutes. Injunctions may also be used in national emergency disputes under the Taft-Hartley Act, postponing a strike for a period of up to eighty days.

Under the *Boys Markets* case, courts have been given the power to enjoin wildcat strikes in situations where the union has obligated itself to arbitrate the dispute.

Though injunctive relief is seldom used, some collective agreements give an arbitrator the power to hold an expedited hearing of any claim that the no-strike or no-lockout clause has been violated. If the claim is found to be valid, the arbitrator may enjoin the violation.

52. Interest Arbitration. The arbitration of the terms of a collective bargaining contract. When contract negotiations reach an impasse and cannot be resolved by collective bargaining, the issues in dispute may be submitted to voluntary arbitration. Several industries have traditionally included provisions for arbitrating new contract terms in their contracts. Even after a strike, the parties may resort to voluntary arbitration.

Although unions and employers have been reluctant to accept arbitration as a means of settling interest disputes, in recent years there has been renewed interest in the idea.

53. Interim Award. Most arbitration statutes in the United States require that arbitration awards be final, and that they determine all of the issues submitted. But where the parties have given expressed or implied consent for an interim award, arbitrators may be authorized to determine some but not all of the issues. Interim awards are sometimes rendered by labor arbitrators in situations where further studies must be made by the parties before the remaining issues can be determined.

54. Judicial Notice. The recognition of a labor arbitrator of certain facts in a case as being self-evident or of common knowledge. A process whereby arbitrators may recognize laws of other jurisdictions, the official acts of governmental agencies, the common practices in collective bargaining, and all other such matters which are so well-known that a party should not be put to the burden of having to establish them by proof.

55. Jurisdiction. The legal power or right to exercise authority. The jurisdiction of the labor arbitrator is defined and limited by the agreement of the parties. From time to time, it has been necessary for courts to decide whether the issues in a dispute lie within the jurisdiction of the arbitrator. But this issue can also be submitted for determination by the arbitrator.

56. Labor Dispute. A conflict which may include a dispute between parties to a collective bargaining agreement over the terms (interests) or the interpretation of the terms (rights) of their contract. The Norris-LaGuardia Act of March 23, 1932, at § 13(c), defines a labor dispute as follows: "The term 'labor dispute' includes any controversy concerning terms or conditions of employment, or concerning the association or representation of persons in negotiating, fixing, maintaining, changing, or seeking to arrange terms or conditions of employment, regardless of whether or not the disputants stand in the proximate relation of employer and employee."

57. Laches. Unreasonable delay in asserting a right which might prevent the enforcement of that right. Arbitrators may consider laches when selecting a remedy to a dispute. An arbitrator might rule that a party who has "slept on its claimed rights" for too long has lost its claim to those rights.

58. Liability of Arbitrator. A labor arbitrator is immune from civil or legal action for any award he may render. Nor is the arbitrator required to explain the reasons for his award, or to testify as to his performance. Without such immunity, a losing party could expose the arbitrator to the hazards of a lawsuit.

59. Locale of Arbitration. The city where the arbitration is held. In labor arbitration, hearings are generally held at some point that is convenient for the union and the employer, often at the plant or a nearby hotel conference room. Reference to AAA rules in the contract permits the AAA to fix the locale when the parties cannot agree. When an arbitrator is appointed, he will decide where and when the hearing is to be held, in accordance with the mutual convenience and desires of the parties.

60. Management Rights. Clauses often appear in collective bargaining contracts which reserve management's right to operate the business. Many labor arbitration cases have involved the definition of "management rights." Some contracts go into some detail in specifying these rights. But disputes nevertheless arise as to whether those rights have been exercised reasonably or whether they have been abandoned through contrary past practice.

61. Mediation. The participation by a third party in dispute negotiations for the purpose of helping the parties resolve their disagreement. The success of this technique depends on the skill of the mediator. The mediator may meet with the parties separately, or may arrange joint conferences. He tries to facilitate the bargaining process by clarifying the issues and helping the parties to discover areas of possible compromise. The mediator may offer suggestions, but he cannot force either party to accept a solution. Sometimes, the mediator may recommend that the parties agree to arbitrate the remaining issues.

62. Merging Seniority Lists. The combining of seniority lists when plants or departments within a company consolidate. Various methods for resolving such seniority issues have been developed, involving principles such as length-of-service, follow-the-work, or the surviving-group. Recently, an increasing number of cases have involved mergers intended to eliminate "islands of discrimination."

63. Merits of a Case. The substantive issues involved in an arbitration case. In its *Trilogy* decisions, the United States Supreme Court ruled that judges are not to consider the merits of the case when they are determining arbitrability or enforcement. Judges should not substitute their judgment for that of the arbitrator.

64. Modifying the Award. In labor arbitration, the arbitrator's award is the terminal point in the resolution of the grievance. Courts are extremely hesitant to order a rehearing by the arbitrator, or to modify or correct the award. Some arbitration statutes authorize the arbitrator to correct miscalculations of figures or mistakes in the identification of the parties. But in correcting such errors, the arbitrator cannot reexamine the merits of the decision.

65. Motion to Compel Arbitration. A form of legal action used by the moving party to petition a court to compel the other party to arbitrate. Where a motion to compel is deemed necessary, the supporting affidavits and documents should provide evidence that there is an agreement to arbitrate, that a dispute exists, and that the opposing party has refused to arbitrate. The court cannot consider the merits of the controversy.

66. Multiple Grievances. The filing of two or more unrelated grievances by the union, to be heard in a single hearing before the same arbitrator. The union's right to file multiple grievances depends upon contract language and past practice.

67. National Academy of Arbitrators. An organization founded in 1947 to foster high standards of knowledge and skill on a professional level among those engaged in the arbitration of industrial disputes. The National Academy is not an agency for the selection or appointment of arbitrators. At its annual meeting, lectures on various aspects of arbitration are delivered, which are published by the Bureau of National Affairs under the title, "Proceedings of the Annual Meeting of the National Academy of Arbitrators."

68. National Labor Relations Board (NLRB). An independent Federal agency created by Congress in 1935 to administer the National Labor Relations Act of July 5, 1935. Under the National Labor Relations Act as amended in 1947 by the Taft-Hartley Act, the NLRB has two primary functions: first, to determine through agency-conducted secret ballot elections which union is to be the exclusive representative of employees for the purpose of collective bargaining; and second, to prevent and remedy unfair labor practices by both labor organizations and employers. Whenever possible, the Board will defer to the parties' existing grievance and arbitration procedures in situations where contractual and unfair labor practice rights are both involved.

69. **National Panel of Labor Arbitrators.** A list of some 2,800 persons skilled in labor arbitration, who are available through the twenty-three regional offices of the AAA to serve as arbitrators throughout the United States. Arbitrators are carefully screened by the AAA for impartiality before being appointed to the panel.

70. **No-Strike Clause.** A clause in a collective bargaining contract under which the union agrees that it will not strike during the life of the contract. In 1957, the United States Supreme Court held, in *Lincoln Mills,* that an agreement to arbitrate grievances in a collective bargaining agreement is the "quid pro quo" for a union's promise not to strike.

71. **Notice of Hearing.** A formal notification of time and place of a hearing. The Rules of the AAA provide that the arbitrator may fix the time and place for each hearing. In doing so, the arbitrator respects the mutual convenience and desires of the parties. Under AAA Rules, such a notice must be mailed at least five days in advance.

72. **Open-End Grievance Procedure.** A grievance procedure which has as its final step the right to strike. Such agreements are increasingly rare. Most contracts now provide for final and binding arbitration.

73. **Opening Statement.** Brief statement made at the opening of a hearing by each advocate, intended to inform the arbitrator of the nature of the dispute and of the evidence they intend to present. It is usual for the claimant to be heard first, but the arbitrator may vary this at his discretion.

74. **Opinion.** A written document in which the arbitrator sets forth the reasons for his award. In most labor cases the parties want the arbitrator to explain his reasoning in order to give them some guidance for similar situations that may arise under the contract. But in other situations the parties may ask the AAA to notify the arbitrator that no opinion will be required. This can substantially reduce the cost and delay of arbitration.

75. **Party-Appointed Arbitrator.** An arbitrator chosen by one of the parties. It is common for such arbitrators to act in a partisan manner. Party-appointed arbitrators are being used less frequently in labor arbitration, as parties recognize the many ambiguities and problems created by their participation. Most modern grievance arbitration systems provide for a single, neutral arbitrator.

76. **Past Practice.** A course of action knowingly followed by a union and a company over a period of time. Where such a pattern exists, the workers involved come to regard it as normal. Past practice becomes significant in arbitration whenever one of the parties submits evidence of it to support its claim. In the *Warrior & Gulf* case, Justice Douglas stated: "The labor arbitrator's source of law is not confined to the express provisions of the contract, as the industrial common law—the practices of the industry and the shop—is equally a part of the collective bargaining agreement although not expressed in it."

77. **Permanent Arbitrator.** An arbitrator who is selected to serve under the terms of a collective bargaining agreement for a specified period of time or for the life of the contract. The duties of the permanent arbitrator are defined in the contract.

78. **Precedent.** The concept that prior decisions serve as a rule which must be followed. Prior opinions are not binding upon a labor arbitrator even though they may be considered in determining the case. Prior decisions on the same point may, of course, be treated as precedent by the parties. This is often done in permanent umpire systems. But the general rule in *ad hoc* arbitration is that the arbitrator is not bound by earlier decisions on the same issue. On the other hand, the arbitrator will often find such opinions relevant and analogous to the case under consideration.

79. **Prehearing Conference.** A meeting of the arbitrator or an AAA representative with the parties prior to the actual hearing, in order to establish appropriate procedural ground rules or to identify the issues to be determined. Such conferences are seldom necessary in labor arbitration cases. Ordinarily, the grievance procedure has afforded the parties ample opportunity to become familiar with the case and to attempt to settle it. It is customary for arbitrators to encounter the issues for the first time at the initial hearing.

80. **Public Employee.** A person who is employed by a municipal, county, state, or Federal agency. Public employees are subject to various public employment relations laws, which generally have the effect of restricting their freedom to engage in work stoppages, often by replacing the right to strike with various impasse settlement mechanisms.

81. **Recognition Clause.** A clause in collective bargaining contracts which commits the employer to dealing with the named union as the bargaining agent for the employees in the unit. Such a commitment is re-

quired by the National Labor Relations Act, which requires an employer to recognize the union that represents a majority of the employees in an appropriate bargaining unit.

82. Reinstatement. The return of a discharged employee to his former job. The crucial issue in discharge cases is whether the discharge was for just cause and whether the penalty was fair and reasonable. An arbitrator may reinstate an employee with full pay for the time lost, or may reduce such back pay by various amounts, or may reinstate the employee with no back pay. Under some contracts, the arbitrator's power to fashion an appropriate remedy has been limited by the parties.

83. Reopening of Hearings. An arbitrator may reopen a hearing on his own motion or at the request of a party. The arbitrator may wish to reopen the hearings to have the parties clarify the issue or present further testimony. A party may request a rehearing for the presentation of new evidence. Before granting such a request, the arbitrator should offer the opposing party the opportunity to present any objections. If reopening the hearings would delay the award beyond the 30-day time limit specified in the AAA Rules, or beyond the contractual time limits, the matter may not be reopened unless both parties agree.

84. Residual Rights. The residual rights doctrine gives management the benefit of the doubt concerning rights and powers on which the contract is silent. An arbitrator will examine the contract to determine whether the employer had agreed to reduce the extent of its traditional management rights.

85. Res Judicata. A legal doctrine to the effect that once an issue has been determined it need not be litigated again. The purpose of the doctrine is to prevent repetitious law suits. Once a case has been properly determined in arbitration, its issues are considered to be *res judicata* as between the parties.

86. Respondent. In labor arbitration, this term is used for the party against whom the demand for arbitration is asserted. Ordinarily this is the employer.

87. Right to Counsel. Each party to a labor arbitration has a right to be represented by an advocate. This right is recognized in the AAA Labor Arbitration Rules. There is no requirement that parties be represented by an attorney. Unions and employers are sometimes represented by lay representatives, persons experienced in labor arbitration.

88. Rotating Panels. A panel of arbitrators selected on a rotating basis for the life of the contract. By this means, parties to a contract seek to expedite the selection process, while still using arbitrators who are familiar with their contract and relationship. If such rotating panels are administered by the AAA, the arbitrations can be held under its Rules.

89. Rules of Evidence. Courtroom rules of evidence are not applicable in arbitration. Under AAA Labor Arbitration Rules, the arbitrator determines whether evidence is relevant and material. He will determine when hearsay may be admitted, when to accept a copy instead of the original document, and when to admit evidence of oral agreements. Before making a ruling on contested evidence, the arbitrator will listen to the parties' arguments on the issue. Ordinarily, labor arbitrators are willing to accept evidence submitted by either party, for whatever probative value it may have. That attitude should not be abused. An arbitrator is unlikely to be persuaded by irrelevant or immaterial evidence. It is unwise to encroach upon the arbitrator's patience.

90. Section 301 Disputes. Section 301 of the Taft-Hartley Act reads as follows: "Suits for violation of contracts between an employer and a labor organization representing employees in an industry affecting commerce as defined in this act, . . . may be brought in any district court of the United States having jurisdiction of the parties, without respect to the amount in controversy or without regard to the citizenship of the parties." In fact, most employers and unions have inserted grievance and arbitration clauses in their contracts in order to eliminate the need for such litigation. The rights created by this Section can be enforced in accordance with the terms of the arbitration clause in the collective bargaining contract.

91. Seniority. The length of service of an employee in his total employment with that employer, or in some particular seniority unit. Comparative seniority often determines the rights of the employee in relation to other employees, as to layoff, to shift preference or to promotion. Benefit seniority can affect the individual's rights as to vacation, severance pay or retirement benefits. The seniority rights of an employee are defined in the collective bargaining contract.

92. Statute of Limitations. A statute which determines the time during which an action may be taken to enforce any legal claim or right. In labor arbitration, the term is also loosely used for the time periods contained in the collective bargaining agreement. These agreements may contain time limitations for performing various acts such as filing a grievance, or appealing the decision of an officer of the company in the grievance procedure. Both courts and arbitrators vary in their treatment of such provisions. The United States Supreme Court in *John Wiley & Sons v. Livingston* held that it is up to the arbitrator to decide whether there was compliance with the time limitations provided in the contract.

93. **Sufficient Ability Clause.** A clause in a labor contract creating a standard for determining which employee shall be awarded a particular job. Sufficient ability clauses create minimum acceptable qualifications for doing the work, provided the employee in question has seniority. The interpretation and application of such provisions are sources of many disputes.

94. **Taft-Hartley Act.** (Labor Management Relations Act, Pub. L. No. 101, 80th Cong. 1st Sess.; 29 U.S.A.C. §§ 141-197)

An act, passed in 1947 over President Truman's veto, which modified the National Labor Relations Act by restricting union activities. The Taft-Hartley Act provided special machinery for handling national emergency disputes. It established the Federal Mediation and Conciliation Service. Title 1 of the Taft-Hartley Act has had particular and specific importance for arbitration since the United States Supreme Court based its landmark decision in *Lincoln Mills* on this section, authorizing the enforcement of the arbitration agreement and of the subsequent award.

95. **Transcript of Hearing.** A verbatim record of an arbitration hearing, in the form of a stenographic report. The use of a reporter in labor arbitration is the exception rather than the rule. A reporter may be used at the request of either party. If only one party asks for a transcript, that party is obliged to pay for it. Otherwise costs are shared by both parties. Since the cost of such transcripts can be substantial, parties are able to sharply reduce the costs of arbitration by eliminating the transcript. Labor arbitrators often use tape recorders to refresh their memory as to evidence in extended cases.

96. **Unfair Labor Practice.** An act on the part of a union or an employer which interferes with the rights of employees to join labor unions and to engage in collective bargaining. Section 8 of the National Labor Relations Act makes such conduct unlawful and empowers the National Labor Relations Board to prevent or to remedy it. State statutes may also declare certain acts to be "unfair labor practices." Arbitrators have no jurisdiction over unfair labor practices except in those cases where such practices also violate collective bargaining agreements.

29. American Arbitration Association Voluntary Labor Arbitration Rules

ROBERT COULSON

Reprinted with permission from *Labor Arbitration—What You Need to Know*, 2d. ed., by Robert Coulson, published by the American Arbitration Association, New York, © 1978.

1. **Agreement of Parties.** The parties shall be deemed to have made these Rules a part of their arbitration agreement whenever, in a collective bargaining agreement or submission, they have provided for arbitration by the American Arbitration Association (hereinafter AAA) or under its Rules. These Rules shall apply in the form obtained at the time the arbitration is initiated.

2. **Name of Tribunal.** Any Tribunal constituted by the parties under these Rules shall be called the Voluntary Labor Arbitration Tribunal.

3. **Administrator.** When parties agree to arbitrate under these Rules and an arbitration is instituted thereunder, they thereby authorize the AAA to administer the arbitration. The authority and obligations of the Administrator are as provided in the agreement of the parties and in these Rules.

4. **Delegation of Duties.** The duties of the AAA may be carried out through such representatives or committees as the AAA may direct.

5. **National Panel of Labor Arbitrators.** The AAA shall establish and maintain a National Panel of Labor Arbitrators and shall appoint arbitrators therefrom, as hereinafter provided.

6. **Office of Tribunal.** The general office of the Labor Arbitration Tribunal is the headquarters of the AAA, which may, however, assign the administration of an arbitration to any of its Regional Offices.

7. **Initiation under an Arbitration Clause in a Collective Bargaining Agreement.** Arbitration under an arbitration clause in a collective bargaining agreement may, under these Rules, be initiated by either party in the following manner:

(a) By giving written notice to the other party of intention to arbitrate (Demand), which notice shall contain a statement setting forth the nature of the dispute and the remedy sought, and

(b) By filing at any Regional Office of the AAA three copies of said notice, together with a copy of the collective bargaining agreement, or such parts thereof as relate to the dispute, including the arbitration provisions. After the Arbitrator is appointed, no new or different claim may be submitted, except with the consent of the Arbitrator and all other parties.

8. **Answer.** The party upon whom the Demand for Arbitration is made may file an answering statement with the AAA within seven days after notice from the AAA, in which event said party shall simultaneously send a copy of its answer to the other party. If no answer is filed within the stated time, it will be assumed that the claim is denied. Failure to file an answer shall not operate to delay the arbitration.

9. **Initiation under a Submission.** Parties to any collective bargaining agreement may initiate an arbitra-

tion under these Rules by filing at any Regional Office of the AAA two copies of a written agreement to arbitrate under these Rules (Submission), signed by the parties and setting forth the nature of the dispute and the remedy sought.

10. **Fixing of Locale.** The parties may mutually agree upon the locale where the arbitration is to be held. If the locale is not designated in the collective bargaining agreement or Submission, and if there is a dispute as to the appropriate locale, the AAA shall have the power to determine the locale and its decision shall be binding.

11. **Qualifications of Arbitrator.** No person shall serve as a neutral Arbitrator in any arbitration in which that person has any financial or personal interest in the result of the arbitration, unless the parties, in writing, waive such disqualification.

12. **Appointment from Panel.** If the parties have not appointed an Arbitrator and have not provided any other method of appointment, the Arbitrator shall be appointed in the following manner: Immediately after the filing of the Demand or Submission, the AAA shall submit simultaneously to each party an identical list of names of persons chosen from the Labor Panel. Each party shall have seven days from the mailing date in which to cross off any names objected to, number the remaining names indicating the order of preference, and return the list to the AAA. If a party does not return the list within the time specified, all persons named therein shall be deemed acceptable. From among the persons who have been approved on both lists, and in accordance with the designated order of mutual preference, the AAA shall invite the acceptance of an Arbitrator to serve. If the parties fail to agree upon any of the persons named or if those named decline or are unable to act, or if for any other reason the appointment cannot be made from the submitted lists, the Administrator shall have power to make the appointment from other members of the Panel without the submission of any additional lists.

13. **Direct Appointment by Parties.** If the agreement of the parties names an Arbitrator or specifies a method of appointing an Arbitrator, that designation or method shall be followed. The notice of appointment, with the name and address of such Arbitrator, shall be filed with the AAA by the appointing party.

If the agreement specifies a period of time within which an Arbitrator shall be appointed, and any party fails to make such appointment within that period, the AAA may make the appointment.

If no period of time is specified in the agreement, the AAA shall notify the parties to make the appointment and if within seven days thereafter such Arbitrator has not been so appointed, the AAA shall make the appointment.

14. **Appointment of Neutral Arbitrator by Party-Appointed Arbitrators.** If the parties have appointed their Arbitrators, or if either or both of them have been appointed as provided in Section 13, and have authorized such Arbitrators to appoint a neutral Arbitrator within a specified time and no appointment is made within such time or any agreed extension thereof, the AAA may appoint a neutral Arbitrator, who shall act as Chairman.

If no period of time is specified for appointment of the neutral Arbitrator and the parties do not make the appointment within seven days from the date of the appointment of the last party-appointed Arbitrator, the AAA shall appoint such neutral Arbitrator, who shall act as Chairman.

If the parties have agreed that the Arbitrators shall appoint the neutral Arbitrator from the Panel, the AAA shall furnish to the party-appointed Arbitrators, in the manner prescribed in Section 12, a list selected from the Panel, and the appointment of the neutral Arbitrator shall be made as prescribed in such Section.

15. **Number of Arbitrators.** If the arbitration agreement does not specify the number of Arbitrators, the dispute shall be heard and determined by one Arbitrator, unless the parties otherwise agree.

16. **Notice to Arbitrator of Appointment.** Notice of the appointment of the neutral Arbitrator shall be mailed to the Arbitrator by the AAA and the signed acceptance of the Arbitrator shall be filed with the AAA prior to the opening of the first hearing.

17. **Disclosure by Arbitrator of Disqualification.** Prior to accepting appointment, the prospective neutral Arbitrator shall disclose any circumstances likely to create a presumption of bias or which he believes might disqualify him as an impartial Arbitrator. Upon receipt of such information, the AAA shall immediately disclose it to the parties. If either party declines to waive the presumptive disqualification, the vacancy thus created shall be filled in accordance with the applicable provisions of these Rules.

18. **Vacancies.** If any Arbitrator should resign, die, withdraw, refuse or be unable or disqualified to perform the duties of the office, the AAA shall, on proof satisfactory to it, declare the office vacant. Vacancies

shall be filled in the same manner as that governing the making of the original appointment, and the matter shall be reheard by the new Arbitrator.

19. **Time and Place of Hearing.** The Arbitrator shall fix the time and place for each hearing. At least five days prior thereto the AAA shall mail notice of the time and place of hearing to each party, unless the parties otherwise agree.

20. **Representation by Counsel.** Any party may be represented at the hearing by counsel or by other authorized representative.

21. **Stenographic Record.** Any party may request a stenographic record by making arrangements for same through the AAA. If such transcript is agreed by the parties to be, or in appropriate cases determined by the arbitrator to be, the official record of the proceeding, it must be made available to the arbitrator, and to the other party for inspection, at a time and place determined by the arbitrator The total cost of such a record shall be shared equally by those parties that order copies.

22. **Attendance at Hearings.** Persons having a direct interest in the arbitration are entitled to attend hearings. The Arbitrator shall have the power to require the retirement of any witness or witnesses during the testimony of other witnesses. It shall be discretionary with the Arbitrator to determine the propriety of the attendance of any other persons.

23. **Adjournments.** The Arbitrator for good cause shown may adjourn the hearing upon the request of a party or upon his own initiative, and shall adjourn when all the parties agree thereto.

24. **Oaths.** Before proceeding with the first hearing, each Arbitrator may take an Oath of Office, and if required by law, shall do so. The Arbitrator has discretion to require witnesses to testify under oath administered by any duly qualified person and, if required by law or requested by either party, shall do so.

25. **Majority Decision.** Whenever there is more than one Arbitrator, all decisions of the Arbitrators shall be by majority vote. The award shall also be made by majority vote unless the concurrence of all is expressly required.

26. **Order of Proceedings.** A hearing shall be opened by the filing of the Oath of the Arbitrator, where required, and by the recording of the place, time and date of hearing, the presence of the Arbitrator and parties, and counsel if any, and the receipt by the Arbitrator of the Demand and answer, if any, or the Submission.

Exhibits, when offered by either party, may be received in evidence by the Arbitrator. The names and addresses of all witnesses and exhibits in order received shall be made a part of the record.

The Arbitrator has discretion to vary the normal procedure under which the initiating party first presents its claim, but in any case shall afford full and equal opportunity to all parties for presentation of relevant proofs.

27. **Arbitration in the Absence of a Party.** Unless the law provides to the contrary, the arbitration may proceed in the absence of any party who, after due notice, fails to be present or fails to obtain an adjournment. An award shall not be made solely on the default of a party. The Arbitrator shall require the other party to submit such evidence as he may require for the making of an award.

28. **Evidence.** The parties may offer such evidence as they desire and shall produce such additional evidence as the Arbitrator may deem necessary to an understanding and determination of the dispute. When the Arbitrator is authorized by law to subpoena witnesses and documents, he may do so upon his own initiative or upon the request of any party. The Arbitrator shall be the judge of the relevancy and materiality of the evidence offered and conformity to legal rules of evidence shall not be necessary. All evidence shall be taken in the presence of all of the Arbitrators and all of the parties except where any of the parties is absent in default or has waived the right to be present.

29. **Evidence by Affidavit and Filing of Documents.** The Arbitrator may receive and consider the evidence of witnesses by affidavit, but shall give it only such weight as the Arbitrator deems proper after consideration of any objections made to its admission.

All documents not filed with the Arbitrator at the hearing but which are arranged at the hearing or subsequently by agreement of the parties to be submitted, shall be filed with the AAA for transmission to the Arbitrator. All parties shall be afforded opportunity to examine such documents.

30. **Inspection.** Whenever the Arbitrator deems it necessary, he may make an inspection in connection with the subject matter of the dispute after written notice to the parties who may, if they so desire, be present at such inspection.

31. Closing of Hearings. The Arbitrator shall inquire of all parties whether they have any further proofs to offer or witnesses to be heard. Upon receiving negative replies, the Arbitrator shall declare the hearings closed and a minute thereof shall be recorded. If briefs or other documents are to be filed, the hearings shall be declared closed as of the final date set by the Arbitrator for filing with the AAA. The time limit within which the Arbitrator is required to make the award shall commence to run, in the absence of other agreement by the parties, upon the closing of the hearings.

32. Reopening of Hearings. The hearings may be reopened by the Arbitrator on his own motion, or on the motion of either party, for good cause shown, at any time before the award is made, but if the reopening of the hearings would prevent the making of the award within the specific time agreed upon by the parties in the contract out of which the controversy has arisen, the matter may not be reopened, unless both parties agree upon the extension of such time limit. When no specific date is fixed in the contract, the Arbitrator may reopen the hearings, and the Arbitrator shall have 30 days from the closing of the reopened hearings within which to make an award.

33. Waiver of Rules. Any party who proceeds with the arbitration after knowledge that any provision or requirement of these Rules has not been complied with and who fails to state objection thereto in writing, shall be deemed to have waived the right to object.

34. Waiver of Oral Hearings. The parties may provide, by written agreement, for the waiver of oral hearings. If the parties are unable to agree as to the procedure, the AAA shall specify a fair and equitable procedure.

35. Extensions of Time. The parties may modify any period of time by mutual agreement. The AAA for good cause may extend any period of time established by these Rules, except the time for making the award. The AAA shall notify the parties of any such extension of time and its reason therefor.

36. Serving of Notices. Each party to a Submission or other agreement which provides for arbitration under these Rules shall be deemed to have consented and shall consent that any papers, notices or process necessary or proper for the initiation or continuation of an arbitration under these Rules and for any court action in connection therewith or the entry of judgment on an award made thereunder, may be served upon such party (a) by mail addressed to such party or its

attorney at its last known address, or (b) by personal service, within or without the state wherein the arbitration is to be held.

37. Time of Award. The award shall be rendered promptly by the Arbitrator and, unless otherwise agreed by the parties, or specified by the law, not later than thirty days from the date of closing the hearings, or if oral hearings have been waived, then from the date of transmitting the final statements and proofs to the Arbitrator.

38. Form of Award. The award shall be in writing and shall be signed either by the neutral Arbitrator or by a concurring majority if there be more than one Arbitrator. The parties shall advise the AAA whenever they do not require the Arbitrator to accompany the award with an opinion.

39. Award upon Settlement. If the parties settle their dispute during the course of the arbitration, the Arbitrator, upon their request, may set forth the terms of the agreed settlement in an award.

40. Delivery of Award to Parties. Parties shall accept as legal delivery of the award the placing of the award or a true copy thereof in the mail by the AAA, addressed to such party at its last known address or to its attorney, or personal service of the award, or the filing of the award in any manner which may be prescribed by law.

41. Release Documents for Judicial Proceedings. The AAA shall, upon the written request of a party, furnish to such party at its expense certified facsimiles of any papers in the AAA's possession that may be required in judicial proceedings relating to the arbitration.

42. Judicial Proceedings. The AAA is not a necessary party in judicial proceedings relating to the arbitration.

43. Administrative Fee. As a nonprofit organization, the AAA shall prescribe an administrative fee schedule to compensate it for the cost of providing administrative services. The schedule in effect at the time of filing shall be applicable.

44. Expenses. The expense of witnesses for either side shall be paid by the party producing such witnesses.

Expenses of the arbitration, other than the cost of the stenographic record, including required traveling and other expenses of the Arbitrator and of AAA representatives, and the expenses of any witnesses or the cost of any proofs produced at the direct request of the Arbitrator, shall be borne equally by the parties unless they agree otherwise, or unless the Arbitrator in the award assesses such expenses or any part thereof against any specified party or parties.

45. **Communication with Arbitrator.** There shall be no communication between the parties and a neutral Arbitrator other than at oral hearings. Any other oral or written communications from the parties to the Arbitrator shall be directed to the AAA for transmittal to the Arbitrator.

46. **Interpretation and Application of Rules.** The Arbitrator shall interpret and apply these Rules insofar as they relate to the Arbitrator's powers and duties. When there is more than one Arbitrator and a difference arises among them concerning the meaning or application of any such Rules, it shall be decided by majority vote. If that is unobtainable, either Arbitrator or party may refer the question to the AAA for final decision. All other Rules shall be interpreted and applied by the AAA.

30. Arbitration from the Arbitrator's View

HERBERT L. MARX, JR.

Labor-management arbitration is the final and binding resolution of a dispute between an employer and a union by a neutral third party. In that simply stated truism, there are two concepts that frequently unsettle and even bewilder the parties directly involved.

The first concept is that of final and binding, which is quite foreign to the continuing concept of collective bargaining in which issues can be raised and reraised in successive negotiations over and over again. The second concept is that of the intrusion of the outside neutral, who is given authority in a situation where that individual may be a relative stranger.

This lack of assurance and confidence in the process is as unfortunate as it is unnecessary because the further simple truth is that the outcome of almost all disputes taken to arbitration depends not on the arbitrator, nor even how expert the parties may be in their presentations to that neutral, but in the facts of the dispute itself.

Before testing this thesis (a fairly well-kept secret in the arbitration field), some preliminary definitions and limitations are necessary.

The conclusion above refers, of course, to *grievance* arbitration or *rights* arbitration—the resolution of a dispute between the employer and the union concerning the meaning or interpretation of an existing collective bargaining agreement. This implies that the parties have an agreement of fixed duration, that they have agreed upon a dispute resolution procedure leading to final and binding arbitration, that they have defined the scope of what issues may or may not be referred to such final adjudication by a neutral, and that such a system is combined inextricably with an undertaking by both sides to forbid strikes or lockouts during the term of the agreement.

From this standard pattern there are some variations that are, however, increasingly rare as collective bargaining relationships achieve the maturity of years and shared experience. In some situations, for example, the parties will exempt certain specific provisions of the agreement from the strike prohibition and/or arbitration procedures.

Occasionally the parties will agree only to an arrangement called *advisory* arbitration, which is not arbitration at all but simply the use of a third party neutral to recommend the resolution of a grievance, with the employer having the right to ignore the advice if it so chooses. This is used occasionally where one or both parties (but usually the employer only) is as yet unwilling to cede the right of final decision to an outsider and appears most frequently in new collective bargaining relationships.

There also is *tripartite* arbitration, in which a neutral arbitrator is joined by representatives of each side to make up an arbitration board. The outcome here is a final and binding settlement that, by the mathematics of the system, depends primarily on the judgment of the neutral member but that supposedly is tempered by the inside expertise of the partisan members of the panel.

825

Of an entirely different nature is *interest* arbitration in which the arbitrator (or an arbitration board) is called upon not to resolve the interpretation of an existing agreement but rather to fashion the terms of a new collective bargaining document. Here there cannot be (despite protestations to the contrary) a stark determination of "right" or "wrong," but rather there is a reasoned evaluation of the various economic and organizational needs of the parties. Interest arbitration and grievance arbitration share in common only the resolution process by a neutral; otherwise, they are fundamentally different in nature and are treated separately in this discussion.

GRIEVANCE ARBITRATION

There are two major categories of cases in grievance arbitration—disciplinary matters and contract interpretation matters. A third category, sharing some of the aspects of the two major types, is composed of grievances concerning the transfer or advancement of employees. Separate characteristics mark the approach to each of these categories.

Disputes Concerning Discipline

The disciplining of employees (including the authority to discharge) is a basic management right. This is a theory supported not only by the employer but in virtually all instances by the union as well. The union has no desire or motivation to sit in judgment of its own members by participating in the initial imposition of discipline. The union may well require, in some instances, the right to be present during disciplinary interviews but it understandably has no wish to share the responsibility for the determination of the propriety of employee conduct. The union, on behalf of those it represents, relies rather on the right to protest after the fact and to insist—through the grievance procedure and before an arbitrator—on clear proof concerning the employee and on fair treatment.

This explains the almost universal brevity of contract language concerning discipline in most collective bargaining agreements, even where other matters are dealt with in meticulous detail. Management typically is limited in its right to discipline only as to "just cause," or even simply "cause." The only other common thread of contract language is a separate provision requiring nondiscriminatory treatment.

When this is understood, it becomes clear why, although a disciplinary grievance is initiated by an employee and/or the union, the issue before the arbitrator is whether or not the employer can prove the case both as to the culpability of the employee and the degree of discipline imposed. Here stands forth most solidly the proposition that the soundness or weakness of the employer's action is determined by what happens before the matter reaches the arbitration table and not at the table itself.

An occasional exception to this theory is found in agreements that list, either in the contract or in published rules of conduct, various offenses and applicable penalties. Here (at least where the list of offenses is included in the agreement) the union has agreed beforehand to certain standards of conduct. This type of case takes a different cast at arbitration in that it revolves around whether the employee's conduct fits the predetermined offenses and, occasionally, whether such standards are enforced uniformly.

The Need for Adequate Communication

The single most important element in disciplinary matters is communication—a word tiresomely overused but having specific meaning here. Is the employee aware of the "rules of the game" as to work performance, attendance, personal conduct, and conduct in relation to other employees and supervisors? If the employer finds the employee deficient in any of these, was the worker made aware of management's criticism? Are oral or written warnings specific as to the offense, timely as to their issuance, and precise as to the consequences of repetition of the offense? Depending on the provisions of the agreement and/or the general philosophy of management, was the union properly advised? Most vital of all, are employee disciplinary records maintained in orderly fashion and available to supervisors for use when they may be called upon to impose discipline? These all are matters within management's control and more often than not determine the outcome of an arbitration.

Arbitrators are careful to observe the difference between two types of disciplinary actions (and the border marking the difference between these two varies from industry to industry). The first type is where discipline is progressive, based on incidents or conduct subject to corrective action. Absenteeism and below-standard work performance are two prime examples. The other type consists of conduct that, standing by itself, may lead the employer to a determination that the individual is not suitable for continued employment. Theft and physical violence are two examples.

Where a dispute in the first type of discipline arises (whether as to a warning notice or an eventual discharge after repeated offenses), the accumulated record and the degree of certainty that the employee has been advised as to the consequences become the essential elements in arbitration. In the second type of case, calling for severe discipline without prior warning, documentation of the incident at the time it occurred becomes the essential basis for a case before the arbitrator.

Put bluntly, the employer has made (or not made) the case in disciplinary matters before the grievance reaches the arbitrator. What remains at the arbitration hearing is the orderly exposition of that case. If the discipline notice is unclear, if records cannot be produced, if consistent treatment cannot be demonstrated, the case will not magically make itself before the arbitrator.

The employer faces one more hurdle in disciplinary cases, however. This goes not to the proof of what the employee did, but whether the penalty imposed can be justified. There is considerable confusion over this. Given the proved facts of a situation, the employer will argue that the judgment of the arbitrator should not be substituted for that of the employer in determining the penalty.

In theory, there is much to be said to support this view. It is not for the arbitrator to decide what would have been done in the same circumstances if that neutral were the employer. But this begs the basic issue. The employer must show just cause not only for any disciplinary action but also for the penalty selected. The parties may agree, tacitly if not openly, that some penalty is appropriate for the employee's repeated tardinesses after repeated warnings. But does this necessarily justify the discharge that the employer imposed? Has the employer been consistent in relation to treatment of other employees? Have mitigating circumstances, of which the employer may not have been aware at the time the penalty was imposed, been considered?

The parties occasionally will agree that the arbitrator should be limited to the single issue of whether or not just cause existed, leaving further resolution of the issue to the parties if just cause is not found. Generally, however, the additional question for the arbitrator's determination is "If not, what is the proper remedy?" Thus the door to alternative resolution of the penalty by the arbitrator is opened. An essential part of each disciplinary arbitration for both parties is to argue whether or not the penalty imposed is appropriate to the misconduct. The more guidance an arbitrator receives on this point from both sides, the less surprising will be the outcome.

Contract Interpretation Grievances

Arbitration involving a dispute over the meaning or interpretation of terms of the agreement is quite a different matter from disciplinary issues. Here, management has acted with a presumption that it is not violating the agreement. The union thinks otherwise, and it thus becomes the union's chief burden to prove its allegation. Unlike disciplinary matters, the records here are quite different: previous grievances and arbitrations under the same agreement dealing with the subject; contract language history as to how the provision in question came into being, along with failed attempts of one or both sides to change the language (giving clues to its present meaning); and previous instances of the same or different management actions involving the same issue.

It needs little emphasis here to say that the arbitrator's first duty is to read and apply the contract as written, and the arbitrator will do so where the language is found to be clear and unambiguous. No amount of argument that the clear language is inefficient, unreasonable, or even unfair can deter the arbitrator from reading it as it is. But many contract interpretation cases involve one or both parties' contentions that the "clear language" is indeed murky or that several different clauses in the agreement provide contradictory meanings. The obligation then is on the union to make its case, using supplementary argument as to history and practice.

Where there is a genuine perceivable issue as to the meaning of a particular clause or clauses, the arbitrator cannot be expected to speculate or to fashion an interpretation. The arbitrator must rely on the adversary arguments advanced by both sides. Some general principles apply. Where there is a general clause in the agreement, followed by more precise provisions on the issue at hand, the more specific carries greater weight. Where exceptions to a rule are listed, then the fact that the issue at hand is not listed as an exception makes it part of the general rule. Where exceptions simply are listed as examples, however, with a phrase like "such as" or similar wording, the principle of exclusion by noninclusion does not necessarily apply.

Still dealing with ambiguous contract language: If it can be shown that one side rather than the other was responsible for the particular wording as a result of previous bargaining, the wording often is considered against the interest of the initiating party; if that party had wished to say it in a different way, presumably it would have done so.

Finally, there is the situation where the meaning of an unclear clause is argued on the basis of past practice. Here the parties frequently come a cropper. What is a "past practice?" Here are some of the things it is *not*: a single previous instance, or instances of such hoary age that they have no present significance; a practice observed by the employer but of which the union can show it had no previous knowledge; or instances where a practice has been challenged previously in the grievance procedure and then resolved specifically "without prejudice" to the effect of future instances. In sum, the past practice that can be relied upon before the arbitrator is one that is known, accepted, and repeated. It becomes even more emphatically so when this has occurred over the course of several contracts (and the parties did not disturb the language in intervening negotiations).

Grievances Concerning Employee Status

A third variety of grievance arbitrations concerns matters of employee status, such as claims of demotion, improper denial of promotion, or changed work assignment or transfer. What often is involved is management's choice of one employee over others for a particular position, or the removal of an employee from a position because of alleged unsatisfactory work performance or failure to meet the requirements of a trial period.

Here, contract language does indeed apply, as in any contract interpretation case. This is especially true where contract language mixes considerations such as length of service, ability, experience, etc. But such instances also resemble disciplinary cases in that it is the employer's judgment that must be defended. Which party has the burden of proof here? The answer is, of course, both—the union to show violation of contract language and the employer to defend the judgment exercised within the constraints of the language. Arbitration procedure in such instances will vary from case to case, but the arbitrator certainly will expect each side to take the initiative and be weighed down with the burden of proof as suggested.

PROCEDURAL OBJECTIONS

Arbitration presentations frequently are not limited to a straightforward fact-finding procedure in which each side sets forth its views of the merits of the case based on what occurred and what the contract says about it. The arbitrator also can be faced with procedural objections. These take two broad forms: (1) a contention that the case is improperly before the arbitrator altogether (questions of arbitrability) or (2) a contention that certain testimony or evidence is offered improperly once the merits are examined (question of relevance).

While such objections may be raised occasionally in a frivolous or inexpert manner, these usually are serious questions for the arbitrator. When raised, how-

ever, they must be defended precisely and forcefully. Considerable time and effort and even emotional involvement have been expended to bring the matter to the arbitration table. To then claim that the matter is moot, improperly handled, or beyond the scope of the arbitrator's authority is at best a jarring occurrence to the grieving party. Nevertheless, such procedural questions deserve the arbitrator's attention and separate resolution, quite apart from the significance of the issue on its merits.

Questions of Arbitrability

The most common instances of questions of arbitrability have to do with the union's alleged failure to meet the procedural requirements of the grievance procedure as detailed in the agreement. This may involve time limits that the agreement says must be observed in raising a grievance or moving it from step to step. The underlying purpose of such time limits is obvious: If there is an issue as to whether the employer violated provisions of the agreement or had just cause for disciplinary action, it is to the advantage of both sides to have the dispute resolved as early as possible. If the employer is found not to have violated the agreement, it is better to have this known sooner rather than later. If the employer is in violation, then prompt settlement not only corrects the situation but also mitigates the possible cost of ameliorating the error. Quite apart from this, time limits on filing and processing grievances have the effect of avoiding the bunching of large numbers of grievances together for tactical purposes.

When unions agree to such time limits, they are fully aware of what they are doing, and in exchange frequently can impose time limits on employer answers or obtain other concessions. The arbitrator therefore will consider seriously an argument that a grievance may not be heard because it is untimely. The contract may state, for example, that a grievance must be filed within ten days of the occurrence or of when the grievant knew or reasonably should have had knowledge of it. Where such language occurs, the objecting party must provide fully adequate proof that the employee (or the union, as the case may be) "should have had knowledge."

Occasionally there are reasonable questions not as to when grievances or their answers were written, but when and how they were received. Again, substantial proof is required before an arbitrator will throw out a grievance based on untimeliness.

Another type of procedural objection occurs when a grievance claims violation of one contract provision but when the matter comes to arbitration, the claim is based on an entirely different provision. A grievance based on missed overtime under the distribution of overtime assignment clause suddenly becomes at the arbitration table a case of alleged discrimination.

There are no pat answers as to how arbitrators will deal with such situations. Sometimes the collective bargaining agreement requires a grievance to specify the exact contract terms allegedly violated; if such is the case, the arbitrator usually will be guided accordingly. If there is no such language, the theoretical approach is that (to use the example cited above) the employer has not had a previous opportunity to answer a charge of discrimination, since the grievance dealt only with overtime distribution. Should not the employer have such opportunity to answer and possibly convince the union of its position before the arbitrator is called upon to rule on the charge? This may have substantial weight in the decision as to whether to entertain the new basis for the grievance.

The arbitrator generally will not permit a union to process a case substantially different from the one previously put forward in the grievance itself and through the grievance procedure. It also is generally true, however, that arbitrators will permit the parties to use contractual language broadly if doing so reasonably supports the known facts of the incident.

Procedural Objections during the Hearing

The other type of procedural objections concerns the method of presenting evidence. It is well established that arbitrators need not and frequently do not follow court rules of evidence, devised primarily to protect an untutored jury. Nevertheless, the arbitrator must deal thoughtfully with objections raised by the parties as to the unreliability of testimony (hearsay), the lack of relevance to the issue at hand, the "leading" of a friendly witness, or the expression of opinion or judgment by nonexpert witnesses. Sometimes such objections are made in good faith simply to alert the arbitrator (on the presumption the arbitrator may not be aware of it) to the dubious character of such testimony or evidence. Frequently, however, the parties genuinely believe that the testimony should not be heard or the evidence not received.

The arbitrator is required to take such objections seriously. But the two sides must bear in mind that the arbitration hearing, unlike many court trials, has not been preceded by pretrial depositions or discovery hearings, nor are the parties necessarily expert in laying the foundation in advance for the testimony or evidence being presented.

What will be of greatest concern to the arbitrator is: Will this help me in deciding the issue that the parties have given me? As a trier of the facts, will I add this to my store of useful knowledge? In arguing in support of or in opposition to a procedural objection, the parties do well to keep these questions in mind.

In addition, the arbitrator will be mindful of the worthy objective of not unduly extending the hearing and sometimes will defer the presentation of questionable testimony until later in the hearing when it can then be determined, for example, if it is indeed relevant or if there is not some better way to receive information than through questionable secondhand or thirdhand sources.

INTEREST ARBITRATION

There is more to be examined concerning grievance arbitration, particularly as to the grievance procedure that precedes the hearing and the aftereffects of the hearing. Before exploring these avenues, however, an examination of an entirely different type of arbitration is in order. This is *interest* arbitration—the setting of the terms of a new or revised collective bargaining agreement between the parties, rather than the resolution of a dispute under an existing contract.

Interest arbitration has taken a more prominent role recently because it is mandated under law in various states for final resolution of public employee labor-management disputes, particularly for public safety workers. There also are instances of the voluntary use of interest arbitration, in health care and elsewhere, particularly where the alternative of a strike—though legal—may be repugnant to, or obviously against the self-interest of, the parties. The Experimental Negotiation Agreement between the major steel companies and the United Steelworkers also calls for ultimate use of binding interest arbitration, although up to 1981 the parties had reached agreement without its use.

Interest arbitration is similar to grievance or rights arbitration simply because it leaves to an outside neutral the final resolution of a dispute and the parties appear and argue before the neutral in an adversary manner. (More often than not, the interest arbitration includes an arbitration panel, with an outside neutral as well as "neutrals" appointed by each party.)

Beyond this, the similarity ends, and employers and unions that participate in both types of arbitration do well to recognize this. Grievance arbitration calls for an interpretation of an existing agreement; the outcome of the case in no way will affect the continuance of the preexisting agreement. Interest arbitration, on the other hand, is not based on establishing the one "right" answer under the contract or whether or not a disciplinary action was taken for just cause. The arbitrator in interest arbitration is weighing the terms and conditions of the future relationship of the two sides. The interest arbitrator seeks not meanings of clauses and history of their application, but rather what changed economic benefits and contract language will be appropriate.

Judgment in this type of situation is based on matters such as comparisons of similar conditions in other agreements under similar circumstances, the ability of the employer to pay, and the effect on employees of general economic conditions. Such judgment will be based on the facts and arguments that the parties set before the interest arbitrator. While the outcome will be just as binding (either by law or by agreement of the parties), the interest arbitration award is based primarily on external factors, while the grievance arbitration award necessarily is based almost exclusively on internal factors (the contract and the employee-employer relationship at the workplace).

One other major difference should be noted: Grievance arbitration is the terminal step of the grievance procedure, during which the parties have met not to compromise (although this may happen) but—by examination of the facts—to determine who is right and who is wrong. There is little room for mutual accommodation. Either the vacation scheduling procedure in the agreement was followed or it wasn't; either the employee is guilty of theft on the job and should be fired, or the employee is not guilty and should not be disciplined.

Interest arbitration, on the other hand, is preceded by extensive bargaining and frequently by third party mediatory efforts—all of which seek to bring a flexibility and compromise to the positions of both sides so that they can agree on new terms. It is not so much a matter of right and wrong, but rather of respective economic strength and comparative status of the parties and their willingness to accommodate each other. Only when this agreement is less than total does interest arbitration take over—and usually only in those areas where tentative agreement has not been reached.

Parties will have their greatest success at the arbitration table by keeping clearly in mind these basic differences between grievance arbitration and interest arbitration and the varying tasks that arbitrators are called upon to complete under each form.

BEFORE THE ARBITRATION

Returning now to grievance arbitration, the significance of the procedure leading up to the arbitration

hearing often is grossly underestimated. The major purpose of the grievance procedure is to resolve disputes bilaterally before they get to arbitration. Too often, this principle is forgotten or disregarded and the parties use the procedure simply as a means either to expedite the dispute to arbitration or to get the one party to concede because it does not wish to undergo the risk, inconvenience, and expense of arbitration.

Fortunately, many employers and unions take the more reasonable course of using the grievance procedure as a means of fact-finding and a forum in which to attempt to convince the other side of the correctness of one's position. In such instances, both parties are less likely to have the issue go to arbitration at all; or, if arbitration is reached, the argument there will be more sharply honed and more closely relevant. As a result, the arbitrator is better able to reach a sound conclusion and one that does not stray beyond the limits within which the parties are comfortable.

As a consequence of this, the grievance procedure can be highly useful in preparing for arbitration (if arbitration is needed). Here are some suggested grievance techniques:

Don't "save it for the arbitrator." Documentary evidence, examples of precedential importance, eyewitness reports—it is far better that such information be part of the grievance procedure, used in an attempt to convince the other party. Where such information is withheld deliberately in the hope of winning the arbitration battle, no such fortuitous effect is likely to ensue.

First, the other party will cry "foul" and will raise emphatic objection to presentation of the "new" evidence to the arbitrator. Unless there is specific contract language to the contrary, arbitrators generally will not refuse to hear such evidence but at the same time often will grant a request for the "surprised" party to consider the effect of the new evidence and, if necessary, to prepare an answer. Thus, nothing is accomplished but delay. The second effect is to weaken the good faith relationship between the parties, with the blame placed on the side withholding the evidence. It shows a lack of trust in the ability of the parties to resolve a grievance by themselves, given all the facts.

Most grievance procedures provide a series of steps in which a management representative hears the complaints (although there are exceptional cases where the hearing at various steps is conducted jointly by union and employer representatives). The employer representative should listen to the presentation as impartially and dispassionately as possible (letting someone else advance the management position in response to the union). This offers a better atmosphere for the employer to recognize error or misjudgment in its case, or for the union to respect and accept the employer representative's answer. Further, this method becomes a helpful trial run for the arbitration hearing itself, if indeed the matter reaches there.

Compromise offers of settlement during the grievance procedure often are appropriate. Too often, they are avoided because of a supposed adverse effect on the offering party's later position before an arbitrator. This is unfortunate, because if the compromise offer is made properly, it may resolve the dispute and, even if not accepted, it should have no ill effect on the arbitration hearing. The proposed compromise should state clearly that if the offer is rejected (for example, reinstatement with a period of unpaid suspension instead of a discharge), the original position of the parties remains in effect. A well-understood principle is that such failed offers are not mentioned to the arbitrator. But even if it does "slip out," the arbitrator is entirely capable of disregarding such information in the deliberations.

A variation of the compromise settlement is an agreement by the parties to modify their positions during the grievance procedure and to agree to submit only the remaining portion of the dispute to arbitration. This, too, is a valuable step in that it reduces the breadth of decision left to a third party.

AFTEREFFECTS OF ARBITRATION

Just as the arbitration has its beginning long before the arbitrator arrives, so too can it have aftereffects of serious consequence quite apart from the opinion and award. To illustrate:

- An employee is discharged for absenteeism after a long series of lesser penalties. Part of the case presented by the employer is testimony from the personnel clerk that he saw the employee on a bus with a department store package at a time the employee was supposed to be at work but had reported off sick.
- In another case, the grievance committee chairman's testimony about alleged past practice is destroyed by extensive and devastating cross-examination by the industrial relations manager, who could as easily have presented a management witness to make the point.
- The union's local representative testifies about a telephone conversation he had with the department head, who confided that the employee had been fired because of insistence from the "front office" and not because the manager wanted to discharge the employee.

In the first two instances, the arbitrator supported the employer's position but in the third case reinstated the discharged employee. But what were the tangential results? The personnel clerk found he no longer could settle minor problems about transfers, insurance benefits, etc., on behalf of individual employees because they now always wanted to see someone else. The number of grievances filed by the grievance committee chairman suddenly doubled. And the union's local representative found it no longer possible to get the ear of anyone in middle management to discuss informally, much less resolve, employee complaints.

Grievance arbitration does require a vigorous presentation by both sides. That is the nature of the proceeding. But mature practitioners also realize that the arbitration process is part of the entire warp and woof of the parties' relationship. The choice of what evidence to select for presentation and the manner in which the parties treat each other across the table may have more profound effects than the arbitration award itself. The arbitrator can do little to control this aspect of the process and is not charged to interfere even when destructive conduct is observed. This is one important aspect of grievance arbitration that only the parties themselves can control.

THE FUTURE OF ARBITRATION

In today's increasingly litigious society, the challenges to arbitration decisions in the courts are increasingly apparent. Management beliefs that arbitrators have exceeded their authority or violated law or controlling legal regulations, grievants' charges that they have not received fair representation, and attempts to stay arbitration altogether (particularly in public sector cases) are but a few recurring examples.

Employees have learned that various other avenues of redress are available, especially in an increasing variety of acts of discrimination. So the arbitrator finds that the grievance (or something closely related to it) has been or will be heard by a court or commission.

In some instances, parties as a matter of course seem to want to explore the possibilities of extending the time between initial hearing of an arbitration case and the award through procedural challenges, hearing transcripts, insistence on extensive testimony and proofs to support known facts that otherwise might be stipulated to, and posthearing briefs and rebuttals.

Need such considerations forecast the end of arbitration as a relatively informal, quick, and efficient means to resolve labor-management disputes? The answer to this question rests with the parties themselves, who create and continue this system of industrial justice every time a new labor-management agreement is signed. In making the continuing determination to utilize arbitration as the guarantor of industrial peace, the parties should not substitute adversary artfulness for the satisfaction and reliability of a self-administered means of dispute resolution.

By and large, arbitration continues to work as a means of resolving genuine disputes between parties who have decided to live together. Only the misuse of the peace-preserving machinery itself to do battle could destroy the effectiveness and unique utility of arbitration.

31. An Overview of Arbitration

MICHAEL G. MACDONALD

The grievance machinery under a collective bargaining agreement is at the very heart of the system of industrial self-government. Arbitration is the means of solving the unforeseeable by molding a system of private law for all problems which may arise and to provide for their solution in a way which will generally accord with the variant needs and desires of the parties. . . . The grievance procedure is, in other words, part of the continuous collective bargaining process. *United Steelworkers of America v. Warrior & Gulf Navigation Co.*, 363 U.S. 574, 581 (1960).

INTRODUCTION

A personnel director of a major teaching hospital recently surprised me by declaring that arbitration was "exclusively" the province of lawyers and was not part of the personnel department's function. Once a case gets to arbitration, said this friend, "it's out of my area and into yours." This is very similar to the statement often heard from physicians that malpractice is a "legal" problem and not a "medical" one. It might be suspected that this personnel director did not have many arbitrations at his hospital or he would have realized how totally incorrect he was in his perception of arbitration in its relationship to the overall administration of personnel policy.

This article demonstrates that arbitration—specifically grievance arbitration—is an inherent part of collective bargaining and of the administration of the collective bargaining agreement and, unlike the judicial system, is not so much a process designed to determine what justice requires, but rather (and very pragmatically) what industrial peace requires. It also demonstrates that arbitration, although the last step in a long chain of events involved in the practical administration of the collective bargaining agreement, is an integral part of those events. It will be shown that the arbitration case begins with the occurrence of the incident giving rise to the arbitration and that management must act with the reference to the common law of industrial relations that has been developed in large part by arbitrators.

EVOLUTION

Some Definitions

It is important to define what is meant by arbitration.

Grievance arbitration, the primary focus of this article, refers to the grievance and arbitration process established to resolve disputes arising under a collective bargaining agreement, such as interpretation of contract terms, the appropriateness of disciplinary action, and so on. In grievance arbitration, once a case has passed through the various stages or steps of the grievance process, a typical arbitration clause would provide that either side then could refer the matter to a third party, usually selected by mutual agreement of the union and the health care institution, from lists of arbitrators, usually provided by the American Arbitration Association. There are no formal pleadings, motions, and the like that tend to clutter court litigation. Grievance arbitration is reasonably swift and fees and expenses are shared equally by the union and the employer. The arbitrator's decision, which is issued soon after the hearing is closed, is binding on all parties—the institution, the union, and the employee. Only with rare exception may a party take the matter to court, either to have the arbitrator's decision reviewed[1] or to initiate an independent action.[2]

Grievance arbitration must be distinguished from contract or interest arbitration, which seeks to resolve disputes over the terms of the collective bargaining agreement itself, i.e., wages, hours, benefits, and other conditions of employment. Until recently, many collective bargaining agreements with state nurses' associations routinely contained interest arbitration clauses. Nurses' associations usually had declared that they would not resort to strikes or other forms of job actions if they were unable to reach agreement in collective bargaining; interest arbitration thus supplied the method for resolution of a negotiating impasse. Even if the agreement is silent on whether the union may strike, the existence of an interest arbitration clause will preclude such action and any threat to walk out in the face of such a provision, as happened in New York City in 1980, may be enjoined and arbitration compelled.[3]

Grievance and interest arbitration must be distinguished from mediation. Mediation is used mostly in connection with collective bargaining for the terms of a collective bargaining agreement and refers to the effort of third parties to bring the disputants together to mediate the disagreements and to facilitate their resolution. The Federal Mediation and Conciliation Service is a federal agency that provides such a service. A mediator's recommendation, if there be one, is not binding on the parties although, of course, the mediator's influence can be substantial, particularly in the health care industry where state and federal reimbursement agencies frequently are involved, usually in an indirect fashion, in the bargaining process.

In addition, the National Labor Relations Act provides for the appointment of a board of inquiry if there is an impasse prior to contract expiration. Typically, both sides will present their cases to the board of inquiry, which then will find the facts. Although the parties are not compelled to abide by these findings, the panel's determinations on such matters as the financial ability of a hospital to pay an increase or the competitiveness of the union's wage scales can be very significant to the ultimate outcome produced by the collective bargaining process.

Grievance Arbitration: Its Central Place

Prior to the enactment of the National Labor Relations Act in 1935, disputes between unions and employers were resolved in ways that to today's generation, nurtured in decades of relative industrial peace, might seem medieval. The muscle of professional strikebreakers hired by management more often than not was met in kind by the unions. The scene was not a pretty one. The judiciary typically allied itself with employers and severely restricted the ability of unions to strike or take other concerted action. The court injunction became a potent weapon that was wielded against the activities of labor groups, which resulted in a number of sweeping decrees issued without any systematic elaboration of national labor policy. But workers persisted in their organizing efforts and the attitude of the courts prompted Congress to enact in 1932 the Norris-LaGuardia Act, which placed severe limitations on the power of the federal judiciary to issue injunctions in labor disputes. It is significant that to this day unions still perceive the courts as being decidedly promanagement. There is no doubt that one of the reasons grievance arbitration has flourished is that unions believe they will receive a more sympathetic hearing from an arbitrator—a person who is subject to their approval and whose paycheck must contain a union signature.

The National Labor Relations (Wagner) Act in 1935 greatly facilitated the development of grievance and arbitration mechanisms in collective bargaining agreements. This act gave workers the right to bargain with management over their working conditions and to take concerted action without fear of reprisal if the negotiating process did not produce satisfactory results. As a consequence, there was a very rapid growth in the number and size of unions and of collective bargaining agreements with grievance and arbitration mechanisms. The acceptance of these mechanisms accelerated during World War II when unions and employers agreed to submit their bargaining disputes to the War Labor Board in lieu of striking. Although this was voluntary, the War Labor Board greatly encouraged arbitration as a means of resolving disputes under collective bargaining agreements. Not only was the Board instrumental in securing the inclusion of grievance and arbitration provisions in contracts, but the favorable practical experience with arbitration that both sides gained rapidly during the war years was an essential ingredient in eliminating distrust of this process and in paving the way to an even broader modern-day acceptance.[4] It is fair to say that today both labor and management generally believe that grievance arbitration represents the best available alternative for resolving disputes arising under collective bargaining agreements.

There is another, complementary reason why arbitration is believed to be the most appropriate alternative of dispute resolution and this explains a good deal about the very practical nature of arbitration. Consider for a moment the subject matter of a grievance arbitration—the collective bargaining agreement.

The Collective Bargaining Agreement

A collective bargaining agreement usually is a relatively short document of 15 or 20 typewritten pages. Yet its scope is enormous. The number of persons it covers often is many thousands, and in some cases many tens of thousands.

In New York City, for example, the collective bargaining agreement between the League of Voluntary Hospitals and Homes and District 1199, and National Union of Hospital & Health Care Employees, AFL-CIO, covers 40,000 employees, from highly skilled professional technicians to janitors and transporters. Given the very complicated structure of hospitals and other health care institutions, many varied and complex labor-management relationships result.

A collective bargaining agreement also covers a vast range of conduct and problems: hiring rates, incumbent rates, differentials, job classifications, hours, health benefits, pensions, layoffs, promotions, subcontracting, hiring, firing, and so on. Yet few of these areas are dealt with at great length in the contract. The number of different problems, factual variations, and unforeseen contingencies that can arise is practically infinite, and the agreement at best can supply only the general framework within which to resolve these issues.

As Prof. Archibald Cox has stated, "the [collective bargaining agreement] . . . is essentially an instrument of governance, . . . the industrial constitution of the enterprise, setting forth the broad general principles upon which the relationship of employer and employee is to be conducted."[5] This philosophy is crucial to understanding why arbitration gradually has emerged as virtually an autonomous system of private industrial dispute resolution.

Congress and the Courts

Although labor arbitration was growing during the 1940s, judicial attitudes lagged behind. Court decisions on such key issues as whether agreements to arbitrate were enforceable and the extent to which courts could independently review arbitrated cases were remarkedly inconsistent. Congress intervened once again and, in 1947, gave grievance arbitration a specific statutory basis with the enactment of the Labor Management Relations Act (Taft-Hartley). Section 301(a) of that act gave federal courts jurisdiction for "suits for violation of [collective bargaining agreements]. . . ."[6]

Immediately controversy swirled around the full meaning of this provision: was it just a procedural rule that did not alter or affect the myriad of inconsistencies that had developed or did it authorize federal courts to develop substantive principles of labor law? After years of uncertainty and litigation, this question was answered finally in 1957 in a famous Supreme Court decision titled *Textile Workers Union of America v. Lincoln Mills of Alabama*.[7] The Supreme Court reversed the lower court's opinion that the courts would not enforce an arbitration provision. In doing so, it made two significant findings:

First, the Court found that section 301(a) "authorizes federal courts to fashion a body of federal law for the enforcement of . . . collective bargaining agreements. . . ." Thus, there would now be a truly federal-labor law in labor matters.

Second, the Court determined that the federal courts could order the enforcement of arbitration provisions in collective bargaining agreements. The Court stated:

Plainly the agreement to arbitrate grievance disputes is the *quid pro quo* for an agreement not to strike. Viewed in this light, the legislation does more than confer jurisdiction in the federal courts over labor organizations. It expresses a federal policy that federal courts should enforce these agreements on behalf of or against labor organizations and that industrial peace can best be obtained only in that way.[8]

It might be argued that the existence of section 301(a) and the Supreme Court's strong decision in *Lincoln Mills* inevitably would place the federal courts at the heart of the arbitration process. This concern was laid to rest in 1960 by the Supreme Court in the famous "trilogy decisions" that placed arbitration squarely at the heart of the collective bargaining process and severely limited the role of the courts in that process.

In the first case, *United Steelworkers of America v. America Mfg. Co.*,[9] an employer refused to arbitrate on the ground that the grievance was "frivolous" and the United States Court of Appeals agreed. The Supreme Court reversed and compelled arbitration:

> The collective bargaining agreement requires arbitration of claims that courts might be unwilling to entertain. In the context of the plant or industry the grievance may assume proportions of which judges are ignorant.

> * * * *

> The courts . . . have no business weighing the merits of the grievance, considering whether there is equity in a particular claim, or determining whether there is particular language in the written instrument which will support the claim. The agreement is to submit all grievances to arbitration, not merely those the court will deem meritorious. The processing of even frivolous claims may have therapeutic values of which those who are not a part of the plant environment may be quite unaware.[10]

In the second of these decisions, the lower court had held, in response to a union suit seeking to compel arbitration, that the collective bargaining agreement excluded the particular grievance from arbitration. The Supreme Court reversed, holding in very broad language:

> [T]he grievance machinery under a collective bargaining agreement is at the very heart of the system of industrial self-government. Arbitration is the means of solving the unforeseeable by molding a system of private law for all the problems which may arise and to provide for their solution in a way which will generally accord with the variant needs and desires of the parties.

> * * * *

> The grievance procedure is, in other words, a part of the continuous collective bargaining process.

> * * * *

> The judiciary sits in these cases to bring into operation an arbitral process which substitutes a regime of peaceful settlement for the older regime of industrial conflict. Whether contracting out in the present case violated the agreement is the question. *It is a question for the arbiter, not the courts.*[11] [Emphasis added.]

And finally, in the last case, the Supreme Court, in sustaining an arbitrator's award that the employer had refused to follow, gave broad support to the power of arbitrators to fashion appropriate remedies, stating: "[T]he courts have no business overruling [the arbitrator] . . . because their interpretation of the contract is different from his. . . ."[12]

The Steelworkers trilogy involved recalcitrant employers who had attempted to circumvent the arbitration process. However, many unions initially took the position that because of the Norris-LaGuardia Act, which restricted the power of courts to enjoin strikes and other work stoppages, a union could strike even though such action concerned a matter that was cognizable under the grievance and arbitration provisions of the collective bargaining agreement. The Supreme Court put this question to rest in 1970 in *The Boys Markets, Inc. v. Retail Clerks, Local 770*,[13] holding that if indeed the incident giving rise to the strike was subject to arbitration, an injunction would issue.

Cooperative Attitude of the NLRB

It also should be noted that in general the National Labor Relations Board (NLRB), which was established to enforce the 1935 Act, will defer to arbitration in its enforcement of the provisions of the Act prohibiting unfair labor practices. The issue here is a bit more clouded than the limitations imposed on judicial review of arbitrators' awards since section 10(a) of the Act vests exclusive jurisdiction to oversee unfair labor practices with the NLRB. Unfair labor practices often involve matters that also are subject to the grievance and arbitration mechanisms in the collective bargaining agreement. Although there is an uneasy tension between the relationship of arbitration and the Board's statutory mandate to enforce the Act's specific proscriptions against unfair labor practices, nonetheless it is fair to say that the NLRB recognizes the fundamental role of arbitration and gives it as full a play as is reasonably possible.[14]

Arbitration thus occupies a central place in the collective bargaining process and provides a realistic and pragmatic means of preserving industrial peace. Arbitrators have fashioned a law of industrial relations that in any particular industry regulates the relationship of management to the union. In areas where unions in the health care industry have existed for some time, there are innumerable arbitrators' awards interpreting and applying virtually every provision of the collective bargaining agreement. With the continued unionization in this industry, management must look increasingly to this body of "law" for guidance in day-to-day personnel decisions. Not only has the process of arbitration become almost the exclusive and final means of contract resolution, but arbitrators' awards increasingly are supplying the substantive norms by which employer-employee behavior is measured.

THE ARBITRATION PROCESS

Now that it has been shown that arbitration has a central role in the relationship of the employer and the union, the question arises: What is arbitration, when can it be invoked, what are its mechanics, and what is involved in preparing and presenting the case? Although the intent here is to provide a general overview of arbitration, the author would like to conclude where he began—in final response to the personnel director friend mentioned at the outset—by connecting the arbitration process itself to overall personnel policy and labor-management relations.

Preliminary Considerations

Is the Case Arbitrable?

One of the first questions is whether the case is arbitrable, i.e., is it subject to the arbitration clause?

It must be noted initially that what is arbitrable and what is not is subject to negotiation and the agreement of the parties pursuant to the collective bargaining process. Many contracts expressly limit the scope of arbitration. In the health care industry, limitations are imposed frequently in agreements with unions of professionals, such as physicians and house staff, where management has achieved the exclusion of a variety of matters from the grievance and arbitration process. Often these excluded areas include such bread-and-butter union issues as layoffs, promotions, and seniority. In addition, agreements with professionals refer issues that can be characterized as "professional" to the medical board in an institution rather than to an outside arbitrator.

In contracts with nonprofessionals, a number of issues are excluded from the arbitration process. This is particularly true of issues that involve management rights where an employer may agree to a certain contract provision but does not wish to have its implementation of that provision subject to third party scrutiny. For example, if an employer agrees to make a good faith effort to schedule every other weekend off for its bargaining unit employees—a traditional management prerogative—the employer will attempt to couple this obligation with a nonarbitrability provision as has been done in many agreements in New York with the state nurses' association. Categories of employees may be excluded from the grievance and arbitration machinery—for example, probationary employees and certain part-time and temporary workers.

Finally, almost all grievance and arbitration provisions contain various time limitations. A typical contract will provide that a grievance must be filed within 10 to 20 days after the incident occurred; once the last step in the grievance process has been completed, the notice of arbitration that initiates the process must be filed within a similar time frame. However, it should be noted that arbitrators are loath to deny a grievant a day in court if an action is untimely, particularly when the filing of arbitrations is controlled by the union and not by the grievant. To protect the employee, arbitrators will strain to find reasons why strict adherence to the specified time periods is not appropriate. An employer that wishes to rely on a lack of timeliness argument must adhere to these provisions consistently and virtually without exception.

Should the Case Go to Arbitration?

Before deciding to go to arbitration, both sides should carefully consider their positions and whether the case should be settled. Many of the considerations that must be evaluated are perhaps self-evident, but it is important to emphasize that these must be analyzed in the context of the overall union-management relationship. Few individual arbitration cases are divorced from these general considerations. The following factors should be evaluated in deciding to let a case go forward to arbitration:

1. What are the strengths and weaknesses of both the management and union cases? What is the probability of success? If total success is not likely, is partial success? How much will it cost in terms of legal fees and management time to take the case forward?
2. What are the consequences of losing? If the case is a matter of contract interpretation, can it be resolved by compromise, by *collective bargaining*, in a way which is reasonably satisfactory to both sides?
3. Can the case be settled on a basis that does not set a precedent? Is this an isolated case that will have little impact on others or will many employees be affected?
4. Does this test a good rule with a bad case? Are there better cases to take forward that would establish the principle the employer seeks to achieve?
5. What impact will arbitrating the case have on preserving good relationships with the union?

(Again, both sides must recognize that arbitration is not total war.)

6. What effect will the arbitration have on morale? Are there more serious problems underlying the arbitration than might be specifically at issue in the arbitration? Is there a possibility that the battle might be won at the risk of widening the war?

7. What effect will the arbitration have on supervisors and on their authority if it is lost?

8. What effect will the arbitration have on the credibility of the grievance process and on the personnel department?

9. What effect will the arbitration have on the credibility of management with the arbitrators who function in this particular industry or with this particular union?

What to Expect, Selection of the Arbitrator

The framework of arbitration has been likened to frontier justice rather than the principled decision making of the courts. As one commentator has stated, it is "rough and ready" and must be dispensed with haste.[15] These surely are exaggerations. Yet it must be remembered constantly that arbitrators are beholden to both parties. It is natural to expect arbitrators in general over a range of cases to attempt to please both sides. Compromises, trade-offs, and "splitting down the middle" all are synonyms to describe the arbitration process. This is particularly true in contract interpretation cases where the language of a particular provision is ambiguous. In this situation, arbitrators often act the way they would in settling a collective bargaining issue. Unlike judges who must decide a case more or less on an all-or-nothing basis, an arbitrator will base a decision on a series of collective bargaining considerations that usually leads to a compromise.

Volumes have been written on how to select the arbitrator. Perhaps the Supreme Court has said it best:

The labor arbitrator is usually chosen because of the parties' confidence in his knowledge of the common law of the shop and their trust in his personal judgment to bring to bear considerations which are not expressed in the contract as criteria for judgment. The parties expect that his judgment of a particular grievance will reflect not only what the contract says but, insofar as the collective bargaining agreement permits, such factors as the effect upon productivity of a particular result, its consequence to the morale of the shop, his judgment whether tensions will be heightened or diminished.[16]

Trust and confidence. These are the key criteria, and whether the parties have trust and confidence in an arbitrator comes only with experience. Some arbitrators tend to be better on certain types of cases than on others. Some arbitrators tend to be more favorably disposed to safeguarding individual rights in discipline cases than are other arbitrators, and some are better at contract interpretation cases. As arbitrator Joseph Wildebush put it:

Arbitrators with legal backgrounds have a tendency to approach the issues with a judicial attitude. College professors sometimes have a quixotic approach to issues. Former labor or management representatives tend to focus on the practical and pragmatic aspects inherent in the issues.[17]

Selection of the arbitrator thus is a key consideration in any arbitration and must be evaluated carefully, based on the parties' practical experience.

Preparation of the Case

General Considerations

Despite the tendencies of arbitration to represent a process of compromise, there is no doubt that thorough preparation and a solid presentation of the case can provide a tremendous advantage.

As noted, at the hearing both sides present their versions of the case and the arbitrator bases the decision on the *evidence* presented. What is meant by evidence? Generally, documents, the testimony of witnesses, and "in-kind" evidence, such as time clocks, photographs of portions of the plant, tools, machines, etc., if such are involved. To illustrate:

Suppose a union employee, a respiratory therapist, is responsible for checking oxygen tanks to make certain they provide the right flow of air to patients and that the tanks do not run down. The employee's supervisor checks the tanks in patient rooms and notices that several are below the safe level. The supervisor cannot locate the employee; he is not where he is supposed to be. The supervisor meets the employee several minutes later in the corridor and asks why the tanks were not checked and changed. The employee says he did check the tanks and that they did not require changing in accordance with institutional policy. The supervisor says that is not the policy and orders the employee to change the tanks. The employee says "get off my back," yells loudly enough to bring several patients and a nurse out into the corridor, and finally walks away. The department head is on vacation and the supervisor waits until his return five days later. They then review the case and decide to fire the employee since "he represents a threat to patient safety exhibited by the failure to change the tanks." The case goes to arbitration.

What documents are to be involved? The collective bargaining agreement containing the grievance procedure, the termination notice, the employee's personnel file and in particular any job evaluations or other warning notices he may have received, written work rules (e.g., any memoranda communicating the policy regarding changing tanks to the employees in the department or any manuals or written industry standards that might be applicable), and the grievance form and notice to arbitrate.

Who will the witnesses be? The supervisor and any other eyewitnesses, such as the nurse, as to what happened on the patient floor; the department head, as to the basis of the decision; possibly the chairman of the appropriate medical department, as to the policy concerning appropriate oxygen levels; and possibly someone from personnel, as to policies regarding progressive discipline.

It is vital to understand that the stuff of which evidence is made is already formed by the time the arbitration is filed. Evidence cannot be manufactured or altered after the fact. The employer cannot rewrite the termination or warning notice to reflect what was really intended because it now is realized that it may be incomplete. The warning notice is like a pleading in that it delineates the issues that are the subject of the arbitration and sets forth the basis for the employer's action (in this case, note that the warning notice is defective because it should have included the additional infractions of failure to be at the proper post, creating a disturbance, and insubordination). A witness cannot be compelled to testify as to facts that did not occur or to deny facts that did occur (for example, how are the witnesses here to support the severity of the discipline on the basis of patient safety when they kept the employee on duty for an additional week after the incident?).

This case also illustrates that the best preparation for arbitration consists of intelligent administration of the collective bargaining agreement and personnel policy. There is simply no substitute for effective, consistent contract administration as the underpinning of an arbitration. Poor supervision, poor documentation, lack of corroboration, failure to properly discipline progressively, and inconsistent application of contract principles are the employer's real nemesis in arbitration. Unless there is an overview of contract administration, these problems will appear with surprising frequency in labor arbitrations. If management does not have this overview, it can rest assured that the union

does and will exploit these weaknesses at arbitration with great skill.

Reviewing the Case, Use of Attorneys

Obviously, the institution wants to present its case in the best light possible and be in a position to attack the union's case effectively. Management must gather all the facts, the bad *and* the good, even though it will not use them all. It is my view that the director of personnel or employee relations must be an integral part of the preparation process, even though the case may be handled by an attorney. Again, this is so because arbitration cannot be divorced from—indeed, it is an essential part of—overall contract administration. For the same reason that it is crucial that the director of personnel or employee relations be involved in the process at the earliest moment to assure that decisions reached are proper and consistent with precedent and other policies of the institution, it is crucial that this person be involved in the case preparation.

After all the relevant documents have been gathered and identified, consideration must be given as to how these will be presented at the arbitration. Although with certain kinds of documents this can be done by stipulation between the parties, documents generally are introduced into the record through witnesses whose responsibilities include the function to which the documents relate or who actually prepared them.

The witnesses should be interviewed as close in time to the occurrence of the incident as possible so that their recollections are fresh and accurate. This may mean that these interviews take place before it is clear that the case will go to arbitration. In the interviews, the witnesses should recite the facts in their own words. This is the only assurance of getting all the relevant facts. It is very unwise to ask leading questions.

After the facts are on the table, the presentation of the case can be structured. Witnesses in particular must be prepared carefully as to what to expect and in general how to present themselves. They should be told to listen carefully to all questions and to respond only to the specifics of the question. They should not volunteer information not solicited by the question or to speculate or to venture opinions. If they do not remember a fact or detail, they should simply say so; witnesses are not expected to have perfect memories. They should be told that if they become flustered or confused to simply take a moment to collect themselves or to ask that if the question is not clear, it be repeated or rephrased.

In preparing the case, it is wise to involve the attorneys, if they are being used, as early as possible in the preparation process. The sooner the facts are obtained, the better the case can be evaluated in the overall context of collective bargaining, and decisions regarding possible settlement made. If the institution does not have in-house counsel, it is crucial that the director of personnel or labor relations develop a close working relationship with outside counsel. In general, the same individual outside attorneys as are used on other matters should work for the institution on labor matters. Knowing and understanding the extremely complex nature of health care institutions as well as the relationship of a particular union to that institution is a process of education that takes time to develop. The institution should avoid becoming the training ground for attorneys who move on to other matters. It also is crucial that the attorney be familiar with the common law of industrial relations as it has developed with respect to the particular union and the particular institution. It has been my experience that the most cost-effective outside attorney is the most qualified partner in the firm, not the least expensive associate who also is likely to be the least experienced.

Order of Presentation

The documents now have been gathered and witnesses "prepped." The case is ready for trial. What happens next?

Burden of Proof

It has become almost universally accepted that in discipline cases the employer proceeds first. In effect, the employer must explain what happened and justify what was done about it. Many believe—and practical experience bears this out—that the employer has the burden of proof in these situations.

It probably is true that the more severe the sanction, the higher the burden of proving the case will be. In addition, the appropriateness of that sanction will be judged in the context of (1) how serious the offense was, (2) how many years the individual has been an employee, and (3) the linkage of the particular sanction to the progressive discipline of the worker. All of these considerations are fundamental to labor-management relations and will be considered carefully by the arbitrator.

In other types of cases, the reverse is true, with the union going first and generally having the burden of proof.

Rules of Evidence

Arbitration is not a court proceeding and the formal rules of evidence do not apply. Rule 28 of the American Arbitration Association's rules simply provides that "the parties may offer such evidence as they desire and shall produce such additional evidence as the arbitrator may deem necessary to an understanding and determination of the dispute. . . . [C]onformity to legal rules of evidence shall not be necessary."

The extent to which a particular arbitrator adheres to the rules of evidence such as, for example, the rule against the admission of hearsay testimony, is important to know in advance. Moreover, although arbitrators frequently take evidence for "whatever it's worth," what the evidence is worth will depend on its authenticity and reliability. It always is best to have testimony from those with firsthand knowledge and to have documents introduced by those who prepared them or who are responsible for the administration of the matters to which they relate.

Opening Statement

The arbitration begins with a preliminary discussion among the parties and the arbitrator to define and delineate the issues. This typically is limited to the scope of the warning notice or grievance form.

Once the issues are agreed upon, counsel or the persons presenting the case for management and the union make opening statements. The opening statement is extremely important since it gives the parties an opportunity to outline the basis of the case in general terms to the arbitrator, who at this point is totally unfamiliar with the facts. It can be used to emphasize the points management believes are important so that the arbitrator will look for them as the case develops.

Sequestration of Witnesses, Court Reporters

Usually all witnesses who will testify remain in the hearing room. However, if there is an issue of credibility—i.e., a possibility that a witness may tailor testimony on the basis of what others have testified to—the witnesses should be sequestered in a separate room. This is discretionary with the arbitrator; the grievant, of course, is permitted to stay.

Often witnesses are not sworn, although this varies from arbitrator to arbitrator and sometimes is subject to the agreement of the parties. In general, the swearing of witnesses seems to give some dignity to the hearing and it usually impresses the witnesses with the need to be truthful. Certainly if there is likely to be an issue of credibility, it always is best to have the witnesses sworn.

A court reporter, i.e., someone who takes down verbatim everything said, is used only where the case is complex or long time intervals may elapse between hearing dates and there thus is a need to have a transcript of the proceedings. Sometimes the presence of a court reporter is useful for purposes of cross-examination of witnesses if great precision is necessary as to what they or others may have said. In general, however, a court reporter represents a formalization of the arbitration process and can impede the progress of a case. For these reasons, court reporters seldom are used.

Testimony, Cross-Examination

Since there usually is no court reporter, it is extremely important to slow the pace of questions so that the arbitrator can absorb what is being said and make appropriate notes. Witnesses should be cautioned to speak slowly, clearly, and audibly and directly to the arbitrator.

The party that starts the case will put its witnesses on the stand to testify by direct examination. On direct examination, witnesses cannot be asked leading questions, that is, questions that contain or imply the answer. Witnesses must tell the story the way they recall it and not the way the attorney leads them to testify.

After each witness testifies, the other side questions the same individual in cross-examination. Here the questions can be leading since the idea is to probe what the witness has said already. Cross-examination is a crucial part of any case since obviously witnesses on direct examination will emphasize only the favorable aspects. Thus, considerable latitude is allowed on cross-examination to develop factual inconsistencies, facts the witness left out, and in general to attempt to impeach the witness's credibility.

After one side presents its witnesses and documents and cross-examination has taken place, the other side presents its case by presenting its witnesses and documents in similar fashion. At the conclusion of this presentation, the first party has an opportunity to offer in rebuttal any testimony or evidence not already in the record.

Closing Summations

Next comes the summation by the attorneys or representatives for each side. Usually the party with the burden of proof sums up first. The purpose of summation is to present the reasons why, based on the record developed at the hearing, the grievance should be sustained or denied. In the summation, each party has a good deal of latitude in reviewing the exact testimony

of the witnesses and in characterizing its probative value or worthlessness. The credibility of the witnesses often is assessed, and errors and inconsistencies are pointed out. Unless posttrial briefs are filed, which is rare, the summation is the last opportunity the parties have to impress the arbitrator with their respective cases.

The hearing then closes and the arbitrator usually takes 30 days or so to issue a written decision.

CONCLUDING COMMENTS

The arbitration process seems relatively straightforward, and indeed it is. In concluding, several very important practical substantive points should be reemphasized:

1. The substance of arbitration is the collective bargaining agreement. Decisions made under the agreement must be made with reference to the common law of industrial relations, which has been developed largely by arbitrators. There are many considerations in deciding whether a case should go to arbitration that involve the broader context of the relationship between the employer and the union. An arbitrator is likely to take a very practical approach to the problem, so both union and management should consider the alternatives to arbitration before plowing ahead. It invariably is better to resolve matters by agreement across the table than by resort to third parties.

2. Health care institutions are divided into a variety of departments and subdepartments and the management structure often is extremely complex. Administration must have an overview of the collective bargaining agreement to assure the consistency of application of the contract principles, including discipline. Inconsistent application, disparate treatment, and similar issues can destroy a case in arbitration.

3. There must be an orderly process of decision making, particularly in disciplinary matters. There must be appropriate documentation of management decisions (there are three rules in disciplinary matters: document, document, document!) and all relevant facts should be gathered and reviewed before actions are taken so that the decisions are correct in the first place. There is nothing more frustrating than to have to compromise a good case because the process of decision making was defective or documentation is inadequate. Evidence is the product of the incident and how it is handled by management. It is

too late to create evidence once the decision is made.

4. Policies and procedures must be written clearly and communicated clearly to employees. These rules must be kept current.

5. Hospitals and other health care providers should embark on educational programs to instruct physicians, nurses, and administrators, particularly those who have line responsibility, as to how to handle disciplinary and other labor-management matters. This is not their area of expertise and they cannot be expected to deal with the myriad of complex issues with any degree of sophistication. It is important that a procedure be established to assure adequate investigation of all incidents and that all relevant persons are involved in deciding the disposition of the case.

It is my belief that implementation of these points should minimize the need to resort to arbitration and, more importantly, lead to a more effectively run institution.

On reflection, I suppose my friend probably ran precisely this sort of personnel/labor relations at his hospital!

NOTES

1. See brief discussion below concerning the deferral policies of the National Labor Relations Board. Rarely will a court review the merits of an arbitrator's decision.

2. An individual does not have the absolute right to have a grievance taken to arbitration. A union, however, has the obligation of "fair representation" of its bargaining unit members and must not act in an arbitrary or capricious way. Only in extreme cases, when the union has breached this duty, will courts permit an employee to pursue independent court action. *See Vaca v. Sipes*, 386 U.S. 171 (1967); *Hines v. Anchor Motor Freight*, 424 U.S. 554 (1976). It must be noted that the existence of a grievance and arbitration process does not prevent an employee from filing a charge of discrimination with the appropriate federal or state agency. *See, e.g., Alexander v. Gardner-Denver*, 415 U.S. 36 (1974), holding that an employee was entitled to a hearing de novo on a charge of racial discrimination and that courts should not defer to arbitration since the arbitrator's task was to construe the law of the shop and not the "law of the land."

3. *The Mount Sinai Hosp. v. New York State Nurses et al.* (S.D.N.Y. 80 Civ. 0727, February 1980).

4. *See* generally Gerald Asken, "History and Development," *Arbitrating Labor Cases* (New York: Practising Law Institute, 1975), p. 11 et seq.

5. Professor Archibald Cox's analysis was accepted by the Supreme Court in the Steelworkers decisions referred to below. *See* Archibald Cox, "Reflections Upon Labor Arbitration," 72 *Harvard Law Review* 1482 (1959).

6. 29 U.S.C. § 185(a).

7. 353 U.S. 448 (1957).

8. 353 U.S. at 455.

9. 363 U.S. 564 (1960).

10. 363 U.S. at 567, 568.

11. *United Steelworkers of America v. Warrior & Gulf Navigation Co.*, 363 U.S. 574, 581, 585 (1960).

12. *United Steelworkers of America v. Enterprise Wheel & Car Corp.*, 363 U.S. 593, 599 (1960).

13. 398 U.S. 235 (1970). And *see Buffalo Forge Co. v. United Steelworkers of America*, 428 U.S. 397 (1976), holding that a sympathy strike could not be enjoined under the theory of *Boys Markets* since the underlying dispute was not subject to the arbitration provisions of the collective bargaining agreement.

14. *See Spielberg Manufacturing Co.*, 112 NLRB 1080 (1955); *Collyer Insulated Wire*, 192 NLRB 837 (1971).

15. Noel Arnold Levin, "Some Practical Considerations and Procedures," *Arbitrating Labor Cases* (New York, Practising Law Institute, 1975), *supra*, p. 100.

16. *United Steelworkers of America v. Warrior & Gulf Navigation Co., supra* at 582.

17. Joseph Wildebush, "What An Arbitrator Looks For," *Arbitrating Labor Cases* (New York: Practising Law Institute, 1975), *supra*, p. 107.

32. How to Discipline: The Positive Approach

NORMAN METZGER

Reprinted with permission from *The Health Care Supervisor's Handbook,* by Norman Metzger, published by Aspen Systems Corporation, Germantown, Md., © 1978.

If you are a supervisor you are going to be faced, almost daily, with the need to effect corrective action when an employee is chronically late, has an absentee problem, disregards a rule or policy of the institution, refuses to follow an order, is unproductive, is uncooperative, or in some ways does not meet the standards of the institution. Taking corrective action is often a euphemism for discipline. On the other hand, the goal of positive discipline is to salvage the employee, to correct the behavioral pattern that is either antisocial or anti-institution.

More often than not, the act of disciplining is conceived of as punishment. Such an approach is referred to as negative discipline. Punishment may be the least effective way to discipline. We shall deal here with the complete spectrum of *constructive* discipline.

A CASE STUDY IN EFFECTIVE DISCIPLINARY ACTION

"You just can't fire anyone here. The union won't permit it." A physician at a large medical center voiced this complaint to the personnel director. The physician referred to "the good old days" when the hospital was run by the doctors and administrators. Now she felt it was run by the union.

The physician was talking specifically about an employee in her department who she felt was beyond redemption. Since she had concluded that she could

not terminate him, she offered a proposal to the personnel director that in effect would "neutralize" the unsatisfactory employee. Instead of releasing him, she was going to keep him in drydock.

Earlier that day a hearing had been held in the personnel director's office in which the union appealed the termination of one of its members, who also happened to be a union delegate. The hearing lasted almost two hours. At the conclusion, the termination was upheld—the union concurred in this decision. But didn't that physician say that you couldn't fire anyone? Wherein lies the difference?

In the first case, a look at the employee's folder revealed no warning notices, no negative performance evaluations, no record of unsatisfactory performance. The physician who headed the department asserted loudly and clearly that the employee was inefficient, often late, often absent, surly, and insubordinate. Yet not a line of documentation existed to support these accusations!

In the case of the union delegate who had been with the institution for three years, the personnel folder contained several warning notices, a notice of suspension, and a final warning notice. In addition, the performance evaluation reflected specific problems—clearly enumerated with dates—regarding attendance, punctuality, and attitude.

The supervisor who said "You can't fire anyone here . . ." was pronouncing a self-fulfilling prophecy. Believing this notion, she documented nothing. She

843

was guilty of the cardinal sin in employee discipline—offering innocuous performance evaluations to escape the unpleasantness of that "chore." Many hospital supervisors will not admit their unwillingness to take the time or effort to discipline, to face the unpleasant job of counseling, issuing warning notices, and confronting the employee in a hearing which could result in a suspension or discharge.

The truth of the matter is that the doctor was right. She was not able to fire anyone for a capricious or arbitrary reason, or where just cause could not be established. For other than clearly overt acts of insubordination, refusal to follow a direct order, or acts which endanger or compromise good patient care, the supervisor has the responsibility of documenting his or her case. *This in no way means that the supervisor is unable to act.* It simply means he or she must show that the employee was fully cognizant of the problems and that a pattern of warnings was used to denote progressive disciplining.

GOOD AND JUST CAUSE

The burden of providing "good and just cause" for discipline rests on administration. If cause has been proved, a penalty imposed by the administration will not be modified by an arbitrator, unless it is shown to have been clearly arbitrary, capricious, discriminatory, or excessive in relation to the offense. The key point to understand about limitation on the right to discipline is that administration may discipline up through discharge *only* for sufficient and appropriate reasons.

It behooves the administration to develop a sound procedure, based upon due process, for the discipline of unionized employees. Even if it is not mandated by a collective bargaining agreement, due process should be available to all employees. Arbitrators will normally support a management action if progressive discipline includes, first, a verbal reprimand and full explanation of what is necessary to remedy the situation, followed by written reprimand for a second infraction and a clear warning of the future penalties that may be imposed. A final warning and suspension may follow, and subsequently the ultimate penalty of discharge.

The arbitrator will also consider whether or not the employee was fully aware of the standards against which his or her behavior was measured. These standards include basic rules and regulations that outline offenses which subject employees to disciplinary action, and the extent of such disciplinary action.

Disciplining has become more juristic and legalistic with the advent of a union, but that does not mean that

it is impossible to discipline employees. It does mean that the administration must record actual events, offenses, and transgressions. You cannot simply wish away problem employees.

Jules Justin, a prominent labor arbitrator, lists some noteworthy rules of corrective discipline:

1. Discipline to be meaningful must be corrective, not punitive.
2. When you discipline one, you discipline all.
3. Corrective discipline satisfies the rule of equality of treatment by enforcing equally among all employees established rules, safety practices, and responsibility on the job.
4. It is the job of the supervisor, not the shop steward, to make the worker toe the line or increase efficiency.
5. Just cause or any other comparable standard for justifying disciplinary action under the labor contract consists of three parts:
   a. Did the employee breach the rule or commit the offense charged against him?
   b. Did the employee's act or misconduct warrant corrective action or punishment?
   c. Is the penalty just and appropriate to the act or offense as corrective punishment?
6. The burden of proof rests on the supervisor. He or she must justify each of the three parts that make up the standard of just cause under the labor contract.[1]

FORMS OF DISCIPLINE

The real purpose of discipline is to correct employees so that unacceptable behavior does not recur. In addition, you wish to deter others from committing the same errors. We have learned a great deal about the need for progressive disciplinary action. Most of what we have learned has come from two sources—the behavioral scientists and arbitrators.

Arbitrators tell us what is required to sustain a discharge. The following points were enunciated by a prominent arbitrator, Milton Friedman, but many other arbitrators have set up similar criteria for the sustaining of discharges.

1. The employer must prove that the alleged acts occurred and were of sufficient gravity to warrant termination.
2. The employer must show that the misconduct was not condoned, but the employee was specifically warned of the consequences through pro-

gressive discipline, such as written warnings and suspension.

3. The evidence must demonstrate that the employee made no genuine effort to heed the warnings although the consequences of continued misconduct were known.
4. The employee cannot be singled out for disparate treatment for offenses that do not subject others to similar discipline.
5. When a long-service employee is involved, there must be sound cause to believe that the events are not transitory, but form a consistent and recurrent pattern that is unlikely to change in the future.

The Oral Reprimand

It is clear that progressive disciplining usually starts with oral reprimands or oral warnings. This function is often handled in a counseling session. What is the purpose of the action? It should be to nip in the bud behavior that is inappropriate to the work area. The necessary ingredients for a successful counseling encounter are complete privacy, a well-planned agenda, enough time to arrive at agreement, and a positive attitude on the part of the supervisor.

In such sessions employees should receive a complete outline of the action in question. Details should not be spared, and dates and times and places should be communicated. The specific institution policy or rule in question should be enunciated. The specific documents (such as a union contract or the personnel policy manual) wherein such rules are contained should be examined. The employee should be given complete freedom to answer the charge, explain his or her behavior, admit or deny the action.

It is obvious that an effective counseling session will develop from the point that the employee *agrees that the action occurred and was inappropriate.* If such an agreement is reached, a plan to improve the employee's performance should be discussed. As I mentioned in an earlier chapter, it is also important at this time to acknowledge the positive aspects of the employee's behavior.

After the counseling session has been completed, anecdotal notes should be prepared by the supervisor and placed in the employee's folder *in the department.* It is not appropriate at this point to forward such notes to the personnel department for inclusion in the employee's personnel folder.

We must repeat that the supervisor who wishes to effect corrective disciplining should be more interested in changing an employee's behavioral patterns and at-

titudes than in reprimanding that employee. Lateiner[2] offers some pointers to the supervisor interested in making criticism more constructive:

1. Don't reprimand a worker who is angry or excited. Wait until he or she has cooled down. Wait until you cool down, too.
2. Don't bawl out someone in front of other people. This is embarrassing and humiliating and is likely to do more harm than good.
3. Find out how the worker feels and thinks about the situation. If you want someone to do something differently, you first have to find out what she or he already knows.
4. When you criticize a person, it is much better to compare her or his performance to department standards than to the performance of another employee. A person is more likely to feel resentful or insecure if she or he is compared unfavorably to a coworker.
5. Most important, if you reprimand constructively, you must show a person how to improve his or her performance. You don't want to destroy an employee's self-confidence. You want to build up confidence by guiding the worker in the direction of a satisfactory performance.

The oral reprimand or warning interview is a useful way for the supervisor to establish a sound relationship with *all* employees—those who require such warnings and those who do not. Employees normally respect supervisors who apply the rules of the institution fairly. Although criticism is often a disturbing element, the need for *constructive* criticism can be fully appreciated by employees.

If the supervisor is to discipline firmly and wisely, it is essential that the employee relations administrator or personnel director fully support the supervisor in those instances where institutional policy is being protected and carried out. It is equally important that the department head or director of the institution provide clear evidence that the supervisor will be backed up at crucial moments. This does not mean that there will never be a situation where the supervisor is overruled, but such incidences should not be based on political pressures, legal technicalities, or sentimentality. The responsibility of meting out discipline is difficult enough without undercutting the first-line supervisor.

Before concluding our discussion of the oral reprimand or warning interview, it should be made clear that the oral reprimand is not appropriate or effective in the face of flagrant offenses such as insubordination, theft, fighting, or carrying firearms. Such actions call for sharper responses—often termination.

Warning Notices

Overt flaunting of institutional rules and appropriate behavior patterns is dealt with by the first-line supervisor either by means of a formal warning notice, suspension, or discharge—if, and only after, a formal warning interview has been held. (This proscription does not apply if the transgression is a major and flagrant one such as those mentioned under exceptions to the oral reprimand.) Some examples of negative behavior which may call for a written warning notice are:

- Insubordination or impertinence
- Unauthorized or chronic absenteeism
- Chronic lateness
- Loafing or sleeping
- Misrepresentation of time cards or records
- Drinking alcoholic beverages
- Dishonesty
- Fighting on the job
- Gambling

The warning notice should not come as a surprise to an employee. It is essentially the second step in the arsenal of weapons used to reverse a poor behavioral pattern. It is often preceded by the oral reprimand, but may directly follow a clear violation of institutional rules and regulations. In preparing the warning notice, the supervisor is again concerned with facts and not with subjective opinions.

The institution normally provides a form to be used for written warning notices. This form usually calls for a clear statement of the specific rule or policy that has been violated. The supervisor may have to refer to the union contract or personnel policy manual or written bulletin containing the specific rule.

Following this reference point, the written warning notice should move toward a description of the act in question. Once again the supervisor is urged to be specific and complete. Dates, time, and, where appropriate, witnesses should be included.

Now we come to the most important part of the warning notice—a statement to indicate that immediate satisfactory improvement must be shown and maintained unless further disciplinary action is to be taken. In many cases, this "immediate satisfactory improvement" can be outlined in detail. For example, suppose an employee has shown a pattern of absenteeism—let us say three days each month for the last six months (many of the days were Mondays, making three-day weekends possible). The supervisor will indicate that the employee's pattern of Monday absences is not acceptable, that the employee's attendance will be monitored over the next two, three,

or four months to gauge improvement, and that if there is no improvement, the employee will be subject to suspension and possible termination.

The warning notice is presented to the employee in private. If possible, the employee should be asked to sign the warning notice, acknowledging receipt. More important than this acknowledgment of the warning form is the employee's acknowledgment that the behavior is inappropriate and that improvement is forthcoming. In some cases—more often than not where unions are involved—employees will refuse to sign a warning notice form. This should be expected and understood, but the supervisor's responsibility does not end here. The supervisor, in order to emphasize the importance of the action and ensure the "legality" of the presentation, should ask another supervisor to witness the actual reading and offer a copy of the warning notice to the employee. This is necessary only if the employee refuses to sign the warning notice form.

Despite the discussion above, it is important to remember that the supervisor's cardinal responsibility in this procedure is to attempt a restructuring of the employee's behavior; it is not the primary responsibility or objective to punish the employee.

One bit of advice is necessary before we explore the final two steps in the disciplinary arsenal of weapons—suspension and termination. There is no easy panacea that can be offered in the area of behavior control. In a few cases oral reprimands or warning notices will never be enough. In still more cases suspensions may be counterproductive. The supervisor must keep in mind that constructive disciplining is a means of achieving the end product—a change in behavior patterns.

Suspension

The suspension is not universally accepted as an effective way to correct behavior patterns. Many employees find the suspension a respite from the stress of the work area. *Some employees even enjoy being out on strike.* For an employee with a chronic absentee record a suspension is certainly not the worst sort of punishment.

A one-day suspension can be as effective as a one-week suspension. The shock of the suspension will usually bring the employee to his or her senses. The length of the suspension has little effect on the probability of rehabilitation. Very often the suspension of an employee causes inordinate difficulties in scheduling and in meeting production quotas. I have come to the conclusion that a one- or two-day suspension is a sufficient final warning to employees before termination.

The suspension should be accompanied with a written warning notice indicating prior attempts, both informal and formal, toward rehabilitation. Most important, the suspension should indicate that it constitutes the final warning.

Termination

In order to sustain a discharge where an arbitration procedure is available, the following minimal requirements must be met. In fact, these requirements should be operative whether or not there is an arbitration procedure, whether or not there is a union.

1. Facts must be presented, clearly indicating that the employee actually committed the offense. Opinion must be separated from hard documentation. Witnesses may be essential.
2. You must be able to display a consistent approach to the offense in question: no playing of favorites.
3. The record should indicate a progressive disciplining ladder, except in the case of blatant and serious offenses.
4. The punishment must fit the crime.

Progressive disciplining normally must precede the discharge of an employee. The procedure for progressive disciplining as outlined above includes a verbal reprimand and a full explanation of what is necessary to remedy the situation. Normally a second infraction calls for a written reprimand with a clear warning of future penalties which may be imposed. A suspension may follow with a final warning and the ultimate penalty is discharge. There is a further consideration in cases that involve discharge—*consistency*. A double standard is often found in health care institutions: one standard for the medical staff and another standard for the other employees. We shall not explore this provocative subject, but the supervisor should be aware of the possibility of employee complaints to the union and to outside agencies of disparate treatment of professionals and nonprofessionals.

DISCIPLINING FOR OPTIMUM RESULTS

Much of the debate over appropriate discipline concerns the spirit, extent, or degree of enforcement that brings optimum results. Pfiffner and Fels put this critical question in proper focus:

Should discipline be strict and severe or tolerant and easygoing? The answer will not be found by locating the optimum point between strict and easy, but rather in the fundamental nature of the social organization which the supervisor must understand as part of his disciplining duties. If the basic mores of an organization are developed in a manner that commands the respect and conformance of its members, disciplining should offer no special problem. The rank and file member will observe the mores either automatically or because of the pressures exerted to do so by other members of the group. That is, he probably will if he has a feeling of belonging and thus recognizing that to belong requires a contribution in accordance with his means and talents. Thus, in essence, the supervisor's attempts to discipline must see discipline as a means not of immediately stopping an undesirable behavior only, but of reaching a goal of desirable citizenship.[3]

Key Points to Effective Disciplining

1. Your primary concern in disciplining employees is to salvage them, *not* to scrap them.
2. Although punishment is part of disciplinary action, it is not the primary part.
3. Direct your attention, and therefore your plan of action, toward correcting improper employee actions.
4. Don't play favorites; be consistent; the rule of equality of treatment should pervade all your disciplinary actions.
5. In the final analysis, you (the supervisor) are responsible for maintaining appropriate employee behavioral patterns and productivity.
6. Whether or not the employees in your department are unionized, *just cause* must be established for all disciplinary action.
7. Be it ever so trite, the punishment must fit the crime.
8. Progressive disciplining includes oral reprimands (including counseling), written warnings, and suspensions; termination is defensible where the infraction or behavior was serious (theft, fighting, carrying firearms) or was preceded by the aforementioned steps.
9. Self-discipline develops where employees trust the supervisor and the management, where employees feel that their job is important and appreciated, where employees feel that they belong.
10. Positive discipline encompasses the following sound supervisory practices:[4]

a. Inform *all* employees of the rules and the penalties. The "why" of the rule is just as important as the "what."

b. Don't play the game of "Do as I say, not as I do." Set a good example. Employees look to their supervisors for fairness in application of the rules.

c. Don't jump before you look. Get all the facts. Keep uppermost in your mind the old adage that there are always *at least* two sides to every story.

d. Beware of incomplete facts or appearances. Judge the act within its context. Look for the least obvious motives and reasons.

e. Move quickly but not hastily. Don't let selected instances of misbehavior develop into habits.

f. Discipline—corrective, that is!—should be meted out in private.

g. Objectivity and fairness are *two* hallmarks of positive, corrective disciplinary action.

h. Consistency is the *third* hallmark.

i. Throughout the disciplinary process, keep your eye on the goal of the process: to correct improper behavior and to salvage the employee.

j. Use punishment as the last resort.

Exhibit 32-1 Checklist for Corrective Action[5]

What is the past record of the employee?	Was the employee disciplined previously for the same type of offense? When? Should he or she receive a more severe penalty than a first offender?
Have you all the facts?	Refer to personnel records. Get concrete facts about this specific situation; refer to rules, standards, and policies; evaluate opinions and feelings. Was there an extenuating reason for the employee's behavior? (Sickness, money trouble, etc.)
Has the employee had a fair chance to improve? When?	Has he or she been given some help, advice, or explanation? Does he or she know what is expected? Did he or she know the rules and standards at the time of the infraction?
When was the employee first given a fair warning of the seriousness of his behavior?	Was a written record made and filed? Who gave the warning?
What action was taken in similar cases?	Are there others in your department who experienced different treatment under similar circumstances? In other departments?
What will be the effect of your action on the group?	Are you fully justified? What will be the effect on groups outside your department?
Are you going to handle this by yourself?	Should you clear with your boss or with the personnel director? Do you need assistance or further information? How is your timing?
What other possible actions are there?	Will your action help the hospital, help improve the work output in your department, and help the employee to improve? Should he or she be warned or suspended?

NOTES

1. Jules J. Justin, *How to Manage with a Union, Book One* (New York: Industrial Relations Workshop Seminars, Inc., 1969), pp. 294–295, 301–302.

2. Alfred R. Lateiner, *Modern Techniques of Supervision* (Stamford, Conn.: Lateiner Publishing), originally appearing in *The Technique of Supervision* by Alfred R. Lateiner (New London, Conn.: National Foreman's Institute, 1954), pp. 28–39.

3. John M. Pfiffner and Marshall Fels, *The Supervision of Personnel,* 3d ed. (Englewood Cliffs, N.J.: Prentice-Hall, Inc., 1964), pp. 111–112.

4. A special note of gratitude to Ms. Rita Hubert, graduate student in the Masters Program for Health Care Administration of Rensselaer Polytechnic Institute.

5. Developed by Dr. Leslie M. Slote.

33. How to Handle Grievances Effectively

NORMAN METZGER

Reprinted with permission from *The Health Care Supervisor's Handbook*, by Norman Metzger, published by Aspen Systems Corporation, Germantown, Md., © 1978.

The handling of employee grievances affords the supervisor the greatest opportunity to win over employee respect and gain employee confidence. The most important employer-employee relationship is the one that exists between the worker and his or her immediate supervisor. It is essential for supervisors to know their people, be genuinely interested in them, and recognize their needs and problems. This good relationship cannot only head off many grievances before they reach the formal grievance stage, but also lead to increased productivity.

The supervisor is often the day-to-day interpreter of institutional policy, rules, and regulations and the administrator of the union contract. If there is a Pandora's box in the day-to-day employer-employee relationship, it is the area of grievances. An unattended accumulation of minor irritations and aggravations may inflate and finally explode in the supervisor's face. A little bit of attention at the beginning will go further than a great deal of harried and pressured attention at the end. As a matter of fact, most complaints can be satisfactorily resolved by the supervisor before they become formal grievances.

A grievance may have some basis in fact or it may be fabricated or exaggerated beyond reality. A grievance may not truly be a grievance as defined in a union contract or under institutional policy. More often than not, it may be a gripe or just information-seeking on the part of the employee. In any case it must be dealt with and resolved.

MINIMIZING GRIEVANCES

Although there is no way to completely eliminate grievances, there are commonsense guidelines that will reduce the number and the cost of grievances. Here are some suggestions:

1. Be alert for common causes of irritation within your department. Correct minor irritations promptly before they explode into major problems.
2. Do not knowingly violate established policy, procedure, or practice. This, of course, requires the supervisor to be completely familiar with all policies and contractual clauses that affect the supervisor-employee relationship.
3. Keep promises. Do not make commitments you cannot keep. Many grievances are over the nonfulfillment of a commitment made by a supervisor.
4. Let your employees know how they are getting along. Don't wait for the formal performance review to keep an employee informed of progress or problems. This will minimize the number of grievances that develop when employees are warned about poor performance after having received positive performance reviews earlier in the year.

5. If an employee doesn't measure up, let that employee know. Find out why there is a problem and provide direction and coaching.
6. Encourage constructive suggestions; act on these suggestions where feasible and give proper recognition to the originators. Participation will go a long way to minimize grievances that may develop because of policy changes.
7. Assign and schedule work impartially; avoid favoritism in respect to working conditions or employee benefits.
8. Be sure your employees understand the meaning of and reasons for your orders and instructions. Use language that is meaningful from their point of view.
9. Be consistent in your words and actions unless there are important reasons for deviation. Where deviation is justified, clearly communicate those reasons to the employees. Explain changes in or deviations from policy, procedure, or established practice.
10. Act promptly on reasonable requests from your employees. Don't keep employees waiting for answers to their questions. Nothing is more destructive than a grievance allowed to grow because of lack of prompt response on the part of the supervisor. Remember, you may have to say "no," but a constructive and sympathetic "no" can do less damage than a harsh "yes."
11. If corrective action must be taken, take it promptly; but do not discipline an employee in public.

HEARING THE GRIEVANCE

Many gripes are not bona fide grievances because they concern situations not specifically covered by a union contract or by an institutional policy. Although a gripe may not qualify as a grievance, the employee should be heard on the subject. If a legalistic attitude is assumed at this stage and the gripes are dismissed summarily, hard feelings will be engendered and another issue properly subject to the grievance machinery will be used to exert pressure. It is not suggested that every petty gripe be given undue importance. However, the employee should not be brushed off without having the complaint fully heard.

Hearing a complaint requires attentive listening—get the complete facts and the underlying attitudes and feelings. Let the employee talk without interruption. Then ask questions until you are satisfied that you understand the specifics of the grievance and the true agenda. Do not become predisposed or argumentative

in response to the employee's answers. Very often complaints reflect dissatisfaction in areas other than those under discussion. It is essential that you find out what is really bothering the employee—the hidden agenda. An excellent approach is to rephrase the employee's statement in your own words. This "reflection" serves four important purposes:

1. The employee is able to correct any misunderstanding you may have.
2. The employee has the opportunity to bring the complaint into closer focus.
3. You and the employee can assume that you understand the situation thoroughly.
4. The employee is assured that both of you are "on the same wave length," that you are empathetic and trying to understand the problem from the employee's point of view.

Further explanation or discussion should be reserved until after the facts have been checked, applicable policies and union contract provisions reviewed, and past practices, grievances, and commitments analyzed. Don't promise anything at this time other than a careful investigation. Specify a time within which an answer will be forthcoming. Don't mislead the employee by promising to do something about the complaint unless you are sure remedial action is in order.

There may be instances where a quick response is indicated. If you are absolutely certain of the facts, an immediate reply is in order. However, in most instances a hasty decision can be disastrous. If you are not sure of the facts, not sure of the appropriate policy provision or contract interpretation, or doubtful that the emotional climate is conducive to resolution, delay your response.

GETTING THE FACTS

After hearing and understanding the complaint, initiate an investigation. A complete investigation includes interviewing other employees who may have been involved, reviewing relevant records, and in general "stepping back" from the problem to gain objectivity. New facts and additional viewpoints are almost always uncovered in this way.

In your investigation, look for information concerning previous settlements of similar grievances and relevant policy or contract interpretations. You may call on other supervisors or the personnel manager. Precedent becomes very important. A hasty decision may provide a precedent with far-reaching impact. Many a supervisor has found that a hasty or careless decision over a relatively minor occurrence becomes important later in a different situation with more serious consequences. It is therefore essential that you investigate before you act.

DECISION-MAKING TIME

After analyzing all the facts uncovered by a thorough investigation, it is time to develop a solution to the problem and an answer to the grievance. It is a good idea to discuss your proposed solution with others. Checking out your hunch, your conclusion or your suggested options with others who are in a position to assess their probable impact is a wise idea. Ask your supervisor, the personnel manager, or other supervisors. Ask how this type of problem has been handled in the past. Consultation is a sign of caution, not indecision. You will not be criticized for reviewing your options with others if you have assembled the facts carefully and approached the grievance objectively.

Now it is time to put your answer in written form. Wherever possible, completely explain the reasons behind your decision. It is important that you deal with the specific complaint and not go beyond that complaint.

COMMUNICATING TO THE EMPLOYEE

Supervisors who admit to their mistakes are more respected than those who cover up mistakes. If a grievance has merit and an error has been made, admit this to the employee and indicate your intention to take immediate corrective action. Make certain that you take such corrective action.

If the complaint has no merit and the grievance is to be denied, a full explanation should be communicated to the employee. Attempt to gain the employee's understanding and acceptance of your decision. If the employee remains dissatisfied, don't get impatient and irritated. Appeals are normally provided for in institutional grievance procedures, and the procedure for such an appeal should be explained to the employee.

THE NEED FOR A WRITTEN RECORD

Whether a grievance is denied, granted, settled by compromise, or handled in another way, it is necessary to prepare a complete statement of all that occurred. Normally grievances are submitted on grievance forms which indicate the "disposition." Once completed, the grievance form should be presented to the employee and a copy kept in the departmental files.

GENERAL GUIDELINES

The following points on effective grievance handling are important for the supervisor to review and accept:

1. There should be a strong desire to resolve dissatisfactions and conflicts before they become real problems.
2. Supervisors should empathize with their employees, try to understand employee problems, and be able and willing to listen in a nonjudgmental fashion.
3. The supervisor should have a sound working knowledge of personnel policy procedures and, where appropriate, the union contract.
4. The supervisor must balance a personal commitment to the interests of the institution with a sense of fair play on behalf of the employees. The supervisor represents the employees to the administration and the administration to the employees.

Broadly speaking, the supervisor's responsibility in grievance procedures embraces four primary functions:

1. investigating the material facts,
2. analyzing the grievance to determine its basic causes,
3. discussing and answering the grievance, and
4. taking action to eliminate present problems and prevent future ones.

If you are to discharge your responsibilities properly, your first task upon receiving a grievance is to investigate, not evaluate.

Here are some of the ways to improve human relations when handling grievances:

1. *Be available.* Know your people are individuals and fit your methods to the individual. Cool off the hothead with patience; sense when something is troubling the quiet worker who keeps anger bottled up until it explodes; calm the sensitive employee who may think he or she is being slighted. You can't solve the problems of strangers, and unless you are approachable, you will have strangers working for you.
2. *Be relaxed.* When employees bring you gripes, real or fancied, let them sound off. If they see

you are listening and will give them a fair hearing, the complaint won't look so big.

3. *Get the facts.* Get the story and get it straight. Ask questions to straighten out inconsistencies. Be objective and sympathetic.

4. *Investigate carefully.* Never accept hearsay. Find out for yourself the answers to such questions as who, what, when, where, and why. Check how the union contract or institutional policy covers the alleged offense, and review your files for precedence.

5. *Be tactful.* Many employees will start to tell a supervisor about unfair treatment only to realize halfway through their story that they don't have a real complaint. If supervisors help such employees "save face," the supervisor makes a friend. You never want a worker to leave the grievance interview humiliated and embarrassed.

6. *Act with deliberation.* Snap judgment leads to impulsive action. Take time to get all the facts. What caused the grievance? Where did it happen? Has the contract been violated? Has an institution policy been violated? Has the employee been unfairly treated? Has there been favoritism, unintentional or deliberate? Was this grievance related to others?

7. *Get the answer.* Maybe it is impossible to address the grievance immediately, but don't give employees the runaround. If you can't get the facts you need to settle this case, say so. If the employee knows you are working on the problem, he or she is likely to be more reasonable.

8. *Consider the consequences of your decision.* Make sure you know the effect your settlement will have, not only on the individual, but on the group.

9. *Admit mistakes.* You are human and make mistakes, so if your decisions are occasionally reversed by higher-ups, admit your error. Don't bear a grudge against the employee who was proved right at your expense.

10. *Sell your decisions.* When you deny an employee's grievance, explain why. A blunt "no" causes resentment. Don't pass the buck by blaming your denial on higher management. Supervision means leadership.[1]

LET'S LOOK AT SOME RESEARCH

First-line supervisors in ten unionized plants were studied by Jennings[2] to determine their attitudes toward the grievance procedure. He was looking at:

1. the significance of grievance handling as a supervisory responsibility,
2. the foremen's responsibilities and activities in grievance handling, and
3. actions taken by other line- and staff-management officials in the grievance process.

He found the following:

1. Supervisors perceive that top management regarded grievance-handling responsibilities as an important aspect of the supervisor's job.
2. Supervisors did not consider the resolution of grievances extremely important.
3. When supervisors spent a great deal of effort resolving grievances, they did not feel they were given much credit for this activity.
4. A majority of the supervisors did not believe that they had the primary responsibility for the grievance procedure.
5. A majority believed that their grievance decisions were usually upheld by higher-level management.
6. A majority of foremen usually consulted the industrial relations representative before responding to a grievance.

What can we learn from the Jennings study? It appears that supervisors are not ranking grievance handling high enough in the total range of supervisory responsibilities. This may well have developed because upper management, although realizing the importance of that aspect of the supervisor's job, has not extended appreciation or recognition for that role. It seems essential that supervisors be given appropriate credit for minimizing and/or resolving grievances. Most arbitration cases (arbitration is usually the last step in a grievance procedure, wherein a third party not connected with the institution or the union judges the merits of the grievance and produces a binding decision) are won or lost on the basis of the supervisor's testimony. It is also obvious from the Jennings findings that communication with staff experts in industrial relations or employee relations is essential to producing consistent and defensible decisions.

A study by Turner and Robinson[3] examined the effect of grievance resolution on union-management relationships. Specifically, they examined the hypothesis that "the greater the number of grievances resolved at the lower steps of the grievance procedure, the more likely is a harmonious union-management relationship." Their findings supported the hypothesis.

To summarize, research indicates that upper management depends significantly on the first-line supervisor to resolve grievances. Yet supervisors seem not to give a high priority to this important responsibility. This would lead us to believe that supervisors do not fully realize that their role is fundamental in minimizing grievances and preventing a grievance from becoming a major dispute. Research data also indicate that the resolution of grievances in the lower steps of the grievance process leads to more harmonious labor-management relationships. The first-line supervisor is key to that improvement.

TIPS FOR HANDLING GRIEVANCES EFFECTIVELY

The principal requirements for handling grievances effectively are:

1. a strong desire to make the personnel policy manual and/or labor contract work, to resolve dissatisfactions and conflicts, and to supervise more effectively;
2. a strong effort on the part of first-line supervisors to settle grievances at the very first step in the grievance procedure;
3. a sound working knowledge of the personnel policy manual and the labor contract, including new interpretations and precedents,
4. a consistent approach to carrying out provisions of the personnel policy manual and/or labor contract.

You, the supervisor, play the key role in the handling of grievances. To be effective in that responsibility, heed the following advice:

1. The people who work for you are just that, people. Treat them as individuals.
2. It is essential that you maintain and preserve the dignity of the employee. This may be difficult when dealing with grievances, but it is at the heart of a sound supervisor-employee relationship.
3. Remember that employees want to be appreciated; they want to know that you recognize their meritorious performance. Give credit where it is due. This will minimize many grievances which spring from a lack of recognition.
4. Look to your employees for suggestions and advice. Give them the feeling that they are in on things. Many grievances arise because the employee is not prepared for change.
5. "A stitch in time. . . ." This old adage is most appropriate in effective grievance handling. Look

around and try to anticipate areas and actions that may cause irritation. By anticipating problems you will minimize them.
6. Employees who are properly trained are less likely to have grievances. Employees who know what they are doing and, therefore, do it well, are less frustrated. This is of particular relevance when dealing with the new employee.
7. Unclear, unexplained orders or instructions can lead to grievances. Make certain that you communicate clearly and back up orders and instructions with a "why."
8. When you must administer discipline, be objective, equitable, and consistent. The majority of grievances stem from real or perceived inequality of treatment.
9. Don't belittle employees or underestimate them. If they have a grievance, it does not really matter whether it falls under the personnel policy manual or the labor contract. It is real to the employee and you must deal with it.

Key Points to Effective Handling of Grievances

1. Employees deserve a complete and empathetic hearing of all grievances they present.
2. The most important job in the handling of grievances is getting at the facts. Therefore, listen attentively, encourage a full discussion, and defer judgment.
3. Look for the hidden agenda. Look beyond the selected incident; judge the grievance in context.
4. Hasty decisions often backfire. On the other hand, the employee deserves a speedy reply. In order to determine the proper disposition of a grievance, ask yourself the following questions.

   a. What actually happened?
   b. Where did it happen?
   c. What should have happened?
   d. When did it happen?
   e. Who was involved?
   f. Were there any witnesses?
   g. Why did the problem develop?[4]

5. While you are investigating the grievance, try to separate fact from opinion or impressions. Consult others when appropriate. Most important, check with your personnel people.
6. After you have come to your decision, promptly communicate that decision to the employee. Remember, a sympathetic "no" is far more effective than a harsh "yes." Therefore, give the

reason for the decision and inform the employee of the right to appeal.

7. Remember that you have to sell your decision. The decision is yours, don't pass the buck by placing the blame on your superiors.

8. There is no substitute for common sense in arriving at a decision.

9. Written records are most important, they serve as a review for the supervisor to ensure consistency.

10. Followup is essential. Even if the employee does not appeal your decision, you should check back to see if the decision "took" or was upheld. There is no better way to win employee respect that to give due recognition to employee problems. A little bit of followup goes a long way.

NOTES

1. This subsection was developed by Joseph Ferentino, Labor Relations Director at The Mount Sinai Medical Center, New York City.

2. Ken Jennings, "Foremen's View of Their Involvement with Other Management Officials in the Grievance Process," *Labor Law Journal* 25, no. 5 (May 1974): 305-316.

3. James T. Turner and James W. Robinson, "A Pilot Study of the Validity of Grievance Settlement Rates as Predictor of Union-Management Relations," *Journal of Industrial Relations* 14, no. 3 (September 1972): 314-322.

4. J. Brad Chapman, "Constructive Grievance Handling," in M. Gene Newport, ed., *Supervisory Management: Tools and Techniques* (St. Paul: West Publishing Co., 1976), p. 268.

Index

857

ABOUT THE EDITOR

Norman Metzger is vice president of The Mount Sinai Medical Center in New York City, responsible for labor relations. He is a director of the League of Voluntary Hospitals and Homes of New York City, which negotiates labor contracts for the voluntary hospitals in New York City. He was president of the league from 1966-1972, and was again elected president and will serve in this capacity for the term 1983-84. He is a professor with tenure in the Department of Health Care Management, Mount Sinai School of Medicine, and a professor in the Graduate Program in Health Care Administration, Baruch College, City University of New York, as well as a professor in the Graduate Program in Health Services Administration at the New School for Social Research.

Mr. Metzger's experience in labor relations and personnel administration spans 30 years in both the health services sector and in industry. He is the author or coauthor of eight books, as well as of close to 100 articles in health care journals. He is a three-time recipient of the American Society for Hospital Personnel Administration's Literature Award.

Hospitals in connection with a series on management effectiveness for two years, and currently is contributing editor for *Modern Healthcare*. Bennett's degrees include a B.S. and an M.S. from New York University and an M.S. (Industrial Engineering) from the Stevens Institute of Technology.

Joel M. Douglas is director of the National Center for the Study of Collective Bargaining in Higher Education, Bernard M. Baruch College, City University of New York. Douglas has been a professor of labor relations and economics at both the graduate and undergraduate levels and is the author of several articles in the fields of labor law, labor relations, contract development, and productivity. In addition, he has been a mediator and arbitrator for the past 12 years and is a member of numerous professional organizations. He received a B.A. from Boston University, an M.A. from State University of New York in Albany, a second M.A. from the New School for Social Research, New York City, and a Ph.D. from New York University, New York City.

Samuel Levey is professor and head of the graduate program in hospital and health administration in the College of Medicine of The University of Iowa. He was founding chairman of the Health Care Administration Department at the City University of New York and has served in Massachusetts health and welfare positions as well as in the field of health planning. He serves on the editorial boards of the *Health Care Management Review* and the *Journal of Long-Term Care Administration* and is the editor of the Spectrum Series on *Health Systems Management*. He currently is chairman of the board of directors of the Association of University Programs in Health Administration. He received his Ph.D. from the University of Iowa, Iowa City, in 1960.

Michael G. Macdonald is vice president and general counsel at The Mount Sinai Medical Center, New York City. In this position he is responsible for handling all legal matters, including labor arbitra-

tions, on behalf of the Medical Center. He graduated from Stanford University, Palo Alto, California, in 1963, where he also received his J.D. degree three years later. He then served as the law clerk for federal Judge Frank M. Johnson, Jr., in Montgomery, Alabama. He is on the faculties of the Mount Sinai School of Medicine of the City University of New York and Brooklyn Law School. Prior to his joining Mount Sinai, he was associated for five years with the New York law firm of Debevoise, Plimpton, Lyons & Gates. He has lectured widely and is the author of many articles in the health care field.

John T. McGervey is the employee relations manager of the northern California region of the Kaiser-Permanente Medical Care Program. In this capacity, he directs the compensation, benefits, equal employment opportunity, personnel, and labor relations functions of the 15,000-employee organization. His labor relations department negotiates and administers 13 collective bargaining agreements covering more than 9,000 employees. Prior to his 11 years with Kaiser-Permanente, he spent 13 years with United States Steel Corporation, where he held a number of positions in industrial relations, industrial engineering, and line management. He received his B.S. in Business Administration in 1951 from the University of California at Berkeley and is a captain in the Naval Intelligence Reserves.

Samuel E. Oberman is president and chief executive officer of Don Rowe Associates, Inc., a personnel, employee, and labor relations consulting firm in Mineola, N.Y. He has conducted seminars and given speeches for the American Hospital Association, American Bankers Association, The National Retail Merchants Association, and many state and local hospital, banking and bar associations. He has served as a member of the faculty of the Graduate School of Banking of The University of Wisconsin. His biographical sketch appears in *Who's Who in America in Finance and Industry*, *Community Leaders of America*, *Who's Who in American Jewry*, and *International Men of Achievement*.

ABOUT THE CONTRIBUTORS

Ralph F. Abbott, Jr., is a graduate of Boston College and the Cornell Law School. He is a partner in the law firm of Skoler, Abbott & Hayes, P.C. He is coauthor of the *Health Care Labor Manual* and is an adjunct professor of Labor Law at Western New England School of Law. He is a member of the American Bar Association and the Massachusetts Bar Association and the Labor Law Sections of both of these associations. He practices before the Supreme Judicial Court of Massachusetts, the First Circuit Court of Appeals, the Federal District Court of Massachusetts, and various state and federal administrative agencies. He has lectured on a variety of labor relations topics to various organizations throughout New England.

Ralph A. Anthenien is regional supervisor of hourly compensation for Kaiser-Permanente Medical Care Program in northern California. He is responsible for the development and administration of the compensation program for more than 12,000 employees covering 13 union groups. He has taught personnel and supervision courses at Holy Names College and San Francisco State College and is an accredited personnel manager of the American Society of Personnel Administrators and is a certified compensation professional of the American Compensation Association. Besides having 13 years of personnel experience, he possesses a B.S. and M.B.A. in industrial relations from the University of California at Berkeley.

Steven H. Appelbaum currently is associate professor of management, faculty of Commerce and Administration, at Concordia University in Montreal, Quebec, Canada. His research and teaching focus upon human resource management, organizational behavior, and stress management. He is an active management-organizational consultant who develops and conducts varied programs dealing with leadership-power-conflict, management by objectives, team building, and organizational development. Over the past eight years, his clients have included The Graduate Hospitals, Union Carbide, Inc., and the Government of Delaware County. He has written more than 60 articles that have appeared in such journals as the *University of Michigan Business Review, Business Society, Academy of Management Proceedings, Personnel Administrator,* and *Health Care Management Review,* and is currently a reviewer for the *Personnel Administrator.* His recently completed book *Stress Management for Health Care Professionals* will be published by Aspen Systems, and he is completing another text *Hospital Survival: Strategies for Success.* He previously served as Manager of Personnel Services for TRW, Inc., manager of Organizational Development for Union Carbide, and assistant professor of Behavioral Sciences, Graduate School of Pace University, New York City. He received his B.S. in Business Administration from Temple University and his M.A. in Social Sciences from St. Joseph's University, both in Philadelphia, Pennsylvania. He was awarded the Ph.D. by the University of Ottawa (Canada) in 1972.

John E. Baer is the founder and president of The Center to Promote Health Care Studies, Inc., a continuing education institute for persons in the health field. He also has served as director of planning for North Center Bronx Hospital, as executive director of the United Cerebral Palsy Association of Nassau County (New York) and its Treatment and Rehabilitation Center, as associate director of The Hospital for Joint Diseases and Medical Center, as assistant director of the Hospital for Special Surgery, as a consultant with Booz-Allen & Hamilton, and as an assistant bureau director for health with the U.S. Civil Service Commission. Baer has teaching affiliations with Columbia University's School of Public Health and New York University's Graduate School of Public Administration. He currently serves as president of the Hospital Executives' Club. He received a D.P.A. from New York University Graduate School of Public Administration.

Lawrence C. Bassett (see Editorial Advisory Board)

Stephen E. Bechtold is associate professor of management, College of Business, The Florida State University at Tallahassee where he has taught courses in operations management, management science, mathematics, and computer science. His previous experience includes positions in quality control, manufacturing engineering, technical sales, and product consultant, all with the Westinghouse Electric Corporation from 1965 through 1969. He has coauthored articles in various management, behavioral, and management science journals which include the *Journal of Management, Journal of Occupational Behavior, Decision Sciences, Omega,* and the *Journal of Operations Management.* He is also a member of the Beta Gamma Sigma and Sigma Iota Epsilon honorary societies and is an active member in the American Institute for Decision Sciences and the Institute of Management Science. He received his D.B.A. from Indiana University.

Thomas R. Beech is an attorney in Houston who has represented numerous clients in the health care industry. He formerly served in the honors program, Office of the General Counsel, National Labor Relations Board, Washington. He has taught courses in labor law and employee rights at South Texas College of Law, Houston. Beech is a member of the American Society of Hospital Attorneys, American Bar Association, and numerous other professional organizations. He received his J.D. degree from the University of Houston in Texas.

Addison C. Bennett (see Editorial Advisory Board)

Gail Ann Bentivegna is assistant to the vice president of Human Resources of Playboy Enterprises. She received an M.A. from the University of Illinois and a Master of Management in industrial relations from the J.S. Kellogg Graduate School of Management. Her human resources responsibilities have included staffing and scheduling research for the U.S. Bureau of Labor Statistics, management of Hospital Industrial Relations Information Services (HIRIS) for the American Hospital Association, and development of a human resource audit for hospital use. Her publications deal with professional union activity, the growth of hospital collective bargaining, and due process in hospital collective bargaining agreements.

Karl R. Birky is the assistant administrator of the Youngstown (Ohio) Hospital Association, North Unit—Tod Babies' and Children's Hospital. Birky has administrative and staff responsibilities for various operating departments in this 974-bed, general, acute care facility. His article grew out of graduate work in hospital and health services administration at The Ohio State University in 1975–77. In 1973 he returned from a two-year position teaching mathematics at Clarendon College in Jamaica, W.I. He now serves on committees of the Ohio Hospital Association, the East Ohio Hospital Association, and a Young Administrators Group of the American College of Hospital Administrators. Birky received his M.S. in hospital and health services administration from Ohio State in 1977, completed his graduate study in business administration in 1974–75 at Kent State University, and received his B.S. in mathematics education in 1971 from Goshen (Ind.) College.

Joan R. Bloom is associate professor, Department of Social and Administrative Health Sciences, School of Public Health, University of California at Berkeley, where she teaches courses in health services and facilities planning and program planning, development, and evaluation. She also is senior health sociologist at Stanford Research International. Prior to obtaining her Ph.D. from Stanford, she was employed as a public health nurse in San Mateo County, California, and taught at the School of Nursing, University of California at San Francisco. She has written a number of articles in the health care field and for the last three years collaborated with coauthors in the field of collective bargaining.

Arthur P. Brief is associate professor of management and organizational behavior in the Graduate School of Business at New York University. He has authored dozens of articles in the human resources management area and several books, including *Managing Job Stress*. Brief, who has extensive experience in the health care field, is active as a management consultant to both private and public sector organizations. In addition, he serves on the editorial boards of the *Academy of Management Journal* and the *Journal of Management*. He received a Ph.D. from the University of Wisconsin in Madison.

Paul E. Brody is a resident in ophthalmology, Long Island Jewish-Hillside Medical Center, New Hyde Park, N.Y. He received his M.D. at the Syracuse University New York Downstate Medical School, Brooklyn. Brody also has an M.B.A. in health care administration from Baruch College-Mount Sinai School of Medicine and received his B.A. in mathematics *summa cum laude* from Yeshiva University, New York. He is an instructor of Administrative Medicine, Division of Health Sciences, Touro College, New York. He has in the past served as admissions coordinator at the Jewish Institute for Geriatric Care, New Hyde Park, New York and was a systems analyst at the central office of the New York City Health and Hospitals Corporation, Ambulatory Care Reimbursements Division. He has published several articles in the field of health care administration as well as ophthalmology.

Jerad D. Browdy is vice president of Witt & Dolan Associates, Inc., Oak Brook, Ill. The firm provides consulting and executive search services to the hospital and health care field. Prior to joining the company in 1973, he was director of employee relations for Oak Forest Hospital, responsible for the complete personnel-employee relations program for the 2,000-bed hospital, which is one of the world's largest institutions for the chronically ill. Browdy received a B.S. degree from Northwestern University in 1951 and an M.S. degree from George Williams College, Downers Grove, Ill., in 1953. He has authored articles on executive compensation and executive recruiting. He was a member of the evening faculty of the Department of Industrial Engineering at the Illinois Institute of Technology, Chicago, and an instructor in management fundamentals with the Midwest Industrial Management Association, West Chester, Ill.

Warren H. Chaney is associate professor of health care administration and management, University of Houston at Clear Lake City in Houston. He also serves as a management consultant to major health care facilities as well as other business and industry organizations such as AT&T, Celanese Chemical Corporation, Western Company of North America, etc. In 1968, following seven years as an officer in the Army Medical Corps, Chaney joined the corporate staff of Frito Lay, Inc., as national training director. From 1972 until 1974 he served on the corporate staff of the Western Company of North America as director of organizational development. With a Ph.D. in behavioral science and a heavy background in industry and health care, Chaney has had broad experience in combating unionization attempts. His basic research into the causes and effects of labor organizations has received wide attention in such publications as the *Labor Law Journal*. He is coauthor of *The Union Epidemic*, and has authored or coauthored more than six books and 36 articles dealing with behavioral topics. Chaney has written for *Colliers Encyclopedia* and has been featured on national television, most recently on the "Today" show and NBC's "Real People." He is a member of the Academy of Management and the Southwest Federation of Academic Disciplines. He received his Ph.D. in Behavioral Sciences from North Texas State University, Dallas, Texas.

William M. Copeland is president of St. Francis-St. George Hospital, Inc., Cincinnati. As the chief executive officer of a two-hospital corporate system, he developed and implemented an organization plan to merge the management and operations of the two facilities to create one hospital at two locations. Copeland has a J.D. degree in law and management. He is the author of "Hospital Responsibility for Basic Care Provided by Medical Staff Members: 'Am I My Brother's Keeper'?" in the *Northern Kentucky Law Review* (1978). He has authored or coauthored numerous articles relating to health care administration. Among other awards, he received the Monsignor Griffin Award for Outstanding Contribution to Hospital Literature, Ohio Hospital Association, 1979. He received his J.D. degree from the Chase College of Law, Northern Kentucky University, and his M.S. degree from the University of Colorado.

Laurence P. Corbett is the senior partner of Corbett, Kane & Berk, with offices in Oakland and San Francisco. The firm specializes in labor and employment law representing employers. Corbett is a former cochairman of the American Bar Association's State Labor Law Development Committee; president-elect of the San Francisco Bar's Labor Law Section; a member of the American Hospital Association's NLRB Committee; a member of the

Federal Mediation and Conciliation Service's Health Advisory Committee; an adjunct professor at Golden Gate University, San Francisco, teaching courses in health care labor law; and the author of articles and papers on collective bargaining, arbitration, and labor law subjects. Corbett received his B.A. degree at Harvard College and his J.D. degree at the Harvard Law School.

Robert Coulson is president of the American Arbitration Association. He is a member of the New York and Massachusetts Bars and a Certified Association Executive (CAE) of the American and New York Societies of Association Executives. He is on the board of directors of the Institute for Mediation and Conflict Resolution, Center for Community Justice, Federation of Protestant Welfare Agencies, Fund for Modern Courts, Edwin Gould Foundation for Children, and National Resource Center for Consumers of Legal Services. Formerly secretary of the Association of the Bar of the City of New York, 1961–1963, he is an Honorary Fellow, Arbitrators' Institute of Canada, and an Honorary Member, American Society of Appraisers. He is the author of *Business Arbitration — What You Need to Know, Labor Arbitration — What You Need to Know,* and *How to Stay Out of Court.* Coulson has written and lectured extensively on the settlement of disputes. He is a graduate of Yale University and Harvard Law School.

Mary Lou Creedon is professional placement director of professional nurses and auxiliary staff, and affirmative action officer for the Mount Sinai Hospital and Mount Sinai Medical School of The Mount Sinai Medical Center, New York City. She is an adjunct faculty member for the surgical nursing program at the Borough of Manhattan Community College and a faculty member in the health administration program at St. Joseph's College. Previously, in addition to other affiliations, she was with the New York City Board of Education in the capacity of senior clinical coordinator for affiliated practical nursing groups at various local hospitals, an instructor in basic sciences, medicine, and surgery, and a basic education/mathematics specialist. She is a member of the Advisory Committee for Projects with Industry of the Institute for Crippled and Disabled. She coauthored the book *Health Careers Curriculum: Behavioral Objectives Model* (1973). She received her M.S. degree in health administration at the Long Island University and her B.S. degree in nursing at Villanova University.

Joel M. Douglas (see Editorial Advisory Board)

Mark W. Dundon is executive director of the Sisters of Charity of Leavenworth Health Services Corporation, a multihospital holding corporation, Leavenworth, Kan. The corporation owns and operates eight hospitals comprising 2,300 beds in five midwestern and western states. Dundon earned his B.S. in biology from St. John's University, Collegeville, Minn., and his M.B.A. in hospital administration from Xavier University, Cincinnati, where he was awarded the Milton Kuttnauer Award as the most outstanding graduate in hospital administration in 1964.

Norbert F. Elbert is an assistant professor of management, College of Business Administration, Northern Arizona University, Flagstaff. He is an accredited personnel specialist with his principal research area being performance appraisal systems. An active management development consultant, he also published articles in numerous academic and professional journals. His primary teaching interests in the management area include personnel administration and organization behavior. He received his Ph.D. from the University of Kentucky.

Wanda L. Ellert is an associate with the law firm of Proskauer Rose Goetz & Mendelsohn in New York City, specializing in labor law. She has instructed seminars at Cornell's New York State School of Industrial and Labor Relations. She received her J.D. degree from the Harvard Law School in 1976.

William J. Emanuel is a Los Angeles attorney and a partner in the law firm of Morgan, Lewis and Bockius. His practice is devoted to the representation and counseling of health care institutions and other employers in labor and employment law matters. Emanuel was a representative of the health care industry in drafting and negotiating the Health Care Amendments to the National Labor Relations Act. He is a member of the Ad Hoc Labor Relations Advisory Committee of the American Hospital Association and the American Society of Hospitals. A frequent writer and lecturer on hospital labor relations issues, he received his A.B. at Marquette University and his J.D. at Georgetown University.

Beth Essig is assistant general counsel at The Mount Sinai Medical Center in New York City. She earned her law degree at the Columbia University School of Law in 1978 after receiving her A.B. degree from Barnard College.

Roger Feldman was born in Wisconsin and studied in London and Rochester, N.Y., where he received his Ph.D. in economics from the University of Rochester. He is an associate professor of health services research and economics at the University of Minnesota. Before joining Minnesota in 1978, he taught at the University of North Carolina at Chapel Hill. Feldman's research centers on the forces that allocate resources in the health services industry. He has studied the economics of medical education, compensation arrangements between hospitals and physicians, and hospital labor unions. He is a consultant to several federal agencies and a reviewer or screener of articles for the *American Economic Review,* the *Southern Economic Journal,* and *Inquiry,* among other journals.

Nancy Connolly Fibish has been a mediator with the Federal Mediation and Conciliation Service (FMCS) in Chicago and Washington since 1968. In June 1977 she was appointed as a national representative to FMCS's Office of Mediation Services in Washington. She serves as coordinator for labor disputes in the health care industry and as the FMCS liaison and chairperson for the national labor-management committee in the private sector of the health care industry. She was assigned to a Detail with the Health Branch, Health and Income Maintenance Division, Office of Management and Budget in Washington, D.C. from September 1980 to March 1981. She was a member of the Labor Relations Task Force, Federal Personnel Management Project in 1977, and was a Congressional Fellow in 1974–75 with experience in labor, health, and appropriations legislation in both Houses of Congress. As a former Fulbright Scholar to the University of Strasbourg, France, she did research in the French mining industry under the auspices of the University's Institute of Labor and the French Department of Health.

Tina Filoromo is the Northeast Regional Recruiter for the Methodist Hospital of Houston, Texas, and a nurse recruitment consultant. A former staff nurse and charge nurse in Intensive Care, she has been a nurse recruiter since 1973, first at Temple University Hospital and then at Pennsylvania Hospital. She is a first vice president of the National Association of Nurse Recruiters and also is a member of the American Nurses Association. She coauthored a book with Dolores Ziff entitled *Nurse Recruitment: Strategies for Success,* published in 1980 by Aspen Systems Corporation. She received her Diploma in Nursing at the Allegheny General Hospital School of Nursing, Pittsburgh, Pa.

Myron D. Fottler is professor of health care management and human resources management in the Graduate School of Business at the University of Alabama, where he teaches courses in health care,

personnel, and labor relations. He received his Ph.D. from Columbia University and formerly taught at the State University of New York at Buffalo and the University of Iowa. He is the author of *Manpower Substitution in the Hospital Industry,* has authored or coauthored some 50 articles dealing with management and health care topics, and serves as a reviewer for numerous scholarly publications. Among other honors, Fottler serves on the executive board of the Personnel/Human Resources Division of the Academy of Management and is listed in numerous bibliographical references.

Inez Greenstadt has been recreational director of The Mount Sinai Medical Center for 20 years. She started the recreational program with nursing students and expanded it to include everyone in the center. She has an M.A. from Teachers College at Columbia University in Student Personnel, and a Sixth Year Certificate from New York University in Vocational Counselling. She also organized the New York City Medical Center Recreational Council. Mrs. Greenstadt supervises recreational interns from four major colleges in the New York area during their placement at Mount Sinai. She is an active member of the New York City Industrial Recreational Directors' Association.

Pat N. Groner is president of Baptist Hospital in Pensacola, Fla., where he has served as the chief executive officer for 30 years. He is past president of the Florida Hospital Association and the Southeastern Hospital Conference; a past member of the board of trustees of the American Hospital Association and the board of regents of the American College of Hospital Administrators; president of the Hospital Research and Development Institute, Inc.; vice president of Voluntary Hospitals of America; and vice president and treasurer of Multihospital Mutual Insurance, Ltd. He is the author of *Cost Containment Through Employee Incentives Program,* as well as numerous articles in professional journals.

Gerald R. Guralnik is president of Woodward Ryan Sharp and Davis, Inc., a 19-year-old New York firm of consulting actuaries and computerized benefit and pension plan consultants. He holds a master's degree from New York University, where he has completed additional credits toward a Ph.D. He has lectured on pension benefit plans and executive compensation subjects. He is a member of the advisory board of the Columbia University Graduate School of Business, and has published several articles in professional journals. Guralnik has testified before the U.S. Senate and House

Labor and Finance Committees on several occasions on matters of ERISA, ADEA, and other benefit subjects. He has contributed to trade associations in studies and position papers on proposed national health insurance and other legislative and regulatory matters affecting benefit plans.

Frances Hoffman Hackbart is administrative associate for nursing at the University of Iowa Hospitals and Clinics in Iowa City. She has taught business topics at the college level, as well as to adults in evening education classes. She has responsibilities in the areas of financial management, personnel, and administration in a department with a staff of approximately 2,000 persons. Ms. Hackbart has a B.A. degree from Carlton College, Northfield, Minn. (1973) and an M.A.T. degree from the University of Iowa, Iowa City (1978).

James D. Hawthorne is an assistant vice president of William A. Mercer, Inc., and manager of its Chicago office communications consulting staff. In the 15 years he has been associated with Mercer he has established communication units in the major metropolitan markets and was responsible nationally for the production of benefit statements. His experience includes print and audiovisual media and considerable work in employee attitude surveys for major corporations. His prior experience includes 15 years with the Jam Handy Organization and Wilding, Inc., audiovisual producers and training consultants, servicing nationally known consumer product and basic industry corporations. He held the positions of writer, director, producer, and account executive with those firms. Hawthorne is a 1949 graduate of Antioch College, where he majored in business administration with a minor in English/drama.

Brian E. Hayes is a graduate of Boston College and Georgetown University Law School. He is a partner in the law firm of Skoler, Abbott & Hayes, P.C. He previously served as a law clerk to the Division of Judges of the National Labor Relations Board and shortly thereafter as counsel to the Chairman of the National Labor Relations Board. He is also an adjunct professor of Law at Western New England Law School where he teaches labor law and collective bargaining. He is also Editor in Chief for the *Health Care Labor Manual*, published by Aspen Systems Corporation. He is a member of the American Bar Association, the Massachusetts Bar Association, the District of Columbia Bar Association, and the Labor Law Section of the American Bar Association. He practices before the First Circuit Court of Appeals, the Federal District Court of Massachu-

setts, and various state and federal administrative agencies.

Thomas A. Helfrich is vice president and associate counsel of the League of Voluntary Hospitals and Homes of New York, where he has represented hospitals and nursing homes in multiemployer bargaining and related matters for the last ten years. A member of the American and New York State Bar Associations' sections on labor and administrative law, Helfrich frequently lectures to graduate students in labor law and labor relations. He is a graduate of New York Law School, where he attained his J.D., *summa cum laude;* he completed his bachelor's degree at Hanover College where he graduated *cum laude* and was awarded departmental honors in economics.

Arthur C. Helton is an associate in the law firm of Mailman & Ruthizer, P.C., New York. He was admitted to the bar in 1977, New York and U.S. District Court, Southern and Eastern Districts of New York; 1978, U.S. Court of Appeals, Second Circuit; and 1980, U.S. Supreme Court. Helton received his A.B. degree at Columbia University, and his J.D. at New York University in New York. From 1976 to 1979, he was Associate Appellate Counsel of the Criminal Appeals Bureau of the Legal Aid Society of New York City. He is a member of the Association of the Bar of the City of New York and the New York State Bar Association (Member: Labor Law Section).

Christine L. Hobart is an associate professor of management at Northeastern University, teaching labor relations in health care and international areas. She is also on the faculty of its School of Nursing and visiting lecturer in labor relations and personnel administration at the Harvard School of Public Health. A panelist of the American Arbitration Association and fact finder and mediator for the Massachusetts Board of Conciliation and Arbitration, she has dealt with both public and private sector cases in the health care industry. She has also had extensive labor relations experience in private industry and has consulted for hospital and professional associations in matters of organizational structure and labor relations. She received her B.A., *cum laude*, from Radcliffe College and her D.B.A. from Harvard Graduate School of Business Administration.

Richard Hoffbeck is a graduate student in economics at the University of Minnesota, where he holds a bachelor's degree in economics. His research involves econometrics, labor, and monetary economics.

Charles L. Joiner is professor, hospital and health administration, and associate dean, School of Community and Allied Health, University of Alabama in Birmingham. He is a graduate of the University of Alabama, where he received his master's in economics and a Ph.D. in business administration. His present responsibilities include graduate courses in human resource management and primary administrative assignments in the areas of finance, personnel, and overall administration. In addition to being author of numerous management presentations and publications, he has served as a consultant and training specialist with numerous health care organizations, particularly in the labor relations and personnel areas.

Hervey A. Juris is professor of Industrial Relations and Urban Affairs in the J.L. Kellogg Graduate School of Management, Northwestern University, where he teaches courses in human resources management and labor management relations. He has published widely in professional journals in the fields of labor relations and in journals for the health industry. He is coauthor of a book on public sector unionism and coeditor of a book on manufacturing unionism in the 1980s. He is an arbitrator and a consultant to industry, government, and health institutions.

Samuel M. Kaynard is regional director of the National Labor Relations Board, Region 29, which has jurisdiction over Brooklyn, Queens, Staten Island, and Nassau and Suffolk Counties in New York State. He is a career employee and has served with the National Labor Relations Board in various capacities both in Washington and in the Regional Office. He is on the faculty of New York University Law School, Fordham University Law School, Brooklyn Law School, Hofstra Law School, and other universities where he teaches courses in Labor Law; Practice and Procedure before the National Labor Relations Board; Strikes, Boycotts, Picketing, and Injunctions; Collective Bargaining; and allied subjects. He lectures extensively in the labor relations field and is the author of various articles in the labor field. He is on the panel of the American Arbitration Association and the New York Public Employment Relations Board.

Theodore W. Kessler has served at the St. Charles Hospital in Toledo, Ohio, since 1975 and currently is director of management services. His prior health care experience was with the Cleveland Clinic Foundation; he previously was associated with the General Electric Company for 20 years in various personnel functions. He received his M.B.A. from Harvard Business School and his B.B.A. from Tulane University in New Orleans.

G. Roger King is a partner in the law firm of Bricker & Eckler of Columbus, Ohio, where his practice is devoted to representing employers in labor relations matters with particular concentration in the health care field. Prior to entering private practice, King served as labor relations counsel to Senator Robert A. Taft, Jr., and as a professional staff counsel to the Senate Committee on Labor. During his tenure with the committee, the 1974 Health Care Amendments to the National Labor Relations Act were developed, and enacted into law. King is a member of the American Society of Hospital Attorneys and the Ad hoc Labor Relations Advisory Committee of the American Hospital Association, and has been an active speaker and author for various health care groups on employment relations matters. He is a graduate of Miami University in Oxford, Ohio, and received his J.D. from Cornell University Law School.

Saul G. Kramer is a member of the New York City law firm of Proskauer Rose Goetz & Mendelsohn. Since 1959 he has specialized in the practice of labor relations law on behalf of management. Kramer was graduated from the Cornell Law School with distinction, was a member of the board of editors of its *Law Quarterly,* and received his B.S. Degree in 1954 from the New York City School of Industrial and Labor Relations at Cornell University and his L.L.B. from Cornell Law School in 1959.

Henry C. LaParo is manager, Management and Administrative Skills Training with Saudi Arabian Airlines in Jiddah, Saudi Arabia. He was formerly director of Training and Personnel Development, New York University Medical Center, where, from 1967–1980, he was responsible for developing and administering a wide spectrum of inservice and education programs ranging from management development to skills training. Previously, he was an educational consultant; director of education, vocation, and avocation of the nation's first Jobs Corps Center (Camp Kilmer, N.J.); and manager, training and education, ITT Laboratories. He holds a patent on an audiovisual apparatus and was an adjunct assistant professor of management at New York University, as well as a lecturer at Cornell and Rutgers. He received his M.Ed. degree from Rutgers University, New Brunswick, N.J.

Harold Laufman, who holds both M.D. and Ph.D. degrees, is emeritus professor of surgery of the Albert Einstein College of Medicine and emeritus director of the Institute for Surgical Studies, a division of the Department of Surgery, Montefiore Hospital and Medical Center in New York. He is a professional lecturer at the Mount Sinai School of Medicine and Columbia University Graduate School of Architecture. As president of Harold Laufman Associates, he is a consultant to many hospitals in the design, equipping, and management of surgical and special care facilities.

Lung-Fei Lee is associate professor of economics at the University of Minnesota, where he has taught applied and theoretical econometrics since 1976. He received his Ph.D. degree in economics from the University of Rochester, New York, in 1976. He has authored or coauthored articles on selectivity problems in econometric models, union decisions, and production functions.

Samuel Levey (see Editorial Advisory Board)

Noel Arnold Levin is a partner in the New York office of Morgan, Lewis & Bockius. A Phi Beta Kappa graduate of Williams College, he received his J.D. from Yale Law School, where he was an editor of the *Yale Law Journal*. Levin is a former president and chairman of the International Foundation of Employee Benefits and currently serves on the executive committee of the board of directors of the American Arbitration Association. He is the author of *ERISA and Labor-Management Benefit Funds, Arbitrating Labor Cases,* and *Successful Labor Relations* and has written columns for *The New York Law Journal, The National Law Journal,* and *Pension World.* Levin has written and lectured extensively on employee benefits, ERISA, and labor relations.

Gary S. Levitz is assistant director and assistant professor in the graduate program in hospital and health administration at the University of Iowa, Iowa City. His teaching interests are organizational behavior, health management, long-term care administration, and health services research. He holds a Ph.D. from the University of Michigan in medical care organization. Currently he is consulting with health organizations on health marketing, organizational analysis, and organizational development.

Robert T. Lyons is vice president of Don Rowe Associates, Mineola, N.Y., an employee relations firm. His activities include supervisory training, organizational development, merger planning, development of personnel policies and procedures, exempt and nonexempt compensation, employee attitude surveys, affirmative action, and a broad range of personnel consulting. Previously, he was an inde-

pendent management consultant in industrial relations, executive recruitment, wage and salary administration, management development and training programs, management information, and production and inventory control systems. He was educated in business administration at LaSalle College, Philadelphia, and the New York Institute of Technology. Lyons is a recognized authority and speaker on topics of personnel management, labor relations, inventory control, and personnel planning.

Michael G. Macdonald (see Editorial Advisory Board)

William A. Maloney is an assistant professor of construction management in the College of Engineering at Ohio State University, where he teaches labor and management problems in construction. After several years of management experience in the construction industry, he received his Ph.D. in business from the University of Michigan and subsequently taught at Arizona State University, Purdue, and the University of Alabama. He is the author of *Productivity Bargaining: A Study in Contract Construction* (1977), as well as articles on labor relations issues. Maloney has had extensive work and consulting experience in productivity bargaining and productivity improvement programs in construction.

Frank J. Malouff holds both academic and administrative appointments at the University of Colorado Health Sciences Center, Denver. In addition to serving on the faculty of the graduate program in health administration, he has served as administrator of both the benefits division and the training division. While responsible for UCHSC's benefits, he administered more than 30 separate benefits programs involving $20 million annually in employee and institutional funds. He also serves as a member of the board of directors of the American Society for Health Manpower Education and Training of the American Hospital Association.

Herbert L. Marx, Jr., is engaged in the practice of arbitration and dispute resolution. Among the permanent arbitration panels on which he serves are the League of Voluntary Hospitals and Homes of New York-District 1199, National Union of Hospital and Health Care Employees; National Railroad Adjustment Board; Board of Education of the City of New York-United Federation of Teachers, AFT; and the U.S. Postal Service-Postal Unions. He is an adjunct lecturer at Pace University Graduate School of Business and an adjunct faculty member of the Institute of Management and Labor Relations at Rutgers.

He is the editor of 13 volumes in the H. W. Wilson Company *Reference Shelf Series,* including *American Labor Unions, American Labor Today,* and *Collective Bargaining for Public Employees,* and has contributed articles to numerous professional and general publications. He is a member of the National Academy of Arbitrators, Society for Professionals in Dispute Resolution, and former president of the New York Chapter, Industrial Relations Research Association.

Earl J. Motzer is senior administrator/operations of Good Samaritan Hospital, a 695-bed referral center of the Samaritan Health Service in Phoenix, Ariz. He formerly was vice president of the Greater Cleveland Hospital Association, an organization providing managerial and shared services for cost containment to 75 health care institutions in Northeast Ohio, and a faculty member of the Cleveland State University College of Business Administration. Motzer has a bachelor's degree in psychology, a master's in hospital administration, and another master's in industrial relations law. He formerly was on the faculty of Xavier University of Cincinnati. He has authored articles on personnel, management, and labor relations. He was appointed in 1974 by the President's Special Assistant as one of the original seven management representatives throughout the U.S. to serve on the Federal Mediation and Conciliation Services Health Care Industry Labor-Management Advisory Committee, which continues to meet periodically.

Charles W. Mueller is an associate professor in the Department of Sociology at the University of Iowa. He received his Ph.D. from the University of Wisconsin (Madison) in 1973. His research interests include race and sex based social inequality and organizational turnover. He is coauthor of *Professional Turnover: The Case of Nurses, Introduction to Factor Analysis,* and *Factor Analysis.* He has authored or coauthored some dozen articles related to his research interests.

Charles A. O'Reilly is assistant professor, School of Business Administration, University of California at Berkeley, where he teaches organizational behavior and human resource management. He also has taught at the Graduate School of Public Health at Berkeley and at the Graduate School of Management at UCLA, where he conducted research and taught in the management of public and not-for-profit organizations. His current research interests include organizational communication and decision making, human resource management, and labor relations in the health sector. He received his Ph.D.

from the School of Business, University of California at Berkeley.

G. Nicholas Parlette is associate dean, School of Public Health, University of California at Berkeley. Prior to this appointment he was executive director of the program of Continuing Education in Public Health, a consortium of the five Western schools of public health. He has published widely in the areas of continuing education, evaluation of professional education, health career patterns, and collective bargaining among health professionals. He is a principal in the management consulting firm Bramson, Parlette, Harrison & Associates. He holds an M.P.H. from the School of Business, University of California at Berkeley.

Richard Pegnetter is an associate professor of industrial relations, College of Business Administration, University of Iowa, where he teaches public and private sector labor relations, labor law, and labor dispute resolution. He is a practicing arbitrator and mediator on various panels, including the American Arbitration Association, the Federal Mediation and Conciliation Service, the Iowa Public Employment Relations Board, the Wisconsin Employment Relations Commission, and the Indiana Education Employment Relations Board. He speaks often on labor relations at conferences and training seminars and has published widely in journals such as the *Industrial and Labor Relations Review* and *Arbitration Journal.* He has served as an editorial referee for the *Public Administration Review,* the *Social Science Quarterly,* and the *Industrial and Labor Relations Review.* He received his Ph.D. from Cornell University's School of Industrial and Labor Relations, and his B.A. and M.A. degrees from Indiana University in Pennsylvania.

Irving Perlmutter is executive director of Health Manpower Management, Inc., the labor and employee relations association of the hospitals in Minneapolis, St. Paul, and throughout Minnesota. He teaches human relations, management, and supervision at Inver Hills Community College, Inver Grove Heights, Minnesota, and at the University of Minnesota. He entered the health care field as assistant director and director of personnel at Montefiore Hospital in Pittsburgh and later joined Montefiore Hospital in the Bronx, New York, as associate director of human resources. Earlier, he spent nine years with the American Cyanamid Company as employee relations manager of the Fibers Division. A graduate of Rutgers University, he earned a B.S. in education and an M.A. in economics. He also served as a coadjutant staff for the Institute of Management and Labor Relations and as faculty for the Rutgers University Extension Division's Management and Labor Relations Departments for more than 15 years.

Dennis D. Pointer is head of the Division of Health Services Management, School of Public Health, at the University of California at Los Angeles. He formerly was assistant director, Department of Teaching Hospitals, Association of American Medical Colleges, and has held academic appointments as an assistant professor in the Department of Administrative Medicine at the Mount Sinai School of Medicine, and the graduate program in health care administration at the City University of New York. While completing his studies at the University of Iowa, where he received his Ph.D., he was a National Institutes of Health Predoctoral Fellow. Pointer is the author of numerous books, articles, and monographs in the health care labor field.

Jay M. Presser is a *cum laude* graduate of Harpur College and George Washington University Law School. He is currently a partner in the firm of Skoler, Abbott & Hayes, P.C., and specializes exclusively in the representation of management in labor relations matters. He previously served in Washington, D.C. as a law clerk to the Division of Judges of the National Labor Relations Board and shortly thereafter as counsel to the National Labor Relations Board's Regional Office in Cincinnati, Ohio. An adjunct professor of Law of Western New England Law School, he teaches collective bargaining. He is also an editor of the *Health Care Labor Manual,* published by Aspen Systems Corporation. He is admitted to practice in Massachusetts, New York, and various federal courts and administrative agencies. He is also a member of the Labor Law Section of the New York Bar Association.

James L. Price is a professor of sociology, Department of Sociology, University of Iowa. His Ph.D. is from Columbia University, and he has taught courses in organizations at the University of Iowa for 14 years. He is the author or coauthor of four books dealing with organizations and has published numerous articles in major journals. Since 1972 he has devoted the bulk of his time to the study of nursing turnover.

Anna M. Rappaport is a vice president of William M. Mercer, Inc., and manager of a benefits consulting unit in its Chicago office. She is an actuary and futurist with 20 years of business experience and a broad background in benefits consulting, corporate research, and life insurance company management. Her special interest in the last few years has been

social change and how it affects the benefits and human resources management in companies. She is the author of many articles and professional papers, and has appeared on many panels. Rappaport previously served as a vice president of the Equitable Life Assurance Society of the United States and as senior vice president and chief actuary of the Standard Security Life Insurance Co. of New York. She is a member of the board of governors of the Society of Actuaries, and previously has served as treasurer of that organization. She is a Fellow in the Society of Actuaries.

Theodore Ruthizer is a member of the law firm of Mailman & Ruthizer, P.C., New York City. He was admitted to the bar in 1973, New York, U.S. District Court, Southern and Eastern Districts of New York, and U.S. Court of Appeals, Second Circuit; 1979, U.S. Supreme Court. He obtained his A.B. at Lafayette College with honors in history, and his J.D. from Columbia Law School, Columbia University. From 1972 to 1975 Ruthizer was a senior appeals attorney for the Legal Aid Society of Nassau County, New York, and was Associate Appellate Counsel, Criminal Appeals Bureau of the Legal Aid Society of New York in 1976. He is a member of the Association of the Bar of the City of New York (Member: Committee on Immigration and Nationality Law); the New York State Bar Association (Member: Labor Law Section); and the Association of Immigration and Nationality Lawyers.

Bernard J. Ryan has more than 15 years of management experience in executive search consulting. Just prior to establishing the firm of Ryan/Smith & Associates, a member firm of the Association of Executive Recruiting Consultants, Inc., he served for four years as National Director of Executive Search Consulting for Coopers & Lybrand. Before that he held the post of treasurer with Railway Express Agency, Inc. He was an executive search consultant for the firm of Peat, Marwick, Mitchell & Co. For three years he was assistant to the Controller of General Public Utilities Corporation. A Certified Public Accountant, Ryan has lectured on recruiting before many professional organizations. He received a B.B.A. at Manhattan College in 1955.

Joseph K. Sapora is a vice president of Woodward Ryan Sharp and Davis, Inc. He leads a team specializing in the health care industry that services several major institutions in the New York Metropolitan area. He is a Fellow in the Society of Actuaries (FSA), a member of the American Academy of Actuaries (MAAA), and an Enrolled Actuary under ERISA. Sapora holds a B.B.A. degree from the University of Wisconsin and a master of science degree from Northeastern University, Boston. He has addressed hospital-industry and professional organizations on benefit plan design, funding, and administration.

Larry E. Shear is vice president of Pacific Health Resources, Los Angeles, where he is responsible for the coordination of consulting efforts in management engineering, quality assurance, hospital operations, and organizational development. He also is a faculty member in health and safety studies at California State University, Los Angeles. Prior to joining PHR in 1975, he was assistant hospital director at the Kings County Hospital Center, Brooklyn. He is the author of a number of articles dealing with cost-effectiveness in health care, and has served as a speaker on national forums on improving hospital organizations. Shear also is president and member of the board of the Hospital Management Systems Society of Southern California.

Jesse Simons is a member of the American Academy of Arbitrators. He was director of the American Arbitration Association's Labor Management Institute. Former positions and assignments were as administrative assistant to Rudolph Hally, President of the City Council in New York City; labor relations and personnel manager, New York Post; consultant in Labor Relations to Esso Petroleum Ltd., London, England; and vice president of labor relations, U.S. Lines. As an arbitrator he was chairman of the Tripartite Personnel Review Board of the New York City Health and Hospitals Corporation; chairman, Public Law Board, Transport Workers Union and AMTRAC; chairman, Public Law Board of AMTRAC and Hotel and Restaurant Workers International Union; designated arbitrator in contract between New York Brewers Board of Trade and Teamsters Locals; Baseball Pay Arbitration Panel; UUP and State University; Board of Education and Teachers Association; State Nurses Association and New York City Voluntary Hospitals; and National Railroad Adjustment Board cases.

Henry P. Sims, Jr., currently is associate professor of Organizational Behavior and academic director of Human Resources Management Program at the Pennsylvania State University. He previously was assistant professor of Administrative and Behavioral Studies at the Graduate School of Business at Indiana University, visiting scholar at the University of California in Irvine, and a research assistant in the Computer Institute of Social Science Research. He has served in a variety of positions with the Ford Motor Company, Dearborn, Mich., ranging from first-line supervision to corporate staff internal consultant. He is president of the Eastern Academy of Management and is a Registered Professional Engineer. His research interests encompass issues of how managerial leadership can influence employee behavior, performance and satisfaction; his research in management and organizational psychology has been published in more than 50 articles in major journals. He has served as consultant, researcher, and/or executive development leader with such organizations as General Motors Corp., B.F. Goodrich, Veterans Administration Hospitals, and others. He received his B.S. at Purdue University (Engineering), his M.B.A. at the University of Detroit (Industrial Relations), and his Ph.D. from Michigan State University (Management).

Michael H. Singer is an assistant general counsel at The Mount Sinai Medical Center in New York City. He was graduated from Fordham University School of Law in 1978 with a J.D., after receiving his B.A. degree at Brandeis University.

Martin E. Skoler is a labor relations attorney who represents hospitals, banks, colleges and universities, and employers in a number of other industries throughout the country. He is counsel to the Vermont Hospital Association. He is also senior partner of the labor relations law firm of Skoler, Abbott & Hayes, P.C., of Springfield and Worcester, Massachusetts. Skoler is author of the *Health Care Labor Manual,* published by Aspen Systems Corporation. Past chairman of the Labor Law Committee of the American Society of Hospital Attorneys, he is a member of the Ad Hoc Committee of the American Hospital Association and was an adjunct professor at Western New England Law School. He is also a former attorney-advisor to John H. Fanning, Chairman of the National Labor Relations Board. Skoler has lectured throughout the United States on labor problems of health care employers.

Joseph T. Small, Jr., is an associate attorney in the law firm of Fulbright & Jaworski, Washington, specializing in litigation, and administrative and labor law. He is a 1975 graduate of the University of Virginia School of Law, where he received his J.D. In addition, Small served as law clerk to U.S. Judge Samuel Conti, of the Northern District of California.

Howard L. Smith is an assistant professor of health care management, R. O. Anderson School of Management, The University of New Mexico. His principal research interests include administrative theory and organizational behavior, and health services administration. He has consulted and published over 40 articles in both academic and professional journals in these areas. He received his Ph.D. at the University of Washington.

Joseph B. Stamm is director of ambulatory care review, New York County Health Services Review Organization. He previously was director of investigation and enforcement for Medicaid for the New York City Department of Health. He has been a guest lecturer on the subjects of ambulatory care and quality assurance at both New York University and Columbia University in New York City. Stamm has presented papers on quality assurance and ambulatory care. He received his M.P.A. degree from New York University and recently completed his doctoral work in public administration at that university.

Paula L. Stamps is associate professor at the University of Massachusetts and visiting professor at Dartmouth Medical School. At the School of Public Health at the University of Massachusetts, she teaches both graduate and undergraduate courses in health administration, including research methods and program evaluation. Stamps is also associated with the Department of Community and Family Medicine at Dartmouth Medical School, where she is the quality assurance coordinator on a federally funded research grant. She is the author of numerous publications and a book in the field of program evaluation. She received her Ph.D. from the University of Oklahoma.

Andrew D. Szilagyi, Jr., is currently associate professor of management in the College of Business Administration at the University of Houston. He also is director of the executive programs for the college which involves administrative responsibility for the Executive MBA Program and all external executive programs. He holds a B.S. degree in Chemical Engineering from Rose-Hulman Institute of Technology, an M.B.A. from Kent State University, and a D.B.A. from Indiana University. He also is a licensed professional engineer in the states of Ohio, Indiana, and Texas and has worked in the chemical industry for some years in a variety of managerial positions in production, engineering, and marketing. Szilagyi is widely published in journals such as the *Academy of Management Journal, Journal of Applied Psychology, Human Relations, Personnel, Organizational Dynamics, Management Review,* and *Hospital Administration.* He has coauthored the successful texts, *Organizational Behavior and Performance—Second Edition* and *Management and Performance.* He is an active consultant on managerial issues, has conducted numerous management

training programs, and has received many teaching excellence awards.

James M. Trono is a graduate of Cornell University's School of Industrial and Labor Relations and Boston University School of Law. Currently an associate in the firm of Skoler, Abbott & Hayes, P.C., he specializes exclusively in the representation of management in labor relations matters. Trono practices before the Supreme Judicial of Massachusetts, various federal courts of Massachusetts, and state and federal administrative agencies. He is an editor of the *Health Care Labor Manual,* published by Aspen Systems Corporation, and has lectured at various colleges and seminars. He is a member of the Massachusetts Bar Association and the Labor Law Section of the American Bar Association.

Carl W. Vogt is a partner in the law firm of Fulbright & Jaworski, Washington, specializing in litigation and administrative and employment law, including equal employment opportunity and occupational safety and health. He is a member of the District of Columbia Bar Association, the State Bar of Texas, the Federal Bar Association, and the American Bar Association. In addition, Vogt is chairman of the Labor Law Committee and the Special Committee on Equal Employment Opportunity Law, Section of Administrative Law, American Bar Association. He is chairman, Labor Law Advisory Committee, National Association of Manufacturers, as well as a member of the Advisory Committee on Labor Law to the General Counsel, American Hospital Association. Vogt has been a member of the U.S. Chamber of Commerce Task Force on Occupational Safety and Health and of the Labor Law Council, Federal Bar Association. He has authored various articles in the field of employment law.

Patricia Vunderink is a program associate, College of Medicine, Graduate Program of Hospital and Health Administration at the University of Iowa, where she works with continuing education programs for health care professionals and research projects involving curriculum models for future health care administrators. She has taught at both the secondary and collegiate levels for more than 12 years. From 1975 to 1978, while on the faculty of the College of Business at Iowa, she taught instructional systems design to persons preparing for careers in education and for training and development in organizational settings. She has authored or coauthored articles for professional journals and has been a member of numerous professional organizations including the Administrative Management Society. She received her Ed.D. from Indiana University, Wilmington, Ind., in 1978.

Robert II. Wilcox is the corporate personnel manager for William H. Mercer, Inc., in Chicago, with responsibility for corporate policies, employee benefit coordination, and corporate programs in equal employment opportunity, compensation, and recruitment. Concurrently, he has been involved as a consultant in a variety of projects in the human resources field, especially in the area of preretirement planning. Previously, he served as a head of a research unit in psychology at the National Naval Medical Center at Bethesda, Md., for four years. He received his Ph.D. from the University of Chicago in 1972. Professional societies of which he is a member include the American Society for Personnel Administration and the American Compensation Association.

Roger W. Williams, Sr., is president of the Center for Health Care Personnel, Weathersfield, Conn. Previously he was senior consultant with Don Rowe Associates, Mineola, N.Y., where he assisted a number of health care institutions in maintaining their union-free status. His special expertise is in the areas of personnel audits, employee opinion surveys, personnel policy and procedures, salary and benefits administration, communication programs, and human resource and organization development. His prior work experience includes a variety of responsibilities in personnel and human resource development. He holds a B.A. degree in psychology from Hartwick College, Oneonta, N.Y., and completed graduate work in industrial psychology and adult education at Michigan State University. He is a charter member of the organization development division of the American Society for Health Manpower Education and Training of the American Hospital Association.

Paul Yager is director of Region One (New York State and all of New England) of the Federal Mediation and Conciliation Service. He earned an M.S. in Industrial and Labor Relations from Cornell University and has been a mediator and executive with FMCS since 1951. When the 1974 health care amendments to the NLRA were passed, Yager became involved actively in the health care industry negotiations throughout his region. He has taught collective bargaining as an adjunct professor at both graduate and undergraduate levels at several universities and has published papers on mediation in the *Labor Law Journal, Proceedings of IRRA, Proceedings of NYU Conference on Labor,* and other professional publications. Yager has served as first vice president of the Society of Professionals in Dispute Resolution and on the executive board of the Industrial Relations Research Association.

Dolores Ziff is director of public relations at Pennsylvania Hospital. She has been in the public relations field for over 25 years, and joined Pennsylvania Hospital in 1966. Under her direction, the institution's public relations department has won 19 awards for outstanding publications and programs. She has been a contributing author to *Hospitals (J.A.H.A.),* and is a past president of the Delaware Valley Health Public Relations Association, the Hospital Association of Pennsylvania and the Philadelphia Public Relations Association. She attended Pennsylvania State University. She coauthored a book with Tina Filoromo entitled *Nurse Recruitment: Strategies for Success,* published in 1980 by Aspen Systems Corporation, Rockville, Maryland.